Textbook of Pediatric HIV Care

Edited by

Steven L. Zeichner
Bethesda, Maryland, USA

Jennifer S. Read
Bethesda, Maryland, USA

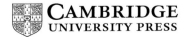

CAMBRIDGE UNIVERSITY PRESS

CAMBRIDGE UNIVERSITY PRESS
Cambridge, New York, Melbourne, Madrid, Cape Town, Singapore, São Paulo

Cambridge University Press
The Edinburgh Building, Cambridge CB2 2RU, UK

Published in the United States of America by Cambridge University Press, New York

www.cambridge.org
Information on this title: www.cambridge.org/9780521821537

First published 2005

Printed in the United Kingdom at the University Press, Cambridge

A catalog record for this book is available from the British Library

Library of Congress Cataloging in Publication data
Textbook of pediatric HIV care / edited by Steven L. Zeichner, Jennifer S. Read.
    p.   cm.
Includes bibliographical references and index.
ISBN 0 521 82153 3 (HB)
1. AIDS (Disease) in children – Patients – Medical care.   2. AIDS (Disease) in children – Treatment.
3. AIDS (Disease) in children.   I. Zeichner, Steven L. (Steven Leonard), 1954–   II. Read, Jennifer S.
[DNLM: 1. HIV Infections – therapy – Adolescent.   2. HIV Infections – therapy – Child.   3. HIV Infections –
complications – Adolescent.   4. HIV Infections – complications – Child, WC 503.2 T355   2004]
RJ387.A25T49   2004
618.92′979206 – dc22   2003063887

ISBN-13 978-0-521-82153-7 hardback
ISBN-10 0-521-82153-3 hardback

For Rachel, Sarah, and Elizabeth

For Alex, Samantha, and Geoffrey

Contents

Part III Antiretroviral therapy

Part IV Clinical manifestations of HIV infection in children

Part V Infectious problems in pediatric HIV disease

Part VI Medical, social, and legal issues

Appendices

Contributors

Elaine J. Abrams,
Department of Pediatrics,
Harlem Hospital Center,
506 Lenox Avenue, MLK 16-119,
New York, NY 10037, USA

Grace M. Aldrovandi,
University of Alabama,
Bevill Biomedical Research,
Building, Room 559,
845 29th Street,
Birmingham, AL 35294, USA

Jane C. Atkinson,
University of Maryland Dental
School,
666 West Baltimore Street,
Baltimore, MD 21201, USA

Andrew Blauvelt,
National Institutes of Health,
1001 Rockville Pike No 1610,
Rockville, MD 20852, USA

Pim Brouwers,
Department of Pediatrics and Neuroscience,
Baylor College of Medicine,
6621 Fannin Street, CCC 1510.12
Houston, TX, USA

Marc Bulterys,
Office of Genetics and Disease
Prevention, Centers for
Disease Control and Prevention,
1600 Clifton Road,
Atlanta, GA 30333, USA

James M. Callahan,
Department of Emergency Medicine,
SUNY – Upstate Medical University,
750 East Adams Street,
Syracuse, NY 13210, USA

Sandra Cely,
Division of Adolescent and Young
Adult Medicine,
Adolescent and Young Adult
Center, 120 Penn Street,
Baltimore, MD 21201, USA

Steven J. Chanock,
Pediatric Oncology Branch,
National Cancer Institute,
National Institutes of Health, Bethesda, MD 20892, USA

Caroline J. Chantry,
University of California
Davis Medical Center,
2516 Stockton Blvd, Ticon II
Suite 334,
Sacramento, CA 95817, USA

Lucy Civitello,
Children's Hospital National
Medical Center,
111 Michigan Avenue NW,
Washington, DC 20010, USA

Gul H. Dadlani,
University of Rochester Medical Center
and Children's Hospital at Strong,
601 Elmwood Avenue,
Box 631,
Rochester, NY 14642, USA

Barry Dashefsky,
Department of Pediatrics
University of Medicine and Dentistry of
New Jersey, Division of Pulmonary, Allergy, Immunology
and Infectious Diseases
185 South Orange Avenue,
MSB F-507A, University Heights, Newark, NJ
07103, USA

Kenneth L. Dominguez,
Division of HIV and AIDS Prevention,
Centers for Disease Control and
Prevention,

1600 Clifton Rd, Mailstop E45,
Atlanta, GA 30333, USA

Daina Dreimane,
Keck School of Medicine
University of South California, Children's Hospital of Los
Angeles, 4650 Sunset Boulevard,
Mailstop 61,
Los Angeles, CA 90027, USA

John Farley,
Department of Pediatrics,
University of Maryland School of
Medicine,
685 West Baltimore St MSTF 314,
Baltimore, MD 21201, USA

Howard F. Fine
Ophthalmology Wilmer Eye Institute, Johns Hopkins
600N Wolfe Drive Wilmer B-20 Baltimore, MD 21205, USA

Courtney V. Fletcher,
Department of Pharmacy Practice,
University of Colorado Health
Sciences Center,
4200 East Ninth, Box C238
Denver, CO 80262, USA

Mitchell E. Geffner,
Keck School of Medicine University of South California,
Children's Hospital of Los
Angeles,
4650 Sunset Boulevard, Mailstop 61,
Los Angeles, CA 90027, USA

Corina E. Gonzalez,
Georgetown University Hospital,
Lombardi Cancer Center,
3800 Reservoir Road NW,
Washington, DC 20007, USA

Heidi J. Haiken,
29 Milton Street,
Metuchen, NJ 08840, USA

Teresa Hammett,
Office of Genetics and Disease
Prevention, Centers for
Disease Control and Prevention,
1600 Clifton Road,
Atlanta, GA 30333, USA

Rohan Hazra,
HIV and AIDS Malignancy Branch,
National Cancer Institute,
National Institutes of Health
Building 10, Room 10S255,
Bethesda, MD 20892-1868, USA

Robert N. Husson,
Division of Infectious Diseases,
Children's Hospital Enders 609,
300 Longwood Avenue,
Boston, MA 02115, USA

Shirley Jankelevich,
Pediatric Medicine Branch,
NIAID, National Institutes of Health,
Room 5224,
6700B Rockledge Drive,
Bethesda, MD 20892, USA

Paul Jarosinksi
Pharmacy Department, Clinical Center, National
Institutes of Health, Building 10,
Room 12C440,
Bethesda, MD 20892, USA

Thomas N. Kakuda,
Medical Liaison (HIV)
Roche Laboratories
Nutley, NJ, USA

Jeffrey B. Kopp,
Metabolic Diseases Branch,
NIDDK, National Institutes of Health,
Building 10,
Room 3N116,
Bethesda, MD 20892, USA

Paul Krogstad,
Departments of Pediatrics and Molecular
and Medical Pharmacology,
UCLA School of Medicine,
10833 Le Conte Avenue,
Los Angeles, CA 90095, USA

Susan S. Lee
National Eye Institute,
National Institutes of Health, Building 10,
Room 10N202,
Bethesda, MD 20892, USA

Sandra Y. Lewis,
77 Orange Road,
Number 72, Montclair, NJ
07042, USA

Mary Lou Lindegren,
Office of Genetics and Disease
Prevention, Centers for
Disease Control and Prevention,
1600 Clifton Road,
Atlanta, GA 30333, USA

Steven E. Lipshultz,
University of Rochester Medical Center
and Children's Hospital at Strong,
601 Elmwood Ave, Box 631,
Rochester, NY 14642, USA

Richard F. Little,
HIV and AIDS Malignancy Branch, National Institutes of
Health,
Building 10,
Room 10S255, MSC 1868,
Bethesda, MD 20892-1868,
USA

Frank Maldarelli,
HIV Drug Resistance Program,
National Cancer Institute, NIH, Building 10,
Room 4A12,
Bethesda, MD 20892, USA

Carolyn McAllaster,
Duke University School of Law,
Box 90360,
Durham, NC 27708, USA

Elizabeth J. McFarland,
Pediatric Infectious Diseases,
University of Colorado Health Sciences Center,
Box C227,
4200 E Ninth Avenue,
Denver, CO 80262, USA

Ross McKinney, Jr.,
Department of Pediatrics,
Duke University School of
Medicine,
P. O. Box 3461,
Durham, NC 27710, USA

James G. McNamara,
Pediatric Medicine Branch,
Division of AIDS, NIAID, National Institutes of Health,
6700B Rockledge Drive,
Bethesda, MD 20892-7620, USA

Ann Melvin,
Children's Hospital and Regional
Medical Center, CH-32,
4800 Sand Point Way,
Seattle, WA 98105, USA

Lynne M. Mofenson,
Pediatric, Adolescent and Maternal AIDS Branch,
National Institutes of Health
6100 Executive Boulevard,
Room 4B11,
Rockville, MD 20852, USA

Rachel Y. Moon,
Department of General Pediatrics,
Children's National Medical Center,
111 Michigan Avenue NW,
Washington, DC 20010, USA

Jack Moye, Jr.,
Pediatric, Adolescent, and Maternal AIDS Branch,
National Institutes of Health,
Building 6100,
Room 4B11 MSC 7510,
Bethesda, MD 20892-7510, USA

Anne O'Connell,
Dept of Public Health and
Dental Health,
Dublin Dental Hospital,
Lincoln Place,
Dublin 2,
Ireland

William C. Owen,
Division of Pediatric Hematology/
Oncology, Children's Hospital
of the King's Daughters,
601 Children's Lane,
Norfolk, VA 23507, USA

Paul Palumbo,
UMDNJ-New Jersey Medical School,
Department of Pediatrics,

185 S Orange Avenue,
F-578 Medical Science Building,
Newark, NJ 07103, USA

Ligia Peralta,
Division of Adolescent and Young
Adult Medicine,
Adolescent and Young Adult
Center, 120 Penn Street,
Baltimore, MD 21201, USA

Stephen C. Piscitelli,
Discovery Medicine-
Antivirals, GlaxoSmithKline,
5 Moore Drive,
Research Triangle Park, NC 27709, USA

Jennifer Read,
Pediatric, Adolescent, and Maternal
AIDS Branch, National Institutes of Health,
Room 4B11F,
6100 Executive Boulevard MSC 7510,
Bethesda, MD 20892-7510, USA

Lisa-Gaye Robinson,
Department of Pediatrics,
Harlem Hospital Center,
506 Lenox Avenue, MLK 16-119,
New York, NY 10037, USA

Michael R. Robinson,
National Eye Institute,
National Institutes of Health, Building 10,
Room 10N202,
Bethesda, MD 20892, USA

Bret J. Rudy,
The Craig Dalsimer
Division of Adolescent Medicine,
Children's Hospital of
Philadelphia, 34th St and Civic Center Boulevard,
Philadelphia, PA 19104-4399, USA

Richard M. Rutstein,
Special Immunology Clinic,
Children's Hospital of
Philadelphia, 34th St & Civic
Center Boulevard,
Philadelphia, PA 19104, USA

Leslie K. Serchuck
Pediatric, Adolescent and Maternal AIDS Branch,
National Institutes of Health,
6100 Executive Boulevard,
Room 4B11,
Rockville, MD 20892–7510, USA

Sherilyn Smith,
Children's Hospital and Regional
Medical Center, CH-32,
4800 Sand Point Way,
Seattle, WA 98105, USA

Stuart E. Starr,
Division of Immunology and Infectious
Diseases, Children's Hospital of
Philadelphia, 34th St & Civic Center Boulevard,
Philadelphia, PA 19104, USA

Somsak Tanawattanacharoen
Metabolic Diseases Branch,
NIDDK, National Institutes of Health,
Building 10,
Room 3N116,
Bethesda, MD 20892, USA

Russell B. Van Dyke
Section of Infectious Diseases,
Department of Pediatrics TB-8,
Tulane University Health Sciences Center,
1430 Tulane Avenue,
New Orleans, LA 70112, USA

Ellen R. Wald,
Division of Allergy, Immunology and Infectious Diseases,
Children's Hospital of Pittsburgh,
3705 Fifth Avenue,
Pittsburgh, PA 15213, USA

Eric J. Werner,
Division of Pediatric Hematology/
Oncology, Children's Hospital
 of the King's Daughters,

601 Children's Lane,
Norfolk, VA 23507, USA

Lori S. Wiener,
HIV and AIDS Malignancy Branch,
National Cancer Institute
National Institutes of Health,
Building 20, Room 10S255,
Bethesda, MD 20892-1868, USA

Harland S. Winter,
Massachusetts General
Hospital for Children,
55 Fruit Street,
Boston, MA 02114, USA

Pamela L. Wolters
HIV and AIDS Malignancy Branch
National Cancer Institute and Medical
Illness Counseling Center, 9030
Old Georgetown Road, Building 82
Room 109, Bethesda, MD 20892–8200,
USA

Lauren V. Wood,
National Institutes of Health,
HIV and AIDS Malignancy Branch,
Building 10, Room 13N240,
Bethesda, MD 20892, USA

Carol J. Worrell,
HIV and AIDS Malignancy Branch,
National Cancer Institute,
Building 10,
Room 10S255,
Bethesda, MD 20892-1868, USA

Steven L. Zeichner
HIV and AIDS Malignancy Branch,
National Cancer Institute,
Bldg 10, Room 10S255,
10 Center Drive, MSC1868,
Bethesda, Maryland 20892-1868, USA

Abbreviations

AAP	American Academy of Pediatrics
ABC	Abacavir
ABCD	Amphotericin B Colloidal Dispersion
ABLC	Amphotericin B Lipid Complex
ACCAP	AIDS Community Care Alternatives Program
ACEI	Angiotensin Enzyme Inhibitors
ACIP	Advisory Committee on Immunization Practices
ACOG	American College of Obstetricians and Gynecologists
ACTG	AIDS Clinical Trials Group
ACTH	Adrenocorticotropin Hormone
ACTIS	AIDS Clinical Trials Information Service
ADCC	Antibody-Dependent Cell-Mediated Cytotoxicity
ADDP	AIDS Drug Distribution Program
ADEC	Association for Death Education and Counseling
ADHD	Attention Deficit/Hyperactivity Disorder
AEGIS	AIDS Education Global Information System
AFB	Acid-Fast Bacilli
AFXB	Association Francois-Xavier Bagnoud
AGCUS	Atypical Glandular Cells of Undetermined Significance
AIDS	Acquired Immune Deficiency Syndrome
ALRI	Acute Lower Respiratory Tract Infection
AmFAR	American Foundation for AIDS Research
AMP	Amprenavir
ANC	Absolute Neutrophil Count
ANRS	Agence Nationale de Recherches sur le SIDA
AOM	Acute Otitis Media
APC	Antigen-Presenting Cell
APV	Amprenavir
ARB	Angiotensin Blockers
ARDS	Acute Respiratory Distress Syndrome

ARF	Acute Renal Failure	CTL	Cytotoxic T Lymphocytes also Cytotoxic Memory T Cells
ARL	AIDS-Related Lymphoma	CVC	Central Venous Catheter
ARN	Acute Retinal Necrosis	CXR	Chest X-Ray
ART	Antiretroviral Therapy	d4T	Stavudine
ASCUS	Atypical Squamous Cells of Undetermined Significance	DC	Dendritic Cells
AST	Aspartate Aminotransferase	DC-SIGN	Dendritic Cell-Specific Intercellular Adhesion Molecule-Grabbing Non-Integrin
ATN	Adolescent Medicine Trials Network	ddC	Zalcitabine
ATP	Adenosine Triphosphate	ddI	Didanosine
ATZ	Atazanavir	DEXA	Dual Energy X-Ray Absorptiometry
AUC	Area Under the Curve	DFA	Direct Fluorescent Antibodies
AZT	Zidovudine (also known as ZDV)	DFA	Direct Immunofluorescence Assay
BAL	Broncheoalveolar Lavage	DHEAS	Dihydroepiandrosterone Sulfate
BBB	Blood–Brain Barrier	DHFR	Dihydrofolate Reductase
BCG	Bacille Calmette–Guerin	DHPS	Dihydropteroate Synthase
βHCG	Serum Beta Human Chorionic Gonadotropin	DHSS	Department of Health and Human Services
BIA	Bioelectrical Impedance Analysis	DIC	Disseminated Intravascular Coagulation
BMC	Bone Mineral Content	DLBCL	Diffuse Large B-Cell Lymphoma
BMD	Bone Mineral Density	DL_{co}	Diffusing Capacity
BMI	Body Mass Index	DLV	Delavirdine
BUN	Blood Urea Nitrogen	DMAC	Disseminated *Mycobacterium Avium* Complex
BV	Bacterial Vaginosis	DMPA	Depot Medroxyprogesterone Acetate
		DNA	Deoxyribonucleic Acid
CARE	Ryan White (Comprehensive AIDS Resources Emergency) Act	dNTPs	Triphosphorylated Nucleosides
CAT	Computerized Axial Tomography	DOT	Directly Observed Therapy
CBC	Complete Blood Count	DOTS	Directly Observed Therapy (Short Course)
CD	Cluster of Differentiation	DSMB	Data Safety Monitoring Board
CDC	Centers for Disease Control and Prevention	DTH	Delayed Type Hypersensitivity
CDC-GAP	Centers for Disease Control and Prevention Global AIDS Program	DTP	Diphtheria–Tetanus–Pertussis
		DTaP	Diphtheria–Tetanus–Acellular Pertussis
CHF	Congestive Heart Failure	DUB	Dysfunctional Uterine Bleeding
Cho	Choline	EBCT	Electron Beam Computed Tomography
CHOP	Cyclophosphamide, Doxorubicin, Vincristine and Prednisone	EBV	Epstein–Barr Virus
CIN	Cervical Intraepithelial Neoplasia	EC	Emergency Contraception **also** Enteric Coated
CIPRA	Comprehensive International Program of Research on AIDS	ECG	Electrocardiogram
Cmax	Maximum Concentration/Peak Blood Concentration	ECHO	Echocardiography
		ED	Emergency Department **also** End Diastolic
CMT	Cervical Motion Tenderness	EEG	Electroencephalogram
CMV	Cytomegalovirus	EFV	Efavirenz
CNS	Central Nervous System	EGPAF	Elizabeth Glaser Pediatric AIDS Foundation
CPAP	Continuous Positive Airway Pressure	EGW	External Genital Warts
CRF	Case Report Form	EIA	Enzyme Immunoassay
CRH	Corticotropin-Releasing Hormone	ELISA	Enzyme-Linked Immunosorbent Assays
CRP	C-Reactive Protein	EMEA	European Agency for the Evaluation of Medicinal Products
CSF	Cerebrospinal Fluid	ENF	Enfuvirtide
CSOM	Chronic Suppurative Otitis Media	Env	Viral Envelope
CT	Computed Tomography		

EP	Extrapulmonary Pneumocytosis		HPA	Hypothalamic-Pituitary-Adrenal
ERCP	Endoscopic Retrograde Cholangiopancreatography		HPTN	HIV Prevention Trials Network
ES	End Systolic		HPV	Human Papillomavirus
ESR	Erythrocyte Sedimentation Rate		HRCT	High-Resolution Computerized Tomography
ESRD	End Stage Renal Disease		HRIG	Human Rabies Immunoglobulin
			HSI	HIV/AIDS and Sexually Transmitted Infections
5-FU	5-Fluorouracil			
FACS	Fluorescent Antibody Cell Sorting		HSV	Herpes Simplex Virus
FAMA	Fluorescent Antibody Membrane Antigen		HTLV-1	Human T Cell Leukemia Virus 1
FDA	Food and Drug Administration		HUS	Hemolytic-Uremic Syndrome
FEV_1	Forced Expiratory Volume in 1 Second			
FFA	Free Fatty Acids		ICASO	International Council of AIDS Services Organizations
FFM	Fat Free Mass		ICD	Immune Complex Dissociated
FRS	Fat Redistribution Syndrome		ICMA	Immunochemiluminescent Assay
FSGS	Focal Segmental Glomerulosclerosis		IDU	Injection Drug Use
FSH	Follicle Stimulating Hormone		IDV	Indinavir
FTC	Emtricitabine		IFA	Immunofluorescence Assay
FTT	Failure to Thrive		IFN	Interferon
FVT	Forced Vital Capacity		Ig	Immunoglobulin
			IGFPB-3	Insulin-Like Growth Factor Binding Protein-3
G-6-PD	Glucose-6-Phosphate Dehydrogenase			
GCP	Good Clinical Practices		IgFBPs	IGF Binding Proteins
g-CSF	Filgrastim		IgF-1	Insulin-Like Growth Factor 1
G-CSF	Granulocyte-Colony Stimulating Factor		IL	Interleukin
GER	Gastroesophageal Reflux		ILD	Interstitial Lung Disease
GH	Growth Hormone		IMCI	Integrated Management of Childhood Illness
GI	Gastro-Intestinal			
GM-CSF	Granulocyte-Macrophage Colony-Stimulating Factor		INH	Isoniazid
			INR	International Normalized Ratio
GnRH	Gonatropin Releasing Hormone		InV	Intravaginal
HAART	Highly Active Antiretroviral Therapy		IP	Interferon Inducible Protein
HAIRAN	Hyperandrogenic-Insulin Resistant Acanthosis Nigricans		IPAA	International Partnership Against AIDS
			IPI	Invasive Pneumococcal Infections
HAMB	HIV and AIDS Malignancy Branch		IPV	Inactivated Polio Vaccine
HAM/TSP	HLTV-1-Associated Myelopathy/Tropical Spastic Paraparesis		IQ	Inhibitory Quotient
			IRB	Institutional Review Board
HAV	Hepatitis A Virus		IRU	Immune Recovery Uveitis
HAZ	Height-for-Age Z-Scores		ISA	Induced Sputum Analysis
hbhA	Heparin-Binding Hemagglutinin Adhesin		ITP	Immune Thrombocytopenia Purpura
HBIG	Heptatitis B Immunoglobulin		IUDs	Intrauterine Devices
HBV	Hepatitis Virus B		IUS	Intrauterine System
HCP	Healthcare Personnel		IVIG	Intravenous Immunoglobulin
HDL	High-Density Lipoprotein			
HDL-C	High-Density Lipoprotein Cholesterol		KOH	Potassium Hydroxide
HHV-6	Human Herpesvirus-6		KS	Kaposi's Sarcoma
HHV-8	Human Herpesvirus-8		KSHV	Kaposi's Sarcoma-Associated Herpesvirus
HIB	*Hemophilus Influenzae* Type B			
HIV	Human Immunodeficiency Virus		LBM	Lean Body Mass
HLA	Human Leukocyte Antigen		LDH	Lactate Dehydrogenase
HMOs	Health Maintenance Organizations		LDL	Low-Density Lipoproteins
^{1}HMRS	Proton Magnetic Resonance Spectroscopy			

LDL-C	Low-Density Lipoprotein Cholesterol		NF-kappa B	Nuclear Factor-kappa B
LFT	Liver Function Test		NFV	Nelfinavir
LGE	Linear Gingival Erythema		NHL	Non-Hodgkin's Lymphoma
LH	Luteinizing Hormone		NIAID	National Institute of Allergy and Infectious Diseases
LIFE	Leadership and Investment in Fighting an Epidemic		NICHD	National Institute of Child Health and Human Development
LIP	Lymphoid Interstitial Pneumonitis		NIH	National Institutes of Health
LIPA	Line Probe Assays		NK	Natural Killer
LP	Lumbar Puncture		NMDA	N-Methyl-D-Aspartate
LPN	Licensed Practical Nurse		NNRTs	Non-Nucleoside Reverse Transcriptase Inhibitors
LPV	Lopinavir		NPA	Nasopharyngeal Aspirate
LPV/r	Lopinavir Plus Ritonavir		nPEP	Non-Occupational Postexposure Prophylaxis
LTNP	Long-Term Non-Progression		NPO	Nothing by Mouth
LTR	(pg 25)		NRTIs	Nucleoside Reverse Transcriptase Inhibitors
LV	Left Ventricular			
			NSAIDs	Non-Steroidal Anti-Inflammatory Drugs
MAC	*Mycobacterium Avium* Complex also Mid-Arm Circumference		NSS	Normal Saline Solution
MACS	Multicenter AIDS Cohort Study		NUG	Necrotizing Ulcerative Gingivitis
MALT	Mucosa-Associated Lymphoid Tissue		NUP	Necrotizing Ulcerative Periodontitis
MAMC	Mid-Arm Muscle Circumference		N/V	Nausea/Vomiting
MCP	Monocyte Chemoattractant Protein			
MDI	Mental Developmental Index **also** Metered Dose Inhaler		17-OHP	17-Hydroxyprogesterone
MDR	Multi-Drug Resistance		OCs	Oral Contraceptives
MEMS	Medication Event Monitoring System		OD	Optical Density
MESA	Myoepithelial Sialadenitis		OGTT	Oral Glucose Tolerance Text
MHC	Major Histocompatibility Complex		OHL	Oral Hairy Leukoplakia
MI	Myo-Inositol		OHRP	Office of Human Research Protections
MIG	Monokine Induced by Interferon Gamma		OIs	Opportunistic Infections
MIP	Macrophage Inflammatory Protein		OLA	Oligonucleotide Ligation Assays
MIRIAD	Mother Infant Rapid Intervention at Delivery		oPEP	Occupational Postexposure Prophylaxis
Mo	Month		OPV	Oral Polio Vaccine
MMR	Measles, Mumps and Rubella		OSHA	Office of Safety and Health
MRI	Magnetic Resonance Imaging			
MRS	Magnetic Resonance Spectroscopy		PACTG	Pediatric AIDS Clinical Trials Group
MRSA	Methicillin-Resistant *Staphylococcus Aureus*		PACTS	Perinatal AIDS Collaborative Transmission Study
MSM	Men Who Had Sex With Men		PAHO	Pan American Health Organization
MTCs	Multilocular Thymic Cysts		PAP	Papanicolaou (Smear)
MTD	Mycobacterium Tuberculosis Direct Test		PBLD	Polymorphic B-Cell Lymphoproliferative Disorder
MTCT	Mother-to-Child Transmission			
			PBMC	Peripheral Blood Mononuclear Cells
NAA	N-Acetyl Aspartate		PCM	Protein–Calorie Malnutrition
NAHC	National Association for Home Care		PCNS	Primary Central Nervous System
NAMs	Nucleoside Associated Mutations		PCOS	Polycystic Ovary Syndrome
NAAT	Nucleic Acid Amplification Tests		PCP	*Pneumocystitis Carinii* Pneumonia and Primary Healthcare Provider
NASBA®	Nucleic Acid Sequence-Based Amplification		P Cr	Plasma Creatinine
NCHS	National Center for Health Statistics			
NCI	National Cancer Institute		PCR	Polymerase Chain Reaction

PCV	Pneumococcal Conjugate Vaccine
PCV7	Heptavalent Pneumococcal Conjugate Vaccine
PEL	Primary Effusion Lymphoma
PENTA	The Pediatric European Network for the Treatment of AIDS
PEP	Postexposure Prophylaxis
PFC	Persistent Fetal Circulation
PFTs	Pulmonary Function Tests
PGE$_2$	Prostaglandin E$_2$
PGP	P-glycoprotein
PHA	Phytohemaglutinin
PHC	Preventive Health Care
PHS	Public Health Service
PI	Pentamidine Isothionate
PIs	Protease Inhibitors
PIC	Pre-Integration Complex
PID	Pelvic Inflammatory Disease
PIT	Pills Identification Test
PJ	*P. Jiroveci*
PLH	Pulmonary Lymphoid Hyperplasia
PMDD	Premenstrual Dysphoric Disorder
PML	Progressive Multifocal Leukoencephalopathy
PMPA	9-[2-(R)-(Phosphonylmethoxy)propyl] Adenine
PMS	Premenstrual Syndrome
PMTCT	Prevention of Mother-to-Child Transmission
P Na	Plasma Sodium
PNS	Peripheral Nervous System
PORN	Progressive Outer Retinal Necrosis
POS	Point of Service
PPD	Purified Protein Derivative
PPOs	Preferred Providers Organizations
PPV	Pneumococcal Polysaccharide Vaccine
PMN	Polymorphonuclear Leukocyte
PRA	Peripheral Renin Activity
PRAMS	Pregnancy Risk Assessment Monitoring System
PSD	Pediatric Spectrum of Disease
PT	Prothrombin Time
PTH	Parathyroid Hormone
PTT	Partial Thromboplatin Time
PTX	Spontaneous Pneumothorax
PWAs	Persons with AIDS
PZA	Pyrazinamide
RAD	Reactive Airway Disease
RBC	Red Blood Cells
RDA	Recommended Dietary Allowance

REACH	Reaching for Excellence in Adolescent Care and Health
RER	Rough Endoplasmic Reticulum
RN	Registered Nurse
RNA	Ribonucleic Acid
rOspA	Recombinant Outer Surface Protein
RPE	Retinal Pigment Epithelium
RR	Relative Risk
RRE	Rev Response Element
RSV	Respiratory Syncytial Virus
RTI	Reverse Transcriptase Inhibitor
RT-PCR	Reverse Transcription-Polymerase Chain Reaction
RTV	Ritonavir
SBIs	Serious Bacterial Infections
Sc	Subcutaneous
SDF	Stromal-Cell Derived Factor
SHBG	Sex Hormone-Binding Globulin
SIADH	Syndrome of Inappropriate Secretion of Antidiuretic Hormone
SILs	Squamous Intraepithelial Lesions
siRNA	Small Interfering Ribonucleic Acids
SIV	Simian Immunodeficiency Virus
SMM	Sooty Mangabey Monkey
SOIs	Sharp Object Injuries
SPECT	Single Photon Emission Computed Tomography
SPNS	Special Projects of National Significance
SQV	Saquinavir
SSDI	Social Security Disability Income
SSI	Supplemental Security Income
SSRIs	Selective Serotonin Reuptake Inhibitors
STIs	Sexually Transmitted Infections
SUDS	Single Use Diagnostic System
3TC	Lamivudine
T4	Free Levothyroxine
TAMS	Thymidine Analogue Mutations
TANF	Temporary Assistance for Needy Families
TAR	Transactivation Responsive
TB	Tuberculosis
TCA	Trichloroacetic Acid
TCR	T Cell Receptors
Td	Tetanus and Diphtheria Toxoids
TDF	Tenofovir Disoproxil Fumarate
TDM	Therapeutic Drug Monitoring
Th	T-Helper
TIG	Tetanus Immunoglobulin
TMP/SMX	Trimethoprim-Sulfamethoxazole
TNF	Tumor Necrosing Factor
TOA	Tubo-Ovarian Abscess

TPN	Total Parenteral Nutrition	VCAM-1	Vascular Cell Adhesion Molecule-1
TREAT	Treatment Regimens Enhancing Adherence in Teens	VGC	Valganciclovir
		VLA-4	Very Late Activation Antigen-4
TRH	Thyrotropin-Releasing Hormone	Vif	Virion Infectivity Factor
TSF	Triceps Skinfold Thickness	VLDL	Very Low Density Lipoprotein
TSH	Thyroid Stimulating Hormone	VZIG	Varicella-Zoster Immunoglobulin
TST	Tuberculin Skin Test	VZV	Varicella-Zoster Virus
TTP	Thrombotic Thrombocytopenia Purpura	WAZ	Weight-for-Age Z-Scores
U Cr	Urine Creatinine	WBCs	White Blood Cells
UDPGT	Uridine Diphosphoglycoronyltransferase	VVC	Vulvovaginal Candidiasis
U Na	Urine Sodium	WHO	World Health Organization
URIs	Upper Respiratory Infections	WITS	Women and Infant Transmission Study
USAID	United States Agency for International Development		
		XR	Extended Release
USPHS	United States Public Health Service		
UTI	Urinary Tract Infection	ZDV	Zidovudine (also Known as AZT)

Foreword

Catherine M. Wilfert, M.D.
Professor Emerita, Department of Pediatrics Duke University Medical Center,
and Scientific Director, Elizabeth Glaser Pediatric AIDS Foundation

More than two decades have passed since this devastating infection was first identified. We have come from a time when no diagnosis could be made and there was no treatment, to an era when the development of multiple therapeutic agents and advances in prevention of HIV infection are commonplace in the developed world. Foremost amongst these accomplishments is our ability to prevent mother to child transmission of HIV infection. Seldom is it possible to chronicle such advances in knowledge which materially affect the lives of thousands of people on a daily basis. All of this speaks to the commitment of scientists and care providers and the rapid evolution of information and technology. There is however, a pervasive recurrent theme of needing to advocate for the health of children infected and affected by HIV infection.

This textbook provides accessible information at a time when the developed world has succeeded in dramatically decreasing the number of children who acquire infection from their mothers. The need for this information is greater now than ever before. First, because the evolution of information continues at a rapid rate. Second, because the complexity of treatment requires expertise and access to the most current information. Third, because the numbers of HIV-infected children have decreased in the USA and the probability that a physician will have cumulative experience with substantive numbers of these children has diminished. It is important that pediatricians continue to be sensitive to the possibility that a child is HIV infected and be attuned to the specific medical needs and support systems required.

There is an index to internet sources of information, convenient summary tables, and eloquent discussions of antiretroviral drugs conveniently separated from therapeutic decision making. The material is readable, concise, and thorough.

I would wish that this information was both accessible, in demand, and essential in the parts of the world where there is so much HIV infection of adults and children. One must reflect on the fact that as many infants are born with HIV infection in sub-Saharan Africa every day as were born in the USA in an entire year prior to the availability of interventions to prevent mother-to-child transmission. Progress is being made to bring these effective interventions to the developing world. We would hope we can entice a new generation of pediatricians, public health authorities, and other providers to devote their lives to addressing the problem as effectively in the developing world as has been done in the developed world. This textbook contributes to the knowledge, and hopefully will provide additional incentive to take these advances to the entire world of children.

Preface

Steven L. Zeichner and Jennifer S. Read

This *Textbook of Pediatric HIV Care* has evolved and grown considerably from its much shorter predecessor, the *Handbook of Pediatric HIV Care*, which was first published in 1999. This definitive new textbook provides a comprehensive clinical reference to the current state of and recommendations for pediatric HIV care. Fully referenced, completely updated and illustrated in depth, it is hoped this will become the standard reference for clinicians and other health-care professionals throughout the world. A much shorter companion volume, summarizing essential clinical information and guidelines, will also be produced which will be more suited for the clinician's pocket and for use in the busy hospital setting.

While we have focused on the management of pediatric HIV disease, we believe that effective management requires a solid understanding of the basic and applied virology, immunology, and pathophysiology of the disease, so that the practitioner can thoughtfully and rationally apply the management information supplied in the other chapters. This textbook therefore gives in-depth coverage to the science behind the disease and uses this standpoint to illuminate and explain clinical management.

The HIV epidemic changes quickly. The authors of the individual chapters have attempted to include a significant amount of new information, including new basic science findings, new information concerning the pathogenesis of the disease and the opportunistic infections that affect children with HIV, descriptions of recently approved drugs and recently developed drugs that may be close to approval, both for HIV and for HIV-related opportunistic infections, new information concerning the management of children infected with HIV, and information concerning the social welfare of children infected with HIV. In some fields, so much new information has become available that we included entirely new chapters in the book.

There are new chapters about the evolutionary biology of antiretroviral drug resistance and the assessment and management of antiretroviral drug resistance, the interruption of mother-to-infant HIV transmission, metabolic complications of HIV infection and antiretroviral therapy, therapeutic drug monitoring for HIV infection, and the gynecology of the HIV-infected adolescent. Whilst HIV vaccines are only in the earliest and experimental stages of clinical development, we felt it was more worthwhile to focus on the basic science, virology, immunology, pathogenesis, and natural history since this fundamental information will help guide vaccine developers to future success. We hope that we will be able to include in a future edition chapters that outline the use of prophylactic and therapeutic vaccines for HIV infection, as they become established in clinical practice.

While the principal focus of the book is on the management of HIV-infected children in the most effective ways possible, ways that tragically may not lie within the financial or technical capabilities of the regions most devastatingly affected by the HIV epidemic, we hope that the information presented in this book may also prove helpful to clinicians practicing in resource-poor countries, who may be able to use the information presented in the book to develop an approach to pediatric HIV disease management suited to their local circumstances. Perhaps, as they read the book, practitioners in resource rich countries can consider the tremendous challenges their colleagues in other parts of the world face every day.

Introduction

Steven L. Zeichner and Jennifer S. Read

Bethesda, MD, USA

Introduction

When we were in training to be pediatricians we diagnosed and treated some of the first children infected with HIV seen in our hospitals. We watched as most of them died quickly, within the first year or two of life, and we saw many of their parents die too. Over the following few years we witnessed the wards of our hospitals fill with children infected with HIV, at least in part because the growing epidemic was not viewed as a serious threat to the population as a whole, a threat that needed to be confronted with the determination and the resources appropriate to the magnitude of that threat.

As the epidemic expanded we initially had few effective therapies, either for HIV infection itself or for the opportunistic infections that complicate the disease. The numbing morbidity and mortality of HIV infection in children grew; we continued to see our patients and their parents die. Slowly, we saw more effective treatments for opportunistic infections and for HIV infection itself come into use. We saw the development of serological tests to diagnose HIV infection, of the first antiretroviral agents and agents for the prevention and treatment of opportunistic infections, of more effective antiretroviral agents, of methods to employ antiviral agents in effective combinations that can drive the viral load to low levels, of assays to determine viral load and methods to use the viral load assays to measure the effectiveness of antiretroviral therapy, of methods to assess whether a patient's virus is resistant to antiretroviral agents and approaches to select optimum combinations of antiretroviral agents, and of therapeutic approaches that dramatically decrease the likelihood that an infected mother will transmit HIV to her newborn.

Now, at least here in the USA and in other rich nations, effective approaches to treat HIV disease and its complications, and to prevent transmission, are in widespread use. Many of our patients are well, our wards are empty, and we have many fewer new patients. We have seen what happens when HIV disease in children is not treated, and we have seen the dramatic benefits that effective therapy for HIV disease can provide. We organized this book in the hope that a clear presentation of the management strategies available for HIV disease and its complications will help healthcare providers offer the most effective management strategies possible to their patients and that a clear presentation of the pathophysiology of HIV disease in children will help providers thoughtfully employ those management strategies.

The first edition of the *Handbook of Pediatric HIV Care* was intended mainly as a ready reference for practitioners who were working together with specialists to care for children with HIV infection. However, both non-specialists and specialists in the care of children with HIV infection seemed to find the book helpful. We hope that this textbook will continue to provide the information that will help non-specialists collaborate with specialists in caring for children with HIV infection, to help educate students, trainees, and others who are new to the pediatric HIV field, and satisfy the needs of specialists who may find the book useful as a ready reference.

The World Health Organization estimates that during 2003 close to one million children were infected with HIV and more than half a million died. These numbers will almost certainly continue to increase. The knowledge and technology now exist to prevent most of those infections and to keep many of the children who are infected alive and healthy for a long time, but the necessary financial, societal, and political resources have not been dedicated toward those goals, so children will continue to be infected and children will continue to die. We hope that at some not too distant time we will not need to edit a revised edition of this book.

PART I

Scientific basis of pediatric HIV care

Normal development and physiology of the immune system

Sherilyn Smith, M.D. and Ann J. Melvin, M.D., M.P.H.

Department of Pediatrics, University of Washington, Division of Pediatric Infectious Disease,
Children's Hospital and Medical Center, Seattle, WA

1.1 Overview

Clinicians involved in the care of children with HIV infection are faced with the dual challenge of understanding the effect of HIV on the immune system and applying this knowledge to patients who, even under normal circumstances, have an immature and changing immune response. Understanding the function of the immune system and the developmental differences in the immune system of children compared with adults will facilitate and improve patient care. This knowledge will aid in effectively interpreting laboratory results, help define disease risk, and improve the understanding of the manifestations and outcome of HIV infection in children. This chapter provides a framework for understanding the unique features of the developing pediatric immune system and how it may affect the course of HIV infection in children.

The functions of the vertebrate immune system include discrimination between self and foreign antigens, the development of a memory response to antigens, recognition of neoplasms and the elimination of pathogens that invade the host. The immune system can be divided into two separate components based on the rapidity and specificity of the response. The "innate arm" of the immune system provides a rapid, non-specific response to pathogens and provides the first line of defense against invading microbes. It also acts as a surveillance system and facilitates the initiation of the antigen-specific phase of the immune system. The major components of innate immunity include barriers (both epithelial and mucosal), complement and other opsonins, the spleen, phagocytes (both of macrophage and neutrophil origins), and NK (natural killer) cells.

The antigen-specific phase of immunity is directed at specific antigens or components of the invading microbe and is a sustained, amplifiable response. The aspects of this inducible portion of the immune system are the cellular and humoral immune response. The interaction of these two components serves to control infection and form long-term immunity against the same or similar organisms. Intact innate and antigen-specific immunity are necessary for full protection from pathogenic microbes and the establishment of long-term immunity induced by vaccinations. Table 1.1 summarizes the major functions of the innate and antigen-specific portions of the immune system and the types of infections that can result from dysfunction of its components.

1.2 Components and function of the immune system

1.2.1 Innate immune system

Barriers

The first line of defense against invading microbes is an intact barrier at both mucosal and epithelial surfaces. The skin, respiratory, gastrointestinal, and urogenital mucosa are the main components of this portion of the immune system. They exclude potential pathogens by forming a relatively impenetrable barrier between the environment and the host. Specialized cells (including ciliated respiratory epithelia that aid in removal of bacteria and particulate matter), and localized chemical barriers (such as stomach acid, the mucus layer in the respiratory and gastrointestinal tracts, and fatty acids in the skin and

Table 1.1 The immune system: functions, developmental aspects and infections associated with dysfunction

Immune system component	Function	Developmental differences	Infections associated with dysfunction
Innate			
Epithelial barriers/mucosal defense	Impede entrance of microorganisms; Present antigen; Sample environment	Epithelial barriers decreased in premature infants; Decreased IgA-adult levels by 6–8 years	Low virulence organisms: coagulase negative staphylococcus, opportunistic gram negative bacteria, fungi
Complement/opsonins	Amplify the immune response; Facilitate phagocytosis; Chemoattractants	Terminal complement levels decreased in neonates	Encapsulated organisms; Recurrent infections with Neisseria species; Recurrent/recalcitrant skin infections
Phagocytes	Engulf and kill microorganisms; Present antigens to T cells (macrophages); Elaborate immune active substances including cytokines and chemotactic factors	Monocytes: decreased chemotaxis, decreased cytokine production – adult function by 6 years; Neutrophils: decreased bone marrow pool in neonates, decreased chemotaxis – adult levels by 1 year	*Staphylococcus aureus*; Low virulence organisms: other staphylococci, gram negative opportunistic bacteria, fungi
Spleen	Filters intravascular organisms; Aids with opsonization; Antibody formation		Encapsulated organisms (*S. pneumoniae*, Salmonella, *H. influenzae*); Develop severe or recurrent infections
Natural killer (NK) cells	Lyse cells presenting "non-self" antigens (e.g. tumor or viral proteins)	Decreased ADCC, decreased cytolytic activity	Recurrent/severe viral infections with members of the Herpes virus family
Dendritic cells	Capture and present antigens to lymphocytes	Decreased ability to present antigen	?
Antigen specific T cells	Cell-mediated immunity; Elaboration of cytokines; Regulation of the immune response; Cytolysis; Increases the efficiency of B cell function by providing "help"	Increased absolute numbers – decline to adult levels by late childhood; Naïve phenotype in neonate (90%) decreased cytokine production, costimulatory molecule expression, and ability to provide "help" to B cells – normalizes throughout infancy with antigenic exposure	Infections with "unusual" organisms: intracellular bacteria (Listeria, mycobacteria); Fungi (Aspergillus, Candida); Viruses (especially HSV, VZV, CMV, HHV-8); Protozoa (Giardia, *Pneumocystis carinii*)
B cells	Humoral immunity (formation of antibody to specific antigens)	Unable to respond to polysaccharide antigens until ~2 years of age	Encapsulated organisms; Enteroviral infections; Recurrent GI or sinopulmonary infections; Inability to respond to vaccines

ADCC – antibody-dependent cell-mediated cytotoxicity; CMV – cytomegalovirus; HHV-8 – human herpesvirus-8; HSV – herpes simplex virus; VZV – varicella-zoster virus.

cerumen) impede entrance of pathogens. Breaches in these barriers may result in disease caused by normally low virulence organisms such as coagulase negative staphylococcus. In most cases the disruption occurs when foreign bodies such as central venous catheters, endotracheal tubes, and indwelling urinary catheters and gastrostomy tubes are placed.

Mucosal immunity
Another component of the innate immune system is a series of lymphoid tissue aggregates (mucosal-associated lymphoid tissues), located at sites that interface with the environment. These lymphoid aggregates (such as Peyer's patches in the intestines) provide a mechanism for continuous sampling of the environment, recognition of foreign antigens, and sites for early initiation of an antigen-specific response [1, 2]. A specific immunoglobulin, secretory IgA, is synthesized in the mucosal associated lymphoid tissues and adds to the local defense in the gastrointestinal and respiratory tracts.

Opsonins
Opsonins are proteins that bind to the surface of bacteria and facilitate phagocytosis. Acute phase reactants (C-reactive protein, fibronectin, etc.), complement, and antibody are the major components of this system. Complement is a collection of proteins that are activated by proteases in a sequential manner. Among its many functions, complement plays an important role in the killing and clearance of invasive bacteria. There are two major methods for activating complement: the classical pathway (antibody binds bacterial antigen which then is complexed with C1, a component of the complement system), which begins a series of proteolytic reactions that activates additional complement components and the alternate pathway (bacterial antigen directly binds the C3b component of the complement pathway) which also activates the cascade. Both pathways converge, and result in formation of a complex that lyses the bacteria. In addition to bacterial clearance, complement is also involved in some of the clinical signs associated with infection including vasodilatation, erythema, and induration [3].

Spleen
The spleen is an important part of the innate immune system and acts as a filter that efficiently removes opsonized bacteria. Absence or dysfunction of the spleen predisposes to overwhelming infection with encapsulated organisms. The spleen is also an important site of antibody production.

Macrophages
Macrophages and monocytes are major effector cells of the innate immune response and are responsible for the killing and clearance of invading microbes. Macrophages, which are present in most tissues, migrate to sites of infection and phagocytose foreign substances. In addition, macrophages elaborate a large number of cytokines (see below) and growth factors. The cytokines may either amplify (e.g. IL-6, TNF-α, IL-1) or dampen (TGF-β) an evolving immune response [4]. Elaborated growth factors may also have direct antimicrobial functions (IFN-α, M-CSF) or induce proliferation and differentiation of nearby T cells.

Neutrophils
Neutrophils are resident blood phagocytes that can adhere to endothelial cells and then migrate between the endothelial cells to sites of infection. They phagocytose microbes that are coated with immunoglobulins or complement. They are particularly important in the host defense against bacteria and fungi. Neutrophils kill phagocytosed pathogens via the respiratory burst (generation of reactive oxygen metabolites) or by degranulation with release of substances that directly kill pathogens or potentiate the effects of the respiratory burst.

Natural killer cells
Natural killer (NK) cells are specialized lymphocytes important in the early recognition of non-self proteins and are particularly important in the early response to viral infections. Viruses often down-regulate host major histocompatibility complex molecules (see below) on the surface of infected cells. The lack of these molecules causes the NK cells to recognize them as foreign, making them targets for lysis.

Dendritic cells
Dendritic cells (DC) are antigen-presenting cells that capture antigen and present it to lymphocytes. DCs are a complex system of bone-marrow derived cells that develop from either lymphoid or myeloid precursors. In general, there are three major DC populations: (a) Langerhans cells, which reside in tissues and migrate to T-cell areas of lymphoid organs after antigen uptake, where they are known as interdigitating cells; (b) myeloid DCs (also known as interstitial or dermal DCs), which become germinal center DCs in lymphoid follicles; and (c) plasmacytoid DCs which reside in the T cell areas of lymphoid tissues [5]. Langerhans cells and myeloid DCs are primarily derived from myeloid progenitor cells while plasmacytoid DCs are derived from lymphoid progenitors [6].

In the tissues, DCs are largely immature and function primarily to take up and process antigen. As they migrate to lymphoid tissues they undergo a maturation process to become effective antigen-presenting cells [5]. The different populations of DCs appear to have different primary functions. Langerhans cells are potent activators of CD8+ cytotoxic T cells [7] and promote T helper type 1 (Th1) responses in CD4+ T cells. Myeloid DCs also promote Th1 responses and are known as DC1 cells, while plasmacytoid DCs induce Th2 responses [8] and are thus known as DC2 cells.

Toll-like receptors

Toll-like receptors are a recently described family of transmembrane proteins that play an important role in the initiation of the innate immune response. To date, there have been 10 Toll-like receptors cloned that are designated TLR1-10. These molecules, first discovered in flies, are conserved across species and serve as an "early warning system" for recognition of microbial antigens. Most studies have focused on the ability of these proteins to recognize whole bacteria (such as *Escherichia coli*, *Staphylococcus aureus* and *Mycobacterium tuberculosis*) or bacterial products (such as lipopolysaccharide or CpG DNA). Toll-like receptors also recognize non-bacterial products such as yeast and respiratory syncytial virus. Activation of toll-like receptors results in the release of chemokines and other inflammatory mediators from dendritic cells and macrophages and modulates the expression of chemokine receptors on dendritic cells [9]. It is likely that several toll-like receptors act in concert to recognize foreign material and induce intracellular reactions that lead to immune activation [10].

1.2.2 Antigen-specific immunity

Cell-mediated immunity

T cells

T lymphocytes, or thymus-dependent lymphocytes, are essential components of the cellular immune system. These cells mediate delayed-type hypersensitivity reactions, regulate the development of antigen-specific antibody responses and provide specific host defense against a variety of organisms. Distinct sub-populations of T lymphocytes that express different cell surface proteins have been identified through the use of monoclonal antibodies. As different monoclonal antibodies may recognize similar cell surface proteins, a system has been developed which uses a cluster of differentiation (CD) nomenclature [11]. The lymphocyte subsets are identified through the use of flow cytometry techniques (fluorescent antibody cell

sorting or FACS analysis). A summary of the function of lymphocytes and commonly used nomenclature is found in Table 1.2.

T cell receptor complex

T lymphocytes bear antigen-specific T cell receptors (TCR), which are required for the recognition and binding of foreign antigen. TCRs are composed of either alpha (α) and beta (β) chains or gamma (γ) and delta (δ) chains. Each of the chains has a variable amino-terminal portion involved in antigen recognition and a carboxy-terminal region that is constant. As the T lymphocytes mature, rearrangement of dispersed segments V (variable), D (diversity, β-chain only), J (joining) and C (constant) of the alpha, beta, gamma and delta chain genes of the TCR occurs so that these gene segments are contiguous [12], creating a unique TCR within each individual T cell with specific capacity to recognize particular antigens. It is through this gene rearrangement that the TCR diversity necessary for the recognition of thousands of antigens is developed. The predominant T cell type in lymphoid organs and in the peripheral circulation express a TCR with α/β chains (α/β T cells). T cells that express the γ/δ TCR chains (γ/δ T cells) are less abundant and located primarily in certain mucosal tissues such as the intestinal epithelium [13].

MHC molecules

Antigen-presenting cells present antigen to T cells in the form of short peptides complexed with major histocompatibility complex (MHC) molecules. These cell surface molecules were initially identified as the major antigens involved in the acceptance or rejection of transplanted tissues. Tissue transplanted from a donor whose cells express different MHC molecules than do the recipient cells will be recognized as "non-self" and be rejected. Similarly, when foreign antigens are complexed with MHC molecules, the complex is recognized as non-self by the TCR and an immune response is initiated [14]. Class I MHC molecules are expressed on the surface of most cells and present endogenous antigens derived from the intracellular compartment of the cell (e.g. protein antigens derived from viruses infecting the host cells). Class II MHC molecules exist primarily on the cell surface of "professional" antigen-presenting cells (monocytes, macrophages, dendritic cells, and B cells) and are able to present proteins which originate outside or within the cell (e.g. proteins derived from phagocytosed bacteria). CD4+ (helper/inducer) T cells preferentially recognize exogenous antigen bound to class II MHC molecules, and CD8+ (cytotoxic) T cells preferentially

Table 1.2 Lymphocyte function and phenotype

Lymphocyte type	Function	Type of antigen receptor	Common cell surface markers
T Lymphocytes			
Helper	Regulation of the immune response Development of "memory" response to antigens	αβ T cell receptor	CD3⁺,CD4⁺, CD8⁻
Th1	Cell-mediated Immunity – control of intracellular pathogens, DTH response Activates macrophages via cytokine elaboration (IFN-γ and IL-2)	αβ T cell receptor	CD3⁺,CD4⁺, CD8⁻
Th2	Stimulates B lymphocyte differentiation and proliferation (humoral immunity) Elaborates cytokines involved primarily in the allergic response (IL-4, IL-5, IL-10)	αβ T cell receptor	CD3⁺,CD4⁺, CD8⁻
Cytotoxic	Lysis of tumor cells, virus-infected cells Stimulates cell-mediated immunity via cytokine production	αβ T cell Receptor	CD3⁺, CD4⁻, CD8⁺
B lymphocytes	Production of antigen-specific immunoglobulins (humoral immune response)	Immunoglobulin molecules (IgG, IgM, IgE, IgA)	Fc receptors, MHC II molecules CD20, CD19
Natural killer (NK) lymphocytes	Lysis of virus-infected cells and tumor cells lacking MHC class I; antibody-dependent cellular cytotoxicity		CD16, CD56

recognize endogenous antigen bound to class I MHC molecules [15].

Antigen presentation

The initiation of a specific immune response to protein antigens begins when the TCR on mature T cells recognizes short peptides that have been processed and bound in a cleft in the MHC molecule of the antigen-presenting cell (APC). The CD3 molecule with which the TCR is invariably associated, mediates signal transduction from the TCR to the interior of the T cell. The TCR/ CD3 complex is essential for proper antigen recognition. Additional molecules expressed by T cells, termed accessory molecules, must also interact with the antigen-presenting cell to insure an appropriate T cell-mediated response [16]. Two of the major accessory molecules expressed by T cells are the CD4 and CD8 molecules. The extracellular portion of these molecules binds to the invariant regions of the class I or class II MCH molecules on antigen-presenting cells. Other molecules including CD28 and members of a class of proteins called integrins act as costimulatory signals for the induction of an appropriate immune response to vaccines and certain pathogens. Through TCR-MHC-antigen interaction, the T cell is activated, further differentiates and initiates the process to respond to the foreign protein. There are surface markers on T cells that change once the T cell TCR has encountered its specific antigen (cognate antigen) [11]. A subset of the adult peripheral CD4⁺ T cells (CD45RA⁺ CD29^low) appear to be naïve cells that have not encountered specific antigen and form the pool of cells capable of responding to novel antigens. It is hypothesized that after an initial encounter with antigen, these cells develop into memory T cells with an altered phenotype (CD45RO[+] CD29[hi]) [17]. These memory T cells are capable of rapid proliferation as well as increased cytokine production after rechallenge with a previously encountered antigen, allowing for a more rapid and expanded secondary host-response.

CD4[+] T cells
The majority of peripheral α/β T cells also express CD4 or CD8 surface antigens. CD4[+] T cells are generally referred to as the helper/inducer subset because of their central role in the induction and regulation of most aspects of the immune response. A major function of CD4[+] T cells is to provide help to B cells for the production of antigen-specific antibody. B cells process internalized antigen and present antigen fragments bound to self-MHC molecules, thus activating CD4[+] T cells. During the cell to cell interaction between B cells and CD4[+] T cells, there is upregulation of various membrane molecules which increase the efficiency of the B cell – T cell interaction [18, 19]. In addition, CD40 ligand appears on the surface of the activated T cell. The interaction between CD40 on the B cell with CD40 ligand on the CD4[+] T cell is essential for a normal humoral immune response [20]. Through both cell–cell contact and the production of cytokines, CD4[+] cells are essential for the development of a normal antibody response including activating B-cells into antibody-secreting cells with the ability to undergo the antibody class switch process (see below). In addition, CD4[+] T cells provide help for the generation of both the cytotoxic (see below) and suppressor function of CD8[+] T cells. Memory T cells which are able to initiate a rapid immune response to previously encountered antigens (see above) are CD4[+] T cells.

Th1 vs Th2 T cells
There appear to be two functionally distinct subsets of CD4 cells that are distinguished primarily by their relative expression of certain cytokines [21]. Th1 cells, which preferentially produce interferon-gamma and IL-2 enhance cellular immunity and macrophage activity. Th1 cells are important in the regulation of delayed-type hypersensitivity responses including granuloma formation and the killing of intracellular pathogens. Th2 cells produce IL-4, IL-5 and IL-10, and are involved in the regulation of humoral immunity. These cytokines play an important role in the development of allergic diseases, as IL-4 is essential for IgE production and IL-5 induces the proliferation and differentiation of eosinophils [22, 16]. Whether naïve CD4[+] T cells differentiate into Th1 or Th2 cells depends on a variety of factors including the cytokine milieu, antigen dose and the nature of the specific antigen.

CD8[+] T cells
CD8[+] T cells are often referred to as the cytotoxic/suppressor subset due to their role as cytotoxic T cells as well as their role in the suppression of various immune responses [15]. The activation of CD8[+] T cells by recognition of antigen bound to class I MHC molecules results in the generation of antigen-specific cytolytic activity. As nearly all host cells express class I MHC molecules, these cytolytic T lymphocytes (CTL) can respond to a viral infection of most host cells [16]. Through the production of several cytokines, particularly IL-2, CD4[+] cells provide help to CD8[+] T cells for the development of an effective CTL response [23].

Cytokines
Cytokines are soluble proteins produced by a variety of cells that modulate the immune response. The cytokines express their effects either locally or systematically by interacting with specific membrane receptors expressed by their target cells. Different cytokines may perform similar functions and affect multiple cell types, and may be functionally linked, either with synergistic or opposing effects. Cytokine functions include: (a) the regulation of lymphocyte growth and differentiation; (b) mediation of inflammation; and (c) the regulation of hematopoesis. Cytokines affecting T cells include the interleukins (IL), interferons, growth factors, and tumor necrosis factor (TNF) [16] (Table 1.3).

Chemokines
Chemokines are a relatively recently discovered family of cytokines whose primary role is regulation of chemotaxis [24]. There are over 40 chemokines grouped into four families. The largest families are comprised of the alpha and beta chemokines. Beta chemokines have two adjacent cysteine residues (CC) and alpha chemokines have one amino acid separating the first two cysteine residues (CXC). Chemokines appear to be produced by almost all cell types, particularly in response to inflammation. Proinflammatory cytokines such as interleukin 1 and TNF alpha [25], lymphokines such as IFN gamma and IL-4 [26], as well as bacterial LPS and viral infection can stimulate chemokine production.

Chemokines bind to specific receptors on the target cells. Most chemokine receptors bind more than one chemokine, however CC chemokine receptors bind only CC chemokines and CXC receptors only CXC chemokines. Different types of leucocytes express different chemokine receptors. Some receptors are restricted to specific cell types, while others are widely expressed (Table 1.4).

Chemokines play an important role in inflammatory disease. The type of inflammatory cells infiltrating the area

Table 1.3 Selected cytokines, cell source and principal effects

Cytokine	Cell source	Target cell/principal effects
IL-2	T cells	T cells: proliferation and differentiation; activation of CTL and macrophages
IL-3	T cells, stem cells	Cell colony stimulating factor
IL-4	T cells	T/B cells: B cell growth factor, isotype selection
IL-6	T/B cells	B cells/hepatocytes: B cell differentiation, acute phase reactant production
IL-8	Monocytes	Granulocytes, basophils, T cells: chemotaxis, superoxide release, granule release
IL-12	Monocytes	T cells: induction of Th1 cells
IFN-gamma	T cells, NK cells	Leukocytes, macrophages: MHC induction, macrophage activation and cytokine synthesis
TNF-alpha	Macrophages, mast cells, lymphocytes	Macrophages, granulocytes: activation of monocytes, granulocytes, increase adhesion molecules, pyrexia, cachexia, acute phase reactant production

IL – interleukin; IFN – interferon; TNF – tumor necrosis factor; CTL – cytolytic T lymphocytes; MHC – major histocompatibility complex.

Table 1.4 Selected chemokines, their receptors and target cells

Chemokine	Receptor	Target cell
MIP-1alpha	CCR1–7	Eosinophils, monocytes, activated T cells, dendritic cells, NK cells
MIP-1beta	CCR1–7	Monocytes, activated T cells, dendritic cells, NK cells
RANTES	CCR1–7	Eosinophils, basophils, monocytes, activated T cells, dendritic cells, NK cells
Fractalkine	CX_3CR1	Monocytes, activated T cells, NK cells
SDF-1	CXCR4	Monocytes, resting T cells, dendritic cells
MIG	CXCR3	Activated T cells, NK cells
IL-8	CXCR1 and 2	Neutrophils
IP-10	CXCR3	Activated T cells
MCP-1	CCR2 and 5	Monocytes, activated T cells, dendritic cells, NK cells
Eotaxin-1	CCR1–3	Eosinophils, basophils

MIP – macrophage inflammatory protein; SDF – stromal-cell derived factor; MIG – monokine induced by interferon gamma; IL – interleukin; IP – interferon inducible protein; MCP – monocyte chemoattractant protein. Adapted from Luster (1998) [24].

of inflammation is determined partly by the subgroup of chemokines expressed by the affected tissue. For example, the concentration of the chemokine IL-8 is increased in alveolar fluid from patients with pneumonia, resulting in an influx of neutrophils [27]. In contrast, in viral meningitis, the concentration of chemokines IP-10 and MCP-1 in the cerebrospinal fluid (CSF) is increased, recruiting monocytes and lymphocytes [28]. The chemokine system provides an important link between the innate and adaptive immune systems. Dendritic cells pick up foreign antigen in the tissues to carry to regional lymph nodes where naïve B and T cells are activated. The activated cells then traffic back to sites of inflammation. The chemokine system regulates this dendritic cell and lymphocyte trafficking – bringing the antigen-loaded dendritic cells and naïve lymphocytes together to generate the adaptive immune response and then delivering the adaptive effector response to sites of inflammation and infection [9].

Humoral immunity

Immunoglobulins

Immunoglobulins (antibodies) are a group of proteins that bind antigen with high affinity and specificity. An immunoglobulin molecule is made up of 2 heavy and 2 light chains, aligned in parallel, and covalently linked by disulfide bonds (IgM is a pentamer of the basic immunoglobulin molecule). The heavy and light chains have both variable (V) and constant regions. The variable regions of the 2 chains (V_H and V_L) form the antigen-binding region of the immunoglobulin. During B cell development, rearrangement of the genes encoding these regions within individual B cells results in the production of a unique antibody with the potential for recognition of one of greater than 10^{12} antigens, imparting enormous diversity and specificity to the humoral immune response [29, 30]. The constant region of the heavy chain determines the antibody isotype: IgG, IgM, IgA, IgE, and IgD. Functions of the immunoglobulin isotypes include: (a) opsonization or binding to a microbe or particle to facilitate phagocytosis or killing (IgM, IgG, IgA, IgE); (b) complement fixation, which involves activation of the complement cascade via the classical pathway (IgM, IgG); (c) direct inactivation of some toxins or viruses (IgG, IgM, IgA); (d) enhanced antigen clearance via the reticuloendothelial system (IgG, IgM); and (e) release of chemical mediators following binding of antibody receptor (IgG, IgE).

B cells

B cells bind antigen via the variable regions of the immunoglobulins that are expressed on the cell surface. Naïve B cells express both IgD and IgM on the cell surface prior to encountering their cognate antigen (the antigen specifically recognized by the immunoglobulin receptor). The surface immunoglobulin is associated with two other proteins, Ig-α and Ig-β, and this complex forms the functional signaling pathway (similar to the TCR/CD3 complex on T cells) [31]. Most B cells require T cell help to become fully activated. T cell help is provided by cytokines secreted by the T cell and direct contact with the T cell that allows interaction of B and T cell costimulatory molecules like CD40 ligand and CD40. Following antigen binding, B cells may terminally differentiate into a plasma cell, which is capable of producing large amounts of specific immunoglobulin after either the initial or a second encounter with its cognate antigen [29].

The primary immune response

The first time the immune system encounters an antigen, few cells specifically recognize the antigen, thus the primary immune response is relatively slow and produces relatively low affinity antibodies [29]. The antigen is endocytosed and processed by an APC (monocyte, macrophage or dendritic cell, usually not B cells), and then it is presented to an antigen-specific T cell. The T cell must then contact and activate B cells specific for the antigen/TCR complex. The B cells then proliferate or differentiate into plasma cells. The antibody produced during this phase of the immune response is typically IgM and has relatively low binding affinity for the antigen. Further refinement of the gene segments encoding the antigen-binding domain of the antibody molecule occurs through a process of somatic hypermutation. B cells expressing antibody with higher affinity for antigen are selected for activation and differentiation. While most B-lymphocytes differentiate into plasma cells, the remainder proliferate in a clonal manner and then revert to memory B cells.

The secondary immune response

When the B cell re-encounters its cognate antigen, the antigen is endocytosed by the memory B cells and loaded onto MHC class II molecules. The peptide is presented on the surface of the B cell by the MHC molecule to CD4 cells that then activate the B cell. The B cells proliferate and undergo further differentiation, including class switching (DNA rearrangement that results in different heavy chain isotypes linked to variable regions). The B cells then are capable of production of different types of high-affinity antigen-specific immunoglobulins – IgG, IgE, or IgA, the specific isotype being influenced by T cell cytokines (e.g. IL4 favors IgE production). The process of clonal proliferation and plasma cell differentiation occurs in an amplified or accelerated manner which results in a rapid production of large amounts of high-affinity antibodies each time the antigen is encountered [19, 30].

1.3 Development and maturation of the immune system

Both the innate and adaptive immune systems are less efficient in infants compared with adults. Mucosal barriers are less effective, particularly in premature infants, placing them at risk for systemic disease from colonizing organisms. Immunoglobulin levels are lower in infants and young children. In addition, the specific immune response is decreased due in part to less effective antigen presentation by dendritic cells and decreased cytokine production by neonatal lymphocytes. Most aspects of the immune system mature with age such that adult-level immune responses are achieved within the first few years of life. The major developmental differences that exist between the adult and neonatal/infant immune systems are summarized in Table 1.1. The immaturity of the infant immune system affects the ability of HIV-infected neonates to control HIV replication and places them at higher risk for opportunistic infections.

1.3.1 Innate immunity

Epithelial barriers/mucosal defenses
The epidermis increases in cell layers and thickness throughout gestation and at term, infant skin is similar to adult skin except that it is thinner. Secretory IgA is undetectable at birth, but is present in various secretions by 2 weeks of age and reaches adult levels by 6–8 years of age. The rate of increase of IgA levels parallels the intensity of antigen exposure [32]. Decreased levels of secretory IgA may allow for greater adherence of pathogenic bacteria to mucosal epithelium.

Complement
Complement synthesis begins early in gestation (6–14 weeks) and by birth the levels and biologic activity of some portions of the complement cascade are equivalent to adult levels. However, some elements of the alternative pathway (C8, C9) are decreased to <20% of adult levels, which may contribute to the age-related susceptibility of young infants to infection with organisms such as *N. meningitidis* [32]. Additionally, infants have decreased levels of C3b that may contribute to increased susceptibility to encapsulated organisms [33, 34].

Phagocytes
Macrophages and monocytes are derived from a common stem cell. The yolk sac is the first site of macrophage development followed by the fetal liver and then the bone marrow after birth. From the bone marrow, mature blood monocytes migrate to the peripheral blood. The monocytes circulate for 1–4 days and then can migrate into tissue where they further differentiate to become resident tissue macrophages. The number of monocytes circulating in the peripheral blood varies, reflecting both egress of cells into tissues, margination of cells along endothelial surfaces and new cells migrating from the bone marrow. Tissue macrophages have a long half-life ranging from 60 days to many years; this cell type is believed to be terminally differentiated.

The absolute number of monocytes is higher in neonates than in adults. The number decreases from early in the neonatal period and reaches adult levels by early childhood. Tissue macrophages from infants may not kill certain pathogens as well as adult macrophages and there are modest differences in the ability of neonatal macrophages to generate reactive oxygen intermediates following phagocytosis [35].

Monocyte function is primed by a number of lymphokines that are released by activated T cells. Neonatal monocytes are less able to support and respond to IFN-γ production by NK and T lymphocytes than adult monocytes, which further diminishes the ability of neonatal T cells and T lymphocytes to produce these molecules [36]. Augmenting this deficit, the production of some cytokines and growth factors (TNF-α, IL-8, IL-6, and G-CSF) from neonatal monocytes/macrophages is reduced [32, 36]. The most striking developmental difference of immature macrophages is decreased chemotaxis to sites of inflammation or infection. Following dermal abrasion there is delayed influx of neonatal monocytes compared with adults, and this difference persists until approximately 6–10 years of age [37].

Neutrophils
Neutrophils arise from stem cells in the bone marrow and differentiate into granulocytes. The development of neutrophils within the bone marrow is highly dependent upon various cytokines and growth factors including granulocyte-colony stimulating factor (G-CSF). Mature neutrophils can be detected as early as 14–16 weeks gestation and the number increases throughout gestation. The blood neutrophil pool is divided into marginated and circulatory components of approximately the same size. In adults, the maturation of neutrophils from stem cells to mature neutrophils takes approximately 9–11 days but can be accelerated by stress or infection.

There is a sharp rise in the number of neutrophils in the peripheral circulation immediately after birth, but the ability to further expand the neutrophil storage pool is limited in neonates [38]. This state may contribute to the inability of infants to increase the number of circulating, mature neutrophils in response to infection. Similar to neonatal monocytes, chemotaxis of neonatal neutrophils to sites of infection is decreased when compared with adults. This deficit is multifactorial, reflecting decreased ability to adhere to vascular endothelium, decreased cytokine production by monocytes, and additional incompletely defined deficiency to move toward chemotactic stimuli [36]. Neutrophil chemotaxis reaches adult competence by 2 years of age [38–42].

Natural killer cells

NK cells make up a significant portion of the lymphocytes in the neonatal liver and can be detected as early as 6 weeks gestation. Neonatal NK cells have reduced cytolytic activity (approximately 50% that of adults) and do not reach adult levels until approximately 9–12 months of age. There is also decreased antibody-dependent cell-mediated cytotoxicity (ADCC). Diminished direct cytolytic activity and ADCC against members of the herpes virus family may contribute to increased susceptibility and infection by herpes simplex virus and cytomegalovirus [32, 43].

Dendritic cells

The reduced ability of neonatal T and B cells to respond to antigens (discussed below) may be due in part to the reduced ability of neonatal dendritic cells to present antigen [44]. Cord blood dendritic cells express fewer MHC and ICAM-1 molecules and are less effective than adult dendritic cells at supporting proliferation of T cells in response to antigenic stimulation [44]. Studies in newborn mice have also demonstrated a defect in the ability of dendritic cells to present specific antigen to T cells which improves with age [45].

1.3.2 Antigen-specific immunity

Cell-mediated immune response

Thymic development

The thymus, which originates from the ventral portions of the third and fourth pharyngeal pouches, descends to its position in the anterior mediastinum between 7–10 weeks gestation. By 10–14 weeks of gestation, the thymus is highly organized and the emigration of mature T cells to the periphery has been established. The thymus is compartmentalized into a cortex, containing immature T-cells, and a medulla into which T cells migrate as they mature. The thymic stromal cells are important for thymic lymphocyte maturation as they play a role in the differentiation, development and selection of T cells [46]. The proper development of T cells bearing the $\alpha\beta$ TCR is absolutely dependent on an intact thymus, while some T cells bearing the $\gamma\delta$ TCR undergo thymus-independent development and maturation [32, 47].

T cell phenotype

Neonatal T cells bear the phenotype of naïve adult T cells (CD45RA$^+$ CD29^{low}) consistent with the limited exposure of the neonate to foreign antigens [48]. The percentage of circulating neonatal T cells of this phenotype is approximately 90%, while the percent in the adult circulation is 60% [17]. This phenotypic difference is significant because

memory T cells (CD45RO$^+$, CD29^{hi}), are able to migrate to sites of inflammation, are less dependent on costimulatory molecules for proper activation, proliferate more rapidly and produce cytokines more efficiently [49]. These attributes allow for a rapidly expanded T cell response with antigenic rechallenge. As the initial encounter with a novel antigen leads to a less robust response, neonates may experience a delayed T cell dependent immune response.

T cell numbers

The number of circulating T cells increases from midgestation until approximately 6 months of age, with a median CD4$^+$ cell count at 6 months of approximately 3000 cells/μL^3. This peak is followed by a gradual decline throughout childhood until adult levels, approximately 1000 cells/μL^3, are reached by late childhood. The changes in CD4% are less dramatic, declining from approximately 50% to 40% between infancy and adulthood. The ratio of CD4$^+$ to CD8$^+$ T cells also changes throughout childhood and the adult ratio of 2:1 is reached at approximately 4 years of age (Figure 1.1) [50].

Cytokine production

The production of some cytokines including TNF-α and GM-CSF is modestly reduced in neonates, while others, critical for a rapid integrated immune response, are markedly decreased in neonates including IFN-γ, IL-3, IL-4, IL-5, and IL-12 [51]. The reduction in cytokine production by neonatal T cells is not global, as IL-2 and TNF-β are produced at near adult levels [52–55]. When stimulated under normal conditions, neonatal CD4$^+$ T cells preferentially develop a Th2 phenotype [56]. However, provision of increased CD28 costimulation results in the production of high levels of Th1 cytokines suggesting that the defect in neonatal T-cells is not intrinsic, but related to the conditions of activation [56]. Additionally, experimental evidence suggests that administration of adult levels of IL-12 can induce an adult-type Th1 response in neonatal animals [57]. The ability to efficiently synthesize cytokines increases with age with TNF-α production normalizing within the first few months of life and IFN-γ and IL-12 production by 1 year of age [32, 51].

T cell help for antibody production

T cells from young infants and neonates are less able than those from adults to provide the necessary help to B cells for activation in most cases. This most likely reflects the naïve phenotype of T cells, reduced cytokine production, particularly Th1 cytokines, and reduced expression

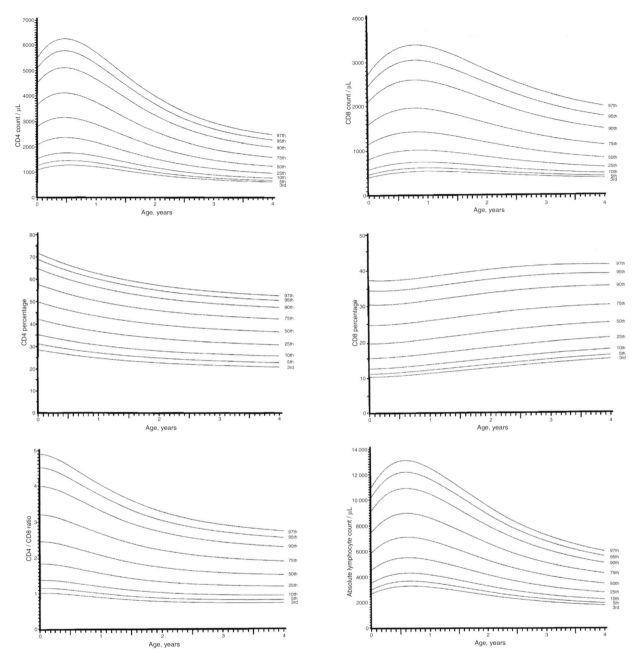

Figure 1.1. Lymphocyte parameters as a function of age. The panels show percentile values for the CD4+ and CD8+ lymphocyte counts and percentages, the CD4+/CD8+ lymphocyte ratio, and the absolute lymphocyte count during the first 4 years of life. Figure modified from reference [66].

of certain costimulatory molecules like CD40 ligand [58]. The practical implications of diminished T cell help for antibody production are delayed responses to certain infections and immunizations compared with adults.

DTH

Delayed type hypersensitivity (DTH) is a method to test the integration of the T lymphocyte with antigen-presenting cells in vivo. At birth, there is no detectable DTH to Candida or tetanus toxoid. The absent DTH response is not solely

Table 1.5 Levels of immunoglobulins in normal subjects by age

| | Total immunoglobulins | | IgG | | | IgM | | IgA |
Age	mg/dl	% of adult level	mg/dl	% of adult level	mg/dl	% of adult level	mg/dl	% of adult level
Newborn	1044 ± 201	67 ± 13	1031 ± 200	89 ± 17	11 ± 5	11 ± 5	2 ± 3	1 ± 2
1–3 mo	481 ± 127	31 ± 9	430 ± 119	37 ± 10	30 ± 11	30 ± 11	21 ± 13	11 ± 7
4–6 mo	498 ± 204	32 ± 13	427 ± 186	37 ± 16	43 ± 17	43 ± 17	28 ± 18	14 ± 9
7–12 mo	752 ± 242	48 ± 15	661 ± 219	58 ± 19	54 ± 23	55 ± 23	37 ± 18	19 ± 9
13–24 mo	870 ± 258	56 ± 16	762 ± 209	66 ± 18	58 ± 23	59 ± 23	50 ± 24	25 ± 12
25–36 mo	1024 ± 205	65 ± 14	892 ± 183	77 ± 16	61 ± 19	62 ± 19	71 ± 37	36 ± 19
3–5 years	1078 ± 245	69 ± 17	929 ± 228	80 ± 20	56 ± 18	57 ± 18	93 ± 27	47 ± 14
6–8 years	1112 ± 293	71 ± 20	923 ± 256	80 ± 22	65 ± 25	66 ± 25	124 ± 45	62 ± 23
9–11 years	1334 ± 254	85 ± 17	1124 ± 235	97 ± 20	79 ± 33	80 ± 33	131 ± 60	66 ± 30
12–16 years	1153 ± 169	74 ± 12	946 ± 124	82 ± 11	59 ± 20	60 ± 20	148 ± 63	74 ± 32
Adult	1457 ± 353	100 ± 24	1158 ± 100	100 ± 26	99 ± 27	100 ± 27	200 ± 61	100 ± 31

Mean values $\pm$ one standard deviation – normal levels may vary at different reference laboratories.
Modified with permission from *Pediatrics*, **37**: (1966), 715–27.

due to naïve T cells, because a normal DTH response cannot be reconstituted with memory cells. Other factors including defective monocyte chemotaxis or decreased numbers of efficient antigen-presenting cells (dendritic cells) compound the defect. The ability to reliably mount a delayed type hypersensitivity response is present after 1–2 years of age [59, 60].

Cytotoxic T lymphocytes (CTL)

While in vitro studies have demonstrated that neonatal T cells are capable of developing into CTL effector cells, the incidence of CTL development and the magnitude of CTL activity are decreased during most natural infections in infants compared with adults. Studies in vaccine trials and from HIV-exposed infants suggest that CTL activity matures within the first year of life [51].

Humoral immune response

Development

Pluripotent stem cells are the primitive precursors of lymphocytes and are found in the yolk sac early in gestation. Early B cell precursors are found in the fetal liver by 7 weeks gestation and stem cells migrate to the bone marrow where they continue to differentiate into B cell precursors by 8–10 weeks gestation. The fetal immune system can mount a humoral immune response by 6–7 months gestation, though the functional capacity of this arm of the immune response does not reach adult competence until after 2 years of age. B cell maturation continues in the bone

marrow throughout life, although only a small fraction of B lymphocytes leave the bone marrow and circulate in the peripheral blood. There is an ongoing process to eliminate any B cells with non-functional immunoglobulins or immunoglobulins that are self-reactive [29, 30, 61].

Immunoglobulins

Neonatal B cells appear to have a similar degree of Ig diversity as adult B cells although there are some heavy-chain variable regions that are expressed in adults that do not appear in the neonatal repertoire. Neonatal B cells have also been shown to undergo somatic mutation at the same rate as adult B cells [62, 63]. There is a gradual rise in the serum concentrations of immunoglobulins with age (Table 1.5) although the repertoire of IgG, especially IgG2a does not achieve an adult phenotype until after 6–12 months of age [51].

B cells

The phenotype of neonatal B cells, including expression of surface markers (CD5[+]) may reflect persistence of cells involved in regulation of the developing immune system. These CD5[+] cells are self-renewing, in contrast to conventional B cells that must be replenished from the bone marrow, and often produce antibodies against self-antigens. Additionally, some neonatal B cells express IgA and IgG on the cell surface in addition to IgM and IgD, the typical pattern of adult B cells. The mechanism and significance of this observation is not known. In most in vitro assay systems, neonatal B cells differentiate into plasma cells that secrete IgM, but not into plasma cells that secrete IgA or IgG. As fetal B cells can be driven to efficiently class switch and make IgG and IgA when provided with T cell help (CD40 ligand) and the appropriate cytokines, the limitation in the capacity of neonatal B cells to produce these isotypes most likely reflects the lack of appropriate T cell help to B cells (discussed above), rather than an inability of B cells to class switch [64, 65].

B cell response to specific antigens

In general, responses to antigens that need T cell help mature faster than the responses that occur independent of T cells. Infection or immunization of neonates with protein antigens (T cell dependent response) generally results in a protective immune response. Infants immunized with tetanus, diphtheria, polio vaccines are protected against infection. Although the response of neonates may not be as rapid or robust as older children, there appears to be rapid maturation of the thymus-dependent phase of the immune response, in many cases by 2 months of age. The magnitude and persistence of IgG antibody responses to protein antigens approaches adult levels after 1 year of age [51]. While T cell dependent immunity rapidly matures postnatally, the response to polysaccharide antigens such as those from *H. influenzae* or *S. pneumoniae* (T cell independent antigens) does not fully mature until 2–3 years of age. The reasons for this delay may include reduced levels of complement receptors on infant B cells, low complement activity (C3d), reduced IgG2a production and immaturity of the splenic marginal zone [51]. These differences help explain the age-specific risk for development of invasive disease with these bacteria.

1.4 Summary

Each component of the immune system matures from conception to adulthood. Some of the components function at adult levels at the time of birth, while others do not fully mature until late childhood. Many factors contribute to the observed immaturity of the developing immune system, including an inability to mount an appropriate antibody response to vaccines, slower institution of antigen-specific immunity, lower levels of some immune-activating substances, and no previous exposure to certain antigens. An awareness of the developmental differences that exist in the various components of the immune system in normal children is key to the understanding of the natural course of HIV infection in children.

REFERENCES

1. Goldblum, R., Hanson, L. & Brandtzaeg, P. The Mucosal Defense System. In E. Steihm (ed.), *Immunologic Disorders in Infants and Children*. Philadelphia, PA: W. B. Saunders (1996), pp. 159–200.
2. Neutra, M., Pingualt, M. & Kraehenhuhl, J. Antigen sampling across epithelial barriers and induction of mucosal immune responses. *Annu. Rev. Immunol.* **14** (1996), 275–300.
3. Johnston, R. The complement system in host defense and inflammation. *Pediatr. Infect. Dis. J.* **12** (1993), 933–41.
4. Johnston, R. Monocytes and macrophages. *New Engl. J. Med.* **318** (1988), 747–52.
5. Gluckman, J.-C., Canque, B. & Rosenzwajg, M. Dendritic cells: a complex simplicity. *Transplantation* **73** (2002), S3–6.
6. Spits, H. J., Couwenberg, F., Bakker, A. Q., Weijer, K. & Uittenbogaart, C. H. Id2 and Id3 inhibit development of CD34+ stem cells into pre-dendritic cells (pre-DC)2 but not into pre-CD1: evidence for a lymphoid origin of pre-DC2. *J. Exp. Med.* **192** (2000), 1785.
7. Ferlazzo, G., Wesa, A., Wei, W. & Galy, A. Dendritic cells generated from either CD34+ progentior cells or from monocytes differ in their ability to activate antigen-specific CD8+ T cells. *J. Immunol.* **163** (1999), 3597.
8. Banchereau, J., Pulendran, B., Steinman, R. & Palucka, K. Will the making of plasmacytoid dendritic cells in vitro help unravel their mysteries? *J. Exp. Med.* **192** (2000), F39.
9. Luster, A. D. The role of chemokines in linking innate and adaptive immunity. *Curr. Opin. Immunol.* **14** (2002), 129–35.
10. Vasselon, T. & Detmers, P. A. Toll receptors: a central element in innate immune responses. *Infect. Immun.* **70** (2002), 1033–41.
11. Bernard, A., Boumsell, L. & Hill, C. In A. Bernard, L. Boumsell, J. Dausett, C. Milstein & S. F. Scholssman (eds.), *Joint Report of the First International Workshop on Human Leucocyte Differentiation Antigens by the Investigators of the Participating Laboratories in Leucocyte Typing*. New York: Springer-Verlag (1984), pp. 9–143.
12. Williams, A. F. & Barclay, A. N. The immunoglobulin superfamily-domains for cell surface recognition. *Ann. Rev. Immunol.* **6** (1988), 381–405.
13. Bucy, R. P., Chan, C.-L. H. & Cooper, M. D. Tissue localization and CD8 accessory molecule expression of Tγδ cells in humans. *J. Immunol.* **142** (1989). 3045–9.
14. Berkower, I. The T cell, maestro of the immune system: receptor acquisition, MHC recognition, thymic selection and tolerance. In S. Sell (ed.), *Immunology, Immunopathology and Immunity, 5th edn.* Stamford, CT: Appleton & Lange (1996), 168–87.
15. Bierer, B. E., Sleckmen, B. P., Ratnofsky, S. E. & Burakoff, S. J. The biological roles of CD2, CD4 and CD8 in T cell activation. *Annu. Rev. Immunol.* **7** (1989), 579–608.
16. Clement, L. T. Cellular interactions in the human immune response. In E. R. Stiehm (ed.), *Immunologic Disorders of*

Infants and Children, 4th edn. Philadelphia, PA: W. B. Saunders (1996), 75–93.

17. Sanders, M., Makgoba, M. & Shaw, S. Human naive and memory T cells: reinterpretation of helper-inducer and suppressor-inducer subsets. *Immunol. Today* **9** (1988), 195–9.

18. Clark, E. & Ledbetter, J. How B and T cells talk to each other. *Nature* **367** (1994), 425–8.

19. Berkower, I. How T cells help B cells make antibodies. In S. Sells (ed.), *Immunology, Immunopathology and Immunity*, 5th edn. Stamford, CT: Appleton & Lange (1996), 188–204.

20. Noelle, R. J., Ledbetter, J. A. & Aruffo, A. CD40 and its ligand, an essential ligand-receptor pair for thymus-dependent B cell activation. *Immunol. Today* **13** (1992), 431–4.

21. Mossman, T. R., Cherwinski, H. M., Bond, M. W., Giedlin, M. A. & Coffman, R. L. Two types of murine helper T cell clones. I. Definition according to profiles of lymphokine activity and secreted proteins. *J. Immunol.* **136** (1986), 2348–57.

22. Gelfand, E. W. & Finkel, T. H. The T-lymphocyte system. In E. R. Stiehm (ed.), *Immunologic Disorders of Infants and Children*, 4th edn. Philadelphia, PA: W. B. Saunders (1996), 14–34.

23. Biddison, W. E., Sharrow, S. O. & Shearer, G. M. T cell subpopulations required for the human cytotoxic T lymphocyte response to influenza virus: evidence for T cell help. *J. Immunol.* **127** (1981), 487–91.

24. Luster, A. D. Chemokines-chemotactic cytokines that mediate inflammation. *New Engl. J. Med.* **338** (1998), 436–45.

25. Baggiolini, M., Dewald, B. & Moser, B. Interleukin 8 and related chemotactic cytokines – CXC and CC chemokines. *Adv. Immunol.* **55** (1994), 97–179.

26. Garcia-Zepeda, E. A., Combadiere, C., Rothenburg, M. E. *et al.* Human monocyte chemoattractant protein (MCP)-4 is a novel CC chemokine with activities on monocytes, eosinophils and basophils induced in allergic and nonallergic inflammation that signals through the CC chemokine receptors (CCR)-2 and -3. *J. Immunol.* **157** (1996), 5613–26.

27. Chollet-Martin, S., Montravers, P., Gibert, C. *et al.* High levels of interleukin-8 in the blood and alveolar spaces of patients with pneumonia and adult respiratory distress syndrome. *Infect. Immunol.* **61** (1993), 4553–9.

28. Lahrtz, F., Piali, L., Nadal, D. *et al.* Chemotactic activity on mononuclear cells in the cerebrospinal fluid of patients with viral meningitis is mediated by interferon-gamma indicible protein-10 and monocyte chemotactic protein-1. *Eur. J. Immunol.* **27** (1997), 2484–9.

29. Cooper, M. B lymphocytes normal development and function. *New Engl. J. Med.* **317** (1987), 1452–6.

30. Parslow, T. Immunoglobulin genes, B cells and the humoral immune response. In D. Stites, A. I. Terr, & T. G. Parslow (eds.), *Basic and Clinical Immunology, 8th edn.* Norwalk, CT: Appleton & Lange (1994), pp. 80–93.

31. Reth, M., Hombach, J., Wienands, J. *et al.* The B-cell antigen receptor complex. *Immunol. Today* **12** (1991), 196–201.

32. Wilson, C., Lewis, D. & Penix, L. The physiologic immunodeficiency of immaturity. In E. R. Stiehm (ed.), *Immunologic Disorders in Infants and Children*, 4th edn. Philadelphia, PA: W. B. Saunders, (1996), pp. 253–95.

33. Davis, C. A., Vollata, E. H. & Forristal, J. Serum complement levels in infancy: age related changes. *Pediatr. Res.* **13** (1979), 1043–6.

34. Norman, M. E., Gall, E. P., Taylor, A., Laster, L. & Nilsson, U. R. Serum complement profiles in infants and children. *J. Pediatr.* **87** (1975), 912–6.

35. Sheldon, W. & Caldwell, J. The mononuclear cell phase of inflammation in the newborn. *Bull. Johns Hopkins Hosp.* **112** (1963), 258–69.

36. Johnston, R. B. Jr. Function and cell biology of neutrophils and mononuclear cells in the newborn infant. *Vaccine* **14/15** (1998), 1363–8.

37. Bullock, J., Robertson, A., Bodenbender, J., Kontras, S. & Miller, C. Inflammatory responses in the neonate reexamined. *Pediatrics* **44** (1969), 58–61.

38. Christensen, R. & Rothstein, G. Exhaustion of mature neutrophils in neonates with sepsis. *J. Pediatr.* **96** (1980), 316–18.

39. Anderson, D., Hughes, B. & Smith, C. Abnormal mobility of neonatal polymorphonuclear leukocytes. *J. Clin. Invest.* **68** (1981), 863–74.

40. Anderson, D., Hughes, B., Wible, L., Perry, G., Smith, C. & Brinkley, B. Impaired mobility of neonatal PMN leukocytes: relationship to abnormalities of cell orientation and assembly of microtubules in chemotactic gradients. *J. Leukocyte Biol.* **36** (1984), 1–15.

41. Pahwa, S., Pahwa, R., Grimes, E. & Smithwick, E. Cellular and humoral components of monocyte and neutrophil chemotaxis in cord blood. *Pediatr. Res.* **11** (1977), 677–80.

42. Rao, S., Olesinski, R., Doshi, U. & Vidyasagar, D. Granulocyte adherence in newborn infants. *J. Pediatr.* **98** (1981), 622–4.

43. Carson, W. & Caliguri, M. Natural killer cell subsets and development. *Methods.* **9** (1996), 327–43.

44. Petty, R. E., & Hunt, D. W. C. Neonatal dendritic cells. *Vaccine* **16** (1998), 1378–82.

45. Muthukkumar, S., Goldstein, J. & Stein, K. E. The ability of B cells and dendritic cells to present antigen increases during ontogeny. *J. Immunol.* **165** (2000), 4803–13.

46. Haynes, B., Martin, M., Kay, H. & Kurtzberg, J. Early events in human T cell ontogeny. Phenotypic characterization and immunohistological localization of T cell precursors in early human fetal tissues. *J. Exp. Med.* **168** (1988), 1061–80.

47. Borst, J., Broom, T., Bos, J. & van Dongen, J. Tissue distribution and repertoire selection of human gd cells: comparison with the murine system. *Curr. Top. Microbiol. Immunol.* **171** (1991), 41–6.

48. Akbar, A., Terry, L., Timms, A., Beverly, P. & Janossy, G. Loss of CD45R and gain of UCHL1 reactivity is a feature of primed T cells. *J. Immunol.* **140** (1988), 2171–8.

49. de Paoli, P., Battistin, S. & Santini, G. Age-related changes in human lymphocyte subsets: progressive reduction of the CD4 CD45R (suppressor-inducer) population. *Clin. Immunol. Immunopathol.* **48** (1988), 290–6.

50. Denny, T., Yogev, R. & Gelman, R. *et al.* Lymphocyte subsets in healthy children during the first 5 years of life. *J. Am. Med. Assoc.* **267** (1992), 1484–8.

51. Siegrist, C. A. Neonatal and early life vaccinology. *Vaccine.* **19** (2001), 3331–46.

52. Ehlers, S. & Smith, K. Differentiation of T cell lymphokine gene expression. The in vitro acquisition of T cell memory. *J. Exp. Med.* **173** (1991), 25–36.

53. English, B., Burchett, S., English, J., Ammann, A., Wara, D. & Wilson, C. Production of lymphotoxin and tumor necrosis factor by human neonatal mononuclear cells. *Pediatr. Res.* **24** (1988), 717–22.

54. Haward, A. Development of lymphocyte responses and interactions in the human fetus and newborn. *Immunol. Rev.* **57** (1981), 62–87.

55. Lewis, D., Yu, C., Meyer, J., English, B., Kahn, S. & Wilson, C. Cellular and molecular mechanisms for reduced interleukin-4 and interferon-gamma production by neonatal T cells. *J. Clin. Invest.* **87** (1991), 194–202.

56. Delespesse, G., Yang, L. P., Ohshima, Y., *et al.* Maturation of human neonatal CD4$^+$ and CD8$^+$ T lymphocytes into Th1/Th2 effectors. *Vaccine.* **16** (1998), 1415–19.

57. Arulanandam, B. P., Van Cleve, V. H. & Metzger, D. IL-12 is a potent neonatal vaccine adjuvant. *Eur. J. Immunol.* **29** (1999), 256–64.

58. Nonoyama, S., Penix, L., Edwards, C., Aruffo, A., Wilson, C. & Ochs, H. Diminished expression of CD40 ligand (gp39) by activated neonatal T cells. *J. Clin. Invest.* **95** (1995), 66–75.

59. Franz, M., Carella, J. & Galant, S. Cutaneous delayed hypersensitivity in a healthy pediatric population: diagnostic value of diptheria-tetanus toxoid. *J. Pediatr.* **88** (1976), 975–8.

60. Kniker, W., Lesourd, B., McBryyde, J. & Corriel, R. Cell-mediated immunity assessed by multitest CMI skin testing in infants and preschool children. *Am. J. Dis. Child.* **134** (1985), 840–5.

61. Burrows, P., Kearney, F. & Schroeder, H. Normal B lymphocyte differentiation. *Baillieres Clin. Haematol.* **6** (1993), 785–806.

62. Hentges, F. B lymphocyte ontogeny and immunoglobulin production. *Clin. Exp. Immunol.* **97S** (1994), 3–9.

63. Duchosal, M. B-cell development and differentiation. *Semin. Hematol.* **34**: 1, Suppl. 1 (1997), 2–12.

64. Banchereau, J., de Paoli, P., Valle Garcia, E. & Rousset, F. Long-term human B cell lines dependent on interleukin-4 and antibody to CD40. *Science* **251** (1991), 70–2.

65. Splawski, J. & Lipsky, P. Cytokine regulation of immunoglobulin secretion by neonatal lymphocytes. *J. Clin. Invest.* **88** (1991), 967–77.

66. European Collaborative Study Age-related standards for T lympohocyte subsets based on uninfected children born to human immunodeficiency virus 1-infected women. *Pediatr. Infect. Dis. J.* **11** (1992), 1018–26.

SUGGESTED READING

Shyur, S. & Hill, H. Immunodeficiency in the 1990's. *Pediatr. Infect. Dis. J.* **10** (1991), 595–611.

Wilson, C., Lewis, D. & Penix, L. The physiologic immunodeficiency of immaturity. In E. R. Stiehm (ed.), *Immunologic Disorders in Infants and Children*, 4th edn. Philadelphia, PA: W. B. Saunders (1996), 253–95.

Fleisher, T. A. Back to basics – immune function. *Pediatr. Rev.* **18** (1997), 351–6.

Adkins, B. T-cell function in newborn mice and humans. *Immunol. Today* **20** (1999), 330–5.

HIV basic virology for clinicians

Steven L. Zeichner, M.D., Ph.D.

HIV and AIDS Malignancy Branch, National Cancer Institute, National Institutes of Health, Bethesda, MD

2.1 Introduction

The molecular details of the HIV replication cycle largely determine the pathogenesis of the diseases caused by HIV and constrain the possible therapeutic strategies. Optimal diagnosis, assessment, and treatment of HIV infection in children thus require knowledge of the viral replication cycle, the viral targets affected by the antiretroviral agents, and the components of the virus detected by the tests used to manage the disease.

2.2 Classification and origin of HIV

HIV-1 is a member of the *Lentivirus* genus of retroviruses (reviewed in [1]). The virus is believed to have entered the human population in Africa about 70 years ago [2], probably as humans hunted and butchered chimpanzees for "bush meat" [3]. The animal virus most closely related to HIV-1, a simian immunodeficiency virus (SIV) designated SIV$_{CPZ}$, is found in chimpanzees, and certain chimpanzee populations continue to harbor large numbers of retroviruses [4]. HIV-2, a less pathogenic relative of HIV-1, infects some human populations in western Africa, with a relatively small number of cases in other parts of the world [5]. HIV-2 is believed to derive from an immunodeficiency virus that infects monkeys. The closest relative to HIV-2 is a simian immunodeficiency virus, SIV$_{SMM}$, with SMM denoting sooty mangabey monkey. HIV-2 has some biological properties that distinguish it from HIV-1, and the disease caused by HIV-2 differs from the disease caused by HIV-1. Untreated, HIV-2 disease is generally a much less fulminant disorder than the disease caused by HIV-1. Some

serological and molecular tests for HIV-1 do not detect HIV-2 well, unless they are specially modified. The HIV-2 reverse transcriptase is not inhibited by the non-nucleoside reverse transcriptase inhibitors effective against HIV-1. The material in this book generally refers to HIV-1, unless otherwise noted, and HIV-1 will usually be referred to simply as HIV.

Lentiviruses that infect other animals include equine infectious anemia virus, bovine immunodeficiency virus, feline immunodeficiency virus, and visna virus of sheep. Other retroviruses that infect humans include human T cell leukemia virus 1 (HTLV-1), the infectious agent implicated in adult acute T cell leukemia/lymphoma, HTLV-1-associated myelopathy/tropical spastic paraparesis (HAM/TSP), and other diseases.

HIV-1 has been phylogenetically divided, using genomic sequence analysis, into several different clades or subtypes, designated A, B, C, D, E, F, G, H, J, and K [1, 6], and three groups, the M (main) group, which includes most of the clades, and the O (outlier) and N (non-M, non-O) groups. Certain clades predominate in certain geographical areas. For example, clade B predominates overwhelmingly in North America, and represents the major subtype in Europe and Australia. Clade A, which has the most heterogeneity, predominates in West Africa, while clade D is the major subtype in Central Africa, and clade C is principally found in southern and eastern Africa and the Indian Subcontinent. Clade E is a major subtype in Thailand and the surrounding area. Some recombinant viruses exist; clade E may be an example of a recombinant virus. While the genetic variation among HIV-1 subtypes may hold greatest interest as a tool to study viral evolution and epidemiology, there are also some important clinical implications, particularly for diagnosis and vaccine development. Some serologic and molecular assays optimized to detect and quantify virus of one clade, for example the clade B that predominates in North America, may not perform optimally when used to detect other clades. Immunologic responses aimed at virus of one clade may not affect virus of other clades, making the development of vaccines capable of inducing effective immunity to many clades a challenge.

2.3 HIV virion structure

HIV shares a common structure with other retroviruses (Figure 2.1) (reviewed in [7]). Table 2.1 lists the proteins of HIV, the genes that encode the proteins, the function of the proteins, and whether the proteins have been the target of antiretroviral drug development. The virion capsid, composed of the viral capsid (CA or p24) protein, encloses two copies of the RNA that comprises the viral genome, together with two copies of the viral reverse transcriptase (RT or p66/p51). Within the capsid, copies of the viral nucleocapsid (NC or p7) protein are complexed with the viral genomic RNA, via sequence-specific interactions between two CCHC zinc finger domains in NC and a specific "packaging signal" (also known as a Ψ-site or encapsidation element) (see below), composed of a particular three-dimensional structure in the viral RNA, and through non-specific charge interactions between the negatively charged RNA and region of positively charged basic amino acid residues in NC. Also within the capsid lie copies of the viral integrase (IN or p31) protein and copies of the viral protease (PR or p11), which also exists in other regions of the viral core. The RT, PR, and IN proteins of the viral core are derived from the gag-pol preprotein precursor (Pr160), which is cleaved into its functional subunits by the viral protease (see below). The other core proteins are derived from the Gag preprotein (Pr55).

The outer region of the viral core includes the HIV matrix (MA or p17) protein. MA lies on the interior face of the virion envelope, and is tethered to the interior side of the envelope through a myristic acid lipid moiety that is covalently attached to a glycine at the N-terminal of MA, and by hydrophobic interactions.

The virion envelope is a lipid bilayer, derived from the plasma membrane of the host cell that produced the virion. Anchored into the lipid bilayer and extending out into extracellular space are the gp41 transmembrane portion of the viral envelope (or Env) glycoprotein (TM or gp41). TM associates non-covalently with the surface gp120

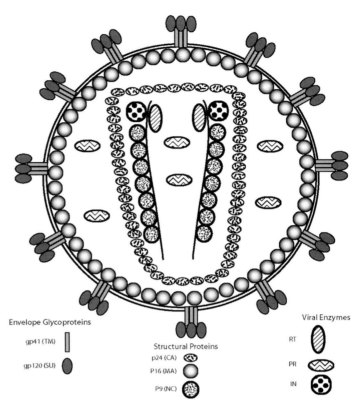

Figure 2.1. A schematic diagram of the HIV virion. Individual viral proteins and their functions are described in detail in the text.

envelope (Env) glycoprotein (SU or gp120); the envelope glycoproteins gp120 and gp41 are processed by cellular proteases from a precursor, gp160, and are highly glycosylated. The gp120 and gp41 remain non-covalently associated with each other after processing from the gp160 precursor. The envelope glycoproteins gp120+gp41 associate with each other as trimers on the outer surface of the virion. The envelope glycoproteins mediate viral entry and syncytium formation. The gp120 glycoprotein has both constant (C) regions, in which the amino acid sequence remains relatively constant from virus to virus, and variable (V) regions, in which the amino acid sequence shows greater variability. One of the variable regions, variable region 3 (also known as the V3 loop), can elicit a strong humoral immune response from the host, but these antibodies are generally ineffectual in controlling the infection.

The virion also contains several macromolecules derived from the host cell, which are incorporated into the virion during virion assembly and budding [8]. Some of these macromolecules play crucial roles in the viral replication cycle. The viral capsid contains cellular lysine transfer RNA

Table 2.1 HIV viral genes and gene products: existing and potential targets for antiretroviral agents

Viral protein	Gene	Function	Inhibitors
P16 (MA)	*gag*	Matrix protein; lies beneath envelope; targeted to membrane via myristoylation; recruits envelope into virion; aids in PI localization to nucleus	Nuclear localization site inhibitors; myristoylation inhibitors; transdominant negative gag mutants
p24 (CA)	*gag*	Capsid protein; viral core	
p9 (NC)	*gag*	Nucleocapsid protein; interacts with viral RNA via zinc fingers	Zinc chelators
p6 (NC)	*gag*		
Protease (PR)	*pol*	Cleaves gag (Pr55) and gag-pol (Pr160) precursor proteins during virion maturation	Protease inhibitors
Reverse Transcriptase (RT)	*pol*	Catalyzes synthesis of viral cDNA from viral genomic RNA	Nucleoside analogue reverse transcriptase inhibitors (NRTIs); nucleotide analogue reverse transcriptase inhibitors (tenofovir); non-nucleoside analogue reverse transcriptase inhibitors (NNRTIs)
Integrase (IN)	*pol*	Catalyzes integration of viral cDNA into host cell genomic DNA to create provirus	Integrase inhibitors
gp120	*env*	Mediate interaction of virus with CD4 and chemokine co-receptors. Initial steps of viral binding and entry.	Chemokine co-receptor inhibitors (e.g. Schering C and D); binding inhibitors (soluble CD4)
gp41	*env*	Integral membrane envelope glycoprotein; contains fusion domain mediating virion envelope-host cell plasma membrane fusion	Fusion inhibitors (e.g enfuvirtide T-20)
Tat	*tat*	Transactivates viral gene expression; binds to TAR structure in nascent viral RNA and cellular kinase leading phosphorylation of celluar RNA polymerase II, increasing processivity	Kinase inhibitors (cellular enzyme); small molecule inhibitors; Tat-TAR interaction blockers; TAR decoys; antisense oligo nucleotides; ribozymes, small interfering RNAs
Rev	*rev*	Mediates nuclear export of singly spliced and unspliced viral RNAs	small molecule inhibitors, inhibitors of Rev-RRE binding (aminoglycosides); RRE decoys; transdominant Rev; antisense oligonucleotides; ribozymes; inhibitors of nuclear export, small interfering RNAs
Vif	*vif*	Viral infectivity factor	
Vpu	*vpu*	gp160/CD4 complex degradation; CD4 downregulation; virus release	
Vpr	*vpr*	Cell cycle arrest; transactivation; ?PIC entry into nucleus	
Nef	*nef*	CD4 downregulation; stimulates cellular signal transduction pathways	

Targets of drugs with current clinical utility (licensed drugs and drugs in advanced clinical development) are shown in **bold**.

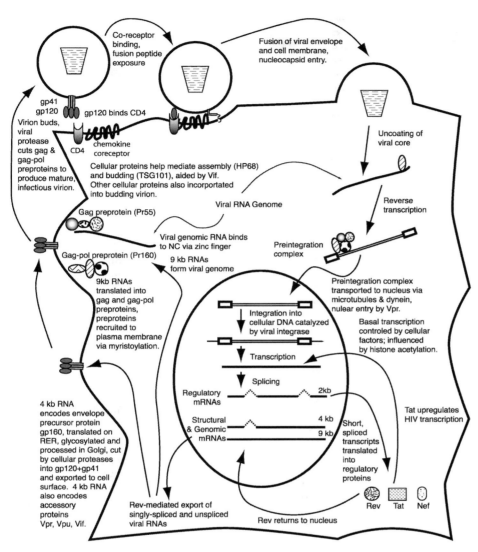

Figure 2.2. A schematic diagram of the HIV replication cycle. The features of the viral life cycle are described in detail in the text.

(tRNA-lys), which serves as the primer for reverse transcription by the viral RT from the viral RNA. The virus contains several host cell proteins, either within the interior of the virion or embedded in the viral envelope. Cyclophilin A physically interacts with one of the viral gag proteins, CA, and appears to be required for viral infectivity. Other cellular proteins that are incorporated into the virion include Class I and Class II HLA histocompatibility antigens, and the cell adhesion molecules LFA-1 and ICAM-1. The lipid bilayer of the viral envelope is derived from the host cell plasma membrane, but the lipids are not completely representative of the plasma membrane because certain lipids appear to be preferentially included and others excluded during virion formation.

2.4 The HIV life cycle

2.4.1 Viral entry into the host cell

Figure 2.2 schematically depicts the HIV life cycle. Infection begins when the virion envelope glycoprotein gp120 binds the viral receptor, the CD4 molecule on the surface of the future host cell (reviewed in [9, 10]). CD4 binding triggers a conformational change in gp120, which facilitates gp120's interaction with a viral co-receptor, generally proteins named CXCR4 or CCR5. Co-receptor triggers a further conformational change in gp41, the viral envelope glycoprotein that is anchored in the viral envelope and is non-covalently associated with gp120. The change in gp41 leads to the insertion of an amino-terminal domain of gp41, the "fusion peptide," into the future host cell's plasma membrane, and to the formation of a specialized structure in gp41, the "six-helix bundle", a hairpin-like structure in gp41, which leads to the close apposition and then fusion of the viral envelope and host cell plasma membrane, releasing the viral capsid into the cytoplasm [11]. This viral envelope–host cell plasma membrane fusion process is similar to the process used by some other viruses, including the well-characterized membrane fusion process used by influenza viruses [10]. The newly developed antiretroviral agent enfuvirtide (T-20, Fuzeon), a peptide composed of 36 amino acids, and related peptides in earlier stages of development (e.g. T-1249) are homologs of part of gp41 [12]. T-20 binds to one of the helices of gp41, instead of the other native gp41 helix, preventing gp41 from undergoing the conformational change and forming the structures that lead to viral envelope–host cell membrane fusion. Some small molecule fusion inhibitors are also under development. Early attempts to block virus binding employed a soluble version of the CD4 viral receptor, with the hope that the soluble CD4 would bind the viral gp120 envelope protein, making it impossible for the virus to bind CD4 on potential host cells. While soluble CD4 can block HIV infection in vitro, it was not effective clinically. Decreasing the expression of CD4 on the surface of cells that would normally support efficient viral replication through, for example, targeting the CD4 messenger RNA for accelerated destruction by interactions with small interfering RNAs (siRNA) can also block in vitro infection [13], but the clinical utility of such approaches, if any, lies far in the future. Cyanonvirin, a small protein derived from a cyanobacterium, can inhibit HIV binding and infection [14]. As a protein, it probably has little utility as a systemic therapeutic agent, but there is some interest in developing it for use as a topical virucide to prevent HIV sexual transmission.

HIV can be distinguished by its tropism for different types of host cells (see also Chapter 5), with virus classified as macrophage-tropic (M-tropic) and T cell-tropic (T-tropic). The co-receptor that the viruses use determines the ability of the virus to infect the different cell types. M-tropic strains can infect macrophages, monocytes, and primary T cells, but are unable to infect $CD4^+$ T cell lines (reviewed in [15]). M-tropic viruses use CCR5 as their co-receptor and so are termed R5 viruses. T-tropic viruses infect $CD4^+$ T cells, but not macrophages and monocytes. T-tropic viruses use CXCR4 as their co-receptor and so are termed X4 viruses.

Some dual tropic (R5X4) viruses also exist. Certain V-region envelope sequences are associated with viral strains that are M-tropic or T-tropic; the interactions of the V regions with the chemokine co-receptors probably mediate these differences in viral tropism. Most patients are usually initially infected with R5 viruses. Later in the disease, often as the amount of circulating virus increases and the $CD4^+$ lymphocyte count declines, the predominant circulating virus undergoes a shift to X4 virus (see Chapter 5 for further details).

The viral coreceptors act, in their native capacity, as chemokine G protein-coupled receptors. As chemokine receptors, they transmit signals from the chemokines into the cell and modify the behavior of the cells via signal transduction pathways, leading to a variety of cellular responses, including cellular activation and chemotaxis, recruiting white blood cells to areas of injury and inflammation.

Chemokines named RANTES, MIP1-α, and MIP1-β bind CCR5, the co-receptor for M-tropic HIV-1 strains. They are termed α-chemokines, or C-C chemokines, for the juxtaposed cysteine residues near their amino terminal end. A chemokine named stromal derived factor 1 (SDF-1) is the native ligand for CXCR4. It is a β- or C-X-C chemokine, named for the cystein-X-cysteine residues near the amino-terminal end of the protein. Several other receptors for chemokines can also serve as HIV co-receptors. These other co-receptors include ones named APJ, BOB (or GPR15), Bonzo (or STRL33), CCR2b, CCR3, and CCR8. The pathogenic significance of many of these co-receptors is unclear, but they may mediate entry of HIV into cells that do not express high levels of the other co-receptors, such as certain cells in the central nervous system (CNS), which may affect the pathogenesis of HIV disease in the CNS. Chemokine co-receptors were first discovered through molecular biological techniques in which potential genes encoding the co-receptors were provided to cells lacking the co-receptors and the genes that led to the expression of the co-receptor and enabled fusion to occur were subsequently identified and sequenced [16]. CXCR4 (also termed "fusin") was the first co-receptor identified, and the identification of other co-receptors quickly followed [17, 18]. An important hint that chemokine co-receptors were involved in HIV binding and entry came with the observation that high concentrations of chemokines, such as those secreted by $CD8^+$ cytotoxic T cells, can inhibit infection in vitro, presumably by competing with HIV for binding to the co-receptor or by causing the potential host cells to down-regulate the amount of CCR5 on their surfaces [19].

Much recent drug development effort has focused on these chemokine co-receptors. Some small molecule competitive inhibitors for chemokine receptor binding inhibit viral replication in vitro and are currently being used in early stage human trials, with some preliminary indications of clinical activity. Small molecule inhibitors generally target only one of the co-receptors. Examples of these small molecule co-receptor inhibitors in development include AMD-3100, which targets CXCR4, and Schering-C and Schering-D, which target CCR5 [20]. Interestingly, when the Schering-C and -D compounds were used in patients, no significant shift in the co-receptor used by the patients' virus, for example from CCR5 to CXCR4, was observed. Such a shift is a theoretical concern for this kind of inhibitor because if the virus rapidly shifted co-receptor usage, the utility of the drug would be limited, and because X4 viruses have been associated with increased pathogenicity (see Chapters 3 and 5). There were some indications of a shift from CXCR4 to CCR5 co-receptor usage in patients treated with AMD-3100.

Some naturally occurring mutations in the viral co-receptors illustrate their key role for viral replication. Individuals with mutations in their co-receptor genes are less likely to become infected with HIV and HIV-infected patients with certain co-receptor mutations tend to have slower disease progression. Some of the HIV-infected patients known as "long-term non-progressors" have co-receptor mutations. For example, some of these long-term non-progressors are heterozygous or homozygous for a 32 base pair deletion in the CCR5 gene (Δ32CCR5) [21, 22]. The Δ32CCR5 does not localize to the cell membrane, so it cannot function as a co-receptor for HIV entry. Cells with the Δ32CCR5, however, are not resistant to infection with T-tropic viruses, since they use the CXCR4 co-receptor. The observation that persons homozygous for the Δ32CCR5 mutation are highly resistant to initial infection supports the model that M-tropic viruses using CCR5 as their co-receptor may be the primary mediators of HIV transmission. Interestingly, individuals with the mutation exhibit no discernible deleterious phenotype. Mutations in the promoter of the CCR5 genes that decrease expression are also seen in long-term non-progressors [23] (see also Chapter 5).

2.4.2 Reverse transcription

After entry, the viral capsid undergoes an incompletely characterized "uncoating" process, releasing the RNA genome, associated with proteins and the tRNA that will prime reverse transcription, into the cytoplasm. RT, encoded by the *pol* gene, catalyzes reverse transcription, the process through which a cDNA copy of the viral genome is produced, prior to the transit of the viral cDNA to the nucleus and integration of the cDNA into the host genome as a provirus (Figure 2.2). RT consists of two subunits p51 and p66, the catalytic subunit, which dimerize to form the functional enzyme. Many effective, licensed drugs target RT, including the nucleoside (or for tenofovir, nucleotide) reverse transcriptase inhibitors (NRTIs), and the non-nucleoside reverse transcriptase inhibitors (NNRTIs). (The process of reverse transcription, the structure and enzymology of RT, and the mechanisms of action of RT inhibitors are described in greater detail in Chapter 21.)

The HIV RNA genome begins at the 5′ end with a sequence termed the "R" (for repeat) region, followed by the U5 (5′ unique) region, the sequences encoding the viral proteins and, at the 3′ end, the U3 (3′ unique) region and another copy of the R region (Figure 2.3) (reviewed in [24]). Using a cellular lysine tRNA molecule carried within the capsid as a primer, the HIV RT synthesizes a minus strand DNA molecule complementary to the plus sense RNA template [25]. Synthesis begins in the 3′ end of the U5 region. When RT reaches the 5′ end of the RNA template, it stops, having produced a short DNA known as "minus strand strong-stop" cDNA. RT's RNase H activity partially degrades the original RNA template, releasing the minus strand strong-stop cDNA. This minus strand strong-stop cDNA then moves to the 3′ end of the viral RNA, where it hybridizes to the complementary R region in the LTR, and RT continues the synthesis of the rest of the minus strand cDNA. Then, through a complicated process that involves strand transfers, and a switch in templates from the genomic RNA to newly synthesized cDNA, RT completes the synthesis of the cDNA. The finished double-stranded cDNA version of the viral genome has two long terminal repeats (LTRs) at either end of the genome. Each LTR consists of the repeated versions of the U3, R, and U5 regions (Figure 2.3).

Reverse transcription constitutes one of the defining features of the retroviridae. RT catalyzes an essential step in the retroviral life cycle and so has been a target for drug development since HIV was first identified. Originally produced as antineoplastic agents, the NRTIs were the earliest drugs for HIV. Following uptake by the cells, NRTIs are converted to the active triphosphate form by cellular kinases and the triphosphate-NRTIs can then compete with native nucleotide triphosphates for use by RT. When RT incorporates the NRTIs into the cDNA, no further nucleotides can be incorporated into the lengthening cDNA, causing a prematurely truncated cDNA. The NRTIs stop the growing cDNA chain because, in the NRTIs, the ribose 3′-OH is replaced by another group incapable of forming a covalent bond with the next nucleotide (Figure 2.4). These drugs are therefore termed "chain terminators." In the case of

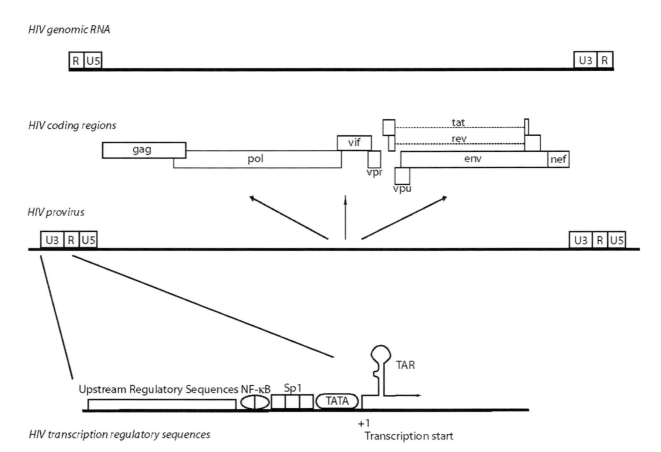

HIV genomic RNA

HIV coding regions

HIV provirus

Upstream Regulatory Sequences NF-κB   Sp1   TATA   TAR

+1
Transcription start

HIV transcription regulatory sequences

Figure 2.3. The genomic organization of HIV. The top of the figure shows the organization of the viral genomic RNA. The middle of the figure shows the HIV provirus, with the reading frames of the different HIV genes identified. The lower portion of the figure shows the location of selected HIV transcription regulatory sites, including both selected sites active in the HIV LTR (NF-kB, Sp1, and TATA), and the TAR site as it exists in the newly transcribed viral RNA.

zidovudine (ZDV or AZT) the 3′-OH is replaced by an azido group. In the case of dideoxyinosine (didanosine, ddI), dideoxycytosine (zalcitabine, ddC), and stavudine (d4T), the 3′-OH group is replaced by a hydrogen. In 3′ thiacytidine (lamivudine, 3TC), the 3′ carbon or the ribose ring is replaced by a sulfur atom, with a single hydrogen in place of the hydroxyl group. Tenofovir has slightly different properties. It is a monophosphate analogue of adenosine. As an analogue of the monophosphate, it bypasses the first phosphorylation step catalyzed by cellular kinases. The kinase activity is decreased in resting cells, so tenofovir may have certain advantages for blocking HIV replication in these cells.

The other class of RT inhibitors is the non-nucleoside RT inhibitors (NNRTIs). There are currently three licensed NNRTIs, efavirenz, nevirapine, and delavirdine, and more are under active development. NNRTIs act via a mechanism distinct from that of the NRTIs. NNRTIs bind a hydrophobic pocket near the active site of the enzyme in the p66 subunit of RT, inhibiting RT. (The process of reverse transcription, the detailed mechanism of action of the NNRTIs and the mutations that confer resistance to the NNRTIs are discussed in more detail in chapter 21.)

RT is an enzyme with "low fidelity." It inserts the wrong base (termed "misincorporation") in the growing cDNA chain every 1 per 1700 to 1 per 4000 bases. In the presence of suboptimal drug concentrations, viral replication can continue. With continued viral replication, some mutant virus will be produced due to misincorporation, and some of the mutations can confer resistance against antiretroviral drugs (see Chapter 21). Because of the very high rates of viral replication and the large amounts of virus seen in infected patients (see Chapter 5), resistance can emerge rapidly, particularly for drugs for which only a single base change in the viral genome confers very high-level resistance, such as lamivudine or the currently available NNRTIs.

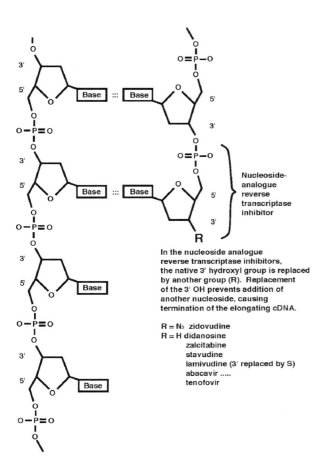

In the nucleoside analogue
reverse transcriptase inhibitors,
the native 3' hydroxyl group is replaced
by another group (R). Replacement
of the 3' OH prevents addition of
another nucleoside, causing
termination of the elongating cDNA.

R = N₃ zidovudine
R = H didanosine
      zalcitabine
      stavudine
      lamivudine (3' replaced by S)
      abacavir .....
      tenofovir

Figure 2.4. The mechanism of action of the nucleoside analogue HIV reverse transcriptase inhibitors. Chain termination occurs when another deoxynucleoside triphosphate cannot add on to the growing viral cDNA.

In fact, due to the high mutation rates and the very large amount of replicating virus, patients may have at least some small amounts of mutant virus present even before beginning to take an antiretroviral agent (see also Chapter 5) The concurrent use of combinations of multiple antiretrovirals that each requires a distinct set of mutations for resistance maximizes the effectiveness of therapy and makes it much less likely that a patient will develop resistant virus.

2.4.3 Nuclear localization and entry

Some retroviruses, such as murine leukemia virus, can only infect dividing cells. HIV, however, can infect both rapidly dividing cells and such terminally differentiated cells as macrophages, and quiescent (non-dividing) CD4⁺ T cells. The quiescent CD4⁺ T cells may make up a large fraction of the cells in a patient infected by HIV and HIV's

ability to infect these quiescent cells may help account for its pathogenicity. HIV's ability to infect these cells depends on its ability to transport the viral cDNA and associated viral proteins to the nucleus, and to enter the nucleus. After reverse transcription, the newly synthesized cDNA exists in close association with several viral proteins, including IN, RT, MA, and NC, the viral accessory protein Vpr, and host cell proteins Ku, INI 1, and HMGa1 (or HMG I(Y)), to form the pre-integration complex (PIC) [26–28]. Some of the components of the PIC, such as IN, which catalyzes integration, are clearly essential for the later steps in the viral replication cycle. Others, such as the cellular proteins, may not be essential, but increase the efficiency of the later steps. Following reverse transcription, the cellular microtubule and dynein machinery transports the PIC to the periphery of the nucleus, probably with help from Vpr [29].

Once transported to the vicinity of the nucleus, the PIC interacts with the nuclear membrane, an interaction mediated at least partly by Vpr docking with a host cell nucleoporin protein, hCG1 [30], leading to the entry of the PIC into the nucleus.

2.4.4 Integration

After the PIC has entered the nucleus, the HIV cDNA integrates into the host cell genomic DNA in a fashion that is not strictly sequence-specific, but may preferentially target regions of the host cell chromosomes that hold genes that are actively being expressed [31]. Soon after reverse transcription, IN first generates a preintegration form of the viral cDNA by removing two or three bases to leave a recessed 3' end. Later, in the nucleus, IN cuts the cellular genomic DNA leaving 5' overhanging ends. The enzyme joins the ends of the cDNA and the cellular DNA, in a process called strand transfer, with IN and cellular enzymes filling in the gaps, leaving the integrated provirus flanked by 5 bp direct repeats derived from the cellular genomic DNA and the dinucleotides TG at the 5' end and CA at the 3' end [32, 33].

The other proteins in the PIC help facilitate integration. For example, one form of the NC protein, the p9 form, enhances the integration in an in vitro model of HIV integration, perhaps by directing the IN protein away from inappropriate sites on the HIV cDNA [34], suggesting that correct and efficient integration of the HIV cDNA must be carefully directed for optimum integration efficiency.

Since integration and formation of the provirus is an essential feature of the retroviral life cycle and since IN is an essential enzyme in HIV replication [35], IN is a very attractive target for drug development [36, 37]. The target is a challenging one, though, because integration is a

Stage 1: Initial Transcription

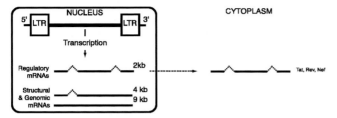

Stage 2: Tat-activated Transcription

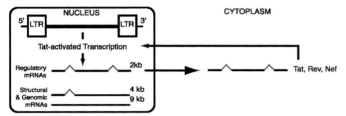

Stage 3: Late Phase Transcription

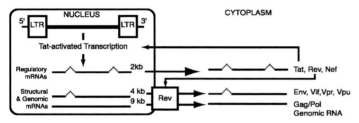

Figure 2.5. Phases of HIV gene expression. Initially, only small amounts of transcription occur and only small quantities of short, multiply spliced viral messages encoding the viral regulatory genes Tat and Rev and the accessory gene Nef are exported to the cytoplasm. When the HIV promoter is activated, more messages are produced and sufficient Tat protein returns to the nucleus to produce a large increase in viral gene expression. Later, when sufficient quantities of Rev are present in the nucleus, the longer singly spliced and unspliced messages encoding the viral structural proteins and comprising the viral genomic RNA are exported to the cytoplasm.

single event that must be completely inhibited for a drug to be judged effective. Nevertheless, several IN inhibitors are in development, including the promising diketo acid class of IN inhibitors, which inhibit strand transfer [38, 39], and which are currently in early stage clinical trials.

2.4.5 Control of viral gene expression

After integration into the host cell's genomic DNA, the HIV provirus behaves, in many ways, as an activatable host cell gene [40]. It can either remain relatively quiescent, directing the production of few transcripts, without rapid

progression to a fully productive infection, or it can begin to generate a larger quantity of viral RNAs that lead to the completion of a productive viral replication cycle. Some of the factors controlling the switch between latency and lytic infection have been described. In vitro, treatment of infected cells with agents that profoundly activate host cell signal transduction pathways, such as phorbol esters, or that alter histone acetylation, such as butyrate [41, 42], or with certain cytokines, such as IL-2, can kindle the completion of a lytic infection cycle in latently infected cells via effects on common signaling pathways often acting through NF-kB [43] (see below). However, the detailed processes that determine the switch between latent and lytic infection in an infected patient remain obscure. The maintenance of latency is clearly an important feature of HIV pathogenesis; the continued presence of large reservoirs of latently infected cells, some in so-called sanctuary sites, is one of the major barriers frustrating the development of a cure for HIV infection (see Chapter 5).

During the progression through the lytic infection cycle, HIV regulates its gene expression at transcriptional and post-transcriptional levels in a tightly controlled, temporally dependent pattern consisting of three phases (Figure 2.5). In the initial phase, only low levels of full-length transcripts are produced because the transcription complex that assembles on the LTR, the HIV promoter, leads the cellular RNA polymerase II to transcribe the HIV RNAs in a highly non-processive fashion: few full length transcripts are produced. The few full length transcripts that are produced are retained in the nucleus until they undergo several splicing reactions and are then exported to the cytoplasm. These short transcripts encode only the viral regulatory proteins, notably Tat. In the second phase, the viral regulatory protein Tat, together with cellular factors, transactivates the transcription of the viral genes, leading to a dramatic increase in viral gene expression. In the third phase, another viral regulatory protein, Rev, mediates the export from the nucleus of unspliced and singly spliced RNAs, which encode the viral structural proteins. The full length, unspliced RNAs also constitute the viral genomic RNAs that will be incorporated in the progeny virions.

Regulation of transcription from the HIV LTR by cellular factors

After proviral integration, the initial production of viral mRNAs is mediated by the cellular transcriptional machinery. The 5′ LTR of the HIV provirus constitutes the viral promoter. It contains several regulatory sites homologous to the regulatory sites in cellular promoters (Figure 2.4) [40, 44]. Some of these sites play a significant role in regulating the basal level of HIV expression in lympho-cytic cells [45], while others may modulate expression in different cell types [46]. Some of the regulatory sequences, while homologous to well-known sequences in some cel-lular genes, may have a less significant effect on HIV gene expression. The regulatory sequences that are criti-cal for fully functional HIV gene expression are the TATA and Sp1 sequences [47–49]. Mutation or deletion of these sequences markedly decreases basal viral gene expression and can cripple viral replication. Mutation or deletion of the NF-κB sequences decreases the basal level of expres-sion and abolishes the ability of the viral promoter to respond to stimulatory signals, such as treatment of the host cell with inflammatory cytokines or phorbol esters. Viruses with mutations in these sequences have substan-tially reduced replication. The TATA sequence lies just 5′ of the transcription initiation site. The TATA element serves as site of assembly for the transcription machin-ery, including various transcription factors and RNA poly-merase II, the enzyme that catalyzes the synthesis of the viral RNA from the integrated proviral cDNA template. Three Sp1 sites lie just upstream from the TATA sequence and, like TATA, are required for wild-type levels of viral gene expression.

HIV clearly requires that the correct, wild-type amounts of all its RNAs be expressed for effective viral replication to proceed. When one or another viral RNA species are tar-geted for destruction, for example by short interfering RNAs (siRNAs), short double-stranded RNAs that lead the cell to destroy RNAs with homologous sequences, HIV repli-cation is diminished [13]. HIV replication is also inhibited when HIV RNAs are targeted in other ways, for example by ribozymes, RNAs which have enzymatic activity and can cleave target RNAs in a sequence-specific fashion [50], or by antisense oligonucleotides, oligonucleotides which are complementary to the targeted RNA and can specifically base pair with the sequence [51]. However, most of these strategies have only been effectively demonstrated in vitro. They all require that the RNAs be introduced into the host cell, either by treating the cell with an agent that causes the RNAs (or a plasmid that can cause the cell to produce the RNAs) to be taken up into the cell, or by genetically altering the cell so that it produces the RNA. Using a gene therapy approach to genetically altering cells such that they pro-duce such RNAs can render the cells resistant to infection, a strategy sometimes termed "intracellular immunization." However, with increased concerns surfacing about gene therapy there has been somewhat less recent interest in such approaches to antiretroviral therapy and the general clinical applicability of such approaches, if they ever arrive, probably lies far in the future.

The NF-κB sites in the HIV LTR respond to a wide variety of signals, leading to increased viral gene expression. The signals can include cytokines that activate T cells, such as TNF-α or IL-1. The transcription factor NF-κB is typically a dimer consisting of two subunits, p50 and p65. NF-κB exists in the cytoplasm in a complex with its inhibitor, IκB [52]. IκB acts to retain NF-κB in the cytoplasm, preventing its transit to the nucleus and so preventing it from acting as a transcription factor, for example mediating an increase in transcription from the HIV LTR. Many stimuli, such as cytokines and growth factors, can induce the phosphory-lation of IκB, which leads to its dissociation from NF-κB, which is then free to enter the nucleus where it can bind to its target sequences, stimulating transcription of genes whose promoters contain those sequences, including the HIV LTR.

Sequences 5′ to the TATA, Sp1, and NF-κB sites can affect HIV gene expression, but their exact function is less clear because they do not make as dramatic a contribution to expression from the HIV LTR. However, some of these sequences at the 5′ end of the LTR are critically important for maximal LTR expression in certain nonlymphocytic cell types [53].

Sequence-specific cellular DNA binding proteins play a key role in regulating expression from the integrated provirus, but expression is also influenced by other factors. One of the more important factors influencing HIV gene expression appears to be chromatin structure. The loca-tion and acetylation state of the histones that organize the DNA into chromatin also play an important part in regulat-ing expression from the integrated provirus [54, 55]. Alter-ing the state of histone acetylation, either non-specifically or through specific histone deacetylase inhibitors [42] can greatly increase expression from the HIV LTR. Histone acetylation has important effects on both the basal pro-moter [55] and in Tat-mediated transcription from the LTR [56].

Regulation of transcription by Tat

Transcription from the LTR initially leads to the appearance of short (2 kb) RNA transcripts. These short transcripts are the product of multiple splicing reactions acting upon the full-length transcribed HIV RNA because, in the absence of Rev (see below), the full-length transcripts cannot leave the nucleus. The short transcripts encode three viral gene prod-ucts, Tat, Rev, and Nef. Tat produces a dramatic increase in expression from the HIV LTR. Rev regulates HIV gene expression post-transcriptionally, by controlling the export of HIV RNA from the nucleus. Nef has a variety of effects on the virus and the host cell (see below).

present simultaneously. With both Tat and TAR-containing RNAs present, Tat binds to the bulge in TAR [59], and then recruits a complex of additional cellular factors called P-TEFb (or TAK, Tat-associated kinase), consisting of the cellular protein kinase CDK9 (also known as PITALRE) and cyclin T [60–62] (Figure 2.6). Cyclin T binds to the TAR loop structure and CDK9 binds to cyclin T. The CDK9 recruited into the complex by Tat can then phosphorylate the C-terminal domain of the RNA polymerase II that is in the transcription complex assembled on the LTR. Phosphorylation of RNA polymerase II makes the enzyme much more processive [63]. Instead of the extremely short, stalled transcripts, the enzyme continues down the length of the proviral template, catalyzing the production of full-length viral RNA. In some circumstances, cyclin T1 appears to interact directly with the LTR through Sp1, leading to an increase in expression from the HIV LTR [64], an activity that may contribute to basal, non-Tat-stimulated LTR-mediated transcription.

Tat has principally been considered a gene product that is produced within a cell and acts within that same cell, but Tat can be secreted from infected cells and taken up into cells when present in the extracellular environment. Secreted and extracellular Tat, acting in a paracrine fashion, can have a variety of effects upon cells [65–67], some of which may make a significant contribution to the pathogenesis of HIV disease.

Inhibition of Tat activity is another potential target for drug development. Tat is essential for efficient viral replication. An early small molecule Tat inhibitor proved clinically useless, but interest in Tat as a drug development target continues. Instead of targeting Tat itself, another approach could involve the development of small molecule inhibitors that block the interaction of Tat and TAR [68]. *In vitro* experiments have shown that inhibitors directed at cdk9 can block Tat activity and inhibit viral replication [69]. Such strategies aimed at the cellular functions essential for viral replication remain intriguing potential therapeutic targets that have not yet been exploited clinically, but the inhibition of cdk9 represents an interesting example of the approach. Although targeting cellular functions may be difficult because it may be hard to develop an inhibitor against important cellular functions that would have an acceptable therapeutic index and toxicity profile, targeting cellular functions may have some advantages. For example, evolution so as to no longer require an important cellular partner may represent a more formidable evolutionary barrier for the virus than simply acquiring a single mutation that changes one amino acid to another that prevents a small molecule inhibitor from effectively blocking the active site of a viral enzyme. Approaches to targeting

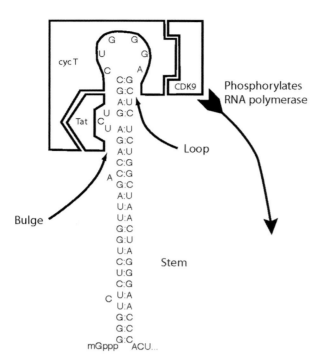

TAR, Tat, cyclin T, and CDK9

Figure 2.6. TAR, Tat, and associated cellular factors. Tat binds to the 'bulge' region of the stem-loop-bulge structure in the TAR RNA. The cellular protein cyclin T interacts with Tat and with the TAR loop region. The cellular kinase cdk9 interacts with cyclin T and then goes on to phosphorylate the C-terminal domain of RNA polymerase II, greatly increasing the processivity of the polymerase, causing a large increase in the expression of the viral RNAs.

Tat acts mainly by binding to a distinctive stem-loop-bulge RNA secondary structure, termed the trans-activation responsive (TAR) region, in newly transcribed HIV RNAs (Figures 2.3 and 2.6), and, by recruiting cellular factors, causes a change in the characteristics of the cellular RNA polymerase II that transcribes the viral RNAs from the HIV proviral template [57, 58]. In the absence of Tat, RNA polymerase II stalls soon after beginning transcription, producing extremely short transcripts that consist of little more than the TAR region. A small number of complete transcripts are made and are spliced down to the small 2 kb size, exported from the nucleus, and translated into protein, including Tat, which can return to the nucleus (Figure 2.5). If the transcription from the LTR is sufficiently active, for example if the cell has been exposed to inflammatory cytokines, there will be enough transcription for Tat and the TAR-containing transcript to be

Tat itself have included "TAR decoys," RNA structures that mimic TAR and bind Tat, making Tat unavailable to the TAR in the viral messages, antisense oligonucleotides, which interfere with the formation of the TAR structure, siRNA (see above), and ribozymes, but these approaches would probably involve gene therapy.

Post-transcriptional regulation of gene expression by Rev

After Tat increases viral gene expression, the long transcripts are subsequently processed into three distinct HIV mRNA species: unspliced, singly spliced, and multiply spliced messages with sizes of 9 kb, 4 kb, and 2 kb (Figure 2.5). As noted above, the 2 kb messages encode the viral regulatory genes, whereas the longer messages encode the viral structural genes and constitute the viral genomic RNA. Rev controls the switch from the early pattern of viral gene expression in which the multiply spliced 2 kb messages are expressed to the late pattern of viral gene expression in which the longer messages are expressed (reviewed in [70]). Rev regulates this switch at a post-transcriptional level [71–73]. These broadly characterized classes of messages can be further subdivided into many additional message species because the virus makes use of many alternative splice sites that give rise to many species of viral messages [1, 74].

Transcription from the integrated HIV provirus produces a full length HIV RNA. The HIV RNA is subject to complicated splicing reactions. If the introns are not spliced out of the RNA, the messages are not readily exported from the nucleus and the 4 kb and 9 kb singly spliced and unspliced messages tend to be retained within the nucleus. Rev enables the export of these singly spliced and unspliced messages from the nucleus. The HIV RNA contains a 250-bp region within the envelope coding sequence that can form a complicated stem-loop secondary structure called the Rev-responsive element or RRE. Rev binds a "bubble" of unpaired RNA in the middle of the RRE. Multiple copies of Rev (as many as eight) bind to the RRE in a cooperative fashion, and when the RRE binds sufficient quantities of Rev, Rev and the longer unspliced messages bound to Rev leave the nucleus. In the absence of Rev, the longer messages are retained within the nucleus, and are subjected to the splicing reactions that produce the short messages.

Rev has two regions, one that determines nuclear localization and binds RNA via an arginine-rich domain, and another region that mediates nuclear export of Rev and the HIV RNA bound to Rev [75–77] (Figure 2.7). Rev-mediated export of the viral RNAs begins with the binding of multiple Revs to the viral RNA RRE. Rev, with the bound HIV RNA, binds to a cellular protein called CRM1, and the CRM1 in the complex binds in turn to another cellular protein, Ran, a

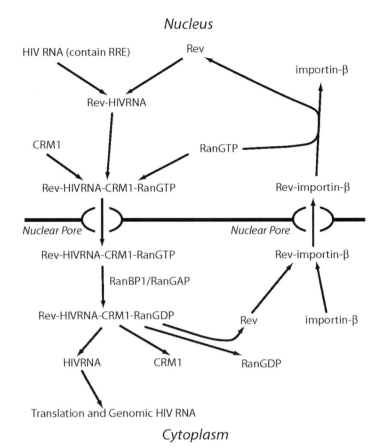

Figure 2.7. Rev and the export of HIV RNA from the host cell nucleus. Singly spliced and unspliced HIV RNAs are exported from the host cell nucleus via a specialized host cell nuclear pore apparatus, after Rev binds to the RRE sequence in the HIV RNA. See text for details.

small GTPase, but only when Ran has bound GTP (this form is called Ran-GTP) [78, 79]. This complex interacts with the nuclear pore and is translocated into the cytoplasm. In the cytoplasm two proteins, Ran GTPase activating protein 1 (Ran GAP1) and Ran binding protein 1 (Ran BP1) leads to the hydrolysis of the GTP bound to Ran, which in turn leads to the dissociation of the complex bound to the HIV RNA, freeing the long HIV RNA for translation or incorporation into virions as viral genomic RNA [80]. The transport out of the nucleus is thus driven by the high energy phosphate bond in the GTP bound to Ran. After discharging its bound HIV RNA, Rev re-enters the nucleus by binding to a cellular protein called importin-β via Rev's nuclear localization signal [81]. Importin-β interacts with the nuclear pores, resulting in the translocation of Rev bound to importin-β back into the nucleus. In the nucleus, Rev is freed from importin-β via another interaction with RanGTP, allowing Rev to bind new molecules of the HIV RNA to start the cycle again. In a sense, Rev and the attached HIV RNAs are exported out of the nucleus down a RanGTP gradient.

Rev is clearly essential for HIV replication. It is an inviting, but as yet relatively unexploited target for antiretroviral drug development. Some small molecules have been shown to inhibit Rev activity in vitro, including small molecules, such as certain aminoglycoside derivatives, that inhibit the interaction of Rev and the RRE [82]. No small molecule inhibitors of Rev function have yet entered clinical development, and targeting the general features of nuclear export and splicing would likely prove quite toxic to uninfected cells, since they also rely on the nuclear import and export apparatus to move macromolecules into and out of the nucleus. Some Rev mutants have been developed that can inhibit Rev function even when present together in a cell with a wild-type version of Rev. When introduced into a cell, these "transdominant negative" Rev mutants inhibit Rev activity and block viral replication [71, 76]. Transdominant negative Rev mutants may constitute another approach to the development of an intracellular immunization strategy to block HIV replication, but suffer from the same potential problems as other gene therapy strategies aimed at inhibiting HIV replication. A small clinical trial showed that inclusion of a transdominant negative Rev mutant in CD4$^+$ lymphocytes given to HIV-infected patients prolonged the survival of the lymphocytes [83], but further work has not been reported.

2.5 Translation of structural (late) viral messages and post-translational modification of the late viral proteins

After Rev directs the change from the early pattern of viral gene expression to the late pattern of viral gene expression with the production of the long singly spliced and unspliced RNAs, the messages that encode the viral structural and enzymatic proteins become available in the cytoplasm (Figure 2.5). A Gag preprotein, Pr55, and a Gag-Pol fusion preprotein, Pr160, are translated from the full-length 9 kb RNA. Certain transdominant negative gag mutants have been identified.

The structural components of the viral capsid, p16 (MA), p24 (CA), p9 (NC), and p6 (NC) are first translated in the form of the Pr55 preprotein, which is subsequently cleaved by the viral protease to form the four proteins during virion maturation. The Gag-Pol fusion protein is also cleaved during virion maturation to form the products of the *pol* gene: RT, IN, and PR.

HIV uses translational mechanisms to regulate the relative amounts of *gag*- and *pol*-derived protein production. In the HIV virion, there are more gag-derived structural proteins than there are pol-derived enzymatic proteins. The virus must modulate translation from the same RNAs so as to produce the optimal ratio of the different protein species. The full-length 9 kb RNA contains two translational reading frames. One reading frame encodes the Pr55 preprotein for the *gag*-derived proteins. A second reading frame, which overlaps the Pr55 reading frame by 200 bp, encodes the Gag-Pol preprotein, Pr160, the precursor for the *pol*-derived proteins. Translation from the first reading frame is more efficient than translation from the second. The ribosome must shift reading frames for the second reading frame to be translated, a shift that occurs at a UUUU-UUA tract in the viral RNA, to ensure the production of the correct ratio of the Gag and Gag-Pol preproteins.

The 4 kb RNA encodes the envelope preprotein gp160 and the HIV accessory proteins Vpr, Vpu, and Vif. gp160 is translated in the rough endoplasmic reticulum (RER). gp160 is glycosylated and transits through the Golgi complex, and is cleaved by cellular proteases of the furin family to form gp41, which remains anchored in the membrane, and gp120, which remains noncovalently associated with gp41 [84, 85]. The pattern of glycosylation may help to influence coreceptor usage by the virus [86]. From the Golgi, gp120/gp41 moves to the external cell surface, anchored in the host cell plasma membrane, where it awaits virion assembly and budding. Envelope protein processing is another critical step in the viral life cycle. If gp160 proteolytic processing is blocked, no infectious virus is produced. While blocking cellular proteases may be an attractive target, producing a drug with an acceptable therapeutic index may be difficult given the widespread involvement of the furin family of proteases in normal cellular physiology.

The glycosylation of the viral envelope glycoprotein also appears to be essential for viral pathogenicity, although perhaps not for viral replication in vitro. Critical, conserved sites, such as the receptor binding sites in the glycosylated proteins, appear to be masked in some way from the host immune response [85]. When the glycosylation sites in the envelope protein are deleted, the envelope glycoproteins become much more immunogenic, and in simian immunodeficiency virus (SIV) monkey models, infection with virus having deleted glycosylation sites produces a much less pathogenic infection, probably because of the more effective immune response the host can mount against the virus lacking a protective cloud of sugar residues guarding critical conserved immunogenic sites in the envelope protein [87, 88]. This requirement for intact glycosylation sites may have interesting implications for vaccine development, but therapeutic strategies involving the inhibition of glycosylation are probably not feasible because they would inhibit glycosylation of cellular proteins, a function critical for the function of many proteins.

In cells expressing CD4, gp160 and CD4 can become non-covalently associated within the RER during translation and processing, preventing the appearance of gp120 and gp41 at the surface. There is also evidence that these gp160/CD4 complexes cause cytopathic effects that range from disruption of normal ER function to interruption of normal nuclear transport. The viral accessory protein Vpu interacts with CD4 in the gp160/CD4 complex and induces its degradation via ubiquitination and proteosome-mediated proteolysis, a specialized degradation process that involves tagging a protein for destruction by the proteosome apparatus with ubiquitin [89]. Gp160 is thus freed from the complex and can be processed into functional envelope glycoproteins. This Vpu-stimulated degradation also results in the downregulation of CD4 at the host cell surface, which may prevent superinfection of the host cell [90].

2.5.1 Virion assembly, budding, and maturation

Assembly of immature virions occurs at the interior face of the host cell's plasma membrane, where the Gag and Gag-Pol preproteins assemble beneath the envelope glycoproteins [91]. Following translation, Gag preproteins are myristoylated on glycine residues at their amino terminal ends: a fatty acid, myristic acid targets the myristoylated to the plasma membrane. Other, somewhat less well-described features of the preprotein amino acid sequence direct the protein to the plasma membrane, as opposed to other membranous organelles [92]. Myristoylation inhibitors have been shown to inhibit HIV replication, but are toxic to cells because many cellular membrane proteins are also myristoylated. A membrane binding domain near the myristoylation domain also contributes to membrane binding. The Gag preprotein does not bind randomly to the plasma membrane. Instead, the preprotein preferentially inserts into cholesterol-rich microdomains or "rafts" in the plasma membrane. The preproteins may individually insert into small rafts that subsequently assemble into larger domains that eventually grow to become the sites where new virions bud out of the host cell membrane [93, 94]. Virion budding through lipid rafts may represent a mechanism through which the viral envelope acquires characteristics distinct from its parental plasma membrane source, including differences in lipid composition and the selective inclusion and exclusion of host cell membrane proteins from the virion envelope. Agents that deplete cholesterol from the plasma membrane, including approved agents like simvastatin, decrease virion production [93], but cholesterol is an obligatory component of many membranes and serves other important functions, and lipid rafts have other important roles in cellular physiology. Inhibiting cholesterol synthesis to the extent necessary to decrease viral production may well produce unacceptable toxicities.

The simple association of Gag with the host cell plasma membrane and insertion of the myristic acid into the lipid rafts in the host cell plasma membrane is not sufficient to drive the formation of a functional virion. Many, perhaps about 1500, Gag molecules must assemble together so that a functional viral core can eventually be formed. A cellular protein called HP68, which normally functions as an inhibitor of the interferon-inducible RNAse L, plays an important part in assembling together the Gag molecules and in promoting the formation of a functional viral core [95].

Other aspects of virion assembly are also mediated by CA. CA contains a domain that enables Gag to form multimers [96], another that functions in the condensation of the viral core, and another that binds the host protein cyclophilin A, which functions as a prolyl isomerase for host cell proteins [97]. Mutations in the multimerization domain or the domain involved in core condensation produce virions with defective morphology. The interaction with cyclophilin A also appears essential for the formation of fully infectious virus, perhaps by ensuring that the CA is optimally folded in the correct tertiary structure within the virion after the Gag precursor is proteolytically processed [98].

The viral RNA genome is recruited to the site of virion formation and packaged into virions by interactions with the Pr55 Gag preprotein [99]. The p9 (NC) region of this preprotein contains the two zinc-finger amino acid motifs (cys-X_2-cys-X_4-his-X_4-cys, where X is any amino acid). These are characterized as CCHC zinc fingers, which are structurally distinct from many cellular zinc finger domains, which also mediate binding of some proteins to nucleic acids, for example binding by transcription factors. The full-length genomic RNA contains a packaging signal sequence (or Ψ site) at the 5' end of the molecule with a distinctive secondary structure, which is necessary for RNA packaging. The sequence is spliced out of the short and intermediate length viral RNAs, preventing them from being packaged into virions. The mechanisms through which viral RNAs are recruited to and packaged into nascent virions is another target for antiretroviral drug development, some of which are in early stages of development. These compounds are zinc chelators, or zinc ejectors. They remove the zinc from the zinc finger or NC, which disrupts the structure of the protein, making it unable to bind the HIV RNA, thus blocking the formation of infectious virions [100, 101]. The compounds can selectively target the retroviral zinc fingers, with little effect on the cellular zinc finger. NC may also play a part in Gag multimerization.

HIV, like other enveloped viruses, requires that the progeny virion bud out from the host cell plasma membrane. While the proteins of HIV are essential for budding, the virus has apparently pirated a cellular pathway, the one used to form the multivesicular body (MVB), a late endosomal compartment [102]. The virus makes use of several of the components of the MVB formation pathway, such as the cellular protein Tsg101, to promote the budding of the progeny virions. The eventual budding from the plasma membrane is aided by an interaction between Gag (the p6 protein) and Tsg101 [103, 104]. Mutant versions of Tsg101 can inhibit virion assembly and so decrease viral replication. p6 is also responsible for recruiting the HIV accessory protein Vpr (see below) for incorporation into new virions. The MA Gag protein has additional functions in virion assembly. Certain point mutations or small deletions in the molecule prevent Env from correctly associating with the assembling viral proteins and being incorporated into budding virions, implying that gp41, the envelope transmembrane subunit, and MA interact in some specific fashion that promotes Env incorporation into the virion [105].

After budding, the newly formed virion must undergo a process of maturation involving the proteolytic processing of the precursor proteins within the viral particle catalyzed by the viral protease. Virions that have not undergone maturation via proteolytic processing are not infectious. During maturation, the viral protease, a derivative of the Gag-Pol preprotein, cleaves Pr55 (Gag) and Pr160 (Gag-Pol) proteins, releasing the capsid structural proteins and enzymatic *pol*-derived proteins to produce the final versions of the proteins that make up the mature virion.

The function of the viral protease is essential for the production of viable, infectious viral particles and has therefore become a favored target for drug development. HIV protease inhibitors (PIs) have proved to be a remarkably effective class of antiretrovirals, providing a key component in many highly active antiretroviral therapy regimens. Resistance to the PIs can develop and is described in more detail, along with detailed descriptions of the mechanisms of action of the PIs, in Chapter 21.

2.5.2 HIV accessory proteins

The HIV accessory proteins, Nef, Vpu, Vif, and Vpr, have important functions in the viral life cycle and can serve to enhance viral pathogenesis. In vitro, mutations in the accessory genes do not completely preclude viral replication but, in vivo, the importance of accessory proteins can be critical.

Vpu enhances virus production by downregulating the HIV receptor, CD4, post-translationally, by binding the cytoplasmic tail of CD4 while CD4 is in the endoplasmic reticulum (ER) [106]. This prevents Env from being trapped in the ER in a complex with CD4. Vpu also enhances virion release via a mechanism that is not well understood [107].

Vif (for virion infectivity factor) appears to be required in certain cell types, but not others, during the late stages of infection to insure the production of infectious virus. Vif is packaged into virions [108]. Some lymphocytes have an innate antiretroviral activity that can act in a dominant negative fashion leading to the production of non-infectious virus. Vif acts to suppress this innate antiretroviral activity. This antiretroviral activity results from a cellular gene, APOBEC 3G (or CEM15), which inhibits the production of infectious virus lacking Vif, but has no effect on the production of infectious virus that has fully effective Vif [109]. APOBEC 3G inhibits the replication of HIV and other retroviruses by deaminating cytosine to uracil in viral minus strand cDNA. This causes plus strand cDNA permutation of guanosine to adenine, which inhibits HIV replication. The cellular protein HP68, which functions in HIV capsid assembly and maturation (see above) also forms a complex with Gag and Vif [95].

Vpr has several functions, in addition to its activity in localizing the PIC to the nucleus and mediating nuclear import of the PIC (see above), which contributes to HIV's ability to infect non-dividing and differentiated cells [110]. Vpr is incorporated in large amounts into virions. Vpr has a modest ability to increase HIV gene expression and alters the expression of some cellular genes, acting mainly through interactions with a cellular transcriptional co-activator CBP/p300 [111], and also perhaps more indirectly via its effects on the cell cycle of the host cell. Cells normally progress through the G_1 (first gap), S (DNA synthesis), G_2 (second gap), and M (mitotic) phases. Vpr alters the progression of the host cell through the cell cycle, causing the host cell cycle to arrest at the G_2 phase [112]. Vpr inhibits the activity of a $p34^{cdc2}$-cyclin B kinase complex, which is required for the cell cycle to progress through G_2 to M. By arresting the host cells in the G_2 phase, Vpr may increase virion production, perhaps by making more precursors available for production of the virions. The HIV LTR may be more active in G_2, and so G_2 arrest may contribute to Vpr's ability to increase HIV gene expression. Vpr has apoptotic activity, via the mitochondria-dependent pathway. The significance of this for viral replication is unclear.

Nef has several activities during viral replication and is incorporated into virions. While not required for viral replication in vitro, Nef is clearly required for the virus to be fully pathogenic, both in SIV monkey models and in humans [113]. Some human cohorts infected with Nef-deleted virus have been described, and they appear to have decelerated disease progression [114]. Some investigators have proposed that Nef-deleted viruses might constitute potential HIV live virus vaccines, but the utility of this approach seems low, since Nef-deleted virus is clearly pathogenic over long periods of time and since Nef-deleted SIV is pathogenic for newborn monkeys [115]. Nef augments the infectivity of HIV virions, induces downregulation of cell surface CD4 molecules [116] by targeting CD4 for incorporation into endosomes through interactions with a cellular protein, β-COP [117], and interacts with cellular signal transduction pathways [118]. Nef also decreases the surface expression of cellular MHC Class 1 molecule by increasing endocytosis [119], which may decrease the chance that an infected cell will be attacked by the host immune system [120].

2.6 Conclusions

Since the discovery of HIV 20 years ago, a notable amount of basic virological information has been obtained. This information has yielded a profound understanding of the pathogenetic strategies of the virus and has led to the development of remarkably effective antiviral agents, agents that have converted a uniformly fatal disease into a chronic, though sometimes difficult-to-manage one. The antiviral agents can block the transmission of HIV from mother to infant, offering the possibility of saving millions of babies from HIV infection. A thorough understanding of the basic features of the HIV life cycle and the mechanisms of action of the antiretroviral will allow the clinician to better understand the pathogenesis of HIV disease in children and employ the available antiretroviral therapies more rationally and effectively.

ACKNOWLEDGMENT

The author would like to thank K. T Jeang for reading the manuscript and providing helpful comments.

REFERENCES

1. Freed, E. & Martin, M. HIVs and their replication. In: D. Knipe, P. Howley, D. Griffin, M. Martin, R. Lamb & B. Roizman (eds.), *Fields Virology*. Philadelphia, PA: Lippincott Williams and Wilkins (2001), pp. 1971–2041.

2. Korber, B., Muldoon, M., Theiler, J. *et al.* Timing the ancestor of the HIV-1 pandemic strains. *Science* **288**: **5472** (2000), 1789–96.

3. Gao, F., Bailes, E., Robertson, D. L. *et al.* Origin of HIV-1 in the chimpanzee *Pan troglodytes troglodytes. Nature* **397** : **6718** (1999), 436–41.

4. Santiago, M. L., Rodenburg, C. M., Kamenya, S. *et al.* SIVcpz in wild chimpanzees. *Science* **295** : **5554** (2002), 465.

5. Pepin, J., Morgan, G., Dunn, D. *et al.* HIV-2-induced immunosuppression among asymptomatic West African prostitutes: evidence that HIV-2 is pathogenic, but less so than HIV-1. *Aids* **5**:**10** (1991), 1165–72.

6. Robertson, D. L., Anderson, J. P., Bradac, J. A. *et al.* HIV-1 nomenclature proposal. *Science* **288** : **5463** (2000), 55–6.

7. Turner, B. G. and Summers, M. F. Structural biology of HIV. *J. Mol. Biol.* **285** : **1** (1999), 1–32.

8. Arthur, L. O., Bess, J. W. J., Sowder, R. C. I. *et al.* Cellular proteins bound to immunodeficiency viruses: implications for pathogenesis and vaccines. *Science* **258** (1992), 1935–8.

9. Bour, S., Geleziunas, R. & Wainberg, M. A. The human immunodeficiency virus type 1 (HIV-1) CD4 receptor and its central role in promotion of HIV-1 infection. *Microbiol. Rev.* **59**:**1** (1995), 63–93.

10. Eckert, D. M. & Kim, P. S. Mechanisms of viral membrane fusion and its inhibition. *Annu. Rev. Biochem.* **70** (2001), 777–810.

11. Golding, H., Zaitseva, M., de Rosny, E. *et al.* Dissection of human immunodeficiency virus type 1 entry with neutralizing antibodies to gp41 fusion intermediates. *J. Virol.* **76** : **13** (2002), 6780–90.

12. Wild, C. T., Shugars, D. C., Greenwell, T. K., McDanal, C. B. & Matthews, T. J. Peptides corresponding to a predictive alpha-helical domain of human immunodeficiency virus type 1 gp41 are potent inhibitors of virus infection. *Proc. Natl. Acad. Sci. U. S. A.* **91** : **21** (1994), 9770–4.

13. Novina, C. D., Murray, M. F., Dykxhoorn, D. M. *et al.* siRNA-directed inhibition of HIV-1 infection. *Nat. Med.* **8** : **7** (2002), 681–6.

14. Mori, T. & Boyd, M. R. Cyanovirin-N, a potent human immunodeficiency virus-inactivating protein, blocks both CD4-dependent and CD4-independent binding of soluble gp120 (sgp120) to target cells, inhibits sCD4-induced binding of sgp120 to cell-associated CXCR4, and dissociates bound sgp120 from target cells. *Antimicrob. Agents Chemother.* **45** : **3** (2001), 664–72.

15. Berger, E. A., Murphy, P. M. & Farber, J. M. Chemokine receptors as HIV-1 coreceptors: roles in viral entry, tropism, and disease. *Annu. Rev. Immunol.* **17** (1999), 657–700.

16. Feng, Y., Broder, C. C., Kennedy, P. E. & Berger, E. A.. HIV-1 entry cofactor: functional cDNA cloning of a seven-transmembrane, G protein-coupled receptor. *Science* **272** : **5263** (1996), 872–7.

17. Choe, H., Farzan, M., Sun, Y. *et al.* The beta-chemokine receptors CCR3 and CCR5 facilitate infection by primary HIV-1 isolates. *Cell* **85**:**7** (1996), 1135–48.

18. Alkhatib, G., Combadiere, C., Broder, C. C. *et al.* CC CKR5: a RANTES, MIP-1alpha, MIP-1beta receptor as a fusion cofactor for macrophage-tropic HIV-1. *Science* **272** : **5270** (1996), 1955–8.

19. Cocchi, F., DeVico, A. L., Garzino-Demo, A., Arya, S. K., Gallo, R. C. & Lusso, P. Identification of RANTES, MIP-1 alpha, and MIP-1 beta as the major HIV-suppressive factors produced by CD8[+] T cells. *Science* **270**:**5243** (1995), 1811–5.

20. Strizki, J. M., Xu, S., Wagner, N. E. *et al.* SCH-C (SCH 351125), an orally bioavailable, small molecule antagonist of the chemokine receptor CCR5, is a potent inhibitor of HIV-1 infection in vitro and in vivo. *Proc. Natl. Acad. Sci. U. S. A.* **98**:**22** (2001), 12718–23.

21. Kostrikis, L. G., Huang, Y., Moore, J. P. *et al.* A chemokine receptor CCR2 allele delays HIV-1 disease progression and is associated with a CCR5 promoter mutation. *Nat. Med.* **4**:**3** (1998), 350–3.

22. Smith, M. W., Dean, M., Carrington, M. *et al.* Contrasting genetic influence of CCR2 and CCR5 variants on HIV-1 infection and disease progression. Hemophilia Growth and Development Study (HGDS), Multicenter AIDS Cohort Study (MACS), Multicenter Hemophilia Cohort Study (MHCS), San Francisco City Cohort (SFCC), ALIVE Study. *Science* **277**:**5328** (1997), 959–65.

23. Kostrikis, L. G., Neumann, A. U., Thomson, B. *et al.* A polymorphism in the regulatory region of the CC-chemokine receptor 5 gene influences perinatal transmission of human immunodeficiency virus type 1 to African-American infants. *J. Virol.* **73**:**12** (1999), 10264–71.

24. Gotte, M., Li, X. & Wainberg, M. A. HIV-1 reverse transcription: a brief overview focused on structure-function relationships among molecules involved in initiation of the reaction. *Arch. Biochem. Biophys.* **365**:**2** (1999), 199–210.

25. Isel, C., Ehresmann, C., Keith, G., Ehresmann, B. & Marquet, R. Initiation of reverse transcription of HIV-1: secondary structure of the HIV-1 RNA/tRNA(3Lys) (template/primer). *J. Mol. Biol.* **247**:**2** (1995), 236–50.

26. Bukrinsky, M. I., Sharova, N., McDonald, T. L., Pushkarskaya, T., Tarpley, W. G. & Stevenson, M. Association of integrase, matrix, and reverse transcriptase antigens of human immunodeficiency virus type 1 with viral nucleic acids following acute infection. *Proc. Natl. Acad. Sci. U.S.A.* **90**:**13** (1993), 6125–9.

27. Farnet, C. M. & Bushman, F. D. HIV-1 cDNA integration: requirement of HMG I(Y) protein for function of preintegration complexes in vitro. *Cell* **88**:**4** (1997), 483–92.

28. Kalpana, G. V., Marmon, S., Wang, W., Crabtree, G. R. & Goff, S. P. Binding and stimulation of HIV-1 integrase by a human homolog of yeast transcription factor SNF5. *Science* **266**:**5193** (1994), 2002–6.

29. McDonald, D., Vodicka, M. A., Lucero, G. *et al.* Visualization of the intracellular behavior of HIV in living cells. *J. Cell Biol.* **159**:**3** (2002), 441–52.

30. Le Rouzic, E., Mousnier, A., Rustum, C. *et al.* Docking of HIV-1 Vpr to the nuclear envelope is mediated by the interaction with the nucleoporin hCG1. *J. Biol. Chem.* **277**:**47** (2002), 45091–8.

31. Schroder, A. R., Shinn, P., Chen, H., Berry, C., Ecker, J. R. & Bushman, F. HIV-1 integration in the human genome favors active genes and local hotspots. *Cell* **110**:**4** (2002), 521–9.

32. Fujiwara, T. & Mizuuchi, K. Retroviral DNA integration: structure of an integration intermediate. *Cell* **54**:**4** (1988), 497–504.

33. Roth, M. J., Schwartzberg, P. L. & Goff, S. P. Structure of the termini of DNA intermediates in the integration of retroviral DNA: dependence on IN function and terminal DNA sequence. *Cell* **58**:**1** (1989), 47–54.

34. Gao, K., Gorelick, R. J., Johnson, D. G. & Bushman, F. Cofactors for human immunodeficiency virus type 1 cDNA integration in vitro. *J. Virol.* **77**:**2** (2003), 1598–603.

35. Englund, G., Theodore, T. S., Freed, E. O., Engleman, A. & Martin, M. A. Integration is required for productive infection of monocyte-derived macrophages by human immunodeficiency virus type 1. *J. Virol.* **69**:**5** (1995), 3216–9.

36. Condra, J. H., Miller, M. D., Hazuda, D. J. & Emini, E. A. Potential new therapies for the treatment of HIV-1 infection. *Annu. Rev. Med.* **53** (2002), 541–55.

37. Craigie, R. HIV integrase, a brief overview from chemistry to therapeutics. *J. Biol. Chem.* **276**:**26** (2001), 23213–6.

38. Hazuda, D. J., Felock, P., Witmer, M. *et al.* Inhibitors of strand transfer that prevent integration and inhibit HIV-1 replication in cells. *Science* **287**:**5453** (2000), 646–50.

39. Grobler, J. A., Stillmock, K., Hu, B. *et al.* Diketo acid inhibitor mechanism and HIV-1 integrase: implications for metal binding in the active site of phosphotransferase enzymes. *Proc. Natl. Acad. Sci. U. S. A.* **99**:**10** (2002), 6661–6.

40. Nabel, G. & Baltimore, D. An inducible transcription factor activates expression of human immunodeficiency virus in T cells [published erratum appears in *Nature* **344**:**6262** (1990 Mar 8), 178]. *Nature* **326**:**6114** (1987), 711–3.

41. Laughlin, M., Zeichner, S., Kolson, D. *et al.* Sodium butyrate treatment of cells latently infected with HIV-1 results in the expression of unspliced viral RNA. *Virology* **196** (1993), 496–505.

42. Sheridan, P. L., Mayall, T. P., Verdin, E. & Jones, K. A. Histone acetyltransferases regulate HIV-1 enhancer activity in vitro. *Genes Dev.* **11**:**24** (1997), 3327–40.

43. Rothe, M., Sarma, V., Dixit, V. M. & Goeddel, D. V. TRAF2-mediated activation of NF-kappa B by TNF receptor 2 and CD40. *Science* **269**:**5229** (1995), 1424–7.

44. Jones, K. A., Kadonaga, J. T., Luciw, P. A. & Tjian, R. Activation of the AIDS retrovirus promoter by the cellular transcription factor, Sp1. *Science* **232**:**4751** (1986), 755–9.

45. Zeichner, S. L., Kim, J. Y. & Alwine, J. C. Linker-scanning mutational analysis of the transcriptional activity of the human immunodeficiency virus type 1 long terminal repeat. *J. Virol.* **65**:**5** (1991), 2436–44.

46. Kim, J., Gonzalez-Scarano, F., Zeichner, S. & Alwine, J. Replication of type 1 human immunodeficiency viruses containing linker substitution mutations in the -201 to -130 region of the long terminal repeat. *J. Virol.* **67** (1993), 1658–62.

47. Berkhout, B. & Jeang, K. T. Functional roles for the TATA promoter and enhancers in basal and Tat-induced expression of the human immunodeficiency virus type 1 long terminal repeat. *J. Virol.* **66**:**1** (1992), 139–49.

48. Harrich, D., Garcia, J., Wu, F., Mitsuyasu, R., Gonazalez, J. & Gaynor, R. Role of SP1-binding domains in in vivo transcriptional regulation of the human immunodeficiency virus type 1 long terminal repeat. *J. Virol.* **63**:**6** (1989), 2585–91.

49. Ross, E. K., Buckler-White, A. J., Rabson, A. B., Englund, G. & Martin, M. A. Contribution of NF-kappa B and Sp1 binding motifs to the replicative capacity of human immunodeficiency virus type 1: distinct patterns of viral growth are determined by T-cell types. *J. Virol.* **65**:**8** (1991), 4350–8.

50. Lustig, B. & Jeang, K. T. Biological applications of hammerhead ribozymes as anti-viral molecules. *Curr. Med. Chem.* **8**:**10** (2001), 1181–7.

51. Dornburg, R. & Pomerantz, R. J. HIV-1 gene therapy: promise for the future. *Adv. Pharmacol.* **49** (2000), 229–61.

52. Baeuerle, P. A. & Baltimore, D. A 65-kappaD subunit of active NF-kappaB is required for inhibition of NF-kappaB by I kappaB. *Genes Dev.* **3**:**11** (1989), 1689–98.

53. Zeichner, S. L., Hirka, G., Andrews, P. W. & Alwine, J. C. Differentiation-dependent human immunodeficiency virus long terminal repeat regulatory elements active in human teratocarcinoma cells. *J. Virol.* **66**:**4** (1992), 2268–73.

54. He, G. & Margolis, D. M. Counterregulation of chromatin deacetylation and histone deacetylase occupancy at the integrated promoter of human immunodeficiency virus type 1 (HIV-1) by the HIV-1 repressor YY1 and HIV-1 activator Tat. *Mol. Cell Biol.* **22**:**9** (2002), 2965–73.

55. El Kharroubi, A., Piras, G., Zensen, R. & Martin, M. A. Transcriptional activation of the integrated chromatin-associated human immunodeficiency virus type 1 promoter. *Mol. Cell Biol.* **18**:**5** (1998), 2535–44.

56. Benkirane, M., Chun, R. F., Xiao, H. *et al.* Activation of integrated provirus requires histone acetyltransferase. p300 and P/CAF are coactivators for HIV-1 Tat. *J. Biol. Chem.* **273**:**38** (1998), 24898–905.

57. Selby, M. J. & Peterlin, B. M. Trans-activation by HIV-1 Tat via a heterologous RNA binding protein. *Cell* **62**:**4** (1990), 769–76.

58. Berkhout, B., Gatignol, A., Rabson, A. B. & Jeang, K. T. TAR-independent activation of the HIV-1 LTR: evidence that tat requires specific regions of the promoter. *Cell* **62**:**4** (1990), 757–67.

59. Berkhout, B., Silverman, R. H. & Jeang, K. T. Tat trans-activates the human immunodeficiency virus through a nascent RNA target. *Cell* **59**:**2** (1989), 273–82.

60. Zhu, Y., Pe'ery, T., Peng, J. *et al.* Transcription elongation factor P-TEFb is required for HIV-1 tat transactivation in vitro. *Genes Dev.* **11**:**20** (1997), 2622–32.

61. Peng, J., Zhu, Y., Milton, J. T. & Price, D. H. Identification of multiple cyclin subunits of human P-TEFb. *Genes Dev.* **12**:**5** (1998), 755–62.

62. Wei, P., Garber, M. E., Fang, S. M., Fischer, W. H. & Jones, K. A. A novel CDK9-associated C-type cyclin interacts directly with HIV-1 Tat and mediates its high-affinity, loop-specific binding to TAR RNA. *Cell* **92**:**4** (1998), 451–62.

63. Parada, C. A. & Roeder, R. G. Enhanced processivity of RNA polymerase II triggered by Tat-induced phosphorylation of its carboxy-terminal domain. *Nature* **384**:**6607** (1996), 375–8.

64. Yedavalli, V. S., Benkirane, M. & Jeang, K. T. Tat and trans-activation-responsive (TAR) RNA-independent induction of HIV-1 long terminal repeat by human and murine cyclin T1 requires Sp1. *J. Biol. Chem.* **278**:**8** (2003), 6404–10.

65. Barillari, G., Sgadari, C., Fiorelli, V. *et al.* The Tat protein of human immunodeficiency virus type-1 promotes vascular cell growth and locomotion by engaging the alpha5beta1 and alphavbeta3 integrins and by mobilizing sequestered basic fibroblast growth factor. *Blood* **94**:**2** (1999), 663–72.

66. Xiao, H., Neuveut, C., Tiffany, H. L. *et al.* Selective CXCR4 antagonism by Tat: implications for in vivo expansion of coreceptor use by HIV-1. *Proc. Natl. Acad. Sci. U. S. A.* **97**:**21** (2000), 11466–71.

67. Nath, A., Conant, K., Chen, P., Scott, C. & Major, E. O. Transient exposure to HIV-1 Tat protein results in cytokine production in macrophages and astrocytes. A hit and run phenomenon. *J. Biol. Chem.* **274**:**24** (1999), 17098–102.

68. Mischiati, C., Jeang, K. T., Feriotto, G. *et al.* Aromatic polyamidines inhibiting the Tat-induced HIV-1 transcription recognize structured TAR-RNA. *Antisense Nucleic Acid Drug Dev* **11**:**4** (2001), 209–17.

69. Chao, S. H., Fujinaga, K., Marion, J. E. *et al.* Flavopiridol inhibits P-TEFb and blocks HIV-1 replication. *J. Biol. Chem.* **275**:**37** (2000), 28345–8.

70. Pollard, V. W. & Malim, M. H. The HIV-1 Rev protein. *Annu. Rev. Microbiol.* **52** (1998), 491–532.

71. Malim, M. H., Tiley, L. S., McCarn, D. F., Rusche, J. R., Hauber, J. & Cullen, B. R. HIV-1 structural gene expression requires binding of the rev trans-activator sequence to its target RNA sequence. *Cell* **60** (1990), 675–83.

72. Malim, M. H., Hauber, J., Le, S.-Y., Maizel, J. V. & Cullen, B. R. The HIV rev transactivator acts through a structured target sequence to activate nuclear export of unspliced viral mRNA. *Nature* **338** (1989), 254–7.

73. Felber, B. K., Hadzopoulou-Cladaras, M., Cladaras, C., Copeland, T. & Pavlakis, G. N. rev protein of human immunodeficiency virus type 1 affects the stability and transport of the viral mRNA. *Proc. Natl. Acad. Sci. U. S. A.* **86**:**5** (1989), 1495–9.

74. Purcell, D. F. & Martin, M. A. Alternative splicing of human immunodeficiency virus type 1 mRNA modulates viral protein expression, replication, and infectivity. *J. Virol.* **67**:**11** (1993), 6365–78.

75. Zapp, M. L., Hope, T. J., Parslow, T. G. & Green, M. R. Oligomerization and RNA binding domains of the type 1 human immunodeficiency virus Rev protein: a dual function for an arginine-rich binding motif. *Proc. Natl. Acad. Sci. U. S. A.* **88**:**17** (1991), 7734–8.

76. Malim, M. H., Bohnlein, S., Hauber, J. & Cullen, B. R. Functional dissection of the HIV-1 Rev trans-activator – derivation of a trans-dominant repressor of Rev function. *Cell* **58**:**1** (1989), 205–14.

77. Malim, M. H. & Cullen, B. R. HIV-1 structural gene expression requires the binding of multiple Rev monomers to the viral RRE: implications for HIV-1 latency. *Cell* **65**:**2** (1991), 241–8.

78. Askjaer, P., Jensen, T. H., Nilsson, J., Englmeier, L. & Kjems, J. The specificity of the CRM1-Rev nuclear export signal interaction is mediated by RanGTP. *J. Biol. Chem.* **273**:**50** (1998), 33414–22.

79. Fornerod, M., Ohno, M., Yoshida, M. & Mattaj, I. CRM1 is an export receptor for leucine-rich nuclear export signals. *Cell* **90** (1997), 1051–60.

80. Gorlich, D. & Mattaj, I. W. Nucleocytoplasmic transport. *Science* **271**:**5255** (1996), 1513–18.

81. Henderson, B. R. & Percipalle, P. Interactions between HIV Rev and nuclear import and export factors: the Rev nuclear localisation signal mediates specific binding to human importin-beta. *J. Mol. Biol.* **274**:**5** (1997), 693–707.

82. Zapp, M. L., Stern, S. & Green, M. R. Small molecules that selectively block RNA binding of HIV-1 Rev protein inhibit Rev function and viral production. *Cell* **74**:**6** (1993), 969–78.

83. Ranga, U., Woffendin, C., Verma, S. *et al.* Enhanced T cell engraftment after retroviral delivery of an antiviral gene in HIV-infected individuals. *Proc. Natl. Acad. Sci. U. S. A.* **95**:**3** (1998), 1201–6.

84. Hallenberger, S., Bosch, V., Angliker, H., Shaw, E., Klenk, H. D. & Garten, W. Inhibition of furin-mediated cleavage activation of HIV-1 glycoprotein gp160. *Nature* **360**:**6402** (1992), 358–61.

85. Decroly, E., Wouters, S., Di Bello, C., Lazure, C., Ruysschaert, J. M. & Seidah, N. G. Identification of the paired basic convertases implicated in HIV gp160 processing based on in vitro assays and expression in CD4(+) cell lines [published erratum appears in *J. Biol. Chem.* **272**:**13** (1997 Mar 28), 8836. *J. Biol. Chem.* **271**:**48** (1996), 30442–50.

86. Ogert, R. A., Lee, M. K., Ross, W., Buckler-White, A., Martin, M. A. & Cho, M. W. N-linked glycosylation sites adjacent to and within the V1/V2 and the V3 loops of dualtropic human immunodeficiency virus type 1 isolate DH12 gp120 affect coreceptor usage and cellular tropism. *J. Virol.* **75**:**13** (2001), 5998–6006.

87. Mori, K., Yasutomi, Y., Ohgimoto, S. *et al.* Quintuple deglycosylation mutant of simian immunodeficiency virus SIVmac239 in rhesus macaques: robust primary replication, tightly contained chronic infection, and elicitation of potent immunity against the parental wild-type strain. *J. Virol.* **75**:**9** (2001), 4023–8.

88. Reitter, J. N., Means, R. E. & Desrosiers, R. C. A role for carbohydrates in immune evasion in AIDS. *Nat. Med.* **4**:**6** (1998), 679–84.

89. Schubert, U., Anton, L. C., Bacik, I., *et al.* CD4 glycoprotein degradation induced by human immunodeficiency virus type 1 Vpu protein requires the function of proteosomes and the ubiquitin-conjugating pathway. *J. Virol.* **72**:**3** (1998), 2280–8.

90. Willey, R. L., Maldarelli, F., Martin, M. A. & Strebel, K. Human immunodeficiency virus type 1 Vpu protein induces rapid degradation of CD4. *J. Virol.* **66**:**12** (1992), 7193–200.

91. Conte, M. R. & Matthews, S. Retroviral matrix proteins: a structural perspective. *Virology* **246**:**2** (1998), 191–8.

92. Ono, A., Orenstein, J. M. & Freed, E. O. Role of the Gag matrix domain in targeting human immunodeficiency virus type 1 assembly. *J. Virol.* **74**:**6** (2000), 2855–66.

93. Ono, A. & Freed, E. O. Plasma membrane rafts play a critical role in HIV-1 assembly and release. *Proc. Natl. Acad. Sci. U. S. A.* **98**:**24** (2001), 13925–30.

94. Nguyen, D. H. & Hildreth, J. E. Evidence for budding of human immunodeficiency virus type 1 selectively from glycolipid-enriched membrane lipid rafts. *J. Virol.* **74**:**7** (2000), 3264–72.

95. Zimmerman, C., Klein, K. C., Kiser, P. K. *et al.* Identification of a host protein essential for assembly of immature HIV-1 capsids. *Nature* **415**:**6867** (2002), 88–92.

96. Gamble, T. R., Yoo, S., Vajdos, F. F. *et al.* Structure of the carboxyl-terminal dimerization domain of the HIV-1 capsid protein. *Science* **278**:**5339** (1997), 849–53.

97. Franke, E. K., Yuan, H. E. & Luban, J. Specific incorporation of cyclophilin A into HIV-1 virions. *Nature* **372**:**6504** (1994), 359–62.

98. Grattinger, M., Hohenberg, H., Thomas, D., Wilk, T., Muller, B. and Krausslich, H. G. In vitro assembly properties of wild-type and cyclophilin-binding defective human immunodeficiency virus capsid proteins in the presence and absence of cyclophilin A. *Virology* **257**:**1** (1999), 247–60.

99. Berkowitz, R., Fisher, J. & Goff, S. P. RNA packaging. *Curr. Top. Microbiol. Immunol.* **214** (1996), 177–218.

100. Basrur, V., Song, Y., Mazur, S. J. *et al.* Inactivation of HIV-1 nucleocapsid protein P7 by pyridinioalkanoyl thioesters. Characterization of reaction products and proposed mechanism of action. *J. Biol. Chem.* **275**:**20** (2000), 14890–7.

101. Huang, M., Maynard, A., Turpin, J. A. *et al.* Anti-HIV agents that selectively target retroviral nucleocapsid protein zinc fingers without affecting cellular zinc finger proteins. *J. Med. Chem.* **41**:**9** (1998), 1371–81.

102. Pornillos, O., Garrus, J. E. & Sundquist, W. I. Mechanisms of enveloped RNA virus budding. *Trends. Cell Biol.* **12**:**12** (2002), 569–79.

103. Demirov, D. G., Ono, A., Orenstein, J. M. & Freed, E. O. Overexpression of the N-terminal domain of TSG101 inhibits HIV-1 budding by blocking late domain function. *Proc. Natl. Acad. Sci. U. S. A.* **99**:**2** (2002), 955–60.

104. Garrus, J. E., von Schwedler, U. K., Pornillos, O. W. *et al.* Tsg101 and the vacuolar protein sorting pathway are essential for HIV-1 budding. *Cell* **107**:**1** (2001), 55–65.

105. Freed, E. O. & Martin, M. A. Domains of the human immunodeficiency virus type 1 matrix and gp41 cytoplasmic tail required for envelope incorporation into virions. *J. Virol.* **70** (1995), 341–51.

106. Bour, S., Schubert, U. & Strebel, K. The human immunodeficiency virus type 1 Vpu protein specifically binds to the cytoplasmic domain of CD4: implications for the mechanism of degradation. *J. Virol.* **69**:**3** (1995), 1510–20.

107. Geraghty, R. J. & Panganiban, A. T. Human immunodeficiency virus type 1 Vpu has a CD4- and an envelope glycoprotein-independent function. *J. Virol.* **67**:**7** (1993), 4190–4.

108. Khan, M. A., Aberham, C., Kao, S. *et al.* Human immunodeficiency virus type 1 Vif protein is packaged into the nucleoprotein complex through an interaction with viral genomic RNA. *J. Virol.* **75** : **16** (2001), 7252–65.

109. Sheehy, A. M., Gaddis, N. C., Choi, J. D. & Malim, M. H. Isolation of a human gene that inhibits HIV-1 infection and is suppressed by the viral Vif protein. *Nature* **418** : **6898** (2002), 646–50.

110. Cohen, E. A., Dehni, G., Sodroski, J. G. & Haseltine, W. A. Human immunodeficiency virus vpr product is a virion-associated regulatory protein. *J. Virol.* **64** : **6** (1990), 3097–9.

111. Felzien, L. K., Woffendin, C., Hottiger, M. O., Subbramanian, R. A., Cohen, E. A. & Nabel, G. J. HIV transcriptional activation by the accessory protein, VPR, is mediated by the p300 coactivator. *Proc. Natl. Acad. Sci. U. S. A.* **95** : **9** (1998), 5281–6.

112. He, J., Choe, S., Walker, R., Di Marzio, P., Morgan, D. O. & Landau, N. R. Human immunodeficiency virus type 1 viral protein R (Vpr) arrests cells in the G2 phase of the cell cycle by inhibiting p34cdc2 activity. *J. Virol.* **69** : **11** (1995), 6705–11.

113. Kestler, H. W. D., Ringler, D. J., Mori, K. *et al.* Importance of the nef gene for maintenance of high virus loads and for development of AIDS. *Cell* **65** : **4** (1991), 651–62.

114. Deacon, N. J., Tsykin, A., Solomon, A. *et al.* Genomic structure of an attenuated quasi species of HIV-1 from a blood transfusion donor and recipients. *Science* **270** : **5238** (1995), 988–91.

115. Baba, T. W., Jeong, Y. S., Pennick, D., Bronson, R., Greene, M. F. & Ruprecht, R. M. Pathogenicity of live, attenuated SIV after mucosal infection of neonatal macaques. *Science* **267** : **5205** (1995), 1820–5.

116. Garcia, J. V. & Miller, A. D. Serine phosphorylation-independent downregulation of cell-surface CD4 by nef. *Nature* **350** : **6318** (1991), 508–11.

117. Piguet, V., Gu, F., Foti, M. *et al.* Nef-induced CD4 degradation : a diacidic-based motif in Nef functions as a lysosomal targeting signal through the binding of beta-COP in endosomes. *Cell* **97** : **1** (1999), 63–73.

118. Collette, Y., Dutartre, H., Benziane, A. *et al.* Physical and functional interaction of Nef with Lck. HIV-1 Nef-induced T-cell signaling defects. *J. Biol. Chem.* **271** : **11** (1996), 6333–41.

119. Schwartz, O., Marechal, V., Le Gall, S., Lemonnier, F. & Heard, J. M. Endocytosis of major histocompatibility complex class I molecules is induced by the HIV-1 Nef protein. *Nat. Med.* **2** : **3** (1996), 338–42.

120. Collins, K. L., Chen, B. K., Kalams, S. A., Walker, B. D. & Baltimore, D. HIV-1 Nef protein protects infected primary cells against killing by cytotoxic T lymphocytes. *Nature* **391** : **6665** (1998), 397–401.

3

The immunology of pediatric HIV disease

Elizabeth J. McFarland, M.D.

Pediatric Infectious Diseases, University of Colorado Health Sciences Center, Denver, CO

HIV-1 infection leads to profound immune dysfunction, resulting in the clinical manifestations of acquired immunodeficiency syndrome (AIDS). The damage that HIV-1 does to the immune system results from the direct, harmful effects that occur when HIV-1 infects a cell, the effects that virions and parts of virions have on cells that do not become infected, and the chronic cell activation that results from infection and the host's response to infection. Abnormal function of HIV-1-affected cells can then lead to dysfunction of other cell types, since the immune system is a highly interconnected system. The main target cells of HIV-1 include cells that are critical in the immune control of the virus, impairing the ability of the host to mount an effective immune response.

3.1 Immunopathogenesis

3.1.1 Primary infection

The majority of adult and adolescent HIV-1 infections are the result of exposure of HIV-1 to mucosal surfaces. This is likely true also for mother-to-child transmission that occurs peripartum and during breastfeeding. Studies of macaques inoculated intravaginally with simian immunodeficiency virus, an animal model for HIV-1, demonstrate the events of primary infection [1]. Dendritic cells, resident in the mucosa, transport HIV-1 to regional lymph nodes within 48 hours of exposure. Within the lymph node, CD4$^+$ T cells become infected through interactions with dendritic cell-associated HIV-1. Subsequently, large numbers of new virions are produced, and infected T cells and free virus can be found in the peripheral blood and in lymph tissue throughout the body approximately 4–11 days after infection.

In adults, and presumably adolescents, the levels of HIV-1 found in the circulation increase rapidly over the first weeks of infection, but then decline dramatically and reach a stable set point at approximately 6 months after infection. The appearance of HIV-1-specific cytotoxic T lymphocytes (CTL) in the peripheral blood is temporally correlated with the initial decline in plasma HIV-1 and may occur as early as 6 weeks after infection (reviewed in [2]). Cytotoxic T-lymphocyte responses appear prior to the detection of neutralizing antibody, suggesting that cell-mediated responses likely are the key immune activities leading to suppression of the initial high levels of viremia. Animal studies using treatments that deplete CD8$^+$ T cells have demonstrated a correlation between the presence of CD8$^+$ cells and increased suppression of viremia [3, 4]. Antibody responses capable of neutralizing virus and antibody-dependent cellular cytotoxicity (ADCC) appear later.

Innate immune responses also contribute to control of plasma HIV-1 levels. CD8$^+$ T cells produce soluble factors that suppress HIV-1 replication in a non-MCH-restricted manner [5]. This response does not require prior exposure to generate the response. A major component of these soluble factors are β-chemokines (RANTES, macrophage inflammatory protein-1) that compete with HIV-1 for binding to co-receptors on monocytes and therefore restrict HIV-1 cell entry [6]. Recently, the alpha-defensins 1, 2, and 3, produced by CD8$^+$ T cells, have been determined to be another important component of the soluble antiviral factors [7].

The immunologic events of perinatal primary infection are less well understood and may differ from those occurring during primary infection in adults. Most infants reach peak viremia at 1–2 months of life but, unlike adults, have only minimal declines in plasma virus over the next several months [8]. Some children with rapid disease progression have no decrease in viral load over the first year of life. Children with slow progression generally have a decline in the number of viral copies/mL but usually not more than 0.5–1 $\log_{10}$.

A number of explanations for the absence of a significant decline in viral load in some vertically infected infants have been proposed. Among these is the possibility that the infant's immature immune system fails to mount an effective response in the newborn period. Studies have demonstrated a delay in the appearance of HIV-1-specific CTL in perinatally infected infants, with responses infrequently detected prior to 6 months of life [9, 10]. Children who have survived to age 2 years, have HIV-1-specific CTL frequencies comparable with those observed in adults [11]. The ADCC responses in infants are also less vigorous [12]. Despite the relative deficiency of some HIV-1-specific immune responses, peripheral blood cells from some infected infants under 6 months of age will suppress the growth of HIV-1 during in vitro culture [13]. This response may be production of the HIV-1-suppressive soluble factors discussed above. Infants with this activity were more likely to have slow progression [13].

Another possible explanation for relatively high viral loads following vertical infection is transmission of virus that has mutated to escape the maternal immune response. Since the infant shares one half of its HLA alleles in common with the mother, virus that has adapted to the mother's immune response may have fewer epitopes that can be recognized in the context of the infant's HLA type. Transmission of this type of escape mutant has been observed [14]. The observation that virus from infants with rapid progression develop fewer new mutations over time also suggests that there is less immune pressure on viral replication in the rapid progressor [15, 16].

3.1.2 Chronic/progressive infection/non-progressive infection

Despite the presence of HIV-1-specific immune responses, HIV-1 continues to replicate, damaging the immune system and leading to the immune abnormalities described below. Lymph nodes during the clinical latency period harbor actively replicating HIV-1 and large quantities of antibody-virus complexes bound to follicular dendritic cells (FDC) in the germinal centers [17]. In vitro studies show that virus bound by the FDCs is highly infectious for

Table 3.1 Mechanisms used by HIV-1 to evade immune responses

Mutations no longer recognized by cytotoxic T lymphocytes (CTL escape mutations)

Mutations no longer recognized by neutralizing antibodies (neutralizing antibody escape mutations)

Inherent resistance to neutralization

Downregulation of MCH class I expression (mediated by viral gene products, e.g. Nef, acting within the infected cell)

Preferential infection and destruction of HIV-1-specific CD4$^+$ T lymphocytes

Dysregulation of cytokine production (IL-2, IFN-γ, IL-12, IL-10)

CD4$^+$ T cells [18]. In advanced HIV-1 infection, lymph node architecture becomes grossly abnormal, with complete loss of the normal germinal center organization. Ongoing viral replication results in generalized immune activation with higher levels of programmed cell death and T cell turnover. There may also be impairment of ability of the thymus to generate new T cells. Eventually the immune system becomes unable to respond to infectious pathogens.

HIV-1 infected adults and children can maintain detectable cytotoxic T cell-mediated immune responses and HIV-1-specific antibody into advanced stages of disease. However, HIV-1-specific lymphoproliferative responses are notably low or absent during chronic, progressive HIV-1 infection. This may be an indication of relative deficiency of CD4$^+$ helper T cell responses (reviewed in [2]). Lack of T cell help may lead to defective effector cell function. High levels of viremia are associated with suppression of HIV-1-specific T cell proliferation by mechanisms that are yet unknown [19]. In addition, CD4$^+$ T cells that are HIV-1-specific are preferentially infected by HIV-1 [20]. Thus, HIV-1 may directly delete some of the T cells required for generating an immune response against it.

HIV-1 may use other mechanisms to evade the immune response (Table 3.1). HIV-1 produces mutant virus at a very high rate, allowing the outgrowth of virus with variant epitopes that fail to be presented by MHC class I and thereby escape recognition by CTL (reviewed in [2]). HIV-1-specific CTL have phenotypes that differ from the phenotype of CTL responding to some other chronic viral infections, raising the possibility that the HIV-1-specific CTL are not fully functional as mature effectors [21–23]. One virus protein, Nef, downregulates expression of MHC class I on HIV-1 infected cells [24]. Expression of MHC class I is critical for CTL recognition and killing of infected cells. HIV-1 is resistant to antibody-mediated neutralization due to inherent characteristics of the HIV-1 envelope protein (reviewed in [25]).

A small number of HIV-1 infected adults and children have no evidence of disease progression for 10 or more years, with generally low levels of HIV-1 in plasma. This course has been termed long-term non-progression (LTNP). Genetic and viral phenotype factors have been associated with LTNP. Some patients have had Nef-deleted mutant virus which may result in a less pathogenic virus [26]. Mutations in cellular molecules that are important in the viral life cycle are associated with slower disease progression (reviewed in [27]). Some HLA alleles are also associated with slower progression [27]. Patients with LTNP are more likely to have HIV-1-specific lymphoproliferative responses as well as a high frequency of HIV-1-specific CTLs [2]. Other qualitative aspects of their immune response may help maintain better virologic control. Studies of the immune response in the persons with LTNP raise the possibility that interventions that enhance the natural HIV-1-specific immune response might render it more effective and delay disease progression.

3.1.3 Effects of antiretroviral therapy

The possibility that the immune response can be improved by therapeutic intervention has been supported in trials of treatment during acute infection of adults. In a small study, patients initiating HIV-1 treatment in the first weeks after infection had markedly higher HIV-1-specific lymphocyte proliferative responses than patients not initiating treatment [28]. Among eight individuals thus treated who have subsequently interrupted antiretroviral therapy in a controlled fashion, five have maintained viral control off treatment over a period of months and appear to have viral set-points that are lower than would be expected based on untreated historical controls. Although the cohort is small and further controlled studies in larger numbers of subjects are needed before firm conclusions are possible, these data are encouraging in that it may be possible to remodel the immune response.

It is unclear whether this scenario will apply to infants receiving early treatment. Infants on antiretroviral treatment with successful viral suppression before 3 months of life do not maintain detectable HIV-1-specific immune responses [10, 29]. Neither HIV-1-specific cell mediated, nor HIV-1 antibody responses, are detected when tested at age 12–15 months. Normal responses to other antigens are found. The infants can generate an HIV-1-specific response, as interruptions of treatment result in rapid appearance of HIV-1-specific antibodies [30]. Infants beginning antiretroviral therapy after 3–6 months have

higher levels of HIV-1-specific CD8+ T cell responses and maintain HIV-1 antibodies (10). Studies of infants who began antiretroviral therapy during acute infection and then subsequently stopped antiretroviral therapy have not been performed.

3.2 Immune abnormalities associated with HIV-1 infection

Both cell-mediated and humoral immune functions are affected during HIV-1 infection, placing patients at risk for a wide variety of pathogens (Table 3.2). (For a description of the normal development of the immune system see Chapter 1).

3.2.1 Cell-mediated immunity

Cell-mediated immunity primarily defends against intracellular pathogens, notably viral infections, and malignancies. Abnormal cell-mediated immunity in HIV-1-infected children leads to more severe or recurrent disease from pathogens such as varicella zoster virus, herpes simplex virus, cytomegalovirus (CMV), *Mycobacterium species*, and *Salmonella species*. Likewise, lymphomas and certain soft tissue malignancies are also more common in HIV-1-infected children. Abnormal cellular immune function also contributes to abnormal humoral immunity.

3.2.2 Defects in helper T-lymphocyte cell function

The hallmark of HIV-1 disease is a decline in the absolute number and percent of helper T lymphocytes (CD4+ T lymphocytes). The CD4 protein found on the surface of helper T lymphocytes is used by HIV-1 as a co-receptor for entry into the cells. As a result, helper T lymphocytes are a main target of HIV-1 infection. It is likely that both direct cytopathic and indirect effects of HIV-1 contribute to the abnormalities in CD4+ T lymphocyte function and number. As the number of CD4+ T lymphocytes declines, the risk of opportunistic infections increases (see Chapters 4 and 5).

Preceding the decline in the absolute number of CD4+ T lymphocytes, alterations in the helper T lymphocyte function are observed. A commonly used laboratory marker of abnormal T-helper cell function is cell proliferation in response to stimulation. Lymphocytes from asymptomatic, HIV-1-infected children have reduced proliferation to common antigenic stimulants (tetanus, diphtheria, Candida) after the age of 2 years or sooner in symptomatic children [31]. As the immunodeficiency of HIV-1 disease progresses, reduced proliferative responses to specific antigens are

Table 3.2 Immunologic abnormalities associated with HIV-1 infection

Cellular
Decreased delayed-type hypersensitivity skin reaction
T-Lymphocytes
   Decreased absolute numbers of CD4 positive (helper) T lymphocytes
   Increased relative numbers of CD8 positive (killer/suppressor) T lymphocytes
   Decreased CD4/CD8 ratio
   Decreased numbers of cells with naïve phenotype (CD45RA+/CD62L+)
   Increased % cells with memory phenotype (CD45RO$^+$)
   Increased % CD8$^+$ cells with diminished proliferative capacity (CD28$^-$; CD95$^+$)
   Increased CD8$^+$ T cells with activated phenotype (CD38$^+$/HLA-DR$^+$)
   Decreased proliferative responses to antigen and mitogens
   Altered cytokine production (see below)
Natural Killer (NK) cells
   Decreased number of NK cells (CD16$^+$/CD56$^+$)
   Decreased cytotoxic activity
Antigen Presenting Cells (monocytes and dendritic cells)
   Decreased stimulation of T cell proliferative response to antigen
   Decreased HLA-DR expression
   Altered cytokine production
Phagocytes
   Monocytes
      Decreased clearance of RBC
      Decreased Fc receptor expression
      Decreased chemotaxis
      Decreased intracellular killing
      Decreased superanion production
   Polymorphonuclear cells
      Neutropenia
      Increased or decreased chemotaxis
      Decreased staphylococcus killing
      Increased or decreased phagocytosis
      Altered surface adhesion proteins and receptors
Humoral
B lymphocytes
   Decreased number of antigen-responsive B cells (CD23$^+$/CD62L$^+$; CD21^{hi})
   Polyclonal activation of B cells
   Increased spontaneous immunoglobulin secretion from B cells
   Decreased immunoglobulin secretion after stimulation of B cells
   Increased IgG, IgA, IgM
Specific antibody responses
   Decreased antibody response to immunization: hepatitis B, HIB conjugate, measles, influenza
   Declining antibody titers to prior immunization: diphtheria, tetanus, Candida, measles
Cytokines
   Decreased production of IL-2, IFN-γ
   Decreased production of IL-12
   Decreased IFN-α
   Increased production of IL-1β, IL-6, and TNF-α
   Increased production of IL-10, transforming growth factor-β

NK – natural killer; RBC – red blood cells.

followed by decreased responses to allo-antigens and, then eventually, diminished responses to mitogens (stimulants which activate all T cells regardless of antigenic specificity) [32].

In HIV-1 disease, helper T lymphocytes also have an abnormal pattern of cytokine secretion (reviewed in [33]). The most prominent defect detected in both adults and children is a decreased post-stimulation production of IL-2 and IFN-γ [34]. Since IL-2 and IFN-γ are important in promoting cell-mediated immune responses, deficient production may contribute to defects in cell-mediated function.

The delayed-type hypersensitivity (DTH) response determined by intradermal skin testing provides a global assessment of cellular immune function. Patients with advanced disease have poor DTH responses to memory antigens such as tetanus, Candida, mumps, and others [35]. Consequently, skin testing for *Mycobacterium tuberculosis* may be unreliable in a patient who has lost DTH responses.

Changes in the phenotype of CD4$^+$ T lymphocytes also occur with HIV-1 infection. The pattern of cell surface protein expression defines lymphocyte phenotype, and phenotype correlates with function. Phenotypic changes can therefore be monitored by determining changes in cell surface protein expression. The most notable phenotypic change is an increase in the proportion of memory CD4$^+$ T lymphocytes (CD45RO$^+$) relative to naïve CD4$^+$ T lymphocytes (CD45RA$^+$CD62L$^+$) [36, 37]. However, due to the overall decline in CD4$^+$ T lymphocyte numbers, the absolute number of both naïve and memory CD4$^+$ T lymphocytes is lower in HIV-1-infected children. The relative increase in memory cells may be the result of stimulation by chronic exposure to HIV-1 or to inability of the thymus to generate naïve cells. Loss of naïve cells may compromise the ability of the immune system to handle new pathogens.

3.2.3 Defects in cytotoxic/suppressor T lymphocyte cell function

Cytotoxic/suppressor T lymphocytes mediate direct cytotoxic activity against pathogen-infected and malignant cells and release soluble factors which inhibit the growth of some pathogens. CD8$^+$ T lymphocytes may play a role in down-regulating the immune response after an infection has been controlled as well.

During acute infection, a large increase in the number of CD8$^+$ T lymphocytes occurs, probably the result of a vigorous CD8-mediated primary immune response to HIV-1. Large expansions of particular CD8$^+$ T cell clones with HIV-1-specificity are identified in acute and chronic infection [38–40]. Subsequently, the absolute number and percent of CD8$^+$ T lymphocytes may remain high, particularly in symptomatic patients. The increased number of CD8$^+$ T lymphocytes can result in a decreased CD4/CD8 ratio (normally > 1), even before significant declines in CD4$^+$ T cell number occurs. In advanced disease, the absolute number of CD8$^+$ T lymphocytes may decline as a result of lymphopenia. The majority of cells accounting for the increase in CD8$^+$ cells are activated (CD38$^+$, HLA-DR$^+$), memory cells (CD45RO$^+$) [41, 42]. A higher proportion of CD8$^+$ T cells in HIV-1 infected people have phenotypic markers of decreased proliferative potential and increased programmed cell death [43–46].

3.2.4 Defects in natural killer lymphocyte cell function

Natural killer (NK) cells are responsible for an early antigen-independent cytolytic response against infected or malignant cells (see Chapter 1). During HIV-1 infection, the number of NK cells is lower than in healthy controls and declines with disease progression [47–49]. Early in HIV-1 infection in both children and adults, laboratory tests reveal decreased NK lytic activity and decreased production of IFN-γ [48, 50, 51]. Exogenous cytokines (IL-2, IL-12, IL-15) can restore these NK cell functions in vitro, suggesting that an altered cytokine milieu may account in part for abnormal function and that the defect might be reversed with immune-based therapies [52].

3.2.5 Defects in antigen-presenting cell function

Antigen-presenting cells (APC), including monocytes, macrophages, and dendritic cells, present antigens in the context of either MHC class I or class II antigens to lymphocytes so that those lymphocytes can mount an immune response against the antigen (see Chapter 1). The mode of presentation and the type of cytokines produced by the APC at the time of interaction with lymphocytes are believed to determine the type of immune response generated. Monocytes express CD4 and the co-receptors used by HIV-1 and can be directly infected with HIV-1, resulting in abnormal function and dissemination of the infection. Dendritic cells express DC-sign, a surface molecule that binds HIV-1 and the association of HIV-1 with dendritic cells facilitates infection of CD4$^+$ T cells [53, 54]. The number of dendritic cells in peripheral blood is decreased in acute and chronic HIV-1 infection in adults [55–57]. Dendritic cells and monocytes from HIV-1-infected patients have a decreased capacity to induce proliferation of T lymphocytes [58, 59].

HIV-1 infection results in abnormal cytokine secretion from monocytes and dendritic cells. Interleukin-12 is a cytokine produced by antigen-presenting cells that promote cellular immune responses. The regulatory pathways for production of IL-12 are altered during HIV-1 infection and the levels of IL-12 produced are low (reviewed in [60]). HIV-1 infection of monocytes in vitro, and presumably in vivo, results in decreased IL-12 production in the infected cells [61]. Moreover, the effects of HIV-1 infection on other cytokines and co-receptors involved in the regulation of IL-12 production result in decreased IL-12 production from cells that are not directly infected with HIV-1 [62–67]. Since IL-12 promotes cellular immunity, decreased production may contribute to defective cell-mediated immunity during HIV-1 infection [68, 69]. HIV-1 infected adults have decreased production of interferon-α (IFN-α) from dendritic cells [55, 70]. Interferon-α is an important component of the innate immune response to pathogens. Increased tumor necrosis factor (TNF)-α serum levels and TNF-α production have been observed in serum, PBMC, brain, and monocytes infected in vitro [71]. Increased serum levels of TNF-α and -β may contribute to wasting disease. Although the correlation with wasting is less clear, high levels do correlate with progressive encephalopathy. HIV-1 patients also have increased plasma levels of pro-inflammatory cytokines (IL-1β, IL-6) and anti-inflammatory cytokines (IL-10, transforming growth factor-β) (reviewed in [33, 71]). Some of these cytokines can enhance HIV-1 replication. The dysregulation of cytokine production is also likely to impair the development of normal immune responses.

3.2.6 Defects in phagocyte cell function

Phagocytes engulf and kill extracellular pathogens (i.e. bacteria and fungi), generate granulomas, and localize infection. Defects in mononuclear phagocyte and polymorphonuclear leukocyte (PMN) function observed during HIV-1 infection include decreased chemotaxis, diminished intracellular killing, and decreased superanion radical production; these defects may contribute to poor granuloma formation observed in HIV-1-infected people [59].

PMNs defend against bacterial and fungal pathogens. Patients with advanced disease often have neutropenia resulting from drug toxicity and the effects of HIV-1 disease. HIV-1-infected patients may also have defects in PMN function such as decreased phagocytosis, decreased bactericidal activity, altered superoxide production, altered chemotaxis, and altered surface adhesion molecules and activation receptors [72–74].

Humoral immunity

Abnormal humoral immunity is observed in HIV-1-infected adults and children, but has more significant clinical effects among HIV-1-infected children. Even at early stages of HIV-1 disease, children have increased rates of minor and invasive bacterial infections. A likely explanation is that HIV-1 has destroyed the ability to produce antibodies against new antigens before the child is exposed to many important pathogens. By contrast, an HIV-1-infected adult may have generated memory B cells to many pathogens prior to HIV-1 infection. These memory cells of adults can then produce protective antibody against many important pathogens upon repeat exposure, at least during the early stages of HIV-1 disease. Hyperglobulinemia is a notable feature of the disease, particularly in many pediatric HIV-1 patients. Hypoglobulinemia can be seen in some pediatric and adult HIV-1 patients.

3.2.7 Defects in B lymphocyte function

B lymphocytes are not infected by HIV-1 but have significantly abnormal function during HIV-1 infection, probably because of direct effects of HIV-1 gp120, altered cytokine levels, and impaired CD4$^+$ T cell mediated immunity. A minority of patients will have hypogammaglobulinemia, usually associated with advanced disease [75]. The more common abnormality is a relatively non-specific polyclonal activation of B lymphocytes, which is observed soon after HIV-1 infection, resulting in hypergammaglobulinemia [76]. Elevated IgG, particularly IgG1 and IgG2 subclasses, is observed by the age of 6 months in the many HIV-1-infected infants (Table 3.3) [77]. Elevated IgA and IgM are also observed, particularly among infants with rapidly progressive disease [77]. Tests of B lymphocytes in vitro reveal increased spontaneous immunoglobulin (Ig) production and cell proliferation, but decreased specific Ig production and cell proliferation in response to stimulation with recall antigens or mitogens specific for B lymphocytes [76]. The majority of the cells produce polyclonal low affinity antibody not directed against a discernible pathogen, although some of the cells (20–40%) make HIV-1-specific antibody [78]. This HIV-1-specific antibody often does not effectively neutralize the HIV-1 found in the plasma contemporaneously although it may neutralize HIV-1 isolated from early times in the infection. There is evidence that gp120 acts as a superantigen for subsets of B lymphocytes that bear a particular variable heavy chain type, resulting in overstimulation of these cells [79]. Increased levels of IL-10 and IL-15 have also been associated with hypergammaglobulinemia [80, 81].

Table 3.3 Serum immunoglobulin levels (median and upper 95% confidence limit) in uninfected, asymptomatic, and symptomatic HIV-1-infected children

		Children		
	Age (months)	Uninfected	Asymptomatic	Symptomatic
IgG (mg/dl)	0–1	554 + 757	836 + 1091	952 + 1122
	1–6	437 + 630	551 + 657	1360 + 1514
	7–12	565 + 711	615 + 918	1893 + 2422
	13–24	725 + 998	774 + 1120	2125 + 2855
IgA (mg/dl)	0–1	16 + 30	16 + 27	54 + 69
	1–6	24 +32	27 + 39	74 + 98
	7–12	27 + 68	26 + 42	141 + 191
	13–24	42 + 69	45 + 89	149 + 188
IgM (mg/dl)	0–1	47 + 78	47 + 77	103 + 152
	1–6	59 + 89	85 + 109	134 + 159
	7–12	79 +104	108 + 134	167 + 183
	13–24	105 + 130	120 + 177	149 + 191

Modified from [77].

3.2.8 Defects in specific antibody production

Despite hypergammaglobulinemia, HIV-1-infected children have functional hypogammaglobulinemia because of diminished ability to produce specific antibody in response to both new and recall soluble antigens. Antibody responses are decreased to both T-independent and T-dependent antigens. In studies of recall responses to tetanus, diphtheria, and Candida, asymptomatic children < 2 years of age had antibody responses similar to uninfected children [31]. After 2 years of age, untreated HIV-1-infected children had decreased antibody responses to these antigens, even with normal CD4+ T lymphocyte numbers [31]. Responses to hepatitis B, measles, influenza, and *Haemophilus influenzae* type B vaccines are decreased in untreated HIV-1-infected infants [82–85]. Disease progression is associated with a decline in B lymphocyte numbers with a preferential loss of B lymphocytes which respond to antigen (CD23+/CD62L+; CD21^low), perhaps leading to decreased production of antigen-specific antibody [86, 87]. The soluble gp120 and presumably HIV infection of CD4+ T cells impairs T cell help for specific B cell responses [88].

3.2.9 Surrogate markers for disease progression: CD4+ T lymphocyte values

Surrogate markers that predict the risk of disease progression before the onset of clinical symptoms are essential for optimal management. Plasma viral RNA quantitation and CD4+ T lymphocyte numbers and percentages have proved to be important and independent markers for progression and response to therapy. CD4+ T lymphocyte numbers are the most useful predictor of the risk of opportunistic infections and are used to make recommendations for the initiation of prophylactic therapy.

3.2.10 Technique for CD4+ T lymphocyte number and percentage determinations

The standard technique for determining CD4+ T lymphocyte number is cell surface marker (i.e. surface protein) analysis performed by flow cytometry, with a concurrent complete blood count (CBC) determined by standard hematology techniques [89]. Peripheral blood cells are incubated with antibodies specific for cell surface proteins that identify the cells of interest. The monoclonal antibodies are conjugated to fluorescent molecules which produce a fluorescent emission of a particular wavelength upon excitation by the light source in the flow cytometer. In the case of CD4+ T cell determinations, the fraction of total lymphocytes that express both cell surface markers CD3 (a protein in the T cell receptor, a marker shared by all T cells) and CD4 (marker of helper T cells) is determined. This value is frequently reported as the percentage of the lymphocytes that are CD4+ (percent CD4+ T cells). Absolute CD4+ T lymphocyte counts are determined by multiplying the percentage of CD3+/CD4+ lymphocytes by the absolute lymphocyte count determined from the white blood cell count (WBC) from the concurrent CBC results:

$$\begin{aligned}
\text{Absolute } &CD4^+ \text{ T lymphocyte count} \\
&= \text{absolute lymphocyte count} \\
&\quad \times \%CD3^+/CD4^+ \text{ lymphocytes} \\
&= WBC \times \%\text{lymphocytes} \\
&\quad \times \%CD3^+/CD4^+ \text{ lymphocytes.}
\end{aligned}$$

In order to standardize $CD4^+$ T lymphocyte determinations, the US Public Health Service has published detailed guidelines for laboratories performing the test [89]. Single platform analysis is an alternative flow cytometric method developed recently that allows direct measurement of the absolute $CD4^+$ T cell count without a separate CBC measurement [90].

Many laboratories determine $CD4^+$ T lymphocyte numbers in the context of a larger panel of cell surface markers, often including killer/suppressor T lymphocytes ($C3^+/CD8^+$ lymphocytes) and B lymphocytes ($CD19^+$ lymphocytes). This permits calculation of the CD4/CD8 ratio. This ratio has been used as an early marker of immunologic abnormality and was once one of the key indicators used to diagnose AIDS, but is now used less frequently in clinical practice.

A number of biologic and analytic factors can introduce variability into $CD4^+$ T lymphocyte test results. The procedure involves calculation of the absolute count based on three separate measurements (the total WBC, percent lymphocytes, and percent CD4 lymphocytes), each of which can introduce a source of error [91]. Biologic sources of variability include diurnal variation, acute illness, immunizations, and drug therapy, particularly corticosteroids [91–94]. The $CD4^+$ T lymphocyte values will vary with the time of day with the lowest values at noon and a peak in the evening. Between 8:00 am and 4:00 pm, the usual clinic hours, an average 19% increase in the $CD4^+$ T lymphocyte count can occur in HIV-1 infected adults [91]. It is best to obtain specimens for $CD4^+$ T lymphocyte determinations on an individual at a consistent time of day. Acute illnesses and immunizations may increase or decrease the total WBC as well as cause transient changes in the percent $CD4^+$ T lymphocytes. Likewise, corticosteroid therapy is associated with decreases in absolute $CD4^+$ T lymphocyte counts, particularly after acute administration (transient decreases from $900/mm^3$ to $300/mm^3$ in adults) [93, 94]. Even without the presence of one of the above conditions, stable patients on average may have a $\pm 22\%$ change in absolute $CD4^+$ T cell counts between specimens [92]. $CD4^+$ T cell percentage values fluctuate less than absolute counts primarily because variations in total white cell count result in changes in absolute counts but do not affect the percentage values [95]. In view of this variability, $CD4^+$ T lymphocyte values which differ substantially from previous values should be evaluated critically especially if obtained during acute illnesses or soon after immunizations.

3.2.11 Interpretation of $CD4^+$ T lymphocyte values

Interpretation of $CD4^+$ T lymphocyte numbers in children requires recognition that the normal number of cells declines with age over the first 6 years of life (see Chapter 1). Normal values for each age have been determined and are used when evaluating $CD4^+$ T lymphocyte numbers in infants and children (see Chapter 1, Figure 1.1). The age-related change is particularly marked for absolute $CD4^+$ T lymphocyte counts; % $CD4^+$ T lymphocyte values change less with age [95].

Routine monitoring of $CD4^+$ T lymphocyte number and percentage is critical to optimal clinical management of HIV-1-infected infants and children as described in more detail in Chapter 9. Pediatric guidelines recommend monitoring both percentage and absolute $CD4^+$ T lymphocyte counts and determining disease staging based on the lowest of the two values. Due to the potential variation in $CD4^+$ T lymphocyte values (see above), major therapeutic decisions, such as changing antiretroviral therapy or initiating prophylaxis, should only be made after the changes have been confirmed with repeat testing and other sources of variability have been ruled out. A sustained decrease of 50% in the absolute $CD4^+$ T cell count or percentage is accepted as significant evidence of disease progression. Smaller changes that are found repeatedly can also be significant if a consistent trend is observed.

3.2.12 Evaluating prognosis and response to therapy using $CD4^+$ T lymphocyte values

HIV-1 infection in children is associated with a progressive decline in $CD4^+$ T lymphocyte values greater than the normal physiologic decline [77, 96]. Cross-sectional and longitudinal studies using healthy controls demonstrate significant decreases in $CD4^+$ T lymphocyte numbers from as early an age as 2 months (Figure 3.1) [96]. These early differences primarily reflect the declines among symptomatic, rapidly progressing children (Table 3.4) [77]. However, by age 13–24 months, $CD4^+$ T lymphocyte values are significantly lower among asymptomatic children compared with uninfected age-matched infants as well (Table 3.4) [77].

$CD4^+$ T lymphocyte numbers and percents and the rate of decline of $CD4^+$ T lymphocyte numbers are useful markers of prognosis in HIV-1-infected children and adults. The staging system for children <13 years published by the Centers for Disease Control (CDC) in 1994 incorporates both

Table 3.4 CD4$^+$ and CD8$^+$ T lymphocyte numbers (mean ± standard deviation) in uninfected, asymptomatic and symptomatic HIV-1-infected children

		Children		
	Age (months)	Uninfected	Asymptomatic	Symptomatic
CD4$^+$ lymphocytes (cells/μL)	0–1	2900 ± 1541	2580 ± 1501	2317 ± 1317
	1–6	3278 ± 1401	3482 ± 1234	1706 ± 1215
	7–12	3051 ± 1285	2769 ± 1326	1951 ± 882
	13–24	2584 ± 1105	2030 ± 1481	1680 ± 1089
CD8$^+$ lymphocytes (cells/μL)	0–1	1418 ± 791	1404 ± 974	1499 ± 1046
	1–6	1626 ± 985	1457 ± 709	1613 ± 958
	7–12	514 ± 300	394 ± 334	523 ± 266
	13–24	1374 ± 663	1902 ± 844	2242 ± 1290

Modified from [77].

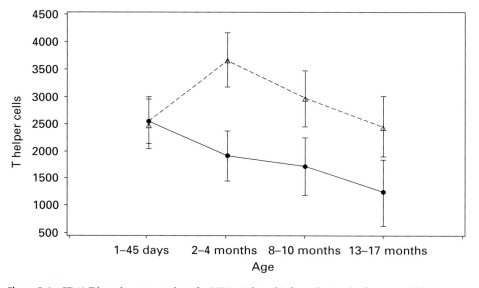

Figure 3.1. CD4$^+$ T lymphocyte numbers for HIV-1-infected infants during the first year of life. Mean and 95% confidence interval for CD4$^+$ T lymphocytes (cells/μL) by HIV-1 status for infants born to HIV-1-infected mothers and followed prospectively. The solid circles represent 31 HIV-1-infected children; the open triangles represent 28 HIV-1-negative (seroreverting) children. The data are represented as the means ± standard errors. For all data comparisons beyond 45 days, a p value of at least 0.05 exists. Reprinted with permission from Shearer *et al. Ann. N. Y. Acad. Sci.* **693** (1993), 35–51, [96].

CD4$^+$ T lymphocyte values and clinical symptoms (see Chapter 5, Table 5.3) [97]. Baseline CD4$^+$ T lymphocyte values and changes with therapy are useful in predicting the risk of disease progression independent of the predictive value of quantitative plasma viral RNA [98–100]. For example, patients with ≥ 1000 cell/mL^3 at age < 12 mo and ≥ 500 at age 12–30 mo are less likely to progress (Figure 3.2) [98].

As described more extensively in Chapter 5, the clinical presentation of HIV-1 infection in infants with vertically acquired disease is bimodal with approximately 30% of infants having rapid progression. Infants with rapid progression often have a lymphocyte phenotype which suggests defective thymus function (markedly decreased CD4$^+$ and CD8$^+$ T lymphocytes and CD5$^+$ B lymphocytes) [101]. They may have precipitous declines in CD4$^+$

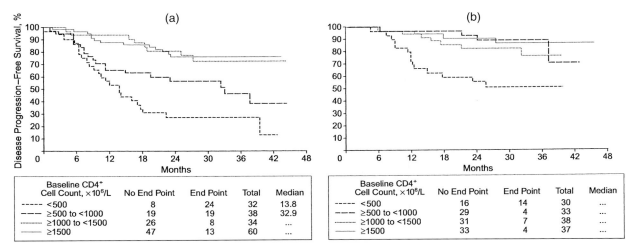

Figure 3.2. Prognostic threshold effects for CD4+ T lymphocyte counts correspond to Centers for Disease Control immunologic categories. Kaplan–Meier estimates of disease progression-free survival utilizing baseline CD4+ T lymphocyte counts. Figure 3.2a depicts infants between 3 and 12 months of age at study entry while Figure 3.2b depicts infants between 12 and 30 months. Approximate quartiles were established for baseline CD4+ T cell counts as represented at the bottom of each figure. Reprinted with permission from Palumbo *et al. J. Am. Med. Assoc.* **279** (1998), 756–61 [98].

T lymphocyte number such that within a 3-month interval their CD4+ T lymphocyte number can decline into the range associated with an increased risk of *Pneumocystis carinii* pneumonia [102]. Infants and children with slow progression have gradual declines in CD4+ T lymphocyte values.

One of the most important uses of CD4+ T lymphocyte determinations has been predicting the risk of specific opportunistic infections. Risk-benefit ratios for prophylaxis of a particular opportunistic infection can then be determined and recommendations for when to initiate such therapy made. Prophylaxis strategies for pediatric HIV-1 patients are described in Chapter 11 .

3.3 Immune restoration after highly active antiretroviral therapy

The immunologic abnormalities described above are associated with untreated, progressive HIV-1 infection. Successful treatment with highly active antiretroviral therapy (HAART) results in reversal of most of the clinical and many of the immunologic signs of disease progression (reviewed in [103, 104]). Patients receiving effective treatment have a lower incidence of opportunistic infections, resolution of HIV-1-related dysfunction of primary organs (i.e. encephalopathy), and improved growth.

The clinical improvements are correlated with increases in CD4+ T cell percentage and absolute cell count. During the first 4–8 weeks after initiating HAART, there are rapid increases in the number of CD4+ T lymphocytes as well as increases in the number of B lymphocytes (Figure 3.3) [105, 106]. The number and percentage of CD4+ T lymphocytes continues to increase over the following 12–18 months. The rapid increases observed early after starting treatment suggests that the initial increases are the result of redistribution of cells that had been sequestered in lymphoid tissue (reviewed in [104]). Phenotypic analysis supports this explanation, as in older children and adults, the increase in CD4+ T cells is largely accounted for by cells with memory phenotype [105]. Younger children have an early increase in naïve cells as well as memory cells, suggesting they may mobilize naïve cells from the thymus earlier after initiation of treatment than older children [105, 107–109]. After the initial rise, the continued increases in CD4+ T cells are almost entirely accounted for by cells with naïve phenotype [105, 106, 110]. Most likely these cells are newly derived from the thymus, although the contribution of proliferation of naïve cells in the peripheral pool cannot be excluded [111, 112].

The predominance of naïve cells after treatment would be expected to allow the generation of responses to new antigens. However, it may also predict that spontaneous reconstitution of responses to recall antigens may not occur. Functional assessments of immune responses have been consistent with this concept. The number of children with delayed type hypersensitivity (DTH) responses to antigens (e.g. Candida) increases after 12–18 months of

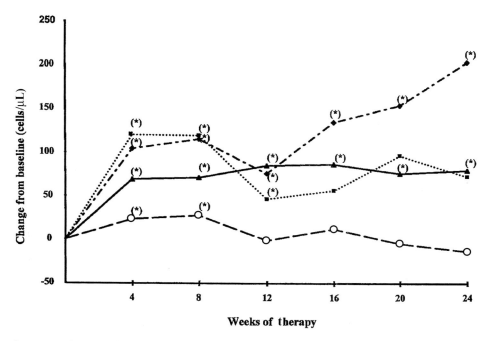

Figure 3.3. Changes in lymphocyte populations after highly active antiretroviral therapy. Median change from entry values of CD8+ T cell (dotted line), CD4+ T cells (dotted-dashed line), B cells (solid line), and NK cells (dashed line) over the course of 24 weeks. Values shown as cells/μL. A statistically significant (P< 0.05) change from baseline is identified with an asterisk. Reprinted with permission from Sleasman *et al. J. Pediat.* **134** (1999), 597–606 [105].

treatment [113]. Likewise, following HAART, lymphoproliferative responses often increase for antigens to which re-exposure is likely to occur (i.e. Candida, CMV, *Mycobacterium avium*) [106, 107, 113–115]. By contrast, proliferative responses to antigens that are not common in the environment, such as tetanus, are less likely to increase with HAART alone [106]. However, preliminary studies indicate that responses to uncommon antigens can be generated through boosting or reimmunization [106, 116]. Further studies of the response to re-immunization in children receiving HAART with a number of the usual childhood vaccines are underway. Adults treated with HAART have decreases in quantitative IgG, IgM, and IgA levels, which are normally elevated during HIV-1 infection, indicating improvements toward a more normal B lymphocyte function [117, 118]. However, not all patients achieve normal levels of immunoglobulins, despite increases in CD4+ T cell parameters and HIV-1 suppression [119]. Studies of the effect of HAART on hypergammaglobulinemia in children are few.

The number of CD8+ lymphocytes increases transiently in the first 8 weeks, but then returns to baseline by 12 weeks (Figure 3.3) [105]. The percentage of CD8+ T cells declines as the relative number of CD4+ T cells increases and the CD4/CD8 ratio normalizes. There are significant changes in phenotype with approximately 40% decrease in the number of cells with cell surface markers for activation and programmed cell death and a modest increase in the number of CD8+ T cells with naïve phenotype [120]. There is a decline in the frequency of CD8+ T cells with HIV-1 specificity [121]. This is likely an adaptation to the decline in viral antigen levels as virus replication is suppressed.

In many children, HAART is associated with effective suppression of plasma HIV-1 RNA to levels that are low or below the limits of detection. However, a substantial number of children will not have durable suppression of viral load, and plasma HIV-1 RNA levels return to near-pretreatment levels [106, 109, 122–124]. Many of these children will have increased CD4+ T cell counts in the face of ongoing viremia. The proportional increases in CD4+ T cell counts may be as great in these so-called virologic non-responders/immunologic responders as in those children who achieve complete viral suppression [122]. Children with ongoing viremia still derive clinical benefit from HAART if their CD4+ T cell counts are increased [124, 125]. The explanation for the ability of the immune system to be at least partially restored in the face of continued high level viral replication is not fully understood. Some evidence points to decreased viral fitness or a switch of virus strain to a less pathogenic phenotype [126–129].

The ability to achieve clinically significant immune restoration appears to be limited by nadir CD4$^+$ T cell counts in adults. Adults with very low CD4$^+$ lymphocyte counts, particularly prolonged, are less likely to show evidence of immune restoration following HAART. This limitation is less apparent for HIV-1-infected children. Even children who have initiated treatment with profoundly suppressed CD4$^+$ T cell counts commonly have had increases to the normal range [108, 113, 126, 130]. Studies comparing children initiating treatment with CD4$^+$ T cell numbers corresponding to CDC category 2 or 3, found that by 18 months, the CD4$^+$ T cell numbers and percentages achieved were comparable in both groups. In these pediatric patients, the slope of increase was greater among children beginning treatment at lower CD4$^+$ T cell values (Figure 3.4) [113]. It is likely that increased thymic function in children contributes to the greater capacity for restoration of T lymphocytes [109, 111, 126]. The lowered incidence of opportunistic infections in these children indicates that the cells are adequate to prevent these infections. Studies to compare immune responses to recall and new antigens between children initiating HAART at high versus low CD4 counts are in progress.

The question of whether the immune system can be restored to a completely normal state after HIV-1 disease has progressed to the point of significant immunodeficiency has occurred remains debatable. It appears that subtle abnormalities persist. The levels of cell activation decrease but remain above normal. The distribution of different T cell receptors may not completely normalize, a possible indication of limited diversity in the T cell population or the persistence of expanded clones [131, 132]. The production of some cytokines remains abnormal [133, 134]. Treatment with a variety of immunologically active agents, such as IL-2, has been proposed as possible interventions to correct these persistent abnormalities. Additional research is needed to determine whether the continuing immune system abnormalities will translate into altered clinical course in the long term.

3.4 Prophylactic HIV-1 vaccination

A prophylactic HIV-1 vaccine is critically needed. As discussed in Chapter 6, new HIV-1 infections continue to occur throughout the world. Although mother-to-child transmission has been reduced to under 2% in resource-

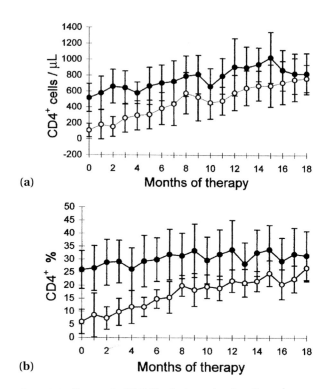

Figure 3.4. Changes in CD4$^+$ T cells depend on baseline values. Changes (mean, SD) in CD4$^+$ T cell counts (a) and CD4$^+$ T cell percentages (b) in patients in CDC category 2 (filled circles) and patients in CDC category 3 (open circles) during 18 months of stavudine, lamivudine, and indinavir treatment. Reprinted with permission from [113].

rich countries, transmission rates may be as high as 30–40% in developing countries because there are many obstacles to implementation of effective interventions to prevent mother-to-child transmission. Even when perinatal interventions are available, many infants continue to be infected through breastfeeding because formula feeding is not possible in many resource-poor areas. An effective vaccine would have a major impact on public health.

The correlates of immune protection from infection with HIV-1 are unknown. In animal models using SIV, sterilizing protection (the absence of any evidence of infection) has been difficult to achieve. High titer neutralizing antibody with activity against the challenge strain can provide sterilizing immunity by active or passive immunization in macaques [135–139]. However, challenges with virus heterologous to the strain on which the candidate vaccine was designed result in infection [139]. Unfortunately, identifying vaccine candidates that induce high titers of neutralizing antibodies required for protection has proven difficult (reviewed in [25, 140]). Although some vaccine strategies used in human trials have generated neutralizing antibody for laboratory strains of virus, no candidate vaccines tested to date have succeeded in generating high titer neutralizing antibody for primary HIV-1 isolates [141–143]. Additional challenges to vaccine design are the inherent heterogeneity and structural resistance to neutralization of the HIV-1 envelope protein [25].

More recently, investigation has focused on induction of HIV-1-specific CTL by candidate vaccines. As discussed earlier in this chapter, HIV-1-specific CTL can suppress viral replication. Vaccines have been designed specifically to induce cell-mediated immunity. The most common strategies use naked DNA vaccines and/or live vector vaccines made by inserting a portion of the HIV-1 genome into attenuated viruses that do not cause disease in humans. These vaccines are being tested alone or in a prime-boost series using various combinations of DNA vaccines, vector vaccines, and protein subunit vaccines [140]. A number have been tested in animal models where it is possible to administer challenge virus after immunization. Vaccines that induce cell-mediated immunity in the absence of neutralizing antibody have failed to provide sterilizing immunity in these animal models. However, when vigorous virus-specific CTL have been induced prior to challenge with large doses of pathogenic virus, the levels of plasma virus and disease progression have been markedly reduced [144–146]. Although sterilizing immunity might be the ultimate goal, a vaccine that could delay disease progression by years or lower viral load and thereby reduce transmission to other contacts would be highly beneficial. It is not yet known whether the results observed in trials with animals will correlate with efficacy in humans.

Several HIV-1 vaccine candidates have completed Phase I and II clinical trials [25, 140]. A protein subunit vaccine did not demonstrate efficacy in a phase III trial. A phase III trial of a recombinant canarypox virus vector with protein subunit boost is underway. HIV-1 envelope protein subunit vaccines have been tested in infants born to HIV-1-infected mothers and found to be immunogenic [147–149]. Since rates of transmission are so high in some countries, a vaccine with only modest efficacy could still have important effects on incidence of infection in regions with rampant epidemics. Although much effort has been focused on HIV-1 vaccine development, the clinical development of effective vaccines is still at an early stage. Unfortunately, HIV-1 vaccines have no current, generally available role in prophylaxis against HIV-1 infection or the management of HIV-1-infected patients.

3.5 Summary

Progressive HIV-1 disease results in cell-mediated and humoral immune defects affecting both the numbers and functions of immune cells. The onset of the immune dysfunction is usually gradual except in infants with rapid progression. The insidious deterioration of immune function leads to increased susceptibility to a wide variety of pathogens and an increased risk of malignancy. The salient feature of the immunodeficiency is reduction in the number of $CD4^+$ T lymphocyte numbers and in the fraction of lymphocytes that are $CD4^+$ T cells. $CD4^+$ T cell counts are useful prognostic markers, which predict risk of progression, risk of particular opportunistic infections, and clinical response to therapy. $CD4^+$ T cell counts should be used in conjunction with plasma viral copy number and clinical manifestations for optimal management of HIV-1 disease. Highly active antiretroviral therapy is associated with improvement in many of the immunologic abnormalities that occur in progressive HIV-1 infection. Strategies that alter HIV-1-specific immunity are areas of active investigation with the hope that long-term outcome can be improved if immune defenses can be enhanced.

ACKNOWLEDGMENTS

The author thanks Tina Yee and Paul Harding for assistance in preparation of the manuscript.

REFERENCES

1. Spira, A. I., Marx, P. A., Patterson, B. K., *et al.* Cellular targets of infection and route of viral dissemination after an intravaginal inoculation of simian immunodeficiency virus into rhesus macaques. *J. Exp. Med.* **183** : **1** ((1996), 215–25.
2. McMichael, A. J. & Rowland-Jones, S. L. Cellular immune responses to HIV. *Nature* **410** (2001), 980–7.
3. Schmitz, J. E., Kuroda, M. J., Santra, S. *et al.* Control of viremia in simian immunodeficiency virus infection by CD8$^+$ lymphocytes. *Science* **283** : **5403** (1999), 857–60.
4. Metzner, K. J., Jin, X., Lee, F. V. *et al.* Effects of in vivo CD8$^{(+)}$ T cell depletion on virus replication in rhesus macaques immunized with a live, attenuated simian immunodeficiency virus vaccine. *J. Exp. Med.* **191** : **11** (2000), 1921–31.
5. Levy, J. A., Hsueh, F., Blackbourn, D. J., Wara, D. & Weintrub, P. S. CD8 cell noncytotoxic antiviral activity in human immunodeficiency virus-infected and -uninfected children. *J. Infect. Dis.* **177** : **2** (1998), 470–2.

6. Barker, E., Bossart, K. N. & Levy, J. A. Primary CD8⁺ cells from HIV-infected individuals can suppress productive infection of macrophages independent of beta-chemokines. *Proc. Natl. Acad. Sci. U.S.A.* **95** : **4** (1998), 1725–9.

7. Zhang, L., Yu, W., He, T. *et al.* Contribution of human alpha-defensin 1, 2, and 3 to the anti-HIV-1 activity of CD8 antiviral factor. *Science* **298** : **5595** (2002), 995–1000.

8. Shearer, W. T., Quinn, T. C., LaRussa, P. *et al.* Viral load and disease progression in infants infected with human immunodeficiency virus type 1. *New Engl. J. Med.* **336** (1997), 1337–42.

9. Luzuriaga, K., Holmes, D., Hereema, A., Wong, J., Panicali, D. L. & Sullivan, J. L. HIV-1-specific cytotoxic T lymphocyte responses in the first year of life. *J. Immunol.* **154** : **1** (1995), 433–43.

10. Spiegel, H. M., Chandwani, R., Sheehy, M. E. *et al.* The impact of early initiation of highly active antiretroviral therapy on the human immunodeficiency virus type-1 specific CD8 T cell response in children. *J. Infect. Dis.* **182**:1 (2000), 88–95.

11. McFarland, E. J., Harding, P. A., Luckey, D., Conway, B., Young, R. K. & Kuritzkes, D. R. High frequency of Gag- and envelope-specific cytotoxic T-lymphocyte precursors in children with vertically-acquired human immunodeficiency virus type-1-infection. *J. Infect. Dis.* **170** (1994), 766–74.

12. Pugatch, D., Sullivan, J. L., Pikora, C. A. & Luzuriaga, K. Delayed generation of antibodies mediating human immunodeficiency virus type 1-specific antibody-dependent cellular cytotoxicity in vertically infected infants. Women and Infants Transmission Study Group. *J. Infect. Dis.* **176** : **3** (1997), 643–8.

13. Pollack, H., Zhan, M. X., Safrit, J. T. *et al.* CD8⁺ T-cell-mediated suppression of HIV replication in the first year of life: association with lower viral load and favorable early survival. *AIDS* **11** : **1** (1997), F9–13.

14. Goulder, P. J., Brander, C., Tang, Y. *et al.* Evolution and transmission of stable CTL escape mutations in HIV infection. *Nature* **412** : **6844** (2001), 334–8.

15. Essajee, S. M., Pollack, H., Rochford, G., Oransky, I., Krasinski, K. & Borkowsky, W. Early changes in quasispecies repertoire in HIV-infected infants: correlation with disease progression. *AIDS Res Human Retroviruses* **16** : **18** (2000), 1949–57.

16. Ganeshan, S., Dickover, R. E., Korber, B. T., Bryson, Y. J. & Wolinsky, S. M. Human immunodeficiency virus type 1 genetic evolution in children with different rates of development of disease. *J. Virol.* **1997** : **71** (1997), 663–77.

17. Haase, A. T. Population biology of HIV-1 infection: viral and CD4⁺ T cell demographics and dynamics in lymphatic tissues. *Ann. Rev. Immunol.* **17** (1999), 625–56.

18. Smith-Franklin, B. A., Keele, B. F., Tew, J. G. *et al.* Follicular dendritic cells and the persistence of HIV infectivity: the role of antibodies and Fcgamma receptors. *J. Immunol.* **168** : **5** (2002), 2408–14.

19. McNeil, A. C., Shupert, W. L., Lyasere, C. A. *et al.* High-level HIV-1 viremia suppresses viral antigen-specific CD4(+) T cell proliferation. *Proc. Natl. Acad. Sci. U.S.A.* **98** : **24** (2001), 13878–83.

20. Douek, D. C., Brenchley, J. M., Betts, M. R. *et al.* HIV preferentially infects HIV-specific CD4⁺ T cells. *Nature* **417** : **6884** (2002), 95–8.

21. Appay, V., Nixon, D. F., Donahoe, S. M. *et al.* HIV-specific CD8(+) T cells produce antiviral cytokines but are impaired in cytolytic function. *J. Exp. Med.* **192** : **1** (2000), 63–75.

22. Champagne, P., Ogg, G. S., King, A. S. *et al.* Skewed maturation of memory HIV-specific CD8 T lymphocytes. *Nature* **410** (2001), 106–11.

23. Miguele, S. A., Laborico, A. C., Shupert, W. L. *et al.* HIV-specific CD8⁺ T cell proliferation is coupled to perforin expression and is maintained in nonprogressors. *Nat. Immunol.* **3** : **11** (2002), 1061–8.

24. Collins, K. L., Chen, B. K., Kalams, S. A., Walker, B. D. & Baltimore, D. HIV-1 Nef protein protects infected primary cells against killing by cytotoxic T lymphocytes. *Nature* **391** : **6665** (1998), 397–401.

25. Letvin, N. L., Barouch, D. H. & Montefiori, D. C. Prospects for vaccine protection against HIV-1 infection and AIDS. *Annu. Rev. Immunol.* **20** (2002), 73–99.

26. Birch, M. R., Learmont, J. C., Dyer, W. B. *et al.* An examination of signs of disease progression in survivors of the Sydney Blood Bank Cohort (SBBC). *J. Clin. Virol.* **22** : **3** (2001), 263–70.

27. Hogan, C. M. & Hammer, S. M. Host determinants in HIV infection and disease. Part 2: genetic factors and implications for antiretroviral therapeutics. *Ann. Int. Med.* **134** : **10** (2001), 978–96.

28. Rosenberg, E. S., Altfeld, M., Poon, S. H. *et al.* Immune control of HIV-1 after early treatment of acute infection. *Nature* **407** (2000), 523–6.

29. Luzuriaga, K., McManus, M., Catalina, M. *et al.* Early therapy of vertical human immunodeficiency virus type 1 (HIV-1) infection: control of viral replication and absence of persistent HIV-1-specific immune responses. *J. Virol.* **74** : **15** (2000), 6984–91.

30. Hainaut, M., Peltier, C. A., Marissens, D., Zissis, G. & Levy, J. Effectiveness of antiretroviral therapy initiated before the age of 2 months in infants vertically infected with human immunodeficiency virus type 1. *Eur. J. Pediatr.* **159** : **10** (2000), 778–82.

31. Borkowsky, W., Rigaud, M., Krasinski, K., Moore, T., Lawrence, R. & Pollack, H. Cell-mediated and humoral immune responses in children infected with human immunodeficiency virus during the first four years of life. *J. Pediatr.* **120** (1992), 371–5.

32. Roilides, E., Clerici, M., De Palma, L., Rubin, M., Pizzo, P. A. & Shearer, G. M. Helper T-cell responses in children infected with human immunodeficiency virus type 1. *J. Pediatr.* **118** (1991), 724–30.

33. Breen, E. C. Pro- and anti-inflammatory cytokines in human immunodeficiency virus infection and acquired immunodeficiency syndrome. *Pharmacol. Therapeut.* **95** : **3** (2002), 295–304.

34. Than, S., Hu, R., Oyaizu, N. *et al.* Cytokine pattern in relation to disease progression in human immunodeficiency virus-infected children. *J. Infect. Dis.* **175** (1997), 47–56.

35. Raszka, W. V., Moriarty, R. A., Ottolini, M. G. *et al.* Delayed-type hypersensitivity skin testing in human immunodeficiency virus-infected pediatric patients. *J. Pediatr.* **129** (1996), 245–50.

36. Ibegbu, C., Spira, T. J., Nesheim, S. *et al.* Subpopulations of T and B cells in perinatally HIV-infected and noninfected age-matched children with those in adults. *Clin. Immunol. Immunopath.* **71**:1 (1994), 27–32.

37. Douglas, S. D., Rudy, B., Muenz, L. *et al.* T-lymphocyte subsets in HIV-infected and high-risk HIV-uninfected adolescents: retention of naive T lymphocytes in HIV-infected adolescents. The Adolescent Medicine HIV/AIDS Research Network. *Arch. Pediatr. Adolesc. Med.* **154**:4 (2000), 375–80.

38. Pantaleo, G., Demarest, J. F., Schacker, T. *et al.* The qualitative nature of the primary immune response to HIV infection is a prognosticator of disease progression independent of the initial level of plasma viremia. *Proc. Natl. Acad. Sci. U.S.A.* **94**:1 (1997), 254–8.

39. McFarland, E. J., Harding, P. A., Striebich, C. C., MaWhinney, S., Kuritzkes, D. R. & Kotzin, B. L. Clonal CD8+ T cell expansions in peripheral blood from human immunodeficiency virus type-1 (HIV-1)-infected children. *J. Infect. Dis.* **186** (2002), 477–85.

40. Than, S., Kharbanda, M., Chitnis, V., Bakshi, S., Gregersen, P. K. & Pahwa, S. Clonal dominance patterns of CD8 T cells in relation to disease progression in HIV-infected children. *J. Immunol.* **162**:6 (1999), 3680–6.

41. Plaeger-Marshall S, Isacescu, V., O'Rourke, S., Bertolli, J., Bryson, Y. J. & Stiehm, E. R. T cell activation in pediatric AIDS pathogenesis: three-color immunophenotyping. *Clin. Immunol. Immunopath.* **71**:1 (1994), 19–26.

42. Gallagher, K., Gorre, M., Harawa, N. *et al.* Timing of lymphocyte activation in neonates infected with human immunodeficiency virus. *Clin. Diagn. Lab. Immunol.* **4**:6 (1997), 742–7.

43. Vigano, A., Pinti, M., Nasi, M. *et al.* Markers of cell death-activation in lymphocytes of vertically HIV-infected children naive to highly active antiretroviral therapy: the role of age. *J. Allergy. Clin. Immunol.* **108**:3 (2001), 439–45.

44. Bohler, T., Wintergerst, U., Linde, R., Belohradsky, B. H. & Debatin, K. M. CD95 (APO-1/Fas) expression on naive CD4(+) T cells increases with disease progression in HIV-infected children and adolescents: effect of highly active antiretroviral therapy (HAART). *Pediatr. Res.* **49**:1 (2001), 101–10.

45. Niehues, T., Ndagijimana, J., Horneff, G. & Wahn, V. CD28 expression in pediatric human immunodeficiency virus infection. *Pediatr. Res.* **44**:2 (1998), 265–8.

46. McCloskey, T. W., Oyaizu, N., Bakshi, S., Kowalski, R., Kohn, N. & Pahwa, S. CD95 expression and apoptosis during pediatric HIV infection: early upregulation of CD95 expression. *Clin. Immunol. Immunopath.* **87**:1 (1998), 33–41.

47. Bruunsgaard, H., Pedersen, C., Siknhof, P. & Pedersen, B. K. Clinical progression of HIV infection: role of NK cells. *Scand. J. Immunol.* **46**:1 (1997), 91–5.

48. Douglas, S. D., Durako, S. J., Tustin, N. B. *et al.* Natural killer cell enumeration and function in HIV-infected and high-risk uninfected adolescents. *AIDS Res. Hum. Retroviruses* **17**:6 (2001), 543–52.

49. Voiculescu, C., Avramescu, C., Balasoiu, M., Turculeanu, A. & Radu, E. Changes of blood CD16/CD56 (NK) and HLA-DR/CD3-positive lymphocyte amounts in HIV-infected children, as related to clinical progression and p24-antigen/p24-antibody presence. *FEMS Immunol. Med. Microbiol.* **9**:3 (1994), 217–21.

50. Scott-Algara, D., Vuillier, F., Cayota, A. & Dighiero, G. Natural killer (NK) cell activity during HIV infection: a decrease in NK activity is observed at the clonal level and is not restored after in vitro long-term culture of NK cells. *Clin. Exper. Immunol.* **90**:2 (1992), 181–7.

51. Ziegner, U., Campbell, D., Weinhold, K., Frank, I., Rutstein, R. & Starr, S. E. Deficient antibody-dependent cellular cytotoxicity against human immunodeficiency virus (HIV)-expressing target cells in perinatal HIV infection. *Clin. Diagn. Lab. Immunol.* **6**:5 (1999), 718–24.

52. Lin, S. J., Roberts, R. L., Ank, B. J., Nguyen, Q. H., Thomas, E. K. & Stiehm, E. R. Human immunodeficiency virus (HIV) type-1 gp120-specific cell-mediated cytotoxicity (CMC) and natural killer (NK) activity in HIV-infected (HIV+) subjects: enhancement with interleukin-2 (IL-2), IL-12, and IL-15. *Clin. Immunol. Immunopath.* **82**:2 (1997), 163–73.

53. Geijtenbeek, T. B., Kwon, D. S., Torensma, R. *et al.* DC-SIGN, a dendritic cell-specific HIV-1-binding protein that enhances trans-infection of T cells. *Cell* **100**:5 (2000), 587–97.

54. Engering, A., Van Vliet, S. J., Geijtenbeek, T. B. & Van Kooyk Y. Subset of DC-SIGN(+) dendritic cells in human blood transmits HIV-1 to T lymphocytes. *Blood* **100**:5 (2002), 1780–6.

55. Chehimi, J., Campbell, D. E., Azzoni, L. *et al.* Persistent decreases in blood plasmacytoid dendritic cell number and function despite effective highly active antiretroviral therapy and increased blood myeloid dendritic cells in HIV-infected individuals. *J. Immunol.* **168**:9 (2002), 4796–801.

56. Pacanowski, J., Kahi, S., Baillet, M. *et al.* Reduced blood CD123+ (lymphoid) and CD11c+ (myeloid) dendritic cell numbers in primary HIV-1 infection. *Blood* **98**:10 (2001), 3016–21.

57. Donaghy, H., Pozniak, A., Gazzard, B. *et al.* Loss of blood CD11c(+) myeloid and CD11c(−) plasmacytoid dendritic cells in patients with HIV-1 infection correlates with HIV-1 RNA virus load. *Blood* **98**:8 (2001), 2574–6.

58. Knight, S. C. Dendritic cells and HIV infection; immunity with viral transmission versus compromised cellular immunity. *Immunobiology* **204**:5 (2001), 614–21.

59. Noel, G. J. Host defense abnormalities associated with HIV infection. *Pediatr. Clin. N. Am.* **38**:1 (1991), 37–43.

60. Ma, X. & Montaner, L. J. Proinflammatory response and IL-12 expression in HIV-1 infection. *J. Leukocyte Biol.* **68**:3 (2000), 383–90.

61. Chougnet, C., Wynn, T. A., Clerici, M. *et al.* Molecular analysis of decreased interleukin-12 production in persons infected with human immunodeficiency virus. *J. Infect. Dis.* **174**:1 (1996), 46–53.

62. Chougnet, C., Thomas, E., Landay, A. L. *et al.* CD40 ligand and IFN-gamma synergistically restore IL-12 production in HIV-infected patients. *Eur. J. Immunol.* **28**:2 (1998), 646–56.

63. Marshall, J. D., Chehimi, J., Gri, G., Kostman, J. R., Montaner, L. J. & Trinchieri, G. The interleukin-12-mediated pathway of immune events is dysfunctional in human immunodeficiency virus-infected individuals. *Blood* **94** : **3** (1999), 1003–11.

64. Ito, M., Ishida, T., He, L. *et al.* HIV type 1 Tat protein inhibits interleukin 12 production by human peripheral blood mononuclear cells. *AIDS Res. Hum. Retroviruses* **14** : **10** (1998), 845–9.

65. Taoufik, Y., Lantz, O., Wallon, C. *et al.* Human immunodeficiency virus gp120 inhibits interleukin-12 secretion by human monocytes: an indirect interleukin -10-mediated effect. *Blood* **89** : **8** (1997), 2842–8.

66. Subauste, C. S., Wessendarp, M., Smulian, A. G. & Frame, P. T. Role of CD40 ligand signaling in defective type 1 cytokine response in human immunodeficiency virus infection. *J. Infect. Dis.* **183** : **12** (2001), 1722–31.

67. Chehimi, J., Starr, S. E., Frank, I. *et al.* Impaired interleukin-12 production in human immunodeficiency virus-infected patients. *J. Exp. Med.* **179** (1994), 1361–6.

68. Uherova, P., Connick, E., MaWhinney, S., Schlichtemeier, R., Schooley, R. T. & Kuritzkes, D. R. In vitro effect of interleukin-12 on antigen-specific lymphocyte proliferative responses from persons infected with human immunodeficiency virus type 1. *J. Infect. Dis.* **174** (1996), 483–9.

69. McFarland, E. J., Harding, P. A., MaWhinney, S., Schooley, R. T. & Kuritzkes, D. R. In vitro effects of interleukin-12 on human immunodeficiency virus type 1 (HIV-1)-specific cytotoxic T-lymphocytes from HIV-1 infected children. *J. Immunol.* **161** (1998), 513–19.

70. Feldman, S., Stein, D., Amrute, S. *et al.* Decreased interferon-alpha production in HIV-infected patients correlates with numerical and functional deficiencies in circulating type 2 dendritic cell precursors. *Clin. Immunol.* **101** : **2** (2001), 201–10.

71. Crammer Bornemann, M. A., Verhoef, J. & Peterson, P. K. Macrophages, cytokines, and HIV. *J. Lab. Clin. Med.* **129** (1997), 10–16.

72. Meddows-Taylor, S., Kuhn, L., Meyers, T. M. & Tiemessen, C. T. Altered expression of L-selectin (CD62L) on polymorphonuclear neutrophils of children vertically infected with human immunodeficiency virus type 1. *J. Clin. Immunol.* **21** : **4** (2001), 286–92.

73. Meddows-Taylor, S., Kuhn, L., Meyers, T. M., Sherman, G. & Tiemessen, C. T. Defective neutrophil degranulation induced by interleukin-8 and complement 5a and down-regulation of associated receptors in children vertically infected with human immunodeficiency virus type 1. *Clin. Diagn. Lab. Immunol.* **8** : **1** (2001), 21–30.

74. Mastroianni, C. M., Lichtner, M., Mengoni, F. *et al.* Improvement in neutrophil and monocyte function during highly active antiretroviral treatment of HIV-1-infected patients. *AIDS* **13** : **8** (1999), 883–90.

75. Maloney, M. J., Guill, M. F., Wray, B. B., Lobel, S. A. & Ebbeling, W. Pediatric acquired immune deficiency syndrome with panhypogammaglobulinemia. *J. Pediatr.* **110** (1987), 266–7.

76. Pahwa, S., Fikrig, S., Menez, R. & Pahwa, R. Pediatric acquired immunodeficiency syndrome: demonstration of B lymphocyte defects in vitro. *Diagn. Immunol.* **4** : **1** (1986), 24–30.

77. de Martino, M., Tovo, P. A., Galli, L. *et al.* Prognostic significance of immunologic changes in 675 infants perinatally exposed to human immunodeficiency virus. *J. Pediatr.* **119** (1991), 702–9.

78. Zouali, M. Nonrandom features of the human immunoglobulin variable region gene repertoire expressed in response to HIV-1. *Appl. Biochem. Biotech.* **61** : **1–2** (1996), 149–55.

79. Muller, S. & Kohler, H. B cell superantigens in HIV-1 infection. *Int. Rev. Immunol.* **14** : **4** (1997), 339–49.

80. Muller, F., Aukrust, P., Nordoy, I. & Froland, S. S. Possible role of interleukin-10 (IL-10) and CD40 ligand expression in the pathogenesis of hypergammaglobulinemia in human immunodeficiency virus infection: modulation of IL-10 and Ig production after intravenous Ig infusion. *Blood* **92** : **10** (1998), 3721–9.

81. Kacani, L., Stoiber, H. & Dierich, M. P. Role of IL-15 in HIV-1-associated hypergammaglobulinaemia. *Clin. Exper. Immunol.* **108** : **1** (1997), 14–18.

82. Rutstein, R. M., Rudy, B., Codispoti, C. & Watson, B. Response to hepatitis B immunization by infants exposed to HIV. *AIDS* **8** (1994), 1281–4.

83. Arpadi, S. M., Markowitz, L. E., Baughman, A. L. *et al.* Measles antibody in vaccinated human immunodeficiency virus type 1-infected children. *Pediatrics* **97** : **5** (1996), 653–7.

84. Gibb, D., Spoulou, V., Giacomelli, A. *et al.* Antibody responses to haemophilus influenzae type b and streptococcus pneumoniae vaccines in children with human immunodeficiency virus infection. *Pediatr. Infect. Dis. J.* **14** (1995), 129–35.

85. Lyall, E. G., Charlett, A., Watkins, P. & Zambon, M. Response to influenza virus vaccination in vertical HIV infection. *Arch. Dis. Child.* **76** : **3** (1997), 215–18.

86. Moir, S., Malaspina, A., Ogwaro, K. M. *et al.* HIV-1 induces phenotypic and functional perturbations of B cells in chronically infected individuals. *Proc. Natl. Acad. Sci. U.S.A.* **98** : **18** (2001), 10362–7.

87. Rodriguez, C., Thomas, J. K., O'Rourke, S., Stiehm, E. R. & Plaeger, S. HIV disease in children is associated with a selective decrease in CD23[+] and CD62L[+] B cells. *Clin. Immunol. Immunopath.* **81** : **2** (1996), 191–9.

88. Chirmule, N., Oyaizu, N., Kalyanaraman, V. S. & Pahwa, S. Inhibition of normal B-cell function by human immunodeficiency virus envelope glycoprotein, gp120. *Blood* **79** : **5** (1992), 1245–54.

89. Centers for Disease Control. 1997 revised guidelines for performing CD4[+] T-cell determinations in persons infected with human immunodeficiency virus (HIV). *MMWR* **46** : **RR-2, RR-2** (1997), 1–29.

90. Centers for Disease Control. Guidelines for performing single-platform absolute CD4[+] T-cell determinations with CD45 gating for persons infected with human immunodeficiency virus. *MMWR* **52** : **RR-2, RR-2** (2003), 1–13.

91. Malone, J. L., Simms, T. E., Gray, G. C., Wagner, K. F., Burge, J. R. & Burke, D. S. Sources of variability in repeated T-helper lymphocyte counts from human immunodeficiency virus type 1-infected patients: total lymphocyte count fluctuations and diurnal cycle are important. *J. AIDS* **3**:2 (1990), 144–51.

92. Hughes, M. D., Stein, D. S., Gundacker, H. M., Valentine, F. T., Phair, J. P. & Volberding, P. A. Within-subject variation in CD4 lymphocyte count in asymptomatic human immunodeficiency virus infection: implication for patient monitoring. *J. Infect. Dis.* **169** (1994), 28–36.

93. Tornatore, K. M., Venuto, R. C., Logue, G. & Davis, P. J. CD4$^+$ and CD8$^+$ lymphocyte and cortisol response patterns in elderly and young males after methylprednisolone exposure. *J. Med.* **29**:3–4 (1998), 159–83.

94. Laurence, J. T-cell subsets in health, infectious disease and idiopathic CD4$^+$ T lymphocytopenia. *Ann. Intern. Med.* **119** (1993), 55–62.

95. Raszka, W. V. J., Meyer, G. A., Waecker, N. J. *et al.* Variability of serial absolute and percent CD4$^+$ lymphocyte counts in healthy children born to human immunodeficiency virus 1-infected parents. *Pediatr. Infect. Dis. J.* **13**:1 (1994), 70–2.

96. Shearer, W. T., Rosenblatt, H. M., Schluchter, M. D. *et al.* Immunologic targets of HIV infection: T cells. *Ann. N. Y. Acad. Sci.* **693** (1993), 35–51.

97. Centers for Disease Control. 1994 revised classification system for human immunodeficiency virus infection in children less than 13 years of age. *MMWR* **43**:RR-12, RR-12 (1994), 1–10.

98. Palumbo, P. E., Raskino, C., Fiscus, S. *et al.* Predictive value of quantitative plasma HIV RNA and CD4 lymphocyte count for disease progression and response to therapy in HIV-infected infants. *J. Am. Med. Assoc.* **279** (1998), 756–61.

99. Mofenson, L. M., Korelitz, J., Meyer, W. A. *et al.* The relationship between serum human immunodeficiency virus type 1 (HIV-1) RNA level, CD4 lymphocyte percent, and long-term mortality risk in HIV-1-infected children. National Institute of Child Health and Human Development Intravenous Immunoglobulin Clinical Trial Study Group. *J. Infect. Dis.* **175**:5 (1997), 1029–38.

100. Mueller, B. U., Zeichner, S. L., Kuznetsov, V. A., Heath-Chiozzi, M., Pizzo, P. A. & Dimitrov, D. S. Individual prognoses of long-term responses to antiretroviral treatment based on virological, immunological and pharmacological parameters measured during the first week under therapy. *AIDS* **12**:15 (1998), F191–6.

101. Kourtis, A. P., Ibegbu, C., Nahmias, A. J. *et al.* Early progression of disease in HIV-infected infants with thymus dysfunction. *New Engl. J. Med.* **335**:19 (1996), 1431–6.

102. Simonds, R. J., Lindegren, M. L., Thomas, P. *et al.* Prophylaxis against *Pneumocystis carinii* pneumonia among children with perinatally acquired human immunodeficiency virus infection in the United States. *Pneumocystis carinii* Pneumonia Prophylaxis Evaluation Working Group. *New Engl. J. Med.* **332**:12 (1995), 786–90.

103. Autran, B., Carcelain, G. & Debre, P. Immune reconstitution after highly active anti-retroviral treatment of HIV infection. *Adv. Exp. Med. Biol.* **495** (2001), 205–12.

104. Lederman, M. M. Immune restoration and CD4$^+$ T-cell function with antiretroviral therapies. *AIDS* **15**:Suppl. 2 (2001), S11–15.

105. Sleasman, J. W., Nelson, R. P., Goodenow, M. M. *et al.* Immunoreconstitution after ritonavir therapy in children with human immunodeficiency virus infection involves multiple lymphocyte lineages. *J. Pediatr.* **134**:5 (1999), 597–606.

106. Essajee, S. M., Kim, M., Gonzalez, C. *et al.* Immunologic and virologic responses to HAART in severely immunocompromised HIV-1-infected children. *AIDS* **13**:18 (1999), 2523–32.

107. Hainaut, M., Ducarme, M., Schandene, L. *et al.* Age-related immune reconstitution during highly active antiretroviral therapy in human immunodeficiency virus type 1-infected children. *Pediatr. Infect. Dis. J.* **22**:1 (2003), 62–9.

108. van Rossum, A. M., Scherpbier, H. J., van Lochem, E. G. *et al.* Therapeutic immune reconstitution in HIV-1-infected children is independent of their age and pretreatment immune status. *AIDS* **15**:17 (2001), 2267–75.

109. Chavan, S., Bennuri, B., Kharbanda, M., Chandrasekaran, A., Bakshi, S. & Pahwa, S. Evaluation of T cell receptor gene rearrangement excision circles after antiretroviral therapy in children infected with human immunodeficiency virus. *J. Infect. Dis.* **183**:10 (2001), 1445–54.

110. Gibb, D. M., Newberry, A., Klein, N., de Rossi, A., Grosch-Woerner, I. & Babiker, A. Immune repopulation after HAART in previously untreated HIV-1-infected children. *Lancet* **355**:9212 (2000), 1331–2.

111. Ometto, L., De Forni, D., Patiri, F. *et al.* Immune reconstitution in HIV-1-infected children on antiretroviral therapy: role of thymic output and viral fitness. *AIDS* **16**:6 (2002), 839–49.

112. Douek, D. C., Koup, R. A., McFarland, R. D., Sullivan, J. L. & Luzuriaga, K. Effect of HIV on thymic function before and after antiretroviral therapy in children. *J. Infect. Dis.* **181**:4 (2000), 1479–82.

113. Vigano, A., Dally, L., Bricalli, D. *et al.* Clinical and immuno-virologic characterization of the efficacy of stavudine, lamivudine, and indinavir in human immunodeficiency virus infection. *J. Pediatr.* **135** (1999), 675–82.

114. Perruzzi, M., Azzari, C., Galli, L., Vierucci, A. & de Martino, M. Highly active antiretroviral therapy restores in vitro mitogen and antigen-specific T-lymphocyte responses in HIV-1 perinatally infected children despite virological failure. *Clin. Exp. Immunol.* **128**:2 (2002), 365–71.

115. Havlir, D. V., Schrier, R. D., Torriani, F. J., Chervenak, K., Hwang, J. Y. & Boom, W. H. Effect of potent antiretroviral therapy on immune responses to *Mycobacterium avium* in human immunodeficiency virus-infected subjects. *J. Infect. Dis.* **182**:6 (2000), 1658–63.

116. Berkelhamer, S., Borock, E., Elsen, C., Englund, J. & Johnson, D. Effect of highly active antiretroviral therapy on the serological response to additional measles vaccinations in human

immunodeficiency virus-infected children. *Clin. Infect. Dis.* **32**:**7** (2001), 1090–4.

117. Notermans, D. W., de Jong, J. J., Goudsmit, J. *et al.* Potent antiretroviral therapy initiates normalization of hypergammaglobulinemia and a decline in HIV type 1-specific antibody responses. *AIDS Res. Hum. Retroviruses* **17**:**11** (2001), 1003–8.

118. Morris, L., Binley, J. M., Clas, B. A. *et al.* HIV-1 antigen-specific and -nonspecific B cell responses are sensitive to combination antiretroviral therapy. *J. Exp. Med.* **188**:**2** (1998), 233–45.

119. Jacobson, M. A., Bashi-Khayam, H., Martin, J. N., Black, D. & Ng, V. Effect of long-term highly active antiretroviral therapy in restoring HIV-induced abnormal B-lymphocyte function. *J. AIDS* **31** (2002), 472–7.

120. Borkowsky, W., Stanley, K., Douglas, S. D. *et al.* Immunologic response to combination nucleoside analogue plus protease inhibitor therapy in stable antiretroviral therapy-experienced human immunodeficiency virus-infected children. *J. Infect. Dis.* **182**:**1** (2000), 96–103.

121. Spiegel, H., DeFalcon, E., Ogg, G. *et al.* Changes in frequency of HIV-1-specific cytotoxic T cell precursors and circulating effectors after combination antiretroviral therapy in children. *J. Infect. Dis.* **180**:**8** (1999), 359–68.

122. Jankelevich, S., Mueller, B. U., Mackall, C. L. *et al.* Long-term virologic and immunologic responses in human immunodeficiency virus type 1-infected children treated with indinavir, zidovudine and lamivudine. *J. Infect. Dis.* **183**:**7** (2001), 116–20.

123. Deeks, S. G., Barbour, J. D., Grant, R. M. & Martin, J. N. Duration and predictors of CD4 T-cell gains in patients who continue combination therapy despite detectable plasma viremia. *AIDS* **16**:**2** (2002), 201–7.

124. Piketty, C., Weiss, L., Thomas, F., Mohamed, A. S., Belec, L. & Kazatchkine, M. D. Long-term clinical outcome of human immunodeficiency virus-infected patients with discordant immunologic and virologic responses to a protease inhibitor-containing regimen. *J. Infect. Dis.* **183**:**9** (2001), 1328–35.

125. Grabar, S., Le Moing, V., Goujard, C. *et al.* Clinical outcome of patients with HIV-1 infection according to immunologic and virologic response after 6 months of highly active antiretroviral therapy. *Ann. Int. Med.* **133**:**6** (2000), 401–10.

126. Nikolic-Djokic, D., Essajee, S., Rigaud, M. *et al.* Immunoreconstitution in children receiving highly active antiretroviral therapy depends on the CD4 cell percentage at baseline. *J. Infect. Dis.* **185**:**3** (2002), 290–8.

127. Stoddart, C. A., Liegler, T. J., Mammano, F. *et al.* Impaired replication of protease inhibitor-resistant HIV-1 in human thymus. *Nat. Med.* **7**:**6** (2001), 712–18.

128. Deeks, S. G., Hoh, R., Grant, R. M. *et al.* CD4$^+$ T cell kinetics and activation in human immunodeficiency virus-infected patients who remain viremic despite long-term treatment with protease inhibitor-based therapy. *J. Infect. Dis.* **185**:**3** (2002), 315–23.

129. Hawley-Foss, N., Mbisa, G., Lum, J. J. *et al.* Effect of cessation of highly active antiretroviral therapy during a discor-dant response: implications for scheduled therapeutic inter-ruptions. *Clin. Infect. Dis.* **33**:**3** (2001), 344–8.

130. Johnston, A. M., Valentine, M. E., Ottinger, J. *et al.* Immune reconstitution in human immunodeficiency virus-infected children receiving highly active antiretroviral therapy: a cohort study. *Pediatr. Infect. Dis. J.* **20**:**10** (2001), 941–6.

131. King, D. J., Gotch, F. M., Larsson-Sciard, E. L. & Pediatric European Network for Treatment of AIDS (PENTA). T-cell re-population in HIV-infected children on highly active anti-retroviral therapy. *Clin. Exp. Immunol.* **125**:**3** (2001), 447–54.

132. Kharbanda, M., Than, S., Chitnis, V. *et al.* Patterns of CD8 T cell clonal dominance in response to change in antiretro-viral therapy in HIV-infected children. *AIDS* **14** (2000), 2229–38.

133. Resino, S., Bellon, J. M., Sanchez-Ramon, S., Gurbindo, D. & Munoz-Fernandez, M. A. Clinical relevance of cytokine pro-duction in HIV-1 infection in children on antiretroviral ther-apy. *Scand. J. Immunol.* **52** (2000), 634–40.

134. Chougnet, C., Jankelevich, S., Fowke, K. *et al.* Long-term pro-tease inhibitor-containing therapy results in limited improve-ment in T cell function not restoration of IL-12 production in pediatric patients with AIDS. *J. Infect. Dis.* **184**:**2** (2001), 201–5.

135. Mascola, J. R., Stiegler, G., VanCott, T. C. *et al.* Protection of macaques against vaginal transmission of a pathogenic HIV-1/SIV chimeric virus by passive infusion of neutralizing anti-bodies. *Nat. Med.* **6** (2000), 207–10.

136. Hofmann-Lehmann, R., Vlasak, J., Rasmussen, R. A. *et al.* Postnatal passive immunization of neonatal macaques with a triple combination of human monoclonal antibodies against oral simian-human immunodeficiency virus challenge. *J. Virol.* **75** (2001), 70–80.

137. Letvin, N. L., Montefiori, D. C., Yasutomi, Y. *et al.* Potent, pro-tective anti-HIV immune responses generated by bimodal HIV envelope DNA plus protein vaccination. *Proc. Natl. Acad. Sci. U.S.A.* **94** (1997), 9378–83.

138. Earl, P. L., Sugiura, W., Montefiori, D. C. *et al.* Immunogenicity and protective efficacy of oligomeric human immunodefi-ciency virus type 1 gp140. *J. Virol.* **75** (2001), 645–53.

139. Cho, M. W., Kim, Y. B., Lee, M. K. *et al.* Polyvalent enve-lope glycoprotein vaccine elicits a broader neutralizing anti-body response but is unable to provide sterilizing protec-tion against heterologous simian/human immunodeficiency virus infection in pigtailed macaques. *J. Virol.* **75** (2001), 2224–34.

140. Graham, B. S. Clinical trials of HIV vaccines. *Annu. Rev. Med.* **53** (2002), 207–21.

141. McElrath, M., Corey, L., Montefiori, D. *et al.* A Phase II study of two HIV Type 1 envelope vaccines, comparing their immuno-genicity in population at risk for acquired HIV type 1 infection. *AIDS Res. Hum. Retroviruses* **16**:**9** (2000), 907–19.

142. Kahn, J., Sinangil, F., Baenziger, J. *et al.* Clinical and immuno-logic responses to human immunodeficiency virus (HIV) type 1SF2gp120 subunit vaccine combined with MF59

adjuvant with or without muramyl tripeptide dipalmitoyl phosphatidylethanolamine in non-HIV-infected human volunteers. *J. Infect. Dis.* **170** (1994), 1288–91.

143. Belshe, R. B., Stevens, C., Gorse, G. J. *et al.* Safety and immunogenicity of a canarypox-vectored human immunodeficiency virus Type 1 vaccine with or without gp120: a phase 2 study in higher and lower risk volunteers. *J. Infect. Dis.* **183**:9 (2001), 1343–52.

144. Allen, T. M., Vogel, T. U., Fuller, D. H. *et al.* Induction of AIDS virus-specific CTL activity in fresh, unstimulated peripheral blood lymphocytes from rhesus macaques vaccinated with a DNA prime/modified vaccinia virus Ankara boost regimen. *J. Immunol.* **164**:9 (2000), 4968–78.

145. Barouch, D. H., Santra, S., Schmitz, J. E. *et al.* Control of viremia and prevention of clinical AIDS in rhesus monkeys by cytokine-augmented DNA vaccination. *Science* **290**:**5491** (2000), 486–92.

146. Amara, R. R., Villinger, F., Altman, J. D. *et al.* Control of a mucosal challenge and prevention of AIDS by a multiprotein DNA/MVA vaccine. *Science* **292**:**5514** (2001), 69–74.

147. McFarland, E. J., Borkowsky, W., Fenton, T. *et al.* Serologic responses to HIV-1 envelope in neonates receiving a HIV-1 recombinant gp120 vaccine. *J. Infect. Dis.* **184** (2001), 1331–5.

148. Borkowsky, W., Wara, D., Fenton, T. *et al.* Lymphoproliferative responses to recombinant HIV-1 envelope antigens in neonates and infants receiving gp120 vaccines. *J. Infect. Dis.* **181** (2000), 890–6.

149. Cunningham, C., Wara, D., Kang, M. *et al.* Safety of two recombinant HIV-1 envelope vaccines in neonates born to HIV-1 infected women. *Clin. Infect. Dis.* **32** (2001), 801–7.

4

The clinical virology of pediatric HIV disease

Paul Palumbo, M.D.

Departments of Pediatrics and of Biochemistry and Molecular Biology, UMDNJ-New Jersey Medical School, Newark, NJ

The advent of potent antiretroviral therapy and effective prophylaxis for opportunistic infections has created a clear need for early diagnosis of HIV infection in pediatric patients and for methods of monitoring disease course and response to therapy. The field has undergone substantial progress within the past decade and innovations continue to emerge. Diagnostic issues will be addressed initially in this chapter, followed by virologic approaches for monitoring disease course and response to therapy.

4.1 Virologic assays for the diagnosis of pediatric HIV infection

4.1.1 Serology

Reports of the isolation of a human immunodeficiency virus (LAV; HTLV-III; later to be known as HIV-1) in 1984 [1–4] were quickly followed by the development of enzyme immunoassays (EIAs) capable of detecting a human antibody response to infection [5, 6]. It soon became clear that reactive EIAs required confirmation by Western blot to verify that the EIA-detected immune response was HIV-specific. While confirmation is essential for all EIA-reactive specimens, it is particularly important in low-risk populations where the positive predictive value of EIA is relatively low [7–10]. This issue has recently resurfaced in the context of rapid antibody tests, which can provide test results soon after the specimen is obtained at the same visit [11]. These rapid diagnostic tests can be performed in 10–30 minutes, an appealing feature for relatively non-compliant populations and for pregnant women at labor and delivery with an unknown HIV infection status. These rapid assays have similar performance characteristics as the standard EIA and thus have a troublesome false positive rate, which varies with the prevalence of HIV infection. Overall, the false positive rate has been estimated by the CDC as 0.4% of all persons tested and as high as 18% of all initial reactive results, particularly in low-prevalence populations. The United States (U.S.) Public Health Service recommends the consideration of this alternative rapid diagnostic approach, i.e. rapid screening with reporting of results during the same clinic visit, followed by confirmatory assays in the event of reactive assays [11]. Currently, there are two rapid tests licensed by the FDA (Murex Single Use Diagnostic System (SUDS) HIV-1 test, Abbott Laboratories, Inc., Abbott Park, ILL; and OraQuick Rapid HIV-1 Antibody Test, OraSure Technologies, Inc., Bethlehem, PA). The former requires an on-site laboratory while the latter is a self-contained system that can be performed at the bedside or in the clinic. There are many additional rapid tests and assay formats which can be performed with relative ease but which have not yet received U.S. regulatory approval. A possible future approach is the confirmation of rapid test results with a second rapid test, allowing same visit results and decision-making with the high sensitivity, specificity, and predictive value of the standard EIA/Western blot approach [12]. Clinical trials evaluating rapid tests during labor and delivery are underway.

The serologic diagnostic approach remains the method of choice for adults and children over 2 years of age, but its utility is critically compromised in young infants due to transplacental passage of HIV antibody from their HIV-infected mothers. Virtually all newborns and infants of such mothers will test positive for HIV antibody, regardless of whether the virus was actually transmitted. Relatively rare exceptions include hypo- or agammaglobulinemia and extreme prematurity (the majority of antibody is transferred during the third trimester). Early in the HIV pandemic, clinicians caring for HIV-exposed infants were limited to following the loss or persistence of antibody over a period as long as 18 months before being able to establish infection status. As with many other perinatal infections, detection of infant IgM antibodies has not proven feasible, while the use of IgA-specific antibody assays are most sensitive after 6 months of age and have not gained wide acceptance[13–18]. Serological assays for diagnosis of HIV infection are discussed in more detail in Chapter 7.

4.1.2 Viral detection

The mainstays of diagnosis during the first 18 months of life are direct virologic detection assays, specifically polymerase chain reaction (PCR), viral culture, and viral p24 antigen detection. While all of these assays have targeted applications, HIV DNA PCR performed on peripheral blood mononuclear cells has become the most widely used due to considerations such as accuracy, cost, and performance time.

Viral culture

In vitro cultivation of HIV from peripheral blood cells was one of the earliest viral detection assays developed and applied to diagnosis in infancy [19–22]. In this approach, peripheral blood mononuclear cells are co-cultivated with an equal number of peripheral blood mononuclear cells (PBMCs) from an uninfected donor. All cells are first stimulated by cultivation with phytohemaglutinin (PHA) to ensure optimum conditions for viral replication. Ideally, five million PBMCs from both patient and donor are co-cultivated for 2–4 weeks in the presence of IL-2. Supernatant from the culture is collected periodically and tested for p24 antigen (see below); p24 detection on two sequential samplings defines a positive result. Fortunately for pediatric applications, the use of fewer cells (1–2 million) has proven reliable for diagnosis in infancy [19]. The majority of positive specimens will be detected within a 7–14 day incubation period, while declaring a culture negative requires 3–4 weeks of total sampling. Culture can also be performed in a quantitative format using serial dilution of PBMCs.

p24 antigen detection

p24 antigen is a protein from the HIV core that can be detected in clinical specimens using a commercially available EIA format. Classically, antibody to p24 antigen is affixed to a solid phase – either a bead or the wells of a plastic microtiter plate. The latter is incubated with a small volume of the patient specimen, usually plasma or serum. If p24 antigen is present in the specimen, an antigen–antibody complex forms, capturing the p24 antigen on the solid phase. Following extensive washing, the antigen–antibody complex can be detected by a second, enzyme-labeled, p24 antigen-specific antibody. While this assay is straightforward and rapid, it has two shortcomings for early pediatric diagnosis: (1) false positives can occur in the first month of life, most probably due to passive transfer of maternal p24 antigen across the placenta without actual infection; and (2) antigen complexed with HIV antibody in the specimen is not detectable with this technique. This is especially problematic in infancy where there is antibody excess due to maternal antibody. This problem can be circumvented by immune complex dissociation prior to p24 antigen detection, which can be accomplished by acid treatment or boiling [23–26] and sensitivity can be enhanced by combination with signal amplification [27, 28]. Currently, there is considerable interest in p24 antigen assays in resource-poor settings for both diagnosis and disease monitoring because it costs less and is simpler to perform than other measures of viral load, but definitive studies assessing the utility of p24 assays in such settings have not been completed.

HIV DNA polymerase chain reaction

HIV DNA polymerase chain reaction (PCR) to detect HIV provirus within peripheral blood mononuclear cells was developed in the late 1980s and has been used extensively for pediatric diagnosis [29]. The PCR process enzymatically copies a targeted gene fragment billions of times, making small amounts of HIV DNA easily detectable. "Primer pairs" – small, synthesized pieces of DNA about 20 nucleotides long – are designed to hybridize specifically to selected regions of the viral target gene and not to other viral or cellular genes. In the assay, the primers are allowed to bind to the target DNA, initiating the synthesis of a copy of the DNA by DNA polymerase. This process is repeated 30–35 times with the newly synthesized DNA copies serving, in turn, as templates for the next round of synthesis, producing an exponential amplification of the target DNA within hours. Diagnostic PCR assays are optimized for extreme sensitivity, and can detect 1–10 viral targets/sample. False positives that can result from specimen contamination with PCR product are a concern. Laboratory procedures and quality controlled commercial reagent kits have been developed which greatly reduce false positive results [30].

The use of blood collected from a heel-stick procedure onto dried filter paper (Guthrie cards) for newborn diagnosis by means of DNA PCR has been studied and validated [31–35]. This approach has appeal for studies conducted in technically challenging environments and may be employed for routine infant screening in the future.

Studies have shown that virus culture and DNA PCR are sensitive and specific [36–38]. The diagnosis of HIV infection in the newborn is discussed in more detail in Chapter 7.

DNA PCR assays were initially developed to detect the prevalent HIV strains (clade B) present in the USA. In recognition of the multiple clades encountered throughout the world, diagnostic PCR kits have been developed incorporating primers that can recognize and bind to target DNAs from essentially all HIV clades. This holds true for disease monitoring HIV RNA quantitation kits (both PCR and other non-PCR-based methodologies such as branched DNA and nucleic acid sequence-based amplification assays – see below). While these disease-monitoring assays are not marketed with performance characteristics, sensitivity, and specificity, optimized for diagnostic use, the assays have been employed for the diagnosis of HIV infection in newborns and infants in some settings due to their widespread availability.

4.2 Viral assays for monitoring HIV infection

4.2.1 HIV RNA quantitation

The introduction of assays capable of accurately quantitating RNA within plasma virions has greatly enhanced the clinician's ability to predict the course of infection and response to therapy. These assays were developed and subsequently introduced in the early 1990s and have since been validated in the clinical setting. The first of these assays was reverse transcription-polymerase chain reaction (RT-PCR) which is commercially available as the Roche Amplicor HIV-1 Monitor® and Amplicor HIV-1 Monitor Ultrasensitive® assays. In these assays reverse transcription of viral RNA into a DNA copy is followed by DNA amplification by means of PCR. An internal control is co-amplified for quantitative purposes. The regular Amplicor HIV-1 Monitor assay has been in use most extensively and has a lower limit of quantitation of 400 viral copies/mL of plasma. More recently, Roche has introduced the Ultrasensitive assay, with a lower quantitation limit of 20–100 copies/mL.

A second assay known as NASBA® (**n**ucleic **a**cid **s**equence-**b**ased **a**mplification) also amplifies target RNA and is commercially available through Organon-Teknika. NASBA is an isothermal amplification reaction which employs three enzymes: reverse transcriptase, RNAse H, and T7 DNA polymerase. It also utilizes internal controls

Table 4.1 Quantitative HIV RNA assays

Assay	Version	Dynamic range	Quantitation limit
RT-PCR	Amplicor HIV-1Monitor	$10^{2.6}$–$10^{5.9}$	400
(Roche)	Amplicor HIV-1Monitor Ultrasensitive	$10^{1.7}$–$10^{5.0}$	50
NASBA	HIV-1 RNA QT	$10^{2.6}$–$10^{7.6}$	400
(Organon-Teknika)	NucliSens	$10^{1.9}$–$10^{7.6}$	80
Branched DNA	Version 1	$10^{4.0}$–$10^{6.2}$	10,000
(Chiron/Bayer)	Version 2	$10^{2.6}$–$10^{6.2}$	400
	Version 3	$10^{1.7}$–??	50

All units are copies/ml.

as quantitation standards, and has a lower limit of quantitation of 1000 copies/mL. A second generation assay – NucliSens® – can quantitate as little as 80–400 copies/mL of plasma, depending on the sample input.

The third commercially available, quantitative assay is the branched DNA assay manufactured by Chiron/Bayer. This assay uses a somewhat different technique than the previous two assays: it amplifies the signal created following capture of viral RNA by nucleic acid hybridization. It is technically the easiest assay to perform, resulting in the highest reproducibility. Unfortunately, the standard assay requires 1 mL of plasma, which makes its use impractical for pediatrics. The initial version of the assay had a quantitation limit of 10000 copies/mL, but newer versions have a lower detection limit of 200 copies/mL.

All of the assays have been extensively tested and validated (see Table 4.1), but there is some sample-to-sample variation in the assays. Samples must show at least a 3-fold ($0.5\log_{10}$) difference for this to be considered significant. For example, two samples from a child drawn 1 month apart are reported as 40 000 and 100 000 copies/mL. These two results are not significantly different from each other since they do not differ by 3-fold. In addition to this performance feature, clinicians should be aware that intercurrent infections and immunizations can activate viral replication and raise RNA levels briefly [39–44]. As with many laboratory tests, clinical decisions should prudently be based on reproducibility between sequential specimens over time and on a composite of clinical and laboratory observations. It would be clinically unwise to make a major change in management on the basis of a single viral load assay.

4.2.2 Kinetics of viral replication

The advent of accurate quantitative RNA assays in combination with potent antiretroviral agents allowed the delineation of viral replication kinetics. Two groups simultaneously reported that the average virion generation time was estimated to be 2.6 days, that plasma virions possess a half life of 6 hours, and that about 10 billion viral particles are produced within an untreated HIV-infected person each day [45, 46]. These rapid kinetics in combination with the tendency of the HIV reverse transcriptase enzyme to introduce mutations when it copies the HIV genome implies that the mutation rate is extraordinarily high: a virus with a mutation at each nucleic acid base within the HIV genome could theoretically be produced within an infected patient each day. These findings argue that antiretroviral drug regimens should produce complete suppression of viral replication to avoid the rapid selection of drug-resistant mutant virus.

In the heady early days following the introduction of HIV protease inhibitors, some postulated that relatively short periods of antiretroviral therapy would be sufficient to eradicate infection. This enthusiasm has been tempered somewhat with the demonstration of long-lived cellular reservoirs in the setting of relatively long-term suppression of plasma virus [46–49]. Individuals in whom plasma virus is non-detectable for years have remained positive for proviral DNA within circulating mononuclear cells and for culturable virus [47, 49–51]. These studies have demonstrated that quiescent memory CD4$^+$ T lymphocytes are the hosts for persistent proviral genomes and their frequency is quite low (1 in 1–10 million cells). While difficult to measure, the calculated decay rates for this cellular reservoir are very slow, with elimination times measured in decades or life times. Treatment methods for eliminating virus from these long-lived reservoirs will almost certainly be necessary if eradication of infection is to be achieved.

4.2.3 Predictive value of quantitative plasma viral RNA

Extensive data have accumulated concerning the predictive value of quantitative plasma RNA for adults with HIV infection – as a prognostic indicator using initial baseline values and after a period of therapy. Some of the earliest and most comprehensive data were generated by Mellors and his colleagues from subsets of the Multicenter AIDS Cohort Study (MACS), which includes data from subjects spanning more than a decade of clinical and laboratory observation [52]. Among 180 men in the Pittsburgh MACS cohort, a 36% reduction in mortality

Table 4.2 Clinical predictive value of plasma RNA concentration – adult cohort series

Study (# of subjects)	Risk reduction (C.I.)	Reference
ACTG 175 (366)	83% (68–92)*	[82]
ACTG 241 (198)	56% (8–79)*	[83]
MACS (180)	36% (25–45)**	[52]
Hopkins IDU (522)	17% (11–22)***	[84]

*Risk reduction for AIDS or death (ACTG 175 and 241: per log decrease);
**for death (MACS: per 3-fold decrease); or ***AIDS (Hopkins: per 3-fold decrease)

risk was observed for every 3-fold reduction in plasma RNA at study enrollment. The strong independent clinical predictive value of plasma RNA at baseline has subsequently been confirmed in the entire MACS cohort and in numerous other epidemiologic and clinical trials (Table 4.2). Plasma RNA determinations, however, cannot entirely predict the clinical outcome; other variables also have significant independent predictive value. Among such factors are the CD4$^+$ lymphocyte count and viral phenotypic properties, including antiretroviral resistance carried by the virus and the propensity of infected cells to form syncytia [53, 54].

Several large pediatric studies have documented significant differences in the natural history of plasma RNA levels compared with adults [55–58] (Figure 4.1). Adults with acute HIV infection have high viral loads that rapidly decline over a few weeks (see also Chapter 5). Vertically infected infants also have initially high viral loads, but they generally continue to maintain prolonged, high circulating viral loads for years. This persistence of high quantities of circulating virus in the first few years of life has been attributed to both an immature immune response and to a relatively increased number of target cells (CD4 lymphocytes) during a period of rapid somatic growth [55, 59, 60].

The implications for this quantitative difference in the natural history of plasma virus evolution during infancy are important. Several pediatric cohort studies have shown that plasma RNA values can independently predict clinical outcomes, as in the adult studies [57, 61, 62]. Interestingly, a linear relationship exists between plasma RNA levels and risk for disease progression that is independent of age [61]. For example, an 8-month-old and an 8-year-old, both with plasma RNA values of 100 000 copies/mL, would have similar risks for future disease progression. The fact that a majority of young infants have relatively high RNA levels is consistent with the clinical observations that a significant proportion of the young infants experience rapid disease progression. Studies have demonstrated that high peak levels attained during infancy and the long length of time that these levels are sustained predict a group at high risk for a poor outcome [56, 58]. Although plasma RNA is a strong independent predictor of the subsequent clinical course, additional variables must be considered, in particular the CD4+ lymphocyte count. Two large pediatric studies have clearly documented that the use of CD4+ lymphocyte count and plasma RNA in combination for prediction purposes is superior to using either alone [57, 61].

Clinicians caring for HIV-infected children and adults had hoped that threshold plasma RNA values would be identified above which disease progression was likely, providing absolute guidelines for decisions about therapy. However, several studies have demonstrated that there is no clear plasma RNA threshold value associated with disease progression. The implication is that the lower the plasma RNA, the lower the risk for disease progression, which strongly supports an aggressive approach to therapy designed to maintain viral loads as low as possible. However, these studies estimate relative risk of disease progression for groups of patients; there can be substantial variation in risk levels for an individual at any given RNA value. Although no clear threshold values for plasma RNA concentrations that predict adverse clinical outcomes have been determined, advisory groups have based therapeutic recommendations on plasma RNA concentrations, combined with CD4+ lymphocyte count thresholds. Unlike plasma RNA levels, certain CD4+ lymphocyte count thresholds do predict adverse clinical outcomes [61]. The US Department of Health and Human Services' (DHHS) *Guidelines for the Use of Antiretroviral Agents in HIV-Infected Adults and Adolescents* recommends antiretroviral treatment for individuals with CD4+ lymphocyte counts < 350 cells/uL and/or for plasma HIV RNA concentrations > 55 000 copies/mL [38]. The U.S. guidelines for initiating therapy in children are somewhat more complicated, and are outlined in detail in Chapter 22. The Pediatric European Network for the Treatment of AIDS (PENTA) [63] recently offered recommendations that include the possibility of deferring therapy for asymptomatic children with CD4+ lymphocyte percents ≥ 25% and plasma HIV RNA concentrations < 15 000 copies. The World Health Organization (WHO) has recently drafted guidelines entitled: *Scaling Up Antiretroviral Therapy in Resource Limited Settings: Guidelines for a Public Health Approach*. The WHO recommendations differentiate between children older and younger than 18 months.

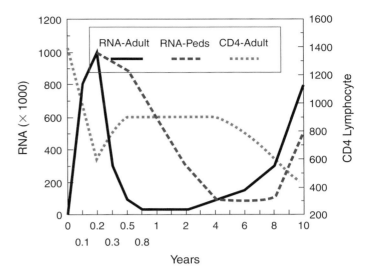

Figure 4.1. Depiction of typical clinical causes for plasma HIV RNA levels and CD4+ lymphocyte counts for children and adults.

However, WHO recommends that all children with AIDS or severe Stage II conditions be treated. WHO recommends that asymptomatic or mildly symptomatic children begin antiretroviral therapy when CD4+ lymphocyte counts fall below 20% (<18 months) or 15% (>18 months). Initiating and changing antiretroviral therapy in non-U.S. contexts is also discussed in more detail in Chapter 22.

4.2.4 Additional quantitative assays

Newer assays that strive to quantitate infected circulating cells have been developed and are reaching commercial availability. These are largely based on DNA PCR and include internal standards to enable accurate quantitation. These assays report "numbers of infected cells" or "copies of viral genomes/microgram of cellular DNA" and may help to monitor viral suppression and the amount of virus in long-lived cellular reservoirs [48, 51].

Qualitative plasma RNA assays are being developed to monitor viral replication breakthrough once individuals attain a non-detectable state. These assays should have excellent sensitivity and relatively low cost and may eventually prove useful for newborn diagnosis. Several investigators have reported that quantitative HIV RNA assays can sometimes permit earlier newborn diagnosis than DNA PCR [55, 64, 65].

Antiretroviral resistance testing may be useful in certain limited clinical situations and is discussed in more detail in Chapter 21.

Table 4.3 Selective list of HIV-related chemokines and their cellular receptors

Chemokine (class)	Chemokine receptor	Interacting virus phenotype
MIP-1α		Macrophage-tropic
MIP-1β	CCR-5	T-lymphotropic
RANTES		Non-syncytium-inducing
SDF-1	CXCR-4	T-lymphotropic
		T-cell lines
		Syncytium-inducing

4.2.5 Chemokines and chemokine receptors

HIV entry into the host cell requires that the virus interact with a chemokine co-receptor and CD4. The chemokines are a large and ubiquitous group of cell signaling molecules (Table 4.3) long known to be involved in inflammation [66]. Three beta-chemokines – MIP-1α, MIP-1β, and RANTES – were discovered to competitively inhibit binding of HIV to cellular targets and suppress viral infection [67]. In parallel, the Berger laboratory identified the alpha-chemokine receptor, CXCR4, as an obligatory second receptor for laboratory strains of HIV adapted to T lymphocyte cell lines [68]. Soon thereafter, a number of research groups identified the beta-chemokine receptor, CCR5, as the second receptor for binding and infection of macrophages and T lymphocytes [69–74]. HIV virions involved in the initial infection event and early asymptomatic infection are generally thought to target CCR-5 receptors while CXCR-4 is the more prevalent receptor involved with infection cycles during progressive disease. While this is almost certainly an overly simplistic picture of the evolution of virus–cell interaction during HIV infection, it has provided a powerful theoretical framework from which new therapeutic approaches are being generated. Natural and synthetic variants of the chemokines and small molecules that interfere with the binding of the virus to its chemokine co-receptors are actively being investigated for their therapeutic potential as competitive inhibitors of HIV binding and entry.

Mutations have been identified in the protein coding regions of CCR-5 and CCR-2 as well as the non-coding, promoter region of CCR-5 [75, 76]. The most extensively studied to date is a 32 base pair deletion within CCR-5. Individuals who are homozygous for the CCR-5 Δ32 mutation are much less likely to become infected with HIV and, if infected, remain well, with low viral loads and limited damage to their immune systems for long periods of time [77–81]. Heterozygosity for CCR-5 Δ32 confers no protection from infection and, in prospective cohort studies, does not provide survival advantage or protection from disease protection.

4.3 Conclusions

Serologic assays for antibodies to HIV have made the blood supply safe and have allowed practitioners to efficiently diagnose HIV infection in most adults, which have produced profound public health benefits. Recently developed rapid HIV serological assays should have further important public health benefits. Viral DNA PCR assays and viral isolation allow for the diagnosis of HIV infection in newborns, with similarly important effects. The various assays for viral RNA provide important prognostic information and help guide antiretroviral therapy. Clinical HIV virological assays play an important part in the prevention and management of HIV disease, and a clear understanding of the technologies involved and the performance characteristics of the assays will enable practitioners caring for patients with HIV to deliver the best possible care.

REFERENCES

1. Barre-Sinoussi, F., Chermann, J. C., Rey, F. *et al.* Isolation of a T-lymphotropic retrovirus from a patient at risk for acquired immune deficiency syndrome (AIDS). *Science* **220** (1983), 868–71.

2. Gallo, R. C., Sarin, P. S., Gelmann, E. P. *et al.* Isolation of human T-cell leukemia virus in acquired immune deficiency syndrome (AIDS). *Science* **220** (1983), 865–7.

3. Gallo, R. C., Salahuddin, S. Z., Popovic, M. *et al.* Frequent detection and isolation of cytopathic retroviruses (HTLV-III) from patients with AIDS and at risk for AIDS. *Science* **224** (1984), 500–3.

4. Levy, J. A., Hoffman, J. D., Kramer, S. M. *et al.* Isolation of lymphocytopathic retroviruses from San Francisco patients with AIDS. *Science* **224** (1984), 840–2.

5. Kalyanaraman, V. S., Cabradilla, C. D., Getchell, J. P. *et al.* Antibodies to the core protein of lymphadenopathy-associated virus (LAV) in patients with AIDS. *Science* **225** (1984), 321–3.

6. Sarngadharan, M. G., Popovic, M., Bruch, L., Schupbach, J. & Gallo, R. C. Antibodies reactive with human T-lymphotropic retroviruses (HTLV-III) in the serum of patients with AIDS. *Science* **224** (1984), 506–8.

7. Centers for Disease Control. Interpretation and use of the western blot assay for serodiagnosis of human immunodeficiency virus type 1 infections. *J. Am. Med. Assoc.* **262** (1989), 3395–7.

8. Centers for Disease Control. Interpretation and use of the western blot assay for serodiagnosis of human immunodeficiency

virus type 1 infections. *Morb. Mortal. Wkly. Rep.* **38** (1989), 1–7.

9. Centers for Disease Control. Interpretive criteria used to report western blot results for HIV-1- antibody testing–United States. *MMWR* **40** (1991), 692–5.

10. Constantine, N. T. Serologic tests for the retroviruses: approaching a decade of evolution. *AIDS* **7** (1993), 1–13.

11. Centers for Disease Control. HIV counseling and testing using rapid tests. *MMWR* **47** (1998), 211–5.

12. Stetler, H. C., Granade, T. C., Nunez, C. A. *et al.* Field evaluation of rapid HIV serologic tests for screening and confirming HIV-1 infection in Honduras. *AIDS* **11** (1997), 369–75.

13. Connor, E., Wang, Z., Stephens, R. *et al.* Enzyme immunoassay for detection of human immunodeficiency virus-specific immunoglobulin A antibodies. *J. Clin. Microbiol.* **31** (1993) 681–4.

14. Kliks, S. C., Wara, D. W., Landers, D. V. & Levy, J. A. Features of HIV-1 that could influence maternal-child transmission. *J. Am. Med. Assoc.* **272** (1994), 467–74.

15. Martin, N. L., Levy, J. A., Legg, H., Weintrub, P. S., Cowan, M. J. & Wara, D. W. Detection of infection with human immunodeficiency virus (HIV) type 1 in infants by an anti-HIV immunoglobulin A assay using recombinant proteins. *J. Pediatr.* **118** (1991), 354–8.

16. McIntosh, K., Comeau, A. M., Wara, D. *et al.* The utility of IgA antibody to human immunodeficiency virus type 1 in early diagnosis of vertically transmitted infection. National Institute of Allergy and Infectious Diseases and National Institute of Child Health and Human Development Women and Infants Transmission Study Group. *Arch. Pediatr. Adolesc. Med.* **150** (1996), 598–602.

17. Quinn, T. C., Kline, R. L., Halsey, N. *et al.* Early diagnosis of perinatal HIV infection by detection of viral- specific IgA antibodies. *J. Am. Med. Assoc.* **266** (1991), 3439–42.

18. Weiblen, B. J., Lee, F. K., Cooper, E. R. *et al.* Early diagnosis of HIV infection in infants by detection of IgA HIV antibodies. *Lancet* **335** (1990), 988–90.

19. Alimenti, A., O' Neill, M., Sullivan, J. L. & Luzuriaga, K. Diagnosis of vertical human immunodeficiency virus type 1 infection by whole blood culture. *J. Infect. Dis.* **166** (1992), 1146–8.

20. Borkowsky, W., Krasinski, K., Pollack, H., Hoover, W., Kaul, A. & Ilmet-Moore, T. Early diagnosis of human immunodeficiency virus infection in children less than 6 months of age: comparison of polymerase chain reaction, culture, and plasma antigen capture techniques. *J. Infect. Dis.* **166** (1992), 616–9.

21. Hollinger, F. B., Bremer, J. W., Myers, L. E., Gold, J. W. & McQuay, L. Standardization of sensitive human immunodeficiency virus coculture procedures and establishment of a multicenter quality assurance program for the AIDS Clinical Trials Group. The NIH/NIAID/DAIDS/ACTG Virology Laboratories. *J. Clin. Microbiol.* **30** (1992), 1787–94.

22. Jackson, J. B., Coombs, R. W., Sannerud, K., Rhame, F. S. & Balfour, H. H., Jr. Rapid and sensitive viral culture method for human immunodeficiency virus type 1. *J. Clin. Microbiol.* **26** (1988), 1416–8.

23. Nishanian, P., Huskins, K. R., Stehn, S., Detels, R. & Fahey, J. L. A simple method for improved assay demonstrates that HIV p24 antigen is present as immune complexes in most sera from HIV-infected individuals. *J. Infect. Dis.* **162** (1990), 21–8.

24. Quinn, T. C., Kline, R., Moss, M. W., Livingston, R. A. & Hutton, N. Acid dissociation of immune complexes improves diagnostic utility of p24 antigen detection in perinatally acquired human immunodeficiency virus infection. *J. Infect. Dis.* **167** (1993), 1193–6.

25. Schupbach, J. & Boni, J. Quantitative and sensitive detection of immune-complexed and free HIV antigen after boiling of serum. *J. Virol. Methods* **43** (1993), 247–56.

26. Schupbach, J., Boni, J., Tomasik, Z., Jendis, J., Seger, R. & Kind, C. Sensitive detection and early prognostic significance of p24 antigen in heat-denatured plasma of human immunodeficiency virus type 1-infected infants. Swiss Neonatal HIV Study Group. *J. Infect. Dis.* **170** (1994) 318–24.

27. Schupbach, J., Flepp, M., Pontelli, D., Tomasik, Z., Luthy, R. and Boni, J. Heat-mediated immune complex dissociation and enzyme-linked immunosorbent assay signal amplification render p24 antigen detection in plasma as sensitive as HIV-1 RNA detection by polymerase chain reaction. *AIDS* **10** (1996), 1085–90.

28. Boni, J., Opravil, M., Tomasik, Z. *et al.* Simple monitoring of antiretroviral therapy with a signal-amplification-boosted HIV-1 p24 antigen assay with heat-denatured plasma. *AIDS* **11** (1997), F47–52.

29. Mullis, K., Faloona, F., Scharf, S., Saiki, R., Horn, G. & Erlich, H. Specific enzymatic amplification of DNA in vitro: the polymerase chain reaction. *Cold Spring Harb. Symp. Quant. Biol.* **51** : **1**(1986), 263–73.

30. Jackson, J. B., Drew, J., Lin, H. J. *et al.* Establishment of a quality assurance program for human immunodeficiency virus type 1 DNA polymerase chain reaction assays by the AIDS Clinical Trials Group. ACTG PCR Working Group, and the ACTG PCR Virology Laboratories. *J. Clin. Microbiol.* **31** (1993), 3123–8.

31. Cassol, S. A., Lapoint, N., Salas, T. *et al.* Diagnosis of vertical HIV-1 transmission using the PCR and dried blood spot specimens. *J. Acquir. Immune Defic. Syndr.* **5** (1992), 113–19.

32. Cassol, S., Salas, T., Gill, M. J. *et al.* Stability of dried blood spot specimens for detection of HIV DNA by PCR. *J. Clin. Microbiol.* **30** (1992), 3039–42.

33. Comeau, A. M., Hsu, H. W., Schwerzler, M., Mushinsky, G. & Grady, G. F. Detection of HIV in specimens from newborn screening programs [letter]. *New Engl. J. Med.* **326** (1992), 1703.

34. Comeau, A. M., Hsu, H. W., Schwerzler, M. *et al.* Identifying human immunodeficiency virus infection at birth: application of polymerase chain reaction to Guthrie cards. *J. Pediatr.* **123** (1993), 252–8.

35. Comeau, A. M., Su, X., Muchinsky, G., Pan, D., Gerstel, J. & Grady, G. F. Quality-controlled pooling strategies for nucleic-acid based HIV screening: using PCR as a primary screen

on dried blood spot specimens in population studies. In 5th Conference on Retroviruses and Opportunistic Infections. Chicago, IL, 1998.

36. Bremer, J. W., Lew, J. F., Cooper, E. *et al.* Diagnosis of infection with human immunodeficiency virus type 1 by a DNA polymerase chain reaction assay among infants enrolled in the Women and Infants' Transmission Study. *J. Pediatr.* **129** (1996), 198–207.

37. Owens, D. K., Holodniy, M., McDonald, T. W., Scott, J. & Sonnad, S. A meta-analytic evaluation of the polymerase chain reaction for the diagnosis of HIV infection in infants. *J. Am. Med. Assoc.* **275** (1996), 1342–8.

38. The Working Group on Antiretroviral Therapy and Medical Management of HIV-Infected Children. *Guidelines for the Use of Antiretroviral Agents in Pediatric HIV Infection, 2001* (http://www.hivatis.org).

39. Stanley, S., Ostrowski, M. A., Justement, J. S. *et al.* Effect of immunization with a common recall antigen on viral expression in patients infected with human immunodeficiency virus type 1. *New Engl. J. Med.* **334** (1996),1222–30.

40. Staprans, S. I., Hamilton, B. L., Follansbee, S. E. *et al.* Activation of virus replication after vaccination of HIV-1-infected individuals. *J. Exp. Med.* **182** (1995), 1727–37.

41. Ramilo, O., Hicks, P. J., Borvak, J. *et al.* T cell activation and human immunodeficiency virus replication after influenza immunization of infected children. *Pediatr. Infect. Dis. J.* **15** (1996), 197–203.

42. O' Brien, W., Grovit-Ferbas, K., Namazi, A. *et al.* Human immunodeficiency virus-type 1 replication can be increased in peripheral blood of seropositive patients after influenza vaccination. *Blood* **86** (1995), 1082–9.

43. Kroon, F. P., van Dissel, J. T., de Jong, J. C. & van Furth, R. Antibody response to influenza, tetanus and pneumococcal vaccines in HIV-seropositive individuals in relation to the number of CD4+ lymphocytes. *AIDS* **8** (1994), 469–76.

44. Brichacek, B., Swindells, S., Janoff, E. N., Pirruccello, S. & Stevenson, M. Increased plasma human immunodeficiency virus type 1 burden following antigenic challenge with pneumococcal vaccine. *J. Infect. Dis.* **174** (1996), 1191–9.

45. Ho, D. D., Neumann, A. U., Perelson, A. S., Chen, W., Leonard, J. M. & Markowitz, M. Rapid turnover of plasma virions and CD4 lymphocytes in HIV-1 infection. *Nature* **373** (1995), 123–6.

46. Wei, X., Ghosh, S. K., Taylor, M. E. *et al.* Viral dynamics in human immunodeficiency virus type 1 infection. *Nature* **373** (1995), 117–22.

47. Wong, J. K., Hezareh, M., Gunthard, H. F. *et al.* Recovery of replication-competent HIV despite prolonged suppression of plasma viremia. *Science* **278** (1997), 1291–5.

48. Finzi, D., Hermankova, M., Pierson, T. *et al.* Identification of a reservoir for HIV-1 in patients on highly active antiretroviral therapy. *Science* **278** (1997), 1295–300.

49. Chun, T., Stuyver, L., Mizell, S. B. *et al.* Presence of an inducible HIV-1 latent reservoir during highly active antiretroviral therapy. *Proc. Natl. Acad. Sci. USA* **94** (1997), 13193–7.

50. Chun, T. W., Carruth, L., Finzi, D. *et al.* Quantification of latent tissue reservoirs and total body viral load in HIV-1 infection. *Nature* **387** (1997), 183–8.

51. Persaud, D., Pierson, T., Ruff, C. *et al.* A stable latent reservoir for HIV-1 in resting CD4(+) T lymphocytes in infected children. *J. Clin. Invest.* **105** (2000), 995–1003.

52. Mellors, J. W., Rinaldo, C. R., Jr., Gupta, P., White, R. M., Todd, J. A. & Kingsley, L. A. Prognosis in HIV-1 infection predicted by the quantity of virus in plasma. *Science* **272** (1996), 1167–70.

53. Coombs, R. W., Welles S. L., Hooper, C. *et al.* Association of plasma human immunodeficiency virus type 1 RNA level with risk of clinical progression in patients with advanced infection. AIDS Clinical Trials Group (ACTG) 116B/117 Study Team. ACTG Virology Committee Resistance and HIV-1 RNA Working Groups. *J. Infect. Dis.* **174** (1996), 704–12.

54. Welles, S. L., Jackson, J. B., Yen-Lieberman, B. *et al.* Prognostic value of plasma human immunodeficiency virus type 1 (HIV-1) RNA levels in patients with advanced HIV-1 disease and with little or no prior zidovudine therapy. AIDS Clinical Trials Group Protocol 116A/116B/117 Team. *J. Infect. Dis.* **174** (1996), 696–703.

55. Palumbo, P. E., Kwok, S., Waters, S. *et al.* Viral measurement by polymerase chain reaction-based assays in human immunodeficiency virus-infected infants. *J. Pediatr.* **126** (1995), 592–5.

56. Shearer, W. T., Quinn, T. C., LaRussa, P. *et al.* Viral load and disease progression in infants infected with human immunodeficiency virus type 1. Women and Infants Transmission Study Group. *N. Engl. J. Med.* **336** (1997), 1337–42.

57. Mofenson, L. M., Korelitz, J., Meyer, W. A., 3rd. *et al.* The relationship between serum human immunodeficiency virus type 1 (HIV-1) RNA level, CD4 lymphocyte percent, and long-term mortality risk in HIV-1-infected children. National Institute of Child Health and Human Development Intravenous Immunoglobulin Clinical Trial Study Group. *J. Infect. Dis.* **175** (1997), 1029–38.

58. Abrams, E. J., Weedon, J., Steketee, R. W. *et al.* Association of human immunodeficiency virus (HIV) load early in life with disease progression among HIV-infected infants. New York City Perinatal HIV Transmission Collaborative Study Group. *J. Infect. Dis.* **178** (1998), 101–8.

59. Zeichner, S. L., Palumbo, P., Feng, Y. *et al.* Rapid telomere shortening in Children. *Blood* **93** (1999), 2824–30.

60. Krogstad, P., Uittenbogaart, C. H., Dickover, R., Bryson, Y. J., Plaeger, S. & Garfinkel, A. Primary HIV infection of infants: the effects of somatic growth on lymphocyte and virus dynamics. *Clin. Immunol.* **92** (1999), 25–33.

61. Palumbo, P. E., Raskino, C., Fiscus, S. *et al.* Predictive value of quantitative plasma HIV RNA and CD4+ lymphocyte count in HIV-infected infants and children. *J. Am. Med. Assoc.* **279** (1998), 756–61.

62. Lindsey, J. C., Hughes, M. D., McKinney, R. E. *et al.* Treatment-mediated changes in human immunodeficiency virus (HIV) type 1 RNA and CD4 cell counts as predictors of weight growth

failure, cognitive decline, and survival in HIV-infected children. *J. Infect. Dis.* **182** (2000), 1385–93.

63. Sharland, M., Gibb, D. & Giaquinto, C. Current evidence for the use of paediatric antiretroviral therapy – a PENTA analysis. Paediatric European Network for the Treatment of AIDS Steering Committee. *Eur. J. Pediatr.* **159** (2000), 649–56.

64. Steketee, R. W., Abrams, E. J., Thea, D. M. *et al.* Early detection of perinatal human immunodeficiency virus (HIV) type 1 infection using HIV RNA amplification and detection. New York City Perinatal HIV Transmission Collaborative Study. *J. Infect. Dis.* **175** (1997), 707–11.

65. Delamare, C., Burgard, M., Mayaux, M. J. *et al.* HIV-1 RNA detection in plasma for the diagnosis of infection in neonates. The French Pediatric HIV Infection Study Group. *J. AIDS Hum. Retrovirol.* **15** (1997), 121–5.

66. Premack, B. A.& Schall, T. J. Chemokine receptors: gateways to inflammation and infection. *Nat. Med.* **2** (1996), 1174–8.

67. Cocchi, F., DeVico, A. L., Garzino-Demo, A., Arya, S. K., Gallo, R. C. & Lusso, P. Identification of RANTES, MIP-1 alpha, and MIP-1 beta as the major HIV- suppressive factors produced by CD8+ T cells. *Science* **270** (1995), 1811–5.

68. Feng, Y., Broder, C. C., Kennedy, P. E. & Berger, E. A.. HIV-1 entry cofactor: functional cDNA cloning of a seven-transmembrane, G protein-coupled receptor. *Science* **272** (1996), 872–7.

69. Berson, J. F., Long, D., Doranz, B. J., Rucker, J., Jirik, F. R. & Doms, R. W. A seven-transmembrane domain receptor involved in fusion and entry of T-cell-tropic human immunodeficiency virus type 1 strains. *J. Virol.* **70** (1996), 6288–95.

70. Deng, H., Liu, R., Ellmeier, W. *et al.* Identification of a major co-receptor for primary isolates of HIV-1. *Nature* **381** (1996), 661–6.

71. Doranz, B. J., Rucker, J., Yi, Y. *et al.* A dual-tropic primary HIV-1 isolate that uses fusin and the beta- chemokine receptors CKR-5, CKR-3, and CKR-2b as fusion cofactors. *Cell* **85** (1996), 1149–58.

72. Dragic, T., Litwin, V., Allaway, G. P. *et al.* HIV-1 entry into CD4+ cells is mediated by the chemokine receptor CC-CKR-5. *Nature* **381** (1996), 667–73.

73. Alkhatib, G., Combadiere, C., Broder, C. C. *et al.* CC CKR5: a RANTES, MIP-1alpha, MIP-1beta receptor as a fusion cofactor for macrophage-tropic HIV-1. *Science* **272** (1996), 1955–8.

74. Choe, H., Farzan, M., Sun, Y. *et al.* The beta-chemokine receptors CCR3 and CCR5 facilitate infection by primary HIV-1 isolates. *Cell* **85** (1996), 1135–48.

75. Liu, R., Paxton, W. A., Choe, S. *et al.* Homozygous defect in HIV-1 coreceptor accounts for resistance of some multiply-exposed individuals to HIV-1 infection. *Cell* **86** (1996), 367–77.

76. Smith, M. W., Dean, M., Carrington, M. *et al.* Contrasting genetic influence of CCR2 and CCR5 variants on HIV-1 infection and disease progression. Hemophilia Growth and Development Study (HGDS), Multicenter AIDS Cohort Study (MACS), Multicenter Hemophilia Cohort Study (MHCS), San Francisco City Cohort (SFCC), ALIVE Study. *Science* **277** (1997), 959–65.

77. Dean, M., Carrington, M., Winkler, C. *et al.* Genetic restriction of HIV-1 infection and progression to AIDS by a deletion allele of the CKR5 structural gene. Hemophilia Growth and Development Study, Multicenter AIDS Cohort Study, Multicenter Hemophilia Cohort Study, San Francisco City Cohort, ALIVE Study. *Science* **273** (1996), 1856–62.

78. Zimmerman, P. A., Buckler-White, A., Alkhatib, G. *et al.* Inherited resistance to HIV-1 conferred by an inactivating mutation in CC chemokine receptor 5: studies in populations with contrasting clinical phenotypes, defined racial background, and quantified risk. *Mol. Med.* **3** (1997), 23–36.

79. Michael, N. L., Chang, G., Louie, L. G. *et al.* The role of viral phenotype and CCR-5 gene defects in HIV-1 transmission and disease progression. *Nat. Med.* **3** (1997), 338–40.

80. Biti, R., French, R., Young, J., Bennetts, B., Stewart, G. & Liang, T. HIV-1 infection in an individual homozygous for the CCR5 deletion allele. *Nat. Med.* **3** (1997), 252–3.

81. Wang, B., Palasanthiran, P., Zeigler, J., Cunningham, A. & Saksena, N. K. CCR5-delta 32 gene deletion in HIV-1 infected patients [letter]. *Lancet* **350** (1997), 742.

The natural history of pediatric HIV disease

Grace M. Aldrovandi, M.D., C.M.

Children's Hospital of Los Angeles, Los Angeles, CA

5.1 Introduction

This chapter will review our current understanding of the natural history of HIV-1 infection in children and adolescents in an effort to provide the clinician with the background needed to rationally treat HIV disease in children. The advent of highly active antiretroviral therapy (HAART) has radically altered the natural history of pediatric HIV infection, transforming it into a chronic manageable disease requiring complex drug regimens and, for now, lifelong therapy.

5.2 Natural history in adults

The natural history of HIV disease was initially described in adults. Knowledge of the natural history of the disease in adults has helped inform pediatric natural history studies and provides a benchmark for the pediatric observations. Infection of adults with HIV-1 is classically followed by three distinct virologic stages: (1) primary or acute infection, (2) clinical latency, and finally (3) progression to AIDS (see Figure 5.1). The time interval between primary infection and the development of AIDS is variable, typically 10 to 11 years [1]. About 20% of individuals will progress in less than 5 years, while a few (< 5%) will remain immunologically normal for over 10 years [2]. The biological basis for this variability is unclear, but undoubtedly reflects differences in viral strains, host immune responses and exposure to other cofactors (microbial or environmental), especially those leading to immune activation.

Several weeks after infection with HIV-1, a variable and non-specific clinical syndrome referred to as primary infection, acute infection syndrome, or acute retroviral syndrome is observed in an unknown proportion of adults (range 10–90%). The degree of symptomatology during this acute phase may have prognostic significance [3–5]. Although classically described as a mononucleosis-like syndrome (fever, pharyngitis or sore throat and cervical adenopathy), in a recent study of over 200 patients with documented symptomatic primary HIV-1 infection only 15% of patients had such a presentation [6]. Fever, myalgias, lethargy and rash were the common presenting symptoms in over 50% of this cohort. Neurologic (meningitis-like syndrome, peripheral neuropathy, encephalitis) or gastrointestinal symptoms can predominate while fever is absent in up to 25% of cases [7]. Regardless of the presentation these symptoms resolve spontaneously over a period of days to weeks. Upon presentation, these persons will often be antibody negative, but will have detectable circulating p24 antigen or HIV RNA (as assessed by assays such as reverse transcription polymerase chain reaction and others; see Chapters 4 and 7). During primary infection, extremely high levels of plasma viremia have been observed, with levels of HIV-1 RNA (viral load) greater than 10^7 copies/mL, dropping to 100 000 copies/mL or less after several weeks [8, 9]. During this period of high viremia, the absolute number of $CD4^+$ lymphocytes decreases, occasionally rather dramatically to below 200 cells/μL. Later, as the level of viremia declines, the $CD4^+$ lymphocyte count increases, often to normal levels. This drop in viral load precedes the development of antibody response and coincides with a measurable cytotoxic lymphocyte (CTL) response directed against HIV [10]. Whether this CTL response causes the decrease in viremia has yet to be resolved. CTL responses do appear to play a key role in suppressing viral replication

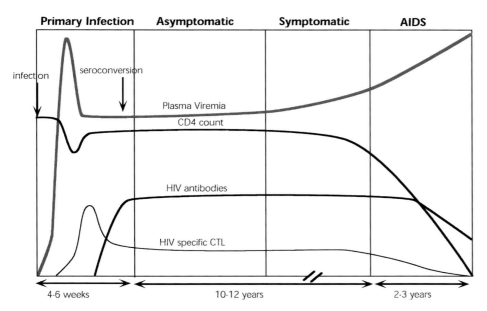

Figure 5.1. Schematic representation of the natural history of HIV-1 infection in adults. The figure shows the typical changes in plasma viremia, CD4$^+$ lymphocyte count, antibodies to HIV, and HIV-specific cytotoxic lymphocyte (CTL) in adult patients following seroconversion.

in long-term non-progressors. After a period of fluctuation, the level of plasma HIV RNA stabilizes around a so-called "set point," usually between 10 000 and 100 000 copies mL (range < 200 copies to > 10 000 000), frequently remaining fairly constant for many years [4]. This period is referred to as clinical latency since patients are clinically asymptomatic. However, much viral replication and destruction of the patient's CD4$^+$ lymphocytes occur during clinical latency. An estimated 10 billion virions, with estimated half-lives of less than 6 hours, are produced daily [11]. Eventually, plasma viral levels increase and levels of CD4$^+$ lymphocytes decrease, heralding the development of advancing immunodeficiency and AIDS [4]. The point of onset of a more rapid fall in CD4$^+$ cells is known as the "inflection point."

5.3 Relationship between plasma viral concentration, CD4$^+$ cell level and disease progression in adults

Assays for the quantification of plasma HIV-1 RNA provide convenient measures of virus replication in infected persons [12, 13]. However, these measurements offer a somewhat imprecise assessment of the viral replication occurring in a patient, since the largest compartment in which virus replication occurs, the lymphoid tissue, is not directly sampled by this measurement [14]. Nevertheless, virus produced in lymphoid tissues appears to be released into the plasma, and plasma HIV-1 RNA concentrations appear to at least indirectly sample viral replication occurring in the lymphoid tissue [15]. Other organ systems in which HIV replication may occur, such as the central nervous system,

the genital tract and breast milk may behave as much more distinct compartments than the lymphoid tissues. Plasma viral RNA levels may not accurately reflect viral replication occurring in these compartments, and virus present in these compartments may be genotypically distinct from the virus found in the peripheral circulation. These distinct viral genotypes may have differing pathogenic properties and differing sensitivities to antiretroviral agents [16–20]. Since antiretroviral agents may not penetrate well into these compartments, they represent a source of resistant virus.

In the absence of antiretroviral therapy (ART), plasma RNA levels can vary widely, depending on the stage of infection and other factors. There is an inverse, but variable, correlation between plasma RNA and the level of CD4$^+$ lymphocytes. At all stages of HIV-1 disease, the plasma RNA level and the absolute CD4$^+$ count are independent prognostic markers. Before HAART became widely available, the steady state level of plasma viral RNA after initial infection ("set point") was the best single predictor of progression to AIDS and death [21, 22]. (Only 8% of adults with low concentrations (< 4350 copies of RNA per ml of plasma) progressed to AIDS within 5 years whereas 62% of those with high plasma RNA concentrations (> 36 270) developed AIDS [21].) Combined use of plasma RNA levels with CD4$^+$ count more accurately predicts prognosis than either marker alone [22]. Use of these variables can define categories of risk for developing AIDS with 3, 6, and 9 years (see Table 5.1).

The use of ART, and especially HAART, often produces decreases in plasma RNA and increases in CD4$^+$ number.

Table 5.1 Relationship between baseline HIV-1 RNA copy number and absolute CD4$^+$ lymphocyte number and probability of developing AIDS

Baseline RNA (copies/mL)	Absolute CD4$^+$ lymphocyte number (cells/μL)	% with AIDS		
		by 3 years	by 6 years	by 9 years
<500	>750	0	1.7	3.6
	<750	3.7	9.6	22.3
501–3000	ND	2	16.6	35.4
3001–10 000	>750	3.2	14.2	40.4
	<750	8.1	37.2	59.7
10 001–30 000	>750	9.5	36.7	62.4
	351–750	16.1	54.9	76.3
	<750	40.1	72.9	86.2
>30 000	>500	32.6	66.8	76.3
	351–500	47.9	77.7	94.4
	201–350	64.4	89.3	92.9
	<200	85.5	97.9	100

HIV-1 RNA was quantified using the bDNA system. Data are derived from [21], with permission.

These changes have clinical and prognostic significance. After the initiation of antiretroviral therapy, progressive decreases in plasma RNA level or increases in CD4$^+$ lymphocyte count predict the development of AIDS more strongly than baseline values [23, 24]. For each 1.0 log$_{10}$ copies/mL (10-fold) decrease in plasma RNA, the risk of disease progression was decreased by 56%, and for every 2-fold higher increase in absolute CD4$^+$ cell count it decreased by 67% [24].

Although ART can have dramatic effects on plasma viremia, a small pool of long-lived latently infected CD4$^+$ lymphocytes persist (reviewed in [25]). Replication competent virus can be recovered from these latently infected cells by the use of sensitive culture techniques. This reservoir is established early in infection and is relatively impervious to the effects of current ART. The rate of turnover of these cells is controversial, with estimates ranging from 6 months to 43 months. In part, this discrepancy may be due to differences in levels of low viral replication even in persons in whom plasma HIV RNA is consistently < 50 copies/mL. Nevertheless the persistence of this compartment represents a major obstacle to the eradication of HIV.

5.4 Factors associated with progression in adults

The determinants of the viral "set point" and the "inflection point" are poorly understood. Individual variation in disease progression is the result of multiple factors. The effectiveness of the host immune response is believed to be a critical determinant of disease progression, but the precise nature of this response has yet to be fully elucidated. The age of an individual at the time of infection can influence the subsequent rate of progression to AIDS [26–29]. As individuals age, the capacity of their immune systems to regenerate declines. Multiple lines of evidence suggest that CD8$^+$ CTL responses play a crucial role in establishing the viral set-point (reviewed in [30]), but ultimately these responses are ineffective in preventing disease progression. Some case reports suggest that even when patients have a vigorous CTL response against HIV and low viral loads, if they are superinfected with another HIV strain, they can fail to control the superinfecting virus, observations that underscore our limited understanding of the immunologic factors that control HIV infection [31, 32].

Certain combinations of HLA genes are associated with either relatively rapid (HLA-B8 or -B35) or delayed (HLA-B27 or -57) progression to AIDS [33, 34]. Locus heterozygosity for any combination of alleles at HLA –A, –B or –C, can significantly delay progression to AIDS compared with individuals who are homozygous for one or more of these loci [33]. It is hypothesized that individuals heterozygous at HLA loci are able to present a greater variety of antigenic peptides to cytotoxic T lymphocytes than are homozygotes. This results in a more effective immune response against a number of pathogens including HIV. Vertically infected children who share HLA haplotypes with their mothers may be at increased risk of progression [35]. A virus that has successfully evaded the maternal HLA class I response would be equipped to evade the infant's CTL response, since identical epitopes would be targeted by the child's immune response.

Inheritance of genes other than HLA have also been implicated in disease progression (see [36, 37] for review). The majority of these studies have been performed in white cohorts. Studies defining immunogenetic factors involved in long-term progression in other racial groups are ongoing. Alterations in the coding or promoter genes of chemokine receptors that serve as co-receptors for entry of HIV-1 into target cells can result in different rates of disease progression in the absence of ART [38–40]. Persons with a 32-base pair deletion in the CCR5 receptor appear to be relatively resistant to infection with certain strains of HIV-1[41–43]. Certain mutations in CCR5 and CCR2 are associated with a 2–4 year delay progression to AIDS. Polymorphisms in the 3′ untranslated region of the gene encoding SDF1 are associated with delays that are several fold stronger than those associated with the CCR5 or CCR2 variants [44]. Mutations in genes for IL-10, Rantes and CX3CR1 also appear to influence disease progression [38, 39, 44–46], but the pathogenic mechanisms have yet to be elucidated.

Other host factors that appear to influence disease progression include co-infection and other sources of immune activation. Since productive replication of HIV-1 can only occur in activated cells, it has been postulated that environmental factors that lead to immune activation increase viral replication and hasten immune deterioration [47]. Exposure to environmental antigens or common infections has been associated with increases in plasma viremia [48–51]. In some HIV-1 infected individuals, immunization with antigens such as influenza and tetanus toxoid has led to transient bursts of viremia followed by a return to baseline plasma RNA levels within 7–10 days [52–54]. These transient increases are not associated with decreases in $CD4^+$ cell levels or increases in proviral DNA. Other studies have found no effect on viremia as a consequence of immunization [55, 56]. The benefits of vaccination preventing infection, which would undoubtedly result in much higher levels of immune activation, outweigh the unproved risks of transient increases in plasma RNA.

Virological factors have also been associated with disease progression. HIV-1 strains have been broadly classified as being M-tropic/NSI (non-syncytium inducing) strains or T-tropic/SI (syncytium inducing). M-tropic strains can replicate in primary $CD4^+$ T cells and macrophages and use the β-chemokine receptor CCR5 (less often CCR3) as their co-receptors (reviewed in [57, 58]). The T-tropic viruses can also replicate in $CD4^+$ T cells but can, in addition, infect established $CD4^+$ T cell lines in vitro via the α-chemokine receptor CXCR4 (fusin). Regardless of the mode of transmission, over 90% of transmitted strains are M-tropic; transmission or systemic establishment of CXCR4-using (T-tropic) strains is rare. However, CXCR4-using strains are especially virulent and once they emerge within an infected person, disease progression is accelerated [59, 60]. At the inflection point, about 50% of adults infected with subtype B will have a switch in the phenotype of the virus from M-tropic viruses to T-tropic viruses [61]. Infection with HIV-1 variants containing genetic defects (e.g. mutations in the *nef* gene) have been documented in a few HIV-1 infected long-term nonprogressors, however, these are rare individuals [62–66].

During its spread among humans, HIV has exhibited extraordinary genetic variation. Phylogenetic analyses of HIV sequences from different regions of the world reveal that HIV can be divided into different clades or subtypes. Most of our understanding of HIV pathogenesis is based on subtype B, the predominant strain in developed countries. However, globally most individuals are infected with non-B subtypes. Whether different subtypes differ in transmissibility, infectivity, and pathogenicity is an important area of active research. Some data suggest that there may be important differences [67]. For example, about 50% of HIV-infected persons harbor subtype C [68], but SI strains of subtype C are very rare, suggesting for this subtype a switch in co-receptor usage is not an important mediator of disease progression.

5.5 Classification of pediatric HIV-1 infection

The Centers for Disease Control and Prevention (CDC) has established a classification system for HIV-infected children into mutually exclusive categories according to their clinical status and immunologic status (see Tables 5.2, 5.3, and 5.4).

The current clinical classification system is based on signs, symptoms, or diagnoses related to HIV-1 infection. In this system, infected children are assigned to one of four mutually exclusive clinical categories: stage N, no signs or symptoms; stage A, mild signs or symptoms; stage B, moderate signs or symptoms; stage C, severe signs or symptoms [69]. All the AIDS-defining illnesses in the 1987 CDC definition of pediatric AIDS are included in stage C, with the exception of LIP (lymphoid interstitial pneumonitis), which is a stage B illness. Although most children pass from stage N to A, B, and C in that order, other children can pass directly from N to B or N to C (see below).

Table 5.2 Conditions associated with clinical categories according to the CDC 1994 Revised HIV Pediatric Classification system

Category A	Category B	Category C
Have 2 or more of the conditions listed below but no category B and C conditions	Examples of conditions in clinical category B	Examples of conditions in clinical category C
Lymphadenopathy (>0.5 cm at more than 2 sites)	Anemia (<8g/dl), neutropenia (<1,000/mm^3), or thrombocytopenia (<1,000,000/mm^3) persisting >30 days	Multiple or recurrent serious bacterial infections (septicemia, pneumonia, meningitis, bone or joint infection, or abscess of an internal organ)
Hepatomegaly	Bacterial meningitis, pneumonia or sepsis (single episode)	Candidiasis, esophageal or pulmonary
Splenomegaly	Candidiasis, oropharyngeal (thrush), persistent (> 2 months) in a child > 6 months	Coccidioimycosis, disseminated
Dermatitis		Cryptococcosis, extrapulmonary
Parotitis	Cardiomyopathy	Cryptosporidiosis or Isosporiasis with diarrhea persisting for >1 month
Recurrent or persistent upper respiratory infection, sinusitis, or otitis media	Cytomegalovirus infection, with onset >1 month of age	Cytomegalovirus disease with onset of symptoms prior to 1 month of age
	Diarrhea, recurrent or chronic	Cytomegalovirus retinitis (with loss of vision)
	Hepatitis,	Encephalopathy in the absence of a concurrent illness other than HIV infection that could explain the findings
	HSV stomatitis, recurrent (>2 episodes within 1 year)	HSV infection causing a mucocutaneous ulcer persisting for >1 month; or as the etiology of bronchitis, pneumonitis or esophagitis
	HSV bronchitis, pneumonitis, or esophagitis with <1 month of age	Histoplasmosis, disseminated
	Herpes zoster involving at >2 distinct episodes or >1 dermatome	Kaposi's sarcoma
	Leiomyosarcoma	Primary CNS lymphoma
	LIP or pulmonary lymphoid hyperplasia	Lymphoma, Burkit's, large cell, or immunoblastic
	Nephropathy	*M. tuberculosis*, disseminated or extrapulmonary
	Nocardiosis	Mycobacterium infections other than tuberculosis, disseminated
	Persistent fever (lasting > 1 month of age)	*Pneumocystis carnii* pneumonia
	Toxoplasmosis, onset < 1 month of age	Progressive multifocal leukoencephalopathy
	Varicella, disseminated	Toxoplasmosis of the brain with onset at >1 month of age
		Wasting syndrome in the absence of a concurrent illness other than HIV infection

Adapted from [69], with permission.

Table 5.3 Immunologic categories according to the CDC 1994 Revised HIV Pediatric Classification

Age of child	No evidence of immune suppression		Evidence of moderate immune suppression		Evidence of severe immune suppression	
	CD4$^+$ lymphocytes (cells/μL)	% CD4$^+$ lymphocytes (cells/μL)	CD4$^+$ lymphocytes (cells/μL)	% CD4$^+$ lymphocytes (cells/μL)	CD4$^+$ lymphocytes (cells/μL)	% CD4$^+$ lymphocytes (cells/μL)
< 1 year	$\geq$1500	$\geq$25	750–1499	15–24	<750	<15
1–5 years	$\geq$1000	$\geq$25	500–999	15–24	<500	<15
6–12 years	$\geq$500	$\geq$25	200–499	15–24	<200	<15

Adapted from [69], with permission.

Table 5.4 HIV pediatric classification incorporating both clinical and immunologic categories

Immunologic categories	Clinical categories			
	N: No signs/ symptoms	A: Mild signs/ symptoms	B: Moderate signs/ symptoms	C: Severe signs/ symptoms
1: No evidence of suppression	N1	A1	B1	C1
2: Evidence of moderate suppression	N2	A2	B2	C2
3: Severe suppression	N3	A3	B3	C3

Adapted from [69], with permission.

The current immunological classification system uses the CD4$^+$ lymphocyte count to assess the degree of immunosuppression. In this immunological classification patients are assigned to mutually exclusive categories characterized by the numbers 1 through 3, with lower CD4$^+$ lymphocyte counts or percent CD4$^+$ cells labeled with higher numbers (Table 5.4). The absolute CD4$^+$ lymphocyte counts associated with different degrees of immunosuppression are similar for all adults. However, for children the normal CD4$^+$ lymphocyte count changes dramatically during the first few years of life. In the first year of life the absolute CD4$^+$ cell count is more than three times that seen in adults and then gradually declines over the first few years of life. Assessing the severity of immune suppression is also complicated because children may develop some opportunistic infections at higher CD4$^+$ cell counts than adults [70] (see Chapters 1 and 3). Thus, the CD4$^+$ lymphocyte counts that define different degrees of immunosuppression vary in an age-dependent fashion.

The current CDC immunologic classification system is based on age-specific CD4$^+$ cell counts using both the absolute CD4$^+$ cell count and the percentage of CD4$^+$ lymphocytes [69] (see Table 5.3). If absolute CD4$^+$ cell count and percentage place a child in different immunologic categories, the more severe category should be used. Children treated with HAART can exhibit significant immune reconstitution, with a much-reduced risk of opportunistic infections. Such immune-reconstituted children may no longer require prophylaxis for certain opportunistic infections (see Chapter 11). However, according to the current system, such an immune-reconstituted child is not reclassified to a less severe category even with higher subsequent CD4$^+$ counts. Any value that results in a change in classification should be confirmed. Since CD4$^+$ cell values (both number and percent) can vary with even mild intercurrent illness, CD4$^+$ cell values are best obtained when the child is clinically well. As in adults, absolute CD4$^+$ cell number best identifies a risk for specific opportunistic infections. However, CD4$^+$ cell percent has less measurement variability and is therefore probably a better marker to follow disease progression.

5.6 Natural history of HIV-1 in children

The pace of HIV disease progression in children is accelerated compared with adults. This difference is presumably a consequence of the acquisition of infection at a time of immunologic immaturity, and/or the availability of increased numbers of susceptible target cells. Older children infected via non-vertical routes may have a course more similar to adults, with longer median time to AIDS diagnosis and death [71, 72].

Vertically infected children exhibit a bimodal pattern of disease progression [73–75]. About 10–25% of infected children develop profound immunosuppression, *Pneumocystitis carinii* pneumonia (PCP), severe encephalopathy, organomegaly, and multiple opportunistic infections in the first few months of life [73, 74]; without treatment few of these children survive more than 2 years [76]. The majority of children have a slower progression to AIDS with mean times of 6–9 years [73, 75, 77–79]. Factors contributing to the variable rates of disease progression include the route and timing of infection [80, 81], the amount and phenotype of the virus, shared maternal HLA types (favoring replication of escape variants), and other host immunogenetic factors. Infection with other pathogens, particularly viruses, has also been suggested as a contributing factor in disease progression [48, 49, 82–84].

Early studies clearly demonstrated that children with early onset of symptoms and an AIDS diagnosis at less than a year of age did not survive as long as those who presented at later ages (see [85] for a review). Investigators hypothesize that these children acquire their infection in utero and are therefore less able to mount an effective immune response [86, 87]. Others have suggested that HIV-1 infection during ontogenic development of the immune system is responsible for a pattern of lymphocyte depletion similar to children with congenital thymic abnormalities [88]. Since the timing of HIV-1 infection cannot be definitively ascertained, a working definition has been proposed wherein in utero transmission is defined as viral detection at less than 48 hours and intrapartum transmission is defined as viral detection at greater than 7 days [81]. Approximately 10–30% of children have detectable virus in the first 2 days of life. Most studies have found that children who fit this in utero definition have a shorter median time to onset of symptoms and death [74, 89] and higher levels of virus as measured by cellular proviral (DNA), p24 antigenemia, and/or plasma RNA levels (29, 34, 73). However, one study found that children with positive cultures in the first 48 hours of life had higher HIV-1 plasma RNA levels than children in whom the virus was detected later, but only for the first few months of life and that this difference disappeared after several months [90]. Children who are vertically infected do not appear to have an acute retroviral infection syndrome.

The most striking difference between the natural history of HIV infection in vertically infected infants and adults is the extremely high levels of plasma viremia observed in vertically infected infants during the first few months of life. The viremia declines substantially in the first year of life and then more slowly over several years [90–92] (see below). At approximately 4–6 years of age RNA levels appear to stabilize at lower levels. These changes in RNA are described in Chapter 4. As discussed above, adults achieve this steady-state or set-point within 6 months of infection. Whether this pattern of slow decline merely reflects the number of available target cells and/or a maturing immune response is unknown. No data are yet available for children infected by routes other than vertical transmission.

5.7 Natural history of HIV-1 infection in children in Africa

The vast majority of HIV-1 infected persons live in sub-Saharan Africa, where seroprevalence rates of over 25% are increasingly common. Over 80% of children infected with HIV live in and over 90% of new pediatric infections occur in this region. Although children account for less than 8% of those infected with HIV world-wide, 20% of deaths due to AIDS have been in children aged less than 15 years [93]. HIV infection has severely increased pediatric morbidity and mortality rates and has begun to reverse the significant gains in child survival that have been achieved during the last few decades. Safe, efficacious, inexpensive, and easy to use interventions to reduce vertical transmission of HIV offer the promise of decreasing pediatric HIV in Africa. However, the challenges of implementing these practices make it likely that African children will continue to be overwhelmingly afflicted by what has become a preventable disease in rich nations.

It had been hypothesized that HIV progression rates are more rapid in Africa than in industrialized countries. The immune activation associated with chronic infection, and the immunosuppression accompanying malnutrition have been postulated to result in higher levels of viremia and a more rapid disease course. Differences in HIV subtype and host genetic factors have also been considered to be important variables. However, more recent data strongly argue that the natural history of HIV infection among adults in Africa is not fundamentally distinct from that of adults in resource-rich settings prior to the advent of ART [94, 95]. Africans, like members of disadvantaged groups in rich countries, tend to present for care later and have much higher levels of general morbidity. Moreover, the burden of infectious diseases such as tuberculosis is much higher. Nevertheless, the median time from seroconversion to AIDS in HIV-infected African adults is 9.4 years, and most die severely immunosuppressed, with clinical features of AIDS [96]. These figures are remarkably similar to those observed in cohorts in the rich countries prior to the availability of effective ART. Levels of plasma viremia are also similar to those observed in rich countries prior to the widespread use of effective antiretroviral therapy [97]. Thus, pathophysiologically, HIV in Africa is not unique.

There are limited data on the natural history of HIV infection in African children. A bimodal pattern of clinical disease progression has been observed in resource-poor countries. Spira *et al.* reported that 17% of HIV-infected children at 1 year of age and 35% of HIV-infected children at 5 years of age had developed AIDS [98]. These rates are similar to those reported in rich countries [77, 99] and other settings [100]. However, the rates of morbidity and mortality are much higher than those reported in rich countries. In Rwanda, by 2 years of age 45% of HIV-infected children had died [98]. In a West African cohort, half the HIV-infected children died before their first birthday [101]. By age 3 years, 89% of the HIV-infected Malawian children had died, 10% were classified as stage B or C and only 1% were asymptomatic (category N) [102]. In contrast, by age 3 years, only 18% of HIV-infected European children had died, 48% were in category B or C, 24% in category A and 10% in category N [78]. These dramatic differences in mortality are likely due to differences in the use of prophylactic treatments, access to medical care, immunizations, nutrition, and antiretroviral use. However, other factors such as more advanced maternal disease, timing of infection, and differences in immunogenetic and/or viral factors cannot be excluded.

5.8 HAART and the natural history of HIV infection

The introduction of HAART in the mid-1990s dramatically reduced the rate of progression to AIDS and HIV-related death in both children and adults. Survival rates of HIV-infected children remained unchanged from 1980 to 1995. Between 1996 (when protease inhibitors were introduced) and 1999, the annual mortality rate among US children enrolled in Pediatric AIDS Clinical Trials Group (PACTG) studies decreased from 5.3% to 0.7% [103]. A similar reduction in mortality was reported in an Italian cohort [104]. Moreover, this study found that while the use of therapy with two ART drugs decreased the risk of death by 30%, treatment with three ART drugs resulted in a 71% decrease [104]. Progression to AIDS is also significantly reduced with HAART compared with mono- or dual therapy [105]. These data are comparable to declines described in adults [106–108].

Unfortunately, many children who initiated HAART were unable to achieve and/or sustain viral suppression. The reason for the lack of suppression is multifactor and may be attributed to higher levels of viremia, sequential use of insufficiently potent ART, inability to achieve adequately high ART levels, and problems with adherence. Many of these children who did not have sustained viral suppression have developed viruses resistant to all the currently available classes of antiretroviral therapy. The prognosis for these children will be significantly worse than for children who achieve good viral suppression unless new, non-cross resistant therapies become available. Although the prognosis is much better for a child who does achieve complete viral suppression, as many as 40% of children treated with HAART who do not achieve virologic suppression appear to derive some immunologic benefit from the therapy, as judged by a sustained CD4$^+$ lymphocyte count increase. These discordant responders with high plasma RNA and high CD4$^+$ cell counts may be infected with less fit (pathogenic) viruses. The prognosis of these children and the need for continued antiretroviral pressure in order to maintain this phenotype is unknown.

The short- and long-term adverse effects attributed to HAART have tempered enthusiasm for aggressive treatment of children. These data raise the disturbing specter of replacing the morbidities associated with immunosuppression with those of antiretroviral toxicity. The metabolic complications of antiretroviral therapy are discussed in detail in Chapter 20.

5.9 Natural history of horizontally acquired HIV infection in pediatrics

Children and youth who acquire HIV infection horizontally appear to have a disease course more similar to adults than perinatally infected infants. Data from the Multicenter AIDS cohort study (MACS), as well as studies in hemophiliac cohorts, have suggested that age of seroconversion is a significant predictor of disease progression [27, 28, 109]. These data indicate that, in the absence of ART, an individual infected at age 13 would develop AIDS at age 24.6 years, or 11.6 years later. The relatively improved prognosis is attributed to more robust immune responses in youth compared with adults. There are also data that suggest that the immune systems of younger persons may have a greater capacity to reconstitute than the immune systems of older persons (see Chapter 1).

Although natural history of HIV per se in adolescent and adult patients with horizontally acquired infection is similar, the pathogenesis of other viral infections in

Table 5.5 Proportion of children progressing to category C disease or death within a 5-year period from the beginning of each stage (before the availability of highly active antiretroviral therapy)

Stage	Percent developing category C disease within a 5-year period from the beginning of each stage	Percent mortality within 5 years from the beginning of each stage
N	50	25
A	58	33
B	60	35
C	–	83

Adapted from [77], with permission.

HIV-infected adolescents appears to be distinct. Adolescent girls appear to be more susceptible to human papilloma virus (HPV) infection than older women. Although HIV-infected young women do not appear to be at increased risk of acquiring this infection, HPV strains persist longer in HIV-infected adolescents and the incidence of squamous intraepithelial lesions is higher. The implications of this are discussed in Chapter 15. The seroprevalence of hepatitis B in HIV-infected youth in the US is much higher than the population at large [110]. Moreover, the serologic response to Hepatitis B vaccine appears to be suboptimal in HIV-infected adolescents and HIV-uninfected adolescents at risk for HIV infection [111]. Thus HIV-infected adolescents may be at greater risk for the Hepatitis B infection and its complications.

The pediatric classification system (Table 5.4) has been used to describe the natural history of HIV-1 disease in the absence of ART. Although a minority exhibit extremely rapid deterioration, most perinatally infected children remain relatively asymptomatic for the first year of life (on average, in one study, 10 months in stage N and 4 months in stage A) [77]. However, in the second year of life, most progress to moderate symptoms (stage B), typically remaining at this stage for over 5 years (mean 65 months). After entering stage C, mean and median survival times are 34 months and 23 months respectively [77]. Within 1 month of developing a category B illness, only 4% of children died, while 21% of children died within a month of a category C illness [78]. Table 5.5 summarizes the percentage of children who progress to stage C from the beginning of each stage and the proportion in each stage surviving at least 5 years [77]. Previously, most children who progressed to stage C in the first few years of life did so on the basis of an opportunistic infection (primarily PCP) [78]. The use of widespread PCP antimicrobial prophylaxis has significantly decreased this manifestation. Encephalopathy or recurrent serious bacterial infections were the next most common indications for category C classification in young children (78). About 50% of children who developed

category C disease in the first year of life had no signs of immune suppression and only 25% had a severe immune deficit (78). In contrast, only 14% of children who developed category C disease after age 1 year had normal immune status, while 59% were severely immunosuppressed [78]. While the mortality rate and clinical progression rate in the first year of life were approximately 10% and 20% respectively, the risk of progression to moderate immunosuppression was 50% and severe immunosuppression was 18%. After age 1 year, the risk of progression was 15% per year to moderate immune suppression and 10% per year to severe immune suppression [78]. Of the children who were alive beyond age 6 years only 2% (1/39) had no signs of immune suppression, 33% (13/39) had moderate suppression and 64% (25/39) had severe suppression [78].

5.10 Relationship between plasma viral concentration, CD4$^+$ cell level, and disease progression in children

A child's plasma RNA concentration appears to be a critical determinant of pediatric disease progression [112] (see also Chapter 4). Patterns of plasma viral RNA kinetics in the first few months of life appear to correlate with disease course. Rapid progressors have marked increases in viral RNA which do not decline [91]. One study found that plasma RNA levels tended to be low at birth (median 10 000 copies/mL for those with early infection), but rapidly increased over the first 2 months of life to very high levels (median approximately 300 000 copies/mL) before slowly declining over a period of several years [90]. Infants with plasma RNA levels above the median had an increased risk of disease progression and death. There was a 44% rate of progression by 24 months for children with an early peak value above 300 000 copies/mL and only a 15% rate of progression for children below this value [90]. Nevertheless, considerable overlap existed in RNA values between rapid

Table 5.6 Relationship between baseline RNA copy number and percentage CD4 and mortality in HIV-1 infected children

Baseline HIV RNA(copies/mL)	Baseline CD4$^+$cell percentage	Number deaths per number patients	Percent mortality
≤100 000	≥15	15/103	15
≤100 000	<15	15/24	63
>100 000	≥15	32/89	36
>100 000	<15	29/36	81

HIV RNA was quantified using the NASBA HIV-1 QT amplification system on samples obtained during the NICHD intravenous immunoglobulin clinical trial. Mean age of subjects was approximately 3 years, and mean follow-up was about 5 years. Data were taken from [113], with permission.

Table 5.7 Relationship between baseline HIV RNA copy number and risk of disease progression or death stratified by age

Baseline HIV RNA(copies/mL)	Number with disease progression or death/number patients	Percent with disease progression or death
Age < 30 Months at Entry		
<1 000–150 000	9/79	11
150 001–500 000	13/66	20
500 001–1 700 000	29/76	38
>1 700 000	42/81	52
Age ≥ 30 months at entry		
<1 000–15 000	0/66	0
15 001–50 000	7/54	13
50 001–150 000	13/80	16
>150 000	22/64	34

HIV RNA was quantified using NASABA HIV-1 QT amplification on samples obtained from children participating in Pediatric AIDS Clinical Trials Group protocol 152. Mean age of children in the < 30 months group was 1.1 years. Mean age of children in the group > 30 months was 7.3 years. All children received ART.
Data taken from [112], with permission.

and non-rapid progressors, and no threshold value could be identified in the first 2 years of life [90]. However, no infant with less than 70 000 copies/mL in the first 4 months of life had rapidly progressive disease [90]. Another study also determined that baseline RNA levels combined with CD4$^+$ lymphocyte percent were predictive of mortality [113] (see Table 5.6). In this study, the association of mortality with HIV-1 RNA levels varied with age; for children under 2 years of age mortality was increased only when the baseline RNA was over 1 million copies/mL, while for children over 2 years of age mortality increased when plasma RNA exceeded 100 000 copies/mL [113]. This is summarized in Table 5.7 and in Chapter 4.

Although most infants are initially infected with M-tropic viral strains, the appearance of T-tropic strains is associated with severe CD4$^+$ depletion and deterioration in clinical status [114–116]. Immunogenetic markers have also been identified which influence vertical transmission and disease progression [117–119].

5.11 Factors associated with disease HIV-infected children

Several clinical factors are associated with disease progression. Age at the time of infection is probably an important factor (see above). Children (over 1 year of age) and adolescents have much slower disease progression than adults [120]. Route of infection during the perinatal period may also be a significant factor. Infants infected by vertical transmission tend to progress more rapidly than those who acquire infection by blood products [71, 72, 121]. Infants born to women with advanced disease and higher viral loads also tend to be rapid progressors [122–124]. Whether this is due to the emergence of more virulent strains in persons with advanced disease and/or a reflection of shared immunogenetic factors is unknown. Finally, certain clinical manifestations of HIV-1 disease appear to be prognostically important in perinatally acquired HIV-1. Children who present at a young age with signs of advanced disease such as PCP or encephalopathy have a worse prognosis than those presenting with lymphoid interstitial pneumonia (LIP) or bacterial infections [76, 99, 125, 126]. Infants with enlarged lymph nodes, hepato- and/or splenomegaly at birth have almost a 40% chance of developing category C disease by 1 year compared with a 15% risk if these signs are absent [74]. Growth failure is another clinical sign of poor prognostic import [127] which has recently been correlated with viral load [128]. Most of these clinical symptoms improve dramatically with HAART. Although none of these clinical findings has been found to be as predictive as the combination of plasma RNA concentration and CD4$^+$ cell percentage, the information is easy and inexpensive to obtain.

5.12 Pediatric long-term non-progressors

Small subsets of adults infected with HIV-1 (< 5 %) are able to maintain normal CD4$^+$ cell counts and low viral loads for periods of greater than 12–15 years without ART. They have been called long-term survivors or long-term non-progressors. In adults, this appellation is restricted to those who have intact immune systems. A few long-term non-progressors appear to be infected with less pathogenic variants of the virus (see above). However, in most cases no progression is believed to be due to host factors.

The definition of a long-term pediatric survivor includes those who have survived more than 8 years and permits inclusion of persons who have received antiretrovirals and are mildly symptomatic. One preliminary study of HIV-1 infected children who were 8 years of age and older found that this was a very diverse group of children with varying stages of disease progression [129]. Only 20% had absolute CD4$^+$ cell counts greater than or equal to 500 cells/μL and no AIDS-defining conditions [129]; reasons for long-term non-progression in children have not been well characterized.

5.13 Transient infection

A few pediatric centers prospectively following HIV-1 seroreverting children have described infants who had transient evidence of HIV infection, including positive DNA and RNA PCR and viral culture, in the immediate postpartum period [130–133]. Others have described the detection of cell-mediated immune responses in seroreverting infants (reviewed in [134]). Studies of macaques infected with simian immunodeficiency virus (SIV) would suggest that transient infection is possible [135]. However, a detailed phylogenetic analysis of such putative human cases could not confirm transient infection [136]. This study strongly suggests that if transient HIV infection occurs it is extremely rare.

5.14 Conclusions

The natural history of pediatric HIV has been radically altered by the use of ART. Our understanding of the dynamics of HIV-1 infection coupled with availability of new antiretroviral agents led many to advocate early aggressive treatment of children. However, the difficulties of adhering to complex regimens and the short- and long-term effects of current therapies dampened enthusiasm for this approach. Balancing benefits of ART and risks of uncontrolled HIV infection in children is the subject of intense research and will undoubtedly provide insights into the natural history of this disease.

ACKNOWLEDGMENTS

We thank Katherine Semrau for helpful discussion and review of the manuscript. Supported in part by grants UO1 AI41025, R01 AI40951, R01 HD39611, R01 HD4775 and R01 HD 40777 from the National Institute of Health, and Contract Number 97PVCL05 from Social & Scientific Systems.

REFERENCES

1. Munoz, A., Wang, M. C., Bass, S. *et al.* Acquired immunodeficiency syndrome (AIDS)-free time after human immunodeficiency virus type 1 (HIV-1) seroconversion in homosexual men. Multicenter AIDS Cohort Study Group. *Am. J. Epidemiol.* **13**c : **3** (1989), 530–9.
2. Munoz, A., Kirby, A. J., He, Y. D. *et al.* Long-term survivors with HIV-1 infection: incubation period and longitudinal patterns of CD4$^+$ lymphocytes. *J. AIDS Hum. Retrovirol.* **8** : **5** (1995), 496–505.

3. Veugelers, P. J., Kaldor J. M., Strathdee, S. A. *et al.* Incidence and prognostic significance of symptomatic primary human immunodeficiency virus type 1 infection in homosexual men. *J. Infect. Dis.* **176** : **1** (1997), 112–17.

4. Lyles, R. H., Munoz, A., Yamashita, T. E. *et al.* Natural history of human immunodeficiency virus type 1 viremia after seroconversion and proximal to AIDS in a large cohort of homosexual men. Multicenter AIDS Cohort Study. *J. Infect. Dis.* **181** : **3** (2000), 872–80.

5. Vanhems, P., Hirschel, B., Phillips, A. N. *et al.* Incubation time of acute human immunodeficiency virus (HIV) infection and duration of acute HIV infection are independent prognostic factors of progression to AIDS. *J. Infect. Dis.* **182** : **1** (2000), 334–7.

6. Vanhems, P., Allard, R., Cooper, D. A. *et al.* Acute human immunodeficiency virus type 1 disease as a mononucleosis-like illness: is the diagnosis too restrictive? *Clin. Infect. Dis.* **24** : **5** (1997), 965–70.

7. Vanhems, P. & Beaulieu, R. Primary infection by type 1 human immunodeficiency virus: diagnosis and prognosis. *Postgrad. Med. J.* **73** : **861** (1997), 403–8.

8. Daar, E. S., Moudgil, T., Meyer, R. D. & Ho, D. D. Transient high levels of viremia in patients with primary human immunodeficiency virus type 1 infection. *New Engl. J. Med.* **324** : **14** (1991), 961–4.

9. Clark, S. J., Saag, M. S., Decker, W. D. *et al.* High titers of cytopathic virus in plasma of patients with symptomatic primary HIV-1 infection. *New Engl. J. Med.* **324** : **14** (1991), 954–60.

10. Rosenberg, E. S., Billingsley, J. M., Caliend, A. M. *et al.* Vigorous HIV-1-specific CD4+ T cell responses associated with control of viremia. *Science* **278** : **5342** (1997), 1447–50.

11. Perelson, A. S., Neumann, A. U., Markowitz, M., Leonard, J. M. & Ho, D. D. HIV-1 dynamics in vivo: virion clearance rate, infected cell life-span, and viral generation time. *Science* **271** : **5255** (1996), 1582–6.

12. Piatak, M., Jr., Saag, M. S., Yang, L. C., *et al.* High levels of HIV-1 in plasma during all stages of infection determined by competitive PCR. *Science* **259** : **5102** (1993), 1749–54.

13. Ho, D. D., Neumann, A. U., Perelson, A. S., Chen, W., Leonard, J. M. & Markowitz, M. Rapid turnover of plasma virions and CD4 lymphocytes in HIV-1 infection. *Nature* **373** : **6510** (1995), 123–6.

14. Haase, A. T., Henry, K., Zupancic, M. *et al.* Quantitative image analysis of HIV-1 infection in lymphoid tissue. *Science* **274** : **5289** (1996), 985–9.

15. Cavert, W., Notermans, D. W., Staskus, K. *et al.* Kinetics of response in lymphoid tissues to antiretroviral therapy of HIV-1 infection. *Science* **276** : **5314** (1997), 960–4.

16. Zhang, H., Dornadula, G., Beumont, M. *et al.* Human immunodeficiency virus type 1 in the semen of men receiving highly active antiretroviral therapy. *New Engl. J. Med.* **339** : **25** (1998), 1803–9.

17. Iversen, A. K., Larsen, A. R., Jensen, T. *et al.* Distinct determinants of human immunodeficiency virus type 1 RNA and DNA loads in vaginal and cervical secretions. *J. Infect. Dis.* **177** : **5** (1998), 1214–20.

18. Delwart, E. L., Mullins, J. I., Gupta, P. *et al.* Human immunodeficiency virus type 1 populations in blood and semen. *J. Virol.* **72** : **1** (1998), 617–23.

19. Poss, M., Rodrigo, A. G., Gosink, J. J. *et al.* Evolution of envelope sequences from the genital tract and peripheral blood of women infected with clade A human immunodeficiency virus type 1. *J. Virol.* **72** : **10** (1998), 8240–51.

20. Panther, L. A., Tucker, L., Xu, C., Tuomala, R. E., Mullins, J. I. & Anderson, D. J. Genital tract human immunodeficiency virus type 1 (HIV-1) shedding and inflammation and HIV-1 env diversity in perinatal HIV-1 transmission. *J. Infect. Dis.* **181** : **2** (2000), 555–63.

21. Mellors, J. W., Kingsley, L. A., Rinaldo, C. R., Jr. *et al.* Quantitation of HIV-1 RNA in plasma predicts outcome after seroconversion. *Ann. Intern. Med.* **122** : **8** (1995), 573–9.

22. Mellors, J. W., Rinaldo, C. R., Jr. & Gupta, P. Prognosis in HIV-1 infection predicted by the quantity of virus in plasma. *Science* **272** : **5265** (1996), 1167–70.

23. O'Brien, W. A., Hartigan, P. M., Daar, E. S., Simberkoff, M. S. & Hamilton, J. D. Changes in plasma HIV RNA levels and CD4+ lymphocyte counts predict both response to antiretroviral therapy and therapeutic failure. VA Cooperative Study Group on AIDS. *Ann. Intern. Med.* **126** : **12** (1997), 939–45.

24. Hughes, M. D., Johnson, V. A., Hirsch, M. S. *et al.* Monitoring plasma HIV-1 RNA levels in addition to CD4+ lymphocyte count improves assessment of antiretroviral therapeutic response. ACTG 241 Protocol Virology Substudy Team. *Ann. Intern. Med.* **126** : **12** (1997), 929–38.

25. Finzi, D. & Siliciano, R. F. Taking aim at HIV replication. *Nat. Med.* **6** : **7** (2000), 735–6.

26. Esterling, B. A., Antoni, M. H., Schneiderman, N. *et al.* Psychosocial modulation of antibody to Epstein-Barr viral capsid antigen and human herpesvirus type-6 in HIV-1-infected and at-risk gay men. *Psychosom. Med.* **54** : **3** (1992), 354–71.

27. Carre, N., Deveau, C., Belanger, F. *et al.* Effect of age and exposure group on the onset of AIDS in heterosexual and homosexual HIV-infected patients. SEROCO Study Group. *Aids* **8** : **6** (1994), 797–802.

28. Rosenberg, P. S., Goedert, J. J. & Biggar, R. J. Effect of age at seroconversion on the natural AIDS incubation distribution. Multicenter Hemophilia Cohort Study and the International Registry of Seroconverters. *AIDS* **8** : **6** (1994), 803–10.

29. Eyster, M. E., Gail, M. H., Ballard, J. O., Al-Mondhiry, H. & Goedert, J. J. Natural history of human immunodeficiency virus infections in hemophiliacs: effects of T-cell subsets, platelet counts, and age. *Ann. Intern. Med.* **107** : **1** (1987), 1–6.

30. Gandhi, R. T. & Walker, B. D. Promises and pitfalls in the reconstitution of immunity in patients who have HIV-1 infection. *Curr. Opin. Immunol.* **14** : **4** (2002), 487–94.

31. Altfeld, M., Allen, T. M., Yu, X. G. *et al.* HIV-1 superinfection despite broad CD8+ T-cell responses containing replication of the primary virus. *Nature* **420** : **6914** (2002), 434–9.

32. Jost, S., Bernard, M.-C., Kaiser, L. *et al.* A patient with HIV-1 superinfection. *New Engl. J. Med.* **347** : **10** (2002), 731–6.

33. Carrington, M., Nelson, G. W., Martin, M. P. *et al.* HLA and HIV-1: heterozygote advantage and B35–Cw04 disadvantage. *Science* **283** : **5408** (1999), 1748–52.

34. Kaslow, R. A., Carrington, M., Apple, R. *et al.* Influence of combinations of human major histocompatibility complex genes on the course of HIV-1 infection. *Nat. Med.* **2** : **4** (1996), 405–11.

35. Goulder, P. J., Brander, C., Tang, Y. *et al.* Evolution and transmission of stable CTL escape mutations in HIV infection. *Nature* **412** : **6844** (2001), 334–8.

36. O'Brien, S. J., Gao, X. & Carrington, M. HLA and AIDS: a cautionary tale. *Trends Mol. Med.* **7** : **9** (2001), 379–81.

37. Dean, M., Carrington, M. & O'Brien, S. J. Balanced polymorphism selected by genetic versus infectious human disease. *Annu. Rev. Genomics Hum. Genet.* **3** (2002), 263–92.

38. Dean, M., Carrington, M., Winkler, C. *et al.* Genetic restriction of HIV-1 infection and progression to AIDS by a deletion allele of the CKR5 structural gene. Hemophilia Growth and Development Study, Multicenter AIDS Cohort Study, Multicenter Hemophilia Cohort Study, San Francisco City Cohort, ALIVE Study. *Science* **273** : **5283** (1996), 1856–62.

39. Smith, M. W., Dean, M., Carrington, M. *et al.* Contrasting genetic influence of CCR2 and CCR5 variants on HIV-1 infection and disease progression. Hemophilia Growth and Development Study (HGDS), Multicenter AIDS Cohort Study (MACS), Multicenter Hemophilia Cohort Study (MHCS), San Francisco City Cohort (SFCC), ALIVE Study. *Science* **277** : **5328** (1997), 959–65.

40. Meyer, L., Magierowska, M., Hubert, J. B. *et al.* Early protective effect of CCR-5 delta 32 heterozygosity on HIV-1 disease progression: relationship with viral load. The SEROCO Study Group. *AIDS* **11** : **11** (1997), F73–8.

41. Liu, R., Paxton, W. A., Choe, S. *et al.* Homozygous defect in HIV-1 coreceptor accounts for resistance of some multiply-exposed individuals to HIV-1 infection. *Cell* **86** : **3** (1996), 367–77.

42. Paxton, W. A., Martin, S. R., Tse, D. *et al.* Relative resistance to HIV-1 infection of CD4 lymphocytes from persons who remain uninfected despite multiple high-risk sexual exposure. *Nat. Med.* **2** : **4** (1996), 412–7.

43. Samson, M., Libert, F., Doranz, B. J. *et al.* Resistance to HIV-1 infection in caucasian individuals bearing mutant alleles of the CCR-5 chemokine receptor gene. *Nature* **382** : **6593** (1996), 722–5.

44. Winkler, C., Modi, W., Smith, M. W. *et al.* Genetic restriction of AIDS pathogenesis by an SDF-1 chemokine gene variant. ALIVE Study, Hemophilia Growth and Development Study (HGDS), Multicenter AIDS Cohort Study (MACS), Multicenter Hemophilia Cohort Study (MHCS), San Francisco City Cohort (SFCC). *Science* **279** : **5349** (1998), 389–93.

45. Shin, H. D., Winkler, C., Stephens, J. C. *et al.* Genetic restriction of HIV-1 pathogenesis to AIDS by promoter alleles of IL10. *Proc. Natl. Acad. Sci. U.S.A.* **97** : **26** (2000), 14467–72.

46. Anzala, A. O., Ball, T. B., Rostron, T., O'Brien, S. J., Plummer, F. A. & Rowland-Jones, S. L. CCR2–64I allele and genotype association with delayed AIDS progression in African women. University of Nairobi Collaboration for HIV Research. *Lancet* **351** : **9116** (1998), 1632–3.

47. Fauci, A. S., Pantaleo, G., Stanley, S. & Weissman, D. Immunopathogenic mechanisms of HIV infection. *Ann. Intern. Med.* **124** : **7** (1996), 654–63.

48. Bush, C. E., Donovan, R. M., Markowitz, N. P., Kvale, P. & Saravolatz, L. D. A study of HIV RNA viral load in AIDS patients with bacterial pneumonia. *J. AIDS Hum. Retrovirol.* **13** : **1** (1996), 23–6.

49. Donovan, R. M., Bush, C. E., Markowitz, N. P., Baxa, D. M. & Saravolatz, L. D. Changes in virus load markers during AIDS-associated opportunistic diseases in human immunodeficiency virus-infected persons. *J. Infect. Dis.* **174** : **2** (1996), 401–3.

50. Stein, D. S. & Drusano, G. L. Modeling of the change in CD4 lymphocyte counts in patients before and after administration of the human immunodeficiency virus protease inhibitor indinavir. *Antimicrob. Agents Chemother.* **41** : **2** (1997), 449–53.

51. Whalen, C., Horsburgh, C. R., Hom, D., Lahart, C., Simberkoff, M. & Ellner, J. Accelerated course of human immunodeficiency virus infection after tuberculosis. *Am. J. Respir. Crit. Care Med.* **151** : **1** (1995), 129–35.

52. Staprans, S. I., Hamilton, B. L., Follansbee, S. E. *et al.* Activation of virus replication after vaccination of HIV-1-infected individuals. *J. Exp. Med.* **182** : **6** (1995), 1727–37.

53. Stanley, S., Ostrowski, M. A., Justement, J. S. *et al.* Effect of immunization with a common recall antigen on viral expression in patients infected with human immunodeficiency virus type 1. *New Engl. J. Med.* **334** : **19** (1996), 1222–30.

54. O'Brien, W. A., Grovit-Ferbas, K., Namazi, A. *et al.* Human immunodeficiency virus-type 1 replication can be increased in peripheral blood of seropositive patients after influenza vaccination. *Blood* **86** : **3** (1995), 1082–9.

55. Fowke, K. R., D'Amico, R., Chernoff, D. N. *et al.* Immunologic and virologic evaluation after influenza vaccination of HIV-1-infected patients. *AIDS* **11** : **8** (1997), 1013–21.

56. Yerly, S., Wunderli, W., Wyler, C. A. *et al.* Influenza immunization of HIV-1-infected patients does not increase HIV-1 viral load. *AIDS* **8** : **10** (1994), 1503–4.

57. Premack, B. A. & Schall, T. J. Chemokine receptors: gateways to inflammation and infection. *Nat. Med.* **2** : **11** (1996), 1174–8.

58. D'Souza, M. P. & Harden, V. A. Chemokines and HIV-1 second receptors. Confluence of two fields generates optimism in AIDS research. *Nat. Med.* **2** : **12** (1996), 1293–300.

59. Connor, R. I., Sheridan, K. E., Ceradini, D., Choe, S. & Landau, N. R. Change in coreceptor use correlates with disease progression in HIV-1–infected individuals. *J. Exp. Med.* **185** : **4** (1997), 621–8.

60. Connor, R. I., Mohri, H., Cao, Y. & Ho, D. D. Increased viral burden and cytopathicity correlate temporally with CD4+

T-lymphocyte decline and clinical progression in human immunodeficiency virus type 1-infected individuals. *J. Virol.* **67** : **4** (1993), 1772–7.

61. Koot, M., van 't Wout, A. B., Kootstra, N. A., de Goede, R. E., Tersmette, M. & Schuitemaker, H. Relation between changes in cellular load, evolution of viral phenotype, and the clonal composition of virus populations in the course of human immunodeficiency virus type 1 infection. *J. Infect. Dis.* **173** : **2** (1996), 349–54.

62. Cao, Y., Qin, L., Zhang, L., Safrit, J. & Ho, D. D. Virologic and immunologic characterization of long-term survivors of human immunodeficiency virus type 1 infection. *New Engl. J. Med.* **332** : **4** (1995), 201–8.

63. Deacon, N. J., Tsykin, A., Solomon, A. *et al.* Genomic structure of an attenuated quasi species of HIV-1 from a blood transfusion donor and recipients. *Science* **270** : **5238** (1995), 988–91.

64. Iversen, A. K., Shpaer, E. G., Rodrigo, A. G. *et al.* Persistence of attenuated *rev* genes in a human immunodeficiency virus type 1-infected asymptomatic individual. *J. Virol.* **69** : **9** (1995), 5743–53.

65. Kirchhoff, F., Easterbrook, P. J., Douglas, N. *et al.* Sequence variations in human immunodeficiency virus type 1 *nef* are associated with different stages of disease. *J. Virol.* **73** : **7** (1999), 5497–508.

66. Michael, N. L., Chang, G., d'Arcy, L. A., Tseng, C. J., Birx, D. L. & Sheppard, H. W. Functional characterization of human immunodeficiency virus type 1 *nef* genes in patients with divergent rates of disease progression. *J. Virol.* **69** : **11** (1995), 6758–69.

67. Neilson, J. R., John, G. C., Carr, J. K. *et al.* Subtypes of human immunodeficiency virus type 1 and disease stage among women in Nairobi, Kenya. *J. Virol.* **73** : **5** (1999), 4393–403.

68. Osmanov, S., Pattou, C., Walker, N., Schwardlander, B. & Esparza, J. Estimated global distribution and regional spread of HIV-1 genetic subtypes in the year 2000. *J. AIDS* **29** : **2** (2002), 184–90.

69. Centers for Disease Control and Prevention. 1994 revised classification system for human immunodeficiency virus infection in children less than 13 years. *MMWR* **43** (1994), 1–19.

70. National Pediatric and Family HIV Resource Center and National Center for Infectious Diseases, Centers for Disease Control and Prevention. 1995 revised guidelines for prophylaxis against *Pneumocystis carinii* pneumonia for children infected with or perinatally exposed to human immunodeficiency virus. *MMWR* **44** : **RR-4** (1995), 1–11.

71. Frederick, T., Mascola, L., Eller, A., O'Neil, L. & Byers, B. Progression of human immunodeficiency virus disease among infants and children infected perinatally with human immunodeficiency virus or through neonatal blood transfusion. Los Angeles County Pediatric AIDS Consortium and the Los Angeles County-University of Southern California Medical Center and the University of Southern California School of

Medicine [see comments]. *Pediatr. Infect. Dis. J.* **13** : **12** (1994), 1091–7.

72. Jones, D. S., Byers, R. H., Bush, T. J., Oxtoby, M. J. & Rogers, M. F. Epidemiology of transfusion-associated acquired immunodeficiency syndrome in children in the United States, 1981 through 1989. *Pediatrics* **89** : **1** (1992), 123–7.

73. Auger, I., Thomas, P., DeGruttola, V. *et al.* Incubation periods for pediatric AIDS patients. *Nature* **336** (1988), 575–7.

74. Mayaux, M. J., Burgard, M., Teglas, J. P. *et al.* Neonatal characteristics in rapidly progressive perinatally acquired HIV-1 disease. The French Pediatric HIV Infection Study Group. *J. Am. Med. Assoc.* **275** : **8** (1996), 606–10.

75. Duliege, A. M., Messiah, A., Blanche, S., Tardieu, M., Griscelli, C. & Spira, A. Natural history of human immunodeficiency virus type 1 infection in children: prognostic value of laboratory tests on the bimodal progression of the disease. *Pediatr. Infect. Dis. J.* **11** : **8** (1992), 630–5.

76. Scott, G. B., Hutto, C., Makuch, R. W. *et al.* Survival in children with perinatally acquired human immunodeficiency virus type 1 infection. *New Engl. J. Med.* **321** : **26** (1989), 1791–6.

77. Barnhart, H. X., Caldwell, M. B., Thomas, P. *et al.* Natural history of human immunodeficiency virus disease in perinatally infected children: an analysis from the Pediatric Spectrum of Disease Project. *Pediatrics* **97** : **5** (1996), 710–16.

78. Blanche, S., Newell, M. L., Mayaux, M. J. *et al.* Morbidity and mortality in European children vertically infected by HIV- 1. The French Pediatric HIV Infection Study Group and European Collaborative Study. *J. AIDS Hum. Retrovirol.* **14** : **5** (1997), 442–50.

79. Galli, L., de Martino, M., Tovo, P. A. *et al.* Onset of clinical signs in children with HIV-1 perinatal infection. Italian Register for HIV Infection in Children. *AIDS* **9** : **5** (1995), 455–61.

80. Pizzo, P. A. Progression of human immunodeficiency virus infection in children is related to the interaction of the virus, the immune system, and then some [editorial; comment]. *Clin. Infect. Dis.* **24** : **5** (1997), 975–6.

81. Bryson, Y. J., Luzuriaga, K., Sullivan, J. L. & Wara, D. W. Proposed definitions for in utero versus intrapartum transmission of HIV-1. *New Engl. J. Med.* **327** : **17** (1992), 1246–7.

82. Doyle, M., Atkins, J. T. & Rivera-Matos, I. R. Congenital cytomegalovirus infection in infants infected with human immunodeficiency virus type 1. *Pediatr. Infect. Dis. J.* **15** : **12** (1996), 1102–6.

83. Nigro, G., Krzysztofiak, A., Gattinara, G. C. *et al.* Rapid progression of HIV disease in children with cytomegalovirus DNAemia. *AIDS* **10** : **10** (1996), 1127–33.

84. Sabin, C. A., Phillips, A. N., Lee, C. A., Janossy, G., Emery, V. & Griffiths, P. D. The effect of CMV infection on progression of human immunodeficiency virus disease is a cohort of haemophilic men followed for up to 13 years from seroconversion. *Epidemiol. Infect.* **114** : **2** (1995), 361–72.

85. Pizzo, P. A. & Wilfert, C. M. Markers and determinants of disease progression in children with HIV infection. The Pediatric AIDS Siena Workshop II. *J. AIDS Hum. Retrovirol.* **8** : **1** (1995), 30–44.

86. Plaeger-Marshall, S., Isacescu, V., O'Rourke, S., Bertolli, J., Bryson, Y. J., Stiehm, E. R. T cell activation in pediatric AIDS pathogenesis: three-color immunophenotyping. *Clin. Immunol. Immunopathol.* **71** : **1** (1994), 19–26.

87. Pollack, H., Zhan, M. X., Ilmet-Moore, T., Ajuang-Simbiri, K., Krasinski, K. & Borkowsky, W. Ontogeny of anti-human immunodeficiency virus (HIV) antibody production in HIV-1-infected infants. *Proc. Natl. Acad. Sci. U.S.A.* **90** : **6** (1993), 2340–4.

88. Kourtis, A. P., Ibegbu, C., Nahmias, A. J. *et al.* Early progression of disease in HIV-infected infants with thymus dysfunction. *New Engl. J. Med.* **335** : **19** (1996), 1431–6.

89. Dickover, R. E., Dillon, M., Gillette, S. G. *et al.* Rapid increases in load of human immunodeficiency virus correlate with early disease progression and loss of CD4 cells in vertically infected infants. *J. Infect. Dis.* **170** : **5** (1994), 1279–84.

90. Shearer, W. T., Quinn, T. C., LaRussa, P. *et al.* Viral load and disease progression in infants infected with human immunodeficiency virus type 1. Women and Infants Transmission Study Group. *New Engl. J. Med.* **336** : **19** (1997), 1337–42.

91. De Rossi, A., Masiero, S., Giaquinto, C. *et al.* Dynamics of viral replication in infants with vertically acquired human immunodeficiency virus type 1 infection. *J. Clin. Invest.* **97** : **2** (1996), 323–30.

92. McIntosh, K., Shevitz, A., Zaknun, D. *et al.* Age- and time-related changes in extracellular viral load in children vertically infected by human immunodeficiency virus. *Pediatr. Infect. Dis. J.* **15** : **12** (1996), 1087–91.

93. UNAIDS/WHO. *AIDS Epidemic Update – December 2002.* Geneva: UNAIDS/WHO, 2002.

94. Cohen, J. Is AIDS in Africa a distinct disease? *Science* **288** : **5474** (2000), 2153–5.

95. Morgan, D. & Whitworth, J. The natural history of HIV-1 infection in Africa. *Nat. Med.* **7** : **2** (2001), 143–5.

96. Morgan, D., Mahe, C., Mayanja, B. & Whitworth, J. A. Progression to symptomatic disease in people infected with HIV-1 in rural Uganda: prospective cohort study. *Br. Med. J.* **324** : **7331** (2002), 193–6.

97. Fideli, U. S., Allen, S. A., Musonda, R. *et al.* Virologic and immunologic determinants of heterosexual transmission of human immunodeficiency virus type 1 in Africa. *AIDS Res. Hum. Retroviruses.* **17** : **10** (2001), 901–10.

98. Spira, R., Lepage, P., Msellati, P. *et al.* Natural history of human immunodeficiency virus type 1 infection in children: a five-year prospective study in Rwanda. Mother-to-Child HIV-1 Transmission Study Group. *Pediatrics* **104** : **5** (1999), e56.

99. Bamji, M., Thea, D. M., Weedon, J. *et al.* Prospective study of human immunodeficiency virus 1-related disease among 512 infants born to infected women in New York City. The New York City Perinatal HIV Transmission Collaborative Study Group. *Pediatr. Infect. Dis. J.* **15** : **10** (1996), 891–8.

100. Lepage, P., Spira, R., Kalibala, S. *et al.* Care of human immunodeficiency virus-infected children in developing countries. International Working Group on Mother-to-Child Transmission of HIV. *Pediatr. Infect. Dis. J.* **17** : **7** (1998), 581–6.

101. Dabis, F., Elenga, N., Meda, N. *et al.* 18-Month mortality and perinatal exposure to zidovudine in West Africa. *AIDS* **15** : **6** (2001), 771–9.

102. Taha, T. E., Graham, S. M., Kumwenda, N. I. *et al.* Morbidity among human immunodeficiency virus-1-infected and -uninfected African children. *Pediatrics* **106** : **6** (2000), E77.

103. Gortmaker, S. L., Hughes, M., Cervia, J. *et al.* Effect of combination therapy including protease inhibitors on mortality among children and adolescents infected with HIV-1. *New Engl. J. Med.* **345** : **21** (2001), 1522–8.

104. de Martino, M., Tovo, P. A., Balducci, M. *et al.* Reduction in mortality with availability of antiretroviral therapy for children with perinatal HIV-1 infection. Italian Register for HIV Infection in Children and the Italian National AIDS Registry. *J. Am. Med. Assoc.* **284** : **2** (2000), 190–7.

105. Resino, S., Bellon, J. M., Sanchez-Ramon, S. *et al.* Impact of antiretroviral protocols on dynamics of AIDS progression markers. *Arch. Dis. Child.* **86** : **2** (2002), 119–24.

106. Mocroft, A., Vella, S., Benfield, T. L. *et al.* Changing patterns of mortality across Europe in patients infected with HIV-1. EuroSIDA Study Group. *Lancet* **352** : **9142** (1998), 1725–30.

107. Detels, R., Munoz, A., McFarlane, G. *et al.* Effectiveness of potent antiretroviral therapy on time to AIDS and death in men with known HIV infection duration. Multicenter AIDS Cohort Study Investigators. *J. Am. Med. Assoc.* **280** : **17** (1998), 1497–503.

108. Palella, F. J., Jr., Delaney, K. M., Moorman, A. C. *et al.* Declining morbidity and mortality among patients with advanced human immunodeficiency virus infection. HIV Outpatient Study Investigators. *New Engl. J. Med.* **338** : **13** (1998), 853–60.

109. Munoz, A., Sabin, C. A. & Phillips, A. N. The incubation period of AIDS. *Aids* **11** : Suppl. A (1997), S69–76.

110. Holland, C. A., Ma, Y., Moscicki, B., Durako, S. J., Levin, L. & Wilson, C. M. Seroprevalence and risk factors of hepatitis B, hepatitis C, and human cytomegalovirus among HIV-infected and high-risk uninfected adolescents: findings of the REACH Study. Adolescent Medicine HIV/AIDS Research Network. *Sex. Transm. Dis.* **27** : **5** (2000), 296–303.

111. Wilson, C. M., Ellenberg, J. H., Sawyer, M. K. *et al.* Serologic response to hepatitis B vaccine in HIV infected and high-risk HIV uninfected adolescents in the REACH cohort. Reaching for Excellence in Adolescent Care and Health. *J. Adolesc. Health.* **29** : **3** Suppl. (2001), 123–9.

112. Palumbo, P. E., Raskino, C., Fiscus, S. *et al.* Predictive value of quantitative plasma HIV RNA and CD4+ lymphocyte count in HIV-infected infants and children. *J. Am. Med. Assoc.* **279** : **10** (1998), 756–61.

113. Mofenson, L. M., Korelitz, J., Meyer, W. A., 3rd. *et al.* The relationship between serum human immunodeficiency virus type 1 (HIV-1) RNA level, CD4 lymphocyte percent, and long-term mortality risk in HIV-1-infected children. National Institute of Child Health and Human Development Intravenous Immunoglobulin Clinical Trial Study Group. *J. Infect. Dis.* **175** : **5** (1997), 1029–38.

114. Balotta, C., Vigano, A., Riva, C. *et al.* HIV type 1 phenotype correlates with the stage of infection in vertically infected children. *AIDS Res. Hum. Retroviruses* **12** : **13** (1996), 1247–53.

115. Spencer, L. T., Ogino, M. T., Dankner, W. M. & Spector, S. A. Clinical significance of human immunodeficiency virus type 1 phenotypes in infected children. *J. Infect. Dis.* **169** : **3** (1994), 491–5.

116. Ometto, L., Zanotto, C., Maccabruni, A. *et al.* Viral phenotype and host-cell susceptibility to HIV-1 infection as risk factors for mother-to-child HIV-1 transmission. *AIDS* **9** : **5** (1995), 427–34.

117. Just, J. J., Casabona, J., Bertran, J. *et al.* MHC class II alleles associated with clinical and immunological manifestations of HIV-1 infection among children in Catalonia, Spain. *Tissue Antigens* **47** : **4** (1996), 313–8.

118. Just, J. J., Abrams, E., Louie, L. G. *et al.* Influence of host genotype on progression to acquired immunodeficiency syndrome among children infected with human immunodeficiency virus type 1. *J. Pediatr.* **127** : **4** (1995), 544–9.

119. Kostrikis, L. G., Neumann, A. U., Thomson, B. *et al.* A polymorphism in the regulatory region of the CC-chemokine receptor 5 gene influences perinatal transmission of human immunodeficiency virus type 1 to African-American infants. *J. Virol.* **73** : **12** (1999), 10264–71.

120. Goedert, J. J., Kessler, C. M., Aledort, L. M. *et al.* A prospective study of human immunodeficiency virus type 1 infection and the development of AIDS in subjects with hemophilia. *New Engl. J. Med.* **321** : **17** (1989), 1141–8.

121. Morris, C. R., Araba-Owoyele, L., Spector, S. A. & Maldonado, Y. A. Disease patterns and survival after acquired immunodeficiency syndrome diagnosis in human immunodeficiency virus-infected children. *Pediatr. Infect. Dis. J.* **15** : **4** (1996), 321–8.

122. Blanche, S., Mayaux, M. J., Rouzioux, C. *et al.* Relation of the course of HIV infection in children to the severity of the disease in their mothers at delivery. *New Engl. J. Med.* **330** : **5** (1994), 308–12.

123. Tovo, P. A., de Martino, M., Gabiano, C. *et al.* AIDS appearance in children is associated with the velocity of disease progression in their mothers. *J. Infect. Dis.* **170** : 4 (1994), 1000–2.

124. Lambert, G., Thea, D. M., Pliner, V. *et al.* Effect of maternal CD4+ cell count, acquired immunodeficiency syndrome, and viral load on disease progression in infants with perinatally acquired human immunodeficiency virus type 1 infection. New York City Perinatal HIV Transmission Collaborative Study Group. *J. Pediatr.* **130** : **6** (1997), 890–7.

125. Krasinski, K., Borkowsky, W. & Holzman, R. S. Prognosis of human immunodeficiency virus infection in children and adolescents. *Pediatr. Infect. Dis. J.* **8** : **4** (1989), 216–20.

126. Blanche, S., Tardieu, M., Duliege, A. *et al.* Longitudinal study of 94 symptomatic infants with perinatally acquired human immunodeficiency virus infection. Evidence for a bimodal expression of clinical and biological symptoms. *Am. J. Dis. Child.* **144** : **11** (1990), 1210–5.

127. McKinney, R. E., Jr. & Wilfert, C. Growth as a prognostic indicator in children with human immunodeficiency virus infection treated with zidovudine. AIDS Clinical Trials Group Protocol 043 Study Group. *J. Pediatr.* **125** : **5** (1994), 728–33.

128. Pollack, H., Glasberg, H., Lee, E. *et al.* Impaired early growth of infants perinatally infected with human immunodeficiency virus: correlation with viral load. *J. Pediatr.* **130** : **6** (1997), 915–22.

129. Nielsen, K., Ammann, A., Bryson, Y. *et al.* A descriptive survey of pediatric HIV-infected long term survivors. In *3rd Conference on Retroviruses and Opportunistic Infections* January 28–February 1 (1996), p. 150. [Abstract].

130. Bryson, Y. J., Pang, S., Wei, L. S., Dickover, R., Diagne, A. & Chen, I. S. Clearance of HIV infection in a perinatally infected infant. *New Engl. J. Med.* **332** : **13** (1995), 833–8.

131. Newell, M. L., Dunn, D., De Maria, A. *et al.* Detection of virus in vertically exposed HIV-antibody-negative children. *Lancet* **347** : **8996** (1996), 213–5.

132. Roques, P. A., Gras, G., Parnet-Mathieu, F. *et al.* Clearance of HIV infection in 12 perinatally infected children: clinical, virological and immunological data. *AIDS* **9** : **12** (1995), F19–26.

133. Bakshi, S. S., Tetali, S., Abrams, E. J., Paul, M. O. & Pahwa, S. G. Repeatedly positive human immunodeficiency virus type 1 DNA polymerase chain reaction in human immunodeficiency virus-exposed seroreverting infants. *Pediatr. Infect. Dis. J.* **14** : **8** (1995), 658–62.

134. Kuhn, L., Meddows-Taylor, S., Gray, G. & Tiemessen, C. Human immunodeficiency virus (HIV)-specific cellular immune responses in newborns exposed to HIV in utero. *Clin. Infect. Dis.* **34** : **2** (2002), 267–76.

135. Miller, C. J., Marthas, M., Torten, J. *et al.* Intravaginal inoculation of rhesus macaques with cell-free simian immunodeficiency virus results in persistent or transient viremia. *J. Virol.* **68** : **10** (1994), 6391–400.

136. Frenkel, L. M., Mullins, J. I., Learn, G. H. *et al.* Genetic evaluation of suspected cases of transient HIV-1 infection of infants. *Science* **280** : **5366** (1998), 1073–7.

The epidemiology of pediatric HIV disease

Mary Lou Lindegren, M.D., Teresa Hammett, MPH, and Marc Bulterys, M.D., Ph.D.

Centers for Disease Control and Prevention, Atlanta, GA

6.1 Introduction

Worldwide, an estimated 2.1 million children were living with HIV infection, and an estimated 2000 new infections in children occurred each day, during 2003 [1]. Mother-to-child transmission (MTCT) of HIV represents the most common means by which children become infected with HIV. In the new millennium, the challenge is to reduce missed opportunities for prevention of transmission of HIV to children in the US and other resource-rich settings, and at the same time to extend the benefits of recent advances in prevention of pediatric HIV infection to resource-poor settings. This chapter will review the current epidemiology of HIV infection in children in the US, and briefly review the growing worldwide impact of HIV on children.

6.2 HIV/AIDS among children in the USA

6.2.1 HIV infection and AIDS reporting

Through June 2001, 8994 US children with AIDS were reported to the US Centers for Disease Control and Prevention (CDC) from all 50 states, Puerto Rico, the District of Columbia, and the US Virgin Islands (Table 6.1) [2]. Fifty-six percent of all cases were reported from only four states: New York (25%), Florida (16%), New Jersey (8%), and California (7%). The majority of AIDS cases (91%) and virtually all new HIV infections resulted from MTCT. Seven percent (7%) of children with AIDS acquired their infection through receipt of contaminated blood or blood products. AIDS also has been reported among children who acquired HIV infection from sexual abuse, mucus membrane exposure to blood,

and percutaneous or cutaneous exposures to blood or contaminated needles during home health care [3]. Only 2% of AIDS cases in US children lack an ascribable risk, usually because of incomplete information about the mother [4]. The majority of children with perinatally acquired AIDS cases were diagnosed at less than 5 years of age (81%), compared with children with hemophilia or transfusion-related AIDS who mostly were diagnosed at 5 years of age or older (95%, 63%, respectively). Black, non-Hispanic and Hispanic children are disproportionately affected by the HIV epidemic. AIDS rates reported in 2000 among black, non-Hispanic (1.7 per 100 000) and Hispanic children (0.3 per 100 000) were 17 and 3 times higher, respectively, than among white, non-Hispanic children (0.1 per 100 000). The racial/ethnic and age distribution of AIDS and HIV infection among children vary by mode of transmission. For example, cases of AIDS resulting from MTCT of HIV have occurred predominantly among black, non-Hispanic (62%) and Hispanic children (23%) while cases attributed to blood or blood-product transfusion are more proportional to the racial/ethnic distribution of the general population.

As of June 2001, HIV infection reporting, using the same methods as for AIDS surveillance, was ongoing in 34 states, the Virgin Islands, and Guam (Table 6.2). As of June 2001, an additional 2206 HIV-infected children have been reported from these areas (Table 6.2) [2]. In many states with HIV reporting, there are over three times as many children living with HIV infection as those living with AIDS (Figure 6.1). Through 2000, there were 2617 children living with AIDS and an additional 1627 children living with HIV infection. National HIV surveillance data are needed to provide critical information on incident cases of HIV infection

Table 6.1 Cumulative pediatric AIDS cases in the US, by mode of transmission*

Characteristic no. (%)	Perinatally acquired AIDS (n = 8207)	Hemophilia/ coagulation disorder (n = 237)	Transfusion (n = 382)	Pediatric risk not reported or identified (n = 168)	Total (n = 8994)
Age at AIDS					
<1 year	3237 (39)	0	29 (8)	38 (23)	3301
1–4 years	3462 (42)	11 (5)	112 (29)	39 (23)	3620
5 + years	1508 (18)	226 (95)	241 (63)	91 (54)	2057
Race/ethnicity					
Black, not Hispanic	5058 (62)	34 (14)	88 (23)	103 (61)	5283
Hispanic	1890 (23)	38 (16)	93 (24)	30 (18)	2051
White, not Hispanic	1185 (14)	159 (67)	190 (50)	30 (18)	1564
Asian/Pacific Islander	34 (<1)	3 (1)	11 (3)	4 (2)	52
American Indian/					
Alaska Native	28 (<1)	2 (1)	–	1 (1)	31
Unknown	12 (<1)	1 (<1)	–	–	13
Sex					
Male	4075 (50)	230 (97)	242 (63)	75 (45)	4622
Female	4132 (50)	7 (3)	140 (37)	93 (55)	4372

*Data reported to CDC National AIDS surveillance through June 2001; [2].

Table 6.2 Pediatric HIV infection cases in the US, by age group, exposure category, race/ethnicity, and gender*

Characteristic no. (%)	Perinatally acquired (n = 1918)	Hemophilia/ coagulation disorder (n = 104)	Transfusion (n = 41)	Pediatric risk not reported or identified (n = 143)	Total (n = 2206)
Age at HIV					
<1 year	934 (49)	2 (2)	0	23 (16)	959
1–4 years	679 (35)	10 (10)	11 (27)	47 (33)	747
5 + years	305 (16)	92 (88)	30 (73)	73 (51)	500
Race/ethnicity					
Black, not Hispanic	1298 (62)	20 (19)	11 (27)	90 (63)	1419
	222 (12)	5 (5)	7 (17)	16 (11)	250
Hispanic					
White, not Hispanic	373 (19)	76 (73)	22 (54)	22 (15)	493
Asian/Pacific Islander	8 (<1)	3 (1)	1 (3)	3 (2)	15
American Indian/					
Alaska Native	9 (<1)	–	–	2 (1)	11
Unknown	8 (<1)	–	–	10 (7)	18
Sex					
Male	908 (47)	102 (98)	17 (41)	70 (49)	1097
Female	1010 (53)	2 (2)	24 (59)	73 (51)	1109

*Data reported to CDC for HIV surveillance through June 2001, from the 36 areas with confidential HIV infection reporting [2].

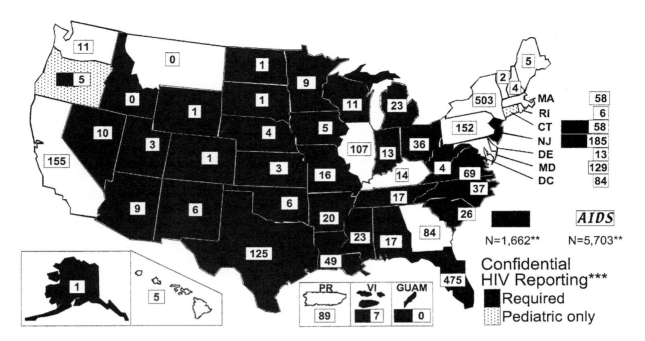

* For areas with confidential HIV infection surveillance reported by patient name. Age based on current age as of December 2000 data reported to CDC.
** Total includes cases missing state of residence data.
*** HIV cases reported by patient name.

Figure 6.1. Children < 13 years of age living with HIV infection* and AIDS, reported through 2000.

in children and the care and treatment needs for this aging group of HIV-infected children. Thirty-three of these areas also collect information on children with perinatal exposure to HIV and follow-up to determine HIV infection and AIDS status, as recommended by the CDC and by the American Academy of Pediatrics (AAP) [5,6]. These states are able to monitor implementation of perinatal prevention recommendations most completely.

6.2.2 Modes of acquisition of HIV infection among US children

Non-perinatal

Blood/blood products

Since the implementation of heat treatment for clotting factors in 1984, nationwide screening of blood and blood products in 1985, and self-deferral of blood donations from high-risk individuals, incident cases of HIV infection attributable to transmission through blood and blood products have been virtually eliminated in the US [7, 8]. Most children with transfusion-acquired AIDS were transfused during infancy because of perinatal problems [8]. As of June 2001, only two children had developed AIDS follow-

ing receipt of blood screened negative for HIV antibody at the time of donation, where the donor later seroconverted [2]. Hemophilia and other clotting disorders accounted for 3% of children diagnosed with AIDS. Nearly all these cases (97%) were in boys (Table 6.1), reflecting the sex-linked transmission of hemophilia.

Sexual transmission

Sexual transmission of HIV infection is the major mode of HIV exposure among adolescents and adults in the US. A number of cases of sexual transmission through sexual abuse have been reported among children [9–11]. Through 1998, population-based HIV/AIDS surveillance was used to describe 26 children who were sexually abused with confirmed (n = 17) or suspected (n = 9) exposure to HIV infection [11]. To date, 29 children have been reported to have acquired HIV infection through sexual abuse, 22 of whom have progressed to AIDS and an additional seven of whom have been diagnosed with HIV infection (CDC, unpubl. data). However, since sexual abuse is likely under-reported, the actual number of children who have acquired HIV infection through sexual abuse is probably larger. Many children are sexually abused in the USA each year; the National

Center on Child Abuse and Neglect reported over 125 000 children who had been sexually abused [12]. Centers for Disease Control and Prevention guidelines for evaluation and treatment of sexually transmitted infections (STIs) recommend that the decision to test for HIV infection among sexually abused children should be made on a case-by-case basis, depending on the likelihood of infection in the assailant [13]. Situations that involve a high risk for STIs, including HIV infection, and in which testing for HIV is strongly recommended, include: if the suspected perpetrator is known to have HIV infection or to be at high risk for HIV infection; if the child has symptoms or signs of HIV infection; or if the prevalence of HIV in the community is high. Other indications for HIV testing include evidence of genital or oral penetration or ejaculation, and STIs in siblings or other children or adults in the household. These recommendations include the need for follow-up testing for HIV after sexual assault to detect seroconversion. Post-exposure antiretroviral prophylaxis for children with potential exposure to HIV, including exposure through sexual abuse, is addressed in Chapter 24.

Other
There have been rare reports of transmission of HIV in households between siblings where opportunities for skin or mucous membranes exposure to HIV-infected blood were present [14–16]. However, of 1167 household contacts (including over 300 children) of HIV-infected individuals who were followed for 1700 person-years in 17 studies conducted in the USA and Europe, none of whom had other risk factors for HIV infection, there were no new HIV infections (upper 95% confidence limit = 0.18 per 100 person-years) [15]. Because of the rare possibility of household transmission, all persons who care for HIV-infected children should be educated about appropriate universal precautions [17]. Policies and procedures should be established to manage potential exposures to blood or blood-containing materials. Additionally there have been rare reports of possible HIV transmission during healthcare practices in the home, e.g. through percutaneous or cutaneous exposure to blood or contaminated needles. These cases also highlight the need for careful attention to proper infection control practices in any setting where exposure to blood is possible. Finally, one instance of intentional inoculation of a child with HIV-infected blood also has been documented [3]. Because HIV transmission is extremely rare in settings such as homes, schools, and day-care centers, and recommendations have been made to prevent exposure in these settings, no need exists to restrict the placement of HIV-infected children in these settings [18,19].

Mother-to-child transmission of HIV
HIV/AIDS among women of childbearing age in the USA
Characteristics of the HIV epidemic in children mirror that of the epidemic in childbearing women. Women account for an increasing proportion of the burden of HIV disease in the USA. Overall, of the 784 032 adult and adolescent cases of AIDS reported to the CDC through June 2001 from the USA, Puerto Rico, District of Columbia, and the US Virgin Islands, 134 845 (17%) cases were among women [2]. The proportion of AIDS cases in women has increased from 12.5% in 1988–1992 to 22.6% in 1996–2000 [20]. Of the 145 753 HIV-infected adolescents and adults in the USA, 29% were women. Finally, among the 5893 HIV-infected adolescents (aged 13–19 years old), 57% were among females, most of whom were infected through heterosexual contact.

The HIV/AIDS epidemic in women is concentrated in the Northeast and in the South, particularly in New York, Florida, Texas, California, and New Jersey. While the highest numbers of women were initially observed in the Northeast, during the past several years the greatest increases appear to have been in the South [21–23]. African-American and Hispanic women are disproportionately affected by the HIV epidemic; in 2000, the highest rates of AIDS were among black, non-Hispanic (46 per 100 000) and Hispanic women (14 per 100 000) compared with white, non-Hispanic women (8 per 100 000). Cumulatively, 40% of AIDS in women is attributable to injection drug use and 41% to heterosexual contact, which surpassed injection drug use in the early 1990s as the predominant mode of transmission among women, particularly among young women [2, 21, 24].

Among young adults and adolescents, aged 13–24 years, 54% of AIDS has been attributable to heterosexual contact. From 1995 to 1999, AIDS diagnoses declined 26% among women compared with 43% among men and then began to level [24]. Declines began later for women than men and the last groups to show a decline were men and women infected through heterosexual contact. The percentage decrease in AIDS diagnoses was smallest among African-American women, women from the South, and men and women infected through heterosexual contact. These patterns reflect differences in HIV incidence in the 1980s and 1990s, HIV testing patterns, and access and adherence to effective therapy [24]. In summary, increasing proportions of persons with AIDS are women, African-American or Hispanic, heterosexuals, and residents of the South. In addition, more than 40% of AIDS diagnoses in 1999 were among residents of the poorest counties in the USA [24]. Among 25 states with HIV reporting to CDC since 1994, HIV diagnosis rates per 100 000 in 1999 were highest for African

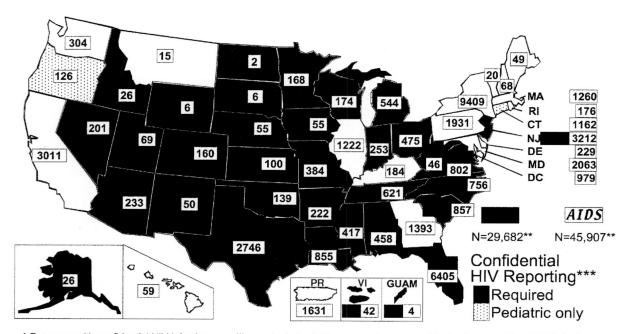

* For areas with confidential HIV infection surveillance. Includes 297 women who were residents of areas without HIV infection surveillance but who were reported by areas with HIV infection surveillance data reported to CDC.
** Totals include cases missing state of residence data.
*** HIV cases reported by patient name.

Figure 6.2. Women 15–44 years of age living with HIV infection* and AIDS, 2000.

American and Hispanic women compared with whites (51.2, 16.3, and 2.5) and 71% of the new HIV infections in 1999 among women were among African-Americans [24].

AIDS surveillance and HIV seroprevalence surveys demonstrated increasing HIV incidence among childbearing women through the 1980s, and then stable seroprevalence from 1989 to 1995 [21, 25]. Trends varied by region, with declining HIV seroprevalence in the Northeast (4.1 to 3.2/1000 childbearing women) and increasing then stable trends in the South (1.6 to 1.9/1000 childbearing women). The stable HIV seroprevalence may have been a combination of stable HIV incidence among childbearing-age women, women aging out of their childbearing years, and reduced fertility among older HIV-infected women due to advanced HIV disease [26]. Particularly high HIV incidence rates (5–6 per 1000 women-years) have been reported from certain institutions which serve an inner-city and high-risk population of women of childbearing age [27, 28].

The number of persons living with AIDS has increased as a result of improved survival of patients receiving potent HAART regimens. In 2000, an estimated 338 978 persons were living with AIDS in the USA, including 69 725 women, a 57% increase since 1996 in the number of women. Between 1993 and 2000, the proportion of persons living

with AIDS who were women increased from 15% to 21%. AIDS prevalence, however, underestimates the number of HIV-infected young women in need of medical and social services. Among the 32 states that report HIV infection among adults as of June 2001, the number of women aged 15–44 years living with HIV infection was two- to three-fold higher than the number living with AIDS in many states (Figure 6.2). More recent estimates indicate that approximately 129 500 to 135 300 women of childbearing age (13–44 years) were living with HIV infection in the USA in 2000, which is substantially higher than the estimated 80 000 HIV-infected women in 1991, reflecting continued HIV incidence and increasing survival of women receiving treatment for HIV infection [29, 30].

Recent data from the Adult/Adolescent Spectrum of HIV Disease Study indicate that pregnancies were less likely to occur among women with advanced HIV disease [31]. Pregnancy rates were significantly higher during the era of widespread use of HAART (1997–2000) compared with 1992–1996. Approximately 6000–7000 HIV-infected women delivered infants each year from 1989 to 1995 [25]. More recent estimates, using a combination of data sources, indicate between 6075 and 6422 infants were born to HIV-infected mothers in 2000 [29].

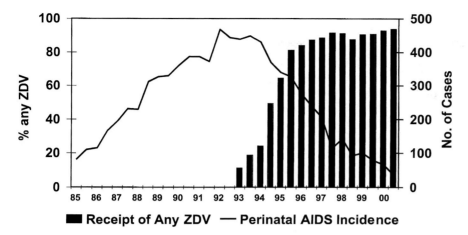

Figure 6.3. Perinatally acquired AIDS by half year of diagnosis (US), and receipt of any zidovudine (ZDV) (prenatal, intrapartum, neonatal) among HIV+ women tested before\at birth: 33 HIV reporting states. Data reported to CDC HIV/AIDS surveillance through June 2001. HIV data from areas with confidential HIV Infection surveillance [2].

An estimated 40 000 new cases of HIV infection occur each year in the USA and more than 10 000 of these new infections are among women [29, 32]. Recent increases in newly diagnosed HIV infections, among heterosexuals as well as men who have sex with men, in several US cities have created concern that HIV incidence may again be on the rise [33]. A new HIV prevention initiative is aimed at reducing barriers to early diagnosis of HIV infection and increasing access to quality medical care and prevention services [30]. Ongoing prevention programs must be targeted at high-risk women, particularly young women, to reduce HIV incidence in this vulnerable group. The increasing number of women living with AIDS and the large and increasing number of childbearing age women living with HIV infection highlight the need for programs to get young HIV-infected women into care and treatment. HIV surveillance is needed in all states to better assess the number of persons in need of care and services [34].

Trends in mother-to-child transmission of HIV
Overall, by year of AIDS diagnosis, adjusted for reporting delay and redistribution of cases with unreported risk [35–38], the number of pediatric AIDS cases in the USA increased rapidly in the 1980s, peaked in 1992, and declined 89% from 1992 (n = 910) to 2000 (n = 104) (Figure 6.3). These declines have been seen in all racial/ethnic groups. The majority of children who acquired HIV infection through MTCT are non-Hispanic blacks and Hispanics, similar to the epidemic in women. Declines were seen in all regions of the US, and in both urban and rural areas. The earliest and largest declines have occurred among children diagnosed before 1 year of age (92%), who represent inci-

dent infection and would reflect recent perinatal prevention efforts earliest, and among children diagnosed at 1–5 years of age (93%). Although treatment of HIV-infected children has likely contributed to the decline in the numbers of pediatric AIDS cases since 1996, when potent combination antiretroviral therapy became standard of care [39], the steep declines in perinatally acquired AIDS cases since 1994, particularly among infants, most likely represent reduced MTCT of HIV. Recent declines in AIDS incidence were substantially greater than could be accounted for by declines in births to HIV-infected women as estimated by the anonymous survey of childbearing women. From 1992 to 1997, the rate per 100 000 births of infants diagnosed with AIDS in the first year of life declined 84% from 9.1 to 1.5 and was greater than expected compared with a decline in births to HIV-infected women [40, 41]. Data from 33 HIV- reporting areas that collect data on perinatally HIV-exposed and infected children, through June 2001, demonstrate declines in rates of MTCT. Of children first evaluated for HIV infection at less than 2 months of age, 22% were HIV-infected in 1993, which declined to 9% in 1997 and then to 4% in 1999.

Rapid implementation of US Public Health Service guidelines regarding use of zidovudine (ZDV) prophylaxis to reduce MTCT of HIV (1994) and regarding universal, routine HIV counseling and voluntary prenatal HIV testing (1995) were associated with the initial decline in the incidence of perinatal HIV infection in the USA, where safe and affordable alternatives to breastfeeding are widely available [42–45]. Data from states with enhanced perinatal HIV surveillance from 1993–1997 indicated an association between receipt by mother–infant pairs of all three components of the ZDV prophylaxis regimen from the AIDS Clinical Trials Group Protocol 076 (ACTG 076) and a 68% reduction in perinatal HIV infection rates [46]. Additional data confirmed the effectiveness of ZDV prophylaxis, with MTCT rates of as low as 5–8% [47–53]. With the introduction of potent combination antiretroviral therapy and cesarean section before labor and ruptured membranes, MTCT rates of less than 2% have been observed [45, 54–56]. Despite dramatic declines, cases of MTCT of HIV continue to occur, especially in populations of women and children who did not receive timely interventions to prevent transmission. For example, of 449 children with perinatally acquired AIDS born in 1995–1997, 35% had mothers who were tested for HIV after birth. Of 227 HIV-infected children born in 1995–1997 in states with enhanced perinatal HIV surveillance, 14% of their mothers had no prenatal care, 20% of their mothers were tested after delivery and 7% at delivery, and only 29% of their mothers had received prenatal care, HIV testing, and all components of the ACTG 076 regimen (including the infant component) [40].

As noted previously, an estimated 6075–6422 infants were born to HIV-infected mothers in the USA in 2000 [29], similar to estimated numbers in the late 1980s and early 1990s from the anonymous survey of childbearing women. Without intervention, a MTCT rate of 25% would result in the birth of an estimated 1500–1750 HIV-infected infants annually in the USA. However, compared with an estimated peak of 1750 HIV-infected infants born in 1991, due to successful perinatal prevention efforts, the estimated number of HIV-infected children born in 2000 declined to 280–379 [29]. If all missed opportunities were eliminated (i.e. all HIV-infected mothers were diagnosed before birth and received optimal management), and assuming a 2% transmission rate, approximately 120–130 HIV-infected infants would be born each year in the USA [29]. Additional prevention efforts are needed, targeting prevention of HIV transmission among those women who remain at high risk for HIV infection, especially substance-using women, young women, and adolescents, to further reduce perinatal HIV transmission.

6.2.3 The perinatal HIV prevention cascade

The most important perinatal prevention strategy is prevention of acquisition of HIV infection in women. Once an HIV-infected woman becomes pregnant, however, a chain of events must take place to prevent HIV transmission to the child. This chain of events provides a useful framework for considering both perinatal HIV prevention interventions and collection of perinatal surveillance data. This chain includes the following: (1) receipt of early prenatal care; (2) provider offering of counseling and testing; (3) pregnant woman's acceptance of testing; (4) HIV-infected pregnant woman's acceptance of one or more interventions to prevent transmission, including antiretroviral prophylaxis, cesarean section before labor and ruptured membranes, and avoidance of breastfeeding; (5) HIV-infected pregnant woman's adherence to an antiretroviral drug regimen and to avoidance of breastfeeding; and (6) follow-up care for both the HIV-infected woman and her infant [57] (see Chapter 8).

Receipt of prenatal care

Compared with the general population, HIV-infected women are much less likely to receive prenatal care [58–60]. Data from the seven states that conducted the enhanced perinatal HIV surveillance project for birth years 1993 to 1996, indicate that 14% (range 3–27%) of women received no or minimal prenatal care and 19% (range 8–23%) initiated prenatal care in the third trimester [59]. This compares with 2% of women in the general population who had late or no prenatal care [61]. As in the general population, prenatal care use among HIV-infected women varied by race and ethnicity with African-American and Hispanic women likely to have fewer prenatal visits. Women who use illicit drugs in pregnancy are at high risk for not receiving prenatal care: 36% had no prenatal care compared to 5% of HIV-infected women who did not use illicit drugs. Among HIV-infected women tested at or within 7 days of delivery, 71% had received no or minimal prenatal care and 67% had substance abuse during pregnancy [59]. Reasons these women may not receive prenatal care include social disruption, fear of criminalization, and lack of access to care. In a recent report from Michigan, a high prevalence of STIs (43%), illegal drug use (33%), and alcohol use (24%) was reported among pregnant HIV-infected women giving birth from 1993–2000, suggesting a need for comprehensive counseling and treatment services to HIV-infected women [60].

Innovative approaches must be developed that address the needs of mothers who receive little or no prenatal care. Most HIV-infected pregnant women in the USA utilize hospitals for delivery, providing a crucial opportunity for rapid screening and intervention [62]. The Mother Infant Rapid Intervention at Delivery (MIRIAD) study is a multicenter project, funded through the CDC, focusing on disadvantaged communities in which many women receive inadequate prenatal care and exhibit relatively high HIV seroprevalence [63]. Funded sites are located in six US metropolitan areas: Atlanta, Baton Rouge, Chicago, Miami, New Orleans, and New York City. The MIRIAD study aims to evaluate (1) innovative approaches for a 24-hour counseling and voluntary rapid HIV-testing program among women in labor presenting with unknown HIV infection status; (2) the feasibility of obtaining informed consent during labor (or, if not feasible, soon after birth); (3) reasons for lack of prenatal care and/or HIV testing among these women; (4) the rapid implementation and assessment of antiretroviral prophylaxis administered at labor and delivery and/or to the neonate; (5) adherence to neonatal therapy; and (6) subsequent receipt of antiretroviral treatment and other services for women identified as HIV-infected. Novel approaches for rapid bedside testing of women in labor and post-test counseling and referral to care for HIV-infected women and their infants are being piloted. Recent data indicate that rapid HIV testing is feasible, accurate and timely with acceptance rates of 84% enabling prompt access to antiretroviral prophylaxis. In cost-effectiveness analyses, rapid HIV testing at labor and delivery appears cost saving to the medical system when HIV prevalence exceeds 0.7 to 1.0% and treatment efficacy exceeds a 5% reduction in perinatal transmission [64, 65].

Offering and acceptance of HIV counseling and testing
Once in prenatal care, women need to be offered and to accept HIV testing. Population-based data on HIV counseling and testing during 1996–1997 were available from 14 states participating in the CDC Pregnancy Risk Assessment Monitoring System (PRAMS) [66]. In 1997, 63–87% of mothers received HIV counseling during pregnancy and 58–81% were tested for HIV infection; the proportions varied by state. Black mothers, mothers with less than a high school education, young mothers, those with public health care providers, and Medicaid recipients were more likely to receive HIV counseling and testing during pregnancy and may reflect targeted testing efforts. Highest rates of testing and increases in testing from 1996–1997 occurred in states with higher HIV seroprevalence among childbearing women.

Updated data from the 1999 PRAMS study, indicate a range of prenatal HIV testing from 61–81% for states that use an "opt in" approach to testing (i.e. women are provided with pre-HIV test counseling and must consent specifically to an HIV antibody test) [67]. Several states, including Arkansas, Texas, Tannessee, and New Mexico, have an "opt-out" testing policy (i.e., women are notified that an HIV test will be included in a standard prenatal battery of tests and that they may refuse testing). In Arkansas, after the law was implemented, prenatal HIV testing rates increased from 57% in 1997 to 71% in 1999. For New York State, prenatal testing rates increased from 69% to 93% after mandatory newborn testing results were

made available within 2 days of delivery [67]. In November 2001, the USPHS issued revised guidelines for HIV testing in pregnancy emphasizing HIV testing as a routine part of prenatal care and strengthening the recommendation that all pregnant women be tested for HIV, including the offering of rapid testing at labor/delivery for women whose status was still unknown at that point [23]. Health care facilities serving women at relatively high risk for HIV should also strongly consider implementing a second voluntary universal HIV test during the third trimester of pregnancy, as is done routinely for syphilis [68]. The AAP and the American College of Obstetricians and Gynecologists (ACOG) have issued recommendations in support of the PHS guidelines [34, 69, 70]. In addition, as part of the new prevention initiative, CDC will further promote recommendations for routine HIV testing of all pregnant women at labor/delivery whose HIV infection status is still unknown, and, as a safety net, for the routine serologic screening after delivery of mothers or infants who were not screened prenatally or at labor/delivery [33].

Data from CDC's active bacterial core surveillance/emerging infectious program network also assessed HIV testing during prenatal care and within 2 days of delivery in a population-based sample of eight US areas in 1998–1999. For opt-in programs prenatal testing rates ranged from 25% to 69%, and in Tennessee where an opt-out testing approach was used, testing rates were 85%. These data suggest that testing rates may be higher with an "opt-out" approach [67].

Population-based data on HIV testing are also available from the Behavioral Risk Factor Surveillance system, a state-specific population-based telephone survey of adults 18 years of age or older [71]. Among women ages 18–44, the proportion of pregnant women tested for HIV in the prior 12 months increased from 1994 to 1996 (41% to 53%), and again from 1997 (52%) to 1998 (60%) [71]. Pregnant women were more likely to be tested if they lived in the South, were not working, were aged 18–24 years, had never been married, or had health insurance.

Additional data indicate that once women are offered HIV testing, acceptance rates are generally high, over 70% in most settings. However, not all women who are offered testing accept it. CDC's Perinatal Guidelines Evaluation Project evaluated reasons women were not tested, and the results indicated some women did not perceive a need for testing since their assessment was that they were not at risk for HIV infection, others knew they had been previously tested for HIV, and finally some women had providers who did not strongly recommend testing [58].

The proportion of pregnant HIV-infected women in whom HIV infection was diagnosed before giving birth is

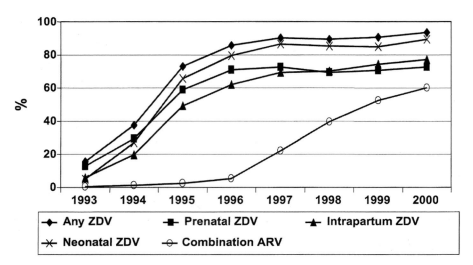

Figure 6.4. Receipt of zidovudine (ZDV) among perinatally exposed children born in 1993–2000 whose mothers tested HIV positive before or at birth – 33 HIV-reporting states (n = 9306). Data reported to CDC HIV/AIDS surveillance through June 2001. HIV data from areas with confidential HIV infection surveillance [2].

high and increasing. In the seven-state enhanced surveillance project, the proportion of HIV-infected women who were tested for HIV before delivery increased from 70% in 1993 to 80% in 1996 [59]. Among women delivering in 1996, approximately half (53%) had their positive HIV test before their pregnancy and half (47%) during their pregnancy. Data from 25 HIV-reporting states in 2000, indicate that 93% of HIV-infected women knew their HIV infection status before delivery [67].

Offering and receipt of antiretroviral drugs
As of June 2001, an increasing proportion of HIV-infected mothers and their infants were prescribed any component of the ACTG 076 perinatal transmission prophylaxis regimen (antepartum, intrapartum, or infant), from 37% of children born in 1994 to 90% or more for children born from 1997–2000 (Figure 6.4). These are population-based data from 33 HIV-reporting areas, using the same methods as AIDS surveillance, involving the monitoring of 9300 HIV-exposed and -infected children born to HIV-infected mothers tested for HIV before or at delivery and then follow-up to determine HIV infection status as well as AIDS status. Receipt of prenatal ZDV increased from almost 30% in 1994 to 71–73% in 1996–1997 and then leveled. An increasing number of HIV-infected women received combination therapy during pregnancy for their own health, from 39% in 1998 to 60% in 2000. Almost two-thirds of mother–infant pairs in 2000 received all three components of the ZDV regimen. The increase in receipt of antiretroviral therapy has resulted in the dramatic decline in perinatally acquired AIDS incidence in the United States (Figure 6.3). Data from

the enhanced perinatal HIV surveillance project in seven states with HIV-infection surveillance also indicated that among women diagnosed before delivery, the proportion offered prenatal ZDV increased from 27% in 1993 to 83% in 1996, the proportion offered intrapartum ZDV increased from 6% to 75%, and the proportion offered ZDV for their infants increased from 8% to 77% [59]. Only 5% of women refused ZDV. Mothers known to be HIV-infected with substance abuse during pregnancy had fewer prenatal care visits and were less likely to receive ZDV [45, 59]. In the Perinatal AIDS Collaborative Transmission Study (PACTS), women with substance abuse, who gave birth preterm, or who had less advanced immunosuppression, were at substantial risk of not receiving all three components of the ACTG 076 perinatal transmission prophylaxis regimen [58].

Cesarean section for the prevention of MTCT of HIV
The American College of Obstetricians and Gynecologists and the USPHS recommends that HIV-infected pregnant women with HIV RNA of 1000 copies/mL or greater be offered elective cesarean section as an adjunct for prevention of perinatal HIV transmission, as cesarean section before onset of labor and rupture of membranes has been shown to decrease the risk of perinatal HIV transmission [72, 73]. Data from the Pediatric Spectrum of HIV Disease Project and Pediatric HIV surveillance indicate that the proportion of HIV-infected mothers who had cesarean sections increased from 20% in 1994–1998 to 44% and almost 50% by 2000, in PSD and surveillance, respectively [74].

for HIV; 69% of HIV-infected women giving birth received ZDV; and 86% of the infants born to HIV-infected women received zidovudine through the program [106]. Lessons learned from Thailand include the importance of providing regular clinical, counseling, and management training related to prevention of MTCT, and using focused monitoring and evaluation data to guide program development, expansion, and improvement. In sub-Saharan Africa during 1999–2000, United Nations-sponsored pilot programs were conducted in nine countries with high HIV-1 prevalence; 82 000 women attended for antenatal care across all sites and HIV prevalence among those tested varied from 13–45% [107]. Of all the women attending antenatal care, only 43% accepted an HIV test. Of the nearly 7000 women who tested positive for HIV infection, 39% were documented to have received ARV prophylaxis. India has implemented a pilot program among 125 000 pregnant women and has recorded testing and antiretroviral prophylaxis acceptance rates comparable to the African rates. Since early 2000, several private foundations such as the Elizabeth Glaser Pediatric AIDS Foundation and the Doris Duke Foundation have funded large-scale perinatal HIV prevention programs in a number of resource-limited settings. Successful programs to reduce MTCT and to expand treatment options for HIV-infected mothers and their families can be achieved only through improved maternal and child health-care services, integrated AIDS prevention and care initiatives, and strong political commitment at all levels [108, 109]. Sexual abuse of children, mainly girls, and forced sexual initiation also appear common in a number of high HIV-prevalence countries in sub-Saharan Africa and South-East Asia, and rape of children is almost universally under-reported [110–114].

6.4 Conclusions

Remarkable changes in the epidemiology of pediatric HIV infection in the USA and similar settings have occurred during the last several years, due primarily to successful efforts to prevent MTCT of HIV. Additionally, advances have been made in the diagnosis and treatment of pediatric HIV infection.

However, the global HIV epidemic among infants, children, and adolescents continues in many parts of the world, where there is an ongoing need to implement effective prevention and treatment programs. HIV infection has already caused a precipitous decline in child survival in resource-poor settings [115]. In such settings, prevention of primary HIV infections among women and adolescent girls, particu-

larly adolescent girls who exhibit the highest HIV incidence rates [104], is critical to the prevention of MTCT of HIV [23].

REFERENCES

1. UNAIDS. http://www.unaids.org/html/pub/Topics/Epidemiology/Slides02_Epicore July 04_en_ppt.ppt.
2. Centers for Disease Control and Prevention. *HIV/AIDS Surveillance Report.* **13**: (2001), 1–41.
3. Centers for Disease Control and Prevention. *HIV/AIDS Surveillance Report.* **12 : 1** (2000), 25.
4. Hammett, T. A., Bush, T. J. & Ciesielski, C. A. Pediatric AIDS cases reported with no identified risk. Presented at the American Public Health Association Meeting, San Francisco, CA. Abstract **1023**, (1993), 19.
5. Centers for Disease Control and Prevention. Guidelines for national human immunodeficiency virus case surveillance, including monitoring for human immunodeficiency virus infection and acquired immunodeficiency syndrome. *MMWR* **48 : RR-13** (1999), 1–31.
6. American Academy of Pediatrics, Committee on Pediatric AIDS. Surveillance of pediatric HIV infection. *Pediatrics* **101 : 2** (1998), 315–19.
7. Selik, R. M., Ward, J. W. & Buehler J. W. Trends in transfusion-associated acquired immune deficiency syndrome in the United States, 1982 through 1991. *Transfusion* **33 : 11** (1993), 890–3.
8. Jones, D. S., Byers, R. H., Bush, T. J., Oxtoby, M. J. & Rogers, M. F. Epidemiology of transfusion-associated acquired immunodeficiency syndrome in children in the United States, 1981 through 1989. *Pediatrics* **89 : 1** (1992), 123–7.
9. Gellert, G. A., Durfee, M. J., Berkowitz, C. D., Higgins, K. V. & Tubiolo, V. C. Situational and sociodemographic characteristics of children infected with human immunodeficiency virus from pediatric sexual abuse. *Pediatrics* **91 : 1** (1993), 39–44.
10. Gutman, L. T., St Claire, K. K., Weedy, C. *et al.* Human immunodeficiency virus transmission by child sexual abuse. *Am. J. Dis. Child.* **145 : 2** (1991), 137–41.
11. Lindegren, M. L., Hanson, I. C., Hammett, T. A., Beil, J., Fleming, P. L. & Ward, J. W. Sexual abuse of children: intersection with the HIV epidemic. *Pediatrics* **102 : 4** (1998), E46.
12. United States Department of Health and Human Services. *Child Maltreatment 1995; Reports from the States to the National Center on Child Abuse and Neglect Data System.* Washington, DC: US Government Printing Office (1998).
13. Centers for Disease Control and Prevention. *Sexually Transmitted diseases: treatment guidelines 2002. MMWR* **51 : RR-6** (2002), 1–84.
14. American Academy of Pediatrics, Committee of Pediatric AIDS and Committee on Infectious Diseases. Issues related to human immunodeficiency virus transmission in schools, child care, medical settings, the home, and community. *Pediatrics* **104 : 2** (1999), 318–24.

15. Simonds, R. J. & Chanock, S. Medical issues related to caring for human immunodeficiency virus-infected children in and out of the home. *Pediatr. Infect. Dis. J.* **12 : 10** (1993), 845–52.

16. Centers for Disease Control and Prevention. Human immunodeficiency virus transmission in household settings – United States. *MMWR* **43 : 19** (1994), 347, 353–347, 356.

17. Centers for Disease Control and Prevention. Update: universal precautions for prevention of transmission of human immunodeficiency virus, hepatitis B virus, and other bloodborne pathogens in health-care settings. *MMWR* **37 : 24** (1988), 377–8.

18. American Academy of Pediatrics: Committee on Pediatric AIDS Education of children with human immunodeficiency virus infection. *Pediatrics* **105 : 6** (2000), 1358–60.

19. Centers for Disease Control and Prevention. Education and foster care of children infected with human T-lymphotropic virus type III/lymphadenopathy-associated virus. *MMWR* **34** (1985), 517–21.

20. Centers for Disease Control and Prevention. HIV and AIDS – United States, 1981–2000. *MMWR* **50 : 21** (2001), 430–4.

21. Wortley, P. M. & Fleming, P. L. AIDS in women in the United States. Recent trends. *J. Am. Med. Assoc.* **278 : 11** (1997), 911–16.

22. Hader, S. L., Smith, D. K., Moore, J. S. & Holmberg, S. D. HIV infection in women in the United States: status at the Millennium. *J. Am. Med. Assoc.* **285 : 9** (2001), 1186–92.

23. Centers for Disease Control and Prevention. Revised recommendations for HIV screening of pregnant women. *MMWR* **50 : RR-19** (2001), 63–85.

24. Karon, J. M. Fleming, P. L., Steketee, R. W. & De Cock, K. M. HIV in the United States at the turn of the century: an epidemic in transition. *Am. J. Public Health* **91 : 7** (2001), 1060–8.

25. Davis, S. F., Rosen, D. H., Steinberg, S., Wortley. P. M., Karon, J. M. & Gwinn, M. Trends in HIV prevalence among childbearing women in the United States, 1989–1994. *J. AIDS Hum. Retrovirol.* **19 : 2** (1998), 158–64.

26. Lee, L. M., Wortley, P. M., Fleming, P. L. & Eldred, L. J. & Gray, R. H. Duration of human immunodeficiency virus infection and likelihood of giving birth in a Medicaid population in Maryland. *Am. J. Epidemiol.* **151 : 10** (2000), 1020–8.

27. Lindsay, M. K., Peterson, H. B., Willis, S. *et al.* Incidence and prevalence of human immunodeficiency virus infection in a prenatal population undergoing routine voluntary human immunodeficiency virus screening, July 1987 to June 1990. *Am. J. Obstet. Gynecol.* **165 : 4** (1991), 961–4.

28. Chirgwin, K. D., Feldman, J., Dehovitz, J. A., Minkoff, H. & Landesman, S. H. Incidence and risk factors for heterosexually acquired HIV in an inner-city cohort of women: temporal association with pregnancy. *J. AIDS Hum. Retrovirol.* **20 : 3** (1999), 295–9.

29. Fleming, P. L., Lindegren, M. L., Byers, R. *et al.* Estimated number of perinatal HIV infections, United States, 2000. In *XIV International Conference, Barcelona, Spain.* (2002). [Abstract TuPeC4773.]

30. Karon, J. M., Rosenberg, P. S., McQuillan, G., Khare, M., Gwinn, M. & Petersen, L. R. Prevalence of HIV infection in the United States, 1984 to 1992. *J. Am. Med. Assoc.* **276 : 2** (1996), 126–31.

31. Blair, J. M., Hanson, D. L., Jones, J. L. *et al.* Trends in pregnancy rates among women with human immunodeficiency virus. *Obstet. Gynecol* **103** : (2004); 663–8.

32. Nakashima, A. K. & Fleming, P. L. HIV/AIDS surveillance in the United States, 1981–2001. *J. AIDS* **32 : Suppl. 1** (2003), S68–85.

33. Centers for Disease Control and Prevention. Advancing HIV prevention: new strategies for a changing epidemic – United States, 2003. *MMWR* **52 : RR-15** (2003), 329–32.

34. Joint statement of the American Academy of Pediatrics and the American College of Obstetricians and Gynecologists. Human immunodeficiency virus screening. *Pediatrics* **104 : 1** (1999), 128.

35. Centers for Disease Control and Prevention. Revision of the CDC surveillance case definition for acquired immunodeficiency syndrome. Council of State and Territorial Epidemiologists; AIDS Program, Center for Infectious Diseases. *MMWR* **36 : Suppl. 1** (1987), 1S–15S.

36. Centers for Disease Control and Prevention. 1994 Revised classification system for human immunodeficiency virus infection in children less than 13 years of age. *MMWR* **43 : RR-12** (1994), 1–10.

37. Green, T. A. Using surveillance data to monitor trends in the AIDS epidemic. *Stat. Med.* **17 : 2** (1998), 143–54.

38. Karon, J., Devine, O. J. & Morgan, W. M. Predicting AIDS incidence by extrapolating from recent trends. In C. Castillo-Chavez (ed.), *Mathematical and Statistical Approaches to AIDS Epidemiology. Lecture Notes in Biomathematics*, Vol. 83. Berlin: Springer-Verlag, (1989), pp. 58–88.

39. Centers for Disease Control and Prevention. Guidelines for the use of antiretroviral agents in pediatric HIV infection. *MMWR* **47 : RR-4** (1998), 1–43.

40. Hammett, T. A., Lindegren, M. L., Byers, R. *et al.* Progress towards elimination of perinatal HIV infection in the United States. In *XIII International Conference on AIDS, Durban, South Africa* (2000). [Abstract MoOrC239.]

41. Lindegren, M. L., Byers, R. H., Jr., Thomas, P. *et al.* Trends in perinatal transmission of HIV/AIDS in the United States. *J. Am. Med. Assoc.* **282 : 6** (1999), 531–8.

42. Centers for Disease Control and Prevention. Recommendation of the U.S. Public Health Service Task Force on the use of zidovudine to reduce perinatal transmission of human immunodeficiency virus. *MMWR* **43 : RR-11** (1994), 1–20.

43. Centers for Disease Control and Prevention. U.S. Public Health Service recommendations for human immunodeficiency virus counseling and voluntary testing for pregnant women. *MMWR* **44 : RR-7** (1995), 1–15.

44. Centers for Disease Control and Prevention. Public Health Service Task Force recommendations for the use of antiretroviral drugs in pregnant women infected with HIV-1 for maternal health and for reducing perinatal HIV-1 transmission in the United States. *MMWR* **47 : RR-2** (1998), 1–30. (Updates available at http://AIDSinfo.nih.gov).

45. Centers for Disease Control and Prevention. Public Health Service Task Force recommendations for the use of antiretroviral drugs in pregnant women infected with HIV-1 for maternal health and for reducing perinatal HIV-1 transmission in the United States. http://www.aidsinfor.nih.gov/guidelines (2002).

46. Lindegren, M. L., Bi, D., Wortley, P. *et al.* Evaluation of zidovudine prophylaxis regimens on perinatal HIV transmission using enhanced perinatal surveillance, 7 states, US. In *XIII International Conference on AIDS, Durban, South Africa* (2000) [Abstract MoPeC2448.]

47. Matheson, P. B., Abrams E. J., Thomas, P. A. *et al.* Efficacy of antenatal zidovudine in reducing perinatal transmission of human immunodeficiency virus type 1. The New York City Perinatal HIV Transmission Collaborative Study Group. *J. Infect. Dis.* **172 : 2** (1995), 353–8.

48. Fiscus, S. A., Adimora, A. A., Schoenbach, V. J. *et al.* Perinatal HIV infection and the effect of zidovudine therapy on transmission in rural and urban countries. *J. Am. Med. Assoc.* **275 : 19** (1996), 1483–8.

49. Simonds, R. J., Steketee, R., Nesheim, S. *et al.* Impact of zidovudine use on risk and risk factors for perinatal transmission of HIV. Perinatal AIDS Collaborative Transmission Studies. *AIDS* **12 : 3** (1998), 301–8.

50. Cooper, E. R., Nugent, R. P., Diaz, C. *et al.* After AIDS clinical trial 076: the changing pattern of zidovudine use during pregnancy, and the subsequent reduction in the vertical transmission of human immunodeficiency virus in a cohort of infected women and their infants. Women and Infants Transmission Study Group. *J. Infect. Dis.* **174 : 6** (1996), 1207–11.

51. Stiehm, E. R., Lambert, J. S., Mofenson, L. M. *et al.* Efficacy of zidovudine and human immunodeficiency virus (HIV) hyperimmune immunoglobulin for reducing perinatal HIV transmission from HIV-infected women with advanced disease: results of Pediatric AIDS Clinical Trials Group protocol 185. *J. Infect. Dis.* **179 : 3** (1999), 567–75.

52. Garcia, P. M., Kalish, L. A., Pitt, J. *et al.* Maternal levels of plasma human immunodeficiency virus type 1 RNA and the risk of perinatal transmission Study Group. *New Engl. J. Med.* **341 : 6** (1999), 394–402.

53. Mofenson, L. M., Lambert, J. S., Stiehm, E. R. *et al.* Risk factors for perinatal transmission of human immunodeficiency virus type 1 in women treated with zidovudine. Pediatric AIDS Clinical Trials Group Study 185 Team. *New Engl. J. Med.* **341 : 6** (1999), 385–93.

54. Dorenbaum, A., Cunningham, C. K., Gelber, R. D. *et al.* Two-dose intrapartum/newborn nevirapine and standard antiretroviral therapy to reduce perinatal HIV transmission: a randomized trial. *J. Am. Med. Assoc.* **288 : 2** (2002), 189–98.

55. Cooper, E. R., Charurat, M., Mofenson, L. *et al.* Combination antiretroviral strategies for the treatment of pregnant HIV-1-infected women and prevention of perinatal HIV-1 transmission. *J. AIDS* **29 : 5** (2002), 484–94.

56. Mandelbrot, L., Landreau-Mascaro, A., Rekacewicz, C. *et al.* Lamivudine-zidovudine combination for prevention of maternal–infant transmission of HIV-1. *J. Am. Med.* Assoc. **285 : 16** (2001), 2083–93.

57. Institute of Medicine. Reducing the Odds. *Preventing Perinatal Transmission of HIV in the United States.* Washington, DC: National Academy Press (1999).

58. Orloff, S. L., Bulterys, M., Vink, P. *et al.* Maternal characteristics associated with antenatal, intrapartum, and neonatal zidovudine use in four US cities, 1994–1998. *J. AIDS* **28 : 1** (2001), 65–72.

59. Wortley, P., Lindegren, M. L. & Fleming, P. L. Successful implementation of perinatal HIV prevention guidelines: a multistate surveillance evaluation. *MMWR* **50 : RR-06** (2001), 17–28.

60. Mokotoff, E. D., Malamud, B. H., Kent, J. B. *et al.* Progress toward elimination of perinatal HIV infection – Michigan, 1993–2000. *MMWR* **51 : 5** (2002), 94–7.

61. Centers for Disease Control and Prevention. Entry into prenatal care – United States, 1989–1997. *MMWR* **49** (2000), 393–8.

62. Minkoff, H. & O'Sullivan, M. J. The case for rapid HIV testing during labor. *J. Am. Med. Assoc.* **279 : 21** (1998), 1743–4.

63. Bulterys, M., Jamieson, D. J., O'Sullivan, M. J. *et al.* Rapid HIV-1 testing during labor: a multicenter study. *J. Am. Med. Assoc.* **292 :** (2004), 219–23.

64. Stringer, J. S. & Rouse, D. J. Rapid testing and zidovudine treatment to prevent vertical transmission of human immunodeficiency virus in unregistered parturients: a cost-effectiveness analysis. *Obstet. Gynecol.* **94 : 1** (1999), 34–40.

65. Grobman, W. A. & Garcia, P. M. The cost-effectiveness of voluntary intrapartum rapid human immunodeficiency virus testing for women without adequate prenatal care. *Am. J. Obstet. Gynecol.* **181 : 5** (1999), 1062–71.

66. Centers for Disease Control and Prevention. Prenatal discussion of HIV testing and maternal HIV testing – 14 states, 1996–1997. *MMWR* **48 : 19** (1999), 401–4.

67. Centers for Disease Control and Prevention. HIV testing among pregnant women – United States and Canada, 1998–2001. *MMWR* **51 : 45** (2002), 1013–16.

68. Sansom, S. L., Jamieson, D. J., Farnham, P. G., Bulterys, M. & Fowler, M. G. Human immunodeficiency virus retesting during pregnancy; costs and effectiveness in preventing perinatal transmission. *Obstet. Gynecol.* **102 : 4** (2003), 782–90.

69. Perinatal human immunodeficiency virus testing. Provisional Committee on Pediatric AIDS, American Academy of Pediatrics. *Pediatrics* **95 : 2** (1995), 303–7.

70. Hale, R. & Zinberg, S. ACOG's position on HIV testing. *ACOG Clin. Rev.* **2 : 1** (1997), 13.

71. Lansky, A., Jones, J. L., Fry, R. *et al.* Trends in HIV testing among pregnant women, United States, 1994–1999. *Am. J. Public Health* **91** (2001), 1291–3.

72. The International Perinatal HIV Group. The mode of delivery and the risk of vertical transmission of human immunodeficiency virus type 1 – a meta-analysis of 15 prospective cohort studies. *New Engl. J. Med.* **340 : 13** (1999), 977–87.

73. The European Mode of Delivery Collaboration. Elective caesarean-section versus vaginal delivery in prevention of vertical HIV-1 transmission: a randomised clinical trial. *Lancet* **353** : **9158** (1999), 1035–9.

74. Dominguez, K. L., Lindegren, M. L., d'Almada, P. J. *et al.* Increasing trend of cesarean deliveries in HIV-infected women in the United States from 1994 to 2000. *J. AIDS* **33** : **2** (2003), 232–8.

75. A report of the Dahlem Workshop on the eradication of infectious diseases. Berlin, March 16–22, 1997. In W. R. Dowdle & D. R. Hopkins (eds.), *The Eradication of Infectious Diseases* Indianapolis, IN: John Wiley & Sons (1997).

76. Centers for Disease Control and Prevention. Perinatal HIV Prevention Program. http://www.cdc.gov/hiv/projects/perinatal/grantees.htm (2003).

77. McNaghten, A. D., Hanson, D. L., Jones, J. L., Dworkin, M. S. & Ward, J. W. Effects of antiretroviral therapy and opportunistic illness primary chemoprophylaxis on survival after AIDS diagnosis. Adult/Adolescent Spectrum of Disease Group. *AIDS* **13** : **13** (1999), 1687–95.

78. Palella, F. J., Jr., Delaney, K. M., Moorman, A. C. *et al.* Declining morbidity and mortality among patients with advanced human immunodeficiency virus infection. HIV Outpatient Study Investigators. *New Engl. J. Med.* **338** : **13** (1998), 853–60.

79. Gortmaker, S. L., Hughes, M., Cervia, J. *et al.* Effect of combination therapy including protease inhibitors on mortality among children and adolescents infected with HIV-1. *New Engl. J. Med.* **345** : **21** (2001), 1522–8.

80. Fleming, P. L., Ward, J. W., Karon, J. M., Hanson, D. L. & De Cock, K. M. Declines in AIDS incidence and deaths in the USA: a signal change in the epidemic. *AIDS* **12** : **Suppl A** (1998), S55–61.

81. Centers for Disease Control and Prevention. Guidelines for the use of antiretroviral agents in HIV-infected adults and adolescents. Department of Health and Human Services and Henry J. Kaiser Family Foundation. *MMWR* **47** : **RR-5** (1998), 43–82.

82. DeMartino, M., Tovo, P. A., Balducci, M. *et al.* Reduction in mortality with availability of antiretroviral therapy for children with perinatal HIV-1 infection. *J. Am. Med. Assoc.* **284** (2000), 190–7.

83. Frederick, T., Mascola, L., Peters, V. *et al.* Trends in HAART use and immune status among HIV-infected infants and children in the pediatric spectrum of disease project, United States, 1994–2000. In *XIV International Conference on AIDS, Barcelona, Spain* (2002). [Abstract TuPeC4735.]

84. Abrams, E. J., Wiener, J., Carter, R. *et al.* Maternal health factors and early pediatric antiretroviral therapy influence the rate of perinatal HIV-1 disease progression in children. *AIDS* **17** : **6** (2003), 867–77.

85. Selik, R. M. & Lindegren, M. L. Changes in deaths reported with human immunodeficiency virus infection among US children less than 13 years old, 1987 through 1999 *Pediatr. Infect. Dis. J.* **22** : **7** (2003), 635–41.

86. Abrams, E. J., Weedon, J., Bertolli, J. *et al.* Aging cohort of perinatally human immunodeficiency virus-infected children in New York City. New York City Pediatric Surveillance of Disease Consortium. *Pediatr. Infect. Dis. J.* **20** : **5** (2001), 511–17.

87. Blanche, S., Mayaux, M. J., Rouzioux, C. *et al.* Relation of the course of HIV infection in children to the severity of the disease in their mothers at delivery. *New Engl. J. Med.* **330** : **5** (1994), 308–12.

88. Matte, C. & Roger, M. Genetic determinants of pediatric HIV-1 infection: vertical transmission and disease progression among children. *Mol. Med.* **7** : **9** (2001), 583–9.

89. Barroga, C. F., Raskino, C., Fangon, M. C. *et al.* The CCR5Delta32 allele slows disease progression of human immunodeficiency virus-1-infected children receiving antiretroviral treatment. *J. Infect. Dis.* **182** : **2** (2000), 413–19.

90. Misrahi, M., Teglas, J. P., N'Go, N. *et al.* CCR5 chemokine receptor variant in HIV-1 mother-to-child transmission and disease progression in children. French Pediatric HIV Infection Study Group. *J. Am. Med. Assoc.* **279** : **4** (1998), 277–80.

91. Centers for Disease Control and Prevention. Guidelines for prophylaxis against *Pneumocystis carinii* pneumonia for children infected with human immunodeficiency virus. *MMWR* **40** : **RR-2** (1991), 1–13.

92. Simonds, R. J., Lindegren, M. L., Thomas, P. *et al.* Prophylaxis against *Pneumocystis carinii* pneumonia among children with perinatally acquired human immunodeficiency virus infection in the United States. *Pneumocystis carinii* Pneumonia Prophylaxis Evaluation Working Group. *New Engl. J. Med.* **332** : **12** (1995), 786–90.

93. Centers for Disease Control and Prevention. 1995 revised guidelines for prophylaxis against *Pneumocystis carinii* pneumonia for children infected with or perinatally exposed to human immunodeficiency virus. National Pediatric and Family HIV Resource Center and National Center for Infectious Diseases, Centers for Disease Control and Prevention. *MMWR* **44** : **RR-4** (1995), 1–11.

94. Kaplan, J. E., Hanson, D., Dworkin, M. S. *et al.* Epidemiology of human immunodeficiency virus-associated opportunistic infections in the United States in the era of highly active antiretroviral therapy. *Clin. Infect. Dis.* **30** : **Suppl. 1** (2000), S5–14.

95. Dankner, W. M., Frederick, T. & Bertolli, J. Infectious complications of pediatric HIV infection. In W. T. Shearer & I. C. Hanson (eds.), *Medical Management of AIDS in Children*. Philadephia: W. B. Saunders Company (2003).

96. Lindegren, M. L., Byers, R., Bertolli, J. *et al.* Increasing numbers of adolescents living with perinatal HIV infection in the United States. In *XIII International Conference on AIDS, Durban, South Africa* (2000). [Abstract TuPeC3351].

97. Centers for Disease Control and Prevention. Pregnancy in perinatally HIV-infected adolescents and young adults – Puerto Rico, 2002. *MMWR* **52** : **8** (2003), 149–51.

98. Walker, N., Schwartlander, B. & Bryce, J. Meeting international goals in child survival and HIV/AIDS. *Lancet* **360** : **9329** (2002), 284–89.

99. De Cock, K. M., Fowler, M. G., Mercier, E. *et al.* Prevention of mother-to-child HIV transmission in resource-poor

countries: translating research into policy and practice. *J. Am. Med. Assoc.* **283** : **9** (2000), 1175–82.

100. Bulterys, M., Fowler, M. G., Shaffer, N. *et al.* Role of traditional birth attendants in preventing perinatal transmission of HIV. *Br. Med. J.* **324** : **7331** (2002), 222–4.

101. Lackritz, E. M., Shaffer, N. & Luo, C. Prevention of mother-to-child HIV transmission in the context of a comprehensive AIDS agenda in resource-poor countries. *J. AIDS* **30** : **2** (2002), 196–9.

102. Nolan, M. L., Greenberg, A. E. & Fowler, M. G. A review of clinical trials to prevent mother-to-child HIV-1 transmission in Africa and inform rational intervention strategies. *AIDS* **16** : **15** (2002), 1991–9.

103. Coovadia, H. & Coutsoudis, A. Problems and advances in reducing transmission of HIV-1 through breastfeeding in developing countries. *AIDScience* **1** (2001), 4.

104. Laga, M., Schwartlander, B., Pisani, E., Sow, P. S. & Carael, M. To stem HIV in Africa, prevent transmission to young women. *AIDS* **15** : **7** (2001), 931–4.

105. Rollins, N. C., Dedicoat, M., Danaviah, S. *et al.* Prevalence, incidence, and mother-to-child transmission of HIV-1 in rural South Africa. *Lancet* **360** : **9330** (2002), 389.

106. Kanshana, S. & Simonds, R. J. National program for preventing mother-child HIV transmission in Thailand: successful implementation and lessons learned. *AIDS* **16** : **7** (2002), 953–9.

107. Mouzin, E., Mercier, E. & Henderson, P. United Nations-sponsored pilot implementation projects on PMTCT: monitoring of intervention uptake in Africa. In *The 3rd Conference on Global Strategies for the Prevention of HIV Transmission from Mothers to Infants*. Kampala, Uganda. (2001). [Abstract 332.]

108. Bulterys, M., Nolan, M. L., Jamieson, D. J., Dominguez, K. L. & Fowler, M. G. Advances in the prevention of mother-to-child HIV-1 transmission: current issues, future challenges. *AIDScience* **2** (2002), 1–18.

109. Mofenson, L. M. Tale of two epidemics – the continuing challenge of preventing mother-to-child transmission of human immunodeficiency virus. *J. Infect. Dis.* **187** : **5** (2003), 721–4.

110. Buga, G. A., Amoko, D. H. & Ncayiyana, D. J. Sexual behaviour, contraceptive practice and reproductive health among school adolescents in rural Transkei. *S. Afr. Med. J.* **86** : **5** (1996), 523–7.

111. Matasha, E., Ntembelea, T., Mayaud, P. *et al.* Sexual and reproductive health among primary and secondary school pupils in Mwanza, Tanzania: need for intervention. *AIDS Care* **10** : **5** (1998), 571–82.

112. Watts, C. & Zimmerman, C. Violence against women: global scope and magnitude. *Lancet* **359** : **9313** (2002), 1232–7.

113. Jewkes, R., Levin, J., Mbananga, N. & Bradshaw, D. Rape of girls in South Africa. *Lancet* **359** : **9303** (2002), 319–20.

114. Bulterys, M. & Davis, L. Child abuse and neglect in Africa: a growing concern. In D. B. Jellifee & E. F. P. Jelliffe (eds.), *Advances in International Maternal and Child Health*. New York: Oxford University Press (1987), pp. 63–9.

115. van Vliet, A. & van Roosmalen, J. Worldwide prevention of vertical human immunodeficiency virus (HIV) transmission. *Obstet. Gynecol. Surv.* **52** : **5** (1997), 301–9.

PART II

General issues in the care of pediatric HIV patients

7

Diagnosis of HIV-1 infection in children

Paul Krogstad, M.D.

Associate Professor, Departments of Pediatrics and Molecular and Medical Pharmacology,
David Geffen School of Medicine at UCLA, University of California, Los Angeles, CA

Effective management of pediatric HIV-1 infection begins with timely and accurate diagnosis. In infants, early diagnosis is essential. Life-threatening immunodeficiency can develop rapidly and unpredictably, and there are no laboratory or clinical characteristics that accurately predict rapid or slow disease progression [1]. Studies in adults and children have shown that very early treatment can slow the progression of immunodeficiency and preserve HIV-1-specific immune responses. Early detection of HIV-1 infection among pregnant women is necessary to optimize medical care for the HIV-1-infected woman and to prevent mother-to-child transmission of HIV-1. This chapter outlines the use of serology, virus culture, and molecular diagnostic methods to detect HIV-1 infection in children.

7.1 HIV-1 diagnostic assays

7.1.1 Detection of antibodies to HIV-1

In 1985, enzyme-linked immunosorbent (ELISA) and immunoblot (Western blot) assays were licensed in the USA for detection of HIV-1-specific IgG antibodies in serum. While other tests are now available, they remain the mainstay for serological diagnosis of infection.

A large number of ELISA-based testing kits for antibody detection of HIV-1 specific antibodies are currently licensed by the US Food and Drug Administration. Early examples employed lysates from HIV-1-infected cell culture to provide HIV-1 antigen material. More recently developed assays often use a mixture of recombinant proteins, and some contain antigens that permit detection of antibodies to HIV-2 as well as antibody responses to HIV-1

(see below). Typically, testing of patient specimens involves adding serum to the wells of a microtiter plate containing HIV-1 antigen, and addition of positive and negative control specimens to additional wells. After incubation and washing steps, an antihuman antibody with an enzyme coupled to it is added to the wells. A chromogenic chemical substrate is modified by the enzyme bound to the antihuman antibody, leading to a color change in the well. The optical density (OD) change produced in this fashion is measured in a spectrophotometer. In order for a test sample to be considered positive (reactive), OD readings from a patient specimen must significantly exceed the "cutoff" value calculated from examination of negative control wells. In general, a serum sample is reported to be reactive only when it has been repeated, and again found to be ELISA positive.

ELISA assays detect all antibodies that react with HIV-1 proteins, and are an excellent method for rapid screening. Moreover, minor modifications, such as dilution of the test samples, allow samples with low antibody titers to be identified. This "detuned ELISA" has been successfully used to identify adults with recently acquired HIV-1 infection [2, 3]. In a high-risk population for HIV-1, the positive predictive value of ELISA testing is reported to exceed 99%. However, false-positive reactions still occur (see below), particularly when used in populations at low risk for HIV-1 infection. As a consequence, ELISA results must be confirmed with an assay of greater specificity, usually immunoblot or immunofluorescence assays [4]. The Western blot assay is used to identify the presence of antibodies in a patient's serum that are directed against specific structural and enzymatic proteins found in HIV-1 particles. In a Western blot assay, HIV-1 proteins are separated by electrophoresis and transferred to a membrane. Patient serum samples are added to the membrane and allowed to bind to HIV-1 proteins, and after washing, a second reagent is added to detect human IgG antibodies. A pattern of "bands" is created, reflecting the presence of antibodies that bind to viral proteins. Some bands represent reactivity to proteins found in the viral core, each identified by their mass (e.g. the 24 kDa capsid protein is known as p24). Others represent reactivity with the 160 kDa envelope glycoprotein, or its 120 kDa and 41 kDa cleavage products (gp160, gp120, and gp41, respectively) [5]. The Association of State and Territorial Public Health Laboratory Directors' criteria are used in the USA as the definition of a positive immunoblot (Western blot) [6]. By these guidelines, a positive Western blot assay reveals the presence of antibodies to any two of the following proteins: p24, gp41, or gp120/gp160. A negative assay shows no reactivity against any HIV-1 proteins. An indeterminate Western blot assay indicates the presence of the patient's antibodies against one or more HIV-1 proteins, but not those required for a positive assay. Most indeterminate assays have bands representing antibodies to p17, p24, p55, or a combination of these proteins. Patients with indeterminate Western blot assays require additional testing to exclude or confirm HIV-1 infection. Generally, the Western blot is repeated soon thereafter, and one or more virological tests are performed as well.

The serological methods described above are complex tests that must be performed by skilled personnel in a medical laboratory. Rapid serological methods to detect IgG antibodies to HIV-1 in blood, saliva, and urine have been developed, and are becoming commercially available [4]. These tests permit HIV-1 antibodies to be detected in as little as 10–20 minutes, without the use of sophisticated equipment, but confirmation by other methods is recommended [7]. Several rapid tests to detect antibodies to HIV-1 in blood and Saliva are now licensed by the US Food and Drug Administration (e.g. the Single Use Diagnostic System (SUDS) HIV-1 Test (Abbott Laboratories) and the Orasure HIV-1 (Orasure Technologies, Inc.)). Rapid serological tests could potentially play an important role in efforts to prevent perinatal transmission of HIV-1, by identifying pregnant women of unknown HIV-1 infection status who present for care at the time of labor and delivery, and their exposed infants [8, 9]. Studies are underway to test the utility of rapid testing methods in this setting.

All results from serologic tests for HIV-1 infection mandate careful clinical interpretation. False negative reactions are found among patients who have not begun to produce antibody (acute antiretroviral syndrome), or, rarely, among those in whom antibodies are no longer

being produced (late stages of HIV-1 infection with resulting hypogammaglobulinemia). Rare cases have been described in which HIV-1 infected individuals with disrupted immunoglobulin production are serologically negative; infection was demonstrated by virological assays (see below). False positive ELISA reactions have been reported among patients with acute DNA viral infections, those with autoimmune disorders, and among multiparous or multiply transfused individuals. Moreover, the shortcomings of serological assays must be born in mind when evaluating infants and young children. The transplacental transfer of maternal IgG antibody during gestation causes all children born to HIV-1-infected women to be seropositive at birth; only a fraction are truly infected [1].

7.1.2 HIV-1 RNA and DNA detection methods

Because HIV-1 is a retrovirus, its genome exists both as an RNA form in virions and in a DNA form in infected cells (see Chapter 2). HIV-1 DNA polymerase chain reaction (PCR) analysis of blood leukocyte DNA is an extremely sensitive assay, and 30–50% of infections in infants can be detected at birth [9–11]. False negative results occur in the first several weeks of age because many infants acquire HIV-1 infection in the immediate peripartum period. However, by 1 month of age, nearly all perinatally acquired infections can be detected (see below).

The amount of virion-packaged HIV-1 RNA in the peripheral blood ("viral load") is an important measure of disease activity and of the effectiveness of antiretroviral therapy. This genomic viral RNA can be measured using reverse transcriptase PCR (RT-PCR) or other RNA quantification techniques such as branched DNA (bDNA) or nucleic acid sequence-based amplification (NASBA). Provided that samples of blood are promptly processed, HIV-1 RNA detection assays are highly sensitive and specific for the diagnosis of HIV-1 infection [12, 13].

PCR assays to detect DNA and RNA are extremely sensitive, and problems can arise if rigorous attention to cross-contamination is not provided. False-positive reactions may also occur owing to sample mix-up and laboratory errors, principally cross-contamination [13, 14].

7.2 Other virological assays

7.2.1 Viral p24 antigen detection

ELISA detection of the presence of the p24 antigen of HIV-1 in serum is an alternative method for diagnosis of HIV-1 infection. In general terms, sera to be tested are allowed to bind to p24-specific antibody that is either bound to a well of a microtiter plate, or to the surface of polystyrene beads. After appropriate incubation and washing steps, the well or beads are incubated with a goat or rabbit antibody that reacts with any p24 antigen captured by the first step. Finally, an anti-goat or anti-rabbit antibody is added, which is coupled to an enzyme that produces a colorimetric reaction in the presence of a chemical substrate. ELISA measurements of the HIV-1 capsid protein (p24), have been used to diagnose HIV-1 infection in all age groups, but have low (30–70%) sensitivity among infants less than 3 months of age [9, 15]. The inability to detect p24 antigen is largely the result of the presence of HIV-1 specific antibodies that in an infant are the result of transplacental transfer. Dissociation of antibody from p24 antigen in serum specimens greatly enhances the sensitivity of the p24 ELISA. In the ICD (immune complex dissociated) p24 assay, serum or plasma samples are treated briefly with acid, which dissociates HIV-1 antibodies from their bound antigens. Following neutralization of the sample, the ELISA is run as described above. However, ICD-p24 antigen testing should not be used for the diagnosis of infection in infants less than a month of age because of an unacceptably high number of false positive results [9, 15]. Other investigators have used heat denaturation of plasma samples to release viral antigen (HD-Ag testing), prior to ELISA. HD-Ag testing appears to be very sensitive for the detection of viremia [16], but a small number of false-positive results occur, compared with PCR testing of the same specimen [17]. Antigen detection methods remain a potentially useful alternative approach to the diagnosis of perinatal HIV infection, with recognition of the need for confirmation of these results.

7.2.2 Culture

Since the initial isolation of HIV-1 in the early 1980s, cultures have been used to detect HIV-1 and to measure the number of HIV-1 infected peripheral blood lymphocytes. In general terms, patient peripheral blood mononuclear cells (PBMCs) are incubated with PBMCs from an HIV-1-seronegative (i.e. uninfected) donor, and cultured for up to 6 weeks in media containing interleukin 2 (IL-2, originally known as T cell growth factor) which activates the PBMCs and facilitates high levels of viral replication within the cells. The growth of HIV-1 in the cells is determined by assaying for capsid protein (p24) by ELISA performed on culture fluid medium. Cultures are designated as positive when significant p24 antigen is detected (usually ≥ 30 pg/mL) [18].

Although cumbersome, time-consuming, and costly to perform, HIV-1 cultures have high specificity and sensitiv-

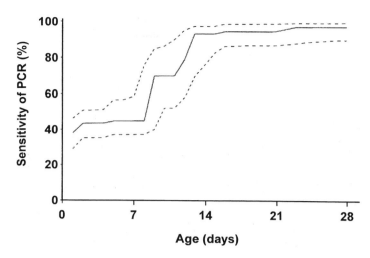

Figure 7.1. Cumulative frequency of PCR detection of perinatally transmitted HIV-1 infection in infants. Broken lines indicate 90% confidence intervals surrounding the mean. Reprinted with permission from [10].

ity. False positive test results are rare and generally result from laboratory errors such as specimen mislabeling. In the absence of antiretroviral treatment, falsely negative cultures are unusual among adult patients, but may exist in early infancy because of small specimen volumes and low amounts of virus soon after perinatal infection. Nonetheless, under optimal conditions, the sensitivity of culture and HIV-1 DNA PCR are equal for detection of HIV-1 infection in infants [9].

7.3 Diagnosing HIV-1 infection in infants and children

Using virological assays, HIV-1 infection can be detected in most infants by 1 month of age, and in nearly all by 6 months of age (Table 7.1) [19]. HIV-1 DNA PCR is currently the diagnostic method of choice for perinatally exposed children under 18 months of age. Umbilical cord specimens must not be used, because contamination of the specimen by maternal blood can occur. Approximately 40% of infants will test positive in the first 24 hours of life. The sensitivity of HIV-1 DNA PCR rises rapidly, and most infants with perinatally acquired infection who test negative at birth will have positive PCR test results by 2 weeks of age. In a meta-analysis of several published studies, the sensitivity of HIV-1 DNA PCR was 93% at 2 weeks of age (95% confidence interval: 76–97%) (Figure 7.1) [10]. The small number of infants who do not have detectable HIV-1 DNA by this time will generally test positive by the end of the second month of life [20]. Early diagnosis of HIV-1 infection

Table 7.1 Detection of HIV-1 infection in infants and children

HIV-1-infected
  a. Child < 18 months known to be seropositive or born to an HIV-1-infected mother with:
      1. Positive results on two separate determinations (excluding cord blood) from one of the
         following detection assays:
         HIV-1 DNA PCR or HIV-1 RNA detection assays
         HIV-1 culture
         HIV-1 p24 antigen (only used in infants above 1 month of age)
         or
      2. Meets the clinical criteria for AIDS diagnosis based on the 1987
         AIDS surveillance case definition
  b. Child ≥ 18 mo with:
      1. Positive HIV-1 antibody detection tests (e.g. repeatedly positive ELISA and confirmatory
         test (Western blot or immunofluorescence assay)
         or
      2. Meets any criteria outlined in (a)

HIV-1-uninfected (seroreverter)
  Child born to an HIV-1-infected mother, who has:
      1. Negative HIV-1 antibody tests (2 or more negative ELISA tests performed one month apart,
         both after 6 months of age)*
         or
      2. No other laboratory evidence of HIV-1 infection (has not had two positive viral detection
         tests, if performed)
         and
      No evidence of an AIDS-defining condition

*In the absence of hypogammaglobulinemia.
Adapted from [19]. (Updates available at www.hivatis.org/guidelines/Pediatric/Dec12_01/peddec.pdf)

is desirable, to allow antiretroviral therapy to be instituted or modified. Testing should be performed within 48 hours of birth, at 1–2 months of age, and again at 4–6 months of age. Any positive tests should be verified as quickly as possible by a second virological test [21].

HIV-1 infection can be excluded with high accuracy when an asymptomatic child has had two or more negative virologic tests, using blood samples drawn at or after 1 month of age, with at least one drawn after 4 months of age. HIV-1 infection also can be excluded when HIV-1 antibodies are not detected in two or more antibody tests (spaced 1 month apart) performed at or after 6 months of age, in a child who has no signs or symptoms of HIV-1 infection. Finally, HIV-1 infection can be ruled out when antibody tests (ELISA or Western blot) are negative, in the absence of hypogammaglobulinemia, in a child at least 18 months of age who lacks any clinical evidence of HIV-1 infection.

HIV-1 infection is diagnosed when two positive HIV-1 virological tests are obtained (HIV-1 RNA or DNA PCR, p24 antigen (for children above 1 month of age), or culture). Separate blood specimens should be used for these tests.

There have been rare reports of infants with positive virological tests, and subsequent negative tests. Although transient HIV-1 infection has been proposed to explain this finding, nearly all such cases are false positive tests resulting from sample mix-up and laboratory error, including PCR contamination [14]. A diagnosis of HIV-1 can be made by serological methods in children 18 months of age or older who have antibodies to HIV-1 detected by ELISA and confirmed by Western blot or immunofluorescence methods.

7.4 Diagnosis of non-subtype B HIV-1 infection

The two human immunodeficiency viruses, HIV-1 and HIV-2, exhibit tremendous genetic heterogeneity, which may complicate PCR-based diagnosis [22]. HIV-1 variants are currently classified into three groups: M (main), O (outlier), and N (non-M/non-O). Within group M, clusters (clades) of related strains have been further classified into subtypes A-D, F-H, J, and K. In addition, inter-subtype recombinants have been identified in several regions of the

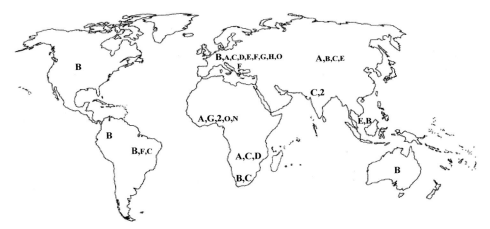

Figure 7.2. Worldwide Geographical Distribution of HIV Variants. Letters indicate the predominate subtypes of HIV-1 found in each area, if known. The presence of HIV-2 in western Africa and India is indicated ("2"). The figure is intended to illustrate the diversity of HIV-1, which has an impact on diagnostic approaches and potential vaccine strategies in an area. This is particularly problematic for the areas most affected by the pandemic: sub-Saharan Africa, India, and Asia. Figure based on data summarized in [20], and updated data found at www.hiv.lanl.gov.

world (Figure 7.2) [22, 23]. A similar classification of HIV-2 subtypes exists.

All of the ELISAs that are currently licensed for use in the USA will detect HIV-1 specific antibodies, but only a subset will detect antibodies to HIV-2. None of these ELISA or confirmatory tests will reliably detect HIV-1 subtype O, and none of the confirmatory tests available will consistently detect HIV-2 antibodies [4]. Fortunately, infections with HIV-1 subtype O and HIV-2 are still rare outside of countries in west central Africa (e.g. Cameroon, Ivory Coast), and commercially available serological tests can be used to detect most infections worldwide.

The genetic diversity of HIV-1 particularly complicates PCR detection of the virus in infants. Subtype B is the most common subtype in the U.S. and Western Europe, and the commercially available Amplicor HIV-1 DNA detection kit (Roche) employs oligonucleotide primers that detect it and the most closely related subtypes (e.g. subtypes D and G) [9, 12, 24]. However, the majority of HIV-1 infections in the world are caused by the other subtypes, which may not be detected (e.g. subtypes A and C) [22, 24]. Alternatives to the use of the Amplicor HIV-1 DNA PCR in these cases include the use of commercial HIV-1 RNA detection methods that include primers with broader specificity (Amplicor HIV-1 Monitor 1.5 or use of NASBA and bDNA assay methods) [25]. These alternative methods should be considered when the maternal history suggests the possibility of infection by an unusual subtype, or when an infant has signs or symptoms of HIV-1 infection, despite negative initial testing. Changes in the worldwide epidemiology of HIV-1 will likely necessitate repeated re-evaluation of methods to detect viral DNA and RNA to ensure detection of HIV-1 in all individuals in a given geographic area.

7.5 Summary

Many assays are commercially available to detect HIV-1 infection in children. In children who are 18 or more months of age, and in adolescents and adults, serologic assays (e.g. ELISA, Western blot) constitute the most cost-effective diagnostic assay for HIV-1 infection. For children younger than 18 months, HIV-1 DNA PCR is the preferred method for early HIV-1 detection. These assays provide clinicians with the opportunity to make a prompt diagnosis of HIV-1 infection, and to initiate antiretroviral therapy as well as prophylaxis against opportunistic infections.

ACKNOWLEDGMENT

The author is an Elizabeth Glaser Scientist sponsored by the Pediatric AIDS Foundation. Elizabeth Glaser is remembered with great admiration for her courage and her work on behalf of all families affected by HIV.

REFERENCES

1. King, S. M.; American Academy of Pediatrics Committee on Pediatric AIDS; American Academy of Pediatrics Infections Diseases and Immunization Committee. Evaluation and treatment of the human immunodeficiency virus-1 exposed infant. *Pediatrics* **114**:**2** (2004), 497–505.

2. Janssen, R. S., Satten, G. A., Stramer, S. L. *et al.* New testing strategy to detect early HIV-1 infection for use in incidence estimates and for clinical and prevention purposes. *J. Am. Med. Assoc.* **280** (1998), 42–8.

3. Machado, D. M., Delwart, E. L., Diaz, R. S. *et al.* Use of the sensitive/less-sensitive (detuned) EIA strategy for targeting genetic analysis of HIV-1 to recently infected blood donors. *AIDS* **16** (2002), 113–19.

4. Centers for Disease Control and Prevention. Revised Guidelines for HIV Counseling, Testing, and Referral. Technical Expert Panel Review of CDC HIV Counseling, Testing and Referral Guidelines. *MMWR* **50: RR-19** (2001), 1–57.

5. Bylund, D. J., Ziegner, U. H. & Hooper, D. G. Review of testing for human immunodeficiency virus. *Clin. Lab. Med.* **12** (1992), 305–33.

6. Centers for Disease Control and Prevention. Interpretation and use of the Western blot assay for serodiagnosis of human immunodeficiency virus type 1 infections. *MMWR* **38** (1989), 1–7.

7. Centers for Disease Control. Update: HIV Counseling and Testing using Rapid Tests – United States, 1995. *MMWR* **11** (1998), 211–15.

8. Minkoff, H. & O'Sullivan, M. J. The case for rapid HIV testing during labor. *J. Am. Med. Assoc.* **279** (1998), 1743–4.

9. Nielsen, K. & Bryson, Y. J. Diagnosis of HIV infection in children. *Pediatr. Clin. North. Am.* **47** (2000), 39–63.

10. Dunn, D. T., Brandt, C. D., Krivine, A. *et al.* The sensitivity of HIV-1 DNA polymerase chain reaction in the neonatal period and the relative contributions of intra-uterine and intra-partum transmission. *AIDS* **9** (1995), F7–11.

11. Shearer, W. T., Quinn, T. C., LaRussa, P. *et al.* Viral load and disease progression in infants infected with human immunodeficiency virus type 1. Women and Infants Transmission Study Group. *New Engl. J. Med.* **336** (1997), 1337–42.

12. Delamare, C., Burgard, M., Mayaux, M. J. *et al.* HIV-1 RNA detection in plasma for the diagnosis of infection in neonates. The French Pediatric HIV Infection Study Group. *J. AIDS Hum. Retrovirol.* **15** (1997), 121–5.

13. Simonds, R. J., Brown, T. M., Thea, D. M. *et al.* Sensitivity and specificity of a qualitative RNA detection assay to diagnose HIV infection in young infants. Perinatal AIDS Collaborative Transmission Study. *AIDS* **12** (1998), 1545–9.

14. Frenkel, L. M., Mullins, J. I., Learn, G. H. *et al.* Genetic evaluation of suspected cases of transient HIV-1 infection of infants. *Science* **280** (1998), 1073–7.

15. Miles, S. A., Balden, E., Magpantay, L. *et al.* Rapid serologic testing with immune-complex-dissociated HIV p24 antigen for early detection of HIV infection in neonates. Southern California Pediatric AIDS Consortium. *New Engl. J. Med.* **328** (1993), 297–302.

16. Schupbach, F. M., Pontelli, D., Tomasik, Z., Luty, R. & Boni, J. Heat-mediated immune complex dissociation and enzyme-linked immunosorbent assay signal amplification render p24 antigen detection in plasma as sensitive as HIV-1 RNA detection by polymerase chain reaction. *AIDS* **10** (1996), 1085–90.

17. Schupbach, B. J., Tomasik, Z., Jendis, J., Seger, R. & Kind, C. Sensitive detection and early prognostic significance of p24 antigen in heat-denatured plasma of human immunodeficiency virus type 1-infected infants. Swiss Neonatal HIV Study Group. *J. Infect. Dis.* **170** (1994), 318–24.

18. Hollinger, F. B., Bremer, J. W., Myers, L. E., Gold, J. W. & McQuay, L. Standardization of sensitive human immunodeficiency virus coculture procedures and establishment of a multicenter quality assurance program for the AIDS Clinical Trials Group. The NIH/NIAID/DAIDS/ACTG Virology Laboratories. *J. Clin. Microbiol.* **30** (1992), 1787–94.

19. Centers for Disease Control and Prevention. 1994 revised classification system for human immunodeficiency virus infection in children less than 13 years of age. *MMWR* **43 : RR-12** (1994), 1–10. (Updates available at http://AIDSInfo.nih.gov).

20. Owens, D. K., Holodniy, M., McDonald, T. W., Scott, J. & Sonnad, S. A meta-analytic evaluation of the polymerase chain reaction for the diagnosis of HIV infection in infants. *J. Am. Med. Assoc.* **275** (1996), 1342–8.

21. Centers for Disease Control and Prevention. Recommendations of the U.S. Public Health Service Task Force on the use of zidovudine to reduce perinatal transmission of human immunodeficiency virus. *MMWR* **44** (1995), 1–20.

22. McCutchan, F. Global diversity in HIV. In K. Crandall (ed.), *Evolution of HIV.* Baltimore, MD: The John Hopkins University Press (1999).

23. Robertson, D. L., Anderson, J. P. & Bradac, J. A. HIV-1 nomenclature proposal. *Science* **288** (2000), 55–6.

24. Bogh, M., Machuca, R. & Gerstoft, J. Subtype-specific problems with qualitative Amplicor HIV-1 DNA PCR test. *J. Clin. Virol.* **20** (2001), 149–53.

25. Rouet, F., Montcho, C. & Rouzioux, C. Early diagnosis of paediatric HIV-1 infection among African breast-fed children using a quantitative plasma HIV RNA assay. *AIDS* **15** (2001), 1849–56.

Prevention of mother-to-child transmission of HIV

Jennifer S. Read, M.D., M.S., M.P.H., D.T.M.&H.

Pediatric, Adolescent, and Maternal AIDS (PAMA) Branch, NIH, Bethesda, MD

8.1 Introduction

Over the past several years, major successes have been achieved in prevention of mother-to-child transmission (MTCT) of human immunodeficiency virus type 1 (HIV). However, these successes have occurred primarily in those countries with the greatest resources and the lowest burden of HIV infection among women and children. Significant challenges remain, particularly in those countries with more limited resources and a greater population burden of HIV infection. Each day an estimated 2000 infants become infected with HIV, virtually all residing in resource-poor settings [1]. In this chapter, the timing and rates of, and risk factors for, MTCT of HIV will be reviewed briefly. Interventions for the prevention of MTCT of HIV will be discussed, both those already shown to be efficacious and those under study. Finally, strategies to prevent MTCT of HIV will be addressed.

8.2 Mother-to-child transmission of HIV: timing and rates

Mother-to-child transmission of HIV can occur during pregnancy, at the time of labor and delivery, and postnatally (through breastfeeding) [2]. Potential mechanisms of antepartum and intrapartum transmission of HIV include transplacental transfer of the virus from mother to fetus before delivery and exposure of the fetus or infant to maternal blood, amniotic fluid, and cervicovaginal secretions during delivery. Evidence for transmission during each of these periods has been elucidated over several years. Evidence for in utero transmission of HIV includes identification of HIV in fetal tissue and blood, in amniotic fluid,

and in placental tissue; and positive viral assays in many HIV-infected infants at birth [3]. Similarly, intrapartum transmission has been suggested by the strong association between longer duration of ruptured membranes and MTCT [4], and has been demonstrated in a randomized clinical trial of cesarean section versus vaginal delivery [5]. Finally, transmission of HIV through breastfeeding has been demonstrated in a randomized clinical trial of formula feeding versus breastfeeding [6]. The risk of MTCT is intermediate to the risk of transmission per exposure event associated with blood transfusion (90%) [7] and with other exposures such as needle sharing among injection drug users (0.67%) [8]. Rates of MTCT of HIV have been calculated in studies conducted around the world in the absence of interventions to decrease transmission [9]. Overall, most studies reported a transmission rate in the range of 25–30% and higher transmission rates were observed in resource-poor settings (13–42%) than in resource-rich settings (14–25%) (Figure 8.1). Although many reasons could explain the differences in observed transmission rates, the relative frequency of breastfeeding among HIV-infected women (essentially universal in the poorest settings; less common, and sometimes quite unusual, in resource-rich settings) is undoubtedly important. Recognition that not all HIV-infected women transmit the infection to their children set the stage for studies aimed at determining the risk factors for MTCT of HIV.

8.3 Risk factors for, and interventions to prevent, mother-to-child transmission of HIV

Numerous risk factors for MTCT of HIV have been identified or are under investigation [10]. General categories of

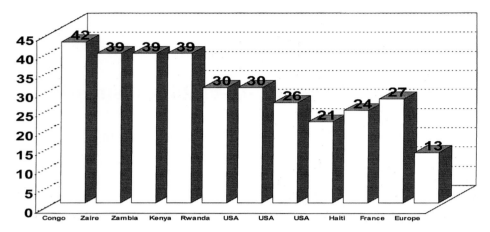

Figure 8.1. Reported mother-to-child transmission rates (percent), without interventions to decrease transmission: Africa, North America, Caribbean, Europe.

risk factors include: the amount of virus to which the child is exposed, the duration of such exposure, factors facilitating the transfer of virus from mother to child, characteristics of the virus, and the child's susceptibility to infection. Identification of risk factors associated with MTCT of HIV is the first step in developing interventions to interrupt such transmission. To date, clinical and public health interventions exist or are under investigation for some, but not all, identified or potential risk factors. More specifically, efficacy has been demonstrated for interventions which decrease maternal viral load and/or decrease the child's susceptibility to infection (antiretroviral prophylaxis regimens), and which decrease the duration of such exposure (intrapartum exposure: cesarean section; postnatal exposure: avoidance of breastfeeding), and other such interventions are under investigation. Interventions to eliminate or ameliorate factors facilitating the transfer of virus from mother to child are under investigation. However, efficacious interventions to affect characteristics of the virus associated with transmission (e.g. viral phenotype [11]) have yet to be identified. Table 8.1 summarizes selected known or potential risk factors for MTCT of HIV, and the associated interventions (already identified or else under investigation) for preventing such transmission. Each risk factor and associated intervention is discussed in greater detail below.

8.3.1 Amount of virus to which the child is exposed

The amount of virus the infant is exposed to is now understood to represent a major risk factor for MTCT of HIV. The greatest amount of information exists regarding maternal viral load in the peripheral bloodstream, but more recent data indicate that the concentrations of virus in cervico-vaginal fluid and breast milk also are important.

Peripheral blood

A higher maternal HIV RNA concentration (viral load) in the peripheral bloodstream is associated with a higher risk of MTCT of HIV [12]. Without receipt of antiretroviral therapy, transmission rates ranged from 5% if maternal cell-free viral load was less than 1000 copies/mL, 15% if viral load was between 1000 and 9999 copies/mL, and 37% if viral load was at or above 10 000 copies/mL. Although the risk of transmission of HIV from mothers with peripheral blood viral loads below the level of assay quantitation is very low, no threshold of peripheral blood viral load below which transmission does not occur has been identified. Although the association between maternal peripheral blood viral load and MTCT remains even among women who received zidovudine prophylaxis [13], receipt of antiretroviral therapy attenuates the relationship between maternal viral load and transmission [12]. Women receiving highly active antiretroviral therapy [14–15] have very low rates of MTCT.

Efficacy of perinatal transmission prophylaxis with antiretroviral drugs

Antiretroviral interventions for the prevention of MTCT of HIV (Table 8.2) began with the success of the AIDS Clinical Trials Group (ACTG) protocol 076, a randomized clinical trial conducted in the USA and France and published in 1994 [16]. Subsequently, the efficacy of other antiretroviral prophylaxis regimens has been demonstrated in different countries around the world. These modified antiretroviral

Table 8.1 Selected known or potential risk factors for, and associated interventions to prevent, MTCT of HIV

Category	Factor	Intervention
Amount of virus	Higher maternal viral load	Decrease maternal viral load and/or provide pre-/post-exposure prophylaxis to the infant
	In peripheral blood	Administer antiretroviral drug(s) to the mother
	In cervicovaginal fluid	Administer antiretroviral drug(s) to the mother
		Administer viricidal agent(s) to the mother (cervicovaginal cleansing) and/or to the newborn
	In breast milk	Administer antiretroviral drug(s) to the mother
		Administer antiretroviral prophylaxis to the infant
		Treat breast milk with heat or chemicals
Duration of exposure	Mode of delivery (vaginal delivery or cesarean section after labor and/or after ruptured membranes)	Cesarean section before labor and before ruptured membranes
	Breastfeeding	Avoid breastfeeding (if safe, affordable, and feasible)
		If breastfeeding unavoidable, early weaning (if possible)
Factors facilitating transfer of the virus from mother to child	Vitamin A deficiency	Administer vitamin A supplementation to the mother and/or infant
	Chorioamnionitis	Administer antibiotics to the mother
	Mixed breastfeeding	Exclusive breastfeeding

prophylaxis regimens have incorporated initiation of antepartum antiretroviral drug(s) as early as 28 weeks gestation and as late as the onset of labor. The duration of antiretroviral prophylaxis administered after delivery to the mother, to the infant, or to both has ranged from none up to 6 weeks. The antiretroviral drugs evaluated have been zidovudine, nevirapine, the combination of zidovudine and lamivudine, and the combination of zidovudine and nevirapine.

ACTG 076 was a randomized, double blind, placebo-controlled trial of a three-part zidovudine regimen administered to HIV-infected women and their infants. Antepartum zidovudine was administered orally beginning at 14–34 weeks of gestation, intrapartum zidovudine was administered intravenously, and oral zidovudine was administered to the infants during the first 6 weeks of life. MTCT was decreased by approximately two-thirds with this regimen of zidovudine [16]. Interestingly, only a small proportion of the protective effect of zidovudine in reducing transmission was explained by lowering of maternal peripheral blood viral load [17]. Data from this trial demonstrating that efficacy was observed irrespective of maternal viral load [17], and, similarly, data from other studies [12, 18], suggested that an important component of protection was pre- and post-exposure prophylaxis of the infant.

Subsequently, the ACTG 076 regimen was modified to address the needs for simplified and cheaper prophylaxis regimens in resource-poor settings. The first simplified antiretroviral prophylaxis trial was conducted in Thailand. This clinical trial demonstrated the efficacy of a shorter, two-part zidovudine regimen involving oral zidovudine administration to the mother beginning at 36 weeks of gestation, and oral zidovudine from the onset of labor until delivery. The infant did not receive zidovudine. Mothers were given infant formula and were asked not to breast-feed. With this regimen, transmission was reduced by 50% in a non-breastfeeding population [19]. Subsequently, two other short-course zidovudine prophylaxis trials were conducted in West Africa among populations of breastfeeding, HIV-infected pregnant women. In a randomized, placebo-controlled trial conducted in the Côte d'Ivoire, the same regimen previously evaluated in Thailand [19] was evaluated. Analysis of transmission rates at 3 months of age demonstrated lesser efficacy (37%) in this breastfeeding population [20]. A different regimen was studied in a randomized, placebo-controlled trial in the Côte d'Ivoire and Burkina Faso. In this trial, zidovudine was initiated at 36–38 weeks gestation and only a single oral dose was given at the onset of labor. In addition, zidovudine was administered to the mother for 1 week after delivery. The infant did not

Table 8.2 Randomized clinical trials: antiretroviral prophylaxis regimens

Drug(s) evaluated	Trial	Location	Breastfeeding	Randomization	Transmission Rates	Efficacy
Zidovudine (ZDV)	Connor 1994 [16]	USA, France	No	*Mother:* Zidovudine 100 mg po 5 times per day beginning at 14–34 weeks gestation, 2 mg/kg IV over a 1 hour period, then 1 mg/kg per hour until delivery *Infant:* 2 mg/kg po q 6 hours for 6 weeks, beginning 8–12 hours after birth Placebo	7.9% (95% CI: 4.1, 11.7) 27.7% (95% CI: 21.2, 34.1)	71%
	Shaffer 1999 [19]	Thailand	No	*Mother:* Zidovudine 300 mg po BID from 36 weeks gestation, q 3 hours from onset of labor until delivery *Infant:* No ZDV Placebo	9.4% (95% CI: 5.2, 13.5) 18.9% (95% CI: 13.2, 24.2)	50%
	Wiktor 1999 [20]	Cote d'Ivoire	Yes (most)	*Mother:* Zidovudine 300 mg po BID from 36 weeks gestation, q 3 hours from onset of labor until delivery *Infant:* No ZDV Placebo	12.2% (1 month) 15.7% (3 months) 21.7% (1 month) 24.9% (3 months)	44% (1 month) 37% (3 months)
	Dabis 1999 [21]	Cote d'Ivoire, Burkina Faso	Yes (most)	*Mother:* Zidovudine 300 mg po BID from 36–38 weeks gestation until labor, 600 mg at beginning of labor, 300 mg po BID × 7 days *Infant:* No ZDV Placebo	18.0% (6 months) 27.5%	38%
	Lallemant 2000 [23]	Thailand	No	All participants: *Mother:* Zidovudine 300 mg po BID until labor, then 300 mg po q 3 hours until delivery *Infant:* Zidovudine 2 mg/kg po q 6 hours with randomization to one of four arms: Long-long: maternal ZDV from 28 weeks, infant ZDV for 6 weeks Short-short: maternal ZDV from 35 weeks, infant ZDV for 3 days	4.1% (interim analysis), 6.5% (4.1, 8.9) (final analysis) 10.5% (interim analysis; enrollment into this arm discontinued)	No statistically significant differences in three arms (long-long, long-short, short-long) Transmission rate among those randomized to arms with longer (from 28 weeks) antepartum ZDV: 1.6% (0.7, 2.6)

	Study	Country	Breastfeeding	Regimen	Transmission rate	Outcome
				Long-short: maternal ZDV from 28 weeks, infant ZDV for 3 days	4.7% (2.4, 7.0) (final analysis)	Transmission rate among those randomized to arms with shorter (from 36 weeks) antepartum ZDV: 5.1% (3.2, 7.0)
				Short-long: maternal ZDV from 35 weeks, infant ZDV for 6 weeks	8.6% (5.6, 11.6) (final analysis)	
ZDV vs. nevirapine (NVP)	Jackson 2003 [24]	Uganda	Yes (most)	Nevirapine 200 mg po at onset of labor (infant NVP 2 mg/kg within 72 hours of birth)	11.8% by 6–8 weeks 13.5% by 14–16 weeks 15.7% by 18 months	41% by 14–16 weeks
				Zidovudine 600 mg po at onset of labor and 300 mg q 3 hours until delivery (infant ZDV 4 mg/kg po BID for 7 days after birth)	20.0% by 6–8 weeks 22.1% by 14–16 weeks 25.8% by 18 months	
ZDV with lamivudine (3TC)	Petra 2002 [26]	South Africa, Tanzania, Uganda	Yes (some)	Antepartum ZDV 300 mg po BID with lamivudine (3TC) 150 mg po BID from 36 weeks gestation Intrapartum ZDV 300 mg × 1, then 300 mg po q 3 hours with 3TC 150 mg × 1, then 150 mg q 12 hours Postpartum (Mother): Zidovudine 300 mg po BID with 3TC 150 mg po BID for 1 week Postnatal (Infant): Zidovudine 4 mg/kg po BID with 3TC 2 mg/kg po BID for 1 week		
				Arm A: Antepartum, intrapartum, and postpartum/postnatal	5.7% at 6 weeks 15% [9–23] at 18 months	No statistically significant differences in transmission rates at 18 months
				Arm B: Intrapartum and postpartum/postnatal only	8.9% at 6 weeks 18% [12–16] at 18 months	
				Arm C: Postpartum/ postnatal only	14.2% at 6 weeks 20% [13–30] at 18 months	
				Placebo	15.3% at 6 weeks 22% [16–30] at 18 months	
	SAINT 2003 [27]	South Africa	Yes (some)	*Mother:* Zidovudine 600 mg po × 1, then 300 mg po q 3 hours until delivery and 300 mg po BID for 1 week after delivery. 3TC 150 mg po × 1, then 150 mg po q12 hours until delivery and 150 mg po BID for 1 week *Infant:* Zidovudine 12 mg po BID for 1 week and 3TC 6 mg po BID for 1 week (if birth weight < 2 kg, then ZDV 4 mg/kg and 3TC 2 mg/kg)	9.3% (7.0, 11.6)	
				Mother: Nevirapine 200 mg po at labor onset, and another dose 48 hours later if still in labor, followed by 200 mg 24–48 hours postpartum	12.3% (9.7, 15.0)	No statistically significant differences in transmission rates

(cont.)

Table 8.2 (*cont.*)

Drug(s) evaluated	Trial	Location	Breastfeeding	Randomization	Transmission Rates	Efficacy
				Infant: Nevirapine 6 mg at 24–48 hours after birth (if birth within 2 hours of the maternal labor dose, another 6 mg dose within 6 hours after delivery)		
NVP	Dorenbaum 2002* [28]	USA, Brazil, Europe, Bahamas	No	*Mother*: Nevirapine 200 mg po after onset of labor	1.4% (0.6, 2.7)	No statistically significant difference in transmission rates
				Infant: Nerivapine 2 mg/kg at 48–72 hours after birth		
				Placebo	1.6% (0.8, 2.9)	
	Lallemant 2002** [29]	Thailand	No	*Mother*: Nevirapine 200 mg po × 1 at the onset of labor		No statistically significant difference in transmission rates between ARM 1 and ARM 2
				Infant: Nevirapine 6 mg po × 1 within 48–72 hours after birth		
				Arm 1: NVP to mother AND NVP to infant	1.9% (0.9, 3.0)	
				Arm 2: NVP to mother AND Placebo to infant	2.8% (1.5, 4.1)	
				Arm 3: Placebo to mother AND placebo to infant	6.5% (enrollment into this arm stopped because transmission significantly higher than in Arm 1	

* All women received at least zidovudine perinatal transmission prophylaxis according to the ACTG protocol 076, and most received combination antiretroviral therapy.

** All women received zidovudine prophylaxis (300 mg po BID) beginning at 28 weeks gestation or as soon as possible thereafter (at least 2 weeks), and 300 mg po every 3 hours from the onset of labor until delivery. Infants received zidovudine prophylaxis for 1 week (or for 4–6 weeks if mothers received less than 4 weeks of zidovudine during pregnancy).

receive zidovudine. Analyses based on infection status at the age of 6 months showed a 38% reduction in transmission [21]. More recently, when data from both trials were combined for analysis of transmission rates by 24 months of age, a statistically significant difference in transmission rates was still observed: 30.2% in the placebo arms versus 22.5% in the zidovudine arms. The risk difference was approximately 8%, and the relative diminution in transmission associated with the treatment arm was approximately 26% [22].

Finally, the relative efficacy of four different zidovudine prophylaxis regimens was evaluated in a randomized clinical trial among non-breastfeeding women in Thailand [23]. The first ('long-long') regimen consisted of maternal zidovudine beginning at 28 weeks gestation, oral zidovudine to the mother during the intrapartum period, and 6 weeks of therapy to the infant. The second ('short-short') regimen involved placebo beginning at 28 weeks gestation, then zidovudine from 35 weeks gestation until the onset of labor, oral zidovudine during the intrapartum period, and only 3 days of drug to the infant (followed by placebo through the sixth week of life). The third and fourth arms were termed the 'long-short' and the 'short-long' arms. The trial's Data Safety Monitoring Board (DSMB) recommended discontinuation of the short-short arm once it was apparent that there was a highly statistically significant difference in transmission rates (4.1% with the long-long regimen and 10.5% with the short-short regimen). The final results of the trial revealed no statistically significant differences in transmission rates in the remaining three arms (long-short, short-long, and long-long). However, in a subanalysis examining the difference in transmission rates among those enrolled in the two arms with a long antepartum course of zidovudine (i.e. zidovudine beginning at 28 weeks) versus those enrolled in the two arms with a short antepartum course of zidovudine (i.e. zidovudine beginning at 35 weeks), there was a statistically significant difference in the in utero transmission rates (1.6% versus 5.1%), suggesting that longer antepartum zidovudine prophylaxis is associated with significantly lower MTCT rates.

HIVNET 012, a randomized, open-label study among a predominantly (98.8%) breastfeeding population of women in Uganda, compared transmission rates with a simple two-dose nevirapine regimen (one dose to the mother at the onset of labor and one dose to the infant within 72 hours of birth) to a very short course zidovudine regimen (600 mg orally to the mother at the onset of labor and 300 mg every 3 hours until delivery, followed by 4 mg/kg orally twice daily to the infant for 7 days after birth) [24]. Transmission rates at 18 months were 25.8% in the zidovu-

dine arm and 15.7% in the nevirapine arm (efficacy: 41%) [25].

The efficacy of a combination of two antiretroviral drugs (zidovudine and lamivudine) for perinatal transmission prophylaxis was evaluated in a randomized, placebo-controlled trial in Uganda, Tanzania, and South Africa [26]. Approximately 75% of enrolled women initiated breastfeeding. In Arm A, prophylaxis with zidovudine and lamivudine was begun at 36 weeks gestation, with oral administration during the intrapartum period. Both mother and baby received prophylaxis for 1 week. In Arm B, prophylaxis began during the intrapartum period and both mother and baby received prophylaxis for 1 week. In Arm C, only oral intrapartum administration occurred. No prophylaxis was administered in the final arm. Early results were encouraging: transmission rates in the 3-part (Arm A) and two-part (Arm B) regimens were significantly lower than in the placebo arm; HIV infection rates at 6 weeks after birth were: 5.7% for Arm A, 8.9% for Arm B, 14.2% for Arm C, and 15.3% for the placebo arm. However, with continued breastfeeding transmission, transmission rates at 18 months after birth were similar: 15% (95% CI: 9–23%) in Arm A, 18% (95% CI: 12–26%) in Arm B, 20% (95% CI: 13–30%) in Arm C, and 22% (95% CI: 16–30%) in the placebo arm.

A randomized, open-label trial in South Africa compared two regimens: nevirapine 200 mg during labor and one dose to the mother and infant 24–48 hours after delivery, and multiple doses of zidovudine and lamivudine during labor and for 1 week to the mother and infant after delivery. Transmission rates were similar in both arms (12.3% in the nevirapine arm and 9.3% in the zidovudine/lamivudine arm; p = 0.11) [27].

A randomized, placebo-controlled trial among non-breastfeeding women was intended to determine the effect of the addition of nevirapine prophylaxis (a 200 mg dose of oral nevirapine to women after the onset of labor and 2 mg/kg dose of oral nevirapine to the infants between 48 and 72 hours after birth) among women already receiving zidovudine prophylaxis and/or other antiretroviral drugs during pregnancy. However, the trial was stopped early because the overall transmission rate was significantly lower than assumed when the trial was designed. There was no statistically significant difference in transmission rates between the nevirapine group (1.4%) and the placebo group (1.6%) [28].

More recently, a multicenter, randomized, three-arm study evaluated the addition of nevirapine to a baseline regimen of zidovudine prophylaxis for HIV-infected pregnant women and their infants [29]. Women received zidovudine prophylaxis beginning at 28 weeks gestation or as soon as possible thereafter (at least 2 weeks), and then 300 mg orally every 3 hours from the onset of labor until delivery. Infants received zidovudine prophylaxis for 1 week (or for 4–6 weeks if mothers received less than 4 weeks of zidovudine during pregnancy). Children were formula-fed. Subjects were randomized into the following groups: Arm (1) addition of one dose (200 mg) of maternal nevirapine at the onset of labor and one dose (6 mg) of infant nevirapine at 48–72 hours after birth; Arm (2) addition of nevirapine to the mother (addition of placebo to the infant); and Arm (3) addition of placebo to the mother and to the infant. At an interim analysis, the trial's DSMB recommended stopping enrollment into Arm 3 because transmission was significantly higher than in Arm 1. Final results of the trial demonstrated very low transmission rates with the addition of maternal nevirapine with (1.9%) or without (2.8%) infant nevirapine.

Important lessons have been learned from these clinical trials of perinatal HIV transmission with antiretroviral drugs. Several different antiretroviral prophylaxis regimens are efficacious, including regimens of zidovudine alone [16, 19–21, 23]; nevirapine alone [24, 25]; zidovudine with lamivudine [26]; and zidovudine with nevirapine [29], although the efficacy of antiretroviral prophylaxis is diminished (or eradicated [26]) in breastfeeding populations, due to continued breastfeeding transmission after prophylactic drug administration has been discontinued. Simplification of the ACTG 076 regimen (oral intrapartum zidovudine, shorter maternal or infant administration) can still result in reductions in MTCT rates similar to those observed with ACTG 076, although longer antepartum courses of zidovudine are associated with lower transmission rates [23]. Not all of the protective effect of antiretroviral drugs is explained by lowering of maternal peripheral blood viral load, and pre- and post-exposure prophylaxis of the infant is also important. Finally, the combination of two antiretroviral drugs (zidovudine with nevirapine) substantially reduces transmission compared with a single drug (zidovudine) [29].

Observational data: receipt of antiretroviral drugs and rates of mother-to-child transmission

More and more HIV-infected women in resource-rich settings are receiving combination antiretroviral therapy, including highly active antiretroviral therapy with three or more drugs, for their own health. Therefore, comparisons of transmission rates among women receiving no therapy, monotherapy with zidovudine or other drugs, and combination therapy with two or more drugs are now possible. For example, an observational study conducted in France evaluated the addition of lamivudine (150 mg twice daily orally) at 32 weeks gestation until delivery and infant lamivudine 2 mg/kg twice daily orally for 6 weeks among French women and their infants receiving zidovudine as per the ACTG 076 regimen [30]. Receipt of both zidovudine and lamivudine was associated with a significantly lower risk of transmission (1.6%) compared with the risk of transmission in historical controls who received zidovudine alone (6.8%). The median decrease in viral load with the combination of zidovudine and lamivudine was 1.24 log_{10}. In the Women and Infants Transmission Study, more potent antiretroviral therapy regimens were associated with lower MTCT rates. Specifically, the following transmission rates were observed: 20% (95% CI: 16.1–23.9%) with no antiretroviral therapy during pregnancy, 10.4% (95% CI: 8.2–12.6%) with zidovudine monotherapy, 3.8% (95% CI: 1.1–6.5%) with dual antiretroviral therapy with no or one highly active drug, and 1.2% (95% CI: 0–2.5%) with highly active antiretroviral therapy [14]. Similar transmission rates were observed in PACTG 367, a descriptive epidemiological study of HIV-infected pregnant women at medical centers throughout the USA. In this cohort, the transmission rate was highest among women with no or unknown antiretroviral therapy during pregnancy (18.5% (95% CI: 13.1–25.0%)), lower among women receiving one antiretroviral drug (5.1% (95% CI: 3–7.9%)), and lowest among those receiving combination antiretroviral therapy (1.3% (95% CI: 0.9–2%)) [15].

Analysis of transmission rates among HIV-infected women who received one or more components (antepartum, intrapartum, and/or postnatal) of the ACTG 076 zidovudine prophylaxis regimen suggested there are reductions in the rates of MTCT of HIV even if abbreviated regimens of zidovudine are received [31–32]. The observed transmission rates (according to when zidovudine prophylaxis was initiated) were: antepartum: 6.1% (95% CI: 4.1–8.9%); intrapartum: 10.0% (95% CI: 3.3–21.8%); 48 hours after birth: 9.3% (95% CI: 4.1–17.5); 3 days or more after birth: 18.4% (95% CI: 7.7, 34.3); and none: 26.6% (95% CI: 21.1–32.7%) [31]. Of those in whom zidovudine administration began within 48 hours after birth, transmission rates were 5.9% if initiated within 12 hours after birth and 25% if initiated 12–24 hours after birth [32].

Cervicovaginal fluid

In addition to peripheral blood viral load, a higher genital tract viral load is independently associated with a higher risk of MTCT of HIV [33–34]. In the Thai study [33], detection of HIV in cervicovaginal lavage specimens was less frequent among women who had received antepartum zidovudine for the preceding 2 weeks than among women who had received placebo. The MTCT rate among women with quantifiable HIV in cervicovaginal lavage specimens and high plasma viral concentrations (over 10 000 copies/mL) was significantly higher (28.7%) than among women without quantifiable HIV in cervicovaginal lavage specimens and with low plasma virus levels ($P < 0.001$). Therefore, peripartum cleansing with virucidal agents has been investigated [35–39].

Prevention of transmission with virucidal cleansing

The utility of cervicovaginal cleansing, with or without immediate surface decontamination of the infant, with virucidal agents such as benzalkonium chloride and chlorhexidine, has been evaluated in several studies in sub-Saharan Africa. A regimen of benzalkonium chloride was evaluated in a small study in West Africa [35]. Self-administered daily vaginal suppositories of 1% benzalkonium chloride or matched placebo beginning at 36 weeks of pregnancy, with an intrapartum dose and bathing of the neonate, was found to be feasible and well-tolerated. There was no statistically significant difference in HIV transmission rates according to treatment group among 103 live-born children [36]. In Malawi, cervicovaginal cleansing with 0.25% chlorhexidine solution every 4 hours during labor, and washing the baby with the same solution at birth, did not reduce MTCT of HIV [37]. However, in a subanalysis, MTCT was significantly lower with chlorhexidine washes in the subgroup of women with duration of ruptured membranes of more than 4 hours. In addition, the intervention was associated with reductions in maternal and neonatal morbidity [40]. Subsequently, another study in Kenya evaluated cervicovaginal lavage with 0.2%, and later 0.4%, chlorhexidine during labor, but this intervention did not decrease either intrapartum only or overall transmission [38]. Finally, the safety and tolerability of different concentrations of chlorhexidine (0.25%, 1%, and 2%) used for peripartum cervicovaginal and infant washes were evaluated in South Africa, and the 1% concentration of chlorhexidine was identified as the highest tolerated concentration [39]. An efficacy trial of 1% chlorhexidine has been proposed.

Breast milk

In addition to the concentration of virus in peripheral blood and cervicovaginal fluid, a higher breast milk viral load is associated with a higher risk of MTCT of HIV [41–43]. If breastfeeding is unavoidable, then it is possible that one or more of the following interventions to decrease the viral load of the breast milk could prevent transmission: administration of antiretroviral drugs to the mother while breastfeeding, antiretroviral prophylaxis administered to the infant, and treatment of breast milk with heat or chemical agents.

Before considering specific interventions to prevent breastfeeding transmission of HIV, it is important to consider the potential effects of breastfeeding on the HIV-infected woman herself. One such potential effect is increased mortality among breastfeeding HIV-infected women. The results of two studies evaluating the risk of mortality among HIV-infected women according to infant feeding modality (breastfeeding compared with formula feeding) have been conflicting. Data from the randomized clinical trial of breastfeeding versus formula feeding in Kenya were analyzed to assess maternal mortality according to infant feeding modality [44]. Analysis of maternal mortality was by intention to treat (i.e., by randomized assignment of mothers to breastfeeding or formula feeding). Maternal mortality over the 2-year period following delivery was higher among those in the breastfeeding group (18 deaths among 197 women, 9%) compared with those in the formula feeding group (six deaths among 200 women, 3%; $P = 0.009$). The cumulative probability of maternal death at 24 months after delivery was 10.5% in the breastfeeding group and 3.8% in the formula group ($P = 0.02$). The relative risk of death for mothers assigned to breastfeeding compared with those assigned to formula feeding was 3.2 (95% CI: 1.3–8.1, $P = 0.01$), and the attributable risk of maternal death due to breastfeeding was 69%. There were significant associations between CD4$^+$ lymphocyte counts and maternal death, as well as between viral load and maternal death. The authors hypothesized that a combination of the metabolic demands of breastfeeding on HIV-infected women (who already could have borderline nutritional status) and of HIV infection itself could be associated with substantial nutritional impairment, which could result in increased risk of death. Indeed, women in the breastfeeding group had greater weight loss postpartum than women in the formula-feeding group.

Data from a second study, a randomized clinical trial of vitamin A supplementation in South Africa, were analyzed to assess maternal mortality among HIV-infected women according to infant feeding modality (breastfeeding or not breastfeeding) [45]. In this trial, mothers chose whether to breastfeed or not (i.e. there was no randomization regarding infant feeding modality). Of 566 mothers whose data were analyzed, 410 breastfed their infants and 156 never breastfed. No differences in maternal mortality rates according to infant feeding modality were observed: over a mean follow-up period of 10 months postpartum, 0.49% (2/410) of women who ever breastfed were known to have died compared with 1.92% (3/156) of those who never breastfed. Morbidity was similar among those who breastfed for more than or less than 3 months.

The reasons for differences in the results of the two studies are not clear. Analyses of mortality among HIV-infected women according to infant feeding modality are underway within the Breastfeeding and HIV International Transmission Study, with a pooled sample size of several thousand HIV-infected women [46].

It is possible that HIV transmission through breastfeeding could be decreased with antiretroviral drugs administered either to the mother or to the infant while breastfeeding. The efficacy of continued administration of antiretroviral prophylaxis to breastfeeding infants is being investigated in several studies in India and in different parts of Africa. These studies are evaluating administration of different antiretroviral drugs to the infant for varying lengths of time (1 week to 6 months). Observational studies and randomized clinical trials involving administration of combinations of antiretroviral drugs to breastfeeding, HIV-infected women in sub-Saharan Africa are being initiated to evaluate the effectiveness and efficacy of maternal combination antiretroviral therapy to prevent MTCT of HIV during breastfeeding. Drugs being evaluated include zidovudine, nevirapine, lamivudine, and didanosine [47].

Treatment of breast milk with either chemical agents or heat to inactivate HIV has been investigated in several studies. Sodium dodecyl sulfate, a microbicidal agent active against HIV and other viruses, does not alter protein content of the milk and can be efficiently removed from breast milk samples [48]. In one study, allowing expressed breast milk to stand at room temperature for 6 hours did not destroy proviral DNA, but boiling expressed breast milk appeared to decrease HIV infectivity of the milk [49]. Pasteurization of breast milk [50, 51], including pasteurization with devices that can be used in a home setting [52–54], can reduce the infectious titer of cell-free HIV and HIV-infected cells by more than 5 logs and 6 logs, respectively [51]. Obviously, utilization of all of these methodologies would not be feasible in many settings. Additionally, while lowering breast milk viral load, these methodologies are unlikely to eliminate HIV from the milk completely. Finally, with any treatment to inactivate HIV, the extent to which the treatment diminishes the protective or nutritional components of breast milk must be carefully assessed.

8.3.2 Duration of exposure to the virus

Intrapartum

It was observed in several studies that HIV-infected women with duration of ruptured membranes of more than 4 hours [55, 56] or more than 12 hours [57] were more likely to transmit HIV to their infants. In a subsequent analysis of 4721 deliveries with duration of ruptured membranes of 24 hours or less (vaginal deliveries as well as cesarean section deliveries after ruptured membranes and/or onset of labor), the risk of MTCT of HIV increased approximately 2% with an increase of 1 hour in the duration of ruptured membranes (adjusted odds ratio [OR] = 1.02 [95% CI: 1.01, 1.04] for each hour increment). Among women diagnosed with AIDS, the estimated probability of transmission increased from 8% to 31% with duration of ruptured membranes of 2 hours and 24 hours, respectively ($P < 0.01$). The results of these analyses supported the importance of duration of ruptured membranes as a risk factor for MTCT of HIV, and suggested a diagnosis of AIDS in the mother at the time of delivery could potentiate the effect of duration of ruptured membranes [4].

Despite the biological plausibility of a decreased risk of transmission of HIV from mother to child with cesarean section delivery before labor and before ruptured membranes (potential mechanisms including avoidance of transfusion of mother's blood to the fetus during labor contractions and/or direct contact of the fetus with infected secretions or blood from the maternal genital tract), early studies of the relationship between mode of delivery and MTCT of HIV had conflicting results; some suggested a lower risk of transmission with cesarean section, but others did not. Thus, an individual patient data meta-analysis was performed to address this issue, incorporating data regarding 8533 mother–child pairs from 15 prospective cohort studies in North America and Europe [58]. In adjusted analyses, the likelihood of MTCT of HIV was approximately 50% lower with cesarean section before labor and delivery, as compared with other modes of delivery (adjusted OR = 0.43 [95% CI: 0.33, 0.56]). The likelihood of transmission was approximately 87% lower among those with cesarean section before labor and delivery and with receipt of antiretroviral therapy during the antepartum, intrapartum, and postnatal periods (most likely zidovudine monotherapy), as compared with other modes of delivery and the absence of such therapy (adjusted OR = 0.13 [95% CI: 0.09, 0.19]). The rates of transmission were lower with cesarean section before labor and delivery than with other modes of delivery whether or not antiretroviral therapy was given. The transmission rate with elective cesarean section without antiretroviral therapy was 10.4%, as compared with a rate of 19.0% with other modes of delivery without antiretroviral therapy. The respective rates with antiretroviral therapy during the antepartum, intrapartum, and postnatal periods were 2.0% and 7.3%.

A randomized clinical trial of mode of delivery among HIV-infected women in Europe documented the efficacy of cesarean section in preventing MTCT [5]. In this trial, in which approximately 400 women were randomized to cesarean section before labor and ruptured membranes

Table 8.3 Randomized clinical trials: mode of delivery and infant feeding modality

Trial	Location	Randomization	Transmission rates	Efficacy
The European Mode of Delivery Collaboration 1999 [5]	Europe	Cesarean section Vaginal delivery	1.8% 10.5%	83%
Nduati *et al.* 2000 [6]	Kenya	Formula feeding Breastfeeding	20.5% (14.0–27.0) 36.7% (29.4–44.0)	44%

or to vaginal delivery, cesarean section decreased transmission (1.8% transmission among those randomized to cesarean delivery versus 10.5% among those randomized to vaginal delivery). The odds ratio for transmission according to allocated mode of delivery (cesarean section compared with vaginal delivery) was: 0.2 (95% CI: 0.1–0.6) (Table 8.3).

Postnatally through breastfeeding

A longer duration of breastfeeding has been associated with an increased risk of HIV transmission [59, 60]. In a meta-analysis of published data from prospective cohort studies of HIV-infected women and their children [61], 499 HIV-infected women who breastfed their children were identified. The estimated risk of breastfeeding transmission of HIV was 16% (95% CI: 9–22%). Among breastfed infants, 47% of HIV infections were attributable to breastfeeding. Breastfeeding transmission occurred in 21% (10–22%) of those with breastfeeding for a median length of 3 or more months, and 13% (95% CI: 4–21%) among infants breastfed for a median of less than 2 months. The cumulative probability of breastfeeding transmission of HIV has been estimated in different studies. In the Breastfeeding and HIV International Transmission Study [46], MTCT of HIV among breastfed children with negative HIV diagnostic test results at 4 weeks of age was assessed. Late postnatal transmission (transmission after 4 weeks of age) occurred throughout breastfeeding, and the risk of such transmission was generally constant through breastfeeding. The cumulative probability of late postnatal transmission was: 1.6% at 3 months of age, 4.2% at 6 months, 6.0 at 9 months, 7.0 at 12 months, 7.2% at 15 months, and 9.3% at 18 months.

A randomized clinical trial of breastfeeding versus formula feeding among HIV-infected women in Kenya demonstrated HIV transmission through breastfeeding and prevention of such transmission with formula feeding [6]. This trial enrolled 425 HIV-infected pregnant women. Compliance was higher in the breastfeeding arm (96%) compared with the formula-feeding arm (70%). The median duration of breastfeeding was 17 months. The cumulative probability of HIV infection in the children at 24 months of age was significantly higher in the breastfed children: 36.7% (95% CI: 29.4–44.0%) in the breastfeeding arm versus 20.5% (95% CI: 14.0–27.0%) in the formula arm ($P = 0.001$) (Table 8.3).

If complete avoidance of breast milk is not possible, early weaning from breast milk (e.g., at 6 months of age), if feasible, would limit exposure to HIV-infected breast milk while allowing the child to experience the benefits of breastfeeding. Breast milk provides the entire nutritional requirements of the infant through the first 4–6 months of life [62, 63]. Although breast milk remains a valuable source of nutrition for many months thereafter, it is possible for children to be successfully weaned from breast milk and provided with other sources of nutrition after 6 months of age. The increased risk of morbidity and mortality associated with replacement feeding (due to malnutrition and infectious diseases other than HIV) is especially high during the first 6 months of life and decreases in magnitude thereafter [64].

For many women, early weaning of their children from breast milk is not possible because of financial or other constraints. Early weaning from breast milk is being evaluated in trials in Zambia [65] and elsewhere.

8.3.3 Factors facilitating transfer of the virus from mother to child

Several factors potentially facilitate transfer of the virus from mother to child, including vitamin A deficiency, chorioamnionitis, mixed breastfeeding, and maternal breast pathology and infant thrush. Modification of these factors in order to decrease the likelihood of MTCT has been or is being evaluated.

Micronutrient deficiencies

A dramatic relationship was observed between maternal vitamin A deficiency and the risk of MTCT of HIV in Africa [66], with lower maternal vitamin A levels associated with higher rates of transmission. This observation stimulated investigations of vitamin A supplementation as a means of decreasing the risk of transmission. More recent data suggest deficiencies of other micronutrients (e.g. selenium) could be associated with the risk of MTCT. For example, in a study in Kenya, selenium deficiency was found among 11% of women and was associated with vaginal or cervical shedding of HIV-infected cells [67].

Results from three completed vitamin A supplementation trials indicated no benefit of supplementation with regard to prevention of MTCT of HIV [68–70]. In Malawi, there was no statistically significant difference in transmission rates according to receipt of vitamin A supplementation from 18–28 weeks gestation until delivery [68], although antenatal vitamin A supplementation increased birth weight and decreased anemia among the infants. In South Africa, HIV-infected women were randomized to receive either placebo or daily vitamin A supplementation during the third trimester of pregnancy and at delivery. There was no statistically significant difference in transmission rates according to treatment arm, but women randomized to vitamin A supplementation were less likely to have preterm delivery [69]. Daily vitamin A supplementation during pregnancy increased the risk of MTCT of HIV in a randomized clinical trial in Tanzania [70]. Enrollment in a fourth vitamin A supplementation trial in Zimbabwe has been completed.

Chorioamnionitis

Following bacterial infection(s) of the placental membranes of HIV-infected women, maternal white blood cells infected with HIV could enter the amniotic fluid, with resultant chorioamnionitis and MTCT of HIV. Placental membrane inflammation (chorioamnionitis and funisitis) has been associated with an increased risk of MTCT of HIV [71–73]. Therefore, a clinical trial of antibiotic treatment to reduce chorioamnionitis in HIV-infected women has begun.

A randomized, placebo-controlled trial of antibiotic treatment during pregnancy to prevent chorioamnionitis-associated MTCT of HIV was initiated at clinical sites in Malawi, Tanzania, and Zambia (HIVNET 024). However, the trial was discontinued after interim analyses suggested no effect.

Mixed breastfeeding

When feeding patterns among infants born to HIV-infected women in Brazil were analyzed, a history of colostrum intake was not associated with transmission, nor was a history of mixed feeding (human milk with other milk, tea, or juice) [74]. However, in South Africa, data from a randomized clinical trial of vitamin A supplementation to prevent MTCT [69] were reanalyzed to evaluate a possible association between feeding patterns among infants of breastfeeding, HIV-infected mothers and the risk of MTCT [75]. In this study, breastfeeding was categorized as exclusive or mixed, i.e. without or with water, other fluids, and

food. Women who chose to breastfeed were counseled to consider exclusive breastfeeding. Follow-up visits after birth, during which an infant feeding history was obtained, occurred at 1 week, 6 weeks, and 3 months of age, and every 3 months thereafter. By 15 months of age, children who ever breastfed were more likely to have become HIV-infected (31.6%) than those children who never breastfed (19.4%), $P = 0.007$. Of children who ever breastfed, those with exclusive breastfeeding until at least 3 months of age but no longer than 6 months of age had a lower estimated transmission point estimate than those with mixed feeding, but the confidence limits for these point estimates overlap (exclusive: 24.7% [95% CI: 16.0–34.4%]; mixed: 35.9% [95% CI: 26.7–45.1%]). The authors proposed that the mechanism of their findings was that contaminated fluids and foods given to infants with mixed breastfeeding damaged the bowel and facilitated the entry of HIV into tissues. The results of this hypothesis-generating study have prompted several investigators to pursue new studies of exclusive breastfeeding to assess more carefully the risk of HIV transmission according to feeding modality.

Exclusive breastfeeding during the first 4–6 months of life is associated with greater benefits than mixed feeding in terms of morbidity and mortality from infectious diseases other than HIV [76, 77]. The suggestive, but not definitive, results of analyses of feeding modality among breastfeeding children of HIV-infected women indicating a possible lower risk of transmission with exclusive breastfeeding compared with mixed breastfeeding [69, 75] have prompted the development of additional studies to evaluate further the role of exclusive versus mixed breastfeeding in MTCT of HIV. For example, data from Zimbabwe suggest mixed breast-feeding is associated with a higher risk of onset of HIV and death [65]. However, exclusive breastfeeding is not the norm in Africa and other parts of the world. For example, only about half of Indian children under 4 months of age are exclusively breastfed [78]. In Zimbabwe, only 39% of infants were exclusively breastfed during the first 3 months of life, and only 7% between 4 and 6 months of age [79]. Despite this, programs to promote exclusive breastfeeding have had some success. For example, the prevalence of exclusive breastfeeding at 5 months of age increased from 6% to 70% with home-based counseling by peer counselors (mothers from the local community with training for 10 days) in Bangladesh [80].

Maternal breast pathology and oral candidiasis in children

An early case report of the temporal association of acquisition of HIV infection by the child of an HIV-infected woman with a breast abscess suggested the ingestion of inflammatory cells related to the bacterial infection of the breast contributes to breastfeeding transmission of HIV [81]. Later studies confirmed the association of transmission of HIV through breastfeeding with maternal breast pathologies such as breast abscesses, mastitis, and nipple lesions. In Kenya, mastitis and breast abscesses were associated with late postnatal transmission of HIV (relative risk [RR] = 21.8 [95% CI: 2.3–211.0] and RR = 51.6 [95% CI: 4.7–571.0], respectively) [34]. In Malawi, women with elevated breast milk sodium levels consistent with subclinical mastitis had higher breast milk viral loads than women without elevated breast milk sodium levels [42]. In another study in Kenya, maternal nipple lesions (OR = 2.3, 95% CI: 1.1–5.0) and mastitis (OR = 2.7, 95% CI: 1.1–6.7) were associated with increased postnatal transmission [82]. Infant oral candidiasis before 6 months of age is associated with late postnatal transmission (OR = 2.8, 95% CI: 1.3–6.2) [82]. Results of a study in Côte d'Ivoire suggested maternal breast abscesses and cracked nipples, as well as oral candidiasis in infants, were risk factors for late postnatal transmission of HIV through breastfeeding [83].

One program underway in Zimbabwe involves education of women who choose to breastfeed following individual counseling regarding exclusive breastfeeding until the infant is 4–6 months of age followed by rapid weaning. Education and counseling also are provided regarding proper positioning during breastfeeding, prompt seeking of medical care if breast problems arise or if the infant develops oral candidiasis or other lesions, avoiding breastfeeding from the affected breast, and safe sex practices while breastfeeding [84].

8.3.4 Summary of studies of interventions to prevent MTCT

Although many different interventions to prevent MTCT of HIV have been and are being investigated, efficacy has been demonstrated to date for only the following: antiretroviral prophylaxis, cesarean section before labor and before ruptured membranes, and avoidance of breastfeeding. In addition to these interventions, observational data strongly suggest that combination antiretroviral therapy, including HAART, is associated with very low rates of transmission.

8.4 Strategies for the prevention of mother-to-child transmission of HIV

Although prevention of MTCT of HIV is often conceptualized as only beginning once an HIV-infected woman is pregnant, prevention of MTCT optimally begins before pregnancy and before acquisition of HIV infection, i.e. through prevention of acquisition of HIV infection by adolescent girls and by women of reproductive age. In

Table 8.4 Prevention of transmission of HIV from pregnant women to their infants

Intervention	Resource-rich settings	Resource-poor settings
Voluntary counseling and testing (VCT)	Yes	Yes
Antiretroviral prophylaxis/ therapy	Yes	Yes (but therapy generally not widely available)
Cesarean section before labor and before ruptured membranes	Yes	Generally No
Complete avoidance of breastfeeding	Yes	Generally No

the absence of primary prevention, then prevention of unwanted pregnancies is important. Assuming an HIV-infected adolescent girl or a woman has become pregnant, then prevention of MTCT of HIV in the USA and other resource-rich settings, where the seroprevalence of HIV among adults is below 1% [85], has incorporated the following interventions: voluntary HIV counseling and testing, complete avoidance of breastfeeding, cesarean section before labor and before ruptured membranes, and antiretroviral drugs (from zidovudine prophylaxis at a minimum, to combination antiretroviral therapy) (Table 8.4). However, in resource-poor settings, where the seroprevalence of HIV among adults is often over 20% [85] and the burden of HIV disease is much greater than in resource-rich settings, complete avoidance of breastfeeding is generally not possible or acceptable, and cesarean delivery for the prevention of MTCT of HIV is generally not feasible due to lack of clinical infrastructure and staffing (Table 8.4). In these settings, efforts to find new, or adapt old, interventions so that they are feasible and affordable to implement remains an urgent priority. Concomitantly there is a growing realization that, if the real goal is to increase the likelihood of children's HIV-free survival (and not just to decrease MTCT rates), it is best for many reasons to work towards optimizing the health of the HIV-infected woman herself since one of the best predictors of children's deaths is their mothers' own deaths. Obviously, provision of treatment for HIV-infected pregnant women is an important goal in and of itself, aside from secondary benefits in terms of lower MTCT rates.

8.4.1 Voluntary HIV counseling and testing

Voluntary HIV counseling and testing has represented an essential component of prevention efforts in the USA [86] and other resource-rich settings, since the greatest effectiveness of current preventive interventions (such as cesarean delivery and antiretroviral drugs) is predicated upon a pregnant woman knowing her HIV infection status before becoming pregnant or else as early as possible during pregnancy. The US Public Health Service recommended that HIV counseling and testing be offered to all pregnant women in 1995 [87]. The proportion of mothers of HIV-exposed or -infected children in the USA whose HIV infection was diagnosed before their child's birth increased from 70% in 1993 (before the original US Public Health Service guidelines were issued in 1995) to 94% in 1997 [88]. However, while a decreasing proportion of the overall population of pregnant women in the US have delayed or no prenatal care (25% in 1989 but 18% in 1997) [89], such may not be the case among HIV-infected women. Additionally, receipt of prenatal care does not guarantee HIV counseling and testing will occur. Data from several studies have indicated missed opportunities for antenatal HIV counseling and testing [90–92]. Such data prompted the US Institute of Medicine to recommend universal, routine testing of pregnant women with patient notification [93]. The US Public Health Service has made similar recommendations [94].

In many resource-poor settings, however, where few or no treatment or prophylactic interventions for HIV-infected individuals exist, acceptance of voluntary HIV counseling and testing (including return to receive results of HIV diagnostic testing) may not be high. For example, only 78% of women receiving antenatal care in Cote d'Ivoire consented to HIV testing and, of these, only 58.4% returned to receive the results [95]. With the use of rapid diagnostic tests (such that results can be made available to the individual being tested on the same day, as opposed to requiring a return visit to the clinic), and with increasing availability of both therapeutic and prevention interventions, it is anticipated that acceptance of voluntary HIV counseling and testing will increase.

8.4.2 Complete avoidance of breastfeeding

Complete avoidance of breastfeeding (e.g. by using infant formula) is an intervention of obvious utility in settings where it is feasible (i.e. where clean water is available), affordable, and culturally acceptable. In resource-rich settings such as the USA, complete avoidance of breastfeeding by HIV-infected women has been advised for several years [96, 97, 98]. Breastfeeding among HIV-infected women is

uncommon in the USA. Estimates of the proportion of HIV-infected women in the USA have ranged from 1–3% before 1994 [99], and less than 1% in 1994 or later [100]. HIV-infected mothers are significantly less likely to breastfeed their children if they are aware of their infection status before delivery [99], highlighting the need for access to prenatal care and HIV counseling and testing.

However, complete avoidance of breastfeeding is not feasible in many resource-poor settings, for reasons including the cost associated with procurement of replacement feeding, the stigma associated with not breastfeeding, and the potential morbidity and mortality associated with replacement feeding. Even in the Nairobi clinical trial of breastfeeding versus formula feeding [6], in which one of the enrollment criteria was access to municipal-treated water, the two groups of children (those whose mothers were randomized to breastfeeding and those whose mothers were randomized to formula feeding) experienced similar rates of mortality during the first 2 years of life [101]. Mortality rates at 24 months of age were 24.4% among children whose mothers were randomized to breastfeeding and 20.0% among those children whose mothers were randomized to formula feeding. Assessment of the feasibility of complete avoidance of breastfeeding or of early weaning involves consideration of an individual woman's situation and local circumstances. The WHO recommends that HIV-infected women who decide to not breastfeed their children, or who decide to wean their children from breast milk early, should receive specific guidance and support during at least the first 2 years of their children's lives to assure adequate replacement feeding [102].

Since complete avoidance of breastfeeding or early weaning may not be possible in many settings, it is extremely important to develop and implement culturally appropriate interventions to prevent breast-milk transmission of HIV in resource-poor settings [102]. Further, in light of the evidence of the association of maternal breast pathologies and breastfeeding transmission, the WHO recommends that HIV-infected women who breastfeed should receive education and counseling to assure good breastfeeding technique to decrease the risk of development of such conditions, and if such conditions arise, they should be treated as quickly and completely as possible [102]. Similarly, oral candidiasis in children should be treated promptly.

8.4.3 Cesarean section before labor and ruptured membranes

Subsequent to the publication of studies demonstrating the efficacy of cesarean section before labor and delivery for the prevention of MTCT [5], and indicating an association between mode of delivery and transmission remained among HIV-infected women receiving antiretroviral therapy (most likely zidovudine prophylaxis) [58], the American College of Obstetricians and Gynecologists [103] and the US Public Health Service [104] issued recommendations that cesarean section as an intervention to prevent transmission should be discussed and recommended for women with peripheral blood viral loads greater than 1000 copies/mL irrespective of receipt of antiretroviral therapy. Cesarean delivery for the prevention of MTCT of HIV has been performed with increasing frequency in clinical centers in the USA and Europe over the past several years [15, 105]. For example, in the USA, cesarean delivery was performed for HIV-infected pregnant women with increasing frequency from 1998 (20%) to 2000 (44–54%) [105]. As noted previously, cesarean delivery as an intervention to prevent MTCT of HIV is generally not feasible in resource-poor settings because of the lack of a skilled attendant during labor and other reasons.

In settings where adequate staffing and infrastructure exist, issues that have been raised regarding use of cesarean section as an intervention to prevent transmission include concerns regarding its effectiveness among women with low viral loads or who are receiving potent antiretroviral therapy, potentially increased maternal and infant morbidity associated with surgical delivery in populations of HIV-infected women, and the risk of healthcare worker infection associated with surgical delivery. Despite the conservative wording of US recommendations [103, 104], more recent data suggest a persistent effect of cesarean section delivery even among those HIV-infected pregnant women with viral loads of less than 1000 copies/mL. For example, in Thailand, cesarean section was associated with a lower risk of MTCT of HIV even after controlling for viral load [106]. Also, data from the European Collaborative Study suggest a lower risk of MTCT among women delivering by cesarean section before labor and ruptured membranes remains despite stratification according to maternal viral load [107]. Finally, delivery by cesarean section was associated with an approximately 70% lower risk of transmission compared with vaginal delivery among a population of women with viral loads less than 1000 copies/mL [18]. Consistent with these results, data from North Carolina suggest that, among women receiving combination antiretroviral therapy, cesarean section before labor and ruptured membranes is associated with a lower risk of transmission compared with vaginal or other cesarean deliveries [108]. It has been estimated that the rate of MTCT of HIV would have to be extremely low before cesarean section would no longer be cost effective in the USA and similar settings [109].

The potential benefit of cesarean section before labor and ruptured membranes for prevention of MTCT of HIV must be weighed against possible deleterious effects of surgical delivery for the mother, for the infant, and for the obstetrician [110, 111]. Cesarean delivery may be associated with a slightly increased risk of postpartum morbidity among HIV-infected women compared with uninfected women, but assessment of currently available data suggest postpartum morbidity rates among HIV-infected women are not sufficiently frequent or severe to outweigh the potential benefit of cesarean section for the prevention of MTCT of HIV [104]. There are no published data regarding the risk of neonatal morbidity according to HIV-infected women's mode of delivery. Finally, although we know the risk must be extremely small, there are essentially no data regarding the relative risk of accidental acquisition of HIV infection by obstetricians or other healthcare workers according to mode of delivery [112]. Some have proposed an increased risk, and others have proposed a decreased risk, with elective cesarean section or vaginal delivery.

8.4.4 Antiretroviral transmission prophylaxis and antiretroviral treatment of HIV-infected pregnant women

Shortly after the release of the results of ACTG 076 [16], the US Public Health Service issued guidelines regarding the use of zidovudine for perinatal HIV transmission prophylaxis [113]. Zidovudine prophylaxis has played a central role in the prevention of MTCT in resource-rich settings for the past several years. For example, the proportion of perinatally HIV-exposed children who received or whose mothers received any zidovudine increased dramatically in the USA from 1993 (7%) to 1997 (91%) [88].

More recently, an increasing number of women in North America, Europe, and Brazil are receiving combination antiretroviral therapy, including HAART, for their own health. For example, recent data indicate 85% of HIV-infected pregnant women in the USA receive combination therapy during the third trimester, while only 2% receive a single antiretroviral drug and 5% receive no antiretroviral drugs [15].

Guidelines for initiation of antiretroviral therapy in adults and adolescents have been developed by several groups, including the US Public Health Service [114]. Criteria for initiation of antiretroviral therapy according to these guidelines include: symptomatic HIV disease, CD4$^+$ lymphocyte count less than 350 cells/mm^3 or less, or plasma HIV RNA levels over 55 000 copies/mL. In addition, guidelines more specifically focused on the use of antiretroviral drugs in pregnant women have been developed by the US

Table 8.5 Recommendations for antiretroviral prophylaxis to prevent MTCT of HIV, according to timing of maternal presentation [104]

Time period at presentation	Previous antiretroviral therapy	Recommendation	Comment/alternatives
Antepartum	No	Women should receive at least the three-part ACTG 076 regimen: *Mother:* Zidovudine 100 mg po 5 times per day beginning at 14–34 weeks gestation, 2 mg/kg IV over a 1 hour period, then 1 mg/kg per hour until delivery *Infant:* Zidovudine 2 mg/kg po q 6 hours for 6 weeks, beginning 8–12 hours after birth	Acceptable alternatives to the maternal regimen in the clinical trial (100 mg orally five times daily) are oral zidovudine (ZDV) administered as 200 mg three times daily or 300 mg twice daily. Combining this zidovudine prophylactic regimen with additional antiretroviral drugs for treatment of the mother's HIV infection is recommended for women whose clinical, immunologic, or virologic status requires treatment [119] or who have peripheral blood viral loads of over 1000 copies/mL. Alternatives to the ACTG 076 prophylactic regimen are (prophylactic regimen initiated during the antepartum period) are listed in Table 8.2: *Mother:* Zidovudine 300 mg po BID from 36 weeks gestation, q 3 hours from onset of labor until delivery [19, 20] *Mother:* Zidovudine 300 mg po BID from 36–38 weeks gestation, 600 mg × 1 at onset of labor, 300 mg po BID for 7 days after delivery [21] *Mother:* Zidovudine 300 mg po BID until onset of labor, then 300 mg po q 3 hours until delivery beginning at 28 weeks gestation; *Infant* 2 mg/kg po q 6 hours for 3 days (6 weeks of infant ZDV if maternal ZDV initiated at/after 35 weeks) [23] *Mother:* Zidovudine/3TC 300 mg/150 mg po BID from 36 weeks gestation; ZDV 300 mg × 1 after onset of labor, then 300 mg po q 3 hours until delivery; 3TC 150 mg × 1 at onset of labor, then 150 mg po q 12 hours until delivery; ZDV/3TC 300/150 mg po BID for 1 week: *Infant:* Zidovudine 4 mg/kg with 3TC 2 mg/kg po BID for 1 week [26, Arm A] *Mother:* ZDV 300 mg po PID beginning at 28 weeks gestation, ZDV 300 mg po 13 hours from onset of labor until delivery, NVP 200 mg po × 1 at the onset of labor; *Infant:* ZDV 2 mg/kg po every 6 hours for 1 week, with or without NVP 6 mg po × 1 within 48–72 hours after birth
Antepartum	Yes	Women should continue therapy if the pregnancy is identified after the first trimester. Zidovudine should be a component of the antepartum regimen after the first trimester if possible. Irrespective of the antepartum regimen,	

Table 8.5 (*cont.*)

Time period at presentation	Previous antiretroviral therapy	Recommendation	Comment/alternatives
		intrapartum and infant ZDV as per the ACTG 076 regimen is recommended. *Mother:* Zidovudine 2 mg/kg IV over a 1 hour period, then 1 mg/kg per hour until delivery *Infant:* Zidovudine 2 mg/kg po q 6 hours for 6 weeks, beginning 8–12 hours after birth	See below for alternative intrapartum and postnatal regimens.
Intrapartum	No	Women/infants should receive at least the intrapartum/postnatal components of the ACTG 076 regimen: *Mother:* Zidovudine 2 mg/kg IV over a 1 hour period, then 1 mg/kg per hour until delivery *Infant:* Zidovudine 2 mg/kg po q 6 hours for 6 weeks, beginning 8–12 hours after birth	*Mother:* NVP 200 mg po × 1 at onset of labor; *Infant:* NVP 2 mg/kg within 48–72 hours of birth [24, 25] *Mother:* ZDV 300 mg × 1 after onset of labor, then 300 mg po q 3 hours until delivery; 3TC 150 mg × 1 at onset of labor, then 150 mg po q 12 hours until delivery; ZDV/3TC 300/150 mg po BID for 1 week; *Infant:* ZDV 4 mg/kg with 3TC 2 mg/kg po BID for 1 week [26, Arm B] Intrapartum zidovudine administered intravenously, followed by 6 weeks of oral zidovudine to the infant, combined with one dose of nevirapine at the onset of the labor and one dose of nevirapine to the infant at 48 hours after birth (intrapartum and infant components of the ACTG 076 regimen, combined with the HIVNET 012 regimen) [29]
Postnatal	No (infant born to mother who did not receive any antiretroviral therapy during the antepartum or intrapartum periods)	Postnatal component of the ACTG 076 regimen: *Infant:* Zidovudine 2 mg/kg po q 6 hours until 6 weeks, beginning 8–12 hours after birth	The efficacy of administering a combination of antiretroviral drugs to the infant for prevention of transmission is under study, and the efficacy is not known at this time.

Public Health Service [104], the British HIV Association [115], and the European Consensus Panel [116]. These guidelines provide generally similar recommendations, although cesarean section before labor and ruptured membranes is emphasized to a greater extent in the British and European guidelines as compared with the US guidelines.

The US Public Health Service guidelines [104] address different groups of HIV-infected women and their infants (Table 8.5). Specifically, the groups addressed are those women who have not received prior antiretroviral therapy, those women who are already receiving antiretroviral therapy during the current pregnancy, those women in labor who have not received therapy previously, and infants born to mothers who have received no antiretroviral therapy during the antepartum or intrapartum periods. It is recommended that *HIV-infected women without previous antiretroviral therapy* receive at least the three-part ACTG 076 regimen (Table 8.2) (although acceptable alternatives to the maternal regimen in the clinical trial [100 mg orally five times daily] are oral zidovudine administered as 200 mg three times daily or 300 mg twice daily). Combining this zidovudine prophylactic regimen with additional antiretroviral drugs for treatment of the mother's HIV infection is recommended for women whose clinical, immunologic, or virologic status requires treatment [114] or who have peripheral blood viral loads of over 1000 copies/mL. *HIV-infected women already receiving antiretroviral therapy* should continue therapy if the pregnancy is identified after the first trimester. Zidovudine should be a component of the antepartum regimen after the first trimester if possible. Irrespective of the antepartum regimen, intrapartum and infant zidovudine as per the ACTG 076 regimen is recommended. Several different regimens of antiretroviral prophylaxis could be administered to *HIV-infected women in labor without previous antiretroviral therapy:* (1) one dose of nevirapine at the onset of labor followed by one dose of nevirapine to the infant at 48 hours after birth (HIVNET 012 regimen); (2) oral zidovudine and lamivudine during labor, followed by 1 week of oral zidovudine and lamivudine for the infant (from the Petra trial); (3) intrapartum zidovudine administered intravenously, followed by 6 weeks of oral zidovudine to the infant (intrapartum and infant components of the ACTG 076 regimen); or (4) intrapartum zidovudine administered intravenously, followed by 6 weeks of oral zidovudine to the infant, combined with one dose of nevirapine at the onset of the labor and one dose of nevirapine to the infant at 48 hours after birth (intrapartum and infant components of the PACTG 076 regimen, combined with the HIVNET 012 regimen). For *infants born to mothers who did not receive any antiretroviral therapy during the antepartum or intrapartum periods,* the 6-week infant zidovudine component of the ACTG 076 regimen should be offered. Zidovudine should be initiated as soon as possible after delivery, preferably within 6–12 hours after birth. The efficacy of administering a combination of antiretroviral drugs to the infant for prevention of transmission is under study, and is not known at this time.

Guidelines for initiation of antiretroviral therapy in adults and adolescents also have been developed by the World Health Organization (WHO) [117]. These guidelines address initiation of therapy if CD4$^+$ lymphocyte testing is or is not available: if CD4 testing is available, initiation of antiretroviral therapy is recommended for those with WHO Stage IV disease; those with WHO Stage III disease and a CD4$^+$ cell count below 350/mm^3; and those with Stage I or II disease and a CD4$^+$ cell count below 200/mm^3. If CD4 testing is unavailable, initiation of antiretroviral therapy is recommended for those with WHO Stage III or IV disease and those with WHO Stage II disease, if the total lymphocyte count is below 1200/mm^3. The use of antiretroviral drugs for treatment of HIV-infected pregnant women and for perinatal transmission prophylaxis in resource-poor settings is currently quite limited in terms of the overall, global need. It is hoped that, with increasing availability of drugs, as well as the infrastructure and staffing for the management of HIV-infected individuals, including pregnant women, this will change.

Important issues to address regarding the use of antiretroviral drugs in general, and their use among pregnant women and infants especially, are the drugs' known toxicities and potential adverse effects, which can affect patients' adherence to the drugs. In turn, poor adherence can facilitate the emergence of antiretroviral drug resistance. Both the known or potential adverse effects of antiretroviral drug use among pregnant women and their infants, and antiretroviral drug resistance as it relates to prevention of MTCT of HIV, have been reviewed in detail [118, 119]. Data from Thailand and elsewhere suggest women who receive intrapartum nevirapine may be less likely to have virologic suppression after 6 months of postpartum treatment with a nevirapine-containing regimen. This issue is being evaluated in large, randomized clinical trials.

Potential safety problems related to antiretroviral prophylaxis for prevention of MTCT can be categorized as follows [118]: fetal toxicity, resulting in adverse pregnancy outcomes such as low birth weight, preterm delivery, congenital anomalies, and fetal/neonatal death; short-term adverse effects on the mother and on the infant, including laboratory abnormalities (e.g. hematologic abnormalities or other laboratory abnormalities suggesting liver or other organ dysfunction) and clinical abnormalities (e.g. rash or other morbidity, mortality); long-term adverse consequences for the child, including mitochondrial toxicity resulting in organ damage or death and development of cancer; and long-term adverse effects on the mother and on the child who becomes infected despite interventions to prevent MTCT, such as more rapid disease progression or development of resistance subsequent to receipt of perinatal transmission prophylaxis with antiretroviral drug(s). Although follow-up of exposed mothers and children should be performed to detect short- and long-term consequences of such exposure, the available data suggest that adverse effects of exposure to antiretroviral drugs for prevention of MTCT are minimal.

Limited data exist regarding antiretroviral prophylaxis regimens and the development of resistance. The US Public Health Service guidelines [104] recommend resistance testing for the same indications in pregnant women as for non-pregnant adults, i.e. acute infection, viral failure or suboptimal viral suppression, or a high likelihood of having resistant views. However, other groups recommend resistance testing for all pregnant women with detectable HIV RNA levels, irrespective of previous receipt of antiretroviral drug(s), in order to maximize the response to antiretroviral therapy [120, 122]. Although MTCT of resistance HIV has been reported [123], it is unknown whether the presence of HIV resistance mutations increases the risk of MTCT. Therefore, it remains controversial whether pregnancy represents a specific indication for resistance testing.

8.5 Conclusions

The field of prevention of MTCT is changing rapidly. For those countries with greater resources and a lower disease burden, utilization of currently available interventions and combination antiretroviral therapy to decrease maternal viral load and to provide pre- and post-exposure prophylaxis has resulted in low transmission rates, but there are ongoing needs. These needs are: to make interventions and therapy more widely available; to address potential problems with existing interventions (e.g. drug toxicity; antiretroviral resistance, postpartum and neonatal morbidity related to surgical delivery); to develop new and better interventions (e.g. passive and active immunization against HIV [124, 125]; and to emphasize primary prevention. However, the great majority of mothers and children affected by HIV in the world reside in those countries with fewer resources with which to fight the disease. In these settings, there is an urgent need to implement known efficacious interventions, to incorporate prevention of MTCT into overall maternal–child health programs, to develop new and better (and simpler, cheaper, and more feasible) interventions, especially with regard to transmission through breastfeeding, and to emphasize primary prevention. Therefore, despite successes in the prevention of MTCT of HIV over the past several years, significant clinical and public health challenges exist.

REFERENCES

1. UNAIDS. AIDS Epidemic Update: December 2003 (http://www.unaids.org).
2. Kourtis, A. P., Bulterys, M., Nesheim, S. R. & Lee, F. K. Understanding the timing of HIV transmission from mother to infant. *J. Am. Med. Assoc.* **285** (2001), 709–12.
3. Mofenson, L. M. Mother–child HIV-1 transmission: timing and determinants. *Obstet. Gynecol. Clin. North Am.* **24** (1997), 759–84.
4. The International Perinatal HIV Group. Duration of ruptured membranes and vertical transmission of HIV-1: a meta-analysis from fifteen prospective cohort studies. *AIDS* **15** (2001), 357–68.
5. The European Mode of Delivery Collaboration. Elective caesarean section versus vaginal delivery in preventing vertical HIV-1 transmission: a randomised clinical trial. *Lancet* **353** (1999), 1035–7.
6. Nduati, R., John, G., Mbori-Ngacha, D., *et al.* Effect of breast-feeding and formula feeding on transmission of HIV-1: a randomized clinical trial. *J. Am. Med. Assoc.* **283** (2000), 1167–74.
7. Donegan, E., Stuart, M., Niland, J. C. *et al.* Infection with human immunodeficiency virus type 1 (HIV-1) among recipients of antibody-positive blood donations. *Ann. Intern. Med.* **113** (1990), 733–9.
8. Kaplan, E. H. & Heimer, R. A model-based estimate of HIV infectivity via needle sharing. *J. AIDS* **5** (1992), 1116–18.
9. Working Group on Mother-to-Child Transmission of HIV. Rates of mother-to-child transmission of HIV-1 in Africa, America, and Europe: results from 13 perinatal studies. *J. AIDS Hum. Retrovirol.* **8** (1995), 506–10.
10. Fowler, M. G., Simonds, R. J. & Roongpisuthipong, A. Update on perinatal HIV transmission. *Pediatr. Clin. N. Am.* **47** (2000), 21–38.
11. LaRussa, P., Magder, L. S., Pitt, J. *et al.* Association of HIV-1 viral phenotype in the MT-2 assay with perinatal HIV transmission. *J. AIDS* **30** (2002), 88–94.
12. Contopoulos-Ioannidis, D. G. & Ioannidis, J. P. A. Maternal cell-free viremia in the natural history of perinatal HIV-1 transmission. *J. AIDS* **18** (1998), 126–35.
13. Mofenson, L. M., Lambert, J. S., Stiehm, E. R. *et al.* Risk factors for perinatal transmission of human immunodeficiency virus type 1 in women treated with zidovudine. Pediatric AIDS Clinical Trials Group Study 185 Team. *New Engl. J. Med.* **341** (1999), 385–93.
14. Cooper, E. R., Charurat, M., Mofenson, L. *et al.* Combination antiretroviral strategies for the treatment of pregnant HIV-1-infected women and prevention of perinatal HIV-1 transmission. *J. AIDS* **29** (2002), 484–94.
15. Shapiro, D., Tuomala, R., Pollack, H. *et al.* Mother-to-child HIV transmission risk according to antiretroviral therapy, mode of delivery, and viral load in 2895 U.S. women (PACTG 367). Eleventh Conference on Retroviruses and Opportunistic Infections (February 2004; San Francisco, CA.), Program and Abstracts. (Abstract S-80).
16. Connor, E. M., Sperling, R. S., Gelber, R. *et al.* Reduction of maternal–infant transmission of human immunodeficiency virus type 1 with zidovudine treatment. *New Engl. J. Med.* **331** (1994), 1173–80.
17. Sperling, R. S., Shapiro, D. E., Coombs, R. W. *et al.* Maternal viral load, zidovudine treatment, and the risk of transmission of human immunodeficiency virus type 1 from mother to infant. *New. Engl. J. Med.* **335** (1996), 1621–9.
18. Ioannidis, J. P. A. Abrams, E. J., Ammann, A. *et al.* Perinatal transmission of human immunodeficiency virus type 1 by

pregnancy women with RNA virus loads < 1000 copies/ml. *J. Infect. Dis.* **183** (2001), 539–45.

19. Shaffer, N., Chuachoowong, R., Mock, P. A. *et al.* Short-course zidovudine for perinatal HIV-1 transmission in Bangkok, Thailand: a randomised controlled trial. *Lancet* **353** (1999), 773–80.

20. Wiktor, S. Z., Ekpini, E., Karon, J. M. *et al.* Short-course zidovudine for prevention of mother-to-child transmission of HIV-1 in Abidjan, Cote d'Ivoire: a randomised trial. *Lancet* **353** (1999), 781–5.

21. Dabis, F., Msellati, P., Meda, N. *et al.* 6-month efficacy, tolerance and acceptability of a short regimen of oral zidovudine to reduce vertical transmission of HIV in breastfed children in Cote d'Ivoire and Burkina Faso: a double-blind placebo-controlled multicentre trial. *Lancet* **353** (1999), 786–92.

22. Leroy, V., Karon, J. M., Alioum, A. *et al.* Twenty-four month efficacy of a maternal short-course zidovudine regimen to prevent mother-to-child transmission of HIV-1 in West Africa. *AIDS* **16** (2002), 631–41.

23. Lallemant, M., Jourdain, G., Le Coeur, S. *et al.* A trial of shortened zidovudine regimens to prevent mother-to-child transmission of human immunodeficiency virus type 1. *New Engl. J. Med.* **353** (2000), 982–91.

24. Guay, L. A., Musoke, P., Fleming, T. *et al.* Intrapartum and neonatal single-dose nevirapine compared with zidovudine for prevention of mother-to-child transmission of HIV-1 in Kampala, Uganda: HIVNET 012 randomised trial. *Lancet* **354** (1999), 795–802.

25. Jackson, J. B., Musoke, P., Fleming, T. *et al.* Intrapartum and neonatal single-dose nevirapine compared with zidovudine for prevention of mother-to-child transmission of HIV-1 in Kampala, Uganda: 18-month follow-up of the HIVNET 012 randomised trial. *Lancet*, **362** (2003), 859–68.

26. The Petra study team. Efficacy of three short-course regimens of zidovudine and lamivudine in preventing early and late transmission of HIV-1 from mother to child in Tanzania, South Africa, and Uganda (Petra study): a randomized, double-blind, placebo-controlled trial. *Lancet* **359** (2002), 1178–86.

27. Moodley, D., Moodley, J., Coovadia, H. *et al.* for the South African Intrapartum Nevirapine Trial (SAINT) Investigators. A multicenter randomized controlled trial of nevirapine versus a combination of zidovudine and lamivudine to reduce intrapartum and early postpartum mother-to-child transmission of human immunodeficiency virus type 1. *J. Infect. Dis.* **187** (2003), 725–35.

28. Dorenbaum, A., Cunningham, C. K., Gelber, R. D. *et al.* Two-dose intrapartum/newborn nevirapine and standard antiretroviral therapy to reduce perinatal HIV transmission: a randomized trial. *J. Am. Med. Assoc.* **288** (2002), 189–98.

29. Lallemant, M., Jourdain, G., Le Coeur, S. *et al.* Single-dose perinatal nevirapine plus standard zidovudine to prevent mother-to-child transmission of HIV-1 in Thailand. *N. Engl. J. Med.*, **351** (2004), 217–28.

30. Mandelbrot, L., Landreau-Mascaro, A., Rekacewicz, C. *et al.* Lamivudine-zidovudine combination for prevention of maternal-infant transmission of HIV-1. *J. Am. Med. Assoc.* **285** (2001), 2083–93.

31. Wade, N. A., Birkhead, G. S., Warren, B. L. *et al.* Abbreviated regimens of zidovudine prophylaxis and perinatal transmission of the human immunodeficiency virus. *New Engl. J. Med.* **339** (1998), 1409–14.

32. Wade, N. A., Birkhead, G. S. & French, P. T. Short courses of zidovudine and perinatal transmission of HIV [letter]. *New Engl. J. Med.* **340** (1999), 1042–3.

33. Chuachoowong, R., Shaffer, N., Siriwasin, W. *et al.* Short-course antenatal zidovudine reduces both cervicovaginal human immunodeficiency virus type 1 RNA levels and risk of perinatal transmission. *J. Infect. Dis.* **181** (2000), 99–106.

34. John, G. C., Nduati, R. W., Mbori-Ngacha, D. A. *et al.* Correlates of mother-to-child human immunodeficiency virus type 1 (HIV-1) transmission: association with maternal plasma HIV-1 RNA load, genital HIV-1 DNA shedding, and breast infections. *J. Infect. Dis.* **182** (2001), 206–12.

35. Msellati, P., Meda, N., Leroy, V. *et al.* Safety and acceptability of vaginal disinfection with benzalkonium chloride in HIV infected pregnant women in west Africa: ANRS 049b phase II randomised, double blinded placebo controlled trial. *Sex. Transm. Infect.* **75** (1999), 420–5.

36. Mandelbrot, L., Msellati, P., Meda, N. *et al.* 15 month follow up of African children following vaginal cleansing with benzalkonium chloride of their HIV infected mothers during late pregnancy and delivery. *Sex. Transm. Infect.* **78** (2002), 267–70.

37. Biggar, R. J., Miotti, P. G., Taha, T. E. *et al.* Perinatal intervention trial in Africa: effect of a birth canal cleansing intervention to prevent HIV transmission. *Lancet* **347** (1996), 1647–50.

38. Gaillard, P., Mwanyumba, F., Verhofstede, C. *et al.* Vaginal lavage with chlorhexidine during labor to reduce mother to child HIV transmission: clinical trial in Mombasa, Kenya. *AIDS* **15** (2001), 389–96.

39. Wilson, C., Gray, G., Read, J. S. *et al.* Tolerance and safety of different concentrations of chlorhexidine for peripartum vaginal and infant washes: HIVNET 025. *J. Acquir. Immune Defic. Syndr.* **35** (2004), 138–43.

40. Taha, T. E., Biggar, R. J., Broadhead, R. L. *et al.* Effect of cleansing the birth canal with antiseptic solution on maternal and newborn morbidity and mortality in Malawi: clinical trial. *Br. Med. J.* **315** (1997), 216–20.

41. Pillay, K., Coutsoudis, A., York, D., Kuhn, L. & Coovadia H. M. Cell-free virus in breast milk of HIV-1-seropositive women. *J. AIDS* **24** (2000), 330–6.

42. Semba, R. D., Kumwenda, N., Hoover, D. R. *et al.* Human immunodeficiency virus load in breast milk, mastitis, and mother-to-child transmission of human immunodeficiency virus type 1. *J. Infect. Dis.* **180** (1999), 93–8.

43. Richardson, B., Stewart-John, G. C., Hughes, J. P. *et al.* Breast-milk infectivity in human immunodeficiency virus type 1-infected mothers. *J. Infect. Dis.* **187** (2003), 736–40.

44. Nduati, R., Richardson, B. A., John, G. *et al.* Effect of breastfeeding on mortality among HIV-1 infected women: a randomised trial. *Lancet* **357** (2001), 1651–5.

45. Coutsoudis, A., Coovadia, H., Pillay, K. & Kuhn, L. Are HIV-infected women who breastfeed at increased risk of mortality? *AIDS* **15** (2001), 653–5.

46. The Breastfeeding and HIV International Transmission Study Group. Late postnatal transmission of HIV-1 in breast-fed children: an individual patient data meta-analysis, *J. Infect, Dis.*, **189** (2004), 2154–66.

47. Gaillard, P., Fowler, M. G., Debis, F. *et al.* Use of antiretroviral drugs to prevent HIV-1 transmission through breast-feeding: from animal studies to randomized clinical trials. *J. Acquir. Immune Defic. Syndr.* **35** (2004), 178–87.

48. Krebs, F. C., Miller, S. R., Malamud, D., Howett, M. K., Wigdahl, B. Inactivation of human immunodeficiency virus type 1 by nonoxynol-9, C31G, or an alkyl sulfate, sodium dodecyl sulfate. *Antiviral Res.* **43** (1999), 157–73.

49. Chantry, C. J., Morrison, P., Panchula, J. *et al.* Effects of lipolysis or heat treatment on HIV-1 provirus in breast milk. *J. AIDS* **24** (2000), 325–9.

50. Eglin, R. P. & Wilkinson, A. R. HIV infection and pasteurisation of breast milk [letter]. *Lancet* **1** (1987), 1093.

51. Orloff, S. L., Wallingford, J. C. & McDougal, J. S. Inactivation of human immunodeficiency virus type 1 in human milk: effects of intrinsic factors in human milk and of pasteurization. *J. Hum. Lact.* **9** (1993), 13–17.

52. Jorgensen, A. F. & Boisen, F. Pasteurization of HIV contaminated breast milk. In *XIII World AIDS Conference* (July 2000; Durban, South Africa). Program and Abstracts, Abstract LbPp122.

53. Jeffery, B. S. & Mercer, K. G. Pretoria pasteurisation: a potential method for reduction of postnatal mother to child transmission of the human immunodeficiency virus. *J. Trop. Pediatr.* **46** (2000), 219–23.

54. Jeffery, B. S., Webber, L., Mokhondo, K. R. & Erasmus, D. Determination of the effectiveness of inactivation of human immunodeficiency virus by Pretoria pasteurization. *J. Trop. Pediatr.* **47** (2001), 345–9.

55. Landesman, S. H., Kalish, L., Burns, D. *et al.* Obstetrical factors and the transmission of human immunodeficiency virus type 1 from mother to child. *New Engl. J. Med.* **334** (1996), 1617–23.

56. Minkoff, H., Burns, D. N., Landesman, S. *et al.* The relationship of the duration of ruptured membranes to vertical transmission of human immunodeficiency virus. *Am. J. Obstet. Gynecol.* **173** (1995), 585–9.

57. Mandelbrot, L., Mayaux, M., Bongain, A. *et al.* Obstetric factors and mother-to-child transmission of human immunodeficiency virus type 1: the French perinatal cohorts. *Am. J. Obstet. Gynecol.* **175** (1996), 661–7.

58. The International Perinatal HIV Group. The mode of delivery and the risk of vertical transmission of human immunodeficiency virus type 1: a meta-analysis of 15 prospective cohort studies. *New Engl. J. Med.* **340** (1999), 977–87.

59. de Martino, M., Tovo, P. A., Tozzi, A. E. *et al.* HIV-1 transmission through breast-milk: appraisal of risk according to duration of feeding. *AIDS* **6** (1992), 991–7.

60. Bobat, R., Moodley, D., Coutsoudis, A. & Coovadia, H. Breastfeeding by HIV-1-infected women and outcome in their infants: a cohort study from Durban, South Africa. *AIDS* **11** (1997), 1627–33.

61. John, G. C., Richardson, B. A., Nduati, R. W., Mbori-Ngacha D. & Kreiss, J. K. Timing of breast milk HIV-1 transmission: a meta-analysis. *East Afr. Med. J.* **78** (2001), 75–9.

62. Woolridge, M. W., Phil, D. & Baum, J. D. Recent advances in breast feeding. *Acta Paediatr. Jpn.* **35** (1993), 1–12.

63. Akre, J. Infant feeding: the physiological basis. *Bull World Health Organ* **67** (1989), 1–108.

64. VanDerslice, J., Popkin, B. & Briscoe, J. Drinking-water quality, sanitation, and breast-feeding: their interactive effects on infant health. *Bull. World Health Organ* **72** (1994), 589–601.

65. Piwoz, E. G., Kasonde, P., Vwalika, C., Shutes, E., Sinkala, M., Kankasa, C., Aldrovandi, G., Kuhn, L., Thea, D. M. The feasibility of early rapid breastfeeding cessation to reduce postnatal transmission of HIV in Lusaka, Zambia. 14th International Conference on AIDS (Barcelona, Spain; July 7–12, 2002), Program and Abstracts, abstract TuPeF5393.

66. Semba, R. D., Miotti, P. G., Chiphangwi, J. D. *et al.* Maternal vitamin A deficiency and mother-to-child transmission of HIV-1. *Lancet* **343** (1994), 1593–7.

67. Baeten, J. M., Mostad, S. B., Hughes, M. P. *et al.* Selenium deficiency is associated with shedding of HIV-1 infected cells in the female genital tract. *J. Acquir. Immune Defic. Syndr.* **26** (2001), 360–4.

68. Kumwenda, N., Miotti, P. G., Taha, T. E. *et al.* Antenatal vitamin A supplementation increases birthweight and decreases anemia, but does not prevent HIV transmission or decrease mortality in infants born to HIV-infected women in Malawi. *Clin. Infect. Dis.* **35** (2002), 618–24.

69. Coutsoudis, A., Pillay, K., Spooner, E. *et al.* Randomized trial testing the effect of vitamin A supplementation on pregnancy outcomes and early mother-to-child HIV-1 transmission in Durban, South Africa. *AIDS* **13** (1999), 1517–24.

70. Fawzi, W. W., Msamanga, G. I., Hunter, D. *et al.* Randomized trial of vitamin supplements in relation to transmission of HIV-1 through breastfeeding and early child mortality. *AIDS* **16** (2002), 1935–44.

71. St. Louis, M., Kamenga, M., Brown, C. *et al.* Risk of perinatal HIV-1 transmission according to maternal immunologic, virologic, and placental factors. *J. Am. Med. Assoc.* **269** (1993), 2853–9.

72. Temmerman, M., O'Nyong's, A., Bwayo, J. *et al.* Risk factors for mother-to-child transmission of human immunodeficiency virus-1 infection. *Am. J. Obstet. Gynecol.* **172** (1995), 700–5.

73. Wabwire-Mangen, F., Gray, R. H., Mmiro F. A. *et al.* Placental membrane inflammation and risks of maternal-to-child transmission of HIV-1 in Uganda. *J. AIDS* **22** (1999), 379–85.

74. Tess, B. H., Rodrigues, L. C., Newell, M. L. *et al.* Infant feeding and risk of mother-to-child transmission of HIV-1 in Sao Paulo State, Brazil. *J. AIDS Hum. Retrovirol.* **19** (1998), 189–94.

75. Coutsoudis, A., Pillay, K., Kuhn, L., Spooner, E., Tsai, W. Y. & Coovadia, H. M. Method of feeding and transmission of HIV-1 from mothers to children by 15 months of age: prospective cohort study from Durban, South Africa. *AIDS* **15** (2001), 379–87.

76. Victora, C. G., Smith, P. G., Vaughan, J. P. *et al.* Evidence for protection by breast-feeding against infant deaths from infectious diseases in Brazil. *Lancet* **2** (1987), 319–22.

77. Brown, K. H., Black, R. E., Lopez de Romana, G. & Creed de Kanashiro, H. Infant-feeding practices and their relationship with diarrheal and other diseases in Huascar (Lima), Peru. *Pediatrics* **83** (1989), 31–40.

78. National Family Health Survey (NFHS-2), India, 1998–1999. Mumbai, India: International Institute for Population Sciences and Calverton, MD: Measure DHS+, ORC MACRO. (2001).

79. Zimbabwe Demographic and Health Survey 1999. Preliminary report. Central Statistical Office, Harare, Zimbabwe. Calverton, MD: Measure DHS+, Macro International Inc. (2000).

80. Haider, R., Ashworth, A., Kabir, I. & Huttly, S. R. Effect of community-based peer counsellors on exclusive breastfeeding practices in Dhaka, Bangladesh: a randomised controlled trial. *Lancet* **356** (2000), 1643–7.

81. Van de Perre, P., Hitimana, D. G., Simonon, A. *et al.* Postnatal transmission of HIV-1 associated with breast abscess. *Lancet* **339** (1992), 1490–1.

82. Embree, J. E., Njenga, S., Datta, P. *et al.* Risk factors for postnatal mother-child transmission of HIV-1. *AIDS* **14** (2000), 2535–41.

83. Ekpini, E. R., Wiktor, S. Z., Satten, G. A. *et al.* Late postnatal mother-to-child transmission of HIV-1 in Abidjan, Côte d'Ivoire. *Lancet* **349** (1997), 1054–9.

84. Tavengwa, N., Piwoz, E., Gavin, L., Zunguza, C., Iliff, P. & Humphrey, J. Development, implementation, and evaluation of a program to counsel women about infant feeding in the context of HIV. In *14th International Conference on AIDS* (July 7–12, 2002; Barcelona, Spain). Program and Abstracts, Abstract MoPeF3881.

85. UNAIDS. 2004 Report on the Global AIDS epidemic (http://www.unaids.org).

86. Read, J. S. Preventing mother-to-child transmission of HIV: the USA experience. *Prenat. Neonat. Med.* **4** (1999), 391–7.

87. Centers for Disease Control and Prevention. U.S. Public Health Service recommendations for human immunodeficiency virus counseling and voluntary testing for pregnant women. *MMWR* **44** : **RR-7** (1995), 1–15.

88. Lindegren, M. L., Byers, R. H. Jr., Thomas, P. *et al.* Trends in perinatal transmission of HIV/AIDS in the United States. *J. Am. Med. Assoc.* **282** (1999), 531–8.

89. Centers for Disease Control and Prevention. Entry into prenatal care – United States, 1989–1997. *MMWR* **49** : **18** (2000), 393–8.

90. Hamm, R. H., Donnell, H. D., Wilson, E., Meredith, K., Louise, S. & Meyerson, B. Prevention of perinatal HIV transmission: beliefs and practices of Missouri prenatal providers. *Mo. Epidemiol.* **March–April** (1996), 5–10.

91. Mills, W. A., Martin, D. L., Bertrand, J. R. & Belongia, E. A. Physicians' practices and opinions regarding prenatal screening for human immunodeficiency virus and other sexually transmitted diseases. *Sex Transm. Dis.* **25** (1998), 169–75.

92. Phillips, K. A., Morrison, K. R., Sonnad, S. S. & Bleecker, T. HIV counseling and testing of pregnant women and women of childbearing age by primary care providers: self-reported beliefs and practices. *J. AIDS Hum. Retrovirol.* **14** (1997), 174–8.

93. Institute of Medicine (IOM). *Reducing the Odds: Preventing Perinatal Transmission of HIV in the United States.* Washington, DC: National Academy Press (1998).

94. Centers for Disease Control and Prevention. Advancing HIV prevention: new strategies for a changing epidemic – United States, 2003. *MMWR* **52** : **15** (2003), 329–32.

95. Cartoux, M., Msellati, P., Meda, N. *et al.* Attitude of pregnant women toward HIV testing in Abidjan, Cote d'Ivoire and Bobo-Dioulasso, Burkina Faso. *AIDS* **12** (1998), 2337–44.

96. Centers for Disease Control. Current recommendations for assisting in the prevention of perinatal transmission of human T-lymphotropic virus type III/lymphadenopathy-associated virus and acquired immunodeficiency syndrome. *MMWR Morb. Mortal. Wkly. Rep.* **34** (1985), 721–6.

97. American Academy of Pediatrics, Committee on Pediatric AIDS. Human milk, breastfeeding, and transmission of human immunodeficiency virus in the United States. *Pediatrics* **96** (1995), 977–9.

98. Read, J. S., and the Committee on Pediatric AIDS, American Academy of Pediatrics. Human milk, breastfeeding, and transmission of human immunodeficiency virus in the United States. *Pediatrics* **112** (2003), 1196–205.

99. Bertolli, J. M., Hsu, H., Frederick, T. *et al.* Breastfeeding among HIV-infected women, Los Angeles and Massachusetts, 1988–1993. In 11th World AIDS Conference, (1996, Vancouver) Abstract We.C.3583.

100. Simonds, R. J., Steketee, R., Nesheim, S. *et al.* Impact of zidovudine use on risk and risk factors for perinatal transmission of HIV. *AIDS* **12** (1998), 301–8.

101. Mbori-Ngacha, D., Nduati, R., John, G. *et al.* Morbidity and mortality in breastfed and formula-fed infants of HIV-1-infected women: a randomized clinical trial. *J. Am. Med. Assoc.* **286** (2001), 2413–20.

102. World Health Organization. Report of the WHO Technical Consultation on Behalf of the UNFPA/UNICEF/WHO/UNAIDS Inter-Agency Task Team on Mother-to-Child Transmission of HIV, October 11–13, 2000. New data on the prevention of mother-to-child transmission of HIV and their policy implications. Geneva, Switzerland: WHO; January 15, 2001 (http://www.unaids.org).

103. American College of Obstetricians and Gynecologists. *Scheduled Cesarean Delivery and the Prevention of Vertical Transmission of HIV Infection. ACOG Committee Opinion Number 234.* Washington, DC: ACOG (May 2000).

104. Centers for Disease Control and Prevention. Public Health Service Task Force recommendations for the use of antiretroviral drugs in pregnant women infected with HIV-1 for maternal health and for reducing perinatal HIV-1 transmission in the United States. *MMWR* 1998; 47 (No. RR-2): 1–30. (updates available at http://AIDSInfo.nih.gov).

105. Dominguez, K. L., Lindegren, M. L., d'Almada, P. J. *et al.* Increasing trend of cesarean deliveries in HIV-infected women in the United States from 1994 to 2000. *J. Acquir. Immune Defic. Syndr.* **33** (2003), 232–8.

106. Shaffer, N., Roongpisuthipong, A., Siriwasin, W. *et al.* Maternal viral load and perinatal HIV-1 subtype E transmission, Thailand. *J. Infect. Dis.* **179** (1999), 590–9.

107. The European Collaborative Study. Maternal viral load and vertical transmission of HIV-1: an important factor but not the only one. *AIDS* **13** (1999), 1377–85.

108. Fiscus, S., Adimora, A., Schoenbach, V. *et al.* Elective c-section may provide additional benefit in conjunction with maternal combination antiretroviral therapy to reduce perinatal HIV transmission. In *XIII World AIDS Conference* (July 2000, Durban, South Africa). Abstract WePpC1388.

109. Mrus, J. M., Goldie, S. J., Weinstein, M. C. & Tsevat, J. The cost-effectiveness of elective Cesarean delivery for HIV-infected women with detectable HIV RNA during pregnancy. *AIDS* **14** (2000), 2543–52.

110. Read, J. S. Cesarean section delivery to prevent vertical transmission of human immunodeficiency virus type 1: associated risks and other considerations. *Ann. N. Y. Acad. Sci.* **918** (2000), 115–21.

111. Read, J. S. Preventing mother to child transmission of HIV: the role of caesarean section. *Sex Transm. Infect.* **76** (2000), 231–2.

112. Ippolito, G., Puro, V., Heptonstall, J., Jagger, J., De Carli, G. & Petrosillo, N. Occupational human immunodeficiency virus infection in health care workers: worldwide cases through September 1997. *Clin. Infect. Dis.* **28** (1999), 365–83.

113. Recommendations of the U.S. Public Health Service Task Force on the use of zidovudine to reduce perinatal transmission of human immunodeficiency virus. *MMWR* **43 : RR-11** (1994), 1–20.

114. Centers for Disease Control and Prevention. Guidelines for the use of antiretroviral agents in HIV-infected adults and adolescents. *MMWR* 47 (1998), 47 (No. RR-5): 43–82 (updates available at http://AIDSInfo.nih.gov).

115. Lyall, E. G. H., Blott, M., de Ruiter, A. *et al.* Guidelines for the management of HIV infection in pregnant women and the prevention of mother-to-child transmission. *HIV Medicine* **2** (2001), 314–34.

116. Newell, M.-L. & Rogers, M. Pregnancy and HIV infection: a European Consensus on management. *AIDS* **16**: (Suppl. 2) (2002), S1–S18.

117. World Health Organization. Scaling up antiretroviral therapy in resource-limited settings: treatment guidelines for a public health approach (2003 revision). (http://www.who.int/3by5/publications/documents/arv_guidelines/en)

118. Mofenson, L. M. & Munderi, P. Safety of antiretroviral prophylaxis of perinatal transmission for HIV-infected pregnant women and their infants. *J. AIDS* **30** (2002), 200–15.

119. Nolan, M., Fowler, M. G. & Mofenson, L. M. Antiretroviral prophylaxis of perinatal HIV-1 transmission and the potential impact of antiretroviral resistance. *J. AIDS* **30** (2002), 216–29.

120. Jourdain, G., Ngo-Giang-Huong, N., Le Coeur, S. *et al.* Intrapartum exposure to nevirapine and subsequent maternal responses to nevirapine-based antiretroviral therapy. *N. Engl. J. Med.* **351** (2004), 229–40.

121. Hirsch, M. S., Brun-Vézinet, F., Clotet, B. *et al.* Antiretroviral drug resistance testing in adults infected with human immunodeficiency virus type 1: 2003 recommendations of an International AIDS Society-USA panel. *Clin. Infect. Dis.* **37** (2003), 113–28.

122. The EuroGuidelines Group for HIV Resistance. Clinical and laboratory guidelines for the use of HIV-1 drug resistance testing as part of treatment management: recommendations for the European setting. *AIDS* **15** (2001), 309–20.

123. Johnson, V. A., Petropoulos, C. J., Woods, C. R. *et al.* Vertical transmission of multi-drug resistance human immunodeficiency virus type 1 (HIV-1) and continued evolution of drug resistance in an HIV-1-infected infant. *J. Infect. Dis.* **183** (2001), 1688–93.

124. Guay, L. A., Musoke, P., Hom, D. L. *et al.* Phase I/II trial of HIV-1 hyperimmune globulin for the prevention of HIV-1 vertical transmission in Uganda. *AIDS* **16** (2002), 1391–400.

125. Biberfeld, G., Buonaguro, F., Lindberg, A., de The, G., Yi, Z. & Zetterstrom, R. Prospects of vaccination as a means of preventing mother-to-child transmission of HIV-1. *Acta Paediatr.* **91** (2002), 241–2.

9

Routine pediatric care

Elaine Abrams, M.D.[1] and Lisa-Gaye Robinson, M.D.[2]

[1] Associate Professor of Clinical Pediatrics, Columbia University, College of Physicians & Surgeons,
Director, Family Care Center, Associate Attending, Harlem Hospital Center, New York, NY
[2] Assistant Professor of Clinical Pediatrics, Columbia University, College of Physicians & Surgeons,
Assistant Attending, Harlem Hospital Center, New York, NY

9.1 Introduction

HIV is a chronic illness with diverse clinical manifestations and psychosocial challenges. The routine care of HIV-infected children demands a dedicated multidisciplinary approach from a variety of health care professionals including medical subspecialists, nurses, psychiatrists, psychologists, dentists, social workers, and case managers. The HIV primary care provider, while ensuring health maintenance and preventing disease, must serve as the coordinator of an array of services crucial to the management of these children in the context of the family. There are important management considerations that are essential to the care of both children who are exposed to HIV but determined to be uninfected and children with HIV infection.

9.2 Care of the HIV-exposed infant

Routine care for the infant born to an HIV-infected mother should begin well before the infant's birth. Pediatric providers should collaborate with the mother's primary care providers to minimize the risk of HIV transmission. Care of the infant after birth includes continued interventions to reduce the risk of HIV infection, as well as HIV diagnostic evaluations and routine infant care (Table 9.1). Care of the HIV-exposed newborn in the hospital begins with a thorough maternal history, including HIV disease status (HIV RNA concentration (viral load), CD4$^+$ lymphocyte count, and HIV-related complications), receipt of interventions to prevent mother-to-child transmission (e.g. antiretroviral prophylaxis, cesarean section delivery before labor and before ruptured membranes), and history of other infections (e.g. syphilis, herpes simplex virus, hepatitis B and C, cytomegalovirus, toxoplasmosis, gonorrhea, or tuberculosis). Psychosocial issues that could affect the child (e.g. substance abuse, homelessness, mental illness, immigration status) should be identified in order to provide any necessary additional services.

9.2.1 Perinatal HIV transmission prophylaxis

Both antiretroviral prophylaxis and cesarean section before the onset of labor and ruptured membranes reduce the risk of transmission of HIV from mothers to their infants [1–7]. In addition, the use of combination antiretroviral therapy for the HIV-infected pregnant woman's own health is associated with a decreased risk of mother-to-child transmission of HIV [8]. Prevention of mother-to-child transmission is discussed in Chapter 8. Independent of the medical and surgical management of the HIV-infected pregnant woman, a 6-week course of oral zidovudine (ZDV) to the infant is recommended [1]. All infants born to HIV-infected women should begin ZDV (2 mg/kg every 6 hours) prophylactic therapy as close to the time of birth as possible (preferably within 12 hours) [5, 9]. Zidovudine should be continued for 6 full weeks unless the infant is identified as being infected at which time it should be immediately discontinued (and the infant should be fully evaluated, see Section 9.3) [10]. Mild reversible anemia is associated with ZDV prophylaxis in the newborn. Therefore, clinicians should check a hemogram at birth and at 2–4 weeks of age to monitor for anemia. Follow-up of ZDV-exposed children and those who received placebo in protocol ACTG 076 have shown no evidence of a higher rate of tumors in

Table 9.1 Care of the HIV-exposed infant

Age	PHC[§]	Immunizations[¶]	Laboratory assays	ZDV prophylaxis[a]	TMP/SMX prophylaxis
Birth	§	Hepatitis B (Hep B) #1	HIV DNA PCR[b]	Begin within 12 hours of birth	
2 weeks	§		HIV DNA PCR[b]		
4 weeks	§	Hep B # 2	HIV DNA PCR[b]		
6 weeks	§			Stop[c]	Begin[d]
2 months	§	DTP, HIB, IPV, Pneumococcal #1			
4 months	§	DTP, HIB, IPV, Pneumococcal #2	HIV DNA PCR[b]		Stop[e]
6 months	§	DTP, HIB, Hep B, Pneumococcal #3 *(Influenza)*[f]			
9 months	§				
12 months	§ TST[h]	MMR, varicella	Hemogram[g] Lead HIV ELISA[i]		

[§] PHC=preventive health care. This includes all the elements of a comprehensive preventive care program recommended by the American Academy of Pediatrics (AAP) for all pediatric patients. All evaluations should include an interval history, assessment of growth and development, anticipatory guidelines and recommended immunizations.

[¶] The immunizations recommended in this table are for HIV-exposed infants who are immunologically normal. Refer to Chapter 10 for routine immunizations in the HIV-infected infant or child.

[a] Zidovudine (ZDV) prophylaxis should be started within 12 hours of birth (regardless of the maternal antiretroviral therapeutic/prophylactic regimen or resistance pattern). Addition of supplementary antiretrovirals should *only* be done in conjunction with an expert in pediatric HIV.

[b] A positive test should be repeated immediately. In addition, a hemogram and lymphocyte subsets should be obtained at that time. Infants suspected of being exposed to a non-subtype B HIV-1 virus (African or Asian origin) may require alternative testing (see text).

[c] ZDV prophylaxis should be discontinued prior to 6 weeks if the infant has laboratory confirmation of HIV infection.

[d] Trimethoprim-sulfamethoxazole (TMP/SMX) should be started prior to 6 weeks of life if the infant has laboratory confirmation of HIV infection and is older than 4 weeks of age.

[e] TMP/SMX prophylaxis should only be discontinued when there is laboratory confirmation that the infant is not infected and is without clinical signs of HIV infection.

[f] Influenza vaccine may be considered for HIV-exposed, uninfected infants as household contacts may be in high-risk groups for whom the vaccine is recommended.

[g] A hemogram is recommended by the AAP for all infants at 12 months of age.

[h] Tuberculin skin test.

[i] Median loss of maternal HIV antibody is at 10 months of life. Documentation of two negative ELISAs to confirm an uninfected status remain a recommendation by the AAP. However, with the low transmission rates in the US and extremely low probability of infection with multiple negative PCR tests, this recommendation may no longer be warranted.

ZDV-exposed children or of abnormalities in development [11]. Eight cases of mitochrondrial disease, including two children with degenerative neurologic disease leading to death, have been reported in France amongst children exposed to ZDV and lamivudine for perinatal prophylaxis [12]. In a large retrospective review of more than 12 000 children exposed to perinatal antiretroviral treatment, no deaths were associated with mitochondrial toxicity [13]. With this in mind, the primary care provider should consider potential complications of antiretroviral exposure as an etiology for unexplained presenting signs and symptoms, especially those with characteristics of mitochrondrial dysfunction. Furthermore, the long-term side-effects of in utero exposure to antiretroviral therapies have not been delineated. Some animal data suggest that several agents have mutagenic potential, and may lead to an increased susceptibility to tumor development as exposed children enter adolescence and early adulthood. (see Chapter 20). Therefore, it is important that the history of antiretroviral exposure remains in a child's medical record and that families understand the importance of this information. Long-term follow-up and surveillance studies continue to investigate whether there are long-term toxicities related to interventions to prevent mother-to-child transmission of HIV.

In addition to ZDV prophylaxis for the infant, avoidance of breastfeeding is another means of decreasing the risk of mother-to-child transmission of HIV. In settings where safe feeding alternatives are available, the biological mother should be counseled during the pregnancy and again in the nursery that breast milk can transmit HIV and that she should not breastfeed.

9.2.2 Diagnosis of HIV infection

All infants born to HIV-infected women should be tested for HIV infection beginning at birth. Such diagnostic testing of the infant should be performed using a DNA polymerase chain reaction (PCR) assay. HIV RNA assays also can be used for diagnosis of HIV infection, though some studies have demonstrated that a low copy number may yield a false positive test during the early months of life which is not substantiated by subsequent tests either by RNA or DNA PCR [14, 15]. If the PCR test result at birth is negative, it should be repeated at 2 weeks and again at 1 month of age. If the 1-month result is negative, a final test should be repeated after 4 months of life. The infant can be considered definitively HIV-uninfected if there are at least 2 negative HIV virologic detection tests, with one test obtained at or after 1 month of age and the second test obtained at or after 4 months of age. The American Academy of Pediatrics (AAP) currently recommends that all patients have HIV antibody tests to confirm absence of infection. The median age at the time of loss of maternal antibody is 10 months. An uninfected infant should no longer have detectable IgG antibody to HIV by 18 months of age. Given the low rate of mother-to-child transmission of HIV in North America, and the extremely low probability of HIV infection in a clinically well infant identified with negative PCR assay results, documentation of loss of maternal antibody may not be warranted [16]. However, parents may request that the test be done and some child welfare and foster care agencies continue to require follow-up antibody testing.

A positive HIV DNA PCR result in any infant should be repeated immediately. Positive results on two separate specimens, not including cord blood, represent definitive laboratory criteria for HIV infection. More than 95% of all HIV-infected infants test positive by 1 month of age [17]. It is important to note that infection with a non-B HIV subtype (e.g. in Africa and Asia) may not be recognized by the commercial HIV DNA PCR routinely available in the USA. Infants born to HIV-infected mothers who could be infected with a non-B subtype may require testing using an alternative test, e.g. the branched-chain DNA (bDNA) test which detects multiple subtypes. This testing should be done in consultation with an expert in pediatric HIV. (See Chapter 7 regarding diagnosis of HIV infection in children.)

9.2.3 Immunizations and prophylaxis for *Pneumocystis carinii* pneumonia

The immunization schedule for the HIV-exposed infants is virtually identical to that for all children (Table 9.1) (see Chapter 10). All infants born to HIV-infected mothers should receive prophylaxis for *Pneumocystis carinii* pneumonia (PCP) beginning at 6 weeks of age, when ZDV is discontinued. Prophylaxis for PCP can be discontinued if the child is confirmed to be HIV-uninfected (usually by 4–6 months). Prophylaxis for PCP should be continued in all infected infants, regardless of CD4$^+$ cell count, throughout the first year of life.

9.2.4 Anticipatory guidance

Anticipatory guidance for the primary caretaker is an important component of the care of an HIV-exposed infant. The caretaker must be advised that it may take several months before the child can be determined to be either uninfected or infected. This often creates significant anxiety. Informing the child's caretaker of the rationale for infant ZDV prophylaxis, as well as for subsequent trimethoprim-sulfamethoxazole (TMP–SMX) PCP prophylaxis will enhance continued adherence to these necessary regimens. The caretaker also should be repeatedly educated about other aspects of HIV disease, including diagnosis, treatment, prognosis, and about signs of infection and symptoms that should cause them to seek immediate medical attention for the infant.

9.3 Care of the HIV-infected pediatric patient

The overall goals of routine care of the HIV-infected pediatric patient are the same as those for all children:

health maintenance and disease prevention. With sophisticated care and new treatments, many children with HIV infection are entering their second and third decade of life. Effective multi-disciplinary care enables them to live with their infection, minimizing disease manifestations and maximizing quality of life. Important aspects of routine care include comprehensive general medical care, HIV disease progression monitoring, treatment of HIV infection, opportunistic infection prophylaxis, mental health evaluation and treatment, and education of and support for both the patient and the family.

9.3.1 Overview – comprehensive general medical care

Routine health maintenance – including assessment of growth, nutrition, development, and mental health; immunizations; evaluation and management of intercurrent illnesses; anticipatory guidance for the prevention of injury and disease; dental referrals; and screening for hearing and vision – should be provided for all children. Sequential assessment of growth and physical development is of particular importance. Growth failure or failure-to-thrive was described as a common finding in children with HIV infection early in the epidemic [18]. A small number are born with low birth weight, but most infected infants grow normally in utero and cannot be distinguished from uninfected infants by size at birth [18, 19]. During the first year of life, some infected infants, particularly those with a more rapid disease course, deviate from their previous growth pattern, and their growth velocity slows significantly [20]. While often associated with disease progression, the etiology of failure-to-thrive is multifactorial, including genetic predisposition, intrauterine environment (drug and alcohol exposure), and medication side-effects [20]. The introduction of combination antiretroviral therapy has decreased the prevalence of failure-to-thrive, but other growth abnormalities have emerged (such as obesity and delayed puberty). Paradoxically, obesity has been noted among some HIV-infected children. Delayed puberty also has been reported [21]. Long-term treatment with combination antiretroviral therapy also appears to put some children at risk for the development of lipodystrophy, a syndrome of abnormal fat distribution and serum lipid elevation [22, 23] (see Chapter 20). All children should have sequential measurements of their growth, and growth charts should be maintained to monitor their patterns and velocity of growth. Special attention should be paid to the timing of pubertal changes and to the distribution of body fat, particularly among children receiving combination antiretroviral therapy.

The immunization schedule for HIV-infected children is generally similar to the routine pediatric immunization schedule [24], but there are important differences. The main differences are a recommendation for yearly influenza vaccine, and cautions regarding the use of live vaccines. Immunocompromised individuals can develop disease from vaccine strains of organisms found in live vaccines. Measles, mumps and rubella should be administered to all infants unless they are severely immunocompromised (CDC class 3). Current data indicate that varicella vaccine is safe, immunogenic and effective in HIV-infected children without evidence of immune suppression (CDC class 1). Children infected with HIV are at increased risk of morbidity from varicella and herpes zoster. Therefore, varicella vaccine should be strongly considered in patients with normal CD4$^+$ cell counts. (See Chapter 10 for more information regarding immunizations for HIV-infected children.)

Patients should have serial assessments of neurological and developmental status. Early in the epidemic, developmental abnormalities were reported in a large proportion of infants and young children [25]. Neurological disorders appear as developmental delays in younger children and as cognitive deficits, behavioral problems, psychiatric manifestations, and school failure in older children and young teens [26]. Neurologic examinations and standard developmental assessments should be a part of routine care for the HIV-infected child. Children with abnormalities on screening should undergo neuropsychological and/or educational testing. See Chapter 17 for more information regarding neurodevelopmental assessment of the HIV-infected pediatric patient.

Some HIV-infected children receive all of their care directly from a team that manages the medical, social, and mental health issues associated with HIV on a daily basis. Alternatively, a general pediatrician provides the bulk of routine care in close consultation with an HIV specialist. The specialist may see a child whose condition is stable two to three times per year, with the general pediatrician providing the remainder of the care. Availability of services and parent preference generally determine the choice of care model. In either model, it is imperative that the child be managed by someone expert in the field.

9.3.2 Initial evaluation of the HIV-infected pediatric patient

The initial evaluation of the HIV-infected pediatric patient should include a comprehensive history, a physical examination, an assessment of the patient's developmental

Table 9.2 Initial evaluation of the HIV-infected pediatric patient

History	Assessment	History	Assessment
Mother's medical history	HIV disease stage CD4$^+$ lymphocyte quantitation Viral load (HIV RNA assay) Clinical stage, complications Receipt of antiretroviral drugs Antiretroviral resistance testing HIV subtype (clade) Drug and alcohol use Labor and delivery history (mode of delivery, duration ruptured membranes, complications)		Family members taking antiretroviral therapy Foster care and adoption history, as appropriate Relationship with biologic family members for children in alternative care settings (foster, adoptive, group homes)
Child's medical history	Gestational age Birth weight Receipt of antiretroviral drugs Neonatal medical problems Breastfeeding history Recurrent symptoms Serious illnesses Age of puberty, menstruation Hospitalizations Chronic medications, allergies Immunizations Growth history Developmental history School history (grade, achievement) Behavioral and mental health history Sexual history	Social history	Primary language in household Disclosure to child and family members Religious and cultural beliefs Legal issues related to guardianship Source of household income Insurance coverage Other caretakers who assist in care
		Physical	A complete comprehensive physical examination including a developmental evaluation
		Laboratory	HIV ELISA and Western blot (if not already done) CBC with differential^a Lymphocyte subsets^a Viral load (HIV RNA assay)^a Blood urea nitrogen, creatinine Liver function tests Cholesterol, triglyceride Urinalysis Hepatitis B and C serologies Cytomegalovirus (CMV), toxoplasmosis, syphilis and varicella serologies^b Tuberculin skin test (TST) with anergy Chest radiograph Brain CT or MRI (if clinically indicated) Electrocardiogram/Echocardiogram^c
Family history	Primary caretaker Family history of illness including HIV, TB Source of care for other family members with HIV		

^{a}The initial results should be repeated within 4 weeks to confirm the results prior to initiating any therapy.
^{b}If the child is < 12 months old, positive serologies should be repeated after 1 year of age to document seroreversion.
^{c}Some centers advocate for baseline electrocardiogram and echocardiogram on all children at the initial evaluation. Insurance funding may not be available to cover these costs.

status, behavioral and mental health issues, as well as baseline laboratory tests as outlined in Table 9.2. A comprehensive evaluation allows the clinician to stage the child clinically, immunologically, and virologically, and to determine the need for therapeutic and/or prophylactic interventions.

The initial evaluation also should include an assessment of the family's adjustment to the diagnosis as well as knowledge and understanding of HIV infection. The initial evaluation also marks the beginning of a dialogue with the child and family about a wide range of social and psychological matters integral to HIV care.

History

A detailed medical history, including the mother's pregnancy, labor, and delivery, and the child's medical, growth, and developmental histories, will enable the provider to assess the clinical stage of disease. However, historical data may be incomplete. Tanner staging and menstrual history should be included for preteens and adolescents. A comprehensive family history should include HIV infection status of other family members, especially siblings. Parents should be encouraged to have the infection status of all the children in the family determined. The initial history also should aim to assess the coping skills and mental health needs of the caregiver and child. A comprehensive social history should be obtained and a family profile developed to determine appropriate assistance and support services. A complete evaluation may not be accomplished during a single visit and may require a number of meetings with different members of the multi-disciplinary team. Over time, disclosure of HIV infection status within the family and community, and to the child, should be explored. Finally, providers should make themselves aware of any cultural and religious beliefs that could influence care and treatment.

Physical examination and laboratory testing

The physical examination should include careful determination of the child's height, weight and, from birth through 2 years of age, head circumference. A comprehensive examination looking for specific organ system involvement is important. Patients should have a thorough neurologic examination and neuropsychologic assessment (see Chapter 17). In some settings, the primary provider may prefer to use a simplified screening tool to assess developmental status and refer only those children with abnormalities on screening for specialized assessments. Similarly, the mental health status and, when appropriate, educational achievement of the child should be assessed, again either by the primary provider or by a specially trained mental health professional.

The diagnostic tests that are suggested for the first evaluation allow the clinician to obtain baseline immunologic and virologic data (CD4 T cell counts, plasma HIV RNA concentration), to assess organ system involvement (complete blood count with differential, serum chemistries, liver and renal function tests, lipid profile, urinalysis, chest radiograph, brain CT and echocardiogram), and to determine exposure to vertically acquired infections and potential opportunistic pathogens (cytomegalovirus, toxoplasmosis, syphilis, varicella, hepatitis B and C serologies). A tuberculin skin test should be placed on all children greater than 1 year of age and all those with a known exposure to an adult with active TB (Table 9.2).

9.3.3 Follow-up evaluations of the HIV-infected pediatric patient

HIV disease progression monitoring

A complete evaluation of the disease status of an HIV-infected infant, child, or adolescent must include immunologic, virologic, and clinical evaluations. The most useful assays for the evaluation of immune function in HIV-infected children are determination of the absolute number and percentage of $CD4^+$ and $CD8^+$ T lymphocytes. $CD4^+$ lymphocyte count is independently predictive of the likelihood of disease progression [27]. Interpretation of $CD4^+$ T cell counts should take into consideration the age of the child, since the normal number of cells declines with age over the first 6 years of life (see Chapter 1). Routine monitoring should be done every 3 months in an otherwise stable child. However, precipitous decreases in the $CD4^+$ lymphocyte absolute count or percentage, changes in plasma HIV RNA concentration, changes in clinical status, or initiation of a new treatment regimen may dictate more frequent measurements.

The plasma HIV RNA concentration (viral load) provides information regarding the child's response to therapy and the child's risk of disease progression [27–31]. It should be monitored every 3–4 months in a stable child, but more frequently for the following groups of children: those with significant increases in viral load measurements, those with significant deteriorations in clinical or immune status, and those whose antiretroviral therapy regimen has changed. There are several different methods available for quantifying HIV RNA, each with different levels of sensitivity (for details, refer to Chapter 4). It is therefore important to use the same assay repeatedly for a given patient as the results of the different assays may be significantly disparate.

All children should be assessed for organ system disease at regular intervals with a thorough history and a complete physical examination. For some organ systems, specific tests may reveal evidence of disease before symptoms develop. Helpful screening assessments (outlined in Table 9.3) include:

- Central nervous system – yearly developmental assessment after 2 years of age, yearly neurologic examination.
- Cardiovascular – chest radiograph, electrocardiogram and echocardiogram every 3–5 years.
- Pulmonary – yearly tuberculin skin test, chest radiograph every 3–5 years.
- Gastrointestinal – liver function testing every 3 months.

Table 9.3 Schedule for follow-up laboratory and diagnostics evaluations for the HIV-infected pediatric patient

Frequency	Assessment
Every 3 months[a]	Complete blood count with differential
	Lymphocyte subsets
	Plasma HIV RNA concentration (viral load)
	Laboratory tests for assessment of toxicities of antiviral and concomitant treatments[b]
Every 6 months	Developmental evaluations to 2 years of age
	Ophthalmologic examination for children with positive cytomegalovirus (CMV) or toxoplasmosis serology and CD4[+] lymphocyte counts placing them at risk for retinitis[c]
Every 12 months	Urinalysis
	CMV and toxoplasma serologies (if previously negative)
	Tuberculin skin test (TST)
	Cholesterol, triglyceride
	Developmental evaluation after 2 years of age
	Dental referral after 1 year of age
	Vision and hearing screen
Every 3–5 years	Chest radiograph
	Electrocardiogram/Echocardiogram[d]

[a]More often if medically indicated.

[b]Laboratory tests that are performed depend on potential toxicities of the specific drugs given. Baseline studies prior to initiation of therapy is warranted.

[c]If the child is < 12 months old, positive serologies should be repeated after 1 year of age to document seroreversion.

[d]Some centers advocate for baseline electrocardiogram and echocardiogram on all children at the initial evaluation. Insurance funding may not be available to cover these costs.

- Renal – yearly urinalysis.
- Hematologic – complete blood count with differential.

Most of the latter tests should be carried out at the suggested intervals in asymptomatic children or at any time when a child presents with a history or symptoms suggestive of disease related to a specific organ system. Patients with advanced disease may require more frequent evaluations dictated by their clinical status. In addition, children receiving antiretroviral therapy will need quarterly routine monitoring for organ system abnormalities (e.g. complete blood count with differential, liver aminotransferases, pancreatic enzymes, and lipid profiles) potentially associated with specific treatments. A schedule for obtaining these tests is provided in Tables 9.2 and 9.3.

Treatment of HIV infection

Pediatric antiretroviral therapy continues to evolve. Those prescribing antiretroviral therapy should be thoroughly familiar with the drugs and how to use them, potential drug toxicities, and drug interactions. Clinicians caring for HIV-infected children should routinely monitor children's response to antiretroviral therapy, as well as adherence to such drug therapy (see Chapters 18, 13, and 21 regarding antiretroviral therapy, adherence, and drug resistance.)

In addition to clinical and laboratory (viral load and CD4[+] T cell counts and percentages) evaluations prior to the initiation of antiretroviral therapy, the family's readiness should be assessed thoroughly. Children sometimes need advance training to ensure that they will adhere adequately to the prescribed regimen. After initiation of a new antiretroviral regimen, viral load assays and CD4[+] T cell counts should be monitored monthly. If viral suppression is achieved, virologic and immunologic evaluations, and laboratory monitoring for toxicity (including complete blood count, liver function tests, lipid profile), can be performed every 3 months. A deterioration in the clinical status may prompt more frequent assessment. Starting and changing antiretroviral therapy is discussed in Chapter 18.

Adherence to antiretroviral therapy is crucial for long-term success of antiretroviral therapy. Adherence is discussed in Chapter 13.

Opportunistic infection prophylaxis

Routine care of HIV-infected children should include prevention of opportunistic infections. The most common opportunistic pathogens include *Pneumocystis carinii*, *Mycobacterium avium* complex (MAC), *Candida* species, cytomegalovirus, and *Toxoplasmosa gondii*. Knowledge of the child's immunologic status based on the CD4$^+$ lymphocyte count or percentage is important in determining the risk for these opportunistic infections and the need for specific prophylaxis. Implementation of guidelines for prophylaxis against PCP in HIV-infected children have led to a significant decline in the incidence of this infection, particularly in young infants [32]. Prophylaxis for MAC infection is recommended for children with advanced immunosuppression based on efficacy studies in adults [33]. Severe candidiasis (esophagitis or severe recurrent thrush) often requires suppressive therapy. (Further information regarding prevention of opportunistic infections can be found in Chapter 11.)

Mental health evaluation and monitoring

A wide variety of mental health needs have been described for HIV-infected children, including emotional, cognitive, learning, and behavioral problems [26, 34]. These children have to grapple with the experience of living with a stigmatizing chronic illness while experiencing the normal developmental milestones of puberty, autonomy, peer relationships, and sexuality. Furthermore, many children and youth with HIV infection are primarily from ethnic minority, socioeconomically disadvantaged families with high rates of substance abuse, psychiatric disorders, chronic stress, and psychological impairment. The complexities of HIV infection in conjunction with extraordinary social inadequacies contribute to the wide variety of diagnoses among HIV-infected children, including developmental delay, school failure, attention deficit disorder, depression, antisocial behavior, and post-traumatic stress syndrome. Increased sensitivity and attention to these issues by the primary provider is essential, and frequent assessments (e.g. at each medical visit) for possible problems should be conducted. The inclusion of mental health professionals within the multi-disciplinary team facilitates evaluation and treatment of this set of problems. Counseling and/or pharmacologic intervention may be appropriate,

if not imperative, for the medical and psychological well-being of the child and their family.

Adolescents with HIV infection represent a particularly challenging population of patients. The care of adolescents with HIV infection is addressed in Chapters 14 and 15.

Education of, and support for, the patient and family

Support and education for HIV-infected children

As HIV-infected children become older, it is important to involve them in their own medical/psychosocial management, including an ongoing dialogue about how HIV infection affects their health and why interventions are instituted. Involvement of the child in the decision-making processes regarding drug regimens will likely enhance adherence. Families should be encouraged to disclose infection status to the child when the child becomes developmentally capable of understanding the information. Many families may be unwilling or unprepared to address issues of disclosure and require ongoing support as they move towards open discussions with their child [35]. As the child approaches adolescence, the issue of disclosure must be resolved to prevent secondary transmission (see Chapter 15).

Family assessment, support, and education

HIV affects multiple family members and reverberates into the local community. All family members are profoundly affected by caring for a child with a chronic illness, especially one with complex medical management, daily medications, and significant social stigma. It is imperative to acknowledge and address the psychological and social needs of all family members to enable them to seek maximal medical and emotional well-being. Young mothers identified as HIV-infected through perinatal testing must face the challenges of caring for a newborn while coping with the stress of learning their infection status. Depression and other psychiatric disorders, limited parenting experience, poor coping skills, and substance abuse may interfere with these mothers' abilities to meet their children's, as well as their own, needs. Parents of older children may require care for their own disease and often continue to struggle with the high risk behaviors, such as alcohol and drug use, which lead to HIV infection. Foster and adoptive parents, who willingly and lovingly took home young infants with HIV, may find themselves overwhelmed by the growing emotional and psychological needs of these children as they enter adolescence. The multi-disciplinary HIV team should be able to assess and address these complex issues and provide appropriate care, case management, and/or referrals to other providers.

The family and child should be engaged in a partnership with the multi-disciplinary team in the management of the child's disease and treatment decisions. Routine care of the child and youth with HIV infection should include ongoing education about the disease: the natural history, clinical signs and symptoms and laboratory evaluations for HIV infection, the risks and benefits of antiretroviral therapy and opportunistic infection prophylaxis, and information about intercurrent illnesses. The need for strict adherence and the identification of barriers to adherence must be discussed frequently. The provider should assess the family's comfort with treatment as well as their personal beliefs and commitment to strict adherence to chronic therapeutic regimens with multiple daily doses.

School and day-care attendance offer special challenges for HIV-infected children. The special problems associated with school and day-care attendance are discussed in Chapter 44.

9.3.4 Subsequent, ongoing care

The clinic visit should serve to deliver routine pediatric care; to monitor the child's disease status, medication adherence, complications of treatment, and mental health wellness; and to provide support and education for the child and family. The schedule for follow-up medical visits will largely depend upon the severity of the child's disease and the complexity and toxicity of the treatment regimen. Children with advanced disease require frequent visits, as often as every 4–6 weeks, while those with more stable disease can be seen quarterly (Table 9.3). For newly diagnosed patients, consideration should be given to shorter intervals between visits during the first 6–9 months after diagnosis. This allows the caregiver time to become familiar with the staff and the concept of attending to the medical needs of a child with a chronic illness. Children beginning new treatment regimens may require weekly visits to reinforce adherence and to closely monitor virologic and immunologic response. Clinically stable children who are not taking antiretroviral medications require less frequent monitoring, every 3–4 months. On the other hand, those with advanced disease who are not receiving antiretroviral medications, generally because of adherence difficulties, should be monitored as often as every 1–2 months.

The interim history should attempt to elicit signs and symptoms of specific organ dysfunction, medication adherence, intolerance and toxicity, and new mental health or behavioral problems. The physical exam should be comprehensive. The laboratory tests that should be obtained at 3-month intervals are outlined in Table 9.3. More frequent testing may be in order for patients with decreasing CD4$^+$ cell counts, increasing HIV RNA copy number and/or deterioration in clinical status. Additionally, antiviral resistance testing (genotypic and/or phenotypic) would be recommended for a patient on antiretroviral therapy with virologic failure who may have developed resistance to specific agents.

Involving the child in the treatment plan as much as possible with age-appropriate education and acknowledgment of the complexities of their medical regimens and social issues will lay a foundation for future ongoing participation in their long-term healthcare. It is important to keep in mind that due to the nature of the illness, most children will remain in care for the duration of their lives.

9.4 Summary

Routine pediatric care of the HIV-exposed and -infected child must be delivered by a primary care provider who is knowledgeable regarding this chronic disease. Co-ordination of medical subspecialities and psychosocial services are needed to deliver optimal routine care. The HIV-exposed infant who is identified as uninfected will require less demanding medical interventions but may continue to demand attention to his or her psychosocial needs by virtue of the nature of this chronic infection within the family unit. The infected child and family will be faced with challenging acute needs and the demands of a chronic and ultimately fatal disease. However, employing a sophisticated multi-disciplinary approach, providing new effective treatment regimens and actively engaging the child and caretaker in the medical/psychosocial care plan will likely enable many HIV-infected children to enter adulthood.

REFERENCES

1. Connor, E. M., Sperling, R. S., Gelber, R. *et al.* Reduction of maternal-infant transmission of human immunodeficiency virus type 1 with zidovudine treatment. *New Engl. J. Med.* **331**:**18** (1994), 1173–80.

2. Shaffer, N., Chuachoowong, R., Mock, P. A. *et al.* Short-course zidovudine for perinatal HIV-1 transmission in Bangkok, Thailand: a randomized controlled trial. *Lancet* **353**:**9155** (1999) 773–80.

3. The PETRA study team. Efficacy of three short-course regimens of zidovudine and lamivudine in preventing early and

late transmission of HIV-1 from mother to child in Tanzania, South Africa, and Uganda (Petra study): a randomised, double- blind, placebo-controlled trial. *Lancet.* **359**:**9313** (2002), 1178–86.

4. Guay, L. A., Musoke, P., Fleming, T. *et al.* Intrapartum and neonatal single-dose nevirapine compared with zidovudine for prevention of mother-to-child transmission of HIV-1 in Kampala, Uganda: HIVNET 012 randomised trial. *Lancet* **354**:**9181** (1999), 795–802.

5. Wade, N. A., Birkhead, G. S., Warren, B. L. *et al.* Abbreviated regimens of zidovudine prophylaxis and perinatal transmission of the human immunodeficiency virus. *New Engl. J. Med.* **339**:**20** (1998), 1409–14.

6. The International Perinatal HIV Group. The mode of delivery and risk of vertical transmission of HIV-1- a meta-analysis of 15 prospective cohort studies. *N. Engl. J. Med.* **340**:**13** (1999), 977–87.

7. The European mode of delivery collaboration. Elective cesarean-section versus vaginal delivery in prevention of vertical HIV-1 transmission: a randomized clinical trial. *Lancet* **353**:**9158** (1999), 1035–9.

8. Cooper, E. R., Charurat, M., Mofenson, L. *et al.* Combination antiretroviral strategies for the treatment of pregnant HIV-1 infected women and prevention of perinatal HIV-1 transmission. *J AIDS* **29**:**5** (2002), 484–94.

9. Wade, N., Birkhead, G. & French, P. T. Short courses of zidovudine and perinatal transmission of HIV. *New Engl. J. Med.* **340** (1999), 1042–3.

10. Centers for Disease Control and Prevention. Guidelines for the use of antiretroviral agents in pediatric HIV infection, 1998. *MMWR* **47** (No. RR-4): 1–43 (updates available at http://AIDSInfo.nih.gov).

11. Hanson, I. C., Antonelli, T. A., Sperling, R. S. *et al.* Lack of tumors in infants with perinatal HIV-1 exposure and fetal/neonatal exposure to zidovudine. *J. AIDS Hum. Retrovirol.* **20**:**5** (1999), 463–7.

12. Blanche, S., Tardieu, M., Rustin, P. *et al.* Persistent mitochondrial dysfunction and perinatal exposure to antiretroviral nucleoside analogues. *Lancet* **354** (1999), 1084–9.

13. The Perinatal Safety Review Working Group. Nucleoside exposure in the children of HIV-infected women receiving antiretroviral drugs: absence of clear evidence for mitochondrial disease in children who died before 5 years of age in five United States cohorts. *J. AIDS* **25** (2000), 261–8.

14. Cunningham, C. K., Charbonneau, T. T., Song, K. *et al.* Comparison of human immunodeficiency virus 1 DNA polymerase chain reaction and qualitative and quantitative RNA polymerase chain reaction in human immunodeficiency virus 1-exposed infants. *Pediatr. Infect. Dis. J.* **18** (1999), 30–5.

15. Delamare, C., Burgard, M., Mayaux, M. J. *et al.* HIV-1 RNA detection in plasma for the diagnosis of infection in neonates. The French Pediatric HIV Infection Study Group. *J. AIDS Hum. Retrovirol.* **15**:**2** (1997), 121–5.

16. Benjamin, D. K., Miller, W. C., Fiscus, S. A. *et al.* Rational testing of the HIV-exposed infant. *Pediatrics* **108**:**1** (2001), E3.

17. Dunn, D. T., Brandt, C. D., Krivine, A. *et al.* The sensitivity of HIV-1 DNA polymerase chain reaction in the neonatal period and the relative contributions of intra-uterine and intra-partum transmission. *AIDS* **9** (1995), F7-11.

18. McKinney, R. E. & Robertson, J. W. Effect of human immunodeficiency virus infection on the growth of young children. Duke Pediatric AIDS Clinical Trials Unit. *J. Pediatr.* **123**:**4** (1993), 579–82.

19. Abrams, E. J., Matheson, P. B., Thomas, P. A. *et al.* Neonatal predictors of infection status and early death among 332 infants at risk of HIV-1 infection monitored prospectively from birth. *Pediatrics* **96** (1995), 451–8.

20. Moye, J., Rich, K. C., Kalish, L. A. *et al.* Natural history of somatic growth in infants born to women infected by human immunodeficiency virus. *J. Pediatr.* **128** (1996), 58–69.

21. DeMartino, M., Tovo, P. A., Galli, L. *et al.* Puberty in perinatal HIV-1 infection: a multicenter longitudinal study of 212 children. *AIDS* **15**:**12** (2001), 1527–34.

22. Arpadi, S. M., Cuff, P. A., Horlick, M., Wang, J. & Kotler, D. P. Lipodystrophy in HIV-infected children is associated with high viral load and low CD4$^+$ -lymphocyte count and CD4$^+$ -lymphocyte percentage at baseline and use of protease inhibitors and stavudine. *J. AIDS* **27**:**1** (2001), 30–4.

23. Melvin, A. J., Lennon, S., Mohan, K. M. & Purnell, J. Q. Metabolic abnormalities in HIV type 1-infected children treated and not treated with protease inhibitors. *AIDS Res. Hum. Retroviruses* **17**:**12** (2001), 1117–23.

24. Centers for Disease Control and Prevention. Recommended Childhood and Adolescent Immunization Schedule-United States, 2004. *MMWR*, **53** (2004), Q1–3.

25. Diamond, G. W. Developmental problems in children with HIV infection. *Ment. Retard.* **27**:**4** (1989), 213–7.

26. Brown, L. K., Lourie, K. J. & Pao, M. Children and adolescents living with HIV and AIDS: a review. *J. Child. Psychol. Psychiatry* **41**:**1** (2000), 81–96.

27. Mofenson, L. M., Korelitz, J., Meyer, W. A. *et al.* The relationship between serum human immunodeficiency virus type 1 (HIV-1) RNA level, CD4 lymphocyte percent, and long-term mortality risk in HIV-1 infected children. National Institute of Child Health and Human Development Intravenous Immunoglobulin Clinical Trial Study Group. *J. Infect. Dis.* **175** (1997), 1029–38.

28. Abrams, E. J., Weedon, J., Steketee, R. W. *et al.* Association of HIV viral load early in life with disease progression among HIV-infected infants. *J. Infect. Dis.* **178** (1998), 101–8.

29. Shearer, W. T., Quinn, T. C., LaRussa, P. *et al.* Viral load and disease progression in infants infected with human immunodeficiency virus type 1. *New Engl. J. Med.* **336** (1997), 1337–42.

30. Palumbo, P. E., Raskino, C., Fiscus, S. *et al.* Predictive value of quantitative plasma HIV RNA and CD4$^+$ lymphocyte count in HIV-infected infants and children. *J. Am. Med. Assoc.* **279**:**10** (1998), 756–61.

31. Dunn, D. HIV Paediatric Prognostic Markers Collaborative Study Group. Short-term risk of disease progression in HIV-1-infected children receiving no antiretroviral therapy or

zidovudine monotherapy: a meta-analysis. *Lancet* **362**:**9396** (2003): 1605–11.

32. Centers for Disease Control and Prevention 1999 revised guidelines for prophylaxis against *Pneumocystis carinii* pneumonia for children infected with or perinatally exposed to human immunodeficiency virus. *MMWR* **48**:**RR-10** (1999).

33. Centers for Disease Control and Prevention 1999 revised guidelines for prophylaxis against *Mycobacterium avium* intracellulare in patients infected with human immunodeficiency virus. *MMWR* **48**:**RR-10** (1999).

34. Havens, J. F., Mellins, C. A. & Hunter, J. Psychiatric aspects of HIV/AIDS in childhood and adolescence. In M. Rutter & E. Taylor (eds.), *Child and Adolescent Psychiatry: Modern Approaches*. Fourth Edition. Oxford, England: Blackwell (2001), pp. 828–41.

35. Mellins, C. A., Brackis-Cott, E., Dolezal, C., Richards, A., Nicholas, S. & Abrams, E. J. Patterns of HIV status disclosure to perinatally infected HIV-positive children and subsequent mental health outcomes. *Clin. Child Psychol. Psychia* **7** (2001), 101–14.

given as pre-exposure prophylaxis. There are three vaccines available in the USA, and five doses (1.0 cm^3 each) are required on days 1, 3, 7, 14, and 28. As antibody response may not be adequate in immunocompromised persons, it is recommended that antibody titers be obtained to assure an appropriate response.

10.3.13 *Rotavirus vaccine*

The original rotavirus vaccine, a live virus vaccine, is contraindicated in HIV-exposed and -infected children [33]. It is no longer available.

10.3.14 *Typhoid vaccine*

Routine typhoid vaccination is not recommended in the USA. If an HIV-infected child is travelling to an area where *Salmonella typhi* is endemic, vaccination with the Vi capsular polysaccharide vaccine or the inactivated vaccine may be given. The Vi capsular polysaccharide vaccine consists of one dose (0.5 cm^3) given intramuscularly, and it should not be given to children less than 2 years old. The inactivated vaccine must be given in two intramuscular doses separated by at least 4 weeks, and should not be given to those less than 6 months of age. Live, attenuated TY21a vaccine is contraindicated in HIV-exposed infants and HIV-infected children [34].

10.3.15 *Varicella vaccine*

Because HIV-infected children are at increased risk for morbidity from varicella infection, the varicella vaccine, a live virus vaccine, should be considered in asymptomatic or mildly symptomatic children in CDC clinical class N1 or A1 with age-specific CD4 percentages $\geq$ 25% [2]. Children should receive two doses of varicella vaccine, 3 months apart. Because vaccinees with impaired cellular immunity may be at increased risk for severe adverse effects from the vaccine, patients should be re-evaluated if they develop a post-vaccination varicella-like rash.

Varicella vaccine can and should be given to susceptible contacts of HIV-infected children [35]. No precautions are needed if the vaccinated contact does not develop a rash. If the vaccinated contact develops a rash, direct contact with susceptible immunocompromised persons should be avoided while the rash is present. However, varicella-zoster immunoglobulin (VZIG) is not indicated in the case of contact with a recent vaccinee.

10.3.16 *Yellow fever vaccine*

While yellow fever vaccine, a live virus vaccine, is not contraindicated in HIV-infected children, there is a theoretical risk of encephalitis in immunosuppressed individuals. If travelling to an endemic area cannot be avoided, patients should be given instructions on avoiding mosquitoes, and asymptomatic HIV-infected persons could be given the option of vaccination [36]. The vaccine is contraindicated for infants under 4 months of age, and ideally vaccination should be postponed until 9–12 months of age.

10.4 Guidelines for immunization in HIV-exposed and HIV-infected infants and children, and their contacts

The US guidelines for immunization in HIV-exposed and -infected infants and their contacts, are shown in Table 10.3.

10.5 Passive immunization

If an HIV-infected patient is directly exposed to a vaccine-preventable disease, he/she should be considered susceptible, regardless of immunization status, and should receive passive immunization. Recommendations for specific diseases follow.

10.5.1 Hepatitis A

Persons who have not been previously immunized with hepatitis A vaccine should be given intramuscular immunoglobulin (IG) if there is recent (less than 2 weeks) exposure to hepatitis A. Such exposures include: (1) household and sexual contacts of patients with serologically confirmed hepatitis A; (2) sharing illicit drugs with someone with serologically confirmed hepatitis A infection; (3) staff and attendees of child care centers/family child care homes if at least one child, one employee, and/or two household contacts of attendees is infected; (4) food handlers working in the same establishment as an hepatitis A-infected food handler [8].

One intramuscular dose of IG (0.02 cm^3/kg) should be given as soon as possible after exposure but not more than 2 weeks after the last exposure. Hepatitis A vaccine can be administered simultaneously with IG.

10.5.2 Hepatitis B

Hepatitis B immunoglobulin (HBIG) should be given to HIV-exposed and -infected children according to the recommended pediatric immunization schedule [1]. Infants with perinatal exposure to Hepatitis B should receive 0.5 cm^3 HBIG within 12 hours of birth concurrently with the first Hepatitis B vaccine. Sexual partners of persons with acute Hepatitis B virus (HBV) infection should receive 0.06 cm^3/kg HBIG and begin the Hepatitis B vaccine series.

Table 10.3 US guidelines for immunization in HIV-exposed and -infected children (and their contacts)

Vaccine	HIV-exposed (infection status indeterminate)	HIV-infected, asymptomatic	HIV-infected, symptomatic	Close contact of HIV-infected individual	Schedule
BCG	No	No	No	No	Not recommended in the US and in areas of low prevalence of tuberculosis; consider in asymptomatic infants in high-prevalence areas
Borrelia burgdorferi (Lyme)	No	No	No	No	Only recommended for persons over 15 years of age who are at high risk of exposure
DTaP/DTP	Yes	Yes	Yes	Yes	2 months, 4 months, 6 months, 12–18 months, 4–6 years
Hepatitis A	If risk factors	If risk factors	If risk factors	If risk factors	Not recommended unless other risk factors (see text)
Hepatitis B	Yes	Yes	Yes	Yes	Birth, 1 month, 6 months
HIB	Yes	Yes	Yes	Yes	2 months, 4 months, 6 months, 12–18 months
Influenza, inactivated	Yes	Yes	Yes	Yes	Each fall after 6 months of age; repeat annually
MMR	Yes	Yes	Yes[a]	Yes	12 months, 1 month after first dose
Plague	No	No	No	No	Not recommended for persons less than 18 year old; only for those at high risk of exposure
Pneumococcal conjugate, 7-valent (PCV-**7**)	Yes	Yes	Yes	Yes	2 months, 4 months, 6 months, 12–15 months
Pneumococcal 23-valent (PPV-23)	N/A	Yes	Yes	No	≥2 years old and ≥2 months after last dose of PCV7; 3–5 years after first dose
Polio, inactivated	Yes	Yes	Yes	Yes	2 months, 4 months, 12–18 months, 4–6 years
Polio, oral	No	No	No	No	
Rabies	Post-exposure	Post-exposure	Post-exposure	Post-exposure	Only for post exposure prophylaxis; days 1, 3, 7, 14, and 28
Rotavirus	No	No	No	No	
Typhoid	No	If travelling to endemic area	If travelling to endemic area	If travelling to endemic area	May be considered if travelling to endemic area. Live, attenuated vaccine should not be given
Varicella	Yes	Yes[b]	No[b]	Yes	At 12 months or older; HIV- positive children receive a 2nd dose 3 months after first dose
Yellow fever	No	If travelling to endemic area	No	Yes	May be considered in asymptomatic persons travelling to endemic areas

[a]MMR should not be given if patient is severely immunocompromised (see text).
[b]Varicella vaccine should be considered in patients in CDC class N-1 and A-1 with age-specific CD-4 percentages ≥ 25% (see text).

HBIG and Hepatitis B vaccination should also be considered when there is direct exposure to blood products that potentially could contain Hepatitis B surface antigen [37].

10.5.3 Measles

Immunoglobulin (IG) should be given within 6 days of exposure. IG should also be given to any measles-susceptible household contacts with asymptomatic HIV infections, especially if they are less than 1 year of age [3]. If the patient has received IVIG within 3 weeks of exposure, IG is not necessary. The dose of IG is:
- Symptomatic HIV-infected: 0.5 mL/kg (maximum 15 mL)
- Asymptomatic HIV-infected or HIV-exposed: 0.25 mL/kg (maximum 15 mL).

10.5.4 Rabies

As in immunocompetent persons, human rabies immunoglobulin (HRIG) should be used concurrently with the first rabies vaccine dose [32]. The recommended dose of HRIG is 20 IU/kg; as much as possible should be used to infiltrate the wound area. The remainder of the dose should be administered intramuscularly using a separate needle and syringe.

10.5.5 Tetanus

As in immunocompetent persons, tetanus immunoglobulin (TIG) should be administered if the patient sustains a tetanus-prone wound (e.g., wounds contaminated with dirt, feces, saliva; puncture wounds; wounds where there is devitalized tissue, such as crush injury, frostbite, or necrosis; bite wounds) [1]. The wound should be thoroughly cleaned and debrided. A dose of 250 units of TIG should be given.

10.5.6 Varicella

Varicella-zoster immunoglobulin should be administered within 96 hours of exposure [1]; VZIG is not necessary if the patient has received IVIG or VZIG within 3 weeks of exposure. The dose of VZIG to be given is one vial (125 units, approximately 1.25 mL)/10 kg, with a minimum 125 units (one vial) and a maximum 625 units (five vials). Patients receiving VZIG are potentially infectious for a period extending from day 8 to day 28 after exposure to infection. Acyclovir may be considered for post-exposure prophylaxis, although data regarding the efficacy in HIV-infected individuals is lacking [5].

10.6 Conclusions

Further research is needed to refine recommendations regarding immunizations in HIV-exposed and HIV-infected children. Assessment of immune response to and clinical efficacy of individual vaccines at the various stages of HIV infection is important in determining specific immunization schedules for HIV-infected children. This should include evaluation of the necessity for booster doses of specific vaccines. In addition, further studies are needed to determine if introduction of antigens via immunization stimulates immune proliferation and adversely affects the clinical course of HIV infection.

REFERENCES

1. Centers for Disease Control and Prevention. Recommendations of the Advisory Committee on Immunization Practices: use of vaccines and immune globulins in persons with altered immunocompetence. *MMWR* **42** : **RR-4** (1993).
2. Centers for Disease Control and Prevention. Prevention of varicella – updated recommendations of the Advisory Committee on Immunization Practices (ACIP). *MMWR* **48** : **RR-6** (1999).
3. Centers for Disease Control and Prevention. Measles, mumps, and rubella – vaccine use and strategies for elimination of measles, rubella, and congenital rubella syndrome and control of mumps: recommendations of the Advisory Committee on Immunization Practices (ACIP). *MMWR* **47** : **RR-8** (1998).
4. Centers for Disease Control and Prevention. The role of BCG vaccine in the prevention and control of tuberculosis in the United States – a joint statement by the Advisory Council for the Elimination of Tuberculosis and the Advisory Committee on Immunization Practices (ACIP). *MMWR* **45** : **RR-4** (1996).
5. Centers for Disease Control and Prevention. 1997 USPHS/IDSA guidelines for the prevention of opportunistic infections in persons infected with human immunodeficiency virus. *MMWR* **46** (1997).
6. Harries, A. D. & Maher, D. *TB/HIV: a Clinical Manual.* Geneva, Switzerland: World Health Organization (1996).
7. World Health Organization. Special Programme on AIDS and expanded programme on immunizations: joint statement – consultation on human immunodeficiency virus (HIV) and routine childhood immunizations. *Wkly. Epidemiol. Rec.* **62** (1987), 297–9.
8. Centers for Disease Control and Prevention. Recommended Childhood and Adolescent Immunization Schedule-United States, 2004. *MMWR* **53** (2004), Q1–4.
9. Centers for Disease Control and Prevention. Prevention of Hepatitis A through active or passive immunization – recommendations of the Advisory Committee on Immunization Practices (ACIP). *MMWR* **48** : **RR-12** (1999).

10. Advisory Committee on Immunization Practices. Prevention and control of influenza – recommendations of the Advisory Committee on Immunization Practices (ACIP). *MMWR* **50**: **RR-4** (2001).

11. O'Brien, W. A., Grovit-Ferbas, K., Namazi, A. *et al.* Human immunodeficiency virus-type 1 replication can be increased in peripheral blood of seropositive patients after influenza vaccination. *Blood* **86** (1995), 1082–9.

12. Ramilo, O., Hicks, P. J., Borvak, J. *et al.* T cell activation and human immunodeficiency virus replication after influenza immunization of infected children. *Pediatr. Infect. Dis. J.* **15** (1996), 197–203.

13. Staprans, S. K., Hamilton, B. L., Follansbee, S. E. *et al.* Activation of virus replication after vaccination of HIV-1 infected individuals. *J. Exp. Med.* **182** (1995), 1727–37.

14. Sullivan, P. S., Hanson, D. L., Dworkin, M. S. *et al.* Effect of influenza vaccination on disease progression among HIV-infected persons. *AIDS* **14** (2000), 2781–5.

15. Kroon, F., van Dissel, J., de Jong, J., Zwinderman, K. & van Furth, R. Antibody response after influenza vaccination in HIV-infected individuals: a consecutive 3-year study. *Vaccine* **18** (2000), 3040–9.

16. King, J. J., Fast, P., Zangwill, K. *et al.* Safety, vaccine virus shedding and immunogenicity of trivalent, cold-adapted, live attenuated influenza vaccine administered to human immunodeficiency virus-infected and noninfected children. *Pediatr. Infect. Dis. J.* **20** (2001), 1124–31.

17. King, J. J., Treanor, J., Fast, P. *et al.* Comparison of the safety, vaccine virus shedding, and immunogenicity of influenza virus vaccine, trivalent, types A and B, live cold-adapted, administered to human immunodeficiency virus (HIV)-infected and non-HIV-infected adults. *J. Infect. Dis.* **181** (2000), 725–8.

18. Centers for Disease Control and Prevention. Using live, attenuated Influenza vaccine for prevention and control of influenza, *MMWR* **52**: **RR-13** (2003).

19. Centers for Disease Control and Prevention, Recommendations for the use of Lyme disease vaccine – recommendations of the Advisory Committee on Immunization Practices (ACIP). *MMWR* **48**: **RR-7** (1999).

20. Angel, J., Udem, S., Snydman, D. *et al.* Measles pneumonitis following measles-mumps-rubella vaccination of a patient with HIV infection, 1993. *MMWR* **45** (1996), 603–6.

21. Monafo, W., Haslam, D., Roberts, R., Zaki, S., Bellini, W. & Coffin, C. Disseminated measles infection after vaccination in a child with a congenital immunodeficiency. *J. Pediatr.* **124** (1994), 273–6.

22. Committee on Infectious Diseases and Committee on Pediatric AIDS, American Academy of Pediatrics. Measles immunization in HIV-infected children. *Pediatrics* **103** (1999), 1057–60.

23. Brunell, P. A., Vimal, V., Sandhu, M., Courville, T. M., Daar, E. & Israele, V. Abnormalities of measles antibody response in human immunodeficiency virus type 1 (HIV-1) infection. *J. AIDS Hum. Retrovirol.* **10** (1995), 540–8.

24. Arpadi, S. M., Markowitz, L. E., Baughman, A. L. *et al.* Measles antibody in vaccinated human immunodeficiency virus type 1-infected children. *Pediatrics* **97** (1996), 653–7.

25. Brena, A. E., Cooper, E. R., Cabral, H. J. & Pelton, S. I. Antibody response to measles and rubella vaccine by children with HIV infection. *J. AIDS* **6** (1993), 1125–9.

26. Centers for Disease Control and Prevention. Prevention of plague – recommendations of the Advisory Committee on Immunization Practices (ACIP). *MMWR* **45**: **RR-14** (1996).

27. Centers for Disease Control and Prevention. Preventing pneumococcal disease among infants and young children – recommendations of the Advisory Committee on Immunization Practices (ACIP). *MMWR* **49**: **RR-9** (2000) .

28. King, J. C., Vink, P. E., Farley, J. J., Smilie, M., Parks, M. & Lichenstein, R. Safety and immunogenicity of three doses of a five-valent pneumococcal conjugate vaccine in children younger than 2 years with and without human immunodeficiency virus infection. *Pediatrics* **99** (1997), 575–80.

29. King, J. C., Vink, P. E. & Farley, J. J. Comparison of the safety and immunogenicity of a pneumococcal conjugate with a licensed polysaccharide vaccine in human immunodeficiency virus and non-human immunodeficiency virus-infected children. *Pediatr. Infect. Dis. J.* **15** (1996), 192–6.

30. Centers for Disease Control and Prevention, Poliomyelitis prevention in the United States – updated recommendations of the Advisory Committee on Immunization Practices (ACIP). *MMWR* **49**: **RR-5** (2000).

31. Technical Consultative Group to the World Health Organization on the Global Eradication of Poliomyelitis. "Endgame" issues for the global poliomyelitis eradication initiative. *Clin. Infect. Dis.* **34** (2002), 72–7.

32. Centers for Disease Control and Prevention. Human rabies prevention – United States, 1999 – recommendations of the Advisory Committee on Immunization Practices (ACIP). *MMWR* **48**: **RR-1** (1999).

33. Centers for Disease Control and Prevention. Rotavirus vaccine for the prevention of Rotavirus gastroenteritis among children – recommendations of the Advisory Committee on Immunization Practices (ACIP). *MMWR* **48**: **RR-2** (1999).

34. Centers for Disease Control and Prevention. Typhoid immunization – recommendations of the Advisory Committee on Immunization Practices (ACIP). *MMWR* **43**: **RR-14** (1994).

35. Centers for Disease Control and Prevention. Update: vaccine side effects, adverse reactions, contraindications, and precautions – recommendations of the Advisory Committee on Immunization Practices (ACIP). *MMWR* **45**: **RR-12** (1996).

36. Centers for Disease Control and Prevention. Health information for international travellers 2001–2002. Atlanta: US Department of Health and Human Services, Public Health Service (2001).

37. Centers for Disease Control and Prevention. Hepatitis B virus: a comprehensive strategy for eliminating transmission in the United States through universal childhood vaccination: recommendations of the Advisory Committee on Immunization Practices (ACIP). *MMWR* **40** (1991).

Prevention of opportunistic infections and other infectious complications of HIV in children

Russell B. Van Dyke, M.D.

Department of Pediatrics, Tulane University Health Sciences Center, New Orleans, LA

11.1 Introduction

AIDS was first recognized in 1981 when an unusual clustering of cases of *Pneumocystis carinii* pneumonia (PCP) occurred among young homosexual men in Southern California, USA. Subsequently, other opportunistic infections were identified in this population, including disseminated mycobacterial infections, toxoplasmosis, and cytomegalovirus retinitis. Soon thereafter, these same opportunistic infections were identified in children. The occurrence of this group of distinctive opportunistic infections remains central to the definition of AIDS. The recognition that HIV-infected individuals are at increased risk for certain specific opportunistic pathogens has stimulated the development of strategies to prevent these infections.

For most HIV-associated opportunistic infections, the risk of infection is correlated with the patient's degree of immunosuppression. Thus, guidelines for initiating prophylaxis are generally based upon the number of circulating CD4$^+$ lymphocytes in the peripheral blood. The normal CD4$^+$ lymphocyte count is substantially higher in infants than in older children and adults, with normal values decreasing over the first few years of life. However, the normal percentage of CD4$^+$ lymphocyte is relatively independent of age. This is reflected in the immune categories of the CDC classification system for HIV infections in children [1] (Table 11.1). Thus, a child of any age with a percentage of CD4$^+$ lymphocytes of less than 15% is considered severely immunosuppressed and a candidate for PCP prophylaxis. In addition, infants have a less effective cellular immune response than do older children (see Chapter 1). Thus, a CD4$^+$ lymphocyte count of 600 cells/μL is normal in an adolescent but represents severe immunosuppression in a 6-month-old infant.

Highly active antiretroviral therapy (HAART) often results in a dramatic increase in the CD4$^+$ lymphocyte count and a decrease in the risk of opportunistic infections. This has led to a dramatic fall in the mortality from AIDS in the USA [2]. Thus, the most effective means of preventing opportunistic infections is to aggressively treat the underlying HIV infection in order to maintain a normal CD4$^+$ lymphocyte count. However, viral resistance or poor adherence to therapy can result in a failure of HAART, leading to a fall in the CD4$^+$ lymphocyte count over time. Thus, it is likely that in the future there will be an increase in the number of opportunistic infections among patients who fail HAART. Certain infections, such as pneumonia, sinusitis, and herpes zoster, occur in HIV-infected children who are not severely immunosuppressed and these are likely to remain common despite HAART.

A number of studies in adults have demonstrated that prophylaxis against PCP, toxoplasmosis, and *Mycobacterium avium* complex (MAC) can be safely discontinued once a patient responds to HAART with a sustained increase in their CD4$^+$ lymphocyte count [3]. There are no data on the safety of discontinuing prophylaxis in children at this time, but many authorities have extrapolated the adult data to children. Currently, a number of studies in adults and children are attempting to characterize the immune reconstitution that results from HAART. Questions such as the need for re-immunization with the childhood vaccines following immune reconstitution remain to be answered.

In both children and adults, PCP remains one of the most commonly reported AIDS-defining diagnoses

Table 11.1 Centers for Disease Control and Prevention immunologic classification of HIV infection in children less than 13 years of age

Immunologic categories	CD4+ lymphocyte count (cells/μL) CD4%		
	< 12 months	1–5 years	6–12 years
1. No evidence of suppression	≥ 1500 ≥ 25%	≥ 1000 ≥ 25%	≥ 500 ≥ 25%
2. Moderate suppression	750–1499 15–24%	500–999 15–24%	200–499 15–24%
3. Severe suppression	< 750 < 15%	< 500 < 15%	< 200 < 15%

Source: Centers for Disease Control and Prevention. *MMWR* **43: RR-12** (1994), 1–10. [1]

[4]. Other common opportunistic infections in children include chronic and recurrent mucosal and esophageal candidiasis, cytomegalovirus infections, non-tuberculous mycobacteria (principally MAC), *Cryptosporidium* enteritis, herpes zoster, and mucocutaneous herpes simplex virus [5] (Table 11.2). HIV-infected children are also at increased risk of common childhood infections such as otitis media, sinusitis, viral respiratory infections, bacterial pneumonia, bacteremia, gastroenteritis, and meningitis.

The remainder of this chapter will focus on selected important infections occurring in HIV-infected children, emphasizing approaches to prevent acquisition of the organism, including chemoprophylaxis. Even when it is not possible to completely suppress HIV replication and maintain a normal CD4+ lymphocyte count, careful attention to opportunistic infection prophylaxis in HIV-infected children can significantly reduce morbidity and mortality. Comprehensive guidelines for the prevention of opportunistic infections in children and adults have been published, as have guidelines for the treatment of opportunistic infections in children [6–7]. These are available on the internet (http://www.hivatis.org/trtgdlns.html) and are updated on a regular basis. They should be consulted for the most up-to-date information.

11.2 *Pneumocystis carinii* pneumonia

Pneumocystis carinii pneumonia remains one of the most common opportunistic infections in HIV-infected children (Table 11.2) (see Chapter 4.2). Prior to the availability of HAART, PCP was the presenting diagnosis in 61% of

Table 11.2 Incidence of opportunistic infections in HIV-infected children in the pre-HAART era (1988–1998)

	Event rate (per 1000 patient years)
Serious bacterial infections	151
Herpes zoster	29
Disseminated *Mycobacterium avium* complex	18
Pneumocystis carinii pneumonia	13
Candidiasis	12
Cryptosporidiosis	6
Cytomegalovirus retinitis	5
Tuberculosis	4
Cytomegalovirus, other than retinitis	2
Fungal, other than Candida	1
Toxoplasmosis	0.6
Progressive multifocal leukoencephalopathy	0.6

Source: [5].

children who were diagnosed with AIDS in the first year of life. In contrast, 19% of older children presented with PCP as their AIDS-defining illness [8]. In childhood, the incidence of PCP peaks at age 4–5 months of age, substantially earlier than do other opportunistic infections. The risk of PCP in the first year of life is 7–20% for HIV-infected infants not receiving PCP prophylaxis.

Pneumocystis carinii pneumonia often progresses rapidly in young infants, with a mortality as high as 50%. The aggressive nature of the infection results from an impaired cellular immune response at this age, in concert with a lack of prior experience with the organism. In adults, PCP generally represents reactivation disease. However, PCP in infancy is likely to result from a primary infection, with the lack of prior immunity to the organism contributing to the severity of the infection.

The epidemiology of *Pneumocystis carinii* is poorly understood. The organism infects a wide range of mammals, including rodents, where it grows in the respiratory tract. However, the strains which infect animals probably do not infect humans. In animals, infection results from airborne transmission. It is unknown whether there is an environmental reservoir of the organism. In humans, asymptomatic infection occurs early in life, with most children having antibody by 4 years of age. There are no effective measures to prevent exposure to the organism.

Table 11.3 Prophylaxis to prevent first episode of opportunistic disease among infants and children infected with human immunodeficiency virus

Pathogen	Indication	Preventive regimen	
		First choice	Alternative
1. Strongly recommended as standard of care			
Pneumocystis carinii[a]	HIV-infected or HIV-indeterminate, infants aged 1–12 months; HIV-infected children aged 1–5 years with CD4$^+$ count of $<$ 500/μL or CD4$^+$ percentages of $<$15%; HIV-infected children aged 6–12 years with CD4$^+$ count of $<$ 200/μL or CD4$^+$ percentages of $<$ 15%	Trimethoprim–sulfamethoxazole (TMP-SMX), 150/750 mg/m^2/day in two divided doses by mouth three times weekly on consecutive days (AII); acceptable alternative dosage schedules: (AII) single dose by mouth three times weekly on consecutive days; two divided doses by mouth daily; or two divided doses by mouth three times weekly on alternate days	Dapsone (children aged $\geq$1 month), 2 mg/kg body weight (max 100 mg) by mouth daily or 4 mg/kg body weight (max 200 mg) by mouth weekly (CII); aerosolized pentamidine (children aged $\geq$ 5 years), 300 mg every month via Respirgard II™ (manufactured by Marquest, Englewood, Colorado) nebulizer (CIII); atovaquone (children aged 1–3 months and $>$24 months, 30 mg/kg body weight by mouth daily; children aged 4–24 months, 45 mg/ kg body weight by mouth daily) (CII)
Mycobacterium tuberculosis Isoniazid-sensitive	Tuberculin skin test (TST) reaction, $\geq$ 5 mm or prior positive TST result without treatment; or contact with any person with active tuberculosis, regardless of TST result	Isoniazid, 10–15 mg/kg body weight (max 300 mg) by mouth daily for 9 mos (AII); or 20–30 mg/kg body weight (max 900 mg) by mouth twice weekly for 9 months (BII)	Rifampin, 10–20 mg/kg body weight (max 600 mg) by mouth daily for 4–6 months (BIII)
Isoniazid-resistant	Same as previous pathogen; increased probability of exposure to isoniazid-resistant tuberculosis	Rifampin, 10–20 mg/kg body weight (max 600 mg) by mouth daily for 4–6 months (BIII)	Uncertain
Multidrug-resistant (isoniazid and rifampin)	Same as previous pathogen; increased probability of exposure to multidrug-resistant tuberculosis	Choice of drugs requires consultation with public health authorities and depends on susceptibility of isolate from source patient	–
Mycobacterium avium complex[b]	For children aged $\geq$ 6 years with CD4$^+$ count of $<$ 50/μL; aged 2–6 years with CD4$^+$ count of $<$ 75/μL; aged 1–2 years with CD4$^+$ count of $<$ 500/μL; aged $<$ 1 year with CD4$^+$ count of $<$ 750/μL	Clarithromycin, 7.5 mg/kg body weight (max 500 mg) by mouth twice daily (AII), or azithromycin, 20 mg/kg body weight (max 1200 mg) by mouth weekly (AII)	Azithromycin, 5 mg/kg body weight (max 250 mg) by mouth daily (AII); children aged $\geq$ 6 years, rifabutin, 300 mg by mouth daily (BI)

(cont.)

Table 11.3 (*cont.*)

Pathogen	Indication	Preventive regimen	
		First choice	Alternative
Varicella-zoster virus[c]	Substantial exposure to varicella or shingles with no history of chickenpox or shingles	Varicella zoster immuno-globulin (VZIG), 1 vial (1.25 mL)/10 kg body weight (max 5 vials) intramuscularly, administered ≤ 96 hours after exposure, ideally in ≤48 hours (AII)	–
Vaccine-preventable pathogens[d]	HIV exposure/infection	Routine immunizations (see Chapter 10)	–
2. Usually recommended			
Toxoplasma gondii[e]	Immunoglobulin G (IgG) antibody to *Toxoplasma* and severe immunosuppression	TMP–SMX, 150/750 mg/m²/day in two divided doses by mouth daily (BIII)	Dapsone (children aged ≥1 mos), 2 mg/kg body weight or 15 mg/m² (max 25 mg) by mouth daily plus pyrimethamine, 1 mg/kg body weight by mouth daily plus leucovorin, 5 mg by mouth every 3 days (BIII); atovaquone, children aged 1–3 months and >24 months, 30 mg/kg body weight by mouth daily; children aged 14–24 months, 45 mg/kg body weight by mouth daily (CIII)
Varicella-zoster virus	HIV-infected children who are asymptomatic and not immunosuppressed	Varicella zoster vaccine (see Chapter 10) (BII)	–
Influenza virus	All patients, annually, before influenza season	Inactivated split trivalent influenza vaccine (see Chapter 10) (BIII)	Oseltamivir (during outbreaks of influenza A or B) for children aged ≥13 years, 75 mg by mouth daily (CIII); rimantadine or amantadine (during out-breaks of influenza A), children aged 1–9 yrs, 5 mg/kg body weight in 2 divided doses (max 150 mg/day) by mouth daily; children aged ≥10 years, use adult doses (CIII)

3. Not recommended for the majority of children; indicated for use only in unusual circumstances

Invasive bacterial infections[f]	Hypogammaglobulinemia (i.e., IgG <400 mg/dL)	Intravenous immunoglobulin (400 mg/kg body weight every 2–4 weeks) (AI)	–
Cryptococcus neoformans	Severe immunosuppression	Fluconazole, 3–6 mg/kg body weight by mouth daily (CII)	Itraconazole, 2–5 mg/kg body weight by mouth every 12–24 hours (CII)
Histoplasma capsulatum	Severe immunosuppression, endemic geographic area	Itraconazole, 2–5 mg/kg body weight by mouth every 12–24 hours (CIII)	–
Cytomegalovirus (CMV)[g]	CMV antibody positivity and severe immunosuppression	Oral ganciclovir, 30 mg/kg body weight by mouth three times daily (CII)	–

Adapted from [6] (Centers for Disease Control and Prevention. *MMWR* **51** : RR-8 (2002))

Notes: Information included in these guidelines might not represent Food and Drug Administration (FDA) approval or approved labeling for products or indications. Specifically, the terms *safe* and *effective* might not be synonymous with the FDA-defined legal standards for product approval. Letters and Roman numerals in parentheses after regimens indicate the strength of the recommendation and the quality of the evidence supporting it (see Ref. #6).

[a] Daily TMP–SMX reduces the frequency of certain bacterial infections. Apparently, TMP–SMX, dapsone-pyrimethamine, and possibly atovaquone (with or without pyrimethamine) protect against toxoplasmosis, although data have not been prospectively collected. When compared with weekly dapsone, daily dapsone is associated with lower incidence of *Pneumocystis carinii* pneumonia (PCP) but higher hematologic toxicity and mortality (*Source:* McIntosh K, Cooper E, Xu J, *et al.* Toxicity and efficacy of daily vs. weekly dapsone for prevention of *Pneumocystis carinii* pneumonia in children infected with human immunodeficiency virus. ACTG 179 Study Team. AIDS Clinical Trials Group. *Pediatr. Infect. Dis. J.* **18** (1999), 432–9). The efficacy of parenteral pentamidine (e.g., 4 mg/kg body weight every 2–4 weeks) is controversial. Patients receiving therapy for toxoplasmosis with sulfadiazine-pyrimethamine are protected against PCP and do not need TMP–SMX.

[b] Substantial drug interactions can occur between rifamycins (i.e., rifampin and rifabutin) and protease inhibitors and non-nucleoside reverse transcriptase inhibitors. A specialist should be consulted.

[c] Children routinely being administered intravenous immunoglobulin (IVIG) should receive varicella–zoster immunoglobulin (VZIG) if the last dose of IVIG was administered > 21 days before exposure.

[d] HIV-infected and exposed children should be immunized according to the childhood immunization schedule (see [6] and Chapter 10), which has been adapted from the January–December 2001 schedule recommended for immunocompetent children by the Advisory Committee on Immunization Practices, the American Academy of Pediatrics, and the American Academy of Family Physicians. This schedule differs from that for immunocompetent children in that both the conjugate pneumococcal vaccine (PCV-7) and the pneumococcal polysaccharide vaccine (PPV-23) are recommended (BII) and vaccination against influenza (BIII) should be offered. Measles, mumps, and rubella should not be administered to severely immunocompromised children (DIII). Vaccination against varicella is indicated only for asymptomatic nonimmunosuppressed children (BII). After an HIV-exposed child is determined not to be HIV-infected, the schedule for immunocompetent children applies.

[e] Protection against toxoplasmosis is provided by the preferred antipneumocystis regimens and possibly by atovaquone. Atovaquone can be used with or without pyrimethamine. Pyrimethamine alone probably provides limited, if any, protection (for definition of severe immunosuppression, see Table 11.1).

[f] Respiratory syncytial virus (RSV) IVIG (750 mg/kg body weight), not monoclonal RSV antibody, can be substituted for IVIG during the RSV season to provide broad anti-infective protection, if this product is available.

[g] Oral ganciclovir and perhaps valganciclovir results in reduced CMV shedding among CMV-infected children. Acyclovir is not protective against CMV.

Antimicrobial prophylaxis is very effective in preventing PCP. Although the principal risk factor for PCP is a decreased CD4$^+$ lymphocyte count, there are several issues to consider when recommending prophylaxis for infants and children. First, as mentioned previously, guidelines for initiating prophylaxis must be based on age-adjusted CD4$^+$ lymphocyte counts [9] (Table 11.3). Second, the CD4$^+$ lymphocyte count of HIV-infected children can fall rapidly in the first year of life with rapid progression of their HIV disease, and PCP can develop before a decrease in the CD4$^+$ lymphocyte count is recognized. Consequently, a child may develop PCP before he is known to be HIV-infected [8]. Thus, in the first year of life, PCP prophylaxis should not be limited to only those children with a documented HIV infection or a decreased CD4$^+$ lymphocyte count. Instead, all infants born to an HIV-infected mother should receive PCP prophylaxis.

Because PCP rarely occurs before 3 months of age, initiation of PCP prophylaxis in HIV-exposed infants can be safely delayed until 6–8 weeks of age, following discontinuation of antiretroviral prophylaxis. This will help to avoid neutropenia which can result from concomitant administration of ZDV and trimethoprim-sulfamethoxazole (TMP–SMX). Once a child is known to be HIV-uninfected, PCP prophylaxis can be discontinued (see Chapter 4.2). Indications for prophylaxis in children over 1 year of age are based upon the CD4$^+$ lymphocyte values (Table 11.3). The decision to continue prophylaxis in an infected child over the age of 1 year who no longer meets criteria for prophylaxis should be made on an individual basis. PCP prophylaxis should also be considered for any HIV-infected child with a rapidly falling CD4$^+$ lymphocyte count.

The drug of choice for PCP prophylaxis is TMP–SMX (Table 11.3). For children who are co-infected with *Toxoplasma gondii*, TMP–SMX is also effective in preventing toxoplasmosis. However, as many as 15% of children are intolerant to TMP–SMX; adverse reactions include rash, fever, neutropenia, anemia, and, rarely, the Stevens–Johnson syndrome. Neutropenia is particularly troublesome in children receiving both TMP–SMX and zidovudine. In adults, the gradual introduction of TMP–SMX in an escalating dose over the first 14 days of therapy reduces the rate of initial adverse reactions [10]. If an adverse reaction is not life-threatening, re-challenge with TMP–SMX is successful in 57–75% of adults. Gradual reintroduction over 1–2 weeks is more likely to be successful than direct re-challenge with the full dose [11]. Successful gradual reintroduction has been reported in a small number of children [12]. If a child develops an adverse reaction to TMP–SMX, the medication should be discontinued. Once the symptoms resolve, if the reaction was not life-threatening, TMP–SMX can be

Table 11.4 Dose escalation of TMP/SMP following resolution of a non life-threatening adverse event

Day	Proportion of full daily dose (%)	Dose (mg/m^2)	Dosing frequency
1	12.5	18.75/93.75	q.d.
2	25	18.75/93.75	b.i.d.
3	37.5	18.75/93.75	t.i.d.
4	50	37.5/187.5	b.i.d.
5	75	37.5/187.5	t.i.d.
6	100	75/375	b.i.d

Note: An antihistamine should be administered during the dose escalation.
Adapted from [11].

gradually reintroduced. This is sometimes termed 'oral desensitization' (Table 11.4). The concomitant use of an antihistamine is recommended. Addition of a nonsteroidal anti-inflammatory agent or corticosteroids may be considered during the reintroduction and for any reactions which develop during ongoing treatment.

Alternatives for PCP prophylaxis in children who cannot tolerate TMP–SMX include dapsone, atovaquone, and pentamidine (Table 11.3). In adults, dapsone, atovaquone, and aerosolized pentamidine have similar efficacy [13, 14]. Dapsone has been shown to be effective in preventing PCP in children. Toxicities include hemolytic anemia, methemoglobinemia, and skin rash [15]. Hematological toxicity is more frequent in children with daily dosing (2 mg/kg/day) than weekly dosing (4 mg/kg/week), although there may be a higher rate of PCP with weekly dosing [16]. Currently, dapsone is not available in a liquid preparation.

Atovaquone is a broad-spectrum antiprotozoan agent with demonstrated efficacy against *P. carinii* and *T. gondii*. Potential advantages of atovaquone include a long half-life, low toxicity, activity against *T. gondii*, and the ability to kill *P. carinii* in an animal model where pentamidine and TMP–SMX only suppress growth of the organism. Atovaquone is well tolerated by children, with mild anemia the principal adverse event. Pharmacokinetic data for the micronized liquid formulation in children has led to an unusual dosing schema (Table 11.3) [17].

Intravenous pentamidine has been commonly used for prophylaxis in young children, despite the lack of efficacy data. Toxicity is common, frequently leading to discontinuation of the drug. The principal adverse events are nephrotoxicity and hypoglycemia. Hypotension, occasionally resulting in death, has been reported with rapid infusions; it is recommended that the drug be infused over 1–2 hours. Less common adverse events include leukopenia, thrombocytopenia, nausea, vomiting, abdominal pain, anorexia, and a bad taste. The dose is 4 mg/kg/dose IV every 2–4 weeks.

The efficacy of aerosolized pentamidine is established in adults, while data in children are lacking [18, 19]. Aerosol delivery does not provide protection against extrapulmonary *P. carinii*, which has been reported in adults receiving aerosol prophylaxis. Sites of involvement include the spleen, lymph nodes, liver, bone marrow, eyes, gastrointestinal tract, thyroid, adrenal glands, and kidney. Older children (generally those 5 years of age or older) can be taught to receive aerosolized pentamidine, and treatment of children as young as 8 months of age has been reported [20]. The principal toxicity of aerosolized pentamidine is irritation of the airways, with cough and wheezing commonly observed. Pre-treatment with a beta-2 agonist may prevent wheezing. In adolescents and adults, the resulting cough can lead to the transmission of unrecognized pulmonary tuberculosis.

Adults who have responded to HAART with an increase in their CD4$^+$ lymphocyte count to greater than 200 cells/μL can safely stop PCP prophylaxis [21, 22]. It is recommended that patients' CD4$^+$ lymphocyte counts be maintained above 200 cells/μL for at least 3 months and that patients have at least partial suppression of their HIV viral load before PCP prophylaxis is discontinued. If the CD4$^+$ lymphocyte count subsequently falls to below 200 cells/μL, then prophylaxis should be restarted. Although the safety of discontinuing PCP prophylaxis in children has not been established, many authorities will discontinue prophylaxis if a child responds to HAART therapy with a sustained suppression in HIV viral load and an increase in CD4$^+$ lymphocytes to CDC immunologic category 1 or 2 for at least 3–6 months.

11.3 Toxoplasmosis

Encephalitis caused by *Toxoplasma gondii* is uncommon in HIV-infected children in the USA. The major route of acquisition of *T. gondii* in children is in utero acquisition from a mother with a primary infection during the pregnancy. In rare cases, an HIV-infected woman with an old *T. gondii* infection can transmit *T. gondii* to the fetus in utero. Congenital toxoplasmosis is uncommon in the USA, with an incidence estimated to be between 1/1000 and 1/12 000 live births. It is not known if the risk of congenital toxoplasmosis is increased among children born to HIV-infected pregnant women. Appropriate management of HIV-infected women, with serologic testing for *T. gondii* and prophylaxis and therapy as appropriate, will prevent congenital toxoplasmosis. Trimethoprim-sulfamethoxazole can be safely administered during pregnancy and is active in preventing reactivation of *T. gondii*. HIV-infected women with a primary *T. gondii* infection or active reactivation disease during pregnancy should receive treatment, in consultation with a specialist in treating toxoplasmosis during pregnancy. Infants born to women infected with both HIV and *T. gondii* should be evaluated for congenital toxoplasmosis.

Older children and adults acquire toxoplasmosis by ingesting cysts in poorly cooked meat, ingesting sporulated oocysts in contaminated food or water, or from contact with infected cats and their feces (e.g. in litter boxes). HIV-infected individuals should avoid eating undercooked meat; meat should be cooked until it is no longer pink inside. Hands should be washed after handling raw meat and after gardening; raw fruits and vegetables should be well washed before eaten raw. Domestic cats are commonly infected with *Toxoplasma*. If the family owns a cat, the litter box should be changed daily, before excreted oocysts have had time to sporulate. Hand washing is essential, and it is best for HIV-infected persons and all pregnant women to avoid changing a litter box. Families need not part with their cat or have the cat tested for *T. gondii*, but should be aware of the risk of cat ownership.

HIV-infected children who are severely immunosuppressed (CDC Immunological Category 3) and infected with *T. gondii* should receive prophylaxis against both toxoplasmosis and PCP. Trimethoprim-sulfamethoxazole, when administered for PCP prophylaxis, also provides prophylaxis against toxoplasmosis. Atovaquone might also provide protection against toxoplasmosis. The child who does not meet criteria for PCP prophylaxis is at low risk for toxoplasmosis and prophylaxis is not necessary. HIV-infected children who meet criteria for PCP prophylaxis, but who are receiving an agent other than TMP–SMX or atovaquone, are not receiving adequate prophylaxis against toxoplasmosis. Therefore, they should have serologic testing for *T. gondii* performed on an annual basis, starting at 12 months of age, to determine if they are infected with *T. gondii*. If seropositive for *T. gondii*, they should receive prophylaxis for both PCP and toxoplasmosis. If the child cannot tolerate TMP–SMX, then atovaquone or dapsone/pyrimethamine/leucovorin are recommended (Table 11.3).

11.4 Cryptosporidium and microsporidiosis

Cryptosporidium parvum, a protozoan, is a common cause of self-limited watery diarrhea in normal infants and children. Transmission is by fecal-oral spread, and outbreaks of *C. parvum* infection are frequent in the day care setting [23]. Large outbreaks in metropolitan areas have resulted from contaminated drinking water and several outbreaks have been associated with public swimming pools. Other sources of infection include contact with infected adults and children, lake and river water, contaminated foods, and young household pets. In children with advanced HIV infection, cryptosporidiosis is characterized by severe and protracted diarrhea with abdominal pain and anorexia. The infection may result in substantial weight loss and even death. The stools are watery in consistency and may contain mucus but lack blood or inflammatory cells. Patients with advanced immunosuppression have protracted infections which rarely clear without immune reconstitution [24]. *Cryptosporidium parvum* has been implicated as a cause of sclerosing cholangitis in HIV-infected persons [25].

Children with severe immunodeficiency should avoid exposure to potential sources of *C. parvum*. Hand washing is recommended following possible exposure. Families may choose to avoid having their child drink tap water; boiling water for one minute will reduce the risk of infection. Drinking bottled water and the use of a submicron personal-use water filter may also reduce the risk of infection; effective filtering of commercial bottled water should be confirmed. Filters should remove particles of one micrometer in diameter in order to remove oocysts. (For detailed information on bottled water and water filters, consult the USPHS/IDSA guidelines [6].)

The most effective means to prevent cryptosporidiosis is to avoid immunosuppression with effective antiretroviral therapy. Chemoprophylaxis for *C. parvum* infection is not recommended. Clarithromycin and rifabutin, when used for MAC prophylaxis, may prevent the development of cryptosporidiosis [26]. This benefit is not seen with azithromycin. However, there are insufficient data to recommend use of these drugs solely to prevent cryptosporidiosis.

Microsporidia is a group of protozoa that causes acute and chronic diarrhea in HIV-infected persons. Infections in humans are zoonotic or waterborne. The incidence of microsporidiosis has declined dramatically with effective antiretroviral therapy. Handwashing and other personal hygiene measures are the only effective means to prevent exposure. Chemoprophylaxis is not available.

11.5 Tuberculosis

The risk of reactivation of latent tuberculosis (TB) is high in HIV-infected individuals (see Chapter 38). Children generally acquire TB from exposure to an infected adult in their immediate environment. A child living in a household with an HIV-infected person is at high risk of being exposed to tuberculosis whether or not the child is HIV-infected. Thus, the incidence of TB disease in HIV-exposed or -infected children in the USA is 10–100 times that of the general population of similar age [27]. The risk is substantially higher in developing countries where tuberculosis is more common. The risk of acquired TB is independent of the child's immune status. The most effective means of preventing TB exposure in children is to identify and treat all adults with TB in the child's environment.

All children born to HIV-infected mothers and all children living in a household with HIV should have a tuberculin skin test (TST, 5-TU PPD) at or before 9–12 months of age, which should be repeated at least annually. In addition, all newly diagnosed HIV-infected children and adolescents should have annual testing. In this setting, 10 mm or more of induration is considered a positive TST. If the child is HIV-infected, has a known TB exposure, or has clinical or radiographic findings compatible with tuberculosis, induration of 5 mm or more is considered a positive test. If the TST is positive, the child should be evaluated for active tuberculosis, including chest radiography. If no evidence of active disease is found, the child should be treated for latent TB. Children living in a household with a TST-positive person should be evaluated for TB. If the child is exposed to a person with active TB, he/she should be treated for latent TB once active disease has been excluded, regardless of the result of their own TST. In HIV-infected children, 9–12 months of isoniazid is recommended for treatment of latent TB unless the child is suspected to be infected with a resistant organism (Table 11.3). Directly observed therapy should be utilized if available (see Chapter 42).

11.6 Disseminated *Mycobacterium avium* complex

Infections with environmental mycobacteria are common in patients with advanced HIV infection (see Chapter 39). More than 85% of these infections are due to the *Mycobacterium avium* complex (MAC). *Mycobacterium avium* complex rarely develops in adults with a CD4$^+$ lymphocyte count greater than 50 cells/μL. An excellent review of this group of organisms has been published [28].

Without prophylaxis, between 10–18% of children with AIDS develop MAC [29, 30]. Prior to the availability of HAART, MAC occurred in children at a rate of 18 cases/1000 patient years (Table 11.2). *Mycobacterium avium* complex is rare in the first year of life but becomes more common with increasing age and decreasing CD4$^+$ lymphocyte count. Among pediatric cases reported to the CDC, the mean age of MAC diagnosis was 3.3 years for children with perinatally acquired HIV infection and 8.7 years for children with transfusion-associated HIV infection [31]. The median CD4+ lymphocyte count in children with MAC was 17 cells/μL, with 70% of children having fewer than 50 cells/μL. However, among children younger than 24 months, MAC occurs at substantially higher CD4+ lymphocyte counts [32]. Members of the *Mycobacterium avium* complex are common in the environment, and are often present in food and water. Person-to-person transmission is not documented. There are no effective means to prevent exposure.

Prophylaxis of disseminated MAC is recommended for children with advanced HIV disease, based upon CD4+ criteria (Table 11.3). Studies in adults have demonstrated the efficacy of rifabutin, clarithromycin, and azithromycin [33–35]. Clarithromycin or azithromycin are the preferred agents. They each also provide some protection against bacterial infections. Rifabutin is associated with many complex drug interactions and its use should be avoided unless a macrolide cannot be used. The combination of clarithromycin and rifabutin should be avoided since it is no more effective than clarithromycin alone and has a higher rate of adverse events than either drug alone [36]. The combination of azithromycin and rifabutin has enhanced efficacy, but frequent drug interactions and lack of a survival benefit argue against its routine use. The safety of discontinuing MAC prophylaxis with immunologic reconstitution following HAART has been demonstrated in adults. In adults, it is recommended that prophylaxis be stopped with an increase in the CD4+ lymphocyte count to greater than 100 cells/μL for at least 3 months [6].

Mycobacterium avium complex prophylaxis has not been evaluated in children. However, based on adult studies, either clarithromycin (7.5 mg/kg/dose [max 500 mg] po bid) or azithromycin (20 mg/kg/dose [max 1200 mg] once weekly) is recommended. The criteria for initiating prophylaxis are based on the CD4+ lymphocyte count (Table 11.3). Before initiating prophylaxis, the patient should be evaluated for active MAC infection, including a blood culture for MAC if symptoms are present, since monotherapy will rapidly lead to drug resistance if infection is present. Although the safety of discontinuing prophylaxis has not been demonstrated in children, many authorities will stop therapy once a child has a sustained increase in the CD4+ lymphocyte count to CDC Immunologic Category 1 or 2 and no longer qualifies for prophylaxis.

Drug interactions are an important consideration when initiating MAC prophylaxis. Clarithromycin is metabolized by the hepatic cytochrome P450 system (CYP3A) (see Chapter 19). While protease inhibitors can increase clarithromycin blood concentrations, dose adjustments are not required. Efavirenz can induce the metabolism of clarithromycin, decreasing the serum concentration and increasing the concentration of the 14-OH clarithromycin, an active metabolite. It is not known whether this reduces the efficacy of clarithromycin. Azithromycin is not metabolized by the cytochrome P450 system, so its metabolism is not altered by antiretroviral therapy. Rifabutin should not be administered to patients receiving certain protease inhibitors and non-nucleoside reverse transcriptase inhibitors because of complex drug interactions which are not well understood [37, 38].

11.7 Bacterial pneumonia, bacteremia, and other invasive bacterial infections

HIV-infected children are at increased risk for common childhood infections such as otitis media and sinusitis. Recurrent sinusitis can be problematic in some children. In addition, HIV-infected children have frequent invasive bacterial infections, including pneumonia, bacteremia, and meningitis (Table 11.2). The organisms causing these infections are generally the same as for normal children, with *Streptococcus pneumoniae* the predominant pathogen [39, 40]. These organisms are common in the community and there is no effective way to limit exposure to them.

All HIV-infected children should be vaccinated with the conjugate *Haemophilus influenzae* type b vaccine and the conjugate polyvalent pneumococcal vaccine according to current guidelines [6]. In addition, all should receive the 23-valent polysaccharide pneumococcal vaccine (PPV) at 24 months of age. A second dose of the PPV should be administered after 3–5 years to children less than 10 years of age, and after 5 years in older children. All HIV-infected children should receive the influenza vaccine yearly starting at 6 months of age [6] (see Chapter 10).

The use of TMP–SMX for PCP prophylaxis results in a reduction in the risk of bacterial infections. There may be an advantage to using daily dosing (150/750 mg/m^2 per day in two divided doses) in children with recurrent infections. Trimethoprim-sulfamethoxazole prophylaxis will not prevent all pneumococcal infections, since the majority of penicillin-resistant strains are also resistant to TMP–SMX. Other antibiotics may be considered for prophylaxis in individual cases, recognizing the risk of promoting drug-resistance with antibiotic prophylaxis.

Monthly infusions of intravenous immunoglobulin (IVIG) (400 mg/kg/dose q month) are effective in preventing recurrent bacterial infections in selected children [39, 40]. (Table 11.3). HIV-infected children have functional hypogammaglobulinemia, despite having elevated immunoglobulin levels. Because of the cost, risk of complications, and discomfort associated with IVIG infusions, the use of IVIG is generally limited to the following indications [7]:

1. Children who experience recurrent bacterial infections despite appropriate antimicrobial prophylaxis and therapy. In children with hypogammaglobulinemia, it may be reasonable to initiate IVIG infusions without attempting antimicrobial prophylaxis. Intravenous immunoglobulin may not provide additional benefit to children receiving daily TMP–SMX prophylaxis [40].

2. Children living in a region with a high prevalence of measles, without detectable antibody to measles despite receiving two measles immunizations.

3. HIV-associated thrombocytopenia (platelet count $< 20\,000/mm^3$ while receiving antiretroviral therapy) (see Chapter 32).

4. HIV-infected children with chronic bronchiectasis who fail to respond to antibiotics and pulmonary care may respond to high-dose IVIG (600 mg/kg/month).

11.8 Bartonellosis

Bartonella henselae is the cause of cat-scratch disease. Severely immunosuppressed HIV-infected persons are at high risk for developing disease caused by infection with *Bartonella*, including bacillary angiomatosis. Cats are the reservoir for human disease, with cats less than 1 year of age most likely to transmit infection. Cat scratches and saliva are believed to be the principal sources of infection. Fleas transmit the organism between cats and may occasionally transmit infection to humans. *Bartonella* infection is very common in cats and serologic testing of cats is not recommended.

HIV-infected children who are severely immunosuppressed should avoid exposure to cats, particularly cats less than 1 year of age. Families should be aware of the risk of cat ownership. Declawing is not advised, but children should avoid rough play with cats, which could result in a bite or scratch. Cats should not be allowed to lick open wounds, and cat-associated wounds should be washed promptly. Families should practice good flea control of cats. Chemoprophylaxis is not recommended.

11.9 Candidiasis

Candida organisms commonly colonize the skin, mucous membranes, and gastrointestinal tract, and infants acquire

the organism early in life. There is no way to avoid exposure to *Candida*. Oral candidiasis is the most common mucocutaneous disease of HIV-infected children. Chronic and recurrent infections of skin and mucous membranes are frequently the presenting infection in HIV-infected children. Judicious use of antibiotics will prevent overgrowth of *Candida* and limit clinical disease. Indwelling venous catheters should be managed with care to avoid contamination and subsequent infection. Fluconazole prophylaxis will prevent mucosal candidiasis but is not generally recommended since treatment is effective and because of concerns about developing resistance, adverse reactions, drug interactions, and cost. However, in selected individuals with severe or frequent recurrent candidiasis, a course of prophylactic fluconazole may be considered (see Chapter 40).

11.10 Cryptococcosis, histoplasmosis, and coccidiodomycosis

Invasive fungal infections are less common in HIV-infected children than in adults, presumably because of less frequent exposure to these pathogens. These organisms are present in the environment and are acquired by inhalation of airborne organisms in contaminated soil. Dissemination may occur in those with severe immunosuppression. There is no evidence that exposure to pigeon droppings increases the risk of cryptococcosis. Histoplasmosis and coccidiodomycosis each have a distinct geographic distribution, and infection is common among persons living in endemic regions. Severely immunosuppressed persons living in or visiting a region endemic for *Histoplasma* should avoid activities known to cause exposure, such as creating dust from soil, cleaning chicken coops, disturbing soil beneath bird roosting sites, remodeling or demolishing old buildings, and exploring caves. Likewise, for *Coccidioides*, severely immunosuppressed persons should avoid exposure to disturbed native soil such as at excavation sites or during dust storms.

Routine skin testing of persons living in endemic regions for *Histoplasma* and *Coccidioides* is not recommended since the results do not predict disease. Fluconazole and itraconazole prophylaxis reduce the frequency of cryptococcal disease among patients with advanced HIV infection (Table 11.3). However, routine antifungal prophylaxis is not recommended because no survival benefit has been shown, infection is uncommon, and therapy is costly, may promote drug resistance, and is associated with drug interactions. Prophylaxis with itraconazole will reduce the frequency of histoplasmosis among patients with advanced

HIV disease living in an endemic region but no improvement in survival has been shown [41]. Primary prophylaxis for coccidiodomycosis has not been shown to be effective. Because these invasive fungal infections are uncommon in children, primary prophylaxis is not recommended.

11.11 Cytomegalovirus

Cytomegalovirus (CMV) infections are common in HIV-infected children (see Chapter 41). However, infection is often asymptomatic and it is difficult to determine the extent to which CMV contributes to disease [42]. Cytomegalovirus disease in children often results from a primary infection rather than reactivation of a past infection, the more common situation in adults. Cytomegalovirus co-infection is likely to accelerate the course of HIV disease in children infected with both viruses [43]. Thus, there may be a benefit to identifying those HIV-infected children who are also CMV-infected.

Most HIV-infected women are co-infected with CMV and both in utero and intrapartum transmission of CMV to the infant can occur. The infant can also acquire CMV through breastfeeding. Intrapartum transmission of CMV, but not in utero infection, may be more common in women co-infected with HIV and CMV than in those infected with CMV alone [44, 45]. The most common route of transmission of CMV during childhood is horizontal spread through contact with saliva or urine. Sexual contact and blood transfusion are less common routes of transmission in childhood. HIV-infected children who are CMV-uninfected or of unknown CMV status and who require a transfusion should receive CMV-seronegative or leukocyte-depleted blood products.

It may be useful to identify which HIV-infected children are co-infected with CMV by doing yearly serologic testing starting at 12 months of age. This will allow a CMV-infected child who is severely immunosuppressed (CDC Immune Category 3) to be evaluated by an experienced ophthalmologist on a regular basis (every 4–6 months) in order to detect early retinitis. Alternatively, children can be screened for CMV once they are severely immunosuppressed. Older children should be taught to recognize "floaters" and changes in visual acuity which could represent retinitis.

Prophylaxis with oral ganciclovir can be considered for CMV-infected children who are severely immunosuppressed, such as those with a CD4$^+$ lymphocyte count < 50 cells/μL [6, 46] (Table 11.3). However, disadvantages of ganciclovir prophylaxis include cost, the toxicity of oral ganciclovir (anemia and neutropenia), limited efficacy data, and

the risk of developing resistant virus. A liquid preparation of ganciclovir for use in children can be prepared from the parenteral preparation; the dose is 30 mg/kg/dose PO TID. Valganciclovir, an oral pro-drug of ganciclovir with much greater bioavailability, is not available in a liquid formulation. It is approved for the treatment of CMV retinitis in adults but is not approved for the prophylaxis of CMV disease in either adults or children.

11.12 Herpes simplex virus

Neonatal herpes simplex virus (HSV) infection is usually acquired during delivery from a mother with an active genital infection (see Chapter 41). It can result in devastating disseminated infection or encephalitis in the newborn. In older infants and children, HSV is acquired by contact. Sexual acquisition is common once an adolescent is sexually active. Recommendations for the prevention of neonatal HSV include delivery by cesarean section if the membranes have not been ruptured for more than 4–6 hours. Oral acyclovir prophylaxis during late pregnancy for women with recurrent genital HSV is a controversial strategy which is recommended by some experts to prevent neonatal HSV. For pregnant women with frequent recurrences of HSV, prophylactic acyclovir might be considered. No fetal toxicity has been reported with acyclovir exposure during pregnancy [47]. HIV-infected children should avoid direct contact with individuals with active HSV infections. Use of latex condoms during all acts of sexual intercourse will reduce the risk of exposure to HSV as well as other sexually transmitted diseases (see Chapter 15).

11.13 Varicella-zoster virus

HIV-infected children who are asymptomatic or mildly symptomatic and not immunosuppressed (i.e., those in CDC class N1 or A1) should receive the live-attenuated varicella vaccine at 12 months of age [48, 49] (Table 11.3). The vaccine should not be administered to other HIV-infected children because of the risk of dissemination of the vaccine virus. Immunization of other children in the household of an HIV-infected child is recommended since this will protect the HIV-infected child from being exposed to varicella-zoster virus (VZV) if he cannot receive the vaccine himself. Any adult in the household who lacks a history of varicella should have serologic testing for VZV and should receive the vaccine if seronegative. There is no contraindication to administering the vaccine to family members of HIV-infected children.

Susceptible HIV-infected children should avoid exposure to persons with varicella or shingles (herpes zoster). If an HIV-infected child who is not known to be immune to VZV is exposed to varicella or zoster, she should receive an injection of varicella-zoster immunoglobulin (VZIG) as soon as possible but within 96 hours of the exposure [50] (1 vial/10 kg body weight intramuscularly up to a maximum of 5 vials) (Table 11.3). The use of oral acyclovir for post-exposure prophylaxis following exposure to VZV is not recommended and should not replace VZIG for the immunosuppressed host. In the healthy HIV-uninfected child who is susceptible to varicella, the live attenuated varicella vaccine can be administered following exposure to VZV to prevent or modify disease. However, in the HIV-infected child, VZIG should be given. The varicella vaccine should not be given with VZIG since antibody may interfere with the activity of the live virus vaccine (see Chapter 10).

11.14 Human herpesvirus 8

Persons co-infected with HIV and human herpesvirus 8 (HHV-8) are at risk for developing Kaposi's sarcoma (KS). Human herpesvirus 8 is transmitted by oral secretions, semen, and the sharing of needles. In regions of the world where HHV-8 is endemic, mother-to-child transmission of HHV-8 is reported, as is horizontal transmission between children [51]. Kaposi's sarcoma is rare in children in developed countries, but is much more common in some regions, particularly sub-Saharan Africa. It is reasonable to recommend that HIV-infected children avoid contact with the oral secretions of an individual with KS. Serologic testing for HHV-8 is not recommended to prevent exposure and no recommendations are available to prevent child-to-child transmission. Use of latex condoms should be effective in reducing the risk of sexual transmission.

11.15 Human papillomavirus

Cutaneous human papillomavirus (HPV) infections are commonly acquired during childhood by person-to-person contact. Warts can be very extensive in HIV-infected individuals. Laryngeal papillomatosis is a rare condition which results from an infant aspirating infectious genital tract secretions during birth. It is not known if this is more likely to occur in a child born to an HIV-infected mother. Anogenital warts are generally acquired through sexual contact but may occasionally result from exposure during birth. Human papillomavirus genital infections are extremely common in sexually active adolescents, frequently leading to cervical dysplasia and the risk of carcinoma. Latex condoms should be used during sexual intercourse, although they are unlikely to completely prevent the transmission of genital HPV, which also can occur as the result of manual innoculation. Sexually active adolescents should be evaluated for genital HPV infection on a regular basis, including, for women, a Pap smear at least once a year. Human papillomavirus vaccines targeting high-risk genotypes are in development.

11.16 Hepatitis B virus and hepatitis C virus

The principal route of acquisition of hepatitis B virus (HBV) in childhood is mother-to-child, with most transmission occurring at the time of delivery. It is not known if HIV co-infection increases the rate of HBV transmission. All pregnant women should be evaluated for HBV infection. All infants born to HIV/HBV co-infected women should receive prophylaxis with hepatitis B immunoglobulin (HBIG) and the hepatitis B vaccine. In older children and adolescents, transmission is by person-to-person exchange of blood and through sexual contact. Immunization of all infants with the hepatitis B vaccine will prevent acquisition of hepatitis B.

Mother-to-child transmission is also the principal route of acquisition of hepatitis C (HCV) in childhood. Maternal risk factors for transmission of HCV to the infant include co-infection with HIV, a higher HCV viral load, and intravenous drug use. The overall rate of transmission from a co-infected mother is 15–22% with rates ranging from 5–36% in different studies. The mode of delivery (vaginal vs cesarean section) and breastfeeding do not influence the rate of transmission [52]. Thus, a cesarean section should not be performed solely to prevent transmission of hepatitis C. All children born to mothers co-infected with HIV and HCV should be evaluated for HCV infection. Since maternal HCV antibody can persist in a child for up to 18 months, serologic testing is not useful in children less than 18 months of age. In this age group, reverse transcriptase-PCR for HCV RNA should be performed to identify virus in the blood. Children infected with HCV, if susceptible, should be vaccinated against hepatitis A virus and hepatitis B virus since infection with a second hepatitis virus can result in fulminant hepatitis. In adolescents and adults, injection drug use is the primary route of HCV transmission; the rate of sexual transmission of HCV is low. Adolescents should avoid injection drug use, body-piercing, and unprotected sexual intercourse.

11.17 Conclusion

Opportunistic infections account for most of the morbidity and mortality resulting from HIV infection. With an understanding of the risk factors predisposing to these infections, we are now able to prevent many of them. In the last decade, effective prophylaxis, in concert with highly active antiretroviral therapy, has dramatically reduced the mortality from HIV, turning it into a chronic disease for most patients. With this change come new questions and challenges. When can we safely stop prophylaxes once a child has responded to antiretroviral therapy? Do children need to be re-immunized with the routine childhood vaccines? With failure of HAART, will we see re-emergence of the classic HIV-associated opportunistic infections? What new infections will we see in patients with chronic HIV infection? What are the toxicities resulting from long-term use of prophylactic agents? Answering these questions are among the challenges facing those of us who care for HIV-infected children.

REFERENCES

1. Centers for Disease Control. 1994 classification system for human immunodeficiency virus infection in children less than 13 years of age. *MMWR* **43**: **RR-12** (1994), 1–10.

2. Palella, F. J., Delaney, K. M., Moorman, A. C., *et al.* Declining morbidity and mortality among patients with advanced human immunodeficiency virus infection. *New Engl. J. Med.* **338** (1998), 853–61.

3. Mussini, C., Pezzotti, P., Govoni, A. *et al.* Discontinuation of primary prophylaxis for *Pneumocystis carinii* pneumonia and toxoplasmic encephalitis in human immunodeficiency virus type-I-infected patients: the changes in opportunistic prophylaxis study. *J. Infect. Dis.* **181** (2000), 1635–42.

4. Centers for Disease Control and Prevention. *HIV/AIDS Surveillance Report.* **9**: 2 (1997), 18.

5. Dankner, W. M., Lindsey, J. C. & Levin, M. J.. Correlates of opportunistic infections in children infected with the human immunodeficiency virus managed before highly active antiretroviral therapy. *Pediatr. Infect. Dis. J.* **20** (2001), 40–8.

6. Centers for Disease Control and Prevention. Guidelines for the prevention of opportunistic infections among HIV-infected persons – 2002 recommendations of the U.S. Public Health Service and the Infectious Diseases Society of America. *MMWR* **51**: **RR-8** (2002), 1–52.

7. Centers for Disease Control and Prevention. Guidelines for the use of antiretroviral agents in pediatric HIV infection. *MMWR* **47**: **RR-4** (1998), 1–43 (updates available at http://AIDSInfo.nih.gov).

8. Simonds, R. J., Oxtoby, M. J., Caldwell, M. B. *et al.* *Pneumocystis carinii* pneumonia among US children with perinatally acquired HIV infection. *J. Am. Med. Assoc.* **270** (1993), 470–3.

9. Centers for Disease Control. 1995 revised guidelines for prophylaxis against *Pneumocystis carinii* pneumonia in children infected with or perinatally exposed to human immunodeficiency virus. *MMWR* **44**: **RR-4** (1995), 1–11.

10. Para, M. F., Finkelstein, D., Becker, S., Dohn, M., Walawander, A. & Black, J. R. Reduced toxicity with gradual initiation of trimethoprim-sulfamethoxazole as primary prophylaxis for *Pneumocystis carinii* pneumonia: AIDS Clinical Trials Group 268. *J. AIDS* **24** (2000), 337–43.

11. Leoung, G. S., Stanford, J. F., Giordano, M. F. *et al.* Trimethoprim-sulfamethoxazole (TMP–SMX) dose escalation versus direct rechallenge for *Pneumocystis carinii* pneumonia prophylaxis in human immunodeficiency virus-infected patients with previous adverse reaction to TMP–SMX. *J. Infect. Dis.* **184** (2001), 992–7.

12. Kletzel, M., Beck, S., Elser, J., Shock, N. & Burks, W. Trimethoprim sulfamethoxazole oral desensitization in hemophiliacs infected with human immunodeficiency virus with a history of hypersensitivity reactions. *Am. J. Dis. Child.* **145** (1991), 1428–9.

13. Chan, C., Montaner, J., Lefebvre, E. A., *et al.* Atovaquone suspension compared with aerosolized pentamidine for prevention of *Pneumocystis carinii* pneumonia in human immunodeficiency virus infected subjects intolerant of trimethoprim or sulfamethoxazole. *J. Infect. Dis.* **180** (1999), 369–76.

14. El-Sadr, W., Murphy, R. L., Yurik, R. M., *et al.* Atovaquone compared with dapsone for the prevention of *Pneumocystis carinii* pneumonia in patients with HIV infection who cannot tolerate trimethoprim, sulfonamides, or both. Community Program for Clinical Research on AIDS and the AIDS Clinical Trials Group. *New Engl. J. Med.* **339** (1998), 1889–95.

15. Stavola, J. J. & Noel, G. J.. Efficacy and safety of dapsone prophylaxis against *Pneumocystis carinii* pneumonia in human immunodeficiency virus-infected children. *Pediatr. Infect. Dis. J.* **12** (1993), 644–7.

16. McIntosh, K., Cooper, E., Xu, J. *et al.* Toxicity and efficacy of daily vs. weekly dapsone for prevention of *Pneumocystis carinii* pneumonia in children infected with human immunodeficiency virus. ACTG 179 Study Team. AIDS Clinical Trials Group. *Pediatr. Infect. Dis. J.* **18** (1999), 432–9.

17. Hughes, W., Dorenbaum, A., Yogev, R., *et al.* Phase I safety and pharmacokinetics study of micronized atovaquone in human immunodeficiency virus-infected infants and children. Pediatric AIDS Clinical Trials Group. *Antimicrob. Agents Chemother.* **42** (1998), 1315–18.

18. Hand, I. L., Wiznia, A. A., Porricolo, M. *et al.* Aerosolized pentamidine for prophylaxis of *Pneumocystis carinii* pneumonia in infants with human immunodeficiency virus infection. *Pediatr. Infect. Dis. J.* **13** (1994), 100–4.

19. Schneider, M. M., Hoepelman, A. I., Eeftinck, Schattenkerk, J. K., *et al.*, and the Dutch AIDS Treatment Group. Controlled trial of aerosolized pentamidine or trimethoprim-sulfamethoxazole as primary prophylaxis against

Pneumocystis carinii pneumonia in patients with human immunodeficiency virus infection. *New Engl. J. Med.* **327** (1992), 1836–41.

20. Katz, B. Z. & Rosen, C.. Aerosolized pentamidine in young children. *Pediatr. Infect. Dis. J.* **12** (1991), 958.

21. Schneider, M. M. E., Borleffs, J. C. C., Stolk, R. P. *et al.* Discontinuation of prophylaxis for *Pneumocystis carinii* pneumonia in HIV-1-infected patients treated with highly active antiretroviral therapy. *Lancet* **353** (1999), 201–3.

22. Lopez Bernaldo de Quiros, J. C., Miro, J. M., Pena, J. M. *et al.* Randomized trial of the discontinuation of primary and secondary prophylaxis against *Pneumocystis carinii* pneumonia after highly active antiretroviral therapy in patients with HIV infection. *New Engl. J. Med.* **344** (2001), 159–67.

23. Cordell, R. L. & Addiss, D. G. Cryptosporidiosis in child care settings: a review of the literature and recommendations for prevention and control. *Pediatr. Infect. Dis. J.* **13** (1994), 310–17.

24. Flanigan, T., Whalen, C., Turner, J. *et al.* Cryptosporidium infection and CD4 counts. *Ann. Internal Med.* **116** (1992), 840–2

25. Cello, J. P.. Acquired immunodeficiency syndrome cholangiopathy: spectrum of disease. *Am. J. Med.* **86** (1989), 539–46.

26. Holmberg, S. D., Moorman, A. C., Von, Bargen, J. C., *et al.* Possible effectiveness of clarithromycin and rifabutin for cryptosporidiosis chemoprophylaxis in HIV disease. *J. Am. Med. Assoc.* **279** (1998), 384–6.

27. Gutman, L. T., Moye, J., Zimmer, B. & Tian, C. Tuberculosis in human immunodeficiency virus-exposed or infected United States children. *Pediatr. Infect. Dis. J.* **13** (1994), 963–8.

28. Inderlied, C. B., Kemper, C. A. & Bermudez, L. E. M. The *Mycobacterium avium* complex. *Clin. Micro. Rev.* **6** (1993), 266–310.

29. Hoyt, L., Oleske, J., Holland, B. & Connor, E. Nontuberculous mycobacteria in children with acquired immunodeficiency syndrome. *Pediatr. Infect. Dis. J.* **11** (1992), 354–60.

30. Rutstein, R. M., Cobb, P., McGowan, K. L. *et al.* *Mycobacterium avium* intracellulare complex infection in HIV-infected children. *AIDS* **7** (1993), 507–12.

31. Horsburgh, C. R. Jr, Caldwell, M. B. & Simons, R. J. Epidemiology of disseminated nontuberculous mycobacterial disease in children with acquired immunodeficiency syndrome. *Pediatr. Infect. Dis. J.* **12** (1993), 219–22.

32. Lindegren, M. L., Hanson, C., Saletan, S. *et al.* *Mycobacterium avium* complex (MAC) in children with AIDS, United States: need for specific prophylaxis guidelines for children less than 6 years old. *Program and Abstracts of the 11th International Conference on AIDS* (July 7–12, 1996, Vancouver, Canada). Abstract no. We.B.420.

33. Nightingale, S. D., Camaron, D. W., Gordin, F. M., *et al.* Two controlled trials of rifabutin prophylaxis against mycobacterium avium complex infection in AIDS. *New Engl. J. Med.* **329** (1993), 828–33.

34. Pierce, M., Crampton, S., Henry, D. *et al.* A randomized trial of clarithromycin as prophylaxis against disseminated *Mycobacterium avium* complex infection in patients with advanced acquired immunodeficiency syndrome. *New Engl. J. Med.* **335** (1996), 384–91.

35. Havlir, D. V., Dube, M. P., Sattler, F. R. *et al.* Prophylaxis against disseminated *Mycobacterium avium* complex with weekly azithromycin, daily rifabutin, or both. *New Engl. J. Med.* **335** (1996), 392–8.

36. Havlir, D. V., Dube, M. P., Sattler, F. R. *et al.* Prophylaxis against disseminated *Mycobacterium avium* complex with weekly azithromycin, daily rifabutin, or both. *New Engl. J. Med.* **335** (1996), 392–8.

37. Centers for Disease Control and Prevention. Guidelines for using antiretroviral agents among HIV-infected adults and adolescents: recommendations of the Panel on Clinical Practices for Treatment of HIV. *MMWR* **51** : **RR-7** (2002), 1–56.

38. Centers for Disease Control and Prevention. Updated guidelines for the use of rifabutin or rifampin for the treatment and prevention of tuberculosis among HIV-infected patients taking protease inhibitors or nonnucleoside reverse transcriptase inhibitors. *MMWR* **49** (2000), 185–9.

39. NICHD IVIG Study Group. Intravenous immune globulin for the prevention of bacterial infection in children with symptomatic human immunodeficiency virus infection. *New Engl. J. Med.* **325** (1991), 73–80.

40. Spector, S. A., Gelber, R. D., McGrath, N. *et al.* A Controlled trial of intravenous immune globulin for the prevention of serious bacterial infections in children receiving zidovudine for advanced human immunodeficiency virus infection. *New Engl. J. Med.* **331** (1994), 1181–7.

41. McKinsey, D. S., Wheat, L. F., Cloud, G. A., *et al.* Itraconazole prophylaxis for fungal infections in patients with advanced human immunodeficiency virus infection: randomized, placebo-controlled, double-blind study. *Clin. Infect. Dis.* **28** (1999), 1049–56.

42. Frenkel, L. D., Gaur, S., Tsolia, M. *et al.* Cytomegalovirus infection in children with AIDS. *Rev. Infect. Dis.* **12**: Supp. 7 (1990), S820–6.

43. Nigro, G., Krzystofiak, A., Gattinara, G. *et al.* Rapid progression of HIV diseases in children with CMV DNAemia. *AIDS* **10** (1996), 1127–33.

44. Mussi-Pinhata, M. M., Yamamoto, Y., Figueiredo, L. T. M., *et al.* Congenital and perinatal cytomegalovirus infection in infants born to mothers infected with human immunodeficiency virus. *J. Pediatr.* **132** (1998), 285–90.

45. Kovacs, A., Schlucter, M., Easley, K. *et al.* Cytomegalovirus infection and HIV-1 disease progression in infants born to HIV-1-infected women. *New Engl. J. Med.* **341** (1999), 77–84.

46. Spector, S. A., McKinley, G. F., Lalezari, J. P. *et al.* Oral ganciclovir for the prevention of cytomegalovirus disease in persons with AIDS. *New Engl. J. Med.* **334** (1996), 1491–7.

47. Centers for Disease Control and Prevention. Pregnancy outcomes following systemic prenatal acyclovir exposure – June 1, 1984–June 30, 1993. *MMWR* **42** (1993), 806–9.

48. Levin, M. J., Gershon, A. A., Weinberg, A. *et al.* Immunization of HIV-infected children with varicella vaccine. *J. Pediatr.* **139** (2001), 305–10.

49. Centers for Disease Control and Prevention. Prevention of Varicella: updated recommendations of the Advisory Committee on Immunization Practices (ACIP). *MMWR* **48 : RR-6** (1999), 1–5.

50. Centers for Disease Control and Prevention. Prevention of varicella: recommendations of the Advisory Committee on Immunization Practices (ACIP). *MMWR* **45 : RR-11** (1996), 20–4.

51. Plancoulaine, S., Abel, L., van Beveren, M. *et al.* Human herpesvirus 8 transmission from mother to child and between siblings in an endemic population. *Lancet* **356** (2000), 1062–5.

52. Yeung, L. T. F., King, S. M. & Roberts, E. A. Mother-to-infant transmission of hepatitis c virus. *Hepatology* **34** (2001), 223–9.

Emergency evaluation and care

James M. Callahan, M.D.

Associate Professor, Department of Emergency Medicine, SUNY – Upstate Medical University, Syracuse, NY

12.1 Introduction

Most pediatric patients with HIV infection in rich countries live in major cities. However, cases have been reported in smaller cities and rural areas. Any clinician who sees sick children in an acute care setting may treat children with HIV and should be familiar with the atypical and sometimes life-threatening diseases that affect these children.

HIV-infected children average 1.2 visits to the emergency department (ED) and 15 ambulatory care visits per year [1]. Children who meet the case definition for pediatric AIDS average 2 ED visits and 18 ambulatory care visits each year [1]. HIV-infected children present to the ED with different complaints, are more likely to have diagnostic or therapeutic procedures performed and are more likely to be admitted to the hospital than uninfected children [2]. HIV status may not be known at the time of an ED visit. Manifestations of HIV infection may not be recognized [3, 4].

Much of the early improvement in HIV-related mortality was related not to new antiretroviral therapies, but to the prompt and effective treatment of the opportunistic infections associated with HIV disease. Even with the wide variety of antiretroviral therapies currently available, the quick recognition and aggressive treatment of the infectious complications of HIV infection in children may be life saving. Initial diagnosis of HIV infection may be made when a child presents with an acute and possibly life-threatening illness. Physicians must know the right questions to ask and the signs to look for. They must also be familiar with the appropriate evaluation and treatment options available to these children.

12.2 Emergency department presentation

12.2.1 History

HIV-infected children, whose diagnosis is not yet known, may first present to the ED. Physicians must be familiar with historical factors that may put a parent or child at risk for HIV infection (Table 12.1). However, the only risk factor for a growing number of HIV-infected persons is unprotected heterosexual intercourse. Today, almost all pediatric patients with HIV infection have acquired that infection perinatally. The incidence of perinatally acquired HIV infection is decreasing. However, improved care has led to longer survival. These patients continue to present to the ED for acute care.

The ED physician must consider HIV infection as a possible cause for poor growth, recurrent infections, or a number of other signs. Clinicians must ask parents about their possible risk factors. Parents may be unaware that they are HIV-infected until the diagnosis is made in their children. The absence of a parent should prompt the physician to inquire about the parents and their health status [5]. Possibly, the parents are deceased or incapacitated as a result of HIV infection.

Pediatric patients with HIV infection can present in many ways. The birth history, birth weight, and histories of poor growth or development may suggest HIV infection. Histories of multiple hospital admissions for invasive bacterial illnesses (e.g. meningitis, cellulitis, sinusitis, and/or pneumonia) [4] and oral thrush unresponsive to treatment or occurring after the first year of life may suggest HIV disease.

Table 12.1 Possible indications of HIV infection from the history

Parental history
    History of HIV infection
    Intravenous drug abuse
    Other substance abuse or addiction
    Sexual contact with intravenous drug user(s)
    Multiple sexual partners
    Prostitution
    Absence of parents (death or inability to care for child
       may be due to parental HIV infection)
Patient history
    Unexplained small-for-gestational age birth
    Unexplained failure to thrive
    Multiple serious (invasive) bacterial infections
    Unexpectedly severe consequences of common viral
       infections
    Recurrent thrush or oral thrush after 12 months of age
    Unexplained developmental delay; loss of milestones
    Persistent or recurrent diarrhea
    Sexually transmitted diseases

A history of otherwise common pediatric problems resistant to usual therapy (e.g. severe eczematous or seborrheic rashes) may also be a sign of HIV disease [5–7]. Patients with sexually transmitted diseases, especially adolescents with recurrent pelvic inflammatory disease should be counseled that they are at risk for HIV infection and should be screened.

In Chapter 6 Lindegren and colleagues describes the epidemiology of pediatric HIV disease; in Chapter 14 Rudy discusses some special considerations for HIV disease in adolescents; and in Chapter 5 Aldrovandi discusses the natural history of pediatric HIV disease.

Some children have long periods of relative wellness with only mild, non-specific signs or symptoms; occasionally the diagnosis may not be made until the child is 6–8 years of age or older. The ED physician must remain open to the possibility that an older child's symptoms or presentation may be due to HIV infection. Children may present with early onset of symptoms, opportunistic infections (especially *Pneumocystis carinii* pneumonia [PCP]), rapid progression and early death [5, 6], or they may have a more indolent course with signs of lymphadenopathy, hepatosplenomegaly, parotid swelling, and recurrent episodes of bacterial illnesses. These children are more likely to have lymphoid interstitial pneumonitis (LIP) and slowly progressive neurologic symptoms. These two types of presentation are not mutually exclusive. Children with

Table 12.2 Physical findings associated with pediatric HIV infection

General
    Failure to thrive; severe wasting
    Extensive and/or persistent lymphadenopathy
    Hepatosplenomegaly
Pulmonary
    Unexplained digital clubbing
    Persistent respiratory distress (especially if hypoxic or
       associated with a reticulonodular pattern or a
       chronic interstitial pneumonia of x-ray)
    Hypoxia out of proportion to respiratory distress
Head and neck
    Oral thrush unresponsive to therapy or in children
       >12 months of age
    Persistent or recurrent parotid swelling
    Severe or recalcitrant otitis media or sinusitis
    Unexplained microcephaly
    Severe stomatitis secondary to herpes simplex virus
Skin
    Unusually severe manifestations of viral illnesses
       (rubeola, varicella)
    Extensive molluscum contagiosum
    Recurrent folliculitis
    Severe or recurrent ulcers to herpes simplex virus
    Severe eczematous or seborrheic dermatitis
    Purpura or petechial rashes
Neurologic
    Unexplained developmental delay or loss of milestones
    Unexplained spasticity

a seemingly slower progression of illness may develop the acute onset of severe symptoms including opportunistic infections.

12.2.2 Physical examination

Table 12.2 lists physical examination findings suggestive of pediatric HIV infection. Many of these findings are non-specific. Their presence should make the physician think about HIV as a possible explanation, although these findings may sometimes occur in other settings. Certainly, a combination of several of these findings (e.g. hepatosplenomegaly, generalized lymphadenopathy, parotid swelling and oral thrush in a 2-year-old) should prompt an evaluation for HIV infection, especially if the child has a history suggestive of HIV disease (see Table 12.1).

Table 12.3 Laboratory and radiologic abnormalities suggestive of HIV infection

Laboratory
  Anemia
  Neutropenia
  Thrombocytopenia
  Increased globulin fraction
  Hematuria, proteinuria
Radiologic
  Chronic, interstitial pneumonitis
  Hilar lymphadenopathy
  Reticulonodular pattern on chest x-ray

Table 12.4 Important history in patients with known HIV infection

Centers for Disease Control and Prevention classification
HIV RNA level
$CD4^+$ count
Antiretroviral therapy
Prophylaxis for opportunistic infections; particularly
  Pneumocystis carinii pneumonia
Past opportunistic infections

12.2.3 Laboratory and radiologic abnormalities

Certain abnormalities (Table 12.3) found on diagnostic testing done in the ED should prompt consideration of HIV as an underlying diagnosis. If these abnormalities are found in a patient with other signs or symptoms of HIV disease or a history suggestive of HIV infection, this diagnosis should be entertained. Hematologic abnormalities associated with HIV infection can include chronic anemia, acute episodes of hemolytic anemia, neutropenia, and immune-mediated thrombocytopenia [5]. Unexplained hematuria or proteinuria or both can be due to HIV-mediated renal disease. Patients who have an elevated serum total protein with a normal or low serum albumin may have an increased globulin fraction owing to the increased production of IgG, particularly in the setting of lymphadenopathy and hepatosplenomegaly.

12.2.4 Presentation of children with known HIV infection

Patients with known HIV infection may present to the ED for related or unrelated complaints. The approach to these patients may have to be modified (e.g. additional diagnostic tests may need to be performed). Disposition and treatment decisions may also need to be modified in patients with known HIV infection. In the ED, HIV-exposed children with indeterminate infection should be treated as if they are HIV-infected [6]. This leads to the safest and most conservative treatment being prescribed.

In obtaining a history in patients with known HIV infection, some key information should be elicited (Table 12.4). If available, the patient's clinical and immunologic Centers for Disease Control and Prevention (CDC) classification, the most recent $CD4^+$ count, and HIV RNA measurement may be helpful. A thorough medication history, including antiretroviral agents and drugs used for the prophylaxis

and treatment of opportunistic infections (e.g. *Mycobacterium avium-intracellulare* infection, cytomegalovirus [CMV] retinitis, PCP, etc.) should be obtained and documented. Even if the ED clinician cannot obtain detailed laboratory, immunologic, or virologic information, a history of opportunistic infections and the use of prophylaxis indicate that the patient is significantly immunocompromised. Patients with evidence of severe immunocompromise and previous episodes of opportunistic infections, especially PCP, are at a much higher risk of developing a new, potentially life-threatening opportunistic infection. However, the absence of these factors does not mean that a patient does not have PCP or another opportunistic infection.

A key component of caring for patients with HIV infection is ensuring good follow-up care. Involvement of the patient's primary care physician in therapeutic decisions is important. This physician knows more about the state of the patient's illness and the home situation than the ED physician does. Also, the primary care physician must be informed of the ED visit, what was done, and when the patient needs to follow up before the patient is discharged from the emergency room.

12.2.5 HIV testing in the emergency department

When a patient presents to the ED with signs or symptoms of possible HIV infection, he or she *must* be tested for HIV. However, the ED may not be the best place to do this. If HIV testing is to be done in the ED, appropriate pre- and post-test counseling must be available there. It must be ensured that the patient can be contacted if he or she does not come back for follow-up. Ideally, the same healthcare provider or providers should see the patient on both visits. There should be adequate time for discussion of test results and their ramifications. In a busy ED where personnel work variable shifts this may be difficult to do. Emergency department social workers may be very helpful in counseling patients or arranging follow-up. If good follow-up, counseling, and patient confidentiality can be

meningitis or those for whom there is a high suspicion of pneumococcal illness, broader coverage, such as the addition of vancomycin or rifampin, should be given. If corticosteroids are to be given in patients with meningitis, rifampin is the preferred additional agent. Antibiotic therapy should be refined when culture and sensitivity results are available.

12.3.4 Evaluation of the child with persistent fevers

Many HIV-infected children have persistent or recurrent fevers as part of their primary illness. Often, extensive workups have already been performed to look for the cause of these fevers. These children should be evaluated thoroughly. Any change in clinical status should prompt a renewed evaluation for possible sources of fever. This includes any change in the frequency or character of the patient's febrile episodes. The clinician best able to make these judgments is the patient's primary care physician. If this physician is unable to see the patient, the ED clinician should at least contact the primary care physician to discuss the patient's clinical presentation and prior workup. The primary concern in evaluating these patients in the ED is to be confident (based upon clinical evaluation and, if necessary, ancillary studies) that a new, acute process is not present.

Causes of chronic fevers in children include infections with toxoplasmosis, intestinal parasites, fungi, mycobacteria including tuberculosis and MAC, Epstein–Barr virus, and CMV. Appropriate studies to look for these causes include large-volume blood cultures, serologic tests, buffy coat examination, urine culture for viruses, purified protein derivative (PPD) with control, and bone marrow biopsy and aspiration for culture [11]. There are no clear guidelines regarding how often these procedures should be performed. If there has not been a change in the patient's clinical condition and the patient does not look acutely ill, these procedures do not need to be done in the ED. This is especially true if they have recently been performed in the ED or by the patient's primary care giver. Close observation of patients with recurrent or persistent fevers is of paramount importance. Any change in the patient's condition warrants not only an investigation to find these less common causes of fever but also laboratory studies to rule out a new, acute process (e.g., bacteremia or pneumonia) as well.

12.4 Respiratory distress

Respiratory distress can be an ominous sign in HIV-infected children. *Pneumocystis carinii* pneumonia is still the most

Table 12.8 Major causes of respiratory distress

Bacterial pneumonia
   Streptococcus pneumoniae, Haemophilus influenzae
     type b, group A streptococci,
   Staphylococcus aureus, Mycoplasma pneumoniae,
     Branhamella catarrhalis,
   Pseudomonas aeruginosa and other Gram negative
     organisms
Common viral pathogens (e.g., respiratory syncytial virus,
   influenza, adenovirus)
Pneumocystis carinii pneumonia
Lymphoid interstitial pneumonitis
Underlying reactive airway disease
Other opportunistic infections (*Mycobacterium avium*
   complex, tuberculosis, aspergillosis, *Legionella*)
Cytomegalovirus pneumonitis
Cardiac disease

common opportunistic infection in these children and a major cause of morbidity [20]. Respiratory infections are the most common cause of mortality in HIV-infected children [21]. Many other causes – both infectious and non-infectious – may be responsible for producing respiratory distress. Respiratory distress in an HIV-infected child should prompt an immediate evaluation and quick treatment.

12.4.1 Causes

The major causes of respiratory distress in children with HIV infections are listed in Table 12.8. Even in HIV-infected children, some of these causes are relatively rare (e.g. opportunistic infections other than PCP and CMV infection). Bacterial pneumonias are common in children with HIV infection. *S. pneumoniae, H. influenzae* type b, group A streptococci, *Staphylococcus aureus, Mycoplasma pneumoniae, Moraxella cattarhalis,* and Gram negative organisms, including *Pseudomonas* sp. have all been found to cause pneumonia. Children may also suffer from infections with common viral pathogens.

Pneumocystis carinii pneumonia is the most worrisome cause of an acute change in a patient's respiratory status. Lymphocytic interstitial pneumonitis is a common finding in children with HIV infection. It may cause a slow but progressive decrease in pulmonary function leading to symptoms. Many children with HIV infection are of African-American or Hispanic descent and live in major urban areas. The prevalence of underlying reactive airway disease is high in this setting. Children with HIV infection

Table 12.9 Emergency evaluation of children with respiratory distress

Complete history and physical examination
Chest radiograph
Complete blood count and differential
Pulse oximetry
Induced sputum or bronchoalveolar lavage to rule out
   Pneumocystis carinii pneumonia (unless another
   diagnosis is definitive)
If indicated:
   Arterial blood gas
   Lactate dehydrogenase (LDH) level
   Blood culture
   Viral studies
   PPD and anergy testing

PPD, purified protein derivative, tuberculin skin test.

may have underlying reactive airway disease as well [22] (see Chapter 31). The impact of HIV infection on other organ systems including the effects of cardiomyopathy may cause respiratory distress. Children may also have respiratory distress due to LIP and other opportunistic infections, including MAC, tuberculosis, aspergillosis, and *Legionella* infection.

12.4.2 Evaluation

The usual evaluation of children with HIV infection and respiratory distress is outlined in Table 12.9. A thorough history and physical examination should be performed in all these patients. Prior history of opportunistic infections (especially PCP) or a bacterial pneumonia should be determined. The purified protein derivative, tuberculin skin test (PPD) status of the patient, family, and contacts should be ascertained [23]. Tuberculosis is relatively rare in children with HIV infection, but when present it requires aggressive therapy. A prior history of reactive airway disease or (LIP) can guide therapy and evaluation.

Children with known reactive airway disease who present with mild, diffuse wheezing, are afebrile and look relatively well may be given a trial of bronchodilator therapy (beta-agonists). If they improve with minimal treatment, are not hypoxic, and continue to look well, no further evaluation needs to be done [22]. Ipratropium may be added to the beta-agonists as it has been shown to decrease admission rates in children without HIV infection and asthma who are having moderate to severe attacks. These children should have close follow-up to be sure that they do not have a

deterioration in their status. Their primary care physician must be informed and follow-up scheduled in 1–2 days.

A chest x-ray and CBC should be done in all other children in addition to pulse oximetry. Children with bacterial pneumonias usually present with acute onset of fever, cough, tachypnea, and varying degrees of respiratory distress [20, 22, 23]. Mild hypoxemia may be present. Many pneumonias in children result from hematogenous seeding of the lung during episodes of occult bacteremia. Respiratory symptoms may be minimal early in the course of these children's illnesses. Chest x-rays usually show lobar or segmental infiltrates [22–24]. There may be associated pleural effusions. Pleurocentesis may provide relief of symptoms and identify an etiologic agent in patients with large pleural effusions. The white blood count is usually elevated, and there is usually a left shift in the differential. Cold agglutinins, if positive, may indicate an infection with *M. pneumoniae*.

Children with HIV infection may also have infection with common respiratory pathogens. When infected with RSV, children with HIV infection are less likely to have wheezing and more likely to present with pneumonia than those without HIV infection [20, 25]. HIV-infected children have prolonged viral shedding. The clinical course is not more severe than in uninfected children. Measles infection may lead to severe pneumonia in children with AIDS [20]. Viral respiratory illnesses may be diagnosed with nasal washings for rapid viral diagnostic tests. Findings are otherwise non-specific. If children have severe symptoms or are not improving as would be expected, simultaneous infection with bacterial pathogens, *Pneumocystis carinii*, or other pathogens may be present.

12.4.3 *Pneumocystis carinii* pneumonia

Children can present with PCP acutely or in a more subtle way. *Pneumocystis carinii* pneumonia can manifest at any age, but 50% of reported cases in children with HIV infection occur in the first 6 months of life [26]. It may be the first manifestation of HIV-related disease and the first presentation may be fatal. Consideration of a PCP diagnosis should trigger the initiation of therapy. Usually, children have acute onset of tachypnea, dyspnea, and cough [6, 20]. However, they may also present with a cough of days to weeks in duration with only slowly progressive tachypnea [22, 23]. Physical examination shows tachypnea, dyspnea, rhonchi, and wheezes. Rales may be present but are rare [22]. These children usually have hypoxia, which is more marked than would be expected from the patient's symptoms. Chest x-rays typically show a diffuse, interstitial pattern, although clear radiographs (especially early in the disease process), hyperinflation, lobar infiltrates, or even severe changes consistent with ARDS have been reported [20, 22]. Lactate dehydrogenase (LDH) levels are usually markedly elevated (>500 IU), and the alveolar–arterial oxygen gradient is usually high (>30 mm Hg) [20, 22, 27]. Definitive diagnosis is made on specimens usually obtained by induced sputum or bronchoalveolar lavage (see Chapter 42 for a detailed discussion of diagnosis and therapy of PCP). Therapy should be started as soon as a diagnosis of PCP is considered and should *not* wait until a definitive diagnosis is made.

12.4.4 Lymphoid interstitial pneumonitis

Lymphoid interstitial pneumonitis (LIP) is a slowly progressive finding in many children with HIV infection and is the most common respiratory complication in these children [23]. Usually, children present after 1 year of age [28]. Patients may have a cough but often present only with mild tachypnea [22]. Digital clubbing is often present. Hypoxia is usually mild but chronic. Often, children with LIP have associated lymphadenopathy, hepatosplenomegaly, and parotid enlargement. They frequently have clear breath sounds, but wheezing and other signs of bronchospasm may be present. Chest x-rays show a diffuse, interstitial process often with a reticulonodular pattern [20, 22, 23, 27, 28]. Lymphoid interstitial pneumonitis and pulmonary lymphoid hyperplasia (PLH) represent a continuum. In PLH, the nodular pattern is more pronounced; LIP–PLH can progress to respiratory failure if not recognized and treated [24]. Lactate dehydrogenase is mildly elevated in these patients (usually 250–500 IU) [22], and there may be some overlap of LDH values with children with PCP (see Chapter 31).

12.4.5 Cytomegalovirus

Many patients with HIV infection have evidence of prior infection with CMV. Cytomegalovirus may reactivate with immune dysfunction, and immunosuppressed patients may have acute infections. Pneumonia may be one manifestation. Retinitis, hepatitis, and colitis may also be seen [22]. Pneumonia accompanied by one of these findings is very suggestive of CMV disease. Pneumonia due to CMV often looks like PCP on chest x-rays. Cytomegalovirus may cause coinfection with PCP and may contribute to a lack of improvement with conventional therapy for PCP [16]. Lung biopsy may be required to definitively diagnose the cause of the patient's respiratory compromise (see Chapter 31).

12.4.6 Therapy

Appropriate treatment for the underlying cause of the patient's respiratory symptoms should be begun quickly. A summary of indicated treatments for specific respiratory

Table 12.10 Treatment of children with respiratory symptoms

Condition	Treatment
Reactive airway disease	Bronchodilators (including ipratropium), corticosteroids
Bacterial pneumonia	Amoxicillin, amoxicillin–clavulanate, or cefuroxime po or cefuroxime IV (if severely ill or accompanied by sepsis, use broader antibiotic coverage)
Bacterial pneumonia in recently hospitalized patients	Ceftriaxone and antistaphylococcal penicillin IV (consider coverage for *Pseudomonas*, e.g. ceftazidime and an aminoglycoside)
Pneumocystis carinii pneumonia	Trimethoprim–sulfamethoxazole or pentamidine IV
Lymphoid interstitial pneumonitis – pulmonary lymphoid hyperplasia	Corticosteroids po (may give IV if critically ill)
Viral processes	Supportive care (consider ribavirin for respiratory syncytial virus, amantadine for influenza, ganciclovir for cytomegalovirus, acyclovir for varicella)

All children should receive supportive care including oxygen, bronchodilator therapy, ventilatory support, and IV fluids as indicated.

conditions in children with HIV infection can be found in Table 12.10. Supportive care, including oxygen therapy, ventilatory support, bronchodilator therapy, and intravenous fluids, should be provided as needed. Patients who may be developing respiratory failure should be kept NPO (nothing by mouth) in anticipation of possible endotracheal intubation. *Pneumocystis carinii* pneumonia can be a rapidly fatal disease in this population. If the diagnosis of PCP is considered, therapy should be begun immediately [5, 20, 22, 23]. Corticosteroids have been shown to be helpful in pediatric patients with PCP and are usually also begun [21, 29–31] (therapy for PCP is covered in detail in Chapter 42).

Afebrile children who present with diffuse wheezing and respiratory distress may be given a trial of bronchodilator therapy. Patients with moderate to severe symptoms often benefit from the addition of ipratropium to beta-agonists in the ED. This therapy may decrease admission rates. Ipratropium is not used as chronic therapy for reactive airway disease. If they improve rapidly and show no signs of a coexisting respiratory infection, they may be discharged to continue bronchodilator therapy at home. Corticosteroids, 1–2 mg/kg/day of prednisone or prednisolone, may be given for 4–5 days. Hypoxia, moderate to severe respiratory distress, or rapidly recurring symptoms are indications for hospital admission just as they are for patients with reactive airway disease without HIV infection (therapy for reactive airway disease in the HIV-infected child is discussed in Chapter 31). Fever, a first episode of wheezing, severe distress, hypoxia, or failure to improve with usual therapy all should prompt the clinician to obtain a chest radiograph. Febrile children with wheezing who have rales, abnormal chest x-rays, or leukocytosis should receive antibiotics as well as therapy for their reactive airway disease [22].

Patients with lobar or segmental infiltrates should be treated for presumed bacterial pneumonia. If the diagnosis is not clear or if the patient is ill-appearing, treatment is often initiated simultaneously for both bacterial infections and PCP while definitive test results are pending. Patients who are only mildly symptomatic, not dehydrated, not hypoxic, and able to tolerate oral medications may be given a trial of oral antibiotics. The patients should be followed up closely. If transportation back to the hospital is not readily available or if the family is unable to adequately monitor the child's progress, the child should be admitted to the hospital for treatment and observation.

Amoxicillin, amoxicillin-clavulanate, and cefuroxime may be good choices for oral therapy, depending on the local pattern of antibiotic resistance, particularly resistant pneumococci. Doubling the usual dose of the antibiotic has been recommended, especially in areas where there is a significant incidence of pneumococci with intermediate sensitivities to beta-lactams [22]. When this is done with amoxicillin-clavulanate, the clinician must be careful not to be giving too high a dose of clavulanate so as not to cause gastrointestinal irritation and diarrhea (see Chapter 37). Trimethoprim–sulfamethoxazole should be reserved for patients with presumed PCP and therefore is not appropriate outpatient therapy in HIV-infected children with pneumonia (all patients with presumed PCP should be admitted). Patients should be re-examined by their primary care physician, if possible, or in the ED within 24 hours. Patients whose clinical status worsens at any time should be admitted for parenteral antibiotics. Patients on oral antibiotics who fail to improve within 24–48 hours should also be admitted for parenteral antibiotic therapy.

Failure to improve should also prompt a serious reconsideration of the underlying diagnosis.

Cefuroxime 100–150 mg/kg/day, divided into three doses, is an excellent choice for otherwise uncomplicated cases in patients requiring parenteral therapy. Patients who have recently been hospitalized should receive broader coverage to include therapy for *S. aureus* and Gram-negative organisms. The combination of ceftriaxone and an anti-staphylococcal penicillin is a good alternative in these patients. If *Pseudomonas* sp. is suspected as a cause, ceftazidime and an aminoglycoside are appropriate. Seriously ill patients should be treated with broader coverage, modified to take into account the clinical details of the patient.

Patients must be monitored closely. Deterioration in clinical status or failure to improve within 24–72 hours should prompt reconsideration of the underlying diagnosis, broadening the spectrum of antibiotic coverage, and additional diagnostic testing. Although it occurs rarely, patients with PCP may have lobar or segmental infiltrates on chest x-ray. The addition of TMP–SMX or pentamidine may be considered.

In children with hypoxia and findings consistent with LIP–PLH, treatment with corticosteroids may be helpful. Prednisone or prednisolone (if a liquid preparation is needed) at 1–2 mg/kg/day is given for several weeks [20, 22, 23]. Chapter 31 discusses therapy for LIP in more detail. Dosages are then slowly tapered as tolerated. Tuberculosis and pulmonary disease with MAC may look similar to LIP–PLH. If the patient has a history of fevers, these should be excluded before the patient is started on corticosteroid therapy [22].

Most viral respiratory infections require only good supportive care. Critically ill children may be treated with specific antiviral agents (e.g. ribavirin for RSV, acyclovir for varicella, ganciclovir for CMV pneumonitis and amantadine for influenza) if a diagnosis is made.

12.5 Gastrointestinal emergencies

12.5.1 Diarrhea

Diarrhea, both acute and chronic, is a common problem in HIV-infected children. In the emergency setting, acute diarrhea can cause dehydration, especially if accompanied by vomiting or fever. Chronic diarrhea and wasting may make an HIV-infected child more prone to dehydration from an intercurrent illness. Dehydration should be treated aggressively with fluids, which may be given intravenously, if necessary. Determining a causative agent may permit specific therapy and more rapid resolution of symptoms.

Table 12.11 Common causes of diarrhea

Bacteria
  Salmonella sp.
  Shigella sp.
  Campylobacter sp.
  Yersinia enterocolitica
  Escherichia coli
  Clostridium difficile
Viruses
  Rotavirus
  Enteroviruses
  Adenovirus
  Cytomegalovirus
Opportunistic infections
  Mycobacterium avium complex
  Giardia lamblia
  Cryptosporidium
  Entamoeba histolytica
  Microsporidia
  Isopora belli
  Cyclospora

Gastrointestinal disorders are discussed more completely in Chapter 33.

Differential diagnosis

Common causes of diarrhea in HIV-infected children are listed in Table 12.11. Bacterial gastroenteritis can be caused by all the agents that cause diarrhea in immunocompetent children. Patients who experience an abrupt onset of diarrhea without preceding vomiting are more likely to have a bacterial infection [32]. Bloody stools are more often seen in children with bacterial gastroenteritis. Although not highly sensitive, the finding of more than five stool leukocytes per high-power field in a stool specimen is indicative of probable bacterial infection.

Patients with emesis of several hours' duration followed by the onset of watery or occasionally mucoid diarrhea frequently have viral gastroenteritis [32]. Children with HIV infection experience infections with routine viral pathogens. However, these agents often cause prolonged symptoms [32, 33]. HIV-infected children may also experience gastroenteritis due to CMV and other uncommon causes.

Opportunistic infections including parasitic diseases and MAC may produce diarrhea in children – often of a chronic nature. Cryptosporidiosis has been reported to cause episodes of severe diarrhea in children with HIV infection, especially in patients with advanced symp-

Table 12.12 Evaluation of children with diarrhea

History
  Possible exposure to infectious agents
  Presence and time course of vomiting
  Nature of diarrhea
  Presence of abdominal pain
  Presence of tenesmus
  Activity level
  Urine output
Physical examination
  Temperature
  Close attention to vital signs
  Signs of dehydration or poor perfusion
  Abdominal tenderness
Laboratory tests
  Complete blood count with differential
  Serum electrolytes and glucose (glucose testing should be done at bedside)
  Blood culture for bacterial pathogens
  Stool examination for leukocytes
  Stool culture for bacterial pathogens
  Stool culture for viral pathogens
  Stool for *Clostridium difficile* toxins
  Stool examination for ova and parasites

toms [34]. Children with prolonged symptoms should be evaluated for these illnesses and treated as outlined in Chapter 33.

Evaluation

The evaluation of the HIV-infected child with diarrhea is outlined in Table 12.12. The clinician should look for signs of dehydration or cardiovascular compromise and attempt to identify a causative agent so that specific therapy can be begun. History of exposure to infectious agents at home or in a day care or school setting can be helpful. Vomiting that precedes diarrhea is often seen with viral infections [32]. Bloody stools are common in bacterial gastroenteritis, especially when *Shigella* sp., *Campylobacter* sp., *Yersinia enterocolitica*, or invasive *Escherichia coli* are the causative agents. *Clostridium difficile*, CMV, and *Entamoeba histolytica* can also cause bloody stools. Tenesmus is common with *Shigella* and *E. histolytica*.

HIV-infected children may be chronically ill and have problems with wasting or failure to thrive. This may make them prone to rapid dehydration with intercurrent illnesses. Caretakers should be asked about the patient's oral intake, activity level, and urine output. On physical examination, lethargy may indicate severe dehydration requiring prompt fluid resuscitation. Signs of dehydration or poor perfusion should also be looked for on physical examination. Tachycardia (especially in the absence of fever), dry mucous membranes, cool extremities, and prolonged capillary refill all are worrisome signs. Decreased activity level may also indicate dehydration. Hypotension is a late sign signaling decompensated shock. Children who progress to this state are near collapse and resuscitation may be difficult. It is imperative to intervene early before this occurs.

Several laboratory studies may be helpful in the evaluation of diarrhea. The presence of fecal leukocytes makes the diagnosis of bacterial gastroenteritis more likely. Sheets of leukocytes are often seen with *Shigella* infections. However, the absence of fecal leukocytes does not exclude bacterial sources as the cause of diarrhea. Children with HIV infection have a higher risk of developing invasive disease due to *Salmonella* sp. and other enteric organisms [32]. Gastroenteritis due to *Salmonella* should be treated with oral or parenteral antibiotics. Any signs of systemic illness (fever, rigors, poor perfusion) in this setting should raise the concern that the patient is bacteremic. Intravenous antibiotics should be administered in addition to rapid fluid resuscitation. If possible, blood cultures should be obtained before antibiotics are given.

A complete blood count may show leukocytosis with a left shift, especially if bacteremia is present. Patients with infections due to *Shigella* sp. often have low or normal total WBCs but a marked bandemia in which band forms often exceed the number of mature neutrophils. Atypical lymphocytes may be seen in children with viral gastroenteritis. Serum electrolytes and glucose should be checked. Marked acidosis may call for bicarbonate replacement. Patients with a history of wasting and decreased body stores may be especially prone to hypoglycemia in the setting of increased losses and decreased intake. In patients with prolonged diarrhea who have negative bacterial cultures and viral antigen tests, stools should be tested for *C. difficile* toxin and examined for ova and parasites and mycobacteria. Enteric cryptosporidiosis can cause severe diarrhea in patients with advanced HIV infection. The diarrhea is secretory in nature and can lead to severe dehydration and weight loss [34]. Recovery was reported in some patients without specific treatment of this entity.

Therapy

The main goal of therapy in the patient with diarrhea is to ensure adequate hydration and end-organ perfusion. Children with mild diarrhea who can tolerate oral fluids may be able to be managed with oral electrolyte solutions or other dietary manipulations. Children who appear more than mildly dehydrated, who have diarrhea accompanied by marked emesis, or who have signs or symptoms of systemic disease that might be consistent with bacteremia should be rapidly rehydrated with intravenous fluids.

Initial fluid therapy consists of 20 ml/kg boluses of isotonic fluid (0.9% normal saline solution [NSS] or Ringer's lactate). Boluses are repeated until signs of decreased perfusion (tachycardia, prolonged capillary refill, decreased urine output) resolve. Urine output should be monitored closely and used as a guide for fluid therapy. In children with signs of decompensated shock (i.e. hypotension), rapid fluid administration is still the first line of therapy. Vasopressor agents should be started if there is no response after 60–80 ml/kg of crystalloid fluids have been administered. Intraosseous needles may be used if intravenous access cannot be obtained. These can be used in all age groups, even in large adolescent patients and adults. The anterior tibial plateau is the preferred site for intraosseous access in young children. The distal, anterior femur may also be used in young infants. In children over 3 years of age and especially in patients greater than 6 years of age, the distal tibia just cephalad to the medial malleolus is the preferred site of insertion. Any fluid or medication (including blood products) which would be administered through a standard intravenous line may be given through an intraosseous site.

Administration of glucose should be guided by serum glucose testing. Boluses of large volumes of glucose-containing fluids should be avoided. Large amounts of intravenous glucose may cause an osmotic diuresis, even in the presence of dehydration, and thus cause further fluid losses. Bedside testing allows for rapid determination of the child's serum glucose. If serum glucose is low, glucose should be administered at a dose of 0.25–0.50 g/kg (2.5–5 ml/kg of 10% dextrose [D_{10}], 1–2 ml/kg of D_{25}, or 0.5–1 ml/kg of D_{50}). Lower concentrations (e.g. D_{10}) are less likely to cause phlebitis or venous irritation leading to a loss of intravenous access.

After fluid resuscitation and the acute treatment of hypoglycemia have been completed, children should be begun on dextrose-containing fluids with saline to slowly replace fluid and electrolyte deficits (e.g. D_5, 0.45% NSS at 1.5 times maintenance). Deficits should be replaced over a period of 24–48 hours (48–72 hours in patients who are hypernatremic).

If a bacterial infection is suspected, antibiotics should be started. Children with mild symptoms who are not dehydrated and appear clinically well may be given oral antibiotics (TMP–SMX is most commonly used for suspected *Salmonella* sp. or *Shigella* sp.). Signs of toxicity, dehydration, poor perfusion, or inability to tolerate oral medications should prompt the institution of intravenous regimens for various suspected pathogens, as outlined in Table 12.13. Cultures should be obtained before antibiotic therapy is begun. After results are available,

Table 12.13 Antibiotics for bacterial gastroenteritis

Suspected agent	Oral antibiotics	Parenteral antibiotics
Salmonella sp.	Amoxicillin TMP–SMX	Ampicillin TMP–SMX Ceftriaxone
Shigella sp.	TMP–SMX Amoxicillin (high rates of resistance in some areas) Tetracycline (in patients >8 years of age)	TMP–SMX Ampicillin Ceftriaxone Chloramphenicol
Campylobacter sp.	Erythromycin Tetracycline (in patients >8 years of age)	Aminoglycosides
Yersinia enterocolitica	TMP–SMX	TMP–SMX Chloramphenicol
Escherichia coli (there are no studies supporting the effectiveness of antibiotics in the treatment of *E. coli* enterocolitis) [36]	TMP–SMX	TMP–SMX
Clostridium difficile	Vancomycin Metronidazole	

TMP–SMX, trimethoprim-sulfamethoxazole
Once available, sensitivity testing should guide antibiotic choice.

sensitivity profiles should be used to guide antibiotic therapy.

Most viral pathogens are not amenable to specific therapy. Cytomegalovirus enteritis, when biopsy confirmed, may be treated with ganciclovir or foscarnet [32, 33]. When identified from specimens, various parasitic and opportunistic infections may be amenable to specific therapies.

12.5.2 Abdominal pain

Differential diagnosis

Children with gastroenteritis may have abdominal pain as part of their constellation of symptoms. Diarrhea or vom-

iting or both may accompany the pain or follow soon after. *Yersinia enterocolitica* infection may cause mesenteric adenitis (inflammation of the mesenteric lymph nodes), which can lead to symptoms of severe abdominal pain, fever, and vomiting. Infections of the mesenteric lymph nodes in MAC infection may also be associated with severe abdominal pain. It may be difficult to distinguish these symptoms from appendicitis or other acute abdominal processes.

Patients with HIV infection may have appendicitis. One study in adults showed that HIV-infected individuals tended to present to the ED relatively late in their course and had a higher appendiceal perforation rate than non-infected controls [35]. Of interest, none of the 26 HIV-infected individuals with appendicitis had an elevated WBC. Patients who present with signs and symptoms of appendicitis should be aggressively evaluated. Surgical intervention must be sought quickly if appendicitis is clearly present. Equivocal findings should prompt evaluation with abdominal and pelvic computed tomography scanning to rule out appendicitis. The WBC may be less useful in evaluating these patients.

Patients with intussusception can present with abdominal pain, vomiting, and varying degrees of lethargy. Intussusception may result from lead points due to various disease processes (e.g. submucosal bleeding in patients with CMV enteritis). Other common causes of abdominal pain such as urinary tract infection and constipation may be seen in HIV-infected children as well. Pneumonia, especially involving the lower lobes may also present with complaints of abdominal pain (and may be accompanied by vomiting). HIV-infected children are also at risk for less common causes of abdominal pain.

Esophagitis due to *Candida* infections may be seen. Usually, these patients have retrosternal or epigastric pain especially with swallowing [32, 33]. Esophagitis may or may not be accompanied by oral thrush. *Herpes simplex* virus (HSV) may lead to esophagitis with similar symptoms. Usually, oral ulcers accompany HSV esophagitis [32]. Young children may refuse to drink or have drooling as presenting signs of these infections.

HIV-infected children have been reported to develop pancreatitis at increased rates [36]. In this group of patients, pancreatitis was associated with the use of pentamidine, especially in patients with very low CD4 counts. *Pneumocystis carinii* pneumonia, CMV, cryptosporidium, and MAC were all associated with pancreatitis. Patients with pancreatitis virtually all have abdominal pain and vomiting. Didanosine (ddI), lamivudine (3TC), stavudine (d4T), and zalcitabine (ddC) are also associated with pancreatitis [21, 37].

Other rare causes of abdominal pain have been reported in children with HIV infections. Splenic abscesses were reported in two patients who had fever and abdominal pain as presenting symptoms [38]. An HIV-infected child with recurrent episodes of abdominal pain was found to have hydrops-like cholecystitis due to cryptosporidial endocholecystitis [39]. In adult patients with HIV infection, hepatobiliary disease is the most common site of extraintestinal involvement with this organism. Extrapulmonary *Pneumocystis carinii* infections can also involve abdominal organs.

Evaluation

Evaluation of the HIV-infected child with abdominal pain begins with a thorough history and physical examination. Other signs and symptoms of gastroenteritis should be sought. Fever may accompany gastroenteritis. Fever is also seen with urinary tract infections, lower lobe pneumonias, and acute abdominal processes such as appendicitis. Many patients with pancreatitis have fever as well. Absence of fever makes infections or suppurative causes of abdominal pain less common but does not exclude them completely.

A medication history may reveal the use of pentamidine, ddI, 3TC, d4T, ddC, or steroids. All of these agents have been associated with pancreatitis. A past history of pancreatitis, urinary tract infections, or recurrent problems with constipation may make one of these processes the most likely diagnosis. Emesis that is not followed by diarrhea within 12–24 hours makes gastroenteritis a less likely cause of abdominal pain. Pancreatitis, intussusception, or acute abdominal processes leading to an ileus or obstruction should be considered. Bilious emesis may be seen with an ileus but should raise the concern of a mechanical obstruction. All children with bilious emesis should have abdominal x-rays with multiple views to rule out an obstruction.

Peritoneal signs should prompt surgical consultation. Right lower quadrant pain and tenderness, rebound tenderness, and guarding are seen with appendicitis. Remember that the WBC count may not be elevated in patients with HIV infection and appendicitis. Abdominal and pelvic CT scans may be helpful. Right upper quadrant tenderness and possibly a mass may be seen with cholecystitis. Periumbilical, epigastric, and flank pain can be seen in children with pancreatitis. Often, the physical signs in children with pancreatitis seem to be less than would be expected from the child's symptoms. Severe pain and emesis are the most common symptoms seen. Intermittent, cramping, severe pain, which may be relieved by episodes of emesis, is more typical of intussusception. A mass may be felt in children with intussusception, usually in the right side of the abdomen. Bloody stools (currant-jelly stools) are a late sign of intussusception indicating mucosal ischemia

and compromise. The goal should be to make this diagnosis before this occurs.

Unless the history and physical examination clearly point to a benign cause of abdominal pain (e.g. constipation) or gastroenteritis, HIV-infected children with abdominal pain should have some screening laboratory and radiologic studies performed. At least two radiologic views of the abdomen to rule out ileus or obstruction should be obtained. A CBC with differential, urinalysis, urine Gram stain and culture may be helpful. Serum transaminases, bilirubin, lipase, and amylase determinations are helpful in the evaluation. Elevated serum lipase is a more sensitive and more specific finding than elevated amylase in patients with pancreatitis. If cholecystitis or other hepatobiliary processes are suspected, serum bilirubin and hepatic transaminases may be elevated. In patients found to have pancreatitis, serum calcium, glucose, and electrolytes should be followed closely.

Specialized studies may be required for diagnosis or treatment in certain situations. Esophagrams or esophagoscopy may be required to make a definitive diagnosis of *Candida* or HSV esophagitis. Ultrasonography may be used to diagnose cholecystitis or monitor patients with pancreatitis for pseudocyst formation. It may also be useful in the diagnosis of appendicitis and some cases of intussusception. Air-contrast or barium enema remains the diagnostic tool of choice as well as the initial treatment for intussusception. Hepatic and splenic abscesses may be found with ultrasound or abdominal computed tomography (CT) scans.

Therapy

The main goal of therapy in HIV-infected children with abdominal pain is to provide good supportive care until the underlying cause can be found. Hydration status should be monitored closely. Intravenous fluids and glucose and electrolytes should be given, if needed. Analgesia should be provided as soon as possible. Delaying the administration of analgesics while diagnostic studies are performed is not necessary. After a diagnosis is made, definitive therapy may be begun.

Children with esophagitis due to *Candida* may be treated with ketoconazole and mycostatin orally [32]. Failure to respond to this therapy in a few days should prompt the institution of parenteral therapy. Amphotericin B or fluconazole are possible alternatives [32] (see Chapter 35).

Treatment of pancreatitis is supportive in nature. Patients should be made NPO and have a nasogastric tube placed and put to low, intermittent suction to effect complete bowel rest. Intravenous fluids and parenteral hyperalimentation should be begun. Nasogastric losses should be replaced. Analgesia with opioids should be provided.

Respiratory status, serum calcium, electrolytes, and glucose should be monitored carefully. Serial ultrasound or abdominal CT scans should be performed to monitor for the development of pancreatic pseudocysts, abscesses, or hemorrhagic complications. Medications that could have caused pancreatitis should be discontinued. Corticosteroids are not indicated and antibiotics should only be given for specific suppurative complications.

Parenchymal abscesses may be treated with antibiotics or antifungal agents if a causative organism is known. However, most parenchymal lesions require surgical drainage at some point [38]. Common causes of abdominal pain should be managed as they would in children without HIV infection (see Chapter 16).

12.6 Neurologic emergencies

Most HIV-infected children have neurologic involvement at some point in their illness [5, 7]. The most common neurologic manifestation of HIV infection in children is an encephalopathy due to primary infection of the CNS [5–7]. Emergency presentations of this encephalopathy are rare except in rapidly progressive cases. However, children with HIV infection may have the acute onset of seizures or a change in mental status that warrants an ED workup and emergency treatment. One case series reports two children in which the initial presentation of their HIV disease was that of seizures accompanying ischemic cerebrovascular accidents [40]. Chapters 17 and 26 contain more detailed discussions of the neurologic and neuropsychologic disorders associated with HIV infection.

12.6.1 Seizures

Differential diagnosis

The encephalopathy associated with HIV infection usually is not associated with seizures [5, 7]. Seizures may be part of the clinical picture if the encephalopathy is rapidly progressive. However, other causes must always be ruled out when an HIV-infected child presents with seizures. The differential diagnosis of seizures in HIV-infected children is found in Table 12.14. Central nervous system infections are a major cause of morbidity. Opportunistic infections of the CNS are seen but are less common than bacterial meningitis in children with HIV infection [7]. The same organisms that are responsible for meningitis in immunocompetent children are often involved. *Streptoccus pneumoniae, H. influenzae* type B, *Escherichia coli*, and *Salmonella* sp. are all seen in these patients [7, 41]. Children with HIV infection may not respond normally to immunizations and, therefore, pneumococcal and HiB disease may be seen even in patients with complete immunizations. Children may

Table 12.14 Differential diagnosis of seizures

Bacterial meningitis
    Streptococcus pneumoniae
    Haemophilus influenzae type b
    Escherichia coli
    Salmonella sp.
    Other bacteria
Opportunistic infections
    Toxoplasma gondii
    Cryptococcus neoformans
    Candida albicans
    Mycobacterium tuberculosis
    Atypical mycobacterium
Viral infections
    Cytomegalovirus
    Herpes simplex virus
CNS malignancy
CNS hemorrhage or infarction
Rapidly progressive HIV encephalopathy

present with fever, headache, lethargy or irritability, nuchal rigidity, and possibly focal deficits. Seizures with fever are a possible presentation.

Opportunistic infections caused by *Toxoplasma gondii, Cryptococcus neoformans, Candida albicans, Mycobacterium tuberculosis*, and atypical mycobacteria may cause focal or generalized seizures in patients with HIV infection. Meningeal signs and signs of increased intracranial pressure may be seen. Viral infections with CMV and HSV as well as common viruses such as enteroviruses may cause meningitis or encephalitis and seizures.

Central nervous system malignancies, usually lymphoma, and hemorrhage or infarction may cause seizures, focal deficits, or an abrupt change in mental status [6, 7, 40, 41]. Central nervous system hemorrhage usually occurs in the setting of immune-mediated thrombocytopenia [6, 7]. A small number of pediatric HIV patients have developed CNS aneurysms [42], and a few develop acquired coagulopathies. Infarctions have been reported in children with HIV encephalopathy and may account for their initial presentation [7, 40]. HIV-infected children may also have seizures due to the same causes seen in other children, including trauma, ingestions, and metabolic derangements. These other causes should also be considered.

Evaluation and treatment

Emergency evaluation and management of HIV-infected children with seizures proceed hand in hand (Figure 12.1). The ED physician should rapidly assess the child's airway,

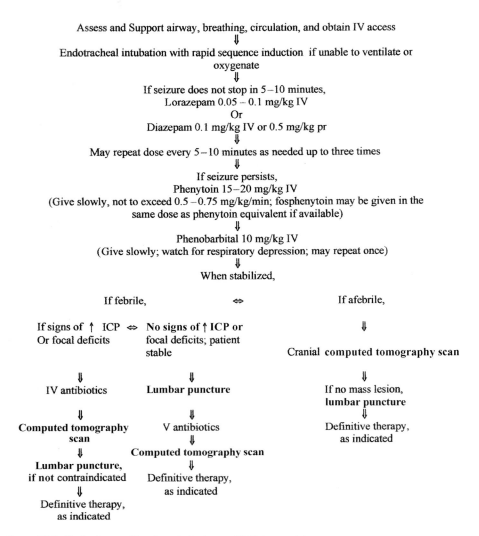

Assess and Support airway, breathing, circulation, and obtain IV access
⇓
Endotracheal intubation with rapid sequence induction if unable to ventilate or
oxygenate
⇓
If seizure does not stop in 5–10 minutes,
Lorazepam 0.05 – 0.1 mg/kg IV
Or
Diazepam 0.1 mg/kg IV or 0.5 mg/kg pr
⇓
May repeat dose every 5–10 minutes as needed up to three times
⇓
If seizure persists,
Phenytoin 15–20 mg/kg IV
(Give slowly, not to exceed 0.5 – 0.75 mg/kg/min; fosphenytoin may be given in the
same dose as phenytoin equivalent if available)
⇓
Phenobarbital 10 mg/kg IV
(Give slowly; watch for respiratory depression; may repeat once)
⇓
When stabilized,

If febrile,   ⇔   If afebrile,

If signs of ↑ ICP ⇔ No signs of ↑ ICP or   ⇓
Or focal deficits   focal deficits; patient
                        stable   Cranial computed tomography scan

⇓   ⇓   ⇓
IV antibiotics   Lumbar puncture   If no mass lesion,
                                           lumbar puncture
⇓   ⇓   ⇓
Computed tomography V antibiotics   Definitive therapy,
scan   ⇓   as indicated
⇓   Computed tomography scan
Lumbar puncture,   ⇓
if not contraindicated Definitive therapy,
⇓   as indicated
Definitive therapy,
as indicated

Figure 12.1. Evaluation and treatment of seizures. ICP, intracranial pressure.

breathing, and circulatory status and support the airway and ventilate, if necessary. Bag-valve-mask ventilation is usually sufficient until the seizure can be controlled. If ventilation is not effective or if prolonged hypoventilation occurs with the use of anticonvulsant medications, endotracheal intubation is indicated. In patients with uncontrolled status epilepticus or signs of increased intracranial pressure, rapid sequence intubation should be considered for cerebral protection. Intravenous access should be obtained. If the clinician is unable to obtain access, intraosseous needles may be used or diazepam may be given per rectum, 0.5 mg/kg, to control seizures.

Seizures that continue for more than a few minutes should be treated with anticonvulsant agents. Benzodiazepines (0.1 mg/kg diazepam IV or 0.05–0.1 mg/kg lorazepam IV) are usually used first. If seizures do not abate

with two to three doses, phenytoin (with a loading dose of 20 mg/kg IV) may be added. Phenytoin does not cause respiratory depression. Phenytoin should be given slowly (no more than 0.5–0.75 mg/kg/min) or hypotension and cardiovascular collapse may occur. Fosphenytoin does not seem to have this untoward side effect. Phenobarbital may also be added, although its respiratory depressive effects are additive to those of the benzodiazepines. Close monitoring of the patient's airway and respiratory effort must be continued.

After the patient has been stabilized, the search for the cause of the seizure must begin. Any signs of increased intracranial pressure (e.g., bulging fontanelle, cranial nerve dysfunction, or papilledema) or focal deficits should prompt emergent neuroradiologic imaging with close monitoring. A prospective study among HIV-infected adolescents and adults in an ED showed that new seizures, depressed or altered orientation, or headaches, different in quality from a usual headache for the patient were all highly associated with the presence of focal lesions on noncontrast head CT [43].

Patients with signs of impending herniation should undergo rapid sequence intubation and hyperventilation and receive mannitol. If the patient is febrile or if bacterial meningitis is suspected for other reasons, antibiotic therapy should be begun. In this situation, antibiotic therapy should not be delayed until CSF is obtained. In febrile patients without signs of increased intracranial pressure or focality, a lumbar puncture can be obtained before CT and then antibiotics can be administered. Cefotaxime or ceftriaxone and vancomycin are an appropriate empiric regimen (see discussion of treatment of bacterial meningitis in Chapters 26 and 37).

Cerebrospinal fluid should be obtained even in the absence of fever. However, cranial CT scans should be performed before lumbar puncture in these cases. Cerebrospinal fluid cell count and differential, glucose and total protein, and Gram stain and bacterial culture and sensitivity should be ordered. Cerebrospinal fluid should also be sent for viral culture, India ink stain or cryptococcal antigen, and fungal cultures. Serum glucose, electrolytes, and calcium levels should be checked in patients with seizures without fevers. Laboratory and radiologic findings in patients with various causes of seizures are outlined in Table 12.15. After the cause of the seizure is determined, specific therapy for bacterial, opportunistic, or viral infections may be begun. Malignancies may be amenable to therapy. Supportive care and possible neurosurgical intervention are indicated for cerebrovascular accidents.

12.6.2 Altered mental status

Children with CNS infections, malignancies, or cerebrovascular accidents may present with an acute alteration in their mental status. The differential diagnosis is similar to that considered for an HIV-infected child who presents with seizures. Once again, signs of increased intracranial pressure or new focal deficits should prompt neuroradiologic imaging. Computed tomography scans are usually more readily available than magnetic resonance imaging (MRI) studies in the acute setting. Patients who are unstable are more easily monitored during CT scans. Computed tomography scans require much less time to complete than MRI studies. A CT scan will reveal major problems (e.g., new mass lesion, acute hemorrhage, etc.) and guide initial management. Magnetic resonance imaging may be done when the patient is more stable. Patients with fever should have a lumbar puncture to exclude CNS infection as a cause of

Table 12.15 Laboratory and radiologic findings for specific causes of seizures

Cause	Laboratory or radiologic findings
Bacterial meningitis	Cerebrospinal fluid (CSF) pleocytosis, low glucose, elevated protein, and positive Gram's stain and culture.
Toxoplasmosis	Single- or multiple-ring-enhancing mass lesions on cranial CT with contrast
Cryptococcal meningitis	Positive India ink stain or cryptococcal antigen in CSF
Viral meningitis/ encephalitis	CSF pleocytosis and elevated protein, *Herpes simplex* virus may give ring-enhancing lesions on cranial CT with contrast
Mycobacterial meningitis	CSF lymphocytic pleocytosis with markedly elevated protein and low glucose; mass lesions may be seen on CT
CNS malignancy	Mass lesion on CT
CNS hemorrhage	Fresh blood on CT
CNS infarction	CT showing edema initially followed by increased lucency over several days
CNS aneurysms	Aneurysms on CT or MRI [42]

CNS, central nervous system; CT, computed tomography; MRI, magnetic resonance imaging.

their deterioration. Opportunistic infections and some viral encephalitides may present without classic signs of meningitis and altered mental status with or without fever may be the only presenting sign. For patients without fever, imaging studies should precede the lumbar puncture. After an underlying diagnosis is found, specific treatment should be begun.

12.7 Summary

Children with HIV infection may present with an acute change in status for a variety of reasons. Sepsis, pulmonary, gastrointestinal, and neurologic emergencies all are major causes of morbidity and mortality. Recognizing the causes of these emergencies and knowing how to treat them are important for any clinician working in the acute care setting. In addition, physicians who work in the emergency department setting must recognize the ways in which HIV infection manifests itself in children. Identifying infected children and referring them for appropriate care can lead to a prolonged survival and an improved quality of life.

REFERENCES

1. Hsia, D. C., Fleishman, J. A., East, J. A. & Hellinger, F. J. Pediatric human immunodeficiency virus infection: recent evidence on the utilization and costs of health services. *Arch. Pediatr. Adolesc. Med.* **149** (1995), 488–96.

2. Friedland, L. R., Bell, L. M. & Rutstein, R. Utilization and clinical manifestations of human immunodeficiency virus type 1-infected children to a pediatric emergency department. *Pediatr. Emerg. Care* **7** (1991), 72–5.

3. Schweich, P. J., Fosarelli, P. D., Duggan, A. K., Quinn, T. C. & Baker, J. L. Prevalence of human immunodeficiency virus seropositivity in pediatric emergency room patients undergoing phlebotomy. *Pediatrics* **86** (1990), 660–5.

4. Fein, J. A., Friedland, L. R., Rutstein, R. & Bell, L. M. Children with unrecognized human immunodeficiency virus infection: an emergency department perspective. *Am. J. Dis. Child.* **147** (1993), 1104–8.

5. Crain, E. F. & Bernstein, L. J. Pediatric HIV infection for the emergency physician: epidemiology and overview. *Pediatr. Emerg. Care* **6** (1990), 6214–18.

6. Walker, A. R. HIV infections in children. *Emerg. Med. Clin. North Amer.* **13** (1995), 147–62.

7. Zuckerman, G., Metrou, M., Bernstein, C. J. & Crain, E. F. Neurologic disorders and dermatologic manifestations in HIV-infected children. *Pediatr. Emerg. Care* **7** (1991), 99–105.

8. Babl, F., Cooper, E. R., Damon, B. *et al.* HIV postexposure prophylaxis for children and adolescents. *Amer. J. Emerg. Med.* **18** (2000), 282–7.

9. Pinkert, H., Harper, M. D., Cooper, T. & Fleisher, G. R. HIV-infected children in the pediatric emergency department. *Pediatr. Emerg. Care* **9** (1993), 265–9.

10. Nicholas, S. W. The opportunistic and bacterial infections associated with pediatric human immunodeficiency virus disease. *Acta. Pediatr.* (Suppl.) **400** (1994), 46–50.

11. Nicholas, S. W. Management of the HIV-positive child with fever. *J. Pediatr.* **119** (1991), S21–4.

12. Larson, T. & Bechtel, L. Managing the child infected with HIV. *Primary Care* **22** (1995), 23–50.

13. Principi, N., Marchisio, P., Tornaghi, R. *et al.* Occurrence of infection in children infected with human immunodeficiency virus. *Pediatr. Infect. Dis. J.* **10** (1991), 190–3.

14. Farley, J. J., King, J. C., Jr., Nair, P. *et al.* Invasive pneumococcal disease among infected and uninfected children of mothers with human immunodeficiency virus infection. *J. Pediatr.* **124** (1994), 853–8.

15. Mao, C., Harper, M., McIntosh, K. *et al.* Invasive pneumococcal infections in human immunodeficiency virus-infected children. *J. Infect. Dis.* **173** (1996), 870–6.

16. Dayan, P. S., Chamberlain, J. M., Arpadi, S. M. *et al. Streptococcus pneumoniae* bacteremia in children infected with HIV: presentation, course, and outcome. *Pediatr. Emerg. Care* **14** (1998), 194–7.

17. Principi, N., Marchisio, P., Tornaghi, R. *et al.* Acute otitis media in human immunodeficiency virus-infected children. *Pediatrics* **88** (1991), 566–71.

18. Barnett, E. D., Klein, J. O., Pelton, S. I. & Luginbuhl, L. M. Otitis media in children born to human immunodeficiency virus-infected mothers. *Pediatr. Infect. Dis. J.* **11** (1992), 360–4.

19. Andiman, W. A., Mezger, J. & Shapiro, E. Invasive bacterial infections in children born to women infected with human immunodeficiency virus type 1. *J. Pediatr.* **124** (1994), 846–52.

20. Bye, M. R. HIV in children. *Clin. Chest. Med.* **17** (1996), 787–96.

21. Harper, M. B. Human immunodeficiency virus infection. In G. R., Fleisher & S. Ludwig (eds.), *Textbook of Pediatric Emergency Medicine*, 4th Edition. Philadelphia, PA: Lippincott, Williams and Wilkins (2000) pp. 795–809.

22. Cunningham, S. J., Crain, E. F. & Bernstein, L. J. Evaluating the HIV-infected child with pulmonary signs and symptoms. *Pediatr. Emerg. Care* **7** (1991), 32–7.

23. Hauger, S. B. Approach to the pediatric patient with HIV infection and pulmonary symptoms. *J. Pediatr.* **119** (1991), S25–33.

24. Cowan, M. J., Shelhamer, J. H. & Levine, S. J. Acute respiratory failure in the HIV-seropositive patient. *Crit. Care. Clin.* **13** (1997), 523–52.

25. King, J. C., Burke, A. R., Clemens, J. D. *et al.* Respiratory syncytial virus illnesses in human immunodeficiency virus- and non-infected children. *Pediatr. Infect. Dis. J.* **12** (1993), 733–9.

26. Simonds, R. J., Oxtoby, M. J., Caldwell, B., Gwinn, M. L. & Rogers, M. F. *Pneumocystis carinii* pneumonia among US children with perinatally acquired HIV infection. *J. Am. Med. Assoc.* **270**: 4 (1993), 470–3.

27. Connor, E., Bagarazzi, M., McSherry, G. *et al.* Clinical and laboratory correlates of *Pneumocystis carinii* pneumonia in children infected with HIV. *J. Am. Med. Assoc.* **265** (1991), 1963–7.

28. Schneider, R. F. Lymphoid interstitial pneumonitis and non-specific interstitial pneumonitis. *Clin. Chest. Med.* **17** (1996), 763–6.

29. Sheikh, S., Bakshi, S. S. & Pahwa, S. G. Outcome and survival in HIV-infected infants with *Pneumocystis carinii* pneumonia and respiratory failure. *Pediatr. AIDS HIV Infect.* **7** (1996), 155–63.

30. Williams, A. J., Duong, T., McNally, L. M. *et al. Pneumocystis carinii* pneumonia and cytomegalovirus infection in children with vertically acquired HIV infection. *AIDS* **15** (2001), 335–9.

31. Sleasman, J. W., Hemenway, C., Klein, A. S. & Barrett, D. J. Corticosteroids improve survival of children with AIDS and

Pneumocystis carinii pneumonia. *Am. J. Dis. Child.* **147** (1993), 30–4.

32. Powell, K. R. Approach to gastrointestinal manifestations in infants and children with HIV infection. *J. Pediatr.* **119** (1991), S34–40.

33. Lewis, J. D. & Winter, H. S. Intestinal and hepatobiliary diseases in HIV-infected children. *Gastroenterol. Clin. N. Am.* **24** (1995), 119–32.

34. Guarino, A., Castaldo, A., Russo, S. *et al.* Enteric cryptosporidiosis in pediatric HIV infection. *J. Pediatr. Gastroenterol. Nutr.* **25** (1997), 182–7.

35. Bova, R. & Meagher, A. Appendicitis in HIV-positive patients. *Aust. N. Z. J. Surg.* **68** (1998), 337–9.

36. Miller, T. L., Winter, H. S., Luginbuhl, L. M. *et al.* Pancreatitis in pediatric human immunodeficiency virus infection. *J. Pediatr.* **120** (1992), 223–7.

37. Love, J. T. & Shearer, W. T. Prevention, diagnosis and treatment of pediatric HIV infection. *Comprehensive Ther.* **22** (1996), 719–26.

38. Smith, M. D., Nio, M., Cawel, J. E. *et al.* Management of splenic abscess in immuno-compromised children. *J. Pediatr. Surg.* **28** (1993), 823–6.

39. Boige, N., Bellaiche, M., Carnet, D. *et al.* Hydrops-like cholecystitis due to cryptosporidiosis in an HIV-infected child. *J. Pediatr. Gastroenterol. Nutr.* **26** (1998), 219–21.

40. Visudtibhan, A., Visudhiphan, P. & Chiemchanya, S. Stroke and seizures as the presenting signs of pediatric HIV infection. *Pediatr. Neurol.* **20** (1999), 53–6.

41. Butler, C., Hittelman, J. & Hauger, S. B. Approach to neurodevelopmental and neurologic complications in pediatric HIV infection. *J. Pediatr.* **119** (1991), S41–6.

42. Husson, R. N., Saini, R., Lewis, L. L. *et al.* Cerebral artery aneurysms in children infected with human immunodeficiency virus. *J. Pediatr.* **121** (1992), 927–30.

43. Rothman, R. E., Keyl, P. M., McArthur, J. C. *et al.* A decision guideline for emergency department utilization of noncontrast head computed tomography in HIV-infected patients. *Acad. Emerg. Med.* **6** (1999), 1010–19.

13

Adherence to antiretroviral therapy in children and youth

John Farley, M.D., M.P.H.

Department of Pediatrics, University of Maryland School of Medicine, Baltimore, MD

Improved health outcomes for HIV-infected children and youth will not be achieved without maximal viral suppression. Highly active antiretroviral therapy (HAART) represents a major breakthrough in HIV management, but not all patients respond optimally to HAART. Non-adherence is well established as a major cause of clinical failure, and intermittent non-adherence is a particular problem. Studies in adults have demonstrated that $\geq$ 95% adherence to HAART is necessary for durable suppression of viral load [1–3]. In the presence of selective pressure by antiretroviral agents, high rates of viral replication and viral mutation lead to the development of drug resistance. Mutations conferring resistance against one antiretroviral agent often confer cross-resistance to other agents; poor adherence can render a whole class of antiretrovirals ineffective.

Although a crucial component of good clinical care, assessment of adherence to HAART in HIV-infected children and youth is challenging and labor intensive. Patient and parent (or other caregiver) characteristics associated with optimal adherence are not well characterized. Studies evaluating interventions to improve adherence in this group are encouraging but few.

13.1 HIV as a chronic illness

Pediatric HIV infection is now referred to as the 'newest chronic illness in childhood' [4, 5]. Chronic illness alters a person's life by creating permanent changes in daily living. The person must adhere to a medical regimen even though there is no cure, often in the absence of visible symptoms. While our understanding of HIV therapy is evolving, life-long treatment will likely be required. Adherence is a major problem in management of patients with all chronic illnesses. Non-adherence with medical regimens occurs with half of all medical recommendations made to chronically ill patients [6].

Pediatric chronic illness presents many unique adherence challenges. Caregivers are responsible for the adherence of children and so have a profound impact on adherence. Children living in families in which the adult caregiver is ill, is subject to significant stress, lacks effective organizational skills, lacks social support, or is not motivated to administer medications will have a high risk of non-adherence. Use of outreach staff to provide additional support for families with such challenges may enhance adherence.

Adherence of children to complex medical regimens is influenced by the parent or caregiver's knowledge of the illness, understanding of the therapeutic recommendations, and duration of treatment [7]. Previous studies of pediatric chronic illnesses have found a relationship between poor adherence and the caregiver's understanding of the prescribed regimen and the complexity of the regimen [8]. Difficulties with adherence are observed with other chronic diseases, such as diabetes. The complexity and numerous demands associated with diabetes treatment often lead to significant declines in adherence over the course of treatment. Periodic non-adherence is often viewed as the rule, rather than the exception [9]. Thus, providers need to emphasize caregiver education, and realize that adherence will likely decrease over time without intervention.

Children's understanding of and reactions to illness change during development through a series of systematic stages that correspond to cognitive abilities [10]. The child's level of cognitive, motor, social, emotional, and psychological functioning affect the course and management of the disease. Their ability to perceive their own illness, approach medical treatment, and respond to interventions is influenced by their developmental level. It is important for care providers to be certain that a child's understanding of his or her illness is periodically updated to keep pace with cognitive and emotional development. Older children assume increasing responsibility for their own care and are influenced by peers and their social setting [8]. Providers need to assess the influence of developmental factors on adherence periodically and adjust interventions to improve adherence as the child matures.

13.2 Models to conceptualize adherence behavior

13.2.1 The Health Belief Model

Although originally developed to understand adherence among chronically ill adults, much of the research on pediatric adherence has been driven by the Health Belief Model [11]. It is the best-known model for predicting an individual's adherence to ongoing medical regimens. The model suggests that an individual's ability to follow through with a recommendation depends upon perceptions of susceptibility to the specific illness, the severity of the condition, perceptions of benefits of the prescribed regimen, and the physical, psychological, financial, and other costs associated with initiating or continuing the recommended treatment [8]. Self-efficacy (believing that one is not hindered by obstacles and has the ability to adhere) was more recently considered a major adherence "determinant," suggesting that perception of vulnerability and an understanding of the disease and its treatment may be necessary, but not sufficient for optimal adherence [12]. (see Figure 13.1). According to this model, the most adherent individuals are those who maintain strong perceptions of vulnerability to disease, view the disease as serious, believe that the regimen will produce positive therapeutic results, and are not hindered by many obstacles to implementing treatment [9]. In a study of 179 HIV-infected adults enrolled in a two-drug combination clinical trial, good adherence was predicted by Health Belief Model premises, in particular the belief that HIV was a serious disease [13].

The Health Belief Model suggests that the caregiver's perspective determines whether or not they will assume responsibility for their child's care and adhere to the specific regimen. However, researchers employing this model have generally not incorporated developmental concerns or the involvement of extended family members. As a result, the relevance of the Health Belief Model in pediatric adherence interventions has been questioned. A

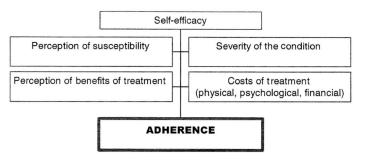

Figure 13.1. Health Belief Model determinants [15, 16].

number of other important determinants such as caregiver stress, psychiatric illness, addictions issues, child behavioral/developmental problems and disclosure of the diagnosis to the child or other family members are not considered in the classic model. For example, depression and ongoing substance abuse are associated with poor adherence among HIV-infected adults, and one would expect a similar association among caregivers of HIV-infected children [2, 14, 15].

13.2.2 The Stages of Change to Model

For newly diagnosed adolescents and some older perinatally infected youth, initiation of HAART and the required adherence is a significant behavioral change. While readiness for behavioral change is unique for each person and may be related to Health Belief Model determinants, the process of behavior change is complex and addressed by the Stages of change to Model. Based on a comparative analysis of major therapy systems [16, 17], the model describes a pattern of movement through five specific stages [18]: individuals are (a) unaware or unwilling to do anything about the problem; (b) consider the possibility of change; (c) become determined and prepared to make the change; (d) take action; and (e) sustain the change over time [19]. They have designated these stages: pre-contemplation, contemplation, preparation, action, and maintenance (see Figure 13.2). It is important to note that the pre-contemplation stage is quite diverse, that an individual frequently recycles or "relapses" several times through different stages, and that an individual may not progress linearly through the stages. The major clinical implications of the model are that providers must carefully assess an individual's readiness for action (i.e. adherence) before prescribing HAART, and that periodic relapse (i.e. non-adherence) is to be expected, necessitating a plan to minimize the clinical impact of non-adherence such as educating the patient to stop all antiretrovirals rather than just some. The TREAT (Treatment Regimens Enhancing Adherence in Teens) Program was developed

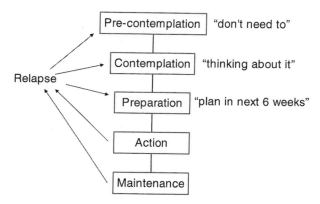

Figure 13.2. The trans-theoretical Stages of Change Model [20–23].

as an adolescent-focused, multi-faceted program, based on the Stages of Change Model, to promote optimal long-term adherence to HAART [20]. TREAT was designed primarily for treatment-naïve HIV-infected youth, and was developed and piloted as part of the REACH (Reaching for Excellence in Adolescent Care and Health) Study for youth infected through sexual activity and injection drug use sponsored by the US National Institutes of Health at multiple sites in the USA.

13.3 Assessment of adherence

A number of methods have been used or proposed to assess adherence in clinical practice and in research studies. Each method has distinctive benefits and drawbacks. The methods include parent interview, pill counts, medication refill records, electronic monitoring, drug level monitoring, monitoring response to therapy, and utilizing records of other health behaviors such as appointment keeping. While it is clear that close to 100% adherence is necessary for sustained viral suppression, the cutoff for an adequate level of adherence does vary somewhat depending upon the assessment method used. The adherence cutoff value may also vary with different antiretroviral therapies. For example, since a single point mutation resulting in a single amino acid change leads to high level resistance to all of the available non-nucleoside reverse transcriptase inhibitors (NNRTIs), regimens including NNRTIs may be less forgiving of adherence lapses than other regimens. A summary of adherence assessment modalities studied in HIV-infected children is shown in Table 13.1.

13.3.1 Caregiver self-report

Caregiver interview or self-report is considered especially subject to bias, as parents may inflate their adherence

report to satisfy clinicians. However, it can be used to identify some poor adherers [21], and these poor adherers can respond to interventions [22]. While useful as a reinforcement tool, parent self-monitoring (i.e. using a calendar to record doses given) is subject to the same bias as caregiver interviews or other approaches to self-report when used as a measurement tool. Caregiver self-report to assess adherence among perinatally HIV-infected children has been utilized with useful but imperfect results. The best-known instrument is the Pediatric AIDS Clinical Trial Group (PACTG) Pediatric Adherence Questionnaire Modules 1 and 2 (http://www.fstrf.org/qol/peds/pedadhere.html). Module 1 of the PACTG Adherence Questionnaire begins with identification of antiretroviral medications and then asks the subject about doses missed during the prior 3 days. Module 2 presents a number of potential problems with adherence and asks the caregiver if any of these potential problems have occurred in the past 14 days.

Good adherence as assessed by self-report instruments is associated with good clinical outcomes. A study using the Pediatric AIDS Clinical Trials Group Protocol (PACTG) instrument in HIV-infected children enrolled in a clinical trial involving a HAART regimen (PACTG 377) found a correlation between the child's virologic outcome and caregiver self-reported adherence during the 3 days prior to the interview [23]. Another larger study (n = 90) using a similar, but not identical self-report questionnaire found that children whose caregivers reported no missed doses in the previous week were more likely to have a viral load < 400 copies/mL [24]. Even though the self-report instruments can predict clinical outcomes, the data obtained using these instruments may not be entirely accurate. Two studies showed that a caregiver self-report questionnaire dramatically overestimated adherence compared with pill count and/or electronic monitoring [25, 26]. It may be possible to improve self-report questionnaires to enhance their accuracy. In one study, participants were more likely to self-report adherence difficulty when questions focused on problems rather than missed doses [26], suggesting a possible strategy for design of alternative self-report instruments and an approach for care providers during patient care visits.

Several variations of self-report instruments have been developed. The Pills Identification Test (PIT) uses a display board with two similar pills for each antiretroviral prescribed and asks patients to identify which pill they are taking. Correct PIT scores have been shown to be associated with adherence in HIV-infected adults [27], suggesting a potential adjunct to self-report for pediatric providers. Audio computer-assisted self-interviewing has been shown

Table 13.1 Adherence assessment modalities studied in HIV-infected children

Reference assessment modality and adherence definition	Number adherent (%)	Number non-adherent (%)	Association with viral load < 400 copies/ml
Watson and Farley [38] (4–6 months follow-up)			
Prescription refill (> 75% all antiretrovirals)	42 (58%)	30 (42%)	$P = 0.001$
Steele *et al.* [25] (3 months follow-up)			
Self-report (< 20% missed doses in prior 3 days)	29 (96.7%)	1 (3.3%)	NS
Pill count (> 80% all antiretrovirals)	18 (69.2%)	8 (30.8%)	NS
MEMS Track Cap™ (> 80% all antiretrovirals)	2 (25%)	6 (75%)	NS
Reddington *et al.* [24] (cross-sectional)			
Self-report (no missed doses in prior week)	50 (57%)	39 (43%)	$P = 0.04$
Van Dyke *et al.* [23] (clinical trial, 6–12 months follow-up)			
Self-report (no missed doses in prior 3 days)	88 (70%)	37 (30%)	$P = 0.02$
Farley *et al.* [26] (6 months follow-up)			
MEMS Track Cap™ (> 80% one antiretroviral)	17 (65%)	11 (35%)	$P < 0.001$
Prescription refill (> 80% all antiretrovirals)	19 (73%)	8 (27%)	$P = 0.002$
Self-report (no missed doses in prior 3 days)	20 (100%)	0 (0%)	NS
Physician assessment (> 80% all antiretrovirals)	14 (74%)	5 (26%)	$P < 0.001$
No missed clinic appointments	18 (69%)	8 (31%)	$P = 0.009$

to encourage more honest answers from patients on sensitive topics than face to face interviews [28]. This approach was utilized in the REACH study to explore risk behaviors, and may be a future alternative to traditional face-to-face interviewing regarding adherence, particularly for older children and adolescents. The evidence concerning the reliability of self-report, particularly outside of the clinical trial setting, is mixed. Care providers should recognize that self-report generally overestimates adherence, and strongly consider incorporating an alternative adherence assessment strategy as part of patient care.

13.3.2 Provider assessment

Physician estimate or clinical judgment of adherence has been studied in adults with chronic illness. Several studies concluded that clinicians do no better than chance when judging whether or not an adult patient is adherent [29–31]. In a study of HIV-infected adults, physician adherence assessment was found to correlate poorly with pill counts [32]. Pediatricians appear to be just as inaccurate as physicians caring for adults when estimating patient adherence [33, 34]. One small study demonstrated an unexpectedly high reliability for provider assessment in HIV-infected children. In this study, physicians relied heavily on pharmacy refill records and virologic response [26], suggesting a useful strategy for clinical practice.

13.3.3 Pill counts

The pill count method to estimate adherence involves a comparison between the amount of medication remaining in the child's bottle and the amount that should be remaining based on the amount and dosage of the initial prescription and the length of time since the patient began using the bottle. This method does provide a measure of adherence over time, but is subject to bias due to "pill dumping" (i.e. the parent may not leave all unused pills in the bottle in an effort to falsely increase the apparent level of adherence and please the clinician), and determining the date when the patient commenced using the current bottle can be a challenge. The PACTG Adherence to Therapy Subcommittee has developed a Pill Count Case Report Form (CRF). The Pill Count CRF can be utilized with either liquid or tablet/capsule formulations, allows calculations to be adjusted if a dose change or drug holiday has occurred in the interval, and minimizes the number of calculations required to complete the form to reduce error. It seems prudent to avoid performing measurements or counts directly in front of the subject. Although labor intensive, pill counts are likely the most practical and readily available non self-report adherence assessment tool. Disappointingly, the one published study to date in HIV-infected children found a poor correlation of pill counts with both electronic monitoring and virologic response.

However, sample sizes were small (n = 8 for electronic monitoring, n = 30 for virologic response) [25]. The utility of this tool in the clinical setting needs to be more widely assessed. The PACTG Pill Count Form, example cases, and an Excel spreadsheet model to easily perform the calculations are available on the public domain portion of the PACTG website: (http://www.fstrf.org/qol/peds/pedadhere.html).

13.3.4 Pharmacy refill records

The chances of pill dumping bias or reporting bias are minimized by using pharmacy medication refill records (i.e. comparing refill data from the pharmacy with the estimated refill requirement if all doses were administered). This method has been utilized in HIV-infected adults (14, 35, 36) and found to correlate with virologic response (35, 37). Pharmacy refill records were utilized in a study of 72 children receiving HAART. Only 42 (58%) were considered adherent (defined as refilling ≥ 75% of protease inhibitor prescriptions and ≥ 75% of all antiretroviral prescriptions in a 6 month interval). Of the 42 children classified as adherent, 22 (52%) achieved and maintained an undetectable viral load (38). This method is less labor intensive than pill counts, but it does require pharmacist collaboration or access to health insurance claims data. The method generally overestimates adherence, since the availability of medication in the home does not necessarily mean the medication was actually administered. However, this method utilized over several months will usually identify adherence problems. Combining this method with periodic pill counts may enhance sensitivity.

13.3.5 Electronic monitoring

Pharmacy refill records and pill counts provide a general assessment of the number of doses taken, but fail to yield any information regarding patterns of poor adherence. Electronic monitoring of adherence offers a more detailed assessment, demonstrating problems with dosing intervals in addition to missed doses. The Medication Event Monitoring System (MEMS, Aprex/Aardex Corp., Menlo Park, CA) uses a microprocessor in the medication container cap to record the date and time of each vial opening. This technology has been utilized in HIV-infected adults to correlate behavioral and virologic data. In a small pilot study of seven HIV-infected adults enrolled in a high-dose study with saquinavir monotherapy, medication adherence was monitored using MEMS Track Caps™. When subjects missed medication for only a few days, most had rapid rises in viral loads and some had evidence suggesting that their virus had developed resistance [39]. Four studies in HIV-infected adults with larger sample sizes demonstrated that

electronic monitoring of adherence was the method of adherence assessment which correlated most robustly with virologic suppression [3, 40–42]. Several groups are utilizing this methodology in ongoing studies of HIV-infected children. A study of 26 perinatally HIV-infected children demonstrated similar findings to the adult studies, with electronic monitoring more robustly associated with virologic response than pharmacy refill records or caregiver self-report [25, 26]. Although improved technology is expected to be available in the near future, MEMS™ electronic monitoring caps are not yet available for bottles containing liquids or powders, so this monitoring approach cannot be practically employed if children are receiving all medications in those formulations. Caregivers or youth who lay out pills in advance or use a pill box storage device are also excluded. Placement of the MEMS™ bottle cap requires caregiver cooperation and/or pharmacist collaboration, and caps may become defective or lost, occasionally resulting in incomplete data. The approximate cost of monitoring is US$100 per patient per year for a single drug. The company has developed a SmartCap™ option which provides patients with a reminder beep when doses are due and an information 'window' telling them when the last time they opened the bottle was. This is attractive as a combined monitor and intervention for older children.

13.3.6 Drug level monitoring

Therapeutic drug monitoring for individual patients is under study in adults and proposed in children with the goal of maintaining levels sufficient to suppress viral load and prevent viral mutation and resistance. Therapeutic drug monitoring is discussed in more detail in Chapter 23. As pediatric therapeutic drug monitoring protocols are developed, it will be important to assess the utility of trough drug levels as an adherence assessment tool. This strategy has been employed in HIV-infected adults [43–45], and has been described in children [46, 47]. Evaluation will require incorporation of other adherence measures for comparison within protocols utilizing therapeutic drug monitoring. An anticipated limitation of drug levels as an adherence assessment tool is that the level will only reflect adherence behavior during a period of time (variable depending on drug metabolism) immediately prior to obtaining the level. Utility in the clinical care setting is limited at this time.

13.3.7 Appointment keeping

In a study of 26 perinatally HIV-infected children over a 6-month period, no missed appointment in the interval was associated with virologic response, but agreement with the adherence rate assessed by electronic monitoring was limited [26]. Further study of the association between adherence and appointment-keeping behavior in a larger population seems warranted, as appointment records are commonly available to providers.

13.4 Improving adherence

An implication of the Stages of Changes Model is that individuals starting therapy prematurely or without adequate preparation may nonetheless benefit from failure, learning lessons that could advance the probability of success on the next attempt. However, this may have serious adverse consequences in the case of HAART therapy. A striking finding of the TREAT Program pilot study was that 39% of the youth currently prescribed HAART were staged in a manner discordant with their treatment status, i.e. they were prescribed HAART, but were staged as precontemplation, contemplation, or preparation [20] and were non-adherent, suggesting care providers need to take more care to assess patient readiness prior to initiating HAART. The pilot suggested that the TREAT intervention was successful in facilitating movement through stages, with 78% of the small number of subjects who completed the full program moving forward [20].

There is clear evidence based on caregiver self-report that poor palatability and unpleasant or inconvenient formulations remain major barriers to excellent adherence in children. In the PACTG 377 study discussed previously, caregivers cited "taste" and "child refuses" as common adherence problems for ritonavir liquid and "taste" and "scheduling interferes with lifestyle" for nelfinavir (dosed 3 times a day in this study) [23]. In the study by Reddington *et al.*, the top two desired interventions caregivers cited as potentially very helpful were: "better tasting medications" (81%) and "take meds fewer times each day" (72%) [24]. Antiretroviral therapy regimens requiring less frequent administration have been associated with better adherence in HIV-infected adults. In a study of 244 patients with adherence assessed by self-report, ≥ 80% adherence to pre-HAART antiretrovirals was associated with once or twice a day dosing on multivariate analysis [48] and this was confirmed in a later HAART study [42]. Thus, providers should choose the least complex and most palatable regimen possible. As an alternative to liquid formulations, some of which are notorious for palatability problems, a procedure for teaching young children to swallow pills was first described in 1984, and is now commonly employed by pediatric HIV care providers [49]. If palatability problems are anticipated, delaying initiation of the regimen while pill-swallowing training is attempted should be considered. If palatability issues are otherwise insurmountable, physicians have occasionally resorted to the placement of gastrostomy tubes for HIV-infected children to improve adherence, with excellent outcomes in one case series [50].

In addition to addressing regimen complexity issues and ongoing education, clinicians need not only to provide caregivers and patients with adherence aids, but more importantly work with patients to plan how adherence will be incorporated in the daily "routine" [51]. Before initiating a regimen, patients and their families should be interviewed about the details of their daily routine and adjustments to the treatment regimen (such as timing of dosing) made to accommodate the routine. Weekends may need to be discussed separately from weekdays. Whenever possible, medication dosing should be "cued" to another regular event such as mealtimes or washing up at bedtime. Medication should be available where the routine event dosing is "cued" to take place (i.e. kitchen or bathroom). Adherence aids such as pill boxes with a compartment for doses for each day and time or an alarm device should be encouraged. The effectiveness of different adherence aids will vary from family to family, and will depend upon the details of the family's routine and the patient's specific drug regimen.

While a falling viral load is a powerful positive reinforcement for caregivers and patients, many providers also utilize a "token economy" as an adherence intervention (i.e. a reward for good adherence is given on a regular basis and then eventually withdrawn with the hope that good adherence will be maintained). While this intervention has not been formally evaluated in this setting, a "token economy" is commonly used to address other pediatric behavioral issues with demonstrated efficacy [52]. For example, a caregiver may give a child with behavior problems interfering with medication administration a reward when the child behaves well. However, many adherence problems are more complex, necessitating targeting both caregiver and child behaviors and requiring a more complex intervention. In addition, eventual withdrawal of the reward must be done carefully to maximize the chance that the desired behavior (i.e. good adherence) will be maintained. Planning and conducting a "token economy" intervention is more complicated than one would assume, and mental health supervision should be considered.

There remains a paucity of data identifying characteristics associated with poor adherence that would facilitate the design and implementation of adherence interventions likely to be efficacious. Nonetheless, a prospective randomized trial of an intensive home-based nursing intervention has been described showing that nursing intervention was associated with improved adherence to HAART and virologic outcome [53]. This suggests that

Table 13.2 Approaches to improving treatment adherence

Prior to prescribing HAART

Assess stage of readiness to be adherent and/or explore Health Belief Model determinants and other potential determinants such as substance abuse or depression

Identify and address potential barriers to adherence such as palatability issues, disclosure, or alternate caregivers

Consider the patient's daily life routine when choosing a regimen and minimize dosing frequency to no more than twice a day if possible

Educate the patient and/or caregiver concerning the importance of adherence, special administration requirements, and possible side effects

Cue dosing to regular life events and offer adherence aids such as a pill box if possible

After initiating HAART

Follow-up frequently during the initial months of therapy

Monitor virologic response. A viral load failing to improve as expected is strongly suggestive of adherence problems

When evaluating adherence, supplement self-report with a second adherence assessment method

Provide positive reinforcement and frequent education boosters

Identify adherence problems early and consider prescribed drug holiday while addressing adherence problems

---

interventions to enhance caregiver knowledge and self-efficacy, overcome child-related barriers to adherence, and provide social support are effective for some caregivers.

Development of new antiretroviral formulations has facilitated the testing of once-daily directly observed therapy, in which a healthcare provider observes the patient taking medication. A clinical trial utilizing this intervention for youth newly initiating HAART is under development. Although highly successful for the treatment of tuberculosis, this expensive and labor-intensive intervention has been utilized in one study among HIV-infected adults, with disappointing results [54].

13.5 Conclusion

While each adherence assessment method has advantages and disadvantages, incorporation of adherence assessment and strategies to optimize adherence into the clinical care of HIV-infected children and youth is essential. A summary of recommendations for clinical practice is shown in Table 13.2. Measuring and improving adherence for children and youth will be even more challenging in the future. In developed countries, an increasing proportion of perinatally HIV-infected children are reaching adolescence, and increasing numbers of adolescents are infected through risk behaviors. A majority of patients cared for by pediatric HIV specialists will soon be adolescents. In a study of HIV-infected pregnant women, being an adolescent was the most robust covariate associated with poor adherence to antiretroviral therapy [14], underscoring the adherence difficulties for this age group. In developing countries, potential adherence barriers unique to this setting will need to be identified and addressed. While challenging, attention to adherence can significantly improve clinical outcomes, leading to longer healthier lives for our patients.

REFERENCES

1. Miller, L. D. & Hays, R. D. Adherence to combination antiretroviral therapy: synthesis of the literature and clinical implications. *AIDS Reader* **10** (2000), 177–85.

2. Gifford, A. L., Bormann, J. E., Shively, M. J., Wright, B. C., Richman, D. D. & Bozzette, S. A. Predictors of self-reported adherence and plasma HIV concentrations in patients on multi-drug antiretroviral regimens. *J. AIDS* **23** (2000), 386–95.

3. Arnsten, J. H., Demas, P. A., Farzadegan, H. *et al.* Antiretroviral therapy adherence and viral suppression in HIV-infected drug users: comparison of self-report and electronic monitoring. *Clin. Infect. Dis.* **33** (2001), 1417–23.

4. Lipson, M. What do you say to a child with AIDS? *Hastings Cent. Rep.* **23** (1993), 6–12.

5. Maieron, M. J., Roberts, M. C. & Prentice-Dunn, S. Children's perception of peers with AIDS. Assessing the impact of contagion information, perceived similarity, and illness conceptualization. *J. of Pediatr. Psychol.* **21** (1996), 321–34.

6. Cameron, K. & Gregor, F. Chronic illness and compliance. *J. Advanced Nurs.* **12** (1987), 671–6.

7. Parrish, J. Parent compliance with medical and behavioral recommendations. In N. Krasnegor, J. Arasteh & M. Cataldo (eds.), *Child Health Behavior.* New York, NY: John Wiley & Sons (1986), pp. 453–501.

8. Thompson, R. J. & Gustafson, K. E. *Adaption to chronic childhood illness.* Washington, DC: American Psychological Association (1996).

9. LaGreca, A. & Schuman, W. B. Adherence to prescribed medical regimens. In M.C. Roberts (ed.), *Handbook of Pediatric Psychology. 2nd edn.* New York, NY: Guilford Press (1995), pp. 55–83.

10. Peterson, L.. Coping by children undergoing stressful medical procedures: some conceptual, methodological, and therapeutic issues. *J. Consult. Clin. Psychol.* **57** (1989), 380–7.

11. Becker, M. H., Maiman, L. A., Kirscht, J. P. *et al.* Patient perceptions and compliance: recent studies of the health belief model. In R. B. Haynes, D. W. Taylor & D. L. Sackett (eds.), *Compliance in Health Care.* Baltimore, MD: Johns Hopkins University Press (1979).

12. Rosenstock, I. M., Strecher, V. J. & Becker, M. H. Social learning theory and the Health Belief Model. *Health Educ. Quart.* **15** (1988), 175–83.

13. Besch, C. L., Morse, E., Simon, P. *et al.* Preliminary results of a compliance study within CPCRA 007 Combination Nucleoside Study. In *Fourth Conference on Retroviruses and Opportunistic Infections* Washington, DC: 1997.

14. Laine, C., Newschaffer, C. J., Zhang, D., Cosler, L., Hauck, W. W. & Turner, B. J. Adherence to antiretroviral therapy by pregnant women infected with human immunodeficiency virus: a pharmacy claims-based analysis. *Obstet. Gynecol.* **95** (2000), 167–73.

15. Gordillo, V., del Amo. J., Soriano, V. & Gonzalez-Lahoz, J. Sociodemographic and psychologic variables influencing adherence to antiretroviral therapy. *AIDS* **13** (1999), 1763–9.

16. Prochaska, J. O. & ? Systems of psychotherapy: A transtheoretical analysis. Homewood IL: Dorsey Press (1979).

17. Prochaska, J. O. & DiClemente, C. C. Stages and processes of self-change of smoking: toward an integrative model of change. *J. Consult. Clinic. Psychol.* **51** (1983), 390–5.

18. Prochaska, J. O., DiClemente, C. C. & Norcross, J. C. In search of how people change: applications to addictive behaviors. *Am. Psychol.* **47** (1992), 1102–14.

19. DiClemente, C. C. Motivational interviewing and the stage of change. In W. R. Miller & S. Rollnick (eds.), *Motivational Interviewing: Preparing People for Change.* New York, NY: Guilford Press (1991).

20. Rogers, A. S., Miller, S., Murphy, D. A., Tanney, M. & Fortune, T. The TREAT (therapeutic regimens enhancing adherence in teens) program: theory and preliminary results. *J. Adoles. Health* **292S** (1991), 30–8.

21. Gordis, L., Markowitz, M. & Lilienfield, A. M. The inaccuracy in using interview to estimate patient reliability in taking medications at home. *Med. Care* **17** (1969), 49–54.

22. Haynes, R. B., Taylor, D. W., Sackett, D. L., Gibson, E. S., Bernholz, C. D. & Mukherjee, J. Can simple clinical measurements detect patient noncompliance? *Hypertension* **2** (1980), 757–64.

23. Van Dyke, R. B., Lee, S., Johnson, G. M. *et al.* Reported adherence as a determinant of response to highly active antiretroviral therapy in HIV-infected children. *Pediatrics* **109** (2002), e61.

24. Reddington, C., Cohen, J., Raldillo, A. *et al.* Adherence to medication regimens among children with human immunodeficiency virus infection. *Pediatr. Infect. Dis. J.* **19** (2000), 1148–53.

25. Steele, R. G., Anderson, B., Rindel, B. *et al.* Adherence to antiretroviral therapy among HIV-positive children: examination of the role of caregiver health beliefs. *AIDS Care* **13** (2001), 617–29.

26. Farley, J. J., Hines, S. E., Musk, A. E., Ferrus, S. & Tepper, V. E. Assessment of adherence to antiviral therapy in HIV-infected children using the medication event monitoring system (MEMS) compared with pharmacy refill, provider assessment, and caregiver self-report. *J. AIDS* **33** (2003), 211–18.

27. Parienti, J. J., Verdon, R., Bazin, C., Bouvet, E., Massari, V. & Larouze, B. The pills identification test: a tool to assess adherence to antiretroviral therapy. *J. Am. Med. Assoc.* **285** (2001), 412.

28. Metzger, D. S., Koblin, B., Turner, C. *et al.* Randomized controlled trial of audio computer-assisted self-interviewing: utility and acceptability in longitudinal studies. HIVNET Vaccine Preparedness Study Protocol Team. *Am. J. Epidemiol.* **152** (2000), 99–106.

29. Caron, H. S. & Roth, H. P. Patient's cooperation with a medical regimen. *J. Am. Med. Assoc.* **203** (1968), 922–6.

30. Davis, M. S. Variations in patients' compliance with doctors' orders: analysis of congruence between survey responses and results of empirical investigations. *J. Med. Educ.* **41** (1966), 1037–48.

31. Mushlin, A. I. & Appel, F. A. Diagnosing potential noncompliance: physician's ability in a behavioral dimension of medical care. *Arch. Intern. Med.* **137** (1977), 318–21.

32. Bangsberg, D. R., Hecht, F. M., Clague, H. *et al.* Provider assessment of adherence to HIV antiretroviral therapy. *J. AIDS* **26** (2001), 435–42.

33. Charney, E., Bynum, R., Eldredge, D. *et al.* How well do patients take oral penicillin? A collaborative study in private practice. *Pediatrics* **40** (1967), 188–95.

34. Wood, H. F., Feinstein, A. R., Taranta, A. *et al.* Rheumatic fever in children and adolescents: a long-term epidemiologic study of subsequent prophylaxis, streptococcal infections, and clinical sequelae. *Ann. Intern. Med.* **60** (suppl.) (1964), 31–46.

35. Maher, K., Klimas, N., Fletcher, M. A. *et al.* Disease progression, adherence, and response to protease inhibitor therapy for HIV infection in an urban Veteran's Affairs medical center. *J. AIDS* **22** (1999), 358–63.

36. Turner, B. J., Newschaffer, C. J., Zhang, D., Cosler, L. & Houch, W. W. Antiretroviral use and pharmacy-based measurement of adherence in post-partum HIV-infected women. *Med. Care* **38** (2000), 911–25.

37. Low-Beer, S., Yip, B., O'Shaughnessy, M. V., Hogg, R. S. & Montaner, J. S. G. Adherence to triple therapy and viral load response. *J. AIDS* **23** (2000), 360–1.

38. Watson, D. C. & Farley, J. J. Efficacy of and adherence to highly active antiretroviral therapy in children infected with human immunodeficiency virus type 1. *Pediatr. Infect. Dis. J.* **18** (1999), 682–9.

39. Vanhove, G. F., Schapiro, J. M., Winters, M. A. *et al.* Patient compliance and drug failure in protease inhibitor monotherapy. *J. Am. Med. Assoc.* **276** (1996), 1955–6.

40. Liu, H., Golin, C. E., Miller, L. G. *et al.* A comparison study of multiple measures of adherence to HIV protease inhibitors. *Ann. Intern. Med.* **134** (2001), 968–77.

41. Bangsberg, D. R., Hecht, F. M., Charlebois, E. D. *et al.* Adherence to protease inhibitors, HIV-1 viral load, and development of drug resistance in an indigent population. *AIDS* **14** (2000), 357–66.

42. Paterson, D. L., Swindells, S., Mohr, J. *et al.* Adherence to protease inhibitor therapy and outcomes in patients with HIV infection. *Ann. Intern. Med.* **133** (2000), 21–30.

43. Tuldra, A., Ferrer, M. J. & Fumaz, C. R. Monitoring adherence to HIV therapy [letter]. *Arch. Intern. Med.* **159** (1999), 1376–7.

44. Samet, J. H., Libman, H. & Steger, K. A. Compliance with zidovudine in patients infected with human immunodeficiency virus, type 1: a cross-sectional study in a municipal hospital clinic. *Am. J. Med.* **92** (1992), 495–502.

45. Murri, R., Ammassari, A., Gallicano, K. *et al.* Patient reported nonadherence to HAART is related to protease inhibitor levels. *J. AIDS* **24** (2000), 123–8.

46. Albano, F., Spagnuolo, M. I., Berni Canani, R. & Guarino, A. Adherence to antiretroviral therapy in HIV-infected children in Italy. *AIDS Care* **11** (1999), 711–14.

47. Kastrissios, H., Suarez, J. R., Hammer, S. *et al.* The extent of non-adherence in a large AIDS clinical trial using plasma dideoxynucleoside concentrations as a marker. *AIDS* **12** (1998), 2305–11.

48. Eldred, L. J., Wu, A. W., Chaisson, R. E. & Moore, R. D. Adherence to antiretroviral and pneumocystis prophylaxis in HIV disease. *J. AIDS* **18** (1998), 117–25.

49. Dahlquist, L. M. & Blount, R. L. Teach a six-year-old girl to swallow pills. *J. Behav. Ther. Exper. Psychiatry* **15** (1984), 171–3.

50. Shingadia, D., Viani, R. M., Yogev, R. *et al.* Gastrostomy tube insertion for improvement of adherence to highly active antiretroviral therapy in pediatric patients with human immunodeficiency virus. *Pediatrics* **105** (2000), e80.

51. Chesney, M. A. Factors affecting adherence to antiretroviral therapy. *Clin. Infect. Dis.* **30** (Suppl. 2) (2000), S171–6.

52. Carney, R. M., Schechter, K. & Davis, T. Improving adherence to blood glucose testing in insulin-dependent diabetic children. *Behav. Ther.* **14** (1983), 247–54.

53. Reynolds, E., Berrien, V., Acosta-Glynn, C. & Salazar, J. Home based, intense, nursing intervention trial improves adherence to HAART in HIV infected children. In *Pediatric Academic Societies 2001 Annual Meeting*. Baltimore, MD (2001).

54. Altice, F. L. Trust and the acceptance of and adherence to antiretroviral therapy. *J. AIDS* **28** (2001), 47–58.

Adolescents and HIV

Bret J. Rudy, M.D.

The Craig Dalsimer Division of Adolescent Medicine, Children's Hospital of Philadelphia, Philadelphia, PA

14.1 Introduction

The HIV epidemic has had a profound impact upon adolescents, both within and outside the USA. Within the USA, as of December 2001, the Centers for Disease Control and Prevention (CDC) estimate that adolescents 13–19 years of age made up less than 1% of persons with AIDS, and young adults from 20–29 years of age accounted for 16% of all reported AIDS cases [1]. This reflects 4428 reported cases in adolescents 13–19 years of age and 28 665 reported in young adults 20–24 years of age. Statistical modeling suggests that one in four new HIV infections occur in persons under the age of 22 [2]. The data suggest that infections are increasing in young women infected through heterosexual transmission and in young men through male-to-male sexual transmission. It is estimated that over 100 000 adolescents are living with HIV in the USA, although most are unaware of their infection [3]. By the end of 2001, it was estimated that worldwide, 11.8 million people aged 15–24 were living with HIV/AIDS. Internationally, more than half of new infections occur in individuals under 25 years of age. Thus, HIV disease in adolescents is a central part of the HIV pandemic.

14.2 Epidemiology

An understanding of the modes of HIV transmission among adolescents provides an essential framework for the design of interventions aimed at decreasing new infections and strategies for treating infected adolescent patients. Male-to-male sexual transmission accounts for the majority of AIDS in young men in the USA. In the 2001 CDC case surveillance data, 35% of AIDS diagnoses in young men from 13–19 was attributable to male-to-male sexual transmission [1]. This rose to 61% in young men from 20–24 years of age. In data from the Young Men's Survey, Valleroy and colleagues studied 3492 men who had sex with men (MSM) aged 15–22 years [4]. The overall prevalence of HIV was 7.2%. The prevalence was highest among African–American and Latino men. Most importantly, only 18% of the 249 HIV-positive men were aware of their infection. Such data calls for the need for enhanced efforts to decrease transmission, and to promote HIV counseling and testing among this population.

Young women are disproportionately affected by HIV compared with older women. In adolescents 13–19 years of age, young women make up 48% of cases through 2001 in the USA, compared with 41% of cases in 20–24-year-olds, and 25% of cases in those over the age of 25 [1]. For young women, heterosexual transmission is the most common mode of transmission in both those 13–19 years old (66%) and 20–24 years old (67%). Injection drug use is less common in women 13–19 years old (19%) compared with young women 20–24 years old (29%). Many young women are unaware of their risk for infection with HIV as they are unaware of the HIV risks of their partners.

Seroprevalence rates for adolescents can vary greatly depending on the testing site. In homeless shelters serving young MSM, seroprevalence can range as high as 16–17% [5]. Sexually transmitted disease (STD) clinics reported rates of 0–3.5%. Minorities are disproportionately affected. In 2001, 61% of AIDS cases in the 13–19-year-olds were among African-Americans, although only 15% of the adolescent population in the US is African-American [1]. This trend appears to be continuing based on reports of HIV infection in states that report HIV.

Table 14.1 Stages of adolescent social and psychosocial development

Adolescent stage Age	Early adolescence 12–14	Mid adolescence 15–17	Late adolescence 18–19
Social orientation	Family oriented	Increasing independence	Adult relationships
Peer relations	Striving for autonomy	Alliance to peer group	Intimacy in friendships
Thought processes	Concrete	Abstract thinking begins; concrete thinking under stress	Abstract thinking; future orientation
Psychosexual development	Concerned about physical development	Sexual experimentation	Romantic relationships

The epidemiology of HIV infection among adolescents in the USA generally mirrors the epidemiology of HIV infection among adolescents in other rich countries. In poor countries, the epidemiology is somewhat different. HIV infection in adolescents in poor countries disproportionately affects young women, who generally become infected via heterosexual contact, often with older men. This chapter emphasizes adolescent HIV infection as seen in the USA, but many of the principles are applicable for patients in other settings.

14.3 Adolescent development

Effective care of the HIV-infected adolescent requires an understanding of the unique psychosocial and physical stages of adolescence. Adolescence can be divided roughly into three stages of intellectual, social, and emotional development: early, middle, and late adolescence [6]. These stages are outlined in Table 14.1. An understanding of adolescent physical development provides essential background for the care of adolescents. The Tanner sexual maturation scale is used to stage sexual maturation [6] (Table 14.2). Girls begin pubertal development between 8–13 years compared with 9.5–13.5 years for boys. Sexual maturation in girls usually begins with thelarche, or breast development; testicular enlargement is the first sign of puberty in boys. Girls begin menstruation around Tanner stage IV; boys begin ejaculation at Tanner stage III, although sperm are produced around Tanner stage IV. It is beyond the scope of this chapter to review physical development in detail; however, understanding the stages of sexual development helps the clinician to understand when there are abnormalities in development that require investigation. Understanding sexual development in the context of psychosocial development helps the clinician guide counseling.

Sexual experimentation often accompanies normal adolescent sexual development, but it can carry a significant

Table 14.2 Stages of adolescent genital development (after Tanner, reviewed in [5]

Stage	Characteristics
Males	
1	Prepubertal
2	Testes become larger, scrotum coarsens, downy hair at base of penis
3	Lengthening of penis, increase in coarseness and amount of pubic hair
4	Penis continues to enlarge, pigmentation of scrotum, adult type hair – not on thighs
5	Adult type hair extending to medial part of thighs
Females	
1	Prepubertal
2	Sparse downy hair on sides of labia
3	Increased amount of hair and increased coarseness
4	Adult type hair not yet on medial part of thighs
5	Adult type hair extending onto medial thighs

risk of HIV infection. The Youth Risk Behavior Survey showed that 45.6% of US high school students report ever having had sexual intercourse, indicating that a very large proportion of youth are potentially at risk for HIV infection [7]. Data from the REACH Project (Reaching for Excellence in Adolescent Care and Health), an observational cohort study of HIV-infected and HIV-uninfected high risk youth, found that 43% of HIV-infected girls and 68% of HIV-infected boys reported eight or more lifetime partners [8]. In the high risk, uninfected group, condom use was sporadic: only 48% of uninfected girls and 56% of uninfected boys reported condom use at last intercourse.

Since HIV presents the greatest risk for young MSM, because HIV transmission via anal intercourse is more efficient than through other kinds of sexual contact, it is essential for the provider to understand that sexual identity formation is a staged process [9]. In the first stage, sensitization, the adolescent feels different from his or her peers and may first sense attraction to the same sex. The next stage, sexual identity confusion, is a stage where the adolescent is confused not about his or her attractions, but rather confused about how to reconcile his or her feelings with negative societal stereotypes. In the sexual identity assumption phase, the adolescent explores his or her own gay identity, and the adolescent considers the options of a homosexual lifestyle. This phase usually lasts several years and may extend beyond late adolescence. In the final stage, integration and commitment, the individual incorporates his or her homosexual identity into a positive self-acceptance. It is during this final stage that an individual is ready not only to accept his or her homosexuality but also to share it with others. Some may never reach this stage and some only reach it in adulthood. Understanding a patient's sexual identity formation stage helps the provider provide optimal care and support the youth through the subsequent stages.

14.4 Counseling and testing

Part of good, comprehensive adolescent care for sexually active and needle-using youth must include HIV counseling and testing. Epidemiologic data indicate that only a fraction of HIV-infected youth have been identified and engaged in care, partly due to the lack of counseling and testing [3, 4]. Often, providers have relied on reported 'high-risk' behavior to identify patients at risk for HIV infection, but studies have shown that many HIV-infected adolescents do not fall into a particular high-risk group. Early in the epidemic, D'Angelo and colleagues found that if only those youth who were perceived to fall into a high-risk group were offered HIV counseling and testing, only 38% of infected youth would be diagnosed [10]. In young pregnant women studied in Atlanta, 59% of those infected reported no risk factor [11]. HIV counseling and testing provides two key benefits. It is the only way to identify HIV-infected adolescents and link them into care and it reduces sexual risk-taking when testing and client-centered prevention counseling are linked [12]. Unfortunately, in a national study sampling 1500 adolescents, only 27% of those who were sexually active reported that they had been tested for HIV [13]

In most jurisdictions in the USA, adolescents can consent to counseling and testing for HIV such as they can for other sexually transmitted diseases.

Key elements that should be included in counseling include the following:
- What HIV/AIDS is.
- How HIV is transmitted.
- How HIV infection is diagnosed.
- What a positive, negative, and indeterminant test really means.
- What will happen if the test is positive.
- Identification of a support person with whom the youth could share their HIV results.
- The adolescent's plans should a test prove positive or negative.

The last point is crucial in HIV counseling of adolescents and young adults. Many adolescents seek care and treatment for conditions during periods of crisis. Assessment for depression and suicide is part of good adolescent primary healthcare. In cases where an adolescent is overwhelmed and an HIV diagnosis could enhance depression and risk for suicide, HIV counseling and testing is not indicated until the adolescent is more emotionally stable. The CDC recommends voluntary HIV counseling and testing for all at-risk patients and in all healthcare settings where the HIV prevalence is >1% or AIDS diagnosis rate 0.1%; thus, many sites who care for at-risk adolescents should make HIV counseling and testing available and developmentally appropriate [14].

Practitioners providing HIV counseling and testing must have a treatment referral plan for patients who are determined to be HIV-infected and should be aware of treatment centers with programs for HIV-infected youth or sites that have providers who have some experience in caring for youth. Adolescents often require tremendous support to link them into care and often require active efforts to engage them at the time of post-test counseling. Youth should ideally be treated in HIV centers with adolescent-specific programs where there are providers versed in adolescent development who can provide the needed psychosocial support.

14.5 Prevention

HIV prevention is an important part of good adolescent healthcare and is key for adolescents who are sexually active, or who use needles for injecting drugs (including steroids), or for tattooing. Although primary health providers are likely to screen adolescents for such things as risk for homicide or suicide and risky behaviors such as smoking and alcohol, risks for HIV such as illicit drug use and lack of condom use are less likely to be addressed [15]. For those adolescents already infected with HIV, prevention is equally important. Infection with new strains of HIV could lead to accelerated disease progression or greater drug resistance problems, and prevention of other STDs is important for potentially immunosuppressed adolescents. Unplanned pregnancies can have a potentially negative impact for the HIV-infected adolescent, both physically and emotionally, and risk infection of an infant. The provision of effective prevention counseling to HIV-infected adolescents can halt further spread of HIV infection. Practitioners must offer intensive psychosocial support to HIV-infected adolescents to help them to negotiate safer sex. Peer support, both one-on-one and in support groups, can serve as an important vehicle for providing adolescents with the ability to negotiate condom use.

All prevention counseling for the HIV-infected adolescent should be done in a caring, supportive atmosphere, rather than in an authoritarian manner. Before beginning prevention counseling for an HIV-infected adolescent, it is often helpful to have a good assessment of the adolescent's living situation. The SHADSSS assessment provides an easy, quick, and effective tool to gain insight into the world of the adolescent.

S = School
H = Home
A = Activities
D = Depression/Self-esteem
S = Substance abuse
S = Sexuality
S = Safety

The SHADSSS assessment provides a framework for discussions of all areas of the life of the adolescent [16], enabling the clinician to provide appropriate counseling and prevention services. In addition, it provides the opportunity to identify particularly troubling areas of the adolescent's life and helps the provider identify services the adolescent may require. For example, if during the interview, a history of substance abuse is noted, it must be dealt with along with issues such as depression to have optimum benefit for the adolescent. Such an assessment provides at least an initial means for the provider to identify key issues related to the adolescent's life, which must be addressed. Problems that may require more extensive interventions, such as alcohol and drug dependence, abusive home relationships, poor self-esteem, and failure at school, are faced by many youth. It is important that the adolescent understands that all information is confidential, except for information that may indicate that the adolescent is a threat to himself or herself, or to another person. Setting the stage for good, confidential counseling is key at every encounter with the adolescent.

Some adolescents are at particular risk for HIV infection. Youths who have run away from home or who live on the street often trade sex for food, housing, and protection. Such survival sex becomes a basic part of that adolescent's existence. Adolescents who survive through the exchange of sex may be unwilling or unable to negotiate safer sex because they fear losing access to their basic needs. These youths must be presented with options, which enable them to provide for themselves without the exchange of sex before issues around safer sex can even begin to be addressed. Similarly, young gay male youths have unique issues related to their sexual orientation. Homosexual identity formation is a process; the youth must gain a degree of acceptance of his sexual orientation before he can begin to plan for safer sex. It is not uncommon to find young gay men involved in relationships with older men, which may add additional barriers to negotiating safer sex [17]. Practitioners must respect the confidentiality of gay youth. Practitioners should also strive to understand the special concerns of gay, lesbian, bisexual, and transgendered youths. Such an understanding is important to provide good healthcare to this group [18].

Clinicians must ensure that adolescents receive counseling concerning safer sex. Abstinence counseling should be provided to all adolescents, even those who are already sexually active. Some adolescents who are sexually active may subsequently decide to refrain from intercourse until they are more comfortable with negotiating safer sex. For these youths, it is helpful to discuss sexual acts such as kissing and touching which hold no risk for disease transmission. Counseling both persons involved in a relationship may help to open up communication between the partners and lead to a more mature and thoughtful attitude. Peer counselors can be particularly helpful in helping adolescents negotiate safer sex. For the provider, it is important to focus not only on knowledge but also on practice. All adolescents should come away from prevention counseling with knowledge of the following: correct use of a condom for oral, vaginal, and anal sex, proper use of an internal or 'female' condom, correct and incorrect lubrication for use with a condom, the common STDs and their symptoms, strategies for negotiating safer sex and not having sex, and the potential consequences of unsafe sex. It is also important for the provider to understand the dynamics of the couple and how that may influence risk taking. Sturdevant and colleagues found that among female adolescents enrolled into the REACH Project, current partners were on average 4–6 years older [19]. This age difference was somewhat greater for the HIV-infected females compared to the uninfected females. Abusive relationships may also pose a particular challenge to the adolescent who is being counseled about how to negotiate safer sex. For the adolescent who continues in high-risk behavior despite counseling, such issues may be pertinent and should be investigated.

All counseling should be done in a supportive, non-judgmental manner. It is also very important for the provider counseling an adolescent to have a clear understanding of the differences between sexuality and sexual behaviors. When counseling about sexuality, it is important to consider emotional as well as the physical dimensions. Discussions of sexuality should include issues related to peer and societal norms, as well as the adolescent's response to feelings as a sexual being. Such discussions can uncover such problems as internalized homophobia, feelings of disempowerment, and issues of abstinence and self-esteem. They require ongoing dialogue between the adolescent and the provider and may call for the input of a psychologist or sex counselor. Sexual curiosity can lead to risk-taking behavior; discussing sex with an adult may help to answer very key questions a young person may feel they can only get from an actual sexual encounter. It has also been shown that discussing sex does not encourage non-sexually active youth to initiate sex. Most providers are more accustomed to discussing sexual behaviors with their adolescent patients. For some youths, the first attempt by the provider to discuss such issues may be poorly received. The provider should explain to the youth why he or she is discussing such issues with them and should also stress the confidentiality of the conversation. The provider must speak in terms understood by the youth and should be as specific as possible to assure the adolescent is learning as much as possible from the session. Repeated reinforcement of the key points of negotiating safer sex is essential.

14.6 Care of the HIV-infected adolescent

The care of the HIV-infected adolescent follows most of the same principles as for children and adults. It is not the intent of this chapter to review all aspects of treatment but rather to address treatment issues that are uniquely pertinent to adolescent care. Good, comprehensive HIV care includes not only the prescribing of antiretroviral medications, but must also include other key elements: general healthcare, care for other sexually transmitted diseases, gynecologic care, family planning, and ongoing psychosocial support and counseling.

In treating any adolescent, it is essential to confirm HIV infection. Uninfected adolescents have presented for HIV care [20]. Retesting provides an opportunity for a thorough discussion concerning HIV infection and AIDS, and the need for good medical care. After confirmation of infection, a comprehensive medical history and physical examination should be performed. The medical history should include a good psychosocial history using the SHADSSS assessment. Although it is often difficult to determine when an adolescent was infected with HIV, an attempt to determine the timing of infection may still be helpful. The history and results of previous HIV tests should be obtained as well as any history of possible acute retroviral infection syndrome. In addition, any history of blood transfusions or other blood products should be obtained because of the possibility that early infection through these routes might present during adolescence. The family history should pay special attention to the health of the parents, since perinatally infected children can, rarely, present during adolescence. Finally, some adolescents are infected with HIV through early childhood sexual abuse; any history of sexual abuse should be included in the assessment.

It is possible that some youths may present with an acute retroviral infection syndrome. It is especially important to diagnose these youths as early as possible, since early initiation of antiretroviral therapy may decrease total viral burden and may theoretically improve the long-term outcome by producing good viral suppression before significant immunologic damage develops. During an acute infection, the ELISA and Western Blot may not detect infection, since it can take up to 6 months from the time of infection until there are sufficient HIV antibodies to yield results. In this situation, another test, such as virus culture, DNA PCR, or an assay for HIV RNA, should be performed to diagnose the patient. Practitioners should stage HIV-infected adolescents, as they stage children and adults, evaluating the CD4$^+$ lymphocyte counts and the HIV viral load. The REACH study studied CD4 cell counts in HIV-uninfected, high-risk, boys and girls [21]. The mean CD4$^+$ lymphocyte count for girls was higher, 871 cells/μL, compared with 736 cells/μL in boys. The impact of age, gender, and racial differences on CD4$^+$ lymphocyte counts, as well as other flow cytometry markers have been evaluated and reported from the REACH Project and is beyond the scope of discussion in this chapter [22].

Appropriate antiretroviral therapy is outlined in Chapters 18 and 22 and in recent guidelines [23]. The decision to treat an adolescent with HAART must take a number of factors into account, including the HIV viral load, CD4$^+$ lymphocyte count, the adolescent's readiness to begin and adhere to a complex treatment regimen, and the side-effects and possible long-term risks from exposure to antiretroviral agents.

Care and treatment of other STDs are essential for the health of the adolescent. Clinicians should take a careful sexual history, which should include questions about oral, vaginal, and anal sex for both men and women, and about the possibility of both receptive and insertive anal sex for MSM. A youth's sexual activities provide an important guide for STD screening. Screening for gonorrhea and chlamydia from the urethra and the cervix can be performed using new technologies such as the ligase chain reaction, or using routine culture techniques. However, at this time, this technology is not approved for use for either pharyngeal or anal infections. When screening these sites, routine culture techniques are recommended. Diagnosing STDs of the anus/rectum or pharynx is important as it may affect treatment regimens, as outlined in recent guidelines [24].

Ensuring that the adolescent patient carefully adheres to prescribed antiretroviral therapy can be difficult. Adolescents may be more likely to adhere to a prescribed regimen when they understand the purpose of the regimen, when they communicate well with the clinician and trust the clinician, when the regimen is simple and requires relatively few doses given at convenient times, and when the regimen produces few unpleasant side-effects. The assessment of adherence and interventions designed to increase adherence are described in detail in Chapter 13.

Clinicians should be careful to prescribe antiretrovirals and agents used for prophylaxis against opportunistic infections correctly. For those adolescents who are either Tanner stage 1 or 2, pediatric dosing should be followed. Adolescents who are Tanner stages 3 and 4 should be closely monitored and pediatric or adult dosing guidelines followed depending on the weight of the young person and comparing the standard adult dose with that based on weight for pediatrics dosing. For adolescents who are Tanner stage 5, the adult dosing guidelines should be followed [23].

Gynecologic care for young women is an integral part of HIV care, and is discussed in detail in Chapter 15. In young men who have sex with men, anal infections with human papilloma virus (HPV) can cause significant disease, including anal warts and cancer. In the REACH Project, anal HPV was found in 48% of the young men [25]. During this study, anal cytology tests were performed using a thin prep technique; anal dysplasia was found in 50% of the young men. In a multivariate analysis of anal HPV infection in males, men with anal HPV were more likely to have both anal warts and to be MSM. Anal dyplasia in males was associated with anal HPV infection and HIV infection. Thus, for young HIV-infected men, concomitant infection with HPV may lead to significant morbidity. Routine screening for anal HPV or anal dysplasia is not included in current treatment guidelines, although some experts advocate such screening. If screening for anal dysplasia is conducted, clinicians should refer patients with anal HPV infection or concerning cytology for anoscopy and biopsy.

The care of HIV-infected adolescents is complex and often requires a team of providers with diverse expertise. Most centers caring for HIV-infected adolescents employ a multi-disciplinary team of providers. Often these teams include case managers and psychologists who can provide ongoing counseling and support and can help address the complex psychosocial issues facing these young people.

Each HIV-infected adolescent may have a unique set of problems, but many share similar concerns. Many young people worry about their ability to have children. HIV-infected adolescents may want to have a child immediately because they fear they may become too ill to have a child or may worry about never having the opportunity to have children. It is important for all young women to understand the risks of perinatal transmission and the risks of pregnancy to their own health. Even in the HIV-infected adolescent, the feelings of invulnerability characteristic of the teenage years may persist and may include unrealistic and inaccurate ideas concerning offspring. Young women must understand the risks of chemoprophylaxis and anti-retroviral therapy during pregnancy and the requirement to test and prophylactically treat the neonate. It is also important for young women to understand that they can live long, healthy lives with HIV and that decisions regarding pregnancy can be made over time. It is important for young men to understand the transmission risks for their partners and the subsequent risks for any children. Ideally, these discussions should take place with both partners.

Disclosure of HIV infection to a sexual partner or partners is often the most challenging and disturbing issue facing the adolescent. All too frequently the sexual partner is the only supportive or loving person in that adolescent's life. The fear of rejection after disclosure can be great. Some youth may be concerned about physical and emotional abuse following disclosure. Disclosure to sexual partners was studied as part of the REACH Project [26]. Of the 242 sexual partners reported by HIV-infected youths enrolled in the study, 47.5% were told of the HIV status of the study subjects. Males and females were equally likely to disclose their HIV status to their partner. Subjects were most likely to disclose to partners whom they considered their 'main' partner and to partners who were also HIV positive, as compared to those who were HIV negative or whose serostatus was uncertain. It is important that the adolescent see the care team as supportive rather than authoritarian, particularly surrounding the problems of disclosure. When the adolescent has accepted disclosure, the team can offer the youth assistance. Some adolescents will want to bring their partners in to see the care team following disclosure to assist with answering questions regarding the disease and transmission. Others may choose to disclose in the clinic setting with a member of the care team present. This can serve several purposes. First, it gives some protection to the adolescent should they fear that the partner might react violently. Second, it provides a good opportunity for counseling the couple as a couple. It is also important that sexual partners be made aware of availability of HIV counseling and testing.

HIV infection presents the adolescent with an as-yet incurable disease. It is essential for the adolescent to understand that HIV can be manageable, given good medical and psychosocial care. HIV-infected youths need a sense of hope and control over their disease, and clinicians need to provide this message.

14.7 Care programs for the HIV-infected adolescent

The care of the HIV-infected adolescent requires a skilled team of providers with broad expertise, including clinicians skilled in medical care and psychological care, and social workers, educators, and case managers who can help the adolescent manage the many bureaucratic and logistical challenges he or she must face. Ideally, these providers can offer basic gynecologic care or have links to gynecologic providers who are also versed in the care of adolescents. Practitioners must emphasize health education and the essential messages concerning safer sex. Health educators can help youths overcome the many barriers to practicing safer sex, help improve self-esteem, and emphasize the critical importance of medication adherence. Peer educators can serve to reinforce information provided by the physicians and professional educators, casting the information in terms better understood by the youths. Many other services are often necessary. Mental healthcare for those youths grappling with depression, substance abuse, or other major mental health disorders is integral to the general care of the adolescent. All too often HIV-infected adolescents are out of school or without jobs. Job readiness training can help the youth to achieve their maximum potential in the work place. Finally, outreach to at-risk youth is essential. Youth need to become aware of their personal risk for HIV and must begin to see how early intervention can help to sustain life. Outreach into the community, partnerships with community service agencies, and work with agencies providing adolescent-specific HIV services can help facilitate entry of youth into HIV counseling, testing, and care.

14.8 Summary

Care of the HIV-infected adolescent requires not only experience with HIV infection but also an understanding of the psychosocial, physical development, and social issues that confront every adolescent. With the help of a dedicated care staff, the adolescent can confront HIV and learn to live with the infection. Through education, support, and understanding, those providing care to the HIV-infected adolescent can help that youth to better care for themselves and live a longer and healthier life.

REFERENCES

1. Centers for Disease Control and Prevention. *HIV/AIDS Surveillance Report* **13** : **2** (2001), 1–44.
2. Rosenberg, P. S., Biggar, R. J. & Goedert, J. J. Declining age at HIV infection in the United States. *New Engl. J. Med.* **330** (1994), 789.
3. Rotheram-Boris, M. J. & Futterman, D. Promoting early detection of HIV infection among adolescents. *Arch. Pediatr. Adolesc. Med.* **154** (2000), 435–9.
4. Valleroy, L. A., MacKellar, D. A., Karon, J. M. *et al.* HIV prevalence and associated risks in young men who have sex with men. *J. Am. Med. Assoc.* **284** (2000), 198–204.
5. Sweeney, P., Lindegren, M. L., Buehler, J. W., Onorato, I. M. & Janssen, R. S. Teenagers at risk of human immunodeficiency virus type I infection. *Arch. Pediatr. Adolesc. Med.* **149** (1995), 521–8.
6. Slap, G. B. Normal physiological and psychosocial growth in the adolescent. *J. Adolesc. Health Care* **7** (1986), 13S–23S.
7. Centers for Disease Control and Prevention. *CDC Surveillance Summaries* **51** : **SS04** (2002), 1–64.
8. Wilson, C. M., House, J., Partlow, C. *et al.* The REACH (Reaching for Excellence in Adolescent Care and Health) Project: study design, methods, and population profile. *J. Adolesc. Health* **29** : **3S** (2001), 8–18.
9. Troiden, R. R. Homosexual identify development. *J. Adolesc. Health Care* **9** (1988), 105–13.
10. D'Angelo, L. J., Getson, P. R., Luban, N. L. C. & Gayle, H. D. Human immunodeficiency virus infection in urban adolescents: can we predict who is at risk? *Pediatrics* **88** (1991), 982–6.
11. Lindsay, M. K., Johnson, N., Peterson, H. B., Willis, S., Williams, H. & Klein, L. Human immunodeficiency virus infection among inner-city adolescent parturients undergoing routine voluntary screening, July 1987 to March 1991. *Am. J. Obstet. Gynecol.* **167** : **4** (1992), 1096–9.
12. Futterman, D. C., Peralta, L., Rudy, B. J. *et al.* The ACCESS (Adolescents Connected to Care, Evaluation, and Special Services) Project: social marketing to promote HIV testing to adolescents, methods and first year results from a six city campaign. *J. Adolesc. Health* **29** : **3S** (2001), 19–29.
13. Kaiser Family Foundation. *National Survey of Teens on HIV/AIDS* (2000), pp. 1–8.

14. Centers for Disease Control and Prevention. Recommendations for HIV testing services for in-patients and outpatients in acute care hospital settings. *MMWR* **42** (1993), 1–17.

15. Centers for Disease Control and Prevention. HIV testing among populations at risk for HIV in nine cities: Results from the HIV Testing Survey (HITS) 1995–96. *MMWR* **47** (1998), 1086–91.

16. Clark, L. R. & Ginsburg, K. R. How to talk to your teenage patients. *Contemp. Adolesc. Gynecol.* **1** (1995–96), 23–7.

17. Remafedi, G. Adolescent homosexuality: psychosocial and medical implications. *Pediatrics* **79** (1987), 331–7.

18. Ginsburg, K. R., Winn, R. J., Rudy, B. J., Crawford, J., Zhao, H. & Schwarz, D. F. How to reach sexual minority youth in the health care setting: The teens offer guidance. *J. Adolesc. Health* **31** (2002), 407–16.

19. Sturdevant, M. S., Belzer, M., Weissman, G. *et al.* The relationship of unsafe sexual behavior and the characteristics of sexual partners of HIV infected and HIV uninfected adolescent females. *J. Adolesc. Health* **29** : **3S** (2001), 64–71.

20. Joseph-Di Caprio, J. & Remafedi, G. J. Adolescents with factitious HIV disease. *J. Adolesc. Health Care* **21** (1997), 102–6.

21. Douglas, S. D., Rudy, B., Muenz, L. *et al.* Peripheral blood mononuclear cell markers in antiretroviral naïve HIV-infected and high risk seronegative adolescents. *AIDS* **13** (1999), 1629–35.

22. Rudy, B. J., Wilson, C. M., Durako, S., Moscicki, A. B., Muenz, L. & Douglas, S. D. Peripheral blood lymphocyte subsets in adolescents: a longitudinal analysis from the REACH Project. *Clin. Diagn. Lab. Immunol.* **9** : **5** (2002), 959–65.

23. DHHS Panel on Clinical Practices for Treatment of HIV Infection. Guidelines for use of antiretroviral agents in HIV-infected adults and adolescents (2001). (http://www.aidsinfo.nih.gov/)

24. Centers for Disease Control and Prevention. Sexually transmitted diseases treatment guidelines 2002. *MMWR* **51** : **RR-6** (2002), 1–79.

25. Moscicki, A. B., Houser, J., Ma, Y., Murphy, D. & Wilson, C. M. Adolescent males and females with HIV at high risk for anal squamous intraepithelial lesions. In *XIII International AIDS Conference*. Durban, South Africa, July 9–14 (2000).

26. D'Angelo, L. J., Abdalian, S. E., Sarr, M., Hoffman, N., Belzer, M. & The Adolescent Medicine HIV/AIDS Research Network. Disclosure of serostatus by HIV infected youth: The experience of the REACH Study. *J. Adolesc. Health* **29** : **3S** (2001), 72–9.

Adolescent reproductive health and HIV

Ligia Peralta, M.D.[1] and Sandra Cely, M.D.[2]

[1] Associate Professor, Chief, Division of Adolescent Medicine, Director, Adolescent HIV Program, University of Maryland School of Medicine, Department of Pediatrics, Baltimore, MD

[2] Assistant Professor, University of Maryland School of Medicine, Department of Pediatrics, Baltimore, MD

15.1 Introduction

Reproductive and gynecological conditions common among adolescent girls, in general and among HIV-infected girls specifically, include delayed puberty; menstrual disorders, such as abnormal uterine bleeding (amenorrhea, hyperandrogenism, oligomenorrhea, and dysfunctional uterine bleeding [DUB]); dysmenorrhea; premenstrual syndrome; and pregnancy. Infectious gynecological conditions include vulvovaginal candidiasis, bacterial vaginosis (BV), trichomoniasis, atypical infections of the female genital tract, cervicitis, pelvic inflammatory disease (PID), human papillomavirus infection (HPV), and herpes simplex virus (HSV) infection. This chapter addresses common reproductive health disorders among HIV-infected adolescents, and also includes a description of risk factors unique to adolescents that contribute to the acquisition of sexually transmitted infections as well as age-appropriate recommendations for secondary prevention. Most reproductive health disorders among HIV-infected adolescent girls are best managed by an adolescent medicine physician. Certain patients, such as those with delayed puberty, amenorrhea, and hyperandrogenism should be managed in collaboration with an endocrinologist.

15.2 Common non-infectious reproductive and gynecological conditions

HIV-infected adolescents, similar to their uninfected counterparts, may experience delayed puberty and menstrual disorders. In addition to these conditions, we will discuss particular considerations related to contraception and pregnancy.

15.2.1 Delayed puberty

Diagnosing delayed puberty may be difficult due to wide ethnic and regional variations in normal development [1–5]. Pubertal maturation in girls begins with the acceleration of growth followed by onset of breast development (thelarche) between the ages of 8 and 13 years. Later signs of pubertal maturation include development of pubic or axillary hair (adrenarche), which generally occurs after age 8 years (mean age: 12.5 years, range: 10–15 years) and onset of menses (menarche) between 9.1–17.7 years (median 12.8) [1, 6]. The failure to have breast budding by age 13 years or menarche by age 15 years is considered indicative of delayed sexual maturation.

Although delayed onset of puberty is often reported in young women suffering from many chronic conditions including HIV infection, the prevalence of pubertal delay associated with HIV infection in girls has not been firmly established. The effect of chronic illness on pubertal development depends upon the severity and duration of the disease as well as individual factors. In general, the earlier the onset and the longer and more severe the illness, the greater are the repercussions on pubertal development [6, 7].

The mechanism responsible for delayed puberty is not well understood but seems to be multifactorial. Total body weight seems to be an important factor; it is believed that girls must reach a critical body weight of 47.8 kg in order to achieve menarche. However, more important than total body weight is the shift in body composition to a greater percent fat (from 16–23.5%), which in turn is influenced by the nutritional state [7, 8]. This theory is supported by the association between leptin and pubertal onset. Leptin is a peptide secreted in adipose tissue; it circulates in the blood, and acts on the central nervous system neurons, which regulate eating behavior and energy balance. Low leptin levels are present in girls with delayed puberty [9–13]. In addition to leptin, other growth hormone disorders have been associated with nutritional deficiency. For example, it appears that inadequate nutritional intake relative to energy utilization, perhaps aggravated by chronic illness, and resulting in markedly lowered body fat leads to disruption of hypothalamic gonadotropin releasing hormone (GnRH) production. Low body weight results in diminished gonadotropin synthesis and secretion, or hypogonadotropic hypogonadism resulting in a very late and slow pubertal process, which may prevent the completion of sexual maturation. These adolescents may also present with short stature. Abnormalities of the growth hormone (GH)–insulin-like growth factor 1 (IGF-1) axis and gonadotropin secretion have been described in patients with other chronic illnesses such as chronic renal failure, cystic fibrosis, and Crohn's disease. In addition, cytokine production during the course of chronic diseases such as juvenile idiopathic arthritis may affect the GH–IGF-1 axis [14–18].

Although malnutrition associated with HIV infection may lead to delayed puberty with hypogonadotropic hypogonadism, other causes may be ruled out once the body composition is corrected. The differential diagnosis of delayed puberty in girls, including those with HIV infection, can be divided between those processes associated with short stature and those associated with normal stature. The differential diagnosis of delayed puberty is summarized in Table 15.1 [18].

Medical assessment is required for any girl with delayed sexual maturation or with extremely slow pubertal progression (e.g. breast development but persistent amenorrhea for 5 years). The medical evaluation must include a history, physical examination, and laboratory testing. The history must include growth records to determine the timing and form of any deviations from the norm. The family history would determine whether there is a history of later puberty in other family members. The height of parents, siblings, and grandparents should be ascertained as well as the age at menarche of the mother and sisters. Most teens with constitutional delay have a positive family history. The review of systems should concentrate on HIV disease progression and the presence of other chronic conditions. A complete physical examination should include assessment of nutritional status and body measurements (height, weight, body mass index, upper/lower body segment ratios). A normal

Table 15.1 Differential diagnosis of delayed puberty in HIV-infected girls

Pubertal delay with short stature:
1. Chronic diseases: HIV-infected teens with other HIV-associated chronic conditions such as wasting syndrome, chronic infections, respiratory illnesses, chronic anemia, gastrointestinal disease, and renal disturbances may be at highest risk for pubertal delay and short stature
2. Constitutional delay of puberty and normal variant short stature
3. Panhypopituitarism: Congenital or acquired infections; viral infection, tuberculosis, sarcoidosis, histiocytosis, posttraumatic, central tumors, sarcoidosis, and histiocytosis
4. Congenital syndromes: An array of genetic disorders, and syndromes of primary gonadal dysfunction with hypergonadotropic hypogonadism, including Turner and Klinefelter syndromes, and a group of acquired and genetic abnormalities
5. Glucocorticoid excess

Pubertal delay without short stature:
1. Constitutional delay of puberty
2. Chronic diseases: HIV, hyperthyroidism, asthma, inflammatory bowel disease, celiac disease, juvenile rheumatoid arthritis, systemic lupus erythematous
3. Acquired gonadotropin deficiency:
   CNS infections: viral encephalitis, tuberculosis
   Central hypothalamic-pituitary tumors:
      craniopharyngioma, hypothalamic glioma, astrocytoma, pituitary adenomas
   Head trauma
   Histiocytosis X
   Sarcoidosis
4. Congenital gonadal disorders: Klinefelter syndrome, enzyme defects on androgen and estrogen production
5. Androgen receptor defects: 'testicular feminization'

Reference: 18

ratio is usually found in growth hormone deficiency, constitutional delay, and chronic illness states. Sexual maturation rate is important to determine whether puberty has started or is delayed. The clinician should also pay attention to examining the thyroid, the chest for evidence of chronic pulmonary disease, the heart, and abdomen. A pelvic examination is essential. A careful visual examination including ophthalmoscopy and visual fields will help to rule out cranial tumors.

Initial laboratory studies are driven by the history and physical examination; consultation with an endocrinologist is highly recommended. If HIV-associated malnutrition is suspected, the initial assessment should concentrate on nutritional assessment, routine complete blood cell count to evaluate anemia and co-infections, chemistry profile (glucose, creatinine, calcium, phosphorus, serum albumin, protein), and liver function tests. Urinalysis for evidence of renal disease and sedimentation rate should also be included in these studies. Determination of bone age is essential when used in conjunction with height age and chronological age. Delayed bone age can be seen in adolescents with chronic illnesses and hypothyroidism. Basic measurements of gonadotropin levels (luteinizing hormone (LH) and follicle stimulating hormone (FSH)) are obtained if gonadal failure (high levels) or hypothalamic-pituitary failure (low levels) are suspected. Further investigation and other tests such as IGF-1, IGF-binding protein 3, and GnRH should be conducted with the guidance of an endocrinologist [19–21].

The goals of therapy are to induce a pubertal growth spurt, to prevent potential short- and long-term psychological and social handicaps, and to achieve full functional sexual maturation. For a short girl concerned about height, GH therapy to try to enhance height outcome can be considered in consultation with an endocrinologist. Growth hormone has also been used in non-GH deficient patients with good results. In a small randomized trial, non-GH deficient peripubertal girls were treated with GH (0.34 mg/kg each week); a highly significant increment in height occurred in the treated group compared with the control group [22].

When the diagnosis of hypogonadism is made, hormonal substitution therapy can be initiated, in consultation with an endocrinologist, to achieve normal pubertal development (see Chapter 35). In girls, estrogen administration when the girl is emotionally and socially ready for the development of secondary sex characteristics is likely to achieve temporally correct maturational changes. Although estrogen has psychological benefits, it should be used with caution since estrogen accelerates skeletal maturation, which can result in a lower adult height than might otherwise be expected [23–25].

15.2.2 Menstrual disorders

Menstrual disorders are a common problem during adolescence. These disorders may cause significant anxiety for patients and their families. Menstrual disorders among adolescent girls, including HIV-infected girls, include abnormal uterine bleeding, dysmenorrhea, and premenstrual syndrome.

Abnormal uterine bleeding

Abnormal uterine bleeding, defined as a significant variation from normal menstrual bleeding patterns, includes amenorrhea (lack of bleeding), oligomenorrhea (very scanty bleeding), menorrhagia (profuse menstrual bleeding, see Section 15.2.5), and dysfunctional uterine bleeding (DUB; the ultimate diagnosis if the cause of abnormal uterine bleeding is not anatomical). In the first 1–2 years following menarche, menstrual cycles generally conform to a cycle length of 21–40 days, with duration of less than 7 days of menstrual flow. Although abnormal uterine bleeding can occur in women of all ages, it is a particularly common problem for adolescents in those first couple of years and it is mostly caused by immaturity of the hypothalamic-pituitary-ovarian axis, resulting in anovulation. Abnormal uterine bleeding is a common complaint of adolescents and is responsible for approximately 50% of gynecologic visits in this age group [26].

Neither HIV infection nor the associated immunosuppression appear to have clinically relevant effects on menstruation [27]. Most HIV-infected older adolescents and women menstruate about every 25–35 days, suggesting monthly ovulation and an intact hypothalamic-pituitary-ovarian axis. However, HIV-infected women with histories of substance abuse have increased rates of amenorrhea, menstrual cycle intervals greater than 6 weeks in length, and fewer premenstrual breast symptoms than their counterparts [28]. This association may be due to persistent elevation of plasma prolactin levels, reflecting chronic drug-induced derangement in neural dopaminergic regulatory systems [29].

15.2.3 Amenorrhea

There are two types of amenorrhea: primary amenorrhea, or lack of onset of menses age 15 years, and secondary amenorrhea, defined as the absence of menses for a period longer than 3 months at any time after the onset of regular menses. Primary amenorrhea is associated with pubertal delay, discussed earlier, and is likely to be more common among girls with perinatally transmitted HIV infection [30].

Most amenorrhea among HIV-infected adolescent girls is secondary amenorrhea, which falls into two categories: amenorrhea associated with low body weight and wasting syndrome, and amenorrhea common to adolescents in general, associated with pregnancy, with long-acting hormonal contraceptives, and with endocrine and hypothalamic pituitary dysfunction. Amenorrhea associated with low body weight appears to be caused by disruption of the pulsatile release of GnRH, interrupting the release of gonadotropin from the pituitary gland, resulting in inadequate follicular development. Girls with perinatally-acquired HIV infection may be at risk for secondary amenorrhea associated with low levels of body fat, as well as for primary amenorrhea associated with delayed puberty, as discussed earlier. Adolescents with perinatally acquired HIV infection are a newly emerging population; many of these issues remain unstudied. However, most HIV-infected adolescent girls who have acquired HIV during adolescence, are at the early stages in their HIV disease progression, and have not experienced significant body fat loss. They are susceptible to secondary amenorrhea as are their uninfected peers [31–32].

Pregnancy is the most common cause of amenorrhea in sexually active adolescents and the clinician must be suspicious of pregnancy in any adolescent presenting with amenorrhea. The second most common cause of amenorrhea is long-acting hormonal contraceptive use. Endocrine conditions associated with amenorrhea include thyroid dysfunction, hyperprolactinemia, and pituitary tumors. In addition, polycystic ovary syndrome (PCOS), an endocrine disorder frequently associated with obesity, is also associated with amenorrhea. This disorder is characterized by high levels of androgens, which can be converted to estrogens in peripheral and hepatic tissue. The excessive levels of both androgens and estrogens may suppress the hypothalamic-pituitary production of gonadotropins and inhibit follicular development, which may result in the accumulation of multiple small cysts within the ovarian cortex [26]. Marijuana and other illicit drug use blocks release of GnRH and can produce amenorrhea, which is reversible after marijuana use is discontinued [33].

The diagnostic workup for amenorrhea should include, at a minimum, a history, physical examination including a pelvic examination, and a pregnancy test to rule out the most common causes of secondary amenorrhea. The history should include indicators of abnormal growth and development; current, past, or anticipated sexual activity; hormonal contraceptive use and symptoms of pregnancy. Medication or drug use history should include marijuana, heroin, and methadone use. The review of systems includes symptoms of hypo- or hyperthyroidism, galactorrhea, and neurological symptoms. It should be determined if there is any family history of hirsutism or endocrinopathies, and the menstrual histories and fertility of family members also should be described [34].

The physical examination should be directed towards signs of systemic disease or malnutrition. When malnutrition is suspected, plotting the adolescent's height and weight on growth charts is often the key to establishing the diagnosis. A failure to gain weight or a fall-off in both height and weight may be the clue to the diagnosis of nutritional insufficiency producing amenorrhea. Staging of puberty and measurements of breast size with areolar and glandular tissue dimensions are relevant in the patient whose puberty is incomplete. Examination also includes inspection of the skin for signs of androgen excess, including acne, acanthosis nigricans, and hirsutism. The neck should be inspected for goiter and nodularity, and the breasts should be examined for galactorrhea. The pelvic examination includes inspection of the vaginal introitus to assess current estrogen effects including enlargement of the labia minora, thickened and pale pink mucosa, and clear or white vaginal secretions. An enlarged clitoris of more than five millimeters in diameter of the glans implies exposure to androgen excess. A maturation index of a vaginal smear can also be obtained by introducing, if patient permits, a cotton-tipped applicator to the vagina which is then fixed with a Papanicolaou fixative. Superficial cells predominate with increasing estrogen effect and parabasal cells predominate in the absence of estrogen [35]. In adolescent girls who are not sexually active, a speculum exam with a Huffman speculum should be attempted to visualize the vagina and cervix. If the hymenal opening is too small to permit a vaginal bimanual examination, a recto-abdominal examination in the lithotomy position may permit palpation of uterine and adnexal masses. In sexually active girls, a full pelvic examination should be performed, to identify signs of pregnancy such as softening and discoloration (purple or hyperemic) of the cervix and uterine enlargement, in addition to a pregnancy test [30, 36].

Laboratory evaluation of the adolescent with amenorrhea should be based on the differential diagnoses suggested by the history and physical examination. For secondary amenorrhea, the initial screening includes a urine or serum beta human chorionic gonadotropin (βHCG). If the results of the βHCG assay are negative and there is absence of menses for over 6 months, more extensive work up is required to identify androgen excess or hypothalamic-pituitary dysfunction. Evaluation of possible androgen excess or hypothalamic-pituitary dysfunction would ideally be conducted in consultation with an endocrinologist and would involve laboratory tests including serum LH, FSH, LH:FSH ratio, prolactin, testosterone, dihydroepiandrosterone sulfate (DHEAS), estradiol, thyroid stimulating hormone (TSH), and free levothyrroxine (T4). Because stress, eating, sleep, and stimulation of the breast tissue can increase prolactin levels, samples should be drawn in a fasting state and the adolescent should be instructed to avoid stress and breast manipulation. If thyroid function is normal and prolactin is increased (>20 ng/mL), consultation with an endocrinologist is necessary to eliminate prolactin-secreting pituitary hormone and other disorders [37].

In general, more extensive evaluation of amenorrhea is recommended if neoplasia is suspected or if signs and symptoms related to other organ systems accompany the amenorrhea. For example, headache, visual changes, and visual fields abnormalities in the presence of amenorrhea suggest a possible pituitary tumor. In these cases, magnetic resonance imaging (MRI) with gadolinium enhancement is recommended [30].

The diagnosis of amenorrhea can include a challenge test with medroxyprogesterone acetate 10 mg orally for five–ten days to cause withdrawal bleeding and to determine whether the endometrium is responding to hormonal stimulation. A positive response to this challenge indicates the presence of an adequate estrogen level and an intact uterine-vaginal tract. The lack of response to progesterone generally indicates hypothalamic-pituitary dysfunction or PCOS. The combination of the lack of response and a low or normal FSH level indicates hypothalamic-pituitary dysfunction. On the other hand, a high FSH level indicates ovarian failure. In general, the lack of withdrawal from a progesterone challenge is indicative of low levels of estradiol. In these patients, the FSH is usually normal and most do not require an MRI evaluation if their prolactin levels are normal. However, if lack of menses persists despite weight correction, prolactin levels are indicated every 6–12 months [36].

Management of amenorrhea depends on whether it is primary or secondary. Primary amenorrhea should be managed in consultation with an endocrinologist and will not be the focus of this discussion. The management of secondary amenorrhea with normal secondary sexual characteristics varies according to the cause. In young women with amenorrhea associated with weight loss, bone mineral density loss can occur soon after amenorrhea develops. Therefore, these patients may be at highest risk of developing osteoporosis and stress fractures. The efficacy of estrogen replacement therapy in this setting is an area of debate. However, estrogen has beneficial effect on bone and other tissues [32]. The use of combination estrogen and progesterone is indicated after pregnancy and neoplasias have been excluded. In addition to the bone effect, cyclic estrogen and progesterone therapy also can be beneficial through restoration of the menstrual pattern desired by the adolescent. In hypothalamic-pituitary failure and ovarian failure, the cause should be evaluated and corrected if possible. These adolescents also require cyclic estrogen and

progestin therapy and should be managed in collaboration with an endocrinologist [30].

15.2.4 Oligomenorrhea and hyperandrogenism

Oligomenorrhea is usually the result of anovulatory cycles and is defined as abnormal menses that are infrequent or irregular, of variable duration, and characterized by painless scanty bleeding. Oligomenorrhea is one of the signs and symptoms of androgen excess (hyperandrogenism) along with hirsutism, acne, weight gain and, if severe, virilization or masculinization. Hirsutism refers to an increase in length and coarseness of the hair, in a male pattern, in areas such as the upper lip, chin, cheeks, inner thighs, lower back, periareolar, sternal, abdominal, and intergluteal regions. Signs of virilization include hirsutism, deepened voice, increased muscle mass, increased libido, clitoromegaly (more than five millimeters in diameter), hair loss with male pattern, and acne. Adolescents with hyperandrogenism are often worried about their appearance and the potential relationship to infertility. Androgen excess can be associated with metabolic disturbances that include decreased high-density lipoprotein cholesterol level, insulin resistance, decreased sex hormone-binding globulin (SHBG), and alterations in the balance between thromboxane and alpha 2 prostacyclin [38].

The differential diagnosis is summarized in Table 15.2. Polycystic ovary syndrome is the most common cause of hyperandrogenism, accounting for 80–90% of all cases of androgen excess in adolescent girls and women. A diagnosis of PCOS is important, particularly in HIV-infected adolescents, because the metabolic defects of PCOS (glucose intolerance leading to type 2 diabetes and dyslipidemia leading to cardiovascular disease) have major implications for the management of HIV-infected young women on antiretroviral therapy [39–40].

The cause of PCOS is not known but may be related to abnormal hypothalamic-pituitary function, ovarian dysfunction, abnormal adrenal androgen metabolism, or insulin resistance. Genetic factors have been associated with this disorder and it is believed that PCOS has a dominant mode of inheritance and its degree of expression may vary within the same family. Although the insulin receptor genes and the LH beta-subunit gene have been mapped to chromosome 19, chromosomal studies of patients with PCOS have shown no consistent abnormality. Some factors have been associated to the development of PCOS and include: insulin increases at the time of puberty, causing mitogenic effects on the ovaries, and theca cell hyperplasia, leading to excessive androgen production. This in turn produces follicular atresia, impairing estradiol

Table 15.2 Differential diagnosis of hyperandrogenism

Endocrine disorders	Characteristics
Ovarian	
Polycystic ovary syndrome (PCOS)	Chronic anovulation with menstrual irregularities, with or without skin manifestations and absence of other androgen disorders. Supportive labs include LH:FSH ratio >2:1 provided that LH level is <8 mIU/mL; mild elevation of testosterone and DHEAS and hyperprolactinemia (20%)
HAIRAN syndrome	Insulin resistance and acanthosis nigricans. Similar metabolic features of PCOS, myocardial hyperophy, insulin receptor mutations, circulating antibodies to the insulin receptor, postreceptor signaling defects. Fasting basal insulin levels of > 80 μU/mL compared with reference range of about 7–8 μU/mL, peaks of >1000 μU/mL (60 μU/mL in healthy individuals)
Ovarian tumors	Palpation of ovarian mass; testosterone level > 200 ng/ml; DHEAS (levels > 700 μU/mL is suggestive of ovarian or adrenal tumor); non-suppression of androgens with dexamethasone
Adrenal	
Late onset 21-hydroxylase (21-OH)	Presentation similar to PCOS, onset in adolescence. Elevated serum 17-OHP (17-hydroxyprogesterone), large increase after 0.25 mg single-dose injection of adrenocorticotropin hormone (ACTH) is diagnostic. Elevated 11-deoxycortisol or DHEAS and 17-hydroxypregnenolone levels are found in 11-hydroxylase and 3 β-hydroxysteroid dehydrogenase deficiencies
Cushing's syndrome	Lack of cortisol suppression after dexamethasone (0.5 mg q.i.d. for 5–7 days)
Adrenal tumors	Rare and associated with rapid feminization. Palpable mass; elevated 17-KS, DHEAS, and DHEA levels. Subnormal suppression with dexamethasone administration. Mass on ultrasound or CT scan
Other	
Idiopathic hirsutism	Ovulation regularly, normal levels of androgens. Mechanism remains to be determined
Exogenous: androgenic drugs	Anabolic steroids, testosterone, DHEAS, androgenic protestins, danazol, corticotropin, high-dose corticosteroids, metyrapone, derivatives of phenothiazine, acetazolamide
Exogenous: non-androgenic drugs	Phenytoin, valproate, cyclosporine, diazoxide, minoxidil, hexachlorobenzene, psoralens
Central nervous system lesions	Encephalitis

LH, luteinizing hormone; FSH, follicle stimulating hormone; HAIRAN, hyperandrogenic-insulin resistant acanthosis nigricans syndrome; DHEAS, dihydroepiandrosterone sulfate

production. Obesity, a frequent finding in PCOS patients, also is associated with increased peripheral aromatization of androgens to estrogens, decreased levels of sex hormone-binding globulin (SHBG), and hyperinsulinemia [41–44].

Patients with PCOS often present with hirsutism (66–70%), oligomenorrhea (47–64%), obesity (38–43%), acne (11–34%), amenorrhea (16–19%), polymenorrhea (2–4%), and acanthosis nigricans (2%) [39, 44–45]. Polycystic ovary syndrome includes its variant, the hyperandrogenic-insulin resistant acanthosis nigricans (HAIRAN) syndrome.

The HAIRAN syndrome is characterized by acanthosis nigricans, a velvety hyperpigmented change of the crease areas of the skin found mostly in black people, fasting glucose levels that are relatively normal despite extremely high circulating levels of insulin (generally over 80 U/mL in the fasting state and over 300 U/mL following an oral glucose tolerance test [OGTT]), and androgen excess [45].

Polycystic ovary syndrome is often a diagnosis of exclusion after other causes have been ruled out. Criteria for diagnosis include chronic anovulation with a pre-menarcheal onset of menstrual irregularities [46], and biochemical or clinical evidence of androgen excess (primarily ovarian in origin). Polycystic ovary syndrome is usually characterized by an elevated LH : FSH ratio of 2 : 1 or greater (provided that the LH level is not below 8 mIU/mL); elevated circulating levels of free testosterone; a reduction of sex hormone-binding globulin (SHBG); variable increases in total testosterone; abnormally high DHEAS levels (in 50% of patients); and mildly elevated prolactin levels (in 10% of patients). Patients with PCOS also may have elevated levels of cholesterol, triglycerides, and low-density lipoprotein cholesterol (LDL-C), and lower levels of high-density lipoprotein cholesterol (HDL-C) and apolipoprotein A-I. These abnormalities are largely associated to hyperinsulinemia. Approximately 50% of women with PCOS are insulin resistant with or without obesity. The exact pathogenesis is not known but it is believed to be associated to excessive serine phosphorylation of the insulin receptor. The typical histologic changes of the polycystic ovary can be encountered with any size ovary. Therefore, increased size of the ovaries is not a critical feature, nor is it necessary for diagnosis. Although "polycystic ovaries" are common, not all patients with PCOS demonstrate ovaries that are "polycystic," nor are "polycystic ovaries" diagnostic for PCOS [38, 45].

Initial laboratory evaluation includes measurements of LH, FSH, LH : FSH ratio, free testosterone, DHEAS, prolactin, thyroid function tests, glucose and insulin levels, and lipid profile. As a rule, all anovulatory women who are hyperandrogenic should be assessed for insulin resistance and glucose tolerance with measurements of the fasting glucose : insulin ratio; a ratio of less than 4.5 is consistent with insulin resistance. Another assessment includes the 2-hour glucose level after a 75 g glucose load. A value is considered normal if it is less than 140 mg/dL, impaired values are between 140–199 mg/dL, and non-insulin dependent diabetes mellitus is 200 mg/dL or higher. Follow-up evaluation of hyperandrogenic patients requires frequent monitoring of glucose intolerance, insulin resistance, and dyslipidemia. Further evaluation to rule out ovarian or adrenal tumor is required for any girl with severe acne, hirsutism, virilization, or markedly elevated levels of serum testosterone and DHEAS. This evaluation requires a computed tomography (CT) scan or an ultrasound examination of the adrenal glands and ovaries, along with consultation with an endocrinologist [38–39, 45, 47].

The overall goals of treatment include reduction of the production of circulating androgens; protection of the endometrium against the effects of unopposed estrogen; achievement of normal body weight; lowering the risk of cardiovascular disease by reducing hyperinsulinemia and diabetes mellitus; and induction of ovulation.

Specific management strategies for PCOS [39–40, 45, 48–49] include:

1. Weight loss to reduce circulating androgen levels and decrease unbound testosterone. Weight loss can reduce insulin levels, thereby reducing testosterone and subsequently, hirsutism [42].

2. Hormonal management with combination oral contraceptives with low androgenic progestins (norethindrone or norgestimate) for abnormal uterine bleeding and endometrial hyperplasia. Oral contraceptives also decrease androgen production by lowering LH levels, thus decreasing androgen production; increasing SHBG, thereby lowering free androgens; decreasing adrenal androgen production; and decreasing 5 α-reductase activity. Therefore, oral contraceptives may improve hirsutism but the response is slow [38].

3. Management of hirsutism. This can be accomplished with cosmetic approaches such as chemical depilatories, electrolysis, and laser photodermodestruction. In addition to combination oral contraceptives, antiandrogenic agents such as spironolactone can be used. Spironolactone, an aldosterone-antagonist diuretic, competes at the androgen receptor peripherally and inhibits 5 α-reductase. The impact of spironolactone treatment on hirsutism is related to dosage and a better effect is seen with a dose of 200 mg daily. The starting dose is 50 mg/day and can be increased by 25 mg every 1–2 weeks to a maximum of 200 mg/day; after a period of time, a maintenance dose of 25–50 mg daily may be sufficient. Side-effects are mild and include dry mouth, diuresis, fatigue, and menstrual spotting. Because of the possibility of hyperkalemia, this drug should be used with caution in young women with diabetes mellitus. In adolescents, spironolactone is usually indicated when patients find oral contraceptives unacceptable or the response is disappointing [38, 45].

4. Management of diabetes. Insulin-sensitizing agents (antidiabetic agents) can be used for overt diabetes and are the focus of current research. These agents include metformin, a biguanide approved to treat type 2 diabetes, but not currently approved to treat PCOS. Gastrointestinal symptoms are the most common side-effects of this drug. Therefore, clinicians start at a low dose of 500 mg/day and increase the dose by 500 mg per dose at weekly intervals. There is a small risk of lactic acidosis among women taking metformin (< 0.1 cases/per 1000 patient years). Although no clinical trials have evaluated the long-term efficacy of metformin use in adolescents, other short-term trials with metformin have shown promising effects in lowering insulin secretion, improving insulin sensitivity, restoring

normal menstrual cycles, and correcting lipid abnormalities. Primary prevention of diabetes and cardiovascular lifestyle modifications, regular exercise, and a balanced diet are also important, especially for those HIV-infected young women taking highly active antiretroviral therapy (HAART) [38, 49].

5. Treatment with clomiphene to induce ovulation. Such treatment is reserved for patients with infertility. These patients should be referred to a reproductive endocrinologist.

15.2.5 Dysfunctional uterine bleeding

Dysfunctional uterine bleeding (DUB) is defined as irregular, painless bleeding of endometrial origin that can be excessive, prolonged, or unpatterned. The bleeding is related to endometrial sloughing in the absence of structural pathology and is usually due to anovulation. Ovulatory DUB occurs secondary to defects in local endometrial hemostasis. Anovulatory DUB, a systemic disorder occurring secondary to endocrinologic, neurochemical, or pharmacologic mechanisms, is the most common and may result from prolonged amenorrhea leading to endometrial hypertrophy [50–51].

Since DUB is a diagnosis of exclusion, the following diagnostic possibilities must be considered and excluded (Table 15.3) [50]: pregnancy and complications of pregnancy; use of exogenous hormones, leading to anovulatory breakthrough or withdrawal bleeding; infections; local pathology; hormonal imbalance; coagulopathies and hematologic conditions; and neoplasias.

The evaluation involves a thorough history, physical examination, and appropriate laboratory studies. A menstrual and sexual history, a history of hormonal contraceptive use, and a family history, including a history of PCOS or bleeding disorders, should be obtained. The review of systems should include specific questions about tachycardia, palpitations fatigue, lightheadedness, easy bruises, and epistaxis or gum bleeding [51, 53, 54].

The physical examination should include an assessment of hemodynamic stability, i.e. blood pressure in supine, sitting, and standing positions and pulse to identify orthostatic changes. In addition, height, weight, and sexual maturity rating should be evaluated. A skin examination is performed to identify signs of hyperandrogenicity or bleeding disorders; the thyroid should be palpated to detect enlargement and nodularities; and breasts should be examined for galactorrhea. Pelvic examination is essential to identify structural abnormalities and to assess the amount of bleeding. A gross assessment of the severity of the bleeding can be estimated by observing the bleeding from the os,

Table 15.3 Differential diagnosis of dysfunctional uterine bleeding (DUB)

Category	Comments
Pregnancy and complications of pregnancy	Spontaneous and incomplete abortion
	Ectopic pregnancy
Use of exogenous hormones leading to anovulatory breakthrough or withdrawal bleeding	Estrogen breakthrough bleeding that occurs when excess estrogen stimulates the endometrium to proliferate
	Estrogen withdrawal bleeding occurs after stopping exogenous estrogen therapy or just before ovulation in the normal menstrual cycle and is usually self-limited
	Progesterone breakthrough bleeding: occurs when the ratio of progesterone to estrogen is high, the endometrium becomes atrophic and more prone to frequent, irregular bleeding. This occurs with the use of progesterone-only contraceptive methods
Infections	Sexually transmitted infections
Local pathology	Trauma
	Foreign body
	Lesions of the cervix or vagina
Hormonal imbalance	Hypothyroidism
	Hyperthyroidism
	Androgen excess
	Insulin resistance
	Obesity
Coagulopathies and hematologic conditions	Thrombocytopenic disorders related or unrelated to HIV infection
	Idiopathic thrombocytopenic purpura
	Abnormal platelet function due to drugs (aspirin)
	Systemic illness or anticoagulant therapy
	Von Willebrand's disease (diagnosed when patient presents with excessive vaginal bleeding upon menarche)
Neoplasia	Rare, but screening for cervical dysplasia highly recommended

considering the duration of the bleeding, and by obtaining hemoglobin values. Grossly, presence of blood in the vaginal vault and the cervix indicates moderate bleeding but duration should be taken into consideration. Continuous blood dripping from the cervical os usually indicates severe bleeding and the patient may rapidly become anemic [50, 55].

The initial laboratory evaluation of DUB includes assessment of hematologic status with a complete blood count to detect anemia and thrombocytopenia and a pregnancy test to rule out pregnancy. Sexually transmitted disease (STD) screening is indicated for adolescents who have had sexual intercourse. No further laboratory testing is necessary in adolescents with mild anovulatory DUB associated with physiological immaturity. Depending on the history and the physical findings, other tests may be required. Thyroid function tests and other endocrine tests are indicated if endocrinologic dysfunction is suspected. Prothrombin time and partial thromboplastin time should be performed if a coagulopathy is suspected. A bleeding time will help diagnose von Willebrand's disease and should be performed before initiation of any hormonal therapy, since hormonal therapy may slightly prolong bleeding time. Other tests for Von Willebrand's disease include Von Willebrand's factor binding activity and antigen levels, and a multimer analysis of von Willebrand factor subtypes. A transabdominal pelvic ultrasonography is recommended to evaluate uterine and ovarian anatomy in patients who do not tolerate a pelvic examination. Transvaginal ultrasonography is indicated if the pregnancy test is positive or a mass is palpated on pelvic examination and tubo-ovarian abscess (TOA) or ectopic pregnancy should be ruled out. Endometrial sampling is rarely recommended in adolescents [52, 56].

The treatment of DUB depends on the severity of the bleeding. Once DUB is diagnosed, hormonal management with oral contraceptives is frequently successful. Low-dose oral contraceptives are as effective as contraceptives with higher estrogen doses. They establish regular menses with decreased menstrual flow, preventing long intervals of amenorrhea and subsequent endometrial hyperplasia with resultant profuse bleeding. The dosage of combined oral contraceptives is guided by the severity of the bleeding. For immediate treatment of moderate bleeding (moderate flow and Hb levels 10–12 g/dL), oral contraceptives may be administered up to one tablet four times a day, with antiemetics prescribed with these high doses. The dose is reduced slowly based on daily assessment of bleeding. Depot medroxyprogesterone acetate (DMPA) 150 mg intramuscularly every 12 weeks has also been used to produce amenorrhea in these cases but has not been traditionally

the first choice for the initial management of moderate to severe dysfunctional uterine bleeding. Severe bleeding (heavy flow and hemoglobin <10 g/dL) usually requires intravenous estrogen and hospitalization. Surgical management is rarely required and is reserved for situations in which medical therapy has been unsuccessful or is contraindicated [52–53, 56–57].

Hormonal contraceptives are also used in the management of ovulatory DUB involving endometrial hemostasis. The management is directed at decreasing menstrual frequency or inducing endometrial atrophy. Combined OCs (21-day packet), one pill daily continuously, is recommended. Discontinuation of the pill for one week every 3 months prevents excessive endometrial proliferation. Endometrial atrophy also can be induced by administration of DMPA 150 mg IM every 3 months once the endometrial stability has been achieved and the bleeding is controlled. Gonadotropin releasing hormone analogs are reserved for severe cases and should not be used for more than 6 months [51, 54, 56, 58].

Dysmenorrhea

Dysmenorrhea, characterized by lower abdominal pain that is usually cramping in nature, occurs in two types. Primary dysmenorrhea refers to cyclic pain associated with the menstrual flow without evidence of pelvic pathology. It is associated with ovulatory cycles and is due to endometrial contractions induced by prostaglandins originating in the secretory endometrium. Secondary dysmenorrhea refers to pain associated with menses due to organic disease such as endometriosis, outflow tract obstruction, or pelvic infections. Dysmenorrhea is a common gynecological disorder affecting 60% of menstruating adolescents, 14% of whom report it as the cause of school absenteeism [59].

There are no studies of the prevalence of dysmenorrhea in HIV-infected adolescents. However, HIV-infected and -uninfected women have similar prevalences of dysmenorrhea [52], so it is likely that prevalence of dysmenorrhea among HIV-infected adolescents is similar to that among uninfected teens. Among adult HIV-infected women, dysmenorrhea appears to be independent of CD4$^+$ lymphocyte count [52].

The most common type of dysmenorrhea in adolescents is primary dysmenorrhea. It appears within 1–2 years of menarche, when ovulatory cycles have been established, and may persist through adulthood as long as the patient is ovulating. Primary dysmenorrhea is caused by an increased production of prostaglandin $F_{2\alpha}$ and prostaglandin E_2 (PGE$_2$). $F_{2\alpha}$ is the most important cause of dysmenorrhea and produces stimulation of uterine contractions, vasoconstriction, and ischemia, and mediates pain sensation.

Prostaglandin E_2 causes vasodilation and platelet disaggregation. Women with this condition have an increased production of prostaglandins and higher vasopressin concentrations than asymptomatic women. For example, in the late luteal phase, there is a three-fold elevation in $F_{2\alpha}$ and PGE_2 levels, followed by a further increase during menstruation that is more intense in the first 48 hours of menses [60]. This mechanism would account for the observation that the pain of primary dysmenorrhea usually begins a few hours prior to the onset of menstrual bleeding and may last as long as 2–3 days. Increased urinary excretion of leukotrienes, inflammatory mediators known to cause potent vasoconstriction and uterine contractions, also have been found in adolescents with dysmenorrhea [58, 61]. The pain of dysmenorrhea is described as suprapubic cramping and can be accompanied by nausea, vomiting, diarrhea, dizziness or syncope, and lumbosacral back pain. Signs include suprapubic tenderness without rebound on palpation. Bimanual examination reveals uterine tenderness but absence of cervical motion tenderness.

Secondary dysmenorrhea usually develops years after menarche and can occur with anovulatory cycles. This condition is rare in adolescents and pelvic abnormalities such as endometriosis or uterine anomalies may be found in approximately 10% of adolescents with severe dysmenorrhea [62]. Gynecologic disorders, including salpingo-oophoritis, endometriosis, adhesions, imperforate hymen, transverse vaginal septum, cervical stenosis, and uterine anomalies, represent the most common cause of secondary dysmenorrhea in adolescents. Prostaglandins also have been shown to be locally elevated in cases of secondary dysmenorrhea such as endometriosis [63]. The pain of secondary dysmenorrhea can be diffused in the pelvic or localized in areas outside the pelvis such as the rectum or the back. The examination may show cervical motion tenderness such as with PID. Tenderness or nodularity of the uterosacral ligaments and cul-de-sac or ovary can be found in patients with endometriosis [64]. The differential diagnosis of secondary dysmenorrhea also includes less frequent causes such as gastrointestinal disorders (irritable bowel syndrome, ulcerative colitis, and Crohn's disease), genitourinary disorders (ureteral obstruction and pelvic kidney), and neurologic disorders). Musculoskeletal causes are rare, and include scoliosis, kyphosis, spondylolysis, and spondylolisthesis [62].

The diagnosis depends on the history of the cyclic nature of the pain and absence of underlying pelvic pathology as determined by pelvic examination. The onset of pain is usually a key factor. Primary dysmenorrhea starts 6–12 months after menarche or when the cycles become ovulatory, and peaks at age 17 and 18 years. Secondary dysmenorrhea should be considered if the pain starts with the onset of menarche after the age of 20 years. A sexual history including previous STDs helps eliminate infection as a cause. History of cigarette smoking has been associated with increased duration of dysmenorrhea [65]. Associated symptoms include nausea or vomiting (89%), fatigue (85%), nervousness (67%), dizziness, diarrhea and backache (60%), and headache (45%). The review of systems should include a complete review of gastrointestinal, genitourinary, neurological, and musculo-skeletal systems. Screening for pregnancy and for STDs, and obtaining a complete blood cell count and an erythrocyte sedimentation rate, are essential to rule out pregnancy, PID, and inflammatory bowel disease, respectively. Ultrasound is indicated when complications of pelvic infections or a müllerian abnormality are suspected and when masses are palpated [62].

The most effective treatments for primary dysmenorrhea are prostaglandin synthetase inhibitors such as non-steroidal anti-inflammatory drugs (NSAIDs) and OCs; NSAIDs are the most common pharmacologic treatment and are effective in approximately 80% of primary dysmenorrhea cases. They should be taken before or at the onset of pain and then every 6–8 hours for the first 3 days of the menstrual period. This approach prevents the re-formation of prostaglandin by-products. An additional effect may be related to decreased prostaglandins from the platelets participating in menstrual clotting. The benefit depends on dose and duration of treatment. A loading dose of NSAIDs (typically twice the regular dose) should be used as initial treatment for dysmenorrhea in adolescents followed by a regular dose until symptoms abate. The most commonly used class of NSAIDs are the carboxylic acids, of which there are different subgroups: salicylic acids (aspirin); acetic acids (indomethacin); propionic acids (ibuprofen 400 mg q4–6h; naproxen 500 mg initial dose, followed by 250 mg q6–8h, and naproxen sodium 550 mg initial dose, followed by 275 q6–8h); and fenamates (mefenamic acid) and ketoprofen. Mefenamic acid has an additional mechanism of action (competition for prostaglandin binding sites). The typical dosage is 500 mg as an initial dose, followed by 250 mg every 6 hours. For those adolescents who also desire contraception or those who do not respond after 3 months of treatment with NSAIDs, combined OCs represent the agent of choice for treating dysmenorrhea. OCs produce an endometrial proliferation similar to the proliferative phase of the early menstrual cycle when prostaglandin concentrations are lowest. Treatment with desogestrel-containing low-dose OCs has also shown reduced menstrual pain severity and significantly less menstrual cramping in women with dysmenorrhea when compared with those receiving placebo. However, no significant change in bloating, anxiety, weight gain, or acne was reported in the treatment group [66]. If dysmenorrhea is not relieved by the above measures, a trial of up to 6 months is indicated, with necessary changes in doses and medications before the therapy is considered a failure. If symptoms persist after 6 months, the clinician should suspect secondary causes of dysmenorrhea such as endometriosis and the patient should be referred to a gynecologist [58, 62].

Premenstrual syndrome

Premenstrual syndrome (PMS) is characterized by behavioral, somatic, affective, and cognitive disorders appearing in the luteal phase of the menstrual cycle and usually disappearing a few days after the onset of menses. The exact prevalence is unknown but it is estimated that up to 85% of women have some degree of symptoms before menses and that 5–10% have severe symptoms and have restrictions of daily activities [67]. Among adolescents, a longitudinal study reported a prevalence of 14% and was associated with self-reported anxiety, inattention, and poor health [68]. In another study most adolescents reported at least one premenstrual symptom of minimal (96%) or moderate (89%) severity, while many reported symptoms they considered severe (59%) or extreme (43%) [69]. Common complaints of adolescents experiencing PMS include physical symptoms such as abdominal bloating, breast tenderness, weight gain, edema of lower extremities, headaches and joint or muscle pain, fatigue, increased appetite, and food cravings. Psychological symptoms include emotional instability, irritability, anxiety, depression, decreased concentration, clumsiness, insomnia or hypersomnia, tearfulness, a sense of being out of control, social withdrawal, and changes in libido [69].

The exact mechanism of PMS is unknown. However, proposed etiologies include estrogen excess or deficiency, progesterone deficiency, alterations in prolactin, growth hormone, thyroid hormone, adrenal activity, LH, FSH, insulin, antidiuretic hormone, aldosterone, and cortisol. Vitamin (A, E, thiamine, B6), magnesium and zinc deficiencies, as well as alterations in glucose metabolism, also have been implicated as mechanisms. More recently, neuroendocrine studies have contributed to a growing list of findings that suggest an underlying neurobiological vulnerability in PMS and it is believed that women with this condition have an alteration in the delicate equilibrium between sex steroids and central neurotransmitters [70–72].

Premenstrual syndrome can have a major impact on an adolescent's quality of life (e.g. it is a major cause of school absence among adolescent girls). Diagnosis requires tracking the patient's complaints over at least two menstrual cycles along with a thorough physical exam. The diagnosis is made by prospectively charting the cyclic nature of the symptoms, which occur in the luteal phase and resolve within a few days after onset of menses. The symptoms must be recurrent and severe enough to disrupt normal activities. The most severe form of PMS is the premenstrual dysphoric disorder (PMDD), in which the symptoms markedly interfere with work, school, usual activities, or relationships with others, and are not the exacerbation of another disorder [73]. The patient history should include an assessment of the patient's lifestyle, diet, stress level, and a history of previous psychiatric disorders [72].

The differential diagnosis for PMS includes exacerbation of existing psychiatric conditions such as major depression, dysthymia, panic or personality disorders, and medical disorders such as seizures, migraine headaches, irritable bowel syndrome, asthma, and allergies. Clinicians must remember that menstrual exacerbation of existing psychiatric or medical disorders does not constitute PMS [70].

Treatment of PMS may be complex. Because the causes of PMS remain unknown, management can be difficult. Stress management, dietary changes, and increased exercise have relieved symptoms in some adolescents. Treatment to suppress ovulation with combined OCs, depot medroxyprogesterone, and GnRH analogues also have been shown to alleviate PMS symptoms. However, the use of GnRH analogues in adolescents is limited due to the hypoestrogenic effects and the risks of bone density. Selective serotonin reuptake inhibitors (SSRIs) are the drugs of choice for severe PMS and for PMDD. Fluoxetine 20–60 mg/day and sertraline 50–150 mg/day are effective. In some cases, the use of these drugs only during the luteal phase has resulted in improvement of symptoms [72, 74–75].

15.2.6 Contraception and pregnancy

Contraception

Nearly 60% of couples worldwide are now using effective contraception. However, this figure hides wide disparities between the industrialized countries of North America, Western Europe, Australia, and New Zealand, with the highest rates of use, and the developing countries, where many barriers to use of effective contraception result in rates as low as 15% of couples in Africa [76].

An estimated 350 million couples around the world lack information about contraceptives and/or adequate access to effective, acceptable methods and services. There are wide variations in the access of women in the developing world to knowledge regarding where and how to receive family planning services [77].

Adolescents and unmarried women are particularly affected by limited access to contraceptives in many areas and cultures where they are prevented or discouraged from using reproductive health services, including family planning services [76]. The use of modern contraceptives among married adolescents ranges between 1% in sub-Saharan African countries to 60% in Latin America. Only 10% of unmarried adolescents use modern contraceptives in 4 out of 19 sub-Saharan countries. Therefore, unmarried adolescents in these sub-Saharan countries are more likely to use modern contraceptives than those who are married [83].

15.2.7 The clinician's role in adolescent contraception

The many contraceptive choices now available, thanks to advances in contraceptive technology, combined with considerations related to adolescent development, require the adolescent girl's full participation in the process of choosing the most appropriate contraceptive method. In addition to a complete history and physical examination to rule out contraindications to hormonal contraceptives, the clinician must review the young woman's lifestyle, assess whether she has disclosed or plans to disclose her sexual activity to her parents/legal guardians, and evaluate her comfort level with various potential methods and their side-effects. Ideally, the clinician would provide basic unbiased information about the general choices available (daily and long-term hormonal, and barrier methods) including a comparison of advantages, disadvantages, and non-contraceptive health benefits as they relate to the teen. For example, teens with acne or with dysmenorrhea could experience additional benefits from some hormonal contraceptives. The adolescent should be encouraged to share her opinions about what she thinks will work best for her. Finally, the clinician should make recommendations after a careful evaluation of all these factors and after responding to patients' questions or concerns. This patient-focused interactive counseling is likely to encourage adherence to the desired method [79]. Regardless of the contraceptive method chosen, ideally the clinician should discuss emergency contraception options with the adolescent, and together develop a plan for responding to situations in which she may have unprotected sex [80–81]. Adolescents infected with HIV also require intense counseling concerning their reproductive health including their desire for pregnancy, contraceptive practice, and decisions and choices if an unintended pregnancy occurs.

15.3 Types of contraceptive methods

There are numerous types of contraception. Barrier methods include male and female condoms, spermicides, diaphragms, cervical caps, and vaginal sponges. The latter three barrier methods are not widely used in the adolescent population, and will not be addressed in detail in this chapter. Hormonal contraceptives, either combined estrogen/progestin or progestin-only contraceptives, are taken orally, or in certain cases injected. Intrauterine devices (IUDs), natural methods (such as coitus interruptus) as well as voluntary sterilization also exist as contraceptive methods, but are not used often in the adolescent population [26] and will not be addressed in detail in this chapter. Diaphragms, cervical caps, and vaginal sponges leave a portion of the vagina unprotected and their protection against the acquisition of HIV/STDs is still not determined. Even more so, vaginal sponges are not highly recommended due to recent data showing a lower efficacy rate than diaphragms [82]. The risk of adverse affects with IUDs, including increased risk of BV, appear to be higher in adolescents and, therefore, they should be used with caution [83–84]. New, recently approved or soon-to-be approved long-acting hormonal contraceptives offer additional useful options for young women. Recently approved methods include new hormonal monthly injections, contraceptive skin patches, and vaginal rings. Other methods in development include biodegradable implants, pellets, microspheres, and microcapsules [26].

Studies have shown that women who learned through voluntary testing and counseling programs that they were HIV-infected reported lower levels of desired fertility than did women in the general population. Their knowledge about contraception and access to family planning services may be limited. Interventions are needed to offer these women more control over their reproductive lives, and serve as a strategy to prevent perinatal HIV infection [85–86].

15.3.1 Barrier methods

Condoms

Following the advent of the HIV/AIDS epidemic, condoms, which had long been eclipsed in the USA by hormonal and other effective contraceptives, have experienced a resurgence in use, with many women, including adolescents, relying on them for contraception. Additionally, the HIV epidemic, as well as the high prevalence of many serious STDs, mandates that adolescents be informed about and strongly encouraged to use male or female condoms to protect themselves from STDs, including HIV, no matter what other method they may use to prevent pregnancy.

The recommended male condom is made of latex and its integrity should be protected by avoiding use of oil-based lubricants and by educating the patient in proper application techniques, including appropriate lubricants, and storage strategies to prevent punctures and heat damage. The female condom consists of a lubricated polyurethane sheath with loose (15 cm) soft rings at each end; it is available in one size, and should be used in conjunction with a lubricant. The inner ring is placed as high as possible in the vagina. The outer ring covers the perineum and thus provides protection against perineal contact with infectious organisms. Like the male condom, it is designed for one time use, and is sold over the counter. Besides abstinence, only condoms, if used consistently and correctly, offer protection against HIV transmission and may substantially reduce the risk for many STDs. Condoms do not offer as much protection against HPV and genital herpes, which can be transmitted by contact with infected skin areas not covered by the condom [26].

The conscious decision at each episode of sexual activity required for effective use of either male or female condoms for contraception or infection prevention is a major disadvantage. As shown in the REACH study, although growing numbers of young women are choosing to rely on condoms for contraception, pregnancy rates and incidence of STDs among those choosing condoms suggest that many do not use them with each sexual encounter, or have difficulties in using them correctly [85].

Vaginal spermicides

Vaginal spermicides containing nonoxynol-9 (N-9) enhance the contraceptive effectiveness of barrier methods. They are not effective in preventing cervical gonorrhea, chlamydia, and HIV infection. In addition, frequent use of N-9-containing products has been associated with genital lesions and sloughing of endothelial cells, which may be associated with an increased risk of HIV transmission. N-9-containing products have more damaging effects upon the rectal mucosa than upon the vaginal mucosa. Adolescent women who engage in anal intercourse, a strategy sometimes used by young women to avoid the risk of conception or to maintain "technical virginity," should be cautioned against the use of N-9-containing products as sexual lubricants. Both diaphragm and spermicide use has been associated with an increased risk of bacterial urinary tract infection in girls; the sponge has been associated with increased risk of candidiasis [87].

Microbicides

Microbicides are being extensively researched as a means to develop a safe, acceptable chemical barrier to prevent HIV transmission during sexual intercourse. Many of these compounds are in different stages of clinical trials, showing promising results. Issues that are being addressed by these research studies are the maintenance of normal vaginal pH and flora, ease of use, length of effect, potential adverse effect on sperm and integrity of mucosal tissue, and behavioral issues related to acceptability and use in sexual relationships [88].

15.3.2 Hormonal contraception

Hormonal contraceptives include combined or single drug oral contraceptive, long-acting estrogen and progesterone or progesterone only methods, and emergency contraception. Table 15.4 summarizes the currently available hormonal contraceptive methods [81, 89–94].

Oral contraceptives

Oral contraceptives are among the most popular birth control methods among teenagers. They are divided in two groups: (1) combination OCs that include an estrogen and a progestin; and (2) progestin-only pills that contain no estrogen. Combination OCs prevent pregnancy by suppressing FSH and LH. The estrogen alters the secretion and cellular structure of the endometrium, leading to edema and dense cellularity. The progestin prevents ovulation by suppressing LH surge, produces thickening of the cervical mucus and decreases sperm motility [81].

Combination OCs come in monophasic packs that contain the same dosage of estrogen and progestin in every pill and multiphasic packs that contain different dosages of estrogen, progestin, or both during the cycle. The latter offers no significant benefit over the monophasic. The pills are also packaged in 21 and 28-day packs. The 28-day pack contains seven placebo pills and is preferred because adolescents are less likely to lose track of the pill-free interval. New products include a shortened placebo interval followed by a low-dose estrogen to reduce breakthrough bleeding. The estrogen component of most OCs of preparations approved in the USA is ethinyl estradiol at a dose of 20–35 μg per pill. The 20–30 μg pills are usually referred as "low dose" OCs. The progestins in OCs can be classified in two families: (1) the estrane family, including norethindrone, norethindrone acetate, ethynodiol diacetate, and norethynodrel (not available in the USA); and (2) the gonane family, including norgestrel, levonorgestrel, norgestimate, desogestrel, and gestodene (not available in the USA). Norgestimate and desogestrel

Table 15.4 Hormonal contraceptive methods

	Oral contraceptive pill (OCP)	Depot medroxy-progesterone acetate (DMPA) (Depo-Provera)	Monthly injectable Lunelle®	Patch OrthoEvra®	Ring NuvaRing®	Intrauterine System (IUS) Mirena®	Subdermal implants Levonorgestrel Rod Implants®	Emergency contraception (EC)
Description	The two types of OCP are: (1) combination pills containing both estrogen (ethinyl estradiol and menstranol) and progestins (norethindrone, norethindrone acetate, ethynodiol diacetate, norgestrel, levonorgestrel, noretgynodrel, desogestrel, norgestimate, and gestodene); (2) Progestin-only pills.	150 mg depot medroxyprogesterone acetate injections every 3-months	A single 0.5 ml monthly intra-muscular injection with a combination of progestin and estrogen (medroxy-progesterone acetate and estradiol cypionate injectable suspension)	A one-and-three-quarter inch square skin patch consisting of three layers containing progesterone and estrogen. It delivers continuous levels of norelgestromin and ethinyl estradiol for a seven-day period. Each cycle contains three hormone-releasing patches	A flexible, transparent, colorless vaginal ring about 2.1 inches in diameter containing the hormones etonogestrel and ethinyl estradiol. Women insert it into the vagina and leave in place for three weeks. It releases daily doses of progestin and estrogen	A small device that is inserted and left inside the uterus and releases progestin (levonorgestrel)	A two-rod system containing levonorgestrel-filled capsules that are inserted subdermally in the upper arm. A single rod system that contains progestin	A one-time oral contraceptive that can be used after intercourse to prevent pregnancy. Treatment initiated within 72 hours of unprotected intercourse. EC reduces the risk of pregnancy by at least 75%
Efficacy	High	High	High	High	High	High	High	High < 72 hours
Dosing frequency	Daily	Every 3 months	Monthly	Weekly	Monthly	Every 5 years	Every 1–3 years	Once

Office visits	Prescription	Every 3 months	Monthly	Prescription	Prescription	For insertion and removal (requires trained clinicians)	For insertion and removal (requires trained clinicians)	Once
Easy reversibility	Yes	No	Yes	Yes	Yes	Yes	Yes	Yes
User controlled	Yes	No	No	Yes	Yes	No	No	Yes
Discreet	Yes	Yes	Yes	Sometimes	Yes	Sometimes	Sometimes	Yes
Side-effects	In some cases: unwanted menstrual cycle changes, nausea and vomiting, headaches, depression, decreased libido, increased cervical ectopy; risk of cardiovascular disease, glucose intolerance, gallbladder disease acceleration, hepatocellular adenoma	Weight gain, depression, breast tenderness, menstrual irregularities (may take up to 8 months after last injection to discontinue side effects), lipid changes, bone density decreases	Bleeding between periods; weight gain or loss; breast tenderness; nausea – rarely, vomiting; changes in mood or sex drive	Same as oral contraceptives, include nausea; vomiting; mastalgia; headaches; menstrual cramps and abdominal pain; irregular bleeding, and skin irritation	Risks and side-effects are the same as oral contraceptives. Also may include vaginal discharge, vaginitis, and irritation.	Most commonly reported side effects include menstrual changes; lower abdominal pain; mastalgia; headache; vaginal discharge; mood changes, and nausea	Irregular bleeding or spotting, headache, weight gain, breast tenderness	Nausea (30–50%) vomiting (15–25%) menstrual change (10–15%). Also, breast tenderness, headache, abdominal pain, fatigue, dizziness
Protection against HIV and other STDs	No	No	No	No	No	No	No	No

Sources: [80, 90–94, 96, 98]

have the lowest androgenicity effect and have less adverse impact on lipoprotein metabolism than levonorgestrel and norgestrel. These lower androgenic progestins may be more appropriate for youths with hyperandrogenism, excessive acne, and hirsutism [81].

In general, among the various options for hormonal oral contraception, very low-dose OCs containing gonane progestins decrease the incidence of estrogen-related side-effects, and are associated with lower rates of breakthrough bleeding. Low-dose OCs have a low margin for error; pregnancy may result if doses are taken at different times of day or if a dose is missed. Despite the obvious disadvantage of the daily requirement for taking a pill, OCs are popular among teenagers [95]. Additional non-contraceptive benefits of OCs, such as improvement of acne and dysmenorrhea, increase the adherence of adolescents to the method and should always be reviewed with young patients [96].

Progestin-only OCs prevent pregnancy by thickening the cervical mucus and preventing sperm from ascending through the cervical os. There is also alteration of the endometrial lining and some suppression of ovulation. They are usually reserved for those adolescents for whom combination OCs are contraindicated and who do not desire injectable, implantable, or dermal methods. The advantages include lack of interference with breastfeeding quality, or quantity of milk production, in lactating teen mothers; decreased menstrual cramps, menstrual flow, PMS, and breast tenderness. The major disadvantage is that progestin-only OCs have a shorter half-life than do combination OCs, causing unpredictable patterns of menstrual bleeding and breakthrough bleeding, the most common side-effect and reason for discontinuation. This method requires daily dosing without hormone-free intervals. Other side-effects include weight gain, increased appetite with subsequent weight gain, headaches, moodiness, fatigue, and breast enlargement [96].

Long-acting hormonal contraceptive methods

Depot medroxyprogesterone acetate (DMPA, or Depo-Provera) injections administered every 3 months (150 mg) have become a more popular hormonal contraceptive method for both HIV-infected and -uninfected adolescents [97]. It prevents ovulation by suppressing the LH surge, increasing pulses of GnRH, and augmenting both the secretion of FSH and the responsiveness of FSH to GnRH stimulation. In addition, DMPA decreases estradiol secretion, with inhibition of follicular development and maturation. As with OCs, discontinuation rates are high. Adolescents will often discontinue the use of DMPA unless close medical supervision is possible and side-effects are carefully monitored and aggressively managed [85, 97]. Side-effects,

primarily menstrual irregularities (26%) and weight gain (18%), are the primary reasons for DMPA discontinuation reported among adolescents [98]. A significant proportion of adolescents who received at least one injection of DMPA failed to present for subsequent scheduled appointments for additional DMPA injections [98]. Restart rates were observed to be lowest among those who report irregular bleeding (15%), weight gain (9%), and hair loss (10%), and highest among those discontinuing because of missed appointments (87%). High pregnancy rates among those who discontinue DMPA (19%) warrant close follow-up after DMPA discontinuation [98].

The contraceptive patch is a one-and-three-quarter inch square skin patch consisting of three layers containing progesterone and estrogen. It delivers continuous levels of norelgestromin and ethinyl estradiol for a 7-day period. Three hormone-releasing patches, used in successive weeks, comprise one cycle. The patch can be worn in several areas of the body, and it is recommended that different areas of skin be used for consecutive patches, to avoid skin irritation. The patches adhere well to the skin, allowing young women to continue any athletic activities including exercise and swimming. It has demonstrated efficacy, safety, and a side-effect profile similar to that of combination OCs. Additionally, the once-weekly dosing results in statistically better adherence than with OCs. A common complaint among adolescents about the patch is its visibility [92–94].

Hormonal implants involve a two-rod system containing levonorgestrel-filled capsules that are inserted subdermally in the upper arm. A single rod system also contains progestin. Implants are the most effective method of birth control (except for continuous abstinence). Left in place, implants can protect against pregnancy for 5 years. However, implants are not very popular among adolescents because they require insertion, and discontinuation requires removal by a trained clinician [98].

Emergency contraception

Emergency contraception (EC) should be available to adolescents for immediate use in the event that a post-coital method becomes necessary. It provides an option that reduces the number of unplanned pregnancies with little or no long-term risk and, like other contraceptive methods, prevents ovulation, fertilization, and/or implantation. Emergency contraception is extremely safe and highly effective. Two hormone regimens, ethinyl estradiol (100 μg) with levonorgestrel (0.5 mg) or high-dose levonorgestrel (0.75 mg), given within 72 hours of intercourse and repeated 12 hours later, are available for this purpose. These regimens are packaged as labeled USA Food and

Drug Administration dedicated products or they can be adapted for use from standard OCs. Levonorgestrel and mifepristone seem to offer the highest effectiveness with an acceptable side-effect profile. Mifepristone, while effective, is not yet licensed for this use as EC in the USA. One disadvantage of mifepristone is that it causes delays in onset of subsequent menses, which may induce anxiety. However, this seems to be dose-related, and low doses of mifepristone (10 mg dose) minimize this side-effect without compromising effectiveness [80, 99–100]. For young women with a past history of deep vein thrombosis, pulmonary embolism, stroke or heart attack, progestin-only regimens may be the preferred EC method. A history of ectopic pregnancy is not a contraindication for EC use. However, these patients require more careful follow up because they are at risk for repeat ectopic pregnancies. All EC patients require follow up for several reasons, including determination of the success of the EC and provision of additional education about other contraceptive methods [80].

Hormonal contraception and drug interactions

With the numerous medications required by HIV-infected individuals, drug interactions between OCs (estrogen-progestin combinations or progestin-only products) and other drugs, including antiretroviral drugs and drugs for prevention or treatment of opportunistic infections (OIs), are likely. Such interactions can result in either an increase or decrease in plasma concentrations of OCs and other drugs (see Chapter 19).

Hormonal contraception and STDs

Counseling about acquisition and transmission of STDs, including HIV, prior to prescribing and during use of hormonal contraceptive methods is essential to minimize the incidence of STDs. Clinicians should emphasize that hormonal contraceptives do not protect against STDs, including HIV [96].

15.4 Pregnancy

Irrespective of their HIV infection status, pregnant adolescents may confront social stigma, lack of support from partner and/or family, financial difficulties, and other psychosocial stressors. In many cases, the young woman first learns of her HIV infection during her pregnancy, and is coping with a double burden of anxiety, dilemmas and choices, and stress. Some young women with HIV infection incur unplanned pregnancies, and still others actively wish to become pregnant. HIV-infected girls in a national

study of adolescents who acquired HIV through sexual activity or injection drug use (IDU) had pregnancy rates twice as high (20.6 per 100 persons/year) as the national rate among adolescents [81, 101–102]. However, the likelihood of a new pregnancy among adolescent girls with living children was lower among those with HIV infection [81, 102].

The main clinical issues confronting HIV-infected adolescent girls and women regarding pregnancy are: the possibility of transmitting the virus to their child or to their uninfected sexual partner; the potential impact of a pregnancy on disease progression; and the potential effects of HIV treatment on the pregnancy and/or the baby.

Perinatal transmission rates have decreased substantially with the use of antiretroviral drugs, cesarean section before labor and before ruptured membranes, and avoidance of breastfeeding. Ideally, the prospective mother with chronic HIV infection would have already initiated antiretroviral therapy before becoming pregnant. However, the implications of current antiretroviral treatment guidelines, suggesting delay of therapy until particular clinical, immunologic, or virologic parameters have been reached, are that many HIV-infected adolescent girls and women confronting an unplanned pregnancy will not have initiated antiretroviral therapy. Moreover, many women do not discover they are infected until tested during the course of prenatal care. Fortunately, efficacious interventions to prevent mother-to-child transmission of HIV which can be initiated during pregnancy exist. The selection of the particular antiretroviral combination is complex, taking into account the woman's stage of disease progression, history of antiretroviral treatment, co-existing infections or conditions, and other issues; treatment regimens may vary depending on the stage of pregnancy [103]. Some highly effective antiretroviral medications are not suitable for use during pregnancy. It is likely that perinatal transmission among women with known HIV infection could be essentially eliminated if appropriate care is available before pregnancy, and pregnancy is delayed until HIV disease is stabilized. Ideally, they would also be free from other STDs, and be committed to using barrier methods during pregnancy to prevent these infections. Ideally, pregnant, HIV-infected teens should receive prenatal care from providers who specialize in both obstetric and HIV care. Access to such providers is generally limited to areas in which HIV prevalence is particularly high. In other cases, it is essential that there be close collaboration between clinicians managing the HIV infection and those managing the pregnancy and delivery.

Current evidence suggests that pregnancy does not exacerbate the progression of the HIV infection [104]. Many pregnant young women appear to be more conscientious in adhering to HIV treatment regimens than they had been before becoming pregnant, suggesting that pregnancy may indirectly improve their clinical status [104]. On the other hand, HIV infection may affect the pregnancy. HIV-infected mothers may be more likely to spontaneously abort than uninfected mothers [104], and be more likely to deliver low-birth weight babies than uninfected mothers [105]. The risks of preterm birth and low birth weight are higher in those HIV-infected women co-infected with STDs or BV, as may be the risk of transmitting HIV from mother to baby [106–110]. Limited data exist regarding the long-term effects of exposure to antiretroviral drugs on HIV-infected mothers and their children.

The subject of future pregnancy and childbearing should be discussed proactively with any HIV-infected adolescent. Experience with HIV-infected adolescent girls suggests that a number of them become anxious to have a baby after learning their diagnosis, believing themselves to be under a death warrant, and therefore having limited time for motherhood, or believing that it would be much better for them to have a baby sooner rather than later when their disease may be more serious. Family and friends and health care professionals may project the opposite attitudes, that HIV infection should preclude pregnancy and childbearing. A major goal of any comprehensive program for HIV-infected adolescents and young adults is to encourage and facilitate them in living normal lives. Accordingly, clinicians should encourage them to be teens during their teen years – discover who they are, proceed with schooling, get jobs and learn how to handle money, plan and begin to work towards their futures, spend time with friends and have some fun, and delay parenthood until after their teenage years. More than other teens, adolescents with HIV infection need to be encouraged to envision and plan for a future, since many assume they have no future. We emphasize that making decisions is part of growing up, and we respect their right to make their own decisions about pregnancy and childbearing. In that context, we encourage them to consult and work together with their clinician if they do intend to become pregnant, or if they experience an unplanned pregnancy, so that we can help to ensure the best possible outcome for them and their babies [85].

Pregnant HIV-infected adolescents should be counseled about all of their options: (a) childbearing and raising the child; (b) childbearing and placing the child up for adoption; and (c) abortion. Providers can help the adolescent to identify individuals who can be truly supportive in helping her to make a decision and understand the implications of her decision for her and her family [86, 94, 111–112]. It is important to avoid assumptions about the supportive-ness of family members, friends, and partners, especially if the girl is contemplating an abortion, and in some cases when she is planning to continue the pregnancy and raise her child. The adolescent should be referred to appropriate counseling and social service facilities. Close collaboration between an infectious disease specialist and the prenatal care providers is essential throughout the pregnancy and through delivery and the postpartum period, and between an infectious disease specialist and pediatrician during the neonatal period.

In a national study of adolescents with sexually or IDU-acquired HIV infection, the pregnancy rate among HIV-infected adolescents was twice as high as the national rate for American adolescents. No major differences in many variables were found between HIV-infected adolescents and "high-risk" (involved in sexual activity or IDU) uninfected counterparts on many variables, which could influence fertility. Irrespective of HIV infection status, older adolescents and those not using hormonal contraception were more likely to become pregnant. Conversely, those with increased problem-solving capacity and increased spiritual hope were less likely to become pregnant. Spiritual hope was defined as measurements on the Likert Scale involving descriptors such as "prayed hard for a good ending to the situation," "trusted your belief in God," "started going to place of worship more often," and "compromised or bargained with higher being" [86].

15.5 Sexually transmitted diseases

15.5.1 Introduction

An estimated global total of 333 million new STD cases among both males and females ages 15–49 occurred in 1998, with 167 million of these cases occurring in developing countries. The total figure includes 89.1 million cases of chlamydia, 62.2 million cases of gonorrhea, and 12.2 million cases of syphilis. Rates for adolescent girls were not available [113]. In the USA, approximately 3 million teenagers acquire STDs each year with adolescent girls (ages 15–19 years) having the highest gonorrhea and chlamydia rates of any age group [114]. Although rates decrease with the implementation of aggressive screening and treatment policies, chlamydia rates are typically 6–18% among adolescent women. The gonorrhea rates vary depending on both the reporting facility and the population seeking health care. For example, rates of over 15% are reported in STD clinics and juvenile detention facilities while the rate is approximately 3–6% in adolescent clinics. *Trichomonas vaginalis* infection rates are up to 14% in adolescent women and HSV seropositivity is up to 30%; HPV rates are between 33–80% of some clinical samples [114–116]. Similar to the US adolescent population as a whole, HIV-infected adolescent girls have high rates of STDs [117–119]. Reported overall prevalence rates among US girls aged 12–19 years are: gonorrhea (10%), chlamydia (22%), both gonorrhea and chlamydia (6%), *Trichomonas* sp. (13%), and syphilis (9%) [118–119]. The only major difference between the HIV-infected and uninfected girls was a higher prevalence of trichomoniasis among the HIV-infected girls. HIV-infected girls also had high HPV infection rates (77.4%), specifically the high-risk HPV types [115]. Studies of HIV-infected women report somewhat conflicting results, with one study reporting similar rates of infections between HIV-infected and uninfected women [120], and another study reporting higher rates of vaginal infections including BV, vulvovaginal candidiasis, and trichomonal vaginitis in HIV-infected women than among their uninfected counterparts [121].

Sexually transmitted diseases among adolescents, both HIV-infected and -uninfected, have important implications, and present challenges to care providers. Sexually transmitted diseases characterized by inflammation such as gonorrhea and chlamydia can increase vulnerability to HIV infection from sexual activity with an HIV-infected partner; high rates of these STDs among adolescents suggest a high level of risk of HIV infection among adolescents [122–124]. The increased vulnerability to HIV infection caused by inflammatory STDs is also an important issue for adolescents who are already HIV-infected, as they can become super-infected with additional HIV strains, some of which may be resistant to various antiretroviral drugs, seriously complicating effective management of the HIV infection [125–126].

Among HIV-infected youth, STDs can be particularly problematic. Adolescent girls have the highest age-specific rates of complications of STDs; immunosuppression due to HIV dramatically increases the severity of these complications [122–123, 127–129]. For example, gonorrhea and chlamydia are more likely to progress to PID, even in young women who are not severely immunosuppressed [130–133], and PID is likely to be more difficult to diagnose and treat in HIV-infected young women [134]. Human papillomavirus infections among HIV-infected young women (even those not severely immunosuppressed) are more likely to involve strains associated with dysplasia and cervical cancer than those occurring among young women without HIV infection [115, 130]. Not only does the HIV infection affect the body's response to STD infection, but STDs and other infections are associated with increases in viral loads and with decreases in CD4+ lymphocyte counts

as the already challenged immune system confronts additional pathogens.

The health education about their condition, which should be an integral component of primary and HIV care for any HIV-infected adolescent, should include a candid discussion about the serious implications of STDs to their health and to effective management of their HIV infection. The challenges facing many HIV-infected adolescents in using condoms consistently and effectively cannot be overestimated. Effectively encouraging responsible sexual behavior, including consistent condom use, is one of the most difficult challenges facing health care providers for this population. Screening for STDs should be included in routine quarterly examinations of HIV-infected youth, and the youths should also be encouraged to call for appointments at the first sign of STD, rather than waiting in the hopes that it will improve on its own [114, 135].

Adolescents with HIV, particularly those who acquired HIV sexually, are at a greatly increased risk of acquiring other STDs. Practitioners caring for HIV-infected adolescents should make every effort to aggressively educate patients about the special risks STDs pose for HIV patients and urge them to use safe sexual practices or to abstain from sexual activity.

15.5.2 Sexually transmitted diseases and HIV: the role of immunity

The common mucosal immune system contributes to immune defense in the female reproductive tract. Cervical secretions contain high concentrations of intrinsic immune components (e.g. complement and defensins) and immunoglobulins that are the first line of defense against invasive pathogens. Additional protection is provided by cellular immune components. Although the regulation of local immune responses in women is not well understood, precise regulation is presumably critical; uncontrolled immune responses may cause non-specific tissue damage that could alter reproductive function [136–137].

An intricate cytokine feedback mechanism controls both stimulation and inhibition of an immune response. Whether the induced immune response is mediated by antibodies or T-lymphocytes, it may be regulated by timing and by exposure to cytokines secreted either by epithelial cells or by T-helper cells. Two patterns of cytokine production have been described: T-helper cell type 1 (Th1) that produces interleukin 2 (IL-2), lymphotoxin and interferon γ. These cytokines produce a cell-mediated response and are important in the resolution of virus infections or intracellular pathogens. The T-helper cell type 2 (Th2) produces

IL-4, IL-5, IL-6, IL-10, and IL-13; these cytokines produce humoral immune responses. Another important cytokine in this feedback system is interleukin 12 (IL-12), which is produced by dendritic cells and monocytes. IL-12 drives helper T-cells type 0 into a Th1 pathway. Local production of these cytokines may determine which arm of the immune response is stimulated and may influence the magnitude of immune protection available in the genital tract. Many different cytokines have been detected in the cervical and vaginal secretions of women. The constitutive level of cytokine expression suggests that the healthy genital tract has a Th2 type of immune environment. Further studies are necessary to determine whether the cervical cytokine responses of adolescent girls are different from those of women [136–137].

Notable differences are observed between HIV-infected and uninfected adolescent girls in the physiology and local immune system of the genital tract. Studies have shown that genital tract viral infections influence the level of cytokine expression. This effect was evaluated in a study of HIV-infected adolescents examining the association among mucosal cytokine concentrations, HIV infection status, and STDs. Higher levels of IL-10 and IL-12 were found in the HIV-infected adolescent girls compared with uninfected girls. Significant alterations in local cervical cytokine production, including cytokine profiles associated with Th1 or Th2 responses, were also found among the HIV-infected adolescents. The levels of IL-2, IL-10, and IL-12 were not influenced by the age or race of the subjects. When compared by HIV infection status, HIV-infected adolescent girls had significantly higher levels of IL-10 and IL-12; no difference according to HIV infection status was found for IL-2 [136].

Additional differences in genital tract cytokine production distinguish women infected with HIV but who have no HPV infection from those HIV-infected women co-infected with HPV, and also distinguish adolescents from adults [136]. Among HIV-infected adolescents, HPV co-infection was the principal factor predicting the high IL-10 concentration found in this cohort; whereas HPV co-infection and the presence of another STD were associated with high levels of IL-12. These findings were present early in HIV infection with CD4$^+$ T-cell counts above 500 cells/μL. Therefore, in HIV-infected adolescents, local immunity may be altered before significant declines in total peripheral CD4$^+$ T lymphocytes develop. The clinical relevance of these Th1/Th2 cytokine profiles is being examined longitudinally to evaluate the progression of HPV infections in HIV-infected and -uninfected adolescents. Although the data demonstrate that in adolescent girls, co-infection with HIV and HPV

is associated with increased IL-10 concentrations, other STIs do not influence the probability of having increased IL-10 concentrations. Still, HIV-uninfected patients with HPV infection have lower IL-10 concentrations than HIV-infected counterparts, suggesting an appropriate switch away from Th2 responses during viral infection [137, 138].

15.5.3 Sexually transmitted diseases and STD syndromes

Vulvovaginitis

Vulvovaginitis is the inflammation of the vulva and vagina that is characterized by symptoms such as vaginal discharge, odor, irritation, vulvar or vaginal itching, burning, and dyspareunia. It is frequently caused by infection. The primary infectious causes of vulvovaginitis in adolescent girls are BV (*Garderella vaginalis*, anaerobes, and *Mycoplasma hominis*), vulvovaginal candidiasis (VVC) (*Candida* species), and trichomoniasis (*Trichomonas vaginalis*). Given the significant differences in pH, leukocyte count on wet mount (a microscopic examination of a vaginal smear after the addition of one to two drops of normal saline to the specimen), and Gram stain appearance, these three common infections are easy to distinguish and differentiate [106, 114].

Other, non-infectious causes of vulvovaginitis include: physiologic causes such as menses, ovulation, hypoestrogenism, physiologic leukorrhea; foreign bodies; cervicitis [114, 139–141]; hypersensitivity, irritant, or allergic vulvovaginitis, including cases resulting from intravaginal medications or personal hygiene products or cases representing latex condom allergy; idiopathic focal vulvovestibulitis; and cytolytic vaginosis [106]. Vaginal aphthae, like oral and esophageal aphthous lesions, have been described among HIV-infected women [142].

15.5.4 Bacterial vaginosis

Vulvovaginitis due to bacterial vaginosis is common, resulting from overgrowth of bacteria (a mixed flora consisting of *Haemophilus* sp., *Bacteroides* sp., *Gardnerella* sp.) replacing the normal vaginal flora (*Lactobacillus*). The prevalence of BV varies by population, ranging from 10–31% in sexually inexperienced adolescents in the USA [106]. Bacterial vaginosis has been associated with a variety of gynecologic and obstetric complications, including PID, post-abortal infection, vaginal cuff cellulitis, preterm birth, low birth weight, prolonged rupture of membranes, and postpartum endometritis.

The clinical and laboratory characteristics associated with BV are shown in Table 15.5. As many as 50% of young women with BV are asymptomatic. When symptomatic, the primary symptom is malodorous vaginal discharge (nonviscous homogeneous, white, uniformly adherent) with an amine odor that is more noticeable after menses or intercourse. Itching and irritation also are present in 67% of the cases [106].

Bacterial vaginosis can be diagnosed clinically based on three of the four Amsel's criteria [143–144] (Table 15.5). Among patients with BV, this test reveals clue cells and very few white blood cells (WBCs). These simple and inexpensive tests provide the most accurate and efficient results to diagnosis of BV [143–144]. A Gram stain of a vaginal smear is considered more reliable than saline microscopy because it can be saved for later review and is useful for research purposes. However, Gram stains are often not performed in clinical practice. Cultures for *Gardnerella* or *Mycoplasma* species have little use in the diagnosis of BV and more expensive tests are not necessary [114, 145]. As some patients with BV are asymptomatic, screening using pH strips, wet mount and KOH should be performed routinely on HIV-infected adolescent girls.

In longitudinal studies using these clinical criteria, women with HIV infection were more likely than uninfected women to have persistent BV, and those with greater immunosuppression (CD4$^+$ cell counts less than 200 cells/μL) were more likely than those with CD4$^+$ cell counts above 500 cells/μL to have persistent and severe BV infections [146–148]. Because HIV infection may predispose these patients to more severe BV infections, perhaps leading to PID, and because the risk of HIV transmission may be greater among women with BV, clinicians should consider treating asymptomatic BV in HIV-infected adolescent girls [106].

Suggested treatment regimens for BV are shown in Table 15.5. Acceptable treatment options include metronidazole or clindamycin [106, 114]. Because of the interaction between metronidazole and alcohol, adolescents needing treatment for BV should be screened for alcohol abuse, and those who are unlikely to be able to abstain from alcohol as needed, should be treated with an alternative antibiotic, e.g. clindamycin.

Useful preventive approaches are difficult to define due to the poor understanding of microbiologic and host risk factors. Recurrence after treatment has been reported to be as high as 80% [149–156]. Such high recurrence rates could be due to persistence of BV-associated organisms and failure of *Lactobacillus* species flora to recolonize. Prevention includes abstinence and avoidance of douching and/or the use of intravaginal soaps. The results of clinical trials indicate that a woman's response to therapy and the likelihood of relapse or recurrence are not affected by treatment of her sex partner(s). Therefore, routine treatment of sex partners is not recommended [114].

15.5.5 Vulvovaginal candidiasis

Vulvovaginal candidiasis (VVC) remains one of the most common infections of the female genital tract. Although it is uncommon before age 17 years, the incidence increases rapidly with age thereafter; by age 25 years, 55% of college women have been diagnosed with this condition and as many as 20% of women may be colonized with *Candida albicans*. Furthermore, this diagnosis will be confirmed in 30% of symptomatic women by isolation of *Candida* species [157]. Factors that increase the risk of VVC include pregnancy, contraceptive use, diabetes, antibiotics (such as tetracycline, ampicillin, and oral cephalosporins), and sexual activity including receptive oral sex [157]. Vulvovaginal candidiasis is most commonly caused by *C. albicans* (80%) and less frequently by other species such as *C. glabrata, C. parapsilosis, C. tropicalis, C. lusitaniae,* and *Saccharomyces cerevisiae* (20%).

The clinical and laboratory characteristics associated with VVC are shown in Table 15.5. Symptoms include vulvar/vaginal itching and or soreness or discomfort, dysuria, and thick discharge. The thick vaginal discharge is clumpy, white, and resembles cottage cheese. Examination frequently reveals vulvar and/or vaginal inflammation and erythema. The diagnosis of VVC requires the combination of clinical and laboratory (microscopy, culture) findings. Patients with vaginitis symptoms can be diagnosed with VVC by examining the vaginal secretions under the microscope. A wet mount or saline preparation should show yeast cells and mycelia and few WBCs. If large numbers of WBCs are present along with yeast cells and mycelia, there is likely a mixed infection. Patients with signs and symptoms of VVC and negative microscopy should have a vaginal culture. Although vaginal cultures are the most sensitive for detecting *Candida* organisms, a positive test does not indicate that yeast is responsible for the vaginal symptoms since *Candida* organisms are isolated from the lower genital tract of an estimated 20% of asymptomatic healthy women without abnormal discharge. Among women with symptoms of VVC, 29.8% had yeast isolated, confirming the diagnosis of VVC [157]. Patients are treated when there is clinical evidence of yeast infection or when the wet mount test with saline shows budding yeast with pseudohyphae. Culture is expensive and time consuming. The culture may be

Table 15.5 Vulvovaginitis: clinical and laboratory characteristics, and treatment

	Normal	Bacterial vaginosis (BV)	Vulvovaginal candidiasis (VVC)	*Trichomonas vaginalis* infection (Trichomoniasis)
Etiology		Bacterial overgrowth with organisms such as *Haemophilus* sp., *Bacteroides* sp., *Gardnerella* sp.	80% *C. albicans* 20% Other *Candida* sp.	Flagellated anaerobic protozoa
Symptoms		Odor, discharge, pruritus (50% asymptomatic)	Pruritus, discomfort, dysuria, thick discharge, soreness	Pruritus, discharge (50% asymptomatic)
Discharge	Clear to white	Homogeneous, adherent, thin, milky white; Malodorous, 'fishy' odor	Thick, clumpy, white, 'cottage cheese'	Frothy, grey or yellow-green; malodorous
Physical examination findings		More vaginal mucosal inflammation	Inflammation and erythema. More vaginal mucosal inflammation	Cervical petechiae ('strawberry cervix') in 5–10% cases Can cause cervical inflammation
Vaginal pH	3.8–4.2	> 4.5 very sensitive but not specific	≤ 4.5	> 4.5
KOH 'whiff' test	Negative	Positive	Negative	Often positive
	Lactobacilli	Clue cells No/few WBCs	Few white blood cells Pseudohyphae or budding cells	Motile flagellated protozoa Many white blood cells; sensitivity 60%
Diagnostic criteria		Amsel criteria (3 of 4) 1. White adherent discharge 2. pH > 4.5 3. fishy odor; positive KOH whiff 4. > 20% clue cells on microscopy	See text	See text
Treatment strategies		Metronidazole 500 mg PO BID × 7 days, OR 2 g PO in single dose, OR 0.75%, 5 g InV BID × 5 days, OR Clindamycin 2% Cream 5 g InV QHS × 7 days, OR 300 mg PO BID × 7 days *If pregnant:* *No creams or gels* *Can use oral meds*	Treatment of *Candida* vaginitis requires individualization. A new classification of VVC into uncomplicated and complicated vaginitis has simplified choice and duration of antifungal therapy Vaginitis due to *C. albicans* responds well to the available therapy: Oral agent: Fluconazole 150 mg PO in single dose (For severe *Candida* vaginitis: two sequential 150-mg doses of fluconazole given 3 days apart) Topical agents (many to choose from) Miconazole 2% cream 5 g InV for 7 days 200 mg InV (suppository) for 3 days 100 mg InV (suppository) for 7 days Other available agents include butoconazole, clotrimazole, tioconazole, and terconazole (Refer to CDC guidelines [33] for doses and duration)	Metronidazole 2 g PO in single dose, OR 500 mg PO BID × 7 days, OR 250 mg PO TID × 7 days, OR Clindamycin 300 mg PO BID × 7 days *If pregnant, use 2 grams PO in single dose*

InV, Intravaginal. Adapted from [114, 140].

useful in the individual with recurrent symptoms consistent with *Candida* vulvovaginitis but negative results from KOH preparation.

Candida vaginitis infection rates in HIV-infected women are unknown, and reports of refractory fungal vaginitis have not been substantiated [158]. HIV-infected women appear more likely to have non-*C. albicans* isolates than women without HIV infection. In one study, oral and vaginal isolates were recovered prospectively over a period of 2 years. Among those with *C. albicans* isolates, resistance of the isolate to antifungal agents (such as fluconazole) was rare. In contrast, non-*C. albicans* isolates frequently had reduced susceptibility to fluconazole, and subjects with non-*C. albicans* isolates had more infections. The non-*C. albicans* species most closely associated with the development of fluconazole resistance were *C. glabrata* and *C. tropicalis* [159]. HIV infection may or may not enhance susceptibility to vaginal candidiasis. Studies suggest that local immunity is more important than systemic immunity for host defense against *Candida* vaginitis [158].

Treatment options for VVC are listed in Table 15.5. An estimated 5% of women suffer complicated VVC, which is defined as recurrent VVC (more than four episodes per year), severe symptomatology, or infections caused by non-*C. albicans* isolates. This diagnosis should be confirmed by cultures before therapy is instituted. Vaginitis due to *C. albicans* responds well to available therapy. There are also many effective topical agents. All of these azoles treat uncomplicated VVC (i.e. mild-to-moderate, sporadic, non-recurrent disease with normally susceptible *C. albicans*) [114, 140].

In contrast, vaginitis due to *C. glabrata* is associated with a high treatment failure rate [159] and requires a longer duration of therapy (i.e. 10–14 days) with either topical or oral azoles [114, 142]. The management of recurrent VVC requires an induction course of either oral or vaginal antimycotic therapy, which must be continued daily until the patient is completely asymptomatic or the culture becomes negative. Failure to initiate a maintenance regimen will result in a clinical relapse of VVC in 50% of cases. Three maintenance suppressive therapy regimens are effective and include ketoconazole 100 mg daily, 100 mg fluconazole orally once weekly and 500 mg clotrimazole suppositories once a week. The treatment of sexual partners adds no benefit to this regimen and the role of yogurt in preventing VVC remains unproven. Hyposensitization with *Candida* antigen preparations has shown encouraging results in subgroups of patients but further double-blind placebo studies are required [157].

15.5.6 Trichomoniasis

Trichomoniasis vaginalis infection is prevalent in sexually active adolescents, e.g. in 12.6% of HIV-infected adolescents and in 3.4% of HIV-uninfected adolescents [119]. Sexual activity is the most common predisposing factor for *T. vaginalis* infection. Prevalence rates have ranged from 5–10% in women in the general population to as high as 50–60% in incarcerated women and commercial sex workers. An increased risk of this infection is described in women with multiple sexual partners, poor personal hygiene, and low socio-economic status.

The clinical and laboratory characteristics associated with trichomoniasis are delineated in Table 15.5. The symptoms of *T. vaginalis* infection include vaginal itch and frothy, malodorous, and gray or yellow-green colored discharge. In HIV-infected women, *T. vaginalis* also can infect Skene's ducts, Bartholin's glands and the urethra, where organisms may not be susceptible to topical therapy [160]. The clinical manifestations of vaginal trichomoniasis vary from asymptomatic carriage to severe vaginitis. This range of clinic symptoms is influenced by host factors, which vary during the course of the menstrual cycle and may influence the expression of T. *vaginalis* virulence. The proportion of women who have symptoms vary from 20–50% depending on the population, selection criteria, and diagnostic method [161]. Physical examination may demonstrate cervical petechiae ("strawberry cervix") in 5–10% of cases, and the cervix, urethra, and bladder can be inflamed. Definitive diagnosis of *T. vaginalis* infection requires microscopic and/or laboratory examination as other pathogens cause similar symptoms. In addition, women with trichomoniasis are more likely to be colonized by *G. vaginalis* and *Bacteriodes* spp. (90%), *Ureaplasma urealyticum* and/or *Mycoplasma hominis* (over 90%), *N. gonorrhoeae* (30%), yeast (20%), and *C. trachomatis* (15%) than women with normal flora. Culture has greater diagnostic sensitivity than wet mount and DNA probe. A special 'Trich pouch' has been developed to facilitate culturing and isolating *T. vaginalis* in the clinic setting. However, clinicians must still be proficient at microscopic examination. Although *T. vaginalis* may be identified on Pap smear, Pap smears have low levels of sensitivity and specificity for *T. vaginalis* and should not be relied on for diagnosis [161].

Trichomonas vaginalis infection of the lower genital tract may be associated with PID. In an African STD clinic study, trichomoniasis was associated with a significantly higher risk of PID ($P = 0.03$). If *T. vaginalis* infection is present, the risk of PID is significantly higher among HIV-infected compared with uninfected patients ($P = 0.002$) [162].

Treatment regimens for *T. vaginalis* infections are shown in Table 15.5 [114, 163]. Treatment generally involves one of two agents: metronidazole or clindamycin. These agents should not be used together because of possible toxicities. Metronidazole is the treatment of choice for both men and women. If the patient is pregnant, the only approved treatment is a single 2 g PO dose of metronidazole. This treatment is highly effective, with cure rates ranging from 82–88%. Simultaneous therapy for sexual partners increases the cure rate to 95% or more with single-dose treatment. Infected women should avoid sexual intercourse until they are cured. Because *T. vaginalis* often infects the urethra and periurethral glands, systemic therapy is superior to a topical regimen.

Metronidazole can produce malaise, nausea, and occasionally vomiting; the nausea and vomiting may be particularly problematic with the 2 g dose. However, for those who can tolerate the one-time larger dose, malaise tends to disappear quickly, whereas those taking smaller doses for a week may feel varying degrees of malaise during the entire time, a factor likely to interfere with compliance. It is also important to note that metronidazole produces antabuse-like reactions with nausea, flushing, headaches, and convulsions in people who drink any alcohol while taking the medication. Women given the single-dose therapy should be alcohol free for 72 hours afterwards. Those taking the 7-day regimens must be prepared to abstain from alcohol for the entire period and through 72 hours after the last dose [114].

If treatment failure occurs, the patient should be retreated with the same agent and an extra effort should be made to ensure treatment of sex partner(s). If the sexual partner(s) are treated and intercourse has been halted, then oral metronidazole 2 g QD for 3–5 days should be considered for patients experiencing previous treatment failure. Metronidazole resistance is rare. HIV-infected individuals with trichomoniasis are treated in the same manner as HIV-uninfected patients [161].

15.5.7 Atypical infections of the female genital tract

Atypical infections of the female reproductive tract generally are more severe manifestations of infections due to common genital tract infectious agents, e.g. HSV and *Candida* species. As mentioned previously, inflammatory STDs such as gonorrheal and chlamydial infections, and trichomoniasis, appear to be more likely to progress to PID among immunosuppressed women [161, 162, 164]. Opportunistic infections associated with HIV infection or immunosuppression that affect other organ systems can theoretically affect the female genital tract, although cytomegalovirus (CMV) has been the only opportunistic infection reported to date to have gynecological manifestations. Cytomegalovirus disease of the female genital tract can result in significant morbidity, including ulcerations, fever, pain, bleeding, and superinfection [165].

Cervicitis

There are two main types of cervicitis: endocervicitis, also called mucopurulent cervicitis (owing to characteristic yellowish mucopurulent exudates from the endocervix) and ectocervicitis, characterized by inflammation of the outside of the cervix. Ectocervicitis is usually caused by infections with *T. vaginalis* or *Candida* species. Among adolescent girls, ectocervicitis may be easily confused during a gynecologic speculum examination with cervical ectopy, characterized by the columnar epithelium of the endocervix extending beyond the cervical os into the region normally occupied by the squamous epithelium of the ectocervix [114]; the brighter red color of the columnar epithelium can easily be mistaken for inflammation.

Mucopurulent cervicitis, common in sexually active women and adolescent girls, is usually caused by sexually transmitted pathogens, including *C. trachomatis* and *N. gonorrhoeae*. Sexual activity is the main risk factor for cervicitis. Both pathogens infect columnar or transitional epithelium and produce superficial mucosal infections, which may be asymptomatic. Annually in the USA, there are approximately 3 million new infections of *Chlamydia trachomatis* among adolescents, and 650 000 new infections of *Neisseria gonorrhoeae* [114, 139–141, 166]. The majority of cases go undiagnosed because asymptomatic infection is common. In the REACH study, prevalence rates of *C. trachomatis* and *N. gonorrhoeae* were similar between the HIV-infected adolescent girls and the high risk, HIV-uninfected girls [119]. Other pathogens causing cervicitis include *T. vaginalis*, *Candida* species, and HSV.

The clinical and laboratory characteristics of mucopurulent cervicitis are delineated in Table 15.6. A presumptive diagnosis of chlamydial or gonorrheal endocervicitis may be made based on the presence of mucopurulent endocervical discharge, cervical friability, and more than 15 WBCs per high power-field seen on either wet mount or Gram stain of endocervical specimens. The diagnosis is definitive if a culture, direct fluorescent antibodies (DFA), DNA probe, or nucleic acid amplification tests (NAAT) shows positive results for *C. trachomatis* and/or *N. gonorrhoeae*. The latter two are the most sensitive diagnostic tests currently available to detect both pathogens. Ectocervicitis is usually associated with vaginitis and the diagnosis is often made with the identification of *T. vaginalis* and *Candida* species on wet mount. Herpes simplex virus infection is

Table 15.6 Mucopurulent cervicitis: clinical and laboratory characteristics, treatment

	Mucopurulent cervicitis	*Chlamydia trachomatis*	*Neisseria gonorrhoeae*
Etiology	*C. trachomatis, N. gonorrhoeae*		
Symptoms	Women may be symptomatic or asymptomatic. Yellow mucopurulent endocervical exudates	Women may be symptomatic or asymptomatic. Dysuria, yellow mucopurulent vaginal discharge	Abnormal vaginal discharge, spotting, abnormal menses, dysuria. Women may be asymptomatic. Anorectal and pharyngeal infections are common and may or may not be symptomatic
Discharge	1. Yellow, mucopurulent endocervical exudate on white cotton-tipped swab. 2. Presence of increased number of polymorphonuclear leukocytes on Gram stain specimen has low predictive value	Presence of yellow, mucopurulent endocervical exudate on white cotton-tipped swab.	Gram stain is not sensitive and should be confirmed by culture, DNA probe, or NAAT; mucopurulent discharge
Diagnosis	Positive chlamydia (culture, DFA, DNA probe, or NAAT) and gonorrhea (culture, DNA probe, or NAAT) test results	Positive chlamydia test (culture, DFA, DNA probe, or NAAT)	Growth on selective medium demonstrating typical colonial morphology, positive oxidase reaction, and typical Gram stain morphology
Treatment	Based on testing results. If patient is unreliable or in a high prevalence area, treat presumptively covering for both organisms *If pregnant*, avoid tetracycline and quinolones	Azithromycin 1 g PO in a single dose, OR doxycycline 100 mg PO BID for 7 days, OR erythromycin base 500 mg PO QID for 7 days *If pregnant:* Azithromycin 1 g PO × 1, amoxicillin 500 ng PO TID for 7 days, OR erythromycin base 500 mg PO QID for 7 days	Cefixime 400 mg PO in a single dose, OR ceftriaxone 125 mg IM in a single dose, OR ciprofloxacin 500 mg PO in a single dose, OR ofloxacin 400 mg PO in a single dose *If pregnant*, avoid quinolones
Complications	Untreated infections may ascend causing endometritis, salpingitis, and subsequent infertility		10–20% of women develop PID if untreated
Follow-up	As appropriate	No need for retesting after therapy completion unless symptoms persist or reinfection is suspected. Rescreening is recommended in 3–4 months since reinfection is common, especially in adolescents	No need for retesting after therapy for patients with uncomplicated gonorrhea. Treatment failure most likely due to reinfection
Partner treatment	Sex partners should be referred for evaluation and treatment. Referral of partners within the last 60 days is recommended. Sexual intercourse should be avoided until patient and partners are cured	Same	Same

DFA = Direct Immunofluorescence Assay; NAAT = Nucleic Acid Amplification Test. Adapted from [106, 114].

highly correlated with cervical ulcers or necrotic lesions, whereas *T. vaginalis* is correlated with colpitis macularis or "strawberry cervix." A positive cervical culture confirms the diagnosis of HSV cervicitis and viral isolation permits the differentiation between HSV-1 and HSV-2, which has prognostic importance, since HSV-1 is less likely than HSV-2 to produce recurrent episodes [106].

Treatment options for mucopurulent cervicitis due to *C. trachomatis* or *N. gonorrhoeae* are shown in Table 15.6 [114]. If a symptomatic adolescent is an unreliable historian or resides in an area of high prevalence for both *C. trachomatis* and *N. gonorrhoeae*, she should be treated presumptively for both organisms. HIV-infected girls should receive the same treatment as HIV-uninfected girls. It is important that any male sex partner during the 60 days preceding the cervicitis diagnosis be referred for evaluation and treatment. Patients and their partners should refrain from sexual intercourse until their infections have been cured. Treatment of HSV infection and trichomoniasis causing ectocervicitis are addressed elsewhere in this chapter.

When discussing prevention of cervicitis, adolescents should be counseled about the use of spermicides, in particular Nonoxynol-9 (N-9). This spermicide was thought to also have antimicrobial effects against pathogens causing common STDs, and once appeared to have in vitro anti-HIV activity. However, studies of its in vivo effectiveness in preventing HIV infection in women have been inconclusive. Moreover, its repeated use has been associated with increased vulnerability to HIV infection. Finally, no significant effects of N-9 on *N. gonorrhoeae* or *C. trachomatis* infections have been reported. Therefore, this spermicide can no longer be considered a potential method of preventing HIV, and should not be encouraged as an adjuvant protective method against STDs [138].

Pelvic inflammatory disease

Pelvic inflammatory disease (PID) represents an acute clinical syndrome resulting from ascending spread of microorganisms from the vagina or cervix to the endometrium, fallopian tubes, ovaries, and contiguous structures. Pelvic inflammatory disease is the most common serious complication of STDs; with its long-term sequelae including ectopic pregnancy, chronic pelvic pain, and tubal infertility [167]. Over one million women in the USA experience an episode of PID each year, with sexually active adolescents having the highest age-specific rates of PID, with those under 19 years of age accounting for one in five cases of PID [168]. Sexually active adolescents are more vulnerable to PID than older women, with sexually active 15-year-old girls estimated to have 10 times the risk of developing PID in a given year than 24-year-old women in the USA [168,

169]. The higher relative risk of PID for younger women has been attributed to their greater biologic vulnerability (for example, due to the incomplete transition from columnar to epithelial cells in the cervix) and behavioral risk factors. Women with STDs (especially infections due to gonorrhea, chlamydia, and BV) are at greater risk of developing PID; having had a previous PID infection increases the risk of another episode because the body's defenses are often damaged during the initial bout of upper genital tract infection. The more sexual partners an adolescent has, the greater her risk of developing PID. Smoking, alcohol use, and use of other drugs have also been identified as risk factors. Recent data suggest women who douche once or twice a month are more likely to have PID than those who douche less than once a month, as douching may push bacteria into the upper genital tract. Douching also may relieve discharge caused by an infection, leading the woman to delay seeking healthcare [168].

Pelvic inflammatory disease may have a more complicated course in HIV-infected women [161]. HIV-infected women with PID appear to be more likely than women without HIV infection to present with sonographically diagnosed adnexal masses (TOAs) [170], to require hospitalization, and to require surgery for PID [114, 134, 171]. In general, HIV-seropositive women with acute salpingitis respond well to appropriate antibiotic therapy [131, 133]. Duration of hospitalization tends to be longer among women with CD4 percentages of <14% [133]. General immune suppression may contribute to the altered pathogenesis of PID in HIV-infected women, but there also appear to be some specific, local, genital tract defects in host defenses in HIV-infected women that predispose them to more serious PID.

The etiology of PID is usually polymicrobial (both aerobic and anaerobic). The most common organisms detected in cultures of cervical secretions include *C. trachomatis*, *N. gonorrhoeae*, and genital *Mycoplasma* species. Although the prevalence of *C. trachomatis* and *N. gonorrhoeae* is similar between HIV-infected and uninfected women with PID, *Mycoplasma* organisms and streptococci have been isolated more commonly from HIV-infected women with PID than from HIV-uninfected women [170]. In the most serious cases, *N. gonorrhoeae* and *C. trachomatis* have been isolated from the upper genital tract in less than one third of women with PID undergoing laparotomy. Other microorganisms causing PID include anaerobic bacteria (e.g. *Peptococcus*, *Peptostreptococcus*, *Bacteriodes*, and *Provetella* species) and facultative aerobes (e.g. *Escherichia coli*, group B streptococcus, *Gardnerella vaginalis*, and *Haemophilus influenzae*). As discussed earlier, trichomoniasis has also been associated with PID.

Women with PID due to gonorrhea usually present with acute (less than 3 days) and severe symptoms, leading to rapid diagnosis. In contrast, women with PID due to chlamydia may be asymptomatic or have only mild symptoms, resulting in a longer period of time until diagnosis, usually more than one week [168].

Pelvic inflammatory disease can be difficult to diagnose. Diagnostic criteria for PID include the following: uterine or adnexal tenderness or cervical motion tenderness (CMT). Additional criteria for diagnosis include: (1) an oral temperature greater than 38.3 °C (101 °F); (2) mucopurulent cervical or vaginal discharge; (3) WBCs on wet mount preparations of vaginal secretions; (4) elevated erythrocyte sedimentation rate (ESR) or C-reactive protein (CRP) levels; and (5) positive test results for chlamydial infection or for gonorrhea [168].

Most girls with PID have mucopurulent cervical discharge or evidence of WBCs on a vaginal fluid wet mount preparation. If the cervical discharge appears normal and there are no WBCs noted on wet mount, the diagnosis of PID is unlikely and alternative causes of pain should be considered and investigated. Elevated levels of CRP are a more sensitive and specific predictor than an elevated ESR [167, 168].

Additional procedures are required for a definitive diagnosis: ultrasound to view the pelvic area to determine whether the fallopian tubes are enlarged or whether there is an abscess, laparoscopy to allow for visual inspection and to collect specimens for cultures and pathology, laparotomy when scarring or abnormal conditions make laparoscopy technically difficult, and endometrial biopsy to document endometritis. Definitive criteria include: (1) histopathologic evidence of endometritis on endometrial biopsy; (2) thickened fluid-filled fallopian tubes with or without free pelvic fluid or TOA on ultrasound or other radiologic tests; and (3) laparoscopic abnormalities consistent with PID. The most rapid, least invasive definitive diagnostic method is ultrasonography. Sonography is indicated in patients in whom a TOA is suspected. Patients with a palpable adnexal mass or persistent fever should be evaluated for TOA. It is also important to appreciate that many adolescents with PID have unrecognized TOAs [114, 139, 140, 172, 174]. Indications for hospitalization include: (1) the inability to exclude surgical emergencies (i.e. appendicitis, ectopic pregnancy); (2) TOA; (3) pregnancy; (4) immunosuppression; (5) inability to follow or tolerate outpatient oral antibiotic therapy; (6) failure to respond clinically to oral antibiotic therapy; and (7) severe illness including severe nausea and vomiting or high fever.

Treatment regimens for PID are shown in Table 15.7. HIV-infected adolescents who are significantly immunocompromised should be hospitalized for treatment. Inadequate treatment of PID in adolescents may lead to serious complications, long-term sequelae, or recurrent infections. HIV-infected adolescents who are not significantly immunocompromised and who are clinically stable may be treated as outpatients, but the clinician should have a low threshold for hospitalization if the patient's condition fails to improve or if the patient does not adhere to the prescribed outpatient therapy [114, 134, 167].

15.5.8 Human papillomavirus

Human papillomavirus infection is the most prevalent STD in the USA. Human papillomavirus causes external genital warts, cervical intraepithelial and invasive neoplasia, low- and high-grade squamous intraepithelial lesions (SILs), and genital squamous cell cancers. Numerous HPV subtypes have been described and are categorized into low-risk (types 6, 11, 42, 43, and 44) or high-risk (types 16, 18, 31, 33, and 35) types depending on their oncogenic potential. Studies among sexually active adolescent girls have described prevalence rates for HPV infection ranging from 20–83% [116]. HIV-infected women have a higher prevalence of HPV infections [175–179] than uninfected women. Human papillomavirus infections among HIV-infected women and adolescent girls differ from those of uninfected women in several ways: they persist for a longer period of time [178, 180]; they are more likely to involve multiple HPV subtypes [181]; and they are more likely to include oncogenic subtypes, particularly subtypes 16 and 18 [175, 182].

HIV, HPV, and cervical dysplasia

Several varieties of abnormal cervical cytologies are associated with HPV infection, especially in the presence of HIV infection. The risk for the development of SILs among HIV-infected and -uninfected women with HPV is most closely associated with infection by high- and intermediate-risk HPV types. In contrast to dysplasias among women, associated with CD4$^+$ and viral load levels indicative of advanced HIV disease [177, 183–185], the degree of immune suppression is not highly predictive of SIL. HIV-infected and high-risk HIV-uninfected adolescent girls have comparable rates of HPV infection and SILs. However, contrary to findings among women, among HIV-infected adolescent girls, increasing severity of HPV infection, evidenced by dysplasia, appears to be independent of HIV disease progression, indicated by low CD4$^+$ cell counts and high viral loads. Therefore, in adolescents, it appears that HIV infection may have a synergistic effect on the HPV infection through additional mechanisms not directly linked to

Table 15.7 Treatment regimens for pelvic inflammatory disease

Inpatient therapy	
Parenteral regimen A	Cefotetan 2 g IV every 12 hours, OR
	Cefoxitin 2 g IV every 6 hours, PLUS doxycycline 100 mg PO or IV every 12 hours
Parenteral regimen B	Clindamycin 900 mg IV every 8 hours, PLUS gentamicin loading dose IV or IM (2 mg/kg), followed by maintenance dose (1.5 mg/kg) every 8 hours
Alternative regimens	Oflaxacin 400 mg IV every 12 hours, OR
	Levofloxacin 500 mg IV QD WITH OR WITHOUT metronidazole 500 mg IV every 8 hours, OR
	Ampicillin/sulfbactam 3 g IV every 6 hours, PLUS doxycycline 100 mg PO or IV every 12 hours
Comments	Both parenteral regimens (A and B) offer excellent coverage for polymicrobial infections, with Regimen B more appropriate when anaerobic coverage is desired.
	Parenteral therapy may be discontinued 24 hours after patient's condition improves clinically, oral therapy with doxycycline should continue until completion of 14-day course.
	When TOA is present, anaerobic coverage is better achieved by combining use of clindamycin or metronidazole with doxycycline
Outpatient therapy	
Oral regimen A	Oflaxacin 400 mg PO BID for 14 days, OR
	Levofloxacin 500 mg PO QD, WITH OR WITHOUT metronidazole 500 mg PO BID for 14 days
Oral regimen B	Ceftriaxone 250 mg IM once, OR
	Cefoxitin 2 g IM, plus probenicid 1 g PO in a single concurrent dose, OR
	Other parenteral 3rd generation cephalosporin (ceftizoxime or cefotaxime) PLUS doxycycline 100 mg PO BID for 14 days, WITH OR WITHOUT
	metronidazole 500 mg PO BID for 14 days
Comments	Regimen A covers gonorrhea and chlamydia effectively, but also provides excellent anaerobic coverage.
	Patients need to return to clinic in 72 hours to assure improvement has occurred and to assess compliance with therapy

Sources: [114, 168]
TOA, tubo-ovarian abscess.

low CD4$^+$ cell counts, particularly early in the course of HIV infection [115].

HIV-infected women who are highly immunocompromised are more likely to experience progression of their dysplasias than HIV-uninfected women. All HIV-infected women, except those with exceptionally well-controlled disease, are less likely to show regression of dysplasia than uninfected women [184].

Several studies have attempted to explain the association between HIV and HPV infection. For example, the results of a recent study suggest that HIV infection may increase the risk of cervical dysplasia in women who are co-infected with HPV through high levels of HIV expression and/or multiple HPV infections [179]. In another study, the association of HIV and cervical intraepithelial neoplasia (CIN) was fully explained by repeated HPV positivity in HIV-infected women [180]; this suggests that the immune response of those with HIV infection is altered, affecting the immune response to HPV. For example, the histology of the

lymphoid follicles following HPV infection differs in HIV-infected women compared with HIV-uninfected women. Due to these recent findings, it is becoming more evident that HPV infection manifests differently in immunosuppressed HIV-infected women [186].

Uncomplicated human papillomavirus infections

External genital warts (EGW) or condylomata are the most common manifestation of HPV in the vulvar area and are often caused by HPV types 6, 11, and 42–44. These lesions usually manifest as hyperkeratotic or warty type lesions in the vulva and perianal areas, and can easily be detected after the application of 5% acetic acid to the area. After this application, the cells undergo dehydration and this produces the characteristic "acetowhite" changes. Although rare, both vulvar SIL and cancers can occur and can present as hyperpigmented raised lesions in the vulva. This is of particular importance in patients with HIV infection. The treatment of EGW includes application of trichloroacetic acid (TCA) directly into the lesion as first-line therapy. Podophylin is a potent antimitotic agent but TCA seems to work better on keratotic lesions. Self-applied therapy should also be offered to patients. They include imidazoquinolone compounds such as imiquimod (5% cream, single dose packets). It is applied directly to the lesion at bedtime for up to 16 weeks on a schedule of 3 alternate days/week. The cream is washed off in 6–10 hours. These compounds generate proinflammatory cytokines and a Th1 cell-mediated response with the generation of cytotoxic effects. Unfortunately, these therapies are costly and patients may need to wait several weeks to notice an improvement [187].

Invasive cervical cancer in HIV disease

In 1993, the case definition of AIDS was expanded by the Centers for Disease Control and Prevention (CDC) to include invasive cervical cancer. Although high-grade changes in cervical cytology and progression to invasive disease are still relatively uncommon among HIV-infected women [184], there is some evidence that the invasive cervical cancer rate in HIV-infected women is higher than in uninfected women [188–190]. Invasive cervical cancer is more severe in HIV-infected women; HIV-infected women are more likely than uninfected women to have cervical cancer which presents at a younger age [191], presents at more advanced stages, metastasizes to unusual sites (e.g. psoas muscle, clitoris, meninges), responds poorly to standard therapy, has higher recurrence and death rates, and has shorter intervals to recurrence or death [192, 193].

Papanicolaou smear screening and colposcopy

Screening tests include the traditional Papanicolaou (Pap) smear, which has a false negative rate of 10–25%. Newer Pap smear screening techniques, such as those modified to employ liquid-based media and other modifications to increase sensitivity and decrease inadequate smears, help to reduce, but not eliminate, false-negative results. These modified techniques also offer the opportunity to perform direct testing for both oncogenic and non-oncogenic types of HPV. The reliability of Pap testing to detect cervical abnormalities is significantly increased with regular, periodic screening. Results should be reported according to the Bethesda System [194].

HIV-infected women and sexually active adolescents should have a complete gynecologic evaluation including a Pap smear and pelvic exam as part of an initial evaluation when the diagnosis of HIV infection is first made [114, 140]. A Pap smear should then be obtained twice in the first year after the diagnosis of HIV infection. If Pap results are normal, annual examinations are recommended. Indications for more frequent Pap smears are: (1) a previously abnormal Pap smear; (2) an HPV infection; (3) previous treatment of cervical dysplasia; or (4) more advanced HIV disease (including $CD4^+$ cell counts < 200 cells/mm^3. The American College of Obstetricians and Gynecologists (ACOG) recommends Pap smears every 3–4 months for the first year after treatment of pre-invasive cervical lesions, followed by Pap smears every 6 months [195]. The role of anal cytology is currently under study.

Atypical squamous cells of undetermined significance (ASCUS) represent the mildest cytologic abnormality in the Bethesda system. HIV-uninfected patients with an initial report of ASCUS should have a prompt repeat Pap smear. If the repeat Pap smear also shows ASCUS, the patient should be referred for colposcopy. Studies in HIV-infected women with ASCUS have found a higher frequency of underlying dysplasia than in non-infected women [196, 197]. Therefore, in HIV-infected women, colposcopy should be performed with any ASCUS result. Women with a diagnosis of atypical glandular cells of undetermined significance (AGCUS) have a significantly higher risk of underlying pathology than patients with ASCUS. Approximately 17–34% of patients with AGCUS have associated significant intraepithelial or invasive lesions [198–200]. Colposcopy and endocervical and endometrial sampling are indicated with any AGCUS result.

Recent studies suggest that HIV-infected women are at increased risk for the development of invasive vulvar carcinoma. Women with any degree of vulvar abnormality, except for typical exophytic condylomata acuminata, should be referred for colposcopy and biopsy so that pre-invasive or invasive disease can be ruled out. The studies have not targeted specific adolescent female populations, therefore no conclusive adolescent specific data can be given [197]. For HIV-infected women, colposcopy should always include thorough examination of the entire lower genital tract (vagina, vulva, and perianal region).

Management of cervical lesions

High-grade cervical lesions require treatment with standard excisional or ablative therapy. HIV-infected women are more likely to have recurrent disease after treatment (over 50%) than HIV-uninfected women, and HIV-infected women with immunosuppression are even more likely to have recurrent disease [201, 202]. Cryotherapy leads to the highest rate of recurrences and should be avoided if other treatment methods are available. Topical vaginal 5-fluorouracil (5-FU) cream (2 g biweekly for 6 months) has been shown to reduce recurrence rates after standard treatment for high-grade cervical dysplasia in HIV-infected women. Disease has also been shown to recur more slowly in HIV-infected women who receive effective antiretroviral therapy [203]. HIV-infected adolescent girls and young women with a history of abnormal Pap smears or a history of cervical dysplasia should continue to be followed closely for evidence of lower genital tract neoplasia, regardless of antiretroviral therapy or stage of HIV disease.

15.5.9 Herpes simplex virus

There are two herpes simplex virus subtypes that cause genital infections, HSV-1 and HSV-2. Herpes simplex virus infections are discussed in more detail in Chapter 41. Herpes simplex virus infections are the most prevalent cause of genital ulcers in the USA. Approximately 22% of individuals aged 12 years or older in the USA are infected [204]. The majority of genital herpes lesions (60–95%) are caused by HSV-2. Transmission of HSV infections likely occurs through close contact with a person who is shedding the virus, e.g. in genital or oral secretions.

For HIV-infected patients, HSV infections can be more frequent, prolonged, and severe, especially with progressive immunosuppression. Lesions can also be atypical in appearance or location. Viral shedding increases in individuals with lower CD4$^+$ cell counts [205], in those using oral contraceptives or depot-medroxyprogesterone, and in individuals with severe vitamin A deficiency [206].

The lesions are typically single or multiple vesicles that are painful, that ulcerate and heal without scarring, and that can appear anywhere on the genitalia. As with most other herpes viruses, HSV causes lifelong infection. Following a primary infection, the virus can remain latent within cells. The latent virus can reactivate when the patient experiences certain stimuli or triggering events including stress, worsening immunosuppression, or even hormonal changes. Some women experience periodic recurrences in association with menses. The primary, or initial, infection can produce systemic symptoms such as fever, photophobia, malaise, and headache. However, primary infections can be sub-clinical such that an individual could experience a first, clinically apparent infection when antibodies to HSV are present. The lesions accompanying primary infection can last longer (mean duration, 12 days) than those accompanying reactivated disease, and viral shedding following a primary infection can continue for days to weeks or more. Recurrent episodes, representing reactivated disease, are generally milder and shorter, with a mean duration of 4–5 days. They can occur at variable frequency and consist of more localized lesions. Viral shedding and sexual transmission can occur during asymptomatic, latent periods. Reactivated disease can sometimes be quite serious, even life-threatening, in patients with severe immunosuppression. The lesions can sometimes have an atypical appearance, particularly in immunosuppressed patients, so the practitioner should be alert to the possibility of HSV disease [205, 206].

A presumptive diagnosis of HSV infection can be made on the basis of clinical presentation with or without one of the following: direct identification of multinucleated giant cells with intranuclear inclusions on a scraping from a lesion (Tzanck preparation), direct immunofluorescent assay performed on material scraped from lesions, or detection of HSV antigens by monoclonal antibody detection systems. Definitive diagnosis can be made using an HSV tissue culture. Observation of typical HSV morphology with electron microscopy of material scraped from lesions or other clinical specimens can also be used for diagnosis [114].

Systemic administration of antiviral drugs (acyclovir, valacyclovir, and famciclovir) can be used to treat primary and recurrent infections. For troublesome, recurrent disease, the drugs can be used as daily suppressive therapy. However, these drugs neither eradicate latent virus nor affect the risk, frequency, or severity of recurrences after the drug is discontinued [114].

Treatment of HSV infections is outlined in Table 15.8. For severe, clinically apparent infections with HSV (severe infections generally requiring hospitalization such as disseminated infection, pneumonitis, hepatitis, or complications of the central nervous system), if lesions persist or recur in a patient receiving antiviral treatment, HSV resistance should be suspected and a viral isolate obtained for sensitivity testing. Such patients should be managed in consultation with a specialist, and alternate therapy should be administered. The CDC has reported a 6.4% resistance rate to acyclovir among HIV-infected patients, as well as cross-resistance to famciclovir and valacyclovir [207]. Factors associated with acyclovir resistance include low CD4$^+$ counts and long-term acyclovir exposure. Most of these isolates are susceptible to other antiviral drugs such as foscarnet or cidofovir. Foscarnet has several potentially serious side-effects and should only be used in severe cases in consultation with specialists, and patients should be monitored carefully for signs of toxicity. Topical cidofovir gel 1% is not commercially available and must be compounded at a pharmacy [114].

Because HSV infection can recur more frequently and with greater severity in HIV patients, suppressive therapy may be needed. Daily suppressive therapy reduces recurrence frequency by more than 75% among patients who suffer from frequent HSV episodes (i.e. six or more

Table 15.8 Recommended treatment of herpes simplex virus infections

	Drug and dose
First clinical episode	Acyclovir 400 mg PO tid for 7–10 days, or
	Acyclovir 200 mg PO 5×/day for 7–10 days, or
	Famciclovir 250 mg PO tid for 7–10 days, or
	Valacyclovir 1 g PO bid for 7–10 days
Recurrent episodes	Acyclovir 400 mg PO tid for 5 days, or
	Acyclovir 200 mg PO 5×/day for 5 days, or
	Acyclovir 800 mg PO bid for 5 days, or
	Famciclovir 125 mg PO bid for 5 days, or
	Valacyclovir 500 mg PO bid for 3–5 days, or
	Valacyclovir 1 g PO qd for 5 days
Daily suppressive therapy	Acyclovir 400 mg PO bid, or
	Famciclovir 250 mg PO bid, or
	Valacyclovir 500 mg PO qd, or
	Valacyclovir 1 g PO qd
Severe disease	Acyclovir 5–10 mg/kg body weight IV q 8 hours for 5–7 days or until clinical resolution is achieved
Acyclovir-resistant HSV	Foscarnet 40 mg/kg body weight IV q 8 hours or 60 mg/kg IV every 12 hours for 3 weeks
	Cidofovir 1% gel topical application to lesions qd for 5 consecutive days

Source: [114]

recurrences per year). Suppressive therapy can reduce but may not eliminate viral shedding.

15.5.10 Secondary prevention of sexually transmitted diseases

HIV-infected adolescents have high STD rates, suggesting that they continue to engage in risky sexual behaviors. HIV-infected adolescent patients should receive careful counseling on a continuing basis aimed at promoting healthy behaviors and at decreasing their risks for further infections. In counseling HIV-infected adolescents, providers should assess their sexual practices, the presence of substance abuse, and their understanding of their HIV disease and other STDs. Patients should be carefully informed of the risks of STDs and of super-infection with HIV [119, 171, 208].

Many adolescents erroneously believe that, if they have unprotected sexual encounters with a steady sexual partner, they are not at risk for acquiring STDs and, consequently, they do not take precautions against acquiring STDs [117, 208, 209]. When counseling adolescents, providers should carefully assess their mental health. Sub-

stance abuse has been associated with an increased risk of acquiring STDs. Depression and anxiety were associated with frequent alcohol use and with a previous history of unprotected sex [117]. Prevention-oriented interventions aimed at reducing risky behaviors and preventing the development of more significant health, mental health, or substance abuse disorders are needed [117, 208, 209].

Appropriate HIV prevention interventions are based on a solid understanding of developmental, societal, cultural, and gender issues affecting each individual. Gender inequality is an important consideration when, in many cases, adolescent girls feel inferior to adolescent boys. Intimate relationships may then result in increased vulnerability to HIV among the adolescent female. Violence and sexual abuse may also prevent girls from expressing their desires to practice preventative behaviors. Many behavioral interventions involve the development of self-efficacy and equipping the young woman with negotiating skills to encourage condom use or to abstain from sexual intercourse. These approaches may not be appropriate in certain cultures where negotiating is unlikely and unacceptable for girls. Therefore, other means of HIV prevention and behavior interventions must be used. The female condom is becoming more popular because it does not necessarily require negotiation by the female [210].

HIV-infected adolescents have limited knowledge of the impact of HIV on their STDs and vice versa [115]. Clear explanation of these interactions as well as prevention messages, early detection, and management of STDs are crucial elements to improve the health of these adolescents. HIV-seropositive adolescents have little understanding of the concept of secondary infection with new HIV strains and the risk of being secondarily infected with drug-resistant strains of HIV [125, 126]. Reducing the risk of transmission of drug-resistant HIV requires careful assessment of the HIV-infected adolescent's sexual practices and health education messages that include discussion about the possibility of acquiring a new, potentially drug-resistant virus.

15.6 Conclusions

The clinician's approach to detecting gynecological conditions in the HIV-infected adolescent female is guided by a complete medical history and physical examination and the clinician's suspicion of common gynecological disorders. The most practical approach when considering the most common gynecological disorders of HIV-infected adolescents is to identify if the adolescent is sexually active or not. Among non-sexually active girls with perinatally acquired HIV infection, the most common conditions include delayed pubertal development and menstrual disorders related to an immature hypothalamic-pituitary axis. Sexually active HIV-infected adolescents are susceptible to many other conditions as a result of their sexual behavior. The most common conditions among this group are similar to those that affect sexually active, HIV-uninfected adolescents. These conditions include STDs, pregnancy, and abnormal uterine bleeding.

A complete gynecological history including risk behaviors greatly facilitates the diagnosis of these disorders. An adolescent medicine specialist may conduct the evaluation of all these conditions. Endocrinology consultation is necessary for management of pubertal delay and appropriate referrals to obstetricians and gynecologists are required for complications of pregnancy and pelvic infections.

REFERENCES

1. Harlan, W. R., Harlan, E. A. & Grillo, G. P. Secondary sex characteristics of girls 12 to 17 years of age: The U.S. health examination survey. *J. Pediatr.* **96** : **6** (1980), 1074–8.

2. Rogol, A. D., Roemmich, J. N. & Clark, P. A. Growth at puberty. *J. Adolesc. Health* **31** : **6** (Suppl) (2002), 192–200.

3. Wheeler, M. D. Physical changes of puberty. *Endocrinol. Metab. Clin. N. Am.* **20** : **1** (1991), 1–14.

4. Sun, S. S., Schubert, C. M., Chumlea, W. C. *et al.* National estimates of the timing of sexual maturation and racial differences among U.S. Children. *Pediatrics* **110** : **5** (2002), 911–19.

5. Wu, T., Mendola, P. & Buck, G. M. Ethnic differences in the presence of secondary sex characteristics and menarche among U.S. girls: The third national health and nutrition examination survey, 1988–1994. *Pediatrics* **110** : **4** (2002), 752–7.

6. Zacharias, L., Rand, W. M. & Wurtman, R. J. A prospective study of sexual development and growth in American girls: The statistics of menarche. *Obstetr. Gygnecol. Survey.* **31** (1976), 325.

7. Frisch, R. E. & Revelle, R. Menstrual cycles: Fatness as a determinant of minimum weight-for-height for their maintenance or onset. *Science* **185** (1974), 949.

8. MacLure, M., Travis, L. B., Willett, W. & MacMahon, B. A prospective cohort study of nutrient intake and age at menarche. *Am. J. Clin. Nutr.* **54** (1991), 649.

9. Chan, J. L., Bluher, S., Yiannakouris, N., Suchard, M. A., Kratzsch, J. & Mantzoros, C. S. Regulation of circulating soluble leptin receptor levels by gender, adiposity, sex steroids, and leptin: observational and interventional studies in humans. *Diabetes* **51** : **7** (2002), 2105–12.

10. Palacio, A. C., Perez-Bravo F, Santos, J. L., Schlesinger, L. & Monckeberg, F. Leptin levels IgF-binding proteins in malnourished children: effect of weight gain. *Nutrition* **18** : **1** (2002), 17–19.

11. Laimer, M., Ebenbichler, C. F., Kaser, S. *et al.* Weight loss increases soluble leptin receptor levels and the soluble receptor bound fraction of leptin. *Obes. Res.* **10** : **7** (2002), 597–601.

12. Shimizu, H., Shimomura, K., Negishi, M. *et al.* Circulating concentrations of soluble leptin receptor: influence of menstrual cycle and diet therapy. *Nutrition* **18** : **4** (2002), 309–12.

13. Beckett, P. R., Wong, W. W. & Copeland, K. C. Developmental changes in the relationship between IGF-I and body composition during puberty. *Growth. Horm. IGF Res.* **8** : **4** (1998), 283–8.

14. D'Ahmed, M. L., Ong, K. K., Morrell, D. J. *et al.* Longitudinal study of leptin concentrations during puberty: sex differences and relationship to changes in body composition. *J. Clin. Endocrin. Metab.* **84** : **3** (1999), 899–905.

15. Bideci, A., Cinaz, P., Hasanglu, A. & Turner, L. Leptin, insulin-like growth factor (IGF)-I and IGF binding protein-3 levels in children with constitutional delay of growth. *J. Pediatr. Endocrinol. Metab.* **15** : **1** (2002), 41–6.

16. D'Fors, H., Matsuoka, H., Bosaeus, I., Rosberg, S., Wikland, K. A. & Bjarnason, R. Serum leptin levels correlate with growth hormone secretion and body fat in children. *J. Clin. Endocrinol. Metab.* **84** : **10** (1999), 3586–90.

17. Simon, D. Puberty in chronically diseased patients. *Horm. Res.* **57** (Suppl. 2) (2002), 53–6.

18. Sedlmeyer, I. L. & Palmert, M. R. Delayed puberty: analysis of a large case series from an academic center. *J. Clin. Endocrinol. Metab.* **87** : **4** (2002), 1613–20.

19. Albanese, A. & Stanhope, R. Investigation of delayed puberty. *Clin. Endocrinology* **43** (1995), 105–10.

20. Mahoney, C. P. Evaluating the child with short stature. *Pediatr. Clin. N. Am.* **34** (1987), 825–49.

21. Oerter, K. E., Uriarte, M. M., Rose, S. R., Barnes, K. M. & Cutler, G. B. Jr. Gonadotropin secretory dynamics during puberty in normal girls and boys. *J. Clin. Endocrinol. Metab.* **71**:5 (1990), 1251–8.

22. Reiter, E. O. & Lee, P. A. Delayed puberty. *Adolesc. Med.* **13**:1 (2002), 101–18, vii.

23. Finkelstein, J. W., Susman, E. J., Chinchilli, V. M. *et al.* Effects of estrogen or testosterone on self-reported sexual responses and behaviors in hypogonadal adolescents. *J. Clin. Endocrinol. Metab.* **83**:7 (1998), 2281–5.

24. Susman, E. J., Finkelstein, J. W., Chinchilli, V. M. *et al.* The effect of sex hormone replacement on behavior problems and moods in adolescents with delayed puberty. *J. Pediatr.* **133**:4 (1998), 521–5.

25. Palmert, M. R., Malin, H. V. & Boepple, P. A. Unsustained or slowly progressive puberty in young girls: initial presentation and long-term follow-up of 20 untreated patients. *J. Clin. Endocrinol. Metab.* **84** (1999), 415–23.

26. Carpenter, S. *Pediatric and Adolescent Gynecology.* Philadelphia, PA: Lippincott Williams and Wilkins (2000).

27. Chirgwin, K. D., Feldman, J., Muneyyirci-Delale O, Landesman, S. & Minkoff, H. Menstrual function in human immunodeficiency virus-infected women without acquired immunodeficiency syndrome. *J. AIDS Hum. Retrovirol.* **12**:5 (1996), 489–94.

28. Ellerbrock, T. V., Wright, T. C., Bus, T. J., Dole, P, Brudney, K. & Chiasson, M. A. Characteristics of menstruation in women infected with human immunodeficiency virus. *Obstet. Gynecol.* **87**:6 (1996), 1030–4.

29. Mendelson, J. H., Teoh, S. K., Lange, U. *et al.* Anterior pituitary, adrenal, and gonadal hormones during cocaine withdrawal. *Am. J. Psychiatry* **145**:9 (1988), 1094–8.

30. Pletcher, J. R. & Slap, G. B. Menstrual disorders. Amenorrhea. *Pediatr. Clin. N. Am.* **46**:3 (1999), 505–18.

31. Grinspoon, S., Corcoran, C., Miller, K. *et al.* Body composition and endocrine function in women with acquired immunodeficiency syndrome wasting. *J. Clin. Endocrinol. Metab.* **82**:5 (1997), 1332–7J.

32. Golden, N. H. A review of the female athlete triad (amenorrhea, osteoporosis and disordered eating). *Int. J. Adolesc. Med. Health.* **14**:1 (2002), 9–17.

33. Teoh, S. K., Lex, B. W., Mendelson, J. H., Mello, N. K. & Cochin, J. Hyperprolactinemia and macrocytosis in women with alcohol and polysubstance dependence. *J. Stud. Alcohol* **53**:2 (1992), 176–82.

34. Block, R. I., Farinpour, R. & Schlechte, J. A. Effects of chronic marijuana use on testosterone, luteinizing hormone, follicle stimulating hormone, prolactin and cortisol in men and women. *Drug Alcohol Depend.* **28**:2 (1991), 121–8.

35. Efstratiades, M., Panitsa-Faflia, C. & Batrinos, M. Vaginal cytology in endocrinopathies. *Acta Cytol.* **27**:4 (1983), 421–5.

36. Laufer, M. R., Floor, A. E., Parsons, K. E., Kuntz, K. M. & Barbieri, R. L. Hormone testing in women with adult-onset amenorrhea. *Gynecol. Obstet. Invest.* **40**:3 (1995), 200–3

37. Biller, B. M., Luciano, A., Crosignani, P. G. *et al.* Guidelines for the diagnosis and treatment of hyperprolactinemia. *J. Reprod. Med.* **44**:12 (Suppl.) (1999), 1075–84.

38. Speroff, L., Glass, R. H. & Kase, N. G. Anovulation and the polycystic ovary. In ?(eds.) *Clinical Gynecology Endocrinology and Infertility.* Philadephia, PA: Lippincott Williams and Wilkins (1999), pp. 487–513.

39. Lobo, R. A. & Carmina, E. The importance of diagnosing the polycystic ovary syndrome. *Ann. Intern. Med.* **132**:12 (2000), 989–93.

40. Stafford, D. E. & Gordon, C. M. Adolescent androgen abnormalities. *Curr. Opin. Obstet. Gynecol.* **14**:5 (2002), 445–51.

41. Legro, R. S. The genetics of polycystic ovary syndrome. *Am. J. Med.* **98** (1995), 9S.

42. Legro, R. S. Detection of insulin resistance and its treatment in adolescents with polycystic ovary syndrome. *J. Pediatr. Endocrinol. Metab.* **15** (Suppl. 5) (2002), 1367–78.

43. Strauss, J. F. 3rd & Dunaif, A. Molecular mysteries of polycystic ovary syndrome. *Mol. Endocrinol.* **13**:6 (1999), 800–5.

44. Balen, A. Pathogenesis of polycystic ovary syndrome – the enigma unravels? *Lancet.* **18**:354 (9183) (1999), 966–7.

45. McKenna, T. J. Pathogenesis and treatment of polycystic ovary syndrome. *New Engl. J. Med.* **318** (1998), 558.

46. Avyad, C. K., Holeuwerger, R., Silva, V. C., Bordallo, M. A. & Breitenbach, M. M. Menstrual irregularity in the first postmenarchal years: an early clinical sign of polycystic ovary syndrome in adolescence. *Gynecol. Endocrinol.* **15**:3 (2001), 170–7.

47. Carmina, E., Wong, L., Chang, L. *et al.* Endocrine abnormalities in ovulatory women with polycystic ovaries on ultrasound. *Hum. Reprod.* **12**:5 (1997), 905–9.

48. Gordon, C. M. Menstrual disorders in adolescents: excess androgens and the polycystic ovary syndrome. *Pediatr. Clin. N. Am.* **46** (1999), 519–543

49. Arslanian, S. A., Lewy, V., Danadian, K. & Saad, R. Metformin therapy in obese adolescents with polycystic ovary syndrome and impaired glucose tolerance: amelioration of exaggerated adrenal response to adrenocorticotropin with reduction of insulinemia/insulin resistance. *J. Clin. Endocrinol. Metab.* **87**:4 (2002), 1555–9.

50. Bravender, T. & Emans, S. J. Menstrual disorders. Dysfunctional uterine bleeding. *Pediatr. Clin. N. Am.* **46**:3 (1999), 545–53, vii.

51. Munro, M. G. Dysfunctional uterine bleeding: advances in diagnosis and treatment. *Curr. Opin. Obstet. Gynecol.* **13**:5 (2001), 475–89.

52. Shah, P. N., Smith, J. R., Wells, C., Barton, S. E., Kitchen, V. S. & Steer, P. J. Menstrual symptoms in women infected by the human immunodeficiency virus. *Obstet. Gynecol.* **83**:3 (1994), 397–400.

53. Munro, M. G. Abnormal uterine bleeding in the reproductive years. Part I –pathogenesis and clinical investigation. *J. Am. Assoc. Gynecol. Laparosc.* **6**:4 (1999), 393–416.

54. Munro, M. G. Abnormal uterine bleeding in the reproductive years. Part II –medical management. *J. Am. Assoc. Gynecol. Laparosc.* **7** : **1** (2000), 17–35.

55. Kilbourn, C. L. & Richards, C. S. Abnormal uterine bleeding. Diagnostic considerations, management options. *Postgrad. Med.* **109** : **1** (2001), 137–8, 141–4, 147–50.

56. Dealy, M. F. Dysfunctional uterine bleeding in adolescents. *Nurse. Pract.* **23** : **5** (1998), 2–3, 16, 18–20.

57. Minjarez, D. A. & Bradshaw, K. D. Abnormal uterine bleeding in adolescents. *Obstet. Gynecol. Clin. N. Am.* **27** : **1** (2000), 63–78.

58. Speroff, L., Glass, R. H. & Kase, N. G. Dysfunctional uterine bleeding. In *Clinical Gynecology Endocrinology and Infertility*. Philadephia, PA: Lippincott Williams and Wilkins (1999), pp. 575–93.

59. Klein, J. R. & Litt, I. F. Epidemiology of adolescent dysmenorrhea. *Pediatrics* **68** : **5** (1981), 661–4.

60. Eldering, J. A., Nay, M. G., Hoberg, L. M., Longcope, C. & McCracken, J. A. Hormonal regulation of endometrial prostaglandin F_2 alpha production during the luteal phase of the rhesus monkey. *Biol. Reprod.* **49** : **4** (1993), 809–15.

61. Harel, Z., Lilly, C., Riggs, S., Vaz, R. & Drazen, J. Urinary leukotriene (LT) E(4) in adolescents with dysmenorrhea: a pilot study. *J. Adolesc. Health* **27** : **3** (2000), 151–4.

62. Harel, Z. A contemporary approach to dysmenorrhea in adolescents. *Pediatr. Drugs.* **4** : **12** (2002), 797–805.

63. Koike, H., Egawa, H., Ohtsuka, T., Yamaguchi, M., Ikenoue, T. & Mori, N. Correlation between dysmenorrheic severity and prostaglandin production in women with endometriosis. *Prostaglandins Leukot. Essent. Fatty Acids.* **46** : **2** (1992), 133–7.

64. Fedele, L., Bianchi, S., Bocciolone, L., Di Nola, G. & Parazzini, F. Pain symptoms associated with endometriosis. *Obstet. Gynecol.* **79** : **5** (Pt 1) (1992), 767–9.

65. Hornsby, P. P., Wilcox, A. J. & Weinberg, C. R. Cigarette smoking and disturbance of menstrual function. *Epidemiology* **9** : **2** (1998), 193–8.

66. Hendrix, S. L. & Alexander, N. J. Primary dysmenorrhea treatment with a desogestrel-containing low-dose oral contraceptive. *Contraception* **66** : **6** (2002), 393–9.

67. Chakmakjian, Z. H. A critical assessment of therapy for the premenstrual tension syndrome. *J. Reprod. Med.* **28** : **8** (1983), 532–8.

68. Raja, S. N., Feehan, M., Stanton, W. R. & McGee, R. Prevalence and correlates of the premenstrual syndrome in adolescence. *J. Am. Acad. Child. Adolesc. Psychiatry* **31** : **5** (1992), 783–9.

69. Fisher, M., Trieller, K. & Napolitano, B. Premenstrual symptoms in adolescents. *J. Adolesc. Health Care* **10** : **5** (1989), 369–75.

70. Steiner, M. & Pearlstein, T. Premenstrual dysphoria and the serotonin system: pathophysiology and treatment. *J. Clin. Psychiatry* **61** (Suppl. 12) (2000), 17–21.

71. Gianetto-Berruti, A. & Feyles, V. Premenstrual syndrome. *Minerva Ginecol* **54** : **2** (2002), 85–95.

72. Freeman, E. W. Premenstrual syndrome: current perspectives on treatment and etiology. *Curr. Opin. Obstet. Gynecol.* **9** : **3** (1997), 147–53.

73. American Psychiatric Association. *Diagnostic and Statistical Manual of Mental Disorders, Fourth Edition* (DSM-IV), Text Revision. Washington, DC: American Psychiatric Association 2000.

74. Wenning, J. Premenstrual syndrome. In E. McAnarney, R. Kreipe, D. Orr & G. Comerci (eds.), *Textbook of Adolescent Medicine*. Philadelphia, PA: W. B. Saunders Company (1992), pp. 670–1.

75. Johnson, S. R. Premenstrual syndrome therapy. *Clin. Obstet. Gynecol.* **41** : **2** (1998), 405–21.

76. UNFPA. *The State of World Population 1997.* New York: UNFPA 1997.

77. Macro International. *Women's Lives and Experiences: A Decade of Research Findings from the Demographic and Health Surveys Program.* Calverton, MD: Macro International (1994) (footnote).

78. Child and adolescent health and development: Overview of CAH. Available at: http://www.who.int/child-adolescent-health/overview/ahd/adh˙sheer.htm.

79. Guest, F. Education and counseling: factors influencing education and counseling. In D. Kowal (ed.), *Contraceptive Technology*, 17th edn. New York: Ardent Media Inc. (1998), pp. 249–61.

80. Derman, S. & Peralta, L. Postcoital contraception: present and future options. RU486 (Mifepristone). *J. Adolesc. Health* **16** (1995), 6–11.

81. Hatcher, R., Trussel, J., Stewart, F. *et al. Contraceptive Technology*, 17th edn. New York: Ardent Media Inc. (1998).

82. Kuyoh, M. A., Toroitich-Ruto, C., Grimes, D. A., Schulz, K. F. & Gallo, M. F. Sponge versus diaphragm for contraception: a Cochrane review. *Contraception* **67** : **1** (2003), 15–18.

83. Joesoef, M. R., Karundeng, A., Runtupalit, C., Moran, J. S., Lewis, J. S. & Ryan, C. A. High rate of bacterial vaginosis among women with intrauterine devices in Manado, Indonesia. *Contraception.* **64** : **3** (2001), 169–72.

84. Morrison, C. S., Sekadde-Kigondu, C., Sinei, S. K., Weiner, D. H., Kwok, C. & Kokonya, D. Is the intrauterine device appropriate contraception for HIV-1-infected women? *Br. J. Obstet. Gynaecol.* Aug; **108** : **8** (2001), 784–90.

85. Belzer, M., Rogers, A. S., Camarca, M. *et al.* Contraceptive choices in HIV-infected and HIV at-risk adolescent females. *J. Adolesc. Health* **29S** (2001), 93–100.

86. Levin, L., Henry-Reid, L., Murphy, D. A. *et al.* Adolescent Medicine HIV/AIDS Research Network. Incident pregnancy rates in HIV-infected and HIV uninfected at-risk adolescents. *J. Adolesc. Health* **29S** (2001), 101–8.

87. Hatcher, R., Trussel, J., Stewart, F. *et al.* HIV/AIDS and reproductive health. In *Contraceptive Technology*, 17th edn. New York NY: Ardent Media Inc. (1998), pp. 141–78.

88. Stone, A. Microbicides: a new approach to preventing HIV and other sexually transmitted infections. *Nat. Rev. Drug. Discov.* **1** : **12** (2002), 977–85.

89. Everett, S. A., Warrem, C. W., Santelli, J. S., Kann, L., Collins, J. L. & Kolbe, L. J. Use of birth control pills, condoms, and withdrawal among U.S. high school students. *J. Adolesc. Health* **27** : **2** (2000), 12–18.

90. Sivin, I. & Moo-Yong, A. Recent developments in contraceptive implants at the Population Council. *Contraception* **65**:**1** (2002), 113–19.

91. Garceau, R. J., Wajszczuk, C. J. & Kaunitz, A. M. Bleeding patterns of women using Lunelle monthly contraceptive injections (medroxyprogesterone acetate and estradiol cypionate injectable suspension) compared with those of women using Ortho-Novum 7/7/7 (norethindrone/ethinyl estradiol triphasic) or other oral contraceptives. *Contraception* **62**:**6** (2000), 289–95.

92. Audet, M. C., Moreau, M., Koltun, W. D. *et al.* Evaluation of contraceptive efficacy and cycle control of a transdermal contraceptive patch vs an oral contraceptive: a randomized controlled trial. *J. Am. Med. Assoc.* **285**:**18** (2001), 2347–54.

93. Abrams, L. S., Skee, D., Matarajan, J. & Wong, F. A. Pharmacokinetic overview of Ortho Evra/Evra. *Fertil. Steril.* **77**:**2** (Suppl. 2) (2002), S3–12.

94. Smallwood, G. H., Meador, M. L., Lenihan, J. P., Shangold, G. A., Fisher, A. C. & Creasy, G. W. Efficacy and safety of a transdermal contraceptive system. *Obstet. Gynecol.* **98**:**5** (Pt 1) (2001), 799–805.

95. Sobel, J. Vulvovaginal candidiasis. In K. Holmes, F. Sparling, S. Lemon *et al.* (eds.), *Sexually Transmitted Diseases*, 3rd edn. New York, NY: McGraw-Hill (1999), pp. 629–39.

96. Hatcher, R. A. & Guillebaud, J. The Pill: Combined oral contraceptive. In: D. Kowal (ed.), *Contraceptive Technology* 17th edn. New York: Ardent Media Inc. (1998), pp. 405–66.

97. The Alan Guttmacher Institute. *Why is Teenage Pregnancy Declining? The Roles of Abstinence, Sexual Activity and Contraceptive Use.* Occasional Report. New York: Alan Guttmacher Institute; (1999).

98. Hatcher, R. A. Depo-Provera, Norplant, and progestin-only pills (minipills). In D. Kowal (ed.), *Contraceptive Technology* 17th edn. New York: Ardent Media Inc. (1998), pp. 467–509.

99. D'Angelo, L., Belzer, M., Futterman, D., Peralta, L. & Sawyer, M. "Reducing the Odds" at what cost: will routine testing of pregnant adolescents decrease perinatal transmission of HIV? *J. Adolesc. Health.* **27**:**5** (2000), 296–7.

100. Johansson, E., Brache, V., Alvarez, F. *et al.* Pharmacokinetic study of different dosing regimens of levonorgestrel for emergency contraception in healthy women. *Hum. Reprod.* **17**:**6** (2002), 1472–6.

101. Sivin, I., Mishell, D. R. Jr., Victor, A. *et al.* A multicenter study of levonorgestrel-estradiol contraceptive vaginal rings. II-Subjective and objective measures of effects. An international comparative trial. *Contraception* **24**:**4** (1981), 359–76.

102. Chu, S. Y., Hanson, D. L. & Jones, J. L. Pregnancy rates among women infected with human immunodeficiency virus. Adult/Adolescent HIV Spectrum of Disease Project Group. *Obstet. Gynecol.* **87**:**2** (1996), 195–8.

103. van Benthem, B. H. B., Vernazza, P., Coutinho, R. A. and Pris, M. The impact of pregnancy and menopause on CD4 cell counts in European HIV-infected women. Presented at *NIH Conference on Fertility and Systemic Hormones in HIV-infected and At-Risk Women*; (Jan 13–14, 2003). McLean, VA (Abstr).

104. Ahdieh, L. Pregnancy and infection with human immunodeficiency virus. *Clin. Obstet. Gynecol.* **44**:**2** (2001), 154–66.

105. Mwanyumba, P., Claeys, P., Gaillard, C. *et al.* Correlation between maternal and infant HIV infection and low birth weight: A study in Mombasu, Kenya. *J. Obstet. Gynecol.* **21**:**1** (2001), 27–31.

106. Holmes, K. & Stamm, W. Lower genital tract infection syndromes in women. In K. Holmes, F. Sparling, S. Lemon *et al.* (eds.), *Sexually Transmitted Diseases*. 3rd edn. New York, NY: McGraw-Hill (1999), p. 766.

107. Hashemi, F. B., Ghassemi, M., Faro, S., Aroutcheva, A. & Spear, G. T. Induction of human immunodeficiency virus type 1 expression by anaerobes associated with bacterial vaginosis. *J. Infect. Dis.* **181**:**5** (2000), 1574–80.

108. Sturm-Ramirez, K., Gaye-Diallo, A., Eisen, G., Mboup, S. & Kanki, P. J. High levels of tumor necrosis factor-alpha and interleukin-1 beta in bacterial vaginosis may increase susceptibility to human immunodeficiency virus. *J. Infect. Dis.* **182**:**2** (2000), 467–73.

109. Cauci, S., Driussi, S., Guaschino, S., Isola, M. & Quadrifoglio, F. Correlation of local interleukin-1 beta levels with specific IgA response against *Gardnerella vaginalis* cytolysin in women with bacterial vaginosis. *Am. J. Reprod. Immunol.* **47**:**5** (2002), 257–64.

110. Martin, H. L., Richardson, B. A., Nyange, P. M. *et al.* Vaginal lactobacilli, microbial flora, and risk of human immunodeficiency virus type 1 and sexually transmitted disease acquisition. *J. Infect. Dis.* **180** (1999), 1863–8.

111. Conley, L. J., Ellerbrock, T. V., Bush, T. J., Chiasson, M. A., Sawo, D. & Wright, T. C. HIV infection and risk of vulvovaginal and perianal condylomata acuminata and intraepithelial neoplasia: a prospective cohort study. *Lancet* **359** (2002), 108–13.

112. D'Angelo, L. J., Belzer, M. Futterman, D. & Peralta, L. Response to the joint statement on HIV screening. *Pediatrics* **105**:**2** (2000), 467–8.

113. Gerbase, A. C., Rowley, J. T. & Mertens, T. E. Global epidemiology of sexually transmitted diseases. *Lancet* **351** (Suppl. III) (1998), 2–4.

114. Centers for Disease Control and Prevention. Sexually transmitted diseases treatment guidelines 2002. *MMWR* **51: RR-6** (2002), 1–78.

115. Moscicki, A. B., Ellenberg, J. H. & Vermund, S. H. Prevalence of and risks for cervical human papillomavirus infection and squamous intraepithelial lesions in adolescent girls: impact of infection with human immunodeficiency virus. *Arch. Pediatr. Adolesc. Med.* **54**:**2** (2000), 127–34.

116. Jacobson, D., Mizell, S., Peralta, L. *et al.* Concordance of human papilloma virus in the cervix and urine of adolescents with a high prevalence of HPV. *Pediatr. Infect. Dis. J.* **19**:**8** (2000), 722–8.

117. Murphy, D. A., Durako, S. D., Moscicki, A. B. *et al.* and the Adolescent Medicine HIV/AIDS Research Network. No change in health risk behaviors over time among HIV-infected adolescents in care: role of psychological distress. *J. Adolesc. Health* **29S** (2001), 57–63.

118. Peralta, L., Durakos, S. J. & Ma, Y. Correlation between urine and cervical specimens for the detection of cervical *Chlamydia trachomatis* and *Neisseria gonorrhoeae* using ligase chain reaction in a cohort of HIV-infected and uninfected adolescents. *J. Adolesc. Health* **29S** (2001), 87–92.

119. Vermund, S. H., Wilson, C. M., Rogers, A. S., Partlow, C. & Moscicki, A. B. Sexually transmitted infections among HIV-infected and HIV uninfected high-risk youth in the REACH study. *J. Adolesc. Health* **9S** (2001), 49–56.

120. Cu-Uvin, S., Hogan, J. W., Warren, D. *et al.* Prevalence of lower genital tract infections among human immunodeficiency virus (HIV)-seropositive and high-risk HIV-seronegative women. HIV Epidemiology Research Study Group. *Clin. Infect. Dis.* **29**:**5** (1999), 1145–50.

121. Helfgott, A., Eriksen, N., Bundrick, C. M., Lorimor, R. & Van Eckhout, B. Vaginal infections in human immunodeficiency virus-infected women. *Am. J. Obstet. Gynecol.* **183**:**2** (2000), 347–55.

122. Wasserheit, J. N. Epidemiological synergy. Inter-relationships between human immunodeficiency virus infection and other sexually transmitted diseases. *Sex Transm. Dis.* **19**:**2** (1992), 61–77.

123. Laga, M., Manoka, A., Kivuvu, M. *et al.* Non-ulcerative sexually transmitted diseases as risk factors for HIV transmission in women: results from a cohort study. *AIDS* **7**:**1** (1993), 95–102.

124. Fleming, D. T. & Wasserheit, J. N. From epidemiological synergy to public health policy and practice: the contribution of other sexually transmitted diseases to sexual transmission of HIV infection. *Sex Transm. Infect.* **75**:**1** (1999), 3–17.

125. Pilon, R., Sandstrom, P., Burchell, A. *et al.* A Transmitted HIV reverse transcriptase inhibitor resistance mutation stability in ART-naive recent seroconverters: results of the polaris HIV seroconversion study. In *XIV International AIDS Conference* (July 9 2002), Barcelona. (Abstr. Code No. TuPeB4611.)

126. Ostrowski, M. & Gough, K. A transmitted HIV reverse transcriptase inhibitor resistance mutation stability in ART-naive recent seroconverters: Results of the polaris HIV seroconversion study. In *XIV International AIDS Conference* (July 9, 2002), Barcelona.

127. Greendale, G. A., Haas, S. T., Holbrook, K., Walsh, B., Schachter, J. & Phillips, R. S. The relationship of *Chlamydia trachomatis* infection and male infertility. *Am. J. Public Health* **83**:**7** (1993), 996–1001.

128. Robertson, D., McMillan, A. & Young, H. *Clinical Practice in Sexually Transmissible Diseases*, 2nd edn. Edinburgh: Churchill Livingstone (1989).

129. Goldenberg, R. L., Andrews, W. W., Yuan, A. C., MacKay, H. T. & St Louis, M. E. Sexually transmitted diseases and adverse outcomes of pregnancy. *Clin. Perinatal* **24**:**1** (1997), 23–41.

130. Moscicki, A. B., Ma, Y., Holland, C. & Vermund, S. H. Cervical ectopy in adolescent girls with and without human immunodeficiency virus infection. *J. Infect. Dis.* **183**:**6** (2001), 865–70.

131. Irwin, K. L., Moorman, A. C. & O'Sullivan, M. J. Influence of human immunodeficiency virus infection on pelvic inflammatory disease. *Obstet. Gynecol.* **95**:**4** (2000), 525–34.

132. Manfredi, R., Alampi, G., Talo, S. *et al.* Silent oophoritis due to cytomegalovirus in a patient with advanced HIV disease. *Int. J. STD AIDS* **11**:**6** (2000), 410–12.

133. Cohen, C. R., Sinei, S. & Reilly, M. Effect of human immunodeficiency virus type 1 infection upon acute salpingitis: a laparoscopic study. *J. Infect. Dis.* **178**:**5** (1998), 1352–8.

134. Korn, A. P. Pelvic inflammatory disease in women infected with HIV. *AIDS Patient Care STDs* **12**:**6** (1998), 431–4.

135. Ahmed, S., Lutalo, T. & Wawer, M. HIV incidence and sexually transmitted disease prevalence associated with condom use: a population study in Rakai, Uganda. *AIDS* **15**:**16** (2001), 2171–9.

136. Rudy, B. J., Crowley-Nowick, P. A. & Douglas, S. D. Immunology and the REACH study: HIV immunology and preliminary findings. Reaching for Excellence in Adolescent Care and Health. *J. Adolesc. Health* **29**:**3** (Suppl.) (2000), 39–48.

137. Crowley-Nowick, P. A., Ellenberg, J. H., Vermund, S. H., Douglas, S. D., Holland, C. A. & Moscicki, A. B. Cytokine profile in genital tract secretions from adolescent women: impact of HIV, human papilloma virus and other sexually transmitted infections. *J. Infect. Dis.* **181** (2002), 939–45.

138. Van Damme, L., Ramjee, G., Alary, M. *et al.* Effectiveness of COL-1492, a nonoxynol-9 vaginal gel, on HIV transmission in female sex workers: a randomized controlled trial. *Lancet* **360**:**9338** (2002), 971–7.

139. Neinstein, L. S. (ed.) *Adolescent Health Care. A Practical Guide*, 4th edn. Philadelphia, PA: Lippincott Williams and Wilkins (2002).

140. California STD/HIV Prevention Training Center. *Core STD Curriculum: Comprehensive Outlines for Clinical STD Management* (1999).

141. Johnson, R. E., Newhall, W. J. & Papp, J. R. Screening tests to detect *Chlamydia trachomatis* and *Neisseria gonorrhea* infections. *MMWR* **51**:**RR-15** (2002), 1–38 quiz CE1–4.

142. Sobel, J. D., Kapernick, P. S. & Zervos, M. Treatment of complicated Candida vaginitis: comparison of single and sequential doses of fluconazole. *Am. J. Obstet. Gynecol.* **185**:**2** (2001), 363–9.

143. Hillier, S. & Holmes, K. K. Bacterial vaginosis. In K. Holmes, F. Sparling, S. Lemon (eds.), *Sexually Transmitted Diseases*, 3rd edn. New York, NY: McGraw-Hill (1999), pp. 563–86.

144. Amsel, R., Totten, P. A., Spiegel, C. A., Chen, K. C., Eschenbach, D. & Holmes, K. K. Nonspecific vaginitis: Diagnostic criteria and microbial and epidemiologic associations. In K. Holmes, F. Sparling, S. Lemon *et al.* (eds.), *Sexually Transmitted Diseases*, 3rd edn. New York, NY: McGraw-Hill (1999), p. 569.

145. Joesef, M. R., Hillier, S. L., Josodiwondo, S. & Linnan, M. Reproducibility of a scoring system for Gram stain diagnosis of bacterial vaginosis. *J. Clin. Microbiol.* **29**:**8** (1991), 1730–1.

146. Ugwumadu, A., Hay, P. & Taylor-Robinson, D. HIV infection associated with abnormal vaginal flora morphology and bacterial vaginosis. *Lancet* **350** : **9086** (1997), 1251.

147. Ledru, S., Meda, N., Ledru, E., Bazie, A. J. & Chiron, J. P. HIV infection associated with abnormal vaginal flora morphology and bacterial vaginosis. *Lancet* **350** : **9086** (1997), 1251–2.

148. Jamieson, D. J., Duerr, A., Klein, R. S. *et al.* Longitudinal analysis of bacterial vaginosis: findings from the HIV epidemiology research study. *Obstet. Gynecol.* **98** : **4** (2001), 656–63.

149. Schwebke, J. R. Asymptomatic bacterial vaginosis: response to therapy. *Am. J. Obstet. Gynecol.* **183** : **6** (2000), 1434–9.

150. Livengood, C. H. 3rd, Soper, D. E., Sheehan, K. L. *et al.* Comparison of once-daily and twice-daily dosing of 0.75% metronidazole gel in the treatment of bacterial vaginosis. *Sex. Transm. Dis.* **26** : **3** (1999), 137–42.

151. Paavonen, J., Mangioni, C., Martin, M. A. & Wajszczuk, C. P. Vaginal clindamycin and oral metronidazole for bacterial vaginosis: a randomized trial. *Obstet. Gynecol.* **96** : **2** (2000), 256–60.

152. Ransom, S. B., McComish, J. F., Greenburg, R. & Tolford, D. A. Oral metronidazole vs. Metrogel Vaginal for treating bacterial vaginosis. Cost-effectiveness evaluation. *J. Reprod. Med.* **44**: **4** (1999), 359–62.

153. Hanson, J. M., McGregor, J. A., Hillier, S. L. *et al.* Metronidazole for bacterial vaginosis. A comparison of vaginal gel vs. oral therapy. *J. Reprod. Med.* **45** : **11** (2000), 889–96.

154. Bannatyne, R. M. & Smith, A. M. Recurrent bacterial vaginosis and metronidazole resistance in *Gardnerella vaginalis. Sex. Transm. Infect.* **74** : **6** (1998), 455–6.

155. Hay, P. Sr. National guideline for the management of bacterial vaginosis. Clinical Effectiveness Group (Association of Genitourinary Medicine and the Medical Society for the Study of Venereal Diseases). *Sex. Transm. Infect.* **75** (Suppl. 1) (1999), S16-18.

156. McCormack, W. M., Covino, J. M. & Thomason, J. L. Comparison of clindamycin phosphate vaginal cream with triple sulfonamide vaginal cream in the treatment of bacterial vaginosis. *Sex. Transm. Dis.* **28** : **10** (2001), 569–75.

157. Sobel, J. D. Vulvovaginal candidiasis. In K. Holmes, F. Sparling, S. Lemon (eds.), *Sexually Transmitted Diseases*, 3rd edn., New York, NY: McGraw-Hill (1999), pp. 629–39.

158. Sobel, J. D., Ohmit, S. E., Schuman, P. *et al.* The evolution of Candida species and fluconazole susceptibility among oral and vaginal isolates recovered from human immunodeficiency virus (HIV)-seropositive and at-risk HIV-seronegative women. *J. Infect. Dis.* **183** : **2** (2000), 286–93.

159. Sobel, J. D. Treatment of vaginal Candida infections. *Expert Opin. Pharmacother.* **3** : **8** (2002), 1059–65.

160. Jackson, D. J., Rakwar, J. P., Bwayo, J. J., Kreiss, J. K. & Moses, S. Urethral *Trichomonas vaginalis* infection and HIV transmission. *Lancet* **350** : **9084** (1997), 1076.

161. Krieger, J. & Alderete, J. Trichomonas vaginalis and Trichomoniasis. In K. Holmes, F. Sparling, S. Lemon, *et al.* (eds.), *Sexually Transmitted Diseases*, 3rd edn. New York, NY: McGraw-Hill (1999), pp. 587–604.

162. Moodley, P., Wilkinson, D., Connolly, C., Moodley, J. & Sturm, A. W. *Trichomonas vaginalis* is associated with pelvic inflammatory disease in women infected with human immunodeficiency virus. *Clin. Infect. Dis.* **34** : **4** (2002), 519–22.

163. Moodley, P., Connolly, C. & Sturm, A. W. Interrelationships among human immunodeficiency virus type 1 infection, bacterial vaginosis, trichomoniasis, and the presence of yeasts. *J. Infect. Dis.* **185** : **1** (2002), 69–73.

164. Kamenga, M., Kamenga, M. C., De Cock, K. M. *et al.* The impact of human immunodeficiency virus infection on pelvic inflammatory disease: a case-control study in Abidjan, Ivory Coast. *Am. J. Obstet. Gynecol.* **172** : **3** (1995), 919–25.

165. Friedmann, W., Schafer, A., Kretschmer, R. & Lobeck, H. Disseminated cytomegalovirus infection of the female genital tract. *Gynecol. Obstet. Invest.* **31** : **1** (1991), 56–7.

166. Centers for Disease Control and Prevention. *HIV/AIDS Surveillance Report* **2** : **2** (2000), 5–44.

167. Igra, V. Pelvic inflammatory disease in adolescents. *AIDS Patient Care STDs* **12** : **2** (1998), 109–24.

168. Westrom, L. & Eschenbach, D. Pelvic inflammatory disease. In K. Holmes, F. Sparling, S. Lemon (eds.), *Sexually Transmitted Diseases*, 3rd edn. New York, NY: McGraw-Hill (1999), pp.783–809.

169. HRP Annual Technical Report 1995: Executive Summary. Available at: www.who.int/reproductive-health/publications/HRP`ATRs/1995/execsum.html.

170. Irwin, K. L., Moorman, A. C., O'Sullivan, M. J. Influence of human immunodeficiency virus infection on pelvic inflammatory disease. *Obstet. Gynecol.* **95** : **4** (2000), 525–34.

171. Bersoff-Matcha, S. J., Horgan, M. M., Fraser, V. J., Mundy, L. M. & Stoner, B. P. Sexually transmitted disease acquisition among women infected with human immunodeficiency virus type 1. *J. Infect. Dis.* **78** : **4** (1998), 1174–7.

172. Rice, P. A. & Schachter, J. Pathogenesis of pelvic inflammatory disease: What are the questions? *J. Am. Med. Assoc.* **266** : **18** (1991), 2587–93.

173. Slap, G. B., Forke, C. M., Cnaan, A. *et al.* Recognition of tubo-ovarian abscess in adolescents with pelvic inflammatory disease. *J. Adol. Health.* **18** : **6** (1996), 397–403.

174. Walker, C. K., Workowski, K. A., Washington, A. E., Soper, D. & Sweet, R. L. Anaerobes in pelvic inflammatory disease: implications for the Centers for Disease Control and Prevention's guidelines for treatment of sexually transmitted diseases. *Clin. Infect. Dis.* **28** (Suppl. 1) (1999), S29-36.

175. Minkoff, H., Feldman, J., DeHovitz, J., Landesman, S. & Burk, R. A longitudinal study of human papillomavirus carriage in human immunodeficiency virus-infected and human immunodeficiency virus-uninfected women. *Am. J. Obstet. Gynecol.* **178** : **5** (1998), 982–6.

176. Palefsky, J. M., Minkoff, H., Kalish, L. A. *et al.* Cervicovaginal human papillomavirus infection in human immunodeficiency virus-1 (HIV)-positive and high-risk HIV-negative women. *J. Natl. Cancer. Inst.* **91** : **3** (1999), 226–36.

177. Shah, K. V., Munoz, A. & Klein, R. S. Prolonged persistence of genital human papillomavirus infections in HIV-infected women. *Program and Abstracts of the 11th International Conference on AIDS* (July 7–12, 1996). Vancouver, Canada, p. 345 (Abst Tu.C.2466).

178. Sun, X. W., Kuhn, L., Ellerbrock, T. V., Chiasson, M. A., Bush, T. J. & Wright, T. C. Human papillomavirus infection in women infected with the human immunodeficiency virus. *New Engl. J. Med.* **337** : **19** (1997), 1343–9.

179. Jamieson, D. J., Duerr, A., Burk, R. *et al.* Characterization of genital human papillomavirus infection in women who have or who are at risk of having the HIV infection. *Am. J. Obstet. Gynecol.* **186** : **1** (2002), 21–7.

180. Ahdieh, L., Munoz, A., Vlahov, D., Trimble, C., Timpson, L. & Shah, K. Cervical neoplasia and repeated positivity of human papillomavirus infection in human immunodeficiency virus-seropositive and -seronegative women. *Am. J. Epidemiol.* **151** : **12** (2000), 1148–57.

181. Brown, D. R., Bryan, J. T., Cramer, H., Katz, B. P., Handy, V. & Fife, K. H. Detection of multiple human papillomavirus types in condylomata acuminata from immunosuppressed patients. *J. Infect. Dis.* **70** (1994), 759–65.

182. Uberti-Foppa, C., Origoni, M., Maillard, M. *et al.* Evaluation of the detection of human papillomavirus genotypes in cervical specimens by hybrid capture as screening for precancerous lesions in HIV-infected women. *J. Med. Virol.* **56** (1998), 133–7.

183. Garzetti, G. G., Ciavattini, A., Butini, L., Vecchi, A. & Montroni, M. Cervical dysplasia in HIV-seropositive women: role of human papillomavirus infection and immune status. *Gynecol. Obstet. Invest.* **40** : **1** (1995), 52–6.

184. Massad, L. S., Riester, K. A. & Anastos, K. M. Prevalence and predictors of squamous cell abnormalities in Papanicolaou smears from women infected with HIV. Women's Interagency HIV Study Group. *J. AIDS* **21** : **1** (1999), 33–41.

185. Delmas, M. C., Larsen, C. & van Benthem, B. Cervical squamous intraepithelial lesions in HIV-infected women: prevalence, incidence, and regression. *AIDS* **14** : **12** (2000), 1775–84.

186. Kobayashi, A., Darragh, T., Herndier, B. *et al.* Lymphoid follicles are generated in high-grade cervical dysplasia and have differing characteristics depending on HIV status. *Am. J. Pathol.* **160** : **1** (2002), 151–64.

187. Kiviat, N., Kovtsky, L. A. & Paavonen, J. Cervical neoplasia and other STD related genital tract neoplasias. In K. Holmes, F. Sparling, S. Lemon *et al.* (eds.), *Sexually Transmitted Diseases*, 3ʳᵈ edn. New York, NY: McGraw-Hill (1999), pp. 811–31.

188. Chiasson, M. A. Declining AIDS mortality in New York City. New York City Department of Health. *Bull. N. Y. Acad. Med.* **74** : **1** (1997), 151–2.

189. Weber, T., Chin, K., Sidhu, J. S. & Janssen, R. S. Prevalence of invasive cervical cancer among HIV-infected and uninfected hospital patients, 1994–1995. In *Program and Abstracts of the 5th Conference on Retroviruses and Opportunistic Infections.* (Chicago, IL, 1998). Abstract 717.

190. Phelps, R., Smith, D. K., Gardner, L. *et al.* Incidence of lung and invasive cervical cancer in HIV-infected women. In *Program and Abstracts of the 13th International Conference on AIDS*, Durban, South Africa, July 9–14, 2000. [Abstract TuPeB3168].

191. Lomalisa, P., Smith, T. & Guidozzi, F. Human immunodeficiency virus infection and invasive cervical cancer in South Africa. *Gynecol. Oncol.* **77** : **3** (2000), 460–3.

192. Maiman, M., Fruchter, R. G., Serur, E., Remy, J. C., Feuer, G. & Boyce, J. Human immunodeficiency virus infection and cervical neoplasia. *Gynecol. Oncol.* **38** : **3** (1990), 377–82.

193. Klevens, R. M., Fleming, P. L., Mays, M. A. & Frey, R. Characteristics of women with AIDS and invasive cancer. *Obstet. Gynecol.* **88** : **2** (1996), 269–73.

194. Solomon, D., Darvey, D., Kurman, R. *et al.* The 2001 Bethesda System: terminology for reporting results of cervical cytology. *J. Am. Med. Assoc.* **287** : **16** (2002), 2114–19.

195. American College of Obstetricians and Gynecologists. *Cervical Cytology: Evaluation and Management of Abnormalities.* Technical Bulletin No. 183. Practice Guidelines August 1993.

196. Wright, T. C., Moscarelli, R. D., Dole, P., Ellerbrock, T. V., Chiasson, M. A. & Vandevanter, N. Significance of mild cytologic atypia in women infected with human immunodeficiency virus. *Obstet. Gynecol.* **87** : **4** (1996), 515–19.

197. Holcomb, K., Abulafia, O., Matthews, R. P. *et al.* The significance of ASCUS cytology in HIV-infected women. *Gynecol. Oncol.* **75** : **1** (1999), 118–21.

198. Duska, L. R., Flynn, C. F., Chen, A., Whall-Strojwas, D. & Goodman, A. Clinical evaluation of atypical glandular cells of undetermined significance on cervical cytology. *Obstet. Gynecol.* **91** : **2** (1998), 278–82.

199. Kennedy, A. W., Salmieri, S. S., Wirth, S. L., Biscotti, C. V., Tuason, L. J. & Travarca, M. J. Results of the clinical evaluation of atypical glandular cells of undetermined significance (AGCUS) detected on cervical cytology screening. *Gynecol. Oncol.* **63** : **1** (1996), 14–18.

200. Korn, A. P., Judson, P. L. & Zaloudek, C. J. Importance of atypical glandular cells of uncertain significance in cervical cytologic smears. *J. Reprod. Med.* **43** : **9** (1998), 774–8.

201. Fruchter, R., Maiman, M., Sedlis, A., Bartley, L., Camilien, L. & Arrastia, C. D. Multiple recurrences of cervical intraepithelial neoplasia in women with the human immunodeficiency virus. *Obstet. Gynecol.* **87** : **3** (1996), 338–44.

202. Holcomb, K., Matthews, R. P., Chapman, J. E. *et al.* The efficacy of cervical conization in the treatment of cervical intraepithelial neoplasia in HIV-infected women. *Gynecol. Oncol.* **74** : **3** (1999), 428–31.

203. Maiman, M., Watts, D. H., Andersen, J., Clax, P., Merino, M. & Kendall, M. A. Vaginal 5-fluorouracil for high-grade cervical dysplasia in human immunodeficiency virus infection: a randomized trial. *Obstet. Gynecol.* **94** : **6** (1999), 954–61.

204. Fleming, D. T., McQuillan, G. M., Jhonson, R. E. *et al.* Herpes simplex virus type 2 in the United States, 1976 to 1994. *New Engl. J. Med.* **337** : **16** (1997), 1105–11.

205. Augenbraun, M., Feldman, J., Chirgwin, K. *et al.* Increased genital shedding of herpes simplex virus type 2 in HIV-seropositive women. *Ann. Int. Med.* **123** : **11** (1995), 845–7.

206. Mostad, S. B., Kreiss, J. K., Ryncarz, A. J. *et al.* Cervical shedding of herpes simplex virus in human immunodeficiency virus-infected women: effects of hormonal contraception, pregnancy and vitamin A deficiency. *J. Infect. Dis.* **181** : **1** (2000), 58–63.

207. Reyes, M., Graber, J. & Reeves, W. Acyclovir-resistant HSV: Preliminary results from a national surveillance system. Presented at *International Conference on Emerging Infectious Diseases* Mar 10 1998, Atlanta, GA (Abstr. No. 55).

208. Tapert, S. F., Aarons, G. A., Sedlar, G. R. & Brown, S. A. Adolescent substance use and sexual risk-taking behavior. *J. Adolesc. Health* **28** : **3** (2001), 181–9.

209. Boyer, C. B., Shafer, M., Wibbelsman, C. J., Seeberg, D., Teitle, E. & Lovell, N. Associations of sociodemographic, psychosocial and behavioral factors with sexual risk and sexually transmitted diseases in teen clinic patients. *J. Adolesc. Health* **27** : **2** (2000), 102–11.

210. Sanders-Phillips, K. Factors influencing HIV/AIDS in women of color. *Public Health Rep.* **117** (Suppl. 1) (2002), S151–6.

16

Growth, nutrition, and metabolism

Caroline J. Chantry, M.D.[1] and Jack Moye, Jr, M.D.[2]

[1] Assistant Professor of Clinical Pediatrics, University of California Davis Medical Center, Sacramento, CA
[2] Pediatric, Adolescent, and Maternal AIDS Branch, National Institute of Child Health and Human Development, NIH, Bethesda, MD

In recent years, growth, nutrition, and metabolism of HIV-infected children have been receiving increased attention for several reasons. It has been recognized for the past decade that HIV-infected children generally do not grow as well as their uninfected counterparts, but more recent evidence suggests that this is often true even in the face of adequate virologic control. Given also that growth is a predictor of survival, there has been closer scrutiny of nutritional and metabolic factors that can contribute to poor growth. Additionally, potentially serious metabolic complications of HIV infection and/or antiretroviral therapies overlap with nutritional aspects of the infection and have prompted attention to the pathophysiology of malnutrition in these children.

The current state of knowledge regarding the complex interrelationships of nutrition, HIV disease, antiretroviral therapy, and growth is reviewed in this chapter. Recommendations for nutritional monitoring and support are discussed, as are therapies for certain recognized causes of malnutrition in HIV-infected children. Briefly described are the complications and recommended treatments for fat redistribution, hyperlipidemia, insulin resistance, osteonecrosis, and mitochondrial toxicity. Finally, nutritional issues most germane to resource-poor settings are highlighted, as are areas in which further research is needed.

16.1 Definitions: malnutrition and growth failure

Pediatric HIV disease can lead to multiple nutritional deficiencies. Deficiencies of adequate macronutrients (protein or calories) and/or micronutrients (vitamins, minerals) to maintain optimal health status is referred to as undernutrition or, more commonly, *malnutrition*. Many definitions for growth failure or failure to thrive (FTT) exist. In this chapter, the terms are used interchangeably and refer to a child who is failing to grow (gain weight and/or height) as expected for age, or who is losing weight. Children with growth failure or FTT can be further classified into those who have decreased weight for height or length (wasting) and those who have abnormal linear growth or decreasing height or length for age (stunting). Malnutrition by itself initially causes weight loss or weight growth failure. With prolonged malnutrition, linear growth is affected. Mechanistically, growth failure can be defined as any of the following:

1. Serial weight or height measurements which downwardly cross two major centile lines (e.g. 95th, 75th, 50th, etc.) on reference growth charts (freely available for downloading via the Internet from the National Center for Health Statistics at http://www.cdc.gov/nchs/about/major/nhanes/growthcharts/charts.htm), or the equivalent z-score (distance in standard deviation units above or below the reference median z-score of 0.0 [50th percentile] for a given age and sex) decrease of 1.4 or more.
2. Failure of the slope of serial growth measurements to parallel or better the standard growth curve in a child previously below the 5th percentile of weight for age.
3. Loss of 5% or more of body weight.
4. Growth velocity below the 3rd percentile for weight or height measurements taken 6 months apart.
5. Weight for height below the 5th percentile.

The use of growth velocities or z-scores is particularly useful to assess change in children whose growth percentile values are near the tails of the distribution (e.g. below the 5th percentile). Reference curves are available to quantify 6-month growth velocities [1]. A minimum interval of 3 months between measurements is recommended to determine growth velocity, as shorter intervals may not be accurate due to the saltatory nature of growth. Z-scores provide a standardized measure of the relative magnitude of weight or height change, regardless of location on or off the curve. Growth failure is considered clinically significant if the above criteria are met within 3 months in an infant, or within 6 months in a child 1–3 years of age, but even more gradual changes should prompt concern in children at high risk for malnutrition, such as those with HIV infection.

It should be noted that the NCHS reference growth charts represent children in the USA, and may not ideally represent children of all genetic backgrounds. Nevertheless, the World Health Organization (WHO) has adopted them as the international standard, based on evidence that growth patterns of well-nourished preschool children from different ethnic backgrounds are similar, i.e. genetic variations are relatively minor compared with the effects of malnutrition. The World Health Organization has a global database of child growth and malnutrition which details growth data and references from many individual countries. It can be found at www.who.int/nutgrowthhdb/p-child_pdf/index.html.

16.2 Effects of malnutrition

16.2.1 General

The term malnutrition covers a broad array of situations and can present variably, largely dependent upon which nutrients are deficient. Deficiencies can impact a wide variety of metabolic functions. Nutrition plays important roles in immune function, central nervous system (CNS) maturation, and physical growth. Malnutrition can cause a broad array of immunodeficiencies, globally referred to as nutritionally acquired immune deficiency syndromes. Chronic protein-calorie malnutrition (PCM) adversely affects T-lymphocyte number and function, delayed type hypersensitivity, complement levels, and new primary antibody responses, and causes atrophy of lymphoid tissue, especially in children. Single-nutrient deficiencies, particularly of vitamins A and C, and of trace metals iron and zinc, often co-exist with PCM. Alone or in conjunction with PCM, they affect cell-mediated immunity and immunoglobulin G responses [2, 3]. Furthermore, deficiency of nutrients which affect nucleic acid metabolism (vitamin A, zinc, and nucleotides), or protein (essential amino acids, iron, zinc,

selenium, copper, and vitamin C), or eicosanoid (polyunsaturated fatty acids) synthesis also can impair host defenses. Other essential nutrients also have been shown to have an effect on cell-mediated immunity, including arginine, glutamine, and pyridoxine [3].

Malnutrition in the first 2 years of life can cause deficient myelinization and abnormal growth of neurons, potentially resulting in irreversibly impaired intelligence or behavior. Both the CNS and peripheral nervous system (PNS) remain susceptible beyond 2 years of age to PCM as well as to micronutrient deficiencies (most notably of B vitamins).

Caloric deficiency impairs growth. Initially, ponderal (weight) growth alone is affected, but with chronic malnutrition, linear (height) growth also is affected, as is head growth in young children. Micronutrient deficiencies also can result in poor growth, and zinc supplements have been noted to improve both ponderal and linear growth, with greater response seen when initial weight-for-age and height-for-age are more severely affected [4]. Iron, copper, vitamin D, and iodine deficiencies can result in impaired growth. Animal studies report a wider variety of trace element deficiencies resulting in growth retardation (e.g. manganese, cobalt, chromium, and molybdenum) [5].

16.2.2 HIV infection

HIV-infected children can present with FTT. Both weight and height are affected within the first 6 months of life [6–9]. Weight for length is also decreased, but less so than weight and length for age. Brain growth as reflected by head circumference also can be affected in the first months of life. On average, body mass index (BMI) decreases in the first 6 months and then recovers to normal by 12 months. Children with AIDS are more stunted than children with less severe illness [2]. Chronic malnourishment can be associated with pubertal delay during adolescence. Wasting syndrome is an AIDS-defining illness and contributes significantly to morbidity and mortality in HIV-infected children [10].

The immunodeficiency of HIV can be exacerbated by malnutrition. Survival in HIV infection, as in other chronic diseases, is directly related to nutritional status. Survival in HIV-infected adults is correlated with body cell mass [11], visceral protein status [12], and micronutrient status, including zinc inadequacy and copper : zinc ratio [13]. Higher vitamin E levels have been shown to protect against disease progression [14], and reduced vitamin A and B_{12} levels are associated with lower CD4$^+$ cell counts [14, 15]. Magnesium has been shown to have a direct impact on immune response during HIV infection [16].

In HIV-infected children, height growth velocity predicts survival, regardless of plasma viral load, age, or CD4+ cell count [17]. In HIV-infected Ugandan children, low weight-for-age (z-score <-1.5) was associated with a five-fold increase in death, and similar associations with increased disease progression and/or decreased survival have been reported in the USA [18, 19]. An association between weight and disease progression has not been described independent of factors previously considered to confound this effect, such as plasma viral load. Secondary analysis of Pediatric AIDS Clinical Trials Group (PACTG) protocol 300 did describe weight growth velocity as an independent predictor for disease progression or death [20], but this finding was confounded by inclusion of weight growth failure as a clinical endpoint.

Selenium deficiency has been shown to be a significant independent predictor of mortality in HIV-infected children [21]. HIV-infected children have been found to exhibit lower mean serum levels of lycopene, retinol, beta-carotene, and vitamin E and lower plasma glutathione levels, and are more likely to have low serum levels of vitamin B_6, vitamin B_{12}, and zinc compared with uninfected children [22]. Several of these vitamins and minerals in adults can affect CD4+ cell counts. While effects of such deficiencies in children are not entirely clear, lower plasma glutathione levels were associated with higher plasma viral load and lower CD4+ cell counts [23], and beta-carotene levels in children with AIDS were half those of HIV-infected children without AIDS [24]. Glutathione removes hydrogen peroxide from cells, and beta-carotene scavenges free radicals directly, as do vitamins A and E. Increased oxidative stress from these deficiencies can play an indirect role in the immunodeficiency of HIV through multiple mechanisms. For example, tumor necrosis factor-alpha (TNF-α) induces apoptosis, and this effect is mediated by oxidative stress via macrophage activation. Nuclear factor-kappa B (NF-kappa B) promotes HIV replication via a mechanism involving free radicals [24]. Few micronutrient supplementation trials in HIV-infected children have been undertaken. Vitamin A supplements given to children in Tanzania reduced mortality in those with HIV more than in uninfected children [25].

The association between HIV morbidity and malnutrition can be bi-directional. Malnourishment appears to affect progression of HIV disease, but HIV infection can itself affect nutritional status via decreased nutrient intake, malabsorption, increased utilization of nutrients, and/or dysregulation of metabolism, particularly when HIV disease is complicated by opportunistic and other infections.

HIV infection can alter body composition, a more accurate measure of nutritional status than weight growth velocity. An early analysis of children in the Women and Infant Transmission Study (WITS) reported impaired growth in HIV-infected children and decreased body mass index (BMI), a crude measure of body composition [26]. Conflicting data about preservation of lean body mass (LBM) in HIV-infected children exist. Preliminary information indicated that LBM is lost preferentially to fat mass in HIV-infected children [27]. A subsequent study found that although fat free mass (FFM) was less in HIV-infected children than in age-matched controls, FFM as a percentage of body weight was not different between infected and uninfected children (i.e. infected children weigh less than uninfected children but they also are stunted, such that relative lean/fat ratios are unaffected) [28]. A later study examined FFM in HIV-infected children with and without linear growth failure, and found a significant inverse correlation between FFM and viral load, suggesting again that dynamics of viral replication and/or the associated host immune response impair anabolism [29]. Lastly, results to date in WITS demonstrate a trend towards decreased arm muscle mass and resistance index (an indirect measure of total LBM measured by bioelectrical impedance analysis [BIA]) in infected compared with uninfected children [30].

The associations between HIV viral load, antiretroviral therapy, and growth remain ambiguous. Two small studies performed in children not receiving protease inhibitors (PIs) have shown growth velocity to correlate inversely with viral load [29, 31]. Another notes higher viral loads in children with FTT [32]. However, secondary analysis of PACTG 152, a large trial of antiretroviral-naïve children beginning nucleoside reverse transcriptase inhibitor therapy, revealed no significant correlation between weight or height growth velocity and viral load [17], although there was a trend towards improved linear growth with lower viral loads. This is similar to results described in hemophilic children and adolescents, most of whom also were not receiving highly active antiretroviral therapy (HAART, generally combination antiretroviral treatment regimens including a PI). There, baseline plasma viral load and CD4+ cell count correlated with subsequent weight and height. However, plasma viral load was not associated with height velocity independent of CD4+ cell count [33]. On this basis, it is postulated that CD4+ cell count better reflects host pathophysiology (e.g. cytokine milieu) than plasma viral load.

An early study of children on HAART showed declines rather than improvements in weight-for-age z-scores (WAZ) and height-for-age z-scores (HAZ), even in those with the best virologic control [34]. More recently, reports suggest improved linear and ponderal growth on PI therapy. One long-term follow-up study found PI treatment to be associated with statistically, but not clinically, significant per-year z-score gains of 0.13 in height and 0.05 in weight, relative to expected growth on non-PI therapy [35]. Another small study reported improvement in height and weight only for virologic responders on HAART, with this response delayed until 96 weeks on HAART [36]. It is unclear yet whether improved growth sometimes seen with PI therapy is a result of inhibition of human proteases, immune restoration, improved virologic control, or another mechanism.

16.2.3 Importance of prevention and early intervention

Nutritional support should be an integral component of all medical management for children with HIV disease. Recognition of nutrition's central role should result in prevention or early diagnosis and treatment of malnutrition. Nutritional intervention with higher quality supplements begun in asymptomatic HIV-infected adults in Uganda resulted in stabilization of CD4+ cell counts. Earlier research in adults also demonstrated prospectively that nutrient intake was inversely related to the risk of developing AIDS [37]. Anticipation of clinical situations which can impair availability, absorption or utilization of sufficient nutrients is critical.

The goals of nutritional support for the HIV-infected child include maintenance of normal growth and development; provision for catch-up growth as necessary; correction of nutritional deficiencies; prevention of further immunologic compromise; enhancement of a sense of well-being and ability to maintain age-appropriate activities; lessened morbidity from secondary infections; and treatment of underlying gastrointestinal and infectious disease.

Prevention of malnutrition is facilitated by regular nutritional assessment of all HIV-infected children. Prevention of specific causes of malnutrition is important. For example, enteric infections increase metabolic needs and can impair absorption of nutrients and therapeutic agents. Enteric infections can be prevented by avoiding ingesting contaminated water or ice, swimming in contaminated water, and eating undercooked meat, and by carefully following food safety precautions. Fever increases metabolic needs and should be treated aggressively in these children. Other components of prevention include routine provision of up to 200% of the appropriate Dietary Reference Intake (e.g. Recommended Dietary Allowance [the average daily dietary nutrient intake level sufficient to meet the nutrient requirement of nearly all healthy persons in a particular life stage and gender group; RDAs provide a safety factor and exceed the actual requirements of most individuals]), with care not to exceed the Tolerable Upper Intake Level

(the highest average daily nutrient intake level which is likely to pose no risk of adverse health effects in almost all individuals in the general population) for vitamins and minerals and 150% for calories and protein. Cultural and ethnic background of the family is important to consider when assisting with food choices. As developmental delays and multiple caretakers have been reported with greater frequency in children with HIV infection and FTT [38], availability of a primary caretaker and screening for developmental delays can be important components of prevention. If the parent(s) is HIV-infected, anticipation of their healthcare needs, including nutritional support, should be considered as part of the child's management.

16.3 Routine nutritional assessment

Nutritional assessment should begin in infancy and continue regularly in all HIV-infected children, in an effort to prevent malnutrition and growth failure. The baseline nutritional evaluation ideally should be performed by a registered dietitian at the first or second visit. Thorough follow-up evaluation every 4–6 months is sufficient if no signs of faltering growth develop. For children with growth abnormalities, poor intake, vomiting, diarrhea, or disease progression, nutritional follow-up should be more frequent, such as every 1–3 months, depending on clinical severity [39]. Guidelines for nutritional assessment are summarized in Table 16.1.

16.3.1 Anthropometric measurements

Height, weight, head circumference, triceps skinfold thickness (TSF) and mid-arm circumference (MAC) should be measured on a regular basis. Older children should have waist and hip circumferences and truncal (sub-scapular and/or abdominal) skinfolds measured. Serial measurements of height, weight and head circumference (for children less than 3 years old) are essential and should be performed at every routine visit. More frequent weight checks are needed if weight loss or lack of weight gain is present. Skinfold and arm circumference measures evaluate adipose and muscle (somatic protein) mass and should be measured every 4–6 months and any time significant weight loss (>5%) occurs. Reference values for arm circumference and triceps skinfold measurements are found in Table 16.2. For sites unable to measure skinfold thickness, the BMI (calculated as weight (in kg) divided by height (in meters) divided by height (in meters), or (weight in kg)/ [height in meters × height in meters]) gives indirect information about body composition. Normal BMI values for

Table 16.1 Recommended nutritional assessment for HIV-infected children[a,b]

Anthropometric measurements

a. Height, weight, head circumference, TSF, MAC, waist circumference, hip circumference, truncal skin fold (e.g. sub-scapular, abdominal)

b. Weight and height growth velocities, weight and height for age, weight for height

Comprehensive dietary history

a. Calorie and protein intake

b. Symptoms of gastrointestinal disturbances

c. Access to food and food preparation facilities

d. Available diet (including food frequencies)

e. Food safety

Laboratory studies

a. Protein status* (Short term: pre-albumin or retinol-binding protein; Long term: albumin or transferrin)

b. Complete blood count with differential

c. Other studies based on clinical features and dietary history*

Assessment of body composition and fat distribution

a. TSF, MAC, sub-scapular or abdominal skin fold

b. Waist circumference or waist/hip ratio, body mass index calculation

c. BIA and/or DEXA scan

Estimation of energy and protein requirements

---

[a] Abnormal results:

Estimate and counsel regarding requirements

Multi-disciplinary evaluation: intake, loss, requirements

Early intervention*

Nutritional follow-up every 1–3 months.

[b] Normal results:

Anthropometrics and nutritional follow-up every 4–6 months.

* Individualize (see text);

TSF, triceps skinfold thickness;

MAC, midarm circumference;

BIA, bioelectrical impedance analysis;

DEXA, dual energy x-ray absorptiometry.

children are presented in Table 16.3. The child's weight and height growth velocities, weight and height for age, BMI, and fat and muscle mass should be assessed, abnormalities evaluated, and comparisons made with previous measures. Children who are crossing percentile lines downwardly on reference growth charts, or who are below the fifth percentile and not paralleling the curve, need to be identified promptly. Establishing trends in a child's growth, LBM, and

fat stores is more valuable than any individual measurement. Standardized procedures for anthropometric measurement accuracy and reproducibility are available and should be followed uniformly; these guidelines are summarized in Table 16.4.

16.3.2 Comprehensive dietary history

A comprehensive dietary history includes an evaluation of: (1) calorie and protein intake; (2) symptoms of gastrointestinal disturbances (e.g. anorexia, dysphagia, nausea, vomiting, diarrhea, early satiety, heartburn, fever); (3) access to food and food preparation facilities (e.g. electricity, refrigeration, cooking appliances and utensils, resources for food transport); (4) available diet (including type and frequency of food and beverage consumption); and (5) food safety (i.e. knowledge and facilities to provide safe food preparation and storage).

Current nutrient intake can be calculated using a 24-hour dietary recall along with food and beverage frequency questionnaires. Reasons for decreased intake or feeding problems should be explored and an assessment of the parent–child interaction should be made. The dietary history is used as a basis for comparing current intake with estimated energy and protein needs (see 'Estimation of energy and protein requirements' below).

16.3.3 Laboratory studies

Visceral protein status can be assessed by use of short-term markers, such as prealbumin (half-life of 2 days) and retinol-binding protein (half-life of 11 hours) levels, or more long-term markers, such as albumin and transferrin (half-lives of 21 and 20 days) levels. Serum iron, total iron-binding capacity or transferrin, folate and B_{12} levels should be evaluated in patients with anemia. A more extensive laboratory evaluation, guided by history (symptoms, disease progression, and diet including vitamin, mineral, and other dietary supplements) and physical examination findings, can be helpful when sub-optimal nutrition is suspected. For example, children with diarrhea should be monitored for electrolyte imbalance and deficiencies of magnesium and zinc. If there is significant fat malabsorption, vitamin A and E levels should be checked. Additional clinical signs on physical examination that may signal deficiency include dermatitis (vitamin A, zinc, biotin, essential fatty acids), cheilosis (riboflavin, biotin, zinc), or peripheral neuropathy (vitamins B_6 or B_{12}).

Monitoring of micronutrients such as selenium, zinc, copper : zinc ratios, beta-carotene, and vitamins A, B_{12}, and E can be beneficial in patients with evidence of

Table 16.2 Reference arm measurements

Percentiles of upper arm circumference (mm) and estimated upper arm muscle circumference (mm) for whites of the United States Health Examination Survey 1 of 1971–1974

	Arm circumference (mm)						Arm muscle circumference (mm)					
	5th	50th	95th	5th	50th	95th	5th	50th	95th	5th	50th	95th
Age (years)	Males			Females			Males			Females		
1–1.9	142	159	183	138	156	177	110	127	147	105	124	143
2–2.9	141	162	185	142	160	184	111	130	150	111	126	147
3–3.9	150	167	190	143	167	189	117	137	153	113	132	152
4–4.9	149	171	192	149	169	191	123	141	159	115	136	157
5–5.9	153	175	204	153	175	211	128	147	169	125	142	165
6–6.9	155	179	228	156	176	211	131	151	177	130	145	171
7–7.9	162	187	230	164	183	231	137	160	190	129	151	176
8–8.9	162	190	245	168	195	261	140	162	187	138	160	194
9–9.9	175	200	257	178	211	260	151	170	202	147	167	198
10–10.9	181	210	274	174	210	265	156	180	221	148	170	197
11–11.9	186	223	280	185	224	303	159	183	230	150	181	223
12–12.9	193	232	303	194	237	294	167	195	241	162	191	220
13–13.9	194	247	301	202	243	338	172	211	245	169	198	240
14–14.9	220	253	322	214	252	322	189	223	264	174	201	247
15–15.9	222	264	320	208	254	322	199	237	272	175	202	244
16–16.9	244	278	343	218	258	334	213	249	296	170	202	249
17–17.9	246	285	347	220	264	350	224	258	312	175	205	257
18–18.9	245	297	379	222	258	325	226	264	324	174	202	245
19–24.9	262	308	372	221	265	345	238	273	321	179	207	249

Percentiles for triceps skinfold for whites of the United States Health and Nutrition Examination Survey 1 of 1971–1974

	Triceps skinfold percentiles (mm)															
Age (years)	Males								Females							
	N	5	10	25	50	75	90	95	N	5	10	25	50	75	90	95
1–1.9	228	6	7	8	10	12	14	16	204	6	7	8	10	12	14	16
2–2.9	223	6	7	8	10	12	14	15	208	6	8	9	10	12	15	16
3–3.9	220	6	7	8	10	11	14	15	208	7	8	9	11	12	14	15
4–4.9	230	6	6	8	9	11	12	14	208	7	8	8	10	12	14	16
5–5.9	214	6	6	8	9	11	14	15	219	6	7	8	10	12	15	18
6–6.9	117	5	6	7	8	10	13	16	118	6	6	8	10	12	14	16
7–7.9	122	5	6	7	9	12	15	17	126	6	7	9	11	13	16	18
8–8.9	117	5	6	7	8	10	13	16	118	6	8	9	12	15	18	24
9–9.9	121	6	6	7	10	13	17	18	125	8	8	10	13	16	20	22
10–10.9	146	6	6	8	10	14	18	21	152	7	8	10	12	17	23	27
11–11.9	122	6	6	8	11	16	20	24	117	7	8	10	13	18	24	28
12–12.9	153	6	6	8	11	14	22	28	129	8	9	11	14	18	23	27
13–13.9	134	5	5	7	10	14	22	26	151	8	8	12	15	21	26	30
14–14.9	131	4	5	7	9	14	21	24	141	9	10	13	16	21	26	28
15–15.9	128	4	5	6	8	11	18	24	117	8	10	12	17	21	25	32
16–16.9	131	4	5	6	8	12	16	22	142	10	12	15	18	22	26	31
17–17.9	133	5	5	6	8	12	16	19	114	10	12	13	19	24	30	37
18–18.9	91	4	5	6	9	13	20	24	109	10	12	15	18	22	26	30
19–24.9	531	4	5	7	10	15	20	22	1060	10	11	14	18	24	30	34

Adapted from Frisancho A. R. New norms of upper limb fat and muscle areas for assessment of nutritional status. *Am. J. Clin. Nutr.* **34** (1981), 2540.

Table 16.3 Body mass index reference values (percentile values of body mass index)

Age (years)	Percentile						
	5	10	25	50	75	90	95
	Males						
1	14.6	15.4	16.1	17.2	18.5	19.4	19.9
2	14.4	15.0	15.7	16.5	17.6	18.4	19.0
3	14.0	14.6	15.3	16.0	17.0	17.8	18.4
4	13.8	14.4	15.0	15.8	16.6	17.5	18.1
5	13.7	14.2	14.9	15.5	16.3	17.3	18.0
6	13.6	14.0	14.7	15.4	16.3	17.4	18.1
7	13.6	14.0	14.7	15.5	16.5	17.7	18.9
8	13.7	14.1	14.9	15.7	17.0	18.4	19.7
9	14.0	14.3	15.1	16.0	17.6	19.3	20.9
10	14.2	14.6	15.5	16.6	18.4	20.3	22.2
11	14.6	15.0	16.0	17.2	19.2	21.3	23.5
12	15.1	15.5	16.5	17.8	20.0	22.3	24.8
13	15.6	16.0	17.1	18.4	20.8	23.3	25.8
14	16.1	16.6	17.7	19.1	21.5	24.4	26.8
15	16.6	17.1	18.4	19.7	22.2	25.4	27.7
16	17.2	17.8	19.1	20.5	22.9	26.1	28.4
17	17.7	18.4	19.7	21.2	23.4	27.0	29.0
18	18.3	19.1	20.3	21.9	24.0	27.7	29.7
19	19.0	19.7	21.1	22.5	24.4	28.3	30.1
	Females						
1	14.7	15.0	15.8	16.6	17.6	18.6	19.3
2	14.3	14.7	15.3	16.0	17.1	18.0	18.7
3	13.9	14.4	14.9	15.6	16.7	17.6	18.3
4	13.6	14.1	14.7	15.4	16.5	17.5	18.2
5	13.5	14.0	14.6	15.3	16.3	17.5	18.3
6	13.3	13.9	14.6	15.3	16.4	17.7	18.8
7	13.4	14.0	14.7	15.5	16.7	18.5	19.7
8	13.6	14.2	15.0	16.0	17.2	19.4	21.0
9	14.0	14.5	15.5	16.6	18.0	20.8	22.7
10	14.3	15.0	15.9	17.1	19.0	21.8	24.2
11	14.6	15.3	16.2	17.8	19.8	23.0	25.7
12	15.0	15.6	16.7	18.3	20.4	23.7	26.8
13	15.4	16.0	17.1	18.9	21.2	24.7	27.9
14	15.7	16.4	17.5	19.4	21.8	25.3	28.6
15	16.1	16.8	18.0	19.9	22.4	26.0	29.4
16	16.4	17.1	18.4	20.2	22.8	26.5	30.0
17	16.9	17.6	18.9	20.7	23.3	27.1	30.5
18	17.2	18.0	19.4	21.1	23.7	27.4	31.0
19	17.5	18.4	19.8	21.4	24.0	27.7	31.3

From National Health and Nutritional Examination Survey, 1971–1974 (NHANES 1); and Hammer, L. D., Kraemer, H. C., Wilson, D. M. *et al.* Standardized percentile curves of body-mass index for children and adolescents. *Am. J. Dis. Child.* **145** (1991), 972.

malnutrition or disease progression, as deficiencies have been associated with disease progression in children and/or adults. Finally, deficiencies of other micronutrients have been reported among HIV-infected patients, and therefore consideration should be given to monitoring carnitine, as well as vitamins C and D, in addition to those micronutrients mentioned above [40–42]. There is little information and less consensus regarding contribution of most of these deficiencies to clinical manifestations of disease in pediatric patients. One report suggests deficiencies of selenium, zinc, and vitamin A are uncommon among HIV-infected children in the USA [43]. In HIV-infected adults, however, deficiencies of vitamins A, E, B_6, B_{12}, and zinc are reported to be common [44].

Baseline evaluation should be performed when the patient is clinically stable because acute illness can affect levels of these micronutrients. Furthermore, plasma levels are not always indicative of mild deficiency, particularly in the case of zinc. In the case of vitamin A, levels should be obtained in conjunction with retinol-binding protein to assess the cause of abnormal values.

16.3.4 Assessment of body composition and fat distribution

As discussed above (see 'Effects of malnutrition – HIV infection'), the bulk of evidence suggests that children with HIV infection lose LBM early in the course of the disease. Lean body mass is known to correlate with survival in many diseases, including adult HIV infection. Therefore, assessment of body composition should be performed routinely, at least in children with any evidence of malnutrition or other significant symptoms of HIV infection, to see if changes in LBM are beginning to occur. Anthropometric measurements of MAC and TSF provide rough measures of body composition. Bioelectrical impedance analysis (BIA) is another simple, non-invasive method to determine body composition and equations have been developed for use with HIV-infected children [45]. Dual energy x-ray absorptiometry (DEXA) scans are one of the most reliable measures of body composition. While the latter methods are currently used most commonly in research settings, consideration should be given to clinical use of these measures – particularly when deviations from the norm are clinically suspected. For sites unable to measure body composition, calculation of BMI (weight in kg/[height in meters × height in meters]) gives indirect information about body fat. Trends observed in body composition are more important than any single isolated measure.

Body fat distribution also should be monitored. Accumulation of central fat and loss of limb fat can occur

Table 16.4 Anthropometric measurement guidelines

General rules of measurement technique

1. Always document measurement conditions. For example, indicate the scale used, whether a length or height measure was taken, or if a child was unstable or moving during the measurement.
2. Calibrate equipment according to individual facility policy.
3. Remember that accuracy of measurements is directly dependent on subject cooperation.
4. Measurements of weight, height/length, and head circumference should be plotted on NCHS growth charts and followed closely, monitoring trends.

Weight

1. Use an electronic scale or beam scale with non-detachable weights.
2. Zero scale prior to each measure. Calibrate scales when needed.
3. Weigh infants and young children lying down with infants wearing only a dry diaper during measurement and small children in a gown or very light clothing.
4. Weigh children who can stand on a beam scale, preferably ones with "handle bars" for support. Calm children and reduce movement as much as possible for accurate measurements. Take a child's weight while in a gown or very light clothing.
5. For children too large for the infant scale who have disabilities that prevent them from standing on a beam scale, using a bed scale is most accurate. However, if equipment is not available, a staff member or caretaker can hold the child on a beam scale, take his/her own weight on the same scale, and subtract to calculate the child's estimated body weight. When using this method, take the average of two measures.

Length

1. Measure children's recumbent length up to 24 months of age and, for those unable to stand, up to 36 months of age on a calibrated length board with a stable headboard and a sliding footboard.
2. Two people are required to perform an accurate length measurement. One person holds the head in place with two hands while the other slides the footboard and takes the reading. The child's foot should be flat against the footboard with toes pointing straight upward and legs should be straight at the time of measurement.
3. If a child has hypertonicity and cannot be held in the above position, other forms of measurement should be performed (e.g. tibial length, below).

Tibial length (Validated only in children over 3 years of age [117])

1. With child sitting or lying down, use a non-stretchable, flexible measuring tape to measure the distance from the tip (superomedial edge) of the tibia to the lower edge of the medial malleolus. In lay terms, measure the inner lower leg from the middle of the knee where the tibia inserts to the bottom edge of the ankle bone.
2. Measure the left leg whenever possible.
3. Measure to the nearest 0.1 centimeter.
4. Take the average of two measures on the same leg.
5. Calculate estimated height using the following equation:
$S = (3.26 \times TL) + 30.8$
S: Stature in centimeters
TL: Tibial length in centimeters
6. Consistently measure individual patients and plot on NCHS growth charts.
7. In children less than 3 years of age, a crown rump measure can be used:
Using a length board, hold head in place at head board. Have a second measurer slide the foot board up to the infant's buttocks, holding the torso as straight as possible. Average crown rump measures and normal increments are available in the literature [51] or an individual's trends can be used.

(cont.)

Table 16.4 (*cont.*)

Height

1. Once a child is greater than 24 months of age and can stand upright, stature is measured using a calibrated stadiometer.
2. For best results, measure children while he/she wears a gown or clothing in which one can visualize body position. Children need to stand with bare feet close together, body and legs straight, arms at sides, relaxed shoulders, and head, back, buttocks, and heels up against the wall or shaft of the stadiometer.
3. Instruct child to look straight ahead and stand tall, keeping heels on the ground.
4. Bring headboard down to top of the child's head while at eye-to-eye level with child and record measure to nearest 0.1 centimeter.
5. Take the average of three measures.

Head circumference

1. Measure head circumference in children regularly at routine physical exam appointments up until 36 months of age.
2. Have the infant or child sit on caretaker's lap or stand if capable.
3. Remove any hair pieces that could interfere with measurement.
4. Place non-stretchable measuring tape just above the eyebrow and ears and straight around the occipital bulge in the back of the child's head.
5. Compress hair with tape and record measure to the nearest 0.1 centimeter.

Mid-arm circumference

1. Use a non-stretchable centimeter tape, with millimeters delineated. On the non-dominant arm bent at a 90 degree angle with palm facing up, mark the midpoint between the acromion and olecranon processes. Make sure clothing is pushed up above the shoulder or removed if interfering with arm tissue.
2. Measure the distance around the arm at the mark and record to the nearest 0.1 centimeter.

Triceps skinfold thickness

1. Grasp vertical fold of fat about 1–2 centimeter above the midpoint using forefinger and thumb.
2. Measure skinfold with calipers at the midpoint after needle stabilizes while continuing to hold fold with hand.
3. Average three measures.
4. Edematous tissue and very squirmy children are two main factors that prevent accuracy of this measurement.
5. Measure to the nearest 0.5 millimeter.

Mid-arm muscle circumference

1. Use the following equation to calculate mid-arm muscle circumference:

$$MAMC = MAC - (TSF \times 3.14)/10 \quad MAC = \text{Mid-arm circumference in centimeters}$$
$$MAMC = \text{Mid-arm muscle circumference in centimeters}$$
$$TSF = \text{Triceps skinfold thickness in millimeters}$$

in HIV-infected children (see 'Metabolic abnormalities and associated therapies' in this chapter, as well as Chapter 20). In children as in adults, a relative central or abdominal distribution of body fat has been associated with adverse lipid and insulin concentrations independently of weight, height, and age [46]. Truncal fat can be measured by various anthropometric or imaging methodologies. Data are accumulating which suggest that waist circumference itself can be a good measure of central adiposity. Taylor and colleagues noted the 80th percentile for waist circumference was 89% and 87% sensitive in detecting girls and boys with high trunk fat mass (z-score ≥ 1), respectively, and 94% and

92% specific [47]. Freedman *et al.* noted that waist circumference (adjusted for weight, height, and age) showed the most consistent and generally strongest association with adverse risk factors, but the association was similar in magnitude when quantified by waist:hip ratio or comparison of the waist circumference to the sum of hip circumference and triceps skinfold thickness [46]. Differentiation of abdominal and visceral adiposity is aided by measures of abdominal and sub-scapular skinfold thicknesses, in addition to waist circumference, height, and ethnicity [48].

While DEXA accurately measures body composition, it is unable to differentiate between intra-abdominal and subcutaneous fat. Nevertheless, truncal fat mass as measured by DEXA has been shown to strongly correlate with intra-abdominal fat in young children and correlation between lipid profiles and fat distribution is similar whether measured by central fat on DEXA or visceral fat on MRI images.

16.3.5 Estimation of energy and protein requirements

Recommended daily allowances for children infected with HIV are not well established because energy requirements engendered by HIV infection itself are not defined. Asymptomatic HIV-infected adults do have increased resting and total energy expenditure, but clinical experience in children suggests that energy requirements are relatively normal when children are well. Two studies of HIV-infected children confirmed the absence of hypermetabolism during times of well-being [29, 49]. At minimum, there are increased energy requirements during periods of stress such as infection, and these children may not compensate well for these increased needs. Accordingly, some recommend estimating both energy and protein requirements at 150% of the Recommended Dietary Allowance for healthy children. Alternatively, a range can be calculated using weight for actual height as the minimum and median (50th percentile) reference weight for actual age as the maximum.

The following formula can be used to grossly estimate caloric requirements for normal children: 100 kcal/kg for the first 10 kg of body weight; 50 kcal/kg for the second 10 kg of body weight; 20 kcal/kg for each kg over 20 kg of body weight. This simple method produces estimates towards the lower end of the range of normal needs. Alternatively, Table 16.5 offers age-adjusted energy and protein requirements for normal children.

Children often have increased energy and protein requirements during illness, particularly during periods of fever or infection. Approximate increases in caloric needs are as follows: 12% for each degree centigrade rise, 25% for acute diarrhea, and 60% for sepsis. It has been estimated that increasing the Recommended Dietary Allowance for protein by 50–100% will provide for increased protein requirements during periods of fever or infection. These estimates of energy and protein requirements are generic recommendations for children under stressful conditions, and applicability to HIV infection has not been confirmed. Early treatment for fever and infection can limit the metabolic impact. As children recover from illness, they often enter a period of catch-up growth. The following formula can be used to estimate caloric and protein

Table 16.5 Recommended daily energy and protein intake by age

Age/years	Kcal/kg	Protein/kg (grams)
0–0.5	108	2.2
0.5–1	98	1.6
1–3	102	1.2
4–6	90	1.2
7–10	70	1.2
11–14 (males)	55	1.0
11–14 (females)	47	1.0
15–18 (males)	45	0.8
15–18 (females)	40	0.8

From Food and Nutrition Board, National Academy of Sciences National Research Council. Recommended Dietary Allowances. Washington, DC: National Academy Press, 1989.

requirements during this phase:

Daily energy requirement, in kcal per kg of body weight

$$= \frac{(\text{RDA Kcal for weight age}^a) \times (\text{ideal weight for height})^b}{(\text{actual weight})}$$

Daily protein requirement, in grams protein per kg of body weight

$$= \frac{(\text{RDA protein for weight age}^a) \times (\text{ideal weight for height})^b}{(\text{actual weight})}$$

^{a} Weight age is the age at which the patient's present weight would be at the 50th percentile.

^{b} For those children recovering from acute illness who tend to have a weight for height greater than the 50th percentile, the "ideal weight for height" in the catch-up equation can be goal weight based on 90th percentile weight growth velocity averages for age added to current weight. Tables are available for both younger and older children [50, 51].

16.4 Causes of malnutrition and associated therapies

There are many different potential causes of malnutrition in HIV-infected children, such as decreased intake, increased nutrient losses, increased nutrient requirements, and metabolic dysregulation. The relative contribution of each of these to the problem of malnutrition among HIV-infected children is not well understood. Malabsorption, increased energy expenditure, and endocrinopathies have been postulated but not documented as etiologic in most HIV-infected children with growth failure [29, 49, 52, 53]. Specific causes of malnutrition and suggested therapies are summarized in Table 16.6 and are discussed in further detail in the text that follows. Appropriate interventions can be divided into those that treat the underlying problem (e.g. identifying and removing a drug that is causing anorexia), symptomatic interventions (e.g. use of appetite stimulants for anorexia), and supportive interventions (use of nutritional supplements to achieve adequate intake despite anorexia). Understanding the difference between starvation and cachexia can be helpful in determining the appropriate intervention. *Starvation* is weight loss from inadequate intake or malabsorption of nutrients. It normally results in loss of fat mass initially. *Cachexia* is loss of weight or growth retardation with preferential catabolism of LBM over fat mass. Why this occurs is not clear, but it could be secondary to increased cytokine production by macrophages. For example, tumor necrosis factor (TNF) and interleukin-1 (IL-1) have both been shown to result in inefficient use of energy substrates. Tumor necrosis factor specifically causes peripheral lipolysis and resultant increased circulation of free fatty acids which are then cycled from liver back to adipose tissue, i.e. futile cycling. IL-1 has catabolic effects on several tissues including liver and connective tissues, resulting in loss of both visceral and somatic protein stores.

Because malnutrition in this population is often multi-factorial in etiology, a multi-disciplinary team approach to evaluation and management is important. Family-centered care is ideal. The assistance of community agencies is of particular importance. For example, home health nurses and aides, or community organizations that provide services such as meal delivery can be of tremendous benefit.

16.4.1 Decreased oral intake

As noted above, many factors can contribute to malnutrition in HIV-infected children, and often more than one etiology is present in an individual child. Many of these causes result in decreased oral intake. In fact, several studies document reduced energy intake in HIV-infected children [29, 54], with some reports noting an association between decreased energy intake and poor growth [49]. Other authors documented decreased intake but did not observe an association with poor growth, theorizing that inadequate intake during frequent illnesses combined with energy intake inadequate for catch-up growth when

children are well might explain the observed lack of association on cross-sectional examination [49]. One group of investigators examining the effect of viral load on growth noted that the association of decreased energy intake was not independent of viral load, suggesting the effect of viral load on growth could be mediated in part by poor intake [29]. Decreased oral intake, in turn, can result from diverse causes including anorexia, food aversion or refusal (often to avoid symptoms such as vomiting, diarrhea, oral pain, etc.), barriers to food access or preparation, dysgeusia, early satiety, or neurologic dysfunction.

Anorexia is associated with many of the medications used in this population, including reverse transcriptase inhibitors (e.g. zidovudine [ZDV], stavudine [d4T], lamivudine [3TC]), PIs (e.g. ritonavir, indinavir, nelfinavir), dapsone, antifungal drugs (e.g. fluconazole, ketoconazole), and antiviral medications (e.g. ganciclovir, acyclovir). Additionally, clarithromycin has been associated with dysgeusia. If anorexia or other side-effects are debilitating and alternative therapeutic options exist, consideration should be given to changing therapies. Additional causes of anorexia in this population include micronutrient deficiency, pain, and depression.

Several appetite stimulants can be considered for anorectic children. Megestrol acetate (Megace) results in weight gain primarily by increasing body fat mass. Almost no data are available on the use of this progestational hormone in children. Doses of megestrol acetate that have been used to increase weight gain include 7.9 mg/kg/day (median dose) [55], 4–15 mg/kg/day, and 200–400 mg/m^2/day. Megestrol acetate has known glucocorticoid activity [56], and adrenal suppression [57, 58] as well as glucose intolerance [59] has been observed among HIV-infected children receiving this medication. Cyproheptadine (Periactin) (0.25–0.5 mg/kg/day or 8 mg/m^2/day divided in two to three daily doses) has been used with anecdotal reports of limited success. Dronabinol (Marinol; 2.5 mg twice daily before meals) also has been used for appetite stimulation although psychological side-effects may limit its use in children.

Micronutrient deficiencies can exacerbate malnutrition by causing anorexia, dysgeusia, etc. and must be addressed. Excesses as well as deficiencies of micronutrients, particularly zinc, iron, and selenium, are harmful to the immune system, and extremely large doses are not recommended. Recommended doses for some of the more commonly supplemented micronutrients are provided in Table 16.7. Children with low iron-binding capacity should not be given supplemental iron. Caution should be exercised with vitamin A supplements in the presence of low retinol-binding protein.

Table 16.6 Causes of malnutrition and associated therapies

Part 1: Decreased oral intake	
Cause	Intervention
All causes	Referral to registered dietitian
1. Anorexia	Supportive: Increase nutrient density of foods, high kcal infant formula, small frequent meals, calorie boosting instructions, nutritional supplements (per tube if needed). Symptomatic: appetite stimulants*
Nutritional deficiency	Treat deficiency (zinc, carnitine, vitamin A, B_6)
Depression/despair	Treat depression
Pain	Acute and chronic pain management
Drug-induced*	Remove offending agent if possible
Cytokine production	Control primary and secondary infections; cytokine modulators untested
Neurologic dysfunction	See below
2. Food aversion/refusal	
Symptom avoidance: (nausea, vomiting diarrhea, abdominal pain)	Referral to feeding/speech therapy
Drug-induced*	Remove offending agent if possible; medications after or between meals
Infections	Treat infection
Behavioral	Reinforce parenting skills;* self-feeding
Upper gastrointestinal tract lesions	
Oral lesions: gingivitis, aphthous ulcers, stomatitis, dental abscesses	Treat infections (CMV, HSV, *Candida)*; symptomatic relief (see text); meticulous oral hygiene
Esophagitis: reflux, infectious	Antacids, H_2 blockers; soft diet; treat infection (CMV, HSV, *Candida*)
gastritis, duodenitis: infectious, peptic	Treat infection; antacids, H_2 blockers if peptic
3. Barriers to food access or preparation	Co-ordinate with social work; Refer: WIC, soup kitchens, food pantries, food stamps, meal delivery programs
Caretaker limitation	As above; home health assistance
Limited food availability (money, transportation, etc.)	Evaluate food availability*
4. Altered taste (dysgeusia)	
Zinc deficiency	Zinc supplements
Neurologic dysfunction	See below
Drug related*	Remove offending agent if possible
5. Early satiety	Small frequent meals
Cytokine-related +/or dysmotility	Consider trial of agent to improve GI motility
6. Neurologic dysfunction:	
Developmental delay	Modify consistency of food and bottle or spoon feed as necessary; reduce inconsistencies in care; daily routine; 1 or 2 caretakers.
Dysphagia	As above for developmental delay
Dysguesia	As above for developmental delay; consider zinc deficiency
Gastroesophageal reflux	Standard reflux therapies.

(*cont.*)

Table 16.6 (*cont.*)

Part 2: Increased nutrient losses	
Cause	Intervention
All causes	Referral to registered dietitian; parenteral nutrition indicated if enteral nutrition not tolerated
1. Vomiting	
Gastritis	See above
Pancreatitis	Standard supportive care
Drug-related (ddI, ddC, d4T, pentamidine)	Remove offending agent
Infectious (CMV, MAC)	Treat infection
Drug Related*	Remove offending agent as necessary
2. Diarrhea	
Enteric infection*	Treat infection
Drug-related*	Symptomatic: loperamide, Kaopectate; remove agent as necessary
Idiopathic	Symptomatic (as above)
3. Malabsorption*	Dietary management;* antibiotics for bacterial overgrowth
Part 3: Increased nutrient requirements	
Cause	Intervention
All causes	Referral to registered dietitian; supportive care: increase intake to meet requirements as for anorexia
1. Fever	Fever control, identify source
2. Secondary infection	Treat infection
3. End-organ complications (cardiac, neurologic, dermatologic hematologic, renal)	Supportive care
Part 4: Metabolic and endocrine dysregulation	
Cause	Intervention
Cytokine production	Cytokine modulators untested; consider oxandrolone for wasting
TNF, interleukins 1 and 6	Control primary disease (antiretroviral therapy)
Endocrine dysregulation (thyroid,	Treat deficiencies
adrenal, growth hormone, IGF-1)	Growth hormone may improve growth in the absence of deficiency

*See text for further details

CMV, cytomegalovirus; HSV, herpes simplex virus; MAC, *Mycobacterium avium* complex; WIC, Special Supplemental Nutrition Program for Woman, Infants and Children.

The child may eat less to avoid exacerbation of symptoms such as nausea, vomiting, diarrhea, or oral or abdominal pain. One or more of these symptoms can be caused by medications that the child is taking. For example, abdominal pain may be associated with didanosine (ddI), 3TC, zalcitabine (ddC), ritonavir, saquinavir, nelfinavir, indinavir, pentamidine, or antibiotics such as sulfonamides and macrolides. Zidovudine alone can cause nausea, vomiting, and esophageal ulcers. Stomatitis, esophagitis, and gastritis all can be caused by opportunistic infections, in addition to the etiologies in healthy children. Food aversion or refusal can be behavioral in origin, and particular attention should be paid to the parent–child interaction.

Symptomatic relief for painful oral lesions often can be achieved by avoiding irritating foods such as orange juice and hot spices, using a straw to bypass the lesions, giving cold foods such as popsicles before meals, and using topical medications before meals. In older children, viscous

Table 16.7 Recommended therapeutic doses for selected micronutrient deficiencies

Nutrient	Dose	Comments
Zinc	0.5–1.0 mg elemental Zn/kg/day PO with food.	
Selenium	50 μgrams/day	
Carnitine	25–350 mg/kg/day PO ÷ bid-tid (maximum 3 g daily dose)	Begin with 50 mg/kg/day if cardiomyopathy present, 25 mg/kg/day if absent; titrate to clinical response and levels; Consider if suspect mitochondrial toxicity; may give iv for adjunctive therapy for lactic acidosis
Copper	Infants: 2–3 mg copper sulfate/day (400–600 μg copper)	
Folate	Infants: 15 μg/kg/day: max 50 μg/day; children 1 mg/day	(PO, IM, IV, SC)
Magnesium	Mg oxide salt: 65–130 mg/kg/day ÷ qid PO, MgSO4 salt: 100–200 mg/kg/dose qid PO	
Vitamin A	100 000 IU/dose 6–12 months. 200 000 IU/dose >1 year Give 2 doses PO qd × 2 +repeat 1 dose 1–4 weeks later	Malabsorption syndrome prophylaxis: >8 years: 10 000–50 000 IU/day water miscible product
Vitamin B1 (thiamine)	Children: 5 mg PO qd for mild disease; 10 mg PO bid for severe disease	Consider if suspect mitochondrial toxicity; high adult dose is 100 mg/day
Vitamin B2 (riboflavin)	Infants: 0.5 mg PO twice weekly Children: 1 mg PO tid for several weeks Adults: 2 mg PO tid for several weeks	Consider if suspect mitochondrial toxicity; may give iv for adjunctive therapy for lactic acidosis; high adult dose is 50 mg/day
Vitamin B6 (pyridoxine)	5–25 mg/day for 3 weeks	Up to 50 mg/day for drug-induced neuritis; (PO preferred, may give IM or IV).
Vitamin B12	Hematologic signs: 30–50 μg/24 h IM or SC for ≥ 14 days to total of 1000–5000 μg. Follow with maintenance. Neurologic signs: 100 μg/24 h IM or SC qd × 10–15 days then once or twice weekly for several months. Taper to 250–1000 μg monthly by 1 year. Maintenance treatment after deficiency: 100–250 μg/dose IM or SC q 2–4 weeks	
Vitamin C	100–300 mg/day ÷ qd-bid for at least 2 weeks	PO preferred, can give IM, IV, SC
Vitamin E	Preterm and newborn infants: 25–50 IU/day × 6–10 weeks Older children: 1 IU/kg/day PO	1 mg DL-tocopherol acetate = 1 IU, use water miscible form with malabsorption; follow levels
Ubidecarenone (Ubiquinone, Coenzyme Q)	1–10 mg/kg/day PO ÷qd-qid	Consider if suspect mitochondrial toxicity; may give iv for adjunctive therapy for lactic acidosis

lidocaine 2% (20 mg/mL) can be applied directly to the lesions at a maximum dose of 3 mg/kg, not to be repeated before 2 hours. Diphenhydramine syrup can be used as a swish and swallow in the usual dose of 5 mg/kg/day in divided doses before meals.

Additionally, 'non-organic' causes of malnutrition such as food availability should be evaluated (e.g. with the food sufficiency questionnaire [60]), ideally by a visiting nurse in the home, and social service agencies should be involved as necessary. Barriers to food preparation can increase with parental illness common to these families. The absence of a primary caretaker or adequate parenting skills should be noted. Family difficulties and behavioral problems of the child can adversely affect the child's nutritional intake.

Neurologic dysfunction is common in HIV-infected children, and even subtle neurologic involvement can result in feeding difficulties. This can take the form of oral-motor dysfunction or prolonged feeding duration. Frank developmental delay may require significant modification of food consistency and routines.

Regardless of the cause of decreased oral intake, enteral formulas can constitute an important form of supplemental nutritional support and should be considered to supply unmet nutritional requirements. There are many commercially available formulas. The daily quantity of a given enteral feeding formula necessary to provide for the child's caloric or protein needs can be calculated and prescribed. The following factors should be considered when choosing a formula:

- Integrity of the gastrointestinal tract.
- Type of protein, fat, and carbohydrate required.
- Density of protein and energy provided and the relative ratio.
- Sodium, potassium, and phosphorus content (especially for patients with cardiac, renal, or hepatic dysfunction).
- Palatability.
- Taste preference.
- Cost.

Enteral feeding formulas for adults can be used for older children but may have too much sodium or protein for younger children, especially those younger than four years. Instant breakfast powders added to whole milk and supplements such as Ensure, Sustacal, or Nutren have similar nutritional values. These supplements are appropriate for older children with intact gastrointestinal tracts. Supplements with higher protein content, such as Sustacal or Ensure High Protein or Ensure Plus (also more calories) may be necessary. Alternatively, children with high-protein needs can use powdered skim milk or protein supplements (e.g. ProMod, Casee) directly mixed with food or beverages, including supplemental formulas. Toddler formulas are available for use in younger children, such as Kindercal (high in fiber), Pediasure (with or without fiber), and Nutren Jr, and are appropriate for those without specialized nutrient needs. For children with evidence of malabsorption, supplements which maximize absorption should be chosen. Specialized supplements are available with hydrolyzed protein and medium-chain triglycerides with or without lactose or sucrose. These are discussed in more detail below under "Increased nutrient losses."

In addition to commercial supplements, other calorie-boosting tips include use of whole milk or cream rather than water (e.g. when cooking hot cereals or soups) if lactose intolerance is not an issue and use of fats such as peanut butter, cheese, or butter when serving vegetables,

fruits, and breads. Calorie content can be boosted further by direct addition of powdered glucose polymers (e.g. Polycose, Moducal) to food or beverages.

Children who are unable to ingest sufficient calories by mouth may require tube feedings. Tube feedings increase fat mass but may not increase LBM significantly [61]. Such weight gain is associated nonetheless with decreased hospitalization and mortality rates [62]. Nasogastric tube feedings are painful, increase the likelihood of sinusitis, and limit oral intake. However, they can supplement nutritional intake acutely and help to evaluate the potential efficacy of long-term gastrostomy feedings. Gastrostomy tubes generally are better tolerated than nasogastric tube feedings, do not restrict normal activities, and can result in improved quality of life in children with nutritional difficulties.

There are a variety of different feeding progression schedules available, with little information to support one regimen over another. Generally tube feeding is begun with a hypo-osmolar concentration, which is gradually increased to full concentration formula over one to several days. Increases in volume follow, assessing tolerance of bolus volumes by measuring remaining volume in the stomach prior to the next feed. If the residual volume is less than 50% of the prior feed, volume can be increased by 25–30% until the desired volume is attained. Continuous feedings are used if bolus feeds are not tolerated, or for overnight feeding when necessary. Residuals also are checked when advancing continuous feeds, at least every 2–4 hours. If residual volume is greater than that infused during the previous 2 hours, the infusion should be stopped for 1–2 hours. When residuals are not a problem, the volume can be increased one to five mL/hour. An alternative method to begin tube feedings uses very small volumes of full concentration formula from the start, with slow increases in volume thereafter as tolerated [63].

16.4.2 Increased nutrient losses

Despite adequate intake, malnutrition can result from increased nutrient loss as occurs with chronic vomiting, diarrhea, or malabsorption. Nausea, vomiting, and diarrhea are extremely common side-effects of medications used in HIV-infected children. Examples of such drugs are antiretroviral medications (ddI, 3TC, and most of the PIs), antibiotics, antifungal medications, and antiviral drugs. Vomiting also can be an indirect result of drugs via pancreatitis caused by antiretroviral medications or pentamidine. Vomiting and/or diarrhea may be the result of gastrointestinal infections such as gastritis, gastroenteritis, or pancreatitis. Besides organisms that cause vomiting and diarrhea in the normal host, opportunistic pathogens can cause chronic gastrointestinal disease in children with HIV infection. In addition, chronic diarrhea may be either the cause or the result of malabsorption.

Malabsorption occurs more commonly in HIV-infected children than healthy controls. It can result from enteric infections, malnutrition, small bowel bacterial overgrowth, or HIV enteropathy, which is villous atrophy associated with HIV infection in the absence of other detectable pathogens. Drug-induced diarrhea can result in malabsorption if transit time is substantially reduced. Carbohydrate (particularly lactose), fat, and protein malabsorption have been described in 32–40%, 30–39%, and 17% of HIV-infected children, respectively [52, 64, 65]. Although exocrine pancreatic insufficiency is often cited as a possible cause of fat malabsorption in this population, Sentongo and colleagues found adequate pancreatic function in the 39% of their population demonstrating qualitative steatorrhea [52]. The authors recommend that evaluation of fat malabsorption in HIV-infected children focus on other potential causes such as bacterial overgrowth. Cross-sectional analyses have not demonstrated an association between malabsorption and growth failure.

Appropriate dietary therapy or supplementation or both should be instituted for children with evidence of malabsorption. Enteral feeding formulas containing fewer simple carbohydrates present less osmotic load and have better gastrointestinal tolerance. Carbohydrate intolerance requires reduction or removal of the specific sugar from the diet. For lactase deficiency, there are many lactose-free supplements for all ages, such as Kindercal, Nutren Jr, and Pediasure for toddlers and young children, and similarly, Ensure, Sustacal, and Nutren for older children. Alternatively, microbial-derived lactase (e.g. Lactaid) can be added directly to milk and milk products or ingested with meals. Milk containing lactase is commercially available. Formulas with no sucrose are available for those with other (non-lactase) disaccharidase deficiency. Examples are Lactofree and Vivonex Pediatric for younger children and Isocal, Peptamen, and Vivonex for older children.

Children with fat malabsorption should be placed on low-fat diets with medium-chain triglyceride oil used directly as a dietary additive for supplementation or as the primary lipid in supplements modified specifically for them (e.g. Lipisorb). Calories also can be increased in patients with fat malabsorption by addition of glucose polymers (Polycose or Moducal) to the diet. While exocrine pancreatic sufficiency was not the cause in patients with steatorrhea in one report noted previously, it was found in 9% of

the patients not presenting with steatorrhea [52]. Pancreatic enzymes (e.g. Cotazym, Pancrease, and others) can be offered in doses of lipase of 1000 U/kg/meal, generally not to exceed 20 000 U, with frequent evaluation for improvement. Doses can be titrated to eliminate diarrhea and steatorrhea and to avoid signs of excessive dosage, such as perianal irritation, occult gastrointestinal bleeding, hyperuricemia, and others. Enzymes should be discontinued if there has not been symptomatic improvement within 2 weeks of consistent administration with meals and snacks. Fat-soluble vitamins (A, D, E, and K) may be deficient in the presence of fat malabsorption, and annual monitoring of their levels should be considered (particularly those vitamins of which deficiencies are associated with HIV disease progression, i.e. vitamins A and E).

Protein malabsorption generally necessitates supplements with hydrolyzed protein (e.g. Peptamen or Peptamen Jr) or amino acids (e.g. Vivonex, Vivonex Pediatric, or Neonate One Plus), depending on the severity. Specialized infant formulas for carbohydrate, fat, or protein malabsorption are available also. Absorption may be further enhanced by continuous gravity tube feedings, if necessary.

Parenteral nutrition can provide essential nutrition for children unable to maintain growth with enteral support alone. However, because of the expense and risks, including infectious complications, total parenteral nutrition should be used only in children unable to tolerate enteral feedings.

16.4.3 Increased nutrient requirements

The third major category of conditions which may result in malnutrition is increased nutritional requirements. A child may not grow despite apparently adequate intake and absorption of normal requirements if their individual requirements are in excess of the norm.

It has been postulated that total energy expenditure is increased in children with HIV infection secondary to basal metabolic increases, as demonstrated in HIV-infected adults [66]. However, multiple studies have failed to detect increased basal metabolic rates in HIV-infected children when they are well [29, 49]. Specifically, Johann-Liang et al. documented that resting and total energy expenditure in HIV-infected children was not greater than expected for normal children, nor different between HIV-infected children with and without growth failure [48]. Arpadi compared total and resting energy expenditures in HIV-infected children with and without growth failure and was unable to demonstrate a hypermetabolic state in those with growth failure. Rather, there was a trend toward decreased total energy expenditure in the children with poor growth, as occurs with chronic undernutrition [29].

Lack of a demonstrable hypermetabolic state in clinically stable HIV-infected children notwithstanding, increased requirements may occur periodically during acute febrile illnesses to which these children are prone. Marginal intake during well times may not allow for the extra nutrition required for catch-up growth after acute illnesses. Additionally, end-organ complications, such as HIV encephalopathy or cardiomyopathy, may result in extra caloric requirements.

In addition to increasing enteral or parenteral intake to account for increased energy requirements, therapy for malnutrition due to increased requirements should be directed at treatment of the underlying cause (e.g. congestive heart failure). Fevers and infections should be aggressively treated to minimize nutritional impact.

16.4.4 Metabolic and endocrine dysregulation

Poor growth may be a manifestation of endocrine disease, which can complicate HIV infection. In particular, thyroid abnormalities, adrenal insufficiency, and classic growth hormone (GH) deficiency have been described [67–70]. Other abnormalities of the growth hormone axis also occur. Reduced insulin-like growth factor-1 (IGF-1) levels have been described in malnourished adults with AIDS and in HIV-infected children, particularly those with FTT [71]. IGF-1 stimulates protein accretion in normal individuals, as does GH, and is probably the best-integrated indicator of GH action [72]. Insulin-like growth factor-1 actions at the target tissue level are modulated by high-affinity IGF binding proteins (IGFBPs), abnormalities of which have been detected in children with HIV. Specifically, catabolic patients with AIDS have increased proteolysis of and therefore diminished serum levels of IGFBP-3, which tracks with growth [71, 73]. In HIV-infected adolescents, linear growth failure may be due in part to delayed sexual maturation [74]. Therefore, appropriate endocrinologic evaluation should be performed if FTT does not readily respond to nutritional interventions (see Chapter 35).

It is hypothesized that, in some cases, the malnutrition associated with HIV infection in children is secondary to metabolic dysregulation produced by inflammatory cytokines, analogous to HIV wasting syndrome in adults, which has been related to overproduction of tumor necrosis factor [75]. Cytokine-mediated malnutrition may overlap with endocrine dysregulation of the growth hormone axis. Interleukin-6 (IL-6) release from mononuclear cells from HIV-infected children was related to height growth velocity and IGF-1 in one report [76]. A similar report documents increased IL-6 activity and decreased IGF-1 levels in HIV-infected children with growth failure [49]. These findings support the theory that growth failure is related to cytokine overproduction. In turn, diminished IGF-1 availability at the tissue level may impair protein accretion and affect anabolism and growth. One plausible mechanism by which growth stunting could occur in association with increased IL-6 activity is via IGFBP-1; IGFBP-1 production is mediated by proinflammatory cytokines such as interleukin-6 (IL-6) and is known to inhibit somatic linear growth and weight gain. Documentation of increased IGFBP-1 in adult AIDS patients with wasting supports this hypothesis [77], as do recent data that significant decreases in IGFBP-1 occur in HIV-infected children after beginning or changing antiretroviral therapy [78]. Furthermore, IGFBP-1 is strongly associated with insulin sensitivity in conditions associated with insulin resistance [77], and thus could be involved in other metabolic abnormalities related to HIV infection.

Effective therapeutic strategies have yet to be developed for growth failure not amenable to traditional nutritional interventions. Cytokine modulators (e.g. thalidomide) and treatment with IGF-1 could have a role but are untested in children. One report documents tolerability of daily growth hormone injections in five prepubertal children with HIV-associated growth failure but normal growth hormone peaks [79]. Weight, IGF-1, and IGFBP-3 all increased over 28 days. Fat-free mass did not increase in this short trial. The two patients who continued treatment long-term increased height-for-age z-score dramatically. Other trials of growth hormone in HIV-infected children are ongoing. Growth hormone accelerates bone age commensurate with height compared with other anabolic agents, which may accelerate bone age out of proportion to linear growth.

In addition to growth failure, wasting syndrome remains a significant contributor to morbidity and mortality in HIV-infected children. One 3-month trial of oxandrolone in HIV-infected children demonstrated increased average LBM and decreased fat mass [80]. Of note, there was no anabolic response when steroids were given in the setting of inadequate energy intake. Therefore, for children with clearly diminished LBM, consideration can be given to oxandrolone. The maximum recommended pediatric dose is 0.1 mg/kg daily. Therapy can be repeated intermittently, as indicated.

Growth hormone, in supraphysiologic doses, does result in increases in both body weight and LBM in HIV-infected adults [81] and also has been shown to have an anabolic effect in HIV-infected adolescent wasting [82]. Administration of GH to patients with AIDS resulted in increased IGF-1 production in one trial, demonstrating lack of GH resistance [77] but in another small trial hypogonadal patients did have GH resistance that improved upon testosterone administration [83]. The anabolic response to GH in adults with HIV infection decreases with advancing disease. Serum concentrations of soluble TNF-α receptor type 2 have been shown to predict poor anabolic response to GH by muscle protein.

16.5 Metabolic abnormalities and associated therapies

16.5.1 Lipodystrophy syndrome

Fat redistribution has been noted to occur in HIV-infected adults and children. It may be associated with metabolic abnormalities, most notably hyperlipidemia (with increases in low density lipoprotein [LDL], cholesterol, and triglyceride levels) and insulin resistance. This triad of findings has been referred to in adults as the "fat redistribution" or "lipodystrophy" syndrome. There can be lipoatrophy (loss of subcutaneous fat) in the face, buttocks and extremities, with concomitant increase in abdominal visceral fat, increased breast size in women, and sometimes development of a dorsocervical fat pad ("buffalo hump"). Cross-sectional clinical studies find that these signs can occur in isolation, e.g. fat redistribution without metabolic changes and vice versa. Specifically, hyperlipidemias are known to occur with increased frequency in HIV-infected persons, and can occur prior to antiretroviral treatment and without noticeable body shape changes.

Those affected with any or all of the three components (insulin resistance, hyperlipidemia, and visceral adiposity) may be at increased risk of cardiovascular disease, particularly children. The etiology of this syndrome likely is multifactorial, and research continues to search for potential causes, associations and treatments. A complete discussion of the current state of knowledge of these metabolic alterations is beyond the scope of this chapter. More information on these abnormalities, including pathophysiology, is found in Chapter 20.

Studies in children

Research in children thus far has focused primarily on defining the prevalence of these abnormalities and associated clinical findings. Care is needed in interpreting and comparing research findings as different authors use differing definitions. Fat redistribution has been reported with highly variable prevalence (18–100%) in HIV-infected children, depending on population and methodology.

Clinically evident changes have been noted in 8–33% in the same populations [84–88]. The prevalence of hyperlipidemia in HIV-infected children is also highly variable and depends on the definition used. Twenty-six to seventy-three percent of subjects have abnormal lipid values; hypercholesterolemia is much more common than hypertriglyceridemia, and appears to be exaggerated in those patients receiving PI therapy [85–88]. Insulin resistance, measured by fasting glucose, insulin, C-peptide levels and/or insulin:glucose ratios, has been reported in 8–35% of HIV-infected children, depending on the population studied [85, 87, 88].

Potential treatments

No trials in children for treatment of fat redistribution or associated metabolic abnormalities have been reported, nor is there consensus regarding whether and when fat redistribution, insulin resistance without glucose intolerance, or hyperlipidemia should be treated. A variety of treatments have been studied in HIV-infected adults with lipodystrophy syndrome, with varying success. Growth hormone administration improves morphologic abnormalities in adults with fat redistribution syndrome. In addition to increasing LBM, GH (3 mg/day) can reduce excess visceral adipose tissue and buffalo hump size [81]. Wanke and colleagues reported decreased waist:hip ratios and improved mid-thigh circumferences in 10 patients treated with 6 mg daily over 12 weeks [89]. Metformin, an insulin-sensitizing agent, was successful in reducing abdominal adiposity and insulin resistance [90].

Trials of substituting and interrupting PI therapies have been undertaken. One randomized trial of PI substitution led to improvement in lipid levels and decreased intra-abdominal fat, but peripheral lipoatrophy was exacerbated and insulin resistance unchanged [91]. Interruption of therapy for 5–10 weeks was noted to improve lipid levels, but had no effect on insulin resistance or anthropometric measures [92].

Preliminary guidelines for the evaluation and management of dyslipidemias in the HIV-infected adult population have been made by the Adult AIDS Clinical Trials Group Cardiovascular Disease Focus Group [93]. Their recommendations are to evaluate and treat on the basis of existing guidelines for hyperlipidemias in the general population, with the additional caveat that drug interactions with antiretrovirals should be avoided. Dietary interventions have been successful in some patients, and drug therapy with pravastatin had a similar magnitude of effect as with endogenous hyperlipidemia [94]. Atorvastatin also probably is safe in combination with PIs. Experience with these drugs in children is very limited. Fibrates are the drug of choice if hypercholesterolemia and hypertriglyceridemia both are present. Combined aerobic and resistance training in adults over 10 weeks achieved an 18% reduction in cholesterol and 25% reduction in triglyceride levels [95].

16.5.2 Osteopenia and osteonecrosis

Adults and children with HIV infection have been reported to be at increased risk of osteopenia. Specifically, there are three reports of decreased total bone mineral content (BMC) or bone mineral density (BMD) in HIV-infected children, two of which included uninfected children for comparison, controlling for appropriate confounders of age, sex, height, weight, and race [96, 97]. The difference in Arpadi's report was significant at all ages studied (4–17 years), increasing in magnitude with age. There was no association with duration of antiretroviral therapy or use of PIs. Association with NRTI therapy could not be assessed as all of the children were receiving this class of drugs [96]. This contrasts with other studies in adults and children that report increased osteopenia on HAART. In adult HIV-infected men, a doubled relative risk of osteoporosis when receiving PI therapy was reported compared with those not receiving PIs. Osteoporosis did not correlate with fat redistribution in this population [98]. Children on HAART compared with untreated or uninfected children were found by Mora to have decreased adjusted lumbar spine and total body BMD. Further analysis demonstrated that the children with lipodystrophy were those with lessened BMD [97]. O'Brien *et al.* assessed BMC in HIV-infected girls aged 6–15 years, and compared the results to those predicted for height, gender, and ethnicity. Mean total BMC/predicted BMC was 1.1 standard deviations below normal [99].

Decreased BMD may be secondary in part to increased bone resorption as evidenced by increased serum and urine markers of bone turnover, including bone specific alkaline phosphatase, serum N-terminal propeptide of type I procollagen, and urinary N-terminal telopeptide of type I collagen [97]. Increased bone turnover has been reported in HIV-infected adults, both those who are untreated and in association with PI use [100]. Calcium insufficiency may contribute to increased bone resorption [99]. Calcium intake in HIV-infected girls studied by O'Brien was 20–50% below that recommended, with 25% having abnormal increases in 1,25-dihydroxyvitamin D, and 12% having elevated parathyroid hormone. Furthermore, elevated 1,25-dihydroxyvitamin D correlated with urinary N-telopeptide, suggesting that calcium insufficiency does contribute to increased bone resorption. Finally, serum osteocalcin, a protein produced by osteoblasts that correlates histologically with bone formation, has been noted to be increased in HIV-infected children on PI therapy compared with both uninfected children and HIV-infected children not receiving PI agents [101]. The serum concentration of C-telopeptide, a degradation product of type I collagen which correlates histologically to bone resorption, was not different between infected children receiving PI therapy versus those who were not, but was slightly lower in those receiving PI therapy compared with uninfected children.

Possibilities consistent with the above biochemical findings in the face of decreased bone mineral density include: bone resorption is increased to a greater degree than bone formation and C-telopeptide alterations are confounded by altered growth in HIV-infected children, or osteocalcin is increased because the PIs interfere with its degradation. Since osteocalcin is a negative regulator of bone formation, reduced osteocalcin degradation would lead to reduced bone formation. Bone formation and resorption are coupled, and reported decreases in C-telopeptide in children on PI therapy compared with uninfected children may be due to reduced bone resorption subsequent to reduced bone formation.

Osteonecrosis has been described with increased frequency in HIV-infected children and adults compared with the general population. Several reports in adults exist, one documenting an incidence in HIV-infected adults 45 times greater than expected [102]. As with osteopenia, the cause may be multifactorial. There simply may be an increased incidence of risk factors such as hyperlipidemia in HIV-infected individuals, or HIV infection itself may somehow contribute.

The most common form of osteonecrosis in children is Legg–Calvé–Perthes disease, or osteonecrosis of the capital femoral epiphysis. Perinatally infected children have been shown to have a 4.8-fold increase in age-adjusted incidence of Legg–Calvé–Perthes disease [103]. As with studies in adults, there was no clear association with antiretroviral therapy in these children. Abnormal growth has been reported as a risk factor in the general population, and this may explain the increased risk in HIV-infected children. Thrombophilia also can be a risk factor for osteonecrosis [104], and decreased free protein S has been reported to be common in HIV-infected children [105].

16.5.3 Mitochondrial toxicity

An additional metabolic complication noted in HIV-infected patients who receive antiretroviral treatment is mitochondrial toxicity and a subsequent decrease in oxidative phosphorylation. Nucleoside analogue reverse transcriptase inhibitors agents have been established to cause some of their toxicity via inhibition of the human DNA polymerase γ, the enzyme that replicates mitochondrial DNA, leading to depletion of the same. When DNA levels reach approximately 20% of normal, symptoms of hyperlactatemia can develop, e.g. fatigue, weight loss, abdominal pain, nausea, and shortness of breath [106]. Mitochondrial dysfunction may contribute to NRTI side-effects as diverse as lactic acidosis, pancreatitis, proximal renal tubular dysfunction, hepatic steatosis, myopathy, cardiomyopathy, peripheral neuropathy, encephalopathy, developmental delay, hyper- or hypotonia, seizures, ataxia, retinopathy, ophthalmoplegia, deafness, and growth failure [107, 108].

Management of potential mitochondrial toxicity during NRTI therapy remains a challenge. A range of treatments which protect mitochondria have been suggested by in vitro studies. Substitution of better tolerated alternative NRTIs or other classes of drugs for the probable causative agent represents the current mainstay of management for mitochondrial toxicity [109]. However, a multivariate analysis of all cases in the literature described a significantly lower mortality rate among patients with nucleoside-associated lactic acidosis who received therapy with an essential cofactor [110]. Co-factor therapies included thiamine, riboflavin, L-carnitine, prostaglandin E, or coenzyme Q, all of which have been used for congenital mitochondrial diseases. High doses of thiamine and riboflavin in particular have been suggested as potentially useful in secondary prevention of hyperlactatemia [111]. Carnitine specifically interacts with cardiolipin and modifies membrane permeability, protecting mitochondrial function. This is the hypothesized mechanism by which carnitine is able to protect against myopathy induced by NRTI agents [112]. Other antioxidants, e.g. N-acetyl cysteine, also could serve this function.

16.6 Resource-poor settings

Discussed earlier in this chapter (see "Effects of Malnutrition") was the bi-directional association between HIV morbidity and malnutrition, with most data from and recommendations primarily fashioned for resource-rich settings. Discussed below is what is known about the interaction of malnutrition and HIV infection in children in resource-poor settings, both the effect of malnutrition on HIV disease as well as the effect of HIV on malnutrition.

Malnutrition is more common by far in resource-poor compared with resource-rich settings, with associated greater risk of morbidity and mortality. Many of the excess deaths in children under 5 years of age in resource-poor settings, regardless of HIV, are attributed to nutritional immunodeficiencies, and the synergistic effect of malnutrition and infectious diseases [22]. This synergy undoubtedly contributes to more rapid disease progression and heightened mortality among HIV-infected children in resource-poor settings. The probability of death for HIV-infected children in sub-Saharan Africa aged 12 months and 5 years, respectively, is 0.23–0.35 and 0.57–0.68, with malnutrition one of the three most common causes of death. This compares with data from Europe prior to HAART of 0.1 and 0.2, for the same ages.

Relationships between micronutrient status and morbidity and mortality among HIV-infected and uninfected children may be different in resource-poor settings, where deficiencies are more common and/or severe. For example, perinatally HIV-exposed infants in Malawi were more likely to have growth failure or die when their mothers had low plasma vitamin A concentrations, but a study in the USA revealed no association in the general population between vitamin A status and childhood growth or mortality. HIV-infected children in the USA have been shown to have more rapid disease progression when maternal vitamin A stores were lower. As would be expected, results of vitamin A and zinc supplementation trials vary by population and risk of deficiency. Some, but not all, studies of vitamin A supplementation show dramatically reduced mortality. Incidence and severity of infections also vary by site. For example, supplemented children were hospitalized less frequently than control children in Ghana but not in Brazil. There are several trials of vitamin A supplementation in HIV-infected children. Periodic supplementation provided to HIV-infected children in Tanzania resulted in a large reduction in mortality in HIV-infected children [113], and a 50% reduction in diarrheal morbidity in South Africa. Vitamin A, when given prenatally to women in South Africa, had the effect of preventing subsequent deterioration of gut integrity in their HIV-infected infants [114]. Pooled analysis of randomized zinc supplementation trials from resource-poor settings has shown decreased incidence of both diarrhea and pneumonia, but the effect specifically on HIV-infected children has not been reported. Although multivitamin administration to HIV-infected pregnant women in Tanzania was shown to substantially improve CD4+ cell counts, this study has yet to be done in children [115].

HIV infection may alter the presentation of malnutrition in resource-poor settings. Zambian children who were HIV-seropositive had lower weight-for-age scores than their seronegative counterparts, but were also more likely to have marasmus compared with seronegative children, who were more likely to have kwashiorkor. Marasmus was associated with higher mortality [116].

No discussion of nutrition and pediatric HIV infection in resource-poor settings would be complete without mention of the controversy surrounding recommendations for feeding infants of HIV-infected mothers. This topic is beyond the scope of this chapter and is discussed in Chapter 8.

16.7 Future research

Despite the dramatic gains in the past decade in knowledge in many areas of pediatric HIV disease, such as prevention of mother-to-child transmission of HIV and treatment of HIV-infected children with antiretroviral therapy, our understanding of the causes, effects, and appropriate interventions for malnutrition and growth failure in this population remains incomplete.

Little is known about prevalence of micronutrient deficiencies in HIV-infected children, or the effects of such deficiencies on disease progression. Vitamin A supplementation in resource-poor settings has been demonstrated clearly to affect mortality in these children, but it is likely that additional micronutrient and early protein/calorie supplementation could affect disease progression as well. This may be true in both resource-rich and resource-poor settings. Interventions should be studied with the aim to maintain the best possible quality of life for as long as possible.

The pathophysiology of growth failure is elusive. Our understanding even of the major determinants of poor growth remains largely speculative. Conceivably, adjunctive interventions that may improve growth, e.g. anticytokine therapies or treatment with IGF-1, may affect anabolism generally and hence disease progression and survival. More research to understand the mechanisms and consequences of poor growth in HIV-infected children and to identify safe and effective therapies clearly is needed.

The incidence, nature, and etiology of metabolic disturbances related to HIV infection and/or antiretroviral therapy are even less well understood in children than in adults. Hyperlipidemia, glucose intolerance, fat redistribution, and osteopenia all have potential to affect morbidity and mortality significantly in HIV-infected children.

REFERENCES

1. Baumgartner, R. N., Roche, A. F. & Himes, J. H. Incremental growth tables: supplementary to previously published charts. *Am. J. Clin. Nutr.* **43** (1986), 711–22.

2. Miller, T. L. Nutrition in paediatric human immunodeficiency virus infection. *Proc. Nutr. Soc.* **59** (2000), 155–62.

3. Beisel, W. R. Nutrition and immune function: overview. *J. Nutr.* **126** (1996), 2611–15S.

4. Brown, K. H., Peerson, J. M., Rivera, J. & Allen, L. H. Effect of supplemental zinc on the growth and serum zinc concentrations of prepubertal children: a meta-analysis of randomized controlled trials. *Am. J. Clin. Nutr.* **75** (2002), 1062–71.

5. Committee on Nutrition, American Academy of Pediatrics. Trace elements. In R. E. Kleinman (ed.), *Pediatric Nutrition Handbook*, 4th edn. Elk Grove, Ill: American Academy of Pediatrics. (1998), pp. 247–66.

6. McKinney, R. E. & Robertson, W. R. Effect of human immunodeficiency virus infection on the growth of young children. *J. Pediatr.* **123** (1993), 579–82.

7. Miller, T. L., Evans, S., Morris, V., Orav, E. J., McIntosh, K. & Winter, H. S. Growth and body composition in children with human immunodeficiency virus-1 infection. *Am. J. Clin. Nutr.* **57** (1993), 588–92.

8. Moye, J. Jr., Rich, K. C., Kalish, L. A. *et al.* Natural history of somatic growth in infants born to women infected by human immunodeficiency virus. *J. Pediatr.* **128** (1996), 58–67.

9. Saavedra, J. M., Henderson, R. A., Perman, J. A., Hutton, N., Livingston, R. A. & Yolken, R. H. Longitudinal assessment of growth in children born to mothers with human immunodeficiency virus infection. *Arch. Pediatr. Adolesc. Med.* **149** (1995), 497–502.

10. Lindegren, M. L., Steinberg, S. & Byers, R. H. Epidemiology of HIV/AIDS in children. *Pediatr. Clin. N. Am.* **47** (2000), 1–20.

11. Kotler, D. P., Tierney, A. R., Wang, J. & Pierson, R. N. Magnitude of body cell mass depletion and the timing of death from wasting in AIDS. *Am. J. Clin. Nutr.* **50** (1989), 444–7.

12. Chlebowski, R. T., Grosvenor, M. B., Berhard, N. H., Morales, L. S. & Bulcavage, L. M. Nutritional status, gastrointestinal dysfunction, and survival in patients with AIDS. *Amer. J. Gastroenterol.* **84** (1989), 1288–93.

13. Lai, H., Lai, S., Shor-Posner, G., Ma, F., Trapido, E. & Baum, M. K. Plasma zinc, copper, copper:zinc ratio, and survival in a cohort of HIV-1-infected homosexual men. *J. Acquir. Immune. Defic. Syndr.* **27** (2001), 56–62.

14. Tang, A. M., Graham, N. M. H., Semba, R. D. & Saah, A. J. Association between serum vitamin A and E levels and HIV-1 disease progression. *AIDS* **11** (1997), 613–20.

15. Baum, M. K., Shor-Posner G, Lu, Y. *et al.* Micronutrients and HIV-1 disease progression. *AIDS* **9** (1995), 1051–6.

16. Cunningham-Rundles, S., Ahrn, S., Abuav-Nussbaum, R. & Dnistrian, A. Development of immunocompetence: role of micronutrients and microorganisms. *Nutr. Rev.* **60** (2002), S68–72.

17. Chantry, C. J., Byrd, R. S., Englund, J. A. *et al.* Growth, survival and viral load in symptomatic childhood human immunodeficiency virus infection. *Pediatr. Infect. Dis. J.* **22**(12) (2003), 1033–9.

18. McKinney, R. E. Jr. & Wilfert, C. Growth as a prognostic indicator in children with human immunodeficiency virus infection treated with zidovudine. AIDS Clinical Trials Group Protocol 043 Study Group. *J. Pediatr.* **125** (1994), 728–33.

19. Berhane, R., Bagenda, D., Marum, L. *et al.* Growth failure as a prognostic indicator of mortality in pediatric HIV infection. *Pediatrics* **100** (1997), e7.

20. Yong, F. H., Stanley, K., McKinney, R. E., *et al.* Prognostic value of plasma RNA, CD4, and growth markers for clinical disease progression in children with HIV disease. *Intersci. Conf. Antimicrob. Agents Chemother.* (ICAAC) **38** (Sept 24–27, 1998), 364 [Abstract no. I-7].

21. Campa, A., Shor-Posner G, Indacochea, F. *et al.* Mortality risk in selenium-deficient HIV-positive children. *J. Acquir. Immune. Defic. Syndr. Hum. Retrovirol.* **20** (1999), 508–13.

22. Duggan, C. & Fawzi, W. Micronutrients and child health: studies in international nutrition and HIV infection. *Nutr. Rev.* **59** (2001), 358–69.

23. Rodríguez, J. F., Cordero, J., Chantry, C. J. *et al.* Glutathione levels in HIV-infected children. *Pediatr. Infect. Dis. J.* **17** (1998), 236–41.

24. Omene, J. A., Easington, C. R., Glew, R. H., Prosper, M. & Ledlie, S. Serum beta-carotene deficiency in HIV-infected children. *J. Natl. Med. Assoc.* **88** (1996), 789–93.

25. Fawzi, W. W., Mbise, R. L., Hertzmark, E. *et al.* A randomized trial of vitamin A supplements in relation to mortality among human immunodeficiency virus-infected and uninfected children in Tanzania. *Pediatr. Infect. Dis. J.* **18** (1999), 127–33.

26. Moye, J. Jr., Rich, K. C., Kalish, L. A. *et al.* Natural history of somatic growth in infants born to women infected by human immunodeficiency virus. Women and Infants Transmission Study Group. *J. Pediatr.* **128** (1996), 58–69.

27. Miller, T. L., Evans, S., Orav, E. J., Morris, V., McIntosh, K. & Winter, H. S. Growth and body composition in children with human immunodeficiency virus-1 infection. *Am. J. Clin. Nutr.* **57** (1993), 588–92.

28. Fontana, M., Zuin, G., Plebani, A. *et al.* Body composition in HIV-infected children: relations with disease progression and survival. *Am. J. Clin. Nutr.* **69** (1999), 1282–6.

29. Arpadi, S. M., Cuff, P. A., Kotler, D. P. *et al.* Growth velocity, fat-free mass and energy intake are inversely related to viral load in HIV-infected children. *J. Nutr.* **130** (2000), 2498–502.

30. Moye, J., Frederick, M., Chantry, C. *et al.* for the Women and Infants Transmission Study. 10-year follow-up of somatic growth in children born to women infected by human immunodeficiency virus. *8ᵗʰ Conf Retroviruses Opportunistic Infect.* (Feb 4–8 2001) [Abstract 514].

31. Pollack, H., Glasberg, H., Lee, E. *et al.* Impaired early growth of infants perinatally infected with human immunodeficiency virus: Correlation with viral load. *J. Pediatr.* **130** (1997), 915–22.

32. Miller, T. L., Easley, K. A., Zhang, W. *et al.* for the Pediatric Pulmonary and Cardiovascular Complications of Vertically Transmitted HIV Infection (P2C2 HIV) Study Group, National Heart, Lung, and Blood Institute, Bethesda, MD. Maternal and infant factors associated with failure to thrive in children with vertically transmitted human immunodeficiency virus-1 infection: The prospective, P2C2 human immunodeficiency virus multicenter study. *Pediatrics* **108** (2001), 1287–96.

33. Hilgartner, M. W., Donfield, S. M., Lynn, H. S. *et al.* The effect of plasma human immunodeficiency virus RNA and CD4+ T lymphocytes on growth measurements of hemophilic boys and adolescents. *Pediatrics* **107** (2001), e56.

34. Nachman, S. A., Lindsey, J. C., Pelton, S. *et al.* Growth in human immunodeficiency virus-infected children receiving ritonavir-containing antiretroviral therapy. *Arch. Pediatr. Adolesc. Med.* **156** (2002), 497–503.

35. Buchacz, K., Cervia, J. S., Lindsey, J. C. *et al.* for the Pediatric AIDS Clinical Trials Group 219 Study Team. Impact of protease inhibitor-containing combination antiretroviral therapies on height and weight growth in HIV-infected children. *Pediatrics* **108** (2001), e72.

36. Verweel, G., van Rossum, A. M. C., Hartwig, N. G., Wolfs, T. F., Scherpbier, H. J. & de Groot, R. Treatment with highly active antiretroviral therapy in human immunodeficiency virus type-1-infected children is associated with a sustained effect on growth. *Pediatrics* **109** (2002), e25.

37. Abrams, B., Duncan, D. & Hertz-Picciotto, H. A prospective study of dietary intake and acquired immune deficiency syndrome in HIV-seropositive homosexual men. *J. Acquir. Immune. Defic. Syndr.* **6** (1993), 949–58.

38. Dunn, A. M., Cervia, J., Burgess, A. *et al.* Failure to thrive in the HIV-infected child. *11ᵗʰ Int Conf AIDS* **1** (1996), 319 [Abstract 2312].

39. Heller, L. S. Nutritional support for children with HIV/AIDS. *AIDS Reader* **10** (2000), 109–14.

40. Allard, J. P., Aghdassi, E., Chau, J., Salit, I. & Walmsley, S. Oxidative stress and plasma antioxidant micronutrients in humans with HIV infection. *Am. J. Clin. Nutr.* **67** (1998), 1443–7.

41. Mintz, M. Carnitine in human immunodeficiency virus type 1 infection/acquired immune deficiency syndrome. *J. Child. Neurol.* **10** (1995), 2S40–44.

42. Haug, C. J., Aukrust, P., Haug, E., Morkrid, L., Muller, F. & Froland, S. S. Severe deficiency of 1,25-dihydroxyvitamin D3 in human immunodeficiency virus infection: association with immunological hyperactivity and only minor changes in calcium homeostasis. *J. Clin. Endocrinol. Metab.* **83** (1998), 3832–8.

43. Henderson, R. A., Talusan, K., Hutton, N., Yolken, R. H. & Caballero, B. Serum and plasma markers of nutritional status in children infected with the human immunodeficiency virus. *J. Am. Diet. Assoc.* **97** (1997), 1377–81.

44. Skurnick, J. H., Bogden, J. D., Baker, H. *et al.* Micronutrient profiles in HIV-1-infected heterosexual adults. *J. AIDS* **12** (1996), 75–83.

45. Horlick, M., Arpadi, S. M., Bethel, J. *et al.* Bioelectrical impedance analysis models for prediction of total body water and fat-free mass in healthy and HIV-infected children and adolescents. *Am. J. Clin. Nutr.* **76** (2002), 991–9.

46. Freedman, D. S., Serdula, M. K., Srnivasan, S. R. & Berenson, G. S. Relation of circumferences and skinfold thicknesses to lipid and insulin concentrations in children and adolescents: the Bogalusa Heart Study. *Am. J. Clin. Nutr.* **69** (1999), 308–17.

47. Taylor, R. W., Jones, I. E., Williams, S. M. & Goulding, A. Evaluation of waist circumference, waist-to-hip ratio, and the conicity index as screening tools for high trunk fat mass, as measured by dual-energy X-ray absorptiometry, in children aged 3–19 years. *Am. J. Clin. Nutr.* **72** (2000), 490–5.

48. Goran, M. I., Gower, B. A., Treuth, M. & Nagy, T. R. Prediction of intra-abdominal and subcutaneous abdominal adipose tissue in healthy pre-pubertal children. *Int. J. Obes. Relat. Metab. Disord.* **22** (1998), 549–68.

49. Johann-Liang, R., O'Neill, L., Cervia, J. *et al.* Energy balance, viral burden, insulin-like growth factor-1, interleukin-6 and growth impairment in children infected with human immunodeficiency virus. *AIDS* **14** (2000), 683–90.

50. Guo, S., Roche, A. F., Foman, S. J. *et al.* Reference data on gains in weight and length during the first two years of life. *J. Pediatr.* **119** (1991), 355–62.

51. Karlberg, P., Taranger, J., Engstrom, I. *et al.* I. Physical growth from birth to 16 years and longitudinal outcome of the study during the same age period. *Acta. Pediatr. Scand. Suppl.* **258** (1976), 7–76.

52. Sentongo, T. A., Rutstein, R. M., Stettler, N. *et al.* Association between steatorrhea, growth, and immunologic status in children with perinatally acquired HIV infection. *Arch. Pediatr. Adolesc. Med.* **155** (2001), 149–53.

53. Alfaro, M. P., Siegel, R. M., Baker, R. C. & Heubi, J. E. Resting energy expenditure and body composition in pediatric HIV infection. *Pediatr. AIDS HIV Infect.* **6** (1995), 276–80.

54. Henderson, R. A., Talusan, K., Hutton, N., Yolken, R. H. & Caballero, B. Resting energy expenditure and body composition in children with HIV infection. *J. AIDS Hum. Retrovirol.* **19** (1998), 150–7.

55. Clarick, R. H., Hanekom, W. A., Yogev, R. & Chadwick, E. G. Megestrol acetate treatment of growth failure in children infected with human immunodeficiency virus. *Pediatrics*, **99**(3) (1997), 354–7.

56. Mann, M., Koller, E., Murgo, A., Malozowski, S., Bacsanyi, J. & Leinung, M. Glucocorticoid like activity of megestrol: a summary of Food and Drug Administration experience and a review of the literature. *Arch. Intern. Med.* **15** (1997), 1651–6.

57. Stockheim, J., Daaboul, J., Scully, S., Yogev, R. Scully, S. P., Binns, H. J. & Chadwick, E. Adrenal suppression in HIV-infected children treated with megestrol acetate. *J. Pediatr.* **134**(3) (1999), 368–70.

58. Chantry, C., González de Pijem, L., Febo, I. & Lugo, L. Adrenal suppression secondary to megestrol acetate in HIV-infected children. *12th Int. Conf. AIDS* (July 1998), 610 [Abstract 32445].

59. Brady, M. T., Korany, K. I. & Hunkler, J. A. Megestrol acetate for the treatment of anorexia associated with human immunodeficiency virus infection in children. *Pediatr. Inf. Dis. J.* **13** (1994), 754–6.

60. Briefel, R. R. & Woteki, C. E. Development of Food Sufficiency Questions for the Third National Health and Nutrition Examination Survey. *J. Nutr. Educ.* **24** (1992), 24S–8S.

61. Henderson, R. A., Saavedra, J. M., Perman, J. A., Hutton, N., Livingston, R. A. & Yolken, R. H. Effect of enteral tube feeding on growth of children with symptomatic human immunodefi-

ciency virus infection. *J. Pediatr. Gastroenterol. Nutr.* **18** (1994), 429–34.

62. Miller, T. L., Awnetwant, E. L., Evans, S., Morris, V. M., Vazquez, I. M. & McIntosh, K. Gastrostomy tube supplementation for HIV infected children. *Pediatrics* **96** (1995), 696–702.

63. Sinden, A. A., Dillard, V. L. & Sutphen, J. L. Enteral nutrition. In W. A., Walker, P. R., Durie, J. R., Hamilton, J. A., Walker-Smith & J. B. Watkins (eds.), *Pediatric Gastrointestinal Disease.* Philadelphia, PA: *BC Decker, Inc.* (1991), p. 1636.

64. Miller, T. L., Orav, E. J., Martin, S. R. *et al.* Malnutrition and carbohydrate malabsorption in children with vertically-transmitted human immunodeficiency virus-1 infection. *Gastroenterology* **100** (1991), 1296–302.

65. The Italian Pediatric Intestinal/HIV Study Group. Intestinal malabsorption of HIV-infected children: relationship to diarrhea, failure to thrive, enteric micro-organisms and immune impairment. *AIDS* **7** (1993), 1435–40.

66. Mulligan, K., Tai, V. W. & Schambelan, M. Energy expenditure in human immunodeficiency virus infection [letter]. *New Engl. J. Med.* **70** (1997), 70–1.

67. Chiarelli, F., Galli, L., Verrotti, A., diRocco, L., Vierucci, A. & de Martino, M. Thyroid function in children with perinatal human immunodeficiency virus type 1 infection. *Thyroid* **10** (2000), 499–505.

68. Laue, L., Pizzo, P. A., Butler, K. & Cutler, G. B., Jr. Growth and neuroendocrine dysfunction in children with acquired immunodeficiency syndrome. *J. Pediatr.* **117** (1990), 541–5.

69. Jospe, N. & Powell, K. R. Growth hormone deficiency in an 8-year old girl with human immunodeficiency virus infection. *Pediatrics* **86** (1990), 309–12.

70. Cieslak, T. J., Ascher, D. P., Zimmerman, P. A. *et al.* Adrenal insufficiency presenting as HIV wasting syndrome in a child: initial successful response to megestrol. *Pediatr. AIDS HIV Infect.* **2** (1991), 279–83.

71. Frost, R. A., Nachman, S. A., Lang, C. H. & Gelato, M. C. Proteolysis of insulin-like growth factor-binding protein-3 in human immunodeficiency virus-positive children with failure to thrive. *J. Clin. Endocrinol. Metab.* **81** (1996), 2957–62.

72. Guyda, H. J. How do we best measure growth hormone action? *Horm. Res.* **48** (Suppl. 5) (1997), 1–10.

73. Gelato, M. C. & Frost, R. A. IGFBP-3. Functional and structural implications in aging and wasting syndromes. *Endocrine* **7**: 1 (1997), 81–5.

74. Mahoney, E. M., Donfield, S. M., Howard, C., Kaufman, F. & Gerner, J. M. HIV-associated immune dysfunction and delayed pubertal development in a cohort of young hemophiliacs. Hemophilia Growth and Development Study. *J. AIDS* **21** (1999), 333–7.

75. Arnalich, F., Martinez, P., Hernanz, A. *et al.* Altered concentrations of appetite regulators may contribute to the development and maintenance of HIV-associated wasting. *AIDS* **11** (1997), 1129–34.

76. de Martino, M., Galli, L., Chiarelli, F. *et al.* Interleukin-6 release by cultured peripheral blood mononuclear cells inversely correlates with height velocity, bone age, insulin-like growth

factor-I, and insulin-like growth factor binding protein-3 serum levels in children with perinatal HIV-1 infection. *Clin. Immunol.* **94** (2000), 212–18.

77. Mynarcik, D. C., Frost, R. A., Lang, C. H. *et al.* Insulin-like growth factor system in patients with HIV infection: effect of exogenous growth hormone administration. *J. AIDS* **22** (1999), 49–55.

78. Chantry, C., Cervia, J., Hughes, M., Patra, K., Hodge, J., Moye, J. and the PACTG Protocol 1010 Team. Body composition and biochemical changes in children starting or switching combination antiretroviral therapy. *10th Conf. Retroviruses Opportunistic Infect.* 2003 [Abstract No. 775].

79. Pinto, G., Blanche, S., Thiriet, I., Souberbielle, J. C., Goulet, O. & Brauner, R. Growth hormone treatment of children with human immunodeficiency virus-associated growth failure. *Eur. J. Pediatr.* **159** (2000), 937–8.

80. Fox-Wheeler, S., Heller, L., Salata, C. M. *et al.* Evaluation of the effects of oxandrolone on malnourished HIV-positive pediatric patients. *Pediatrics* **104** (1999), e73.

81. Lo, J. C., Mulligan, K., Noor, M. A. *et al.* The effects of recombinant human growth hormone on body composition and glucose metabolism in HIV-infected patients with fat accumulation. *J. Clin. Endocrinol. Metab.* **8** (2001), 3480–7.

82. Dreimane, D., Gallagher, K., Nielsen, K. *et al.* Growth hormone exerts potent anabolic effects in an adolescent with human immunodeficiency virus wasting. *Pediatr. Infect. Dis. J.* **18** (1999), 167–9.

83. Grinspoon, S., Corcoran, C., Stanley, T., Katznelson, L. & Klibanski, A. Effects of androgen administration on the growth hormone-insulin-like growth factor I axis in men with acquired immunodeficiency syndrome wasting. *J. Clin. Endocrinol. Metab.* **83** (1998), 4251–6.

84. Brambilla, P., Bricalli, D., Sala, N. *et al.* Highly active antiretroviral-treated HIV-infected children show fat distribution changes even in absence of lipodystrophy. *AIDS* **15** (2001), 2415–22.

85. Arpadi, S. M., Cuff, P. A., Horlick, M., Wang, J. & Kotler, D. R. Lipodystrophy in HIV-infected children is associated with high viral load and low CD4+-lymphocyte count and CD4+-lymphocyte percentage at baseline and use of protease inhibitors and stavudine. *J. AIDS* **27** (2001), 30–4.

86. Melvin, A. J., Lennon, S., Mohan, K. M. & Purnell, J. Q. Metabolic abnormalities in HIV type 1-infected children treated and not treated with protease inhibitors. *AIDS Res. Hum. Retroviruses* **17** (2001), 1117–23.

87. Amaya, R. A., Kozinetz, C. A., McMeans, A., Schwarzwald, H., & Kline, M. W. Lipodystrophy syndrome in human immunodeficiency virus-infected children. *Pediatr. Infect. Dis. J.* **21** (2002), 405–10.

88. Jaquet, D., Levine, M., Ortega-Rodriguez, E. *et al.* Clinical and metabolic presentation of the lipodystrophic syndrome in HIV-infected children. *AIDS* **14** (2000), 2123–8.

89. Wanke, C., Gerrior, J., Kantaros, J., Coakley, E. & Albrecht, M. Recombinant human growth hormone improves the fat redistribution syndrome (lipodystrophy) in patients with HIV. *AIDS* **13** (1999), 2099–103.

90. Hadigan, C., Corcoran, C., Basgoz, N., Davis, B., Sax, P. & Grinspoon, S. Metformin in the treatment of HIV lipodystrophy syndrome: a randomized controlled trial. *J. Am. Med. Assoc.* **284** (2000), 472–7.

91. Carr, A., Hudson, J., Chuah, J. *et al.* HIV protease inhibitor substitution in patients with lipodystrophy: a randomized, controlled, open-label, multicentre study. *AIDS* **15** (2001), 1811–22.

92. Hatano, H., Miller, K. D., Yoder, C. P. *et al.* Metabolic and anthropometric consequences of interruption of highly active antiretroviral therapy. *AIDS* **14** (2000), 1935–42.

93. Dube, M. P., Sprecher, D., Henry, W. K. *et al.* Preliminary guidelines for the evaluation and management of dyslipidemia in adults infected with human immunodeficiency virus and receiving antiretroviral therapy: recommendations of the Adult AIDS Clinical Trial Group Cardiovascular Disease Focus Group. *Clin. Infect. Dis.* **31** (2000), 1216–24.

94. Moyle, G. J., Lloyd, M., Reynolds, B., Baldwin, C., Mandalia, S. & Gazzord, B. G. Dietary advice with or without pravastatin for the management of hypercholesterolaemia associated with protease inhibitor therapy. *AIDS* **15** (2001), 1503–8.

95. Jones, S. P., Doran, D. A., Leatt, P. B., Maher, B. & Pirmohamed, M. Short-term exercise training improves body composition and hyperlipidaemia in HIV-positive individuals with lipodystrophy. [letter] *AIDS* **15** (2001), 2049–51.

96. Arpadi, S. M., Horlick, M., Thornton, J., Cuff, P. A., Wang, J. & Kotler, D. P. Bone mineral content is lower in prepubertal HIV-infected children. *J. AIDS* **29** (2002), 450–4.

97. Mora, S., Sala, N., Bricalli, D. *et al.* Bone mineral loss through increased bone turnover in HIV-infected children treated with highly active antiretroviral therapy. *AIDS* **15** (2001), 1823–9.

98. Tebas, P., Powderly, W. G., Claxton, S. *et al.* Accelerated bone mineral loss in HIV-infected patients receiving potent antiretroviral therapy. *AIDS* **14** (2000), F63–7.

99. O'Brien, K. O., Razavi, M., Henderson, R. A., Caballero, B. & Ellis, K. J. Bone mineral content in girls perinatally infected with HIV. *Am. J. Clin. Nutr.* **73** (2001), 821–6.

100. Aukrust, P., Haug, C. J., Ueland, T. *et al.* Decreased bone formative and enhanced resorptive markers in human immunodeficiency virus infection: indication of normalization of the bone-remodeling process during highly active antiretroviral therapy. *J. Clin. Endocrinol. Metab.* **84** (1999), 145–50.

101. Tan, B. M., Nelson, R. P., James-Yarish M, Emmanuel, P. J. & Schurman, S. J. Bone metabolism in children with human immunodeficiency virus infection receiving highly active antiretroviral therapy including a protease inhibitor. *J. Pediatr.* **139** (2001), 447–51.

102. Brown, P. & Crane, L. Avascular necrosis of bone in patients with human immunodeficiency virus infection: report of 6 cases and review of the literature. *Clin. Infect. Dis.* **32** (2001), 1221–6.

103. Gaughan, D. M., Mofenson, L. M. & Hughes, M. D. Ostenecrosis of the hip (Legg–Calve–Perthes Disease) in human immunodeficiency virus-infected children. *Pediatrics* **109** (2002), e74.

104. Sugerman, R. W., Church, J. A., Goldsmith, J. C. & Ens, G. E. Acquired protein S deficiency in children infected with

human immunodeficiency virus. *Pediatr. Infect. Dis. J.* **15** (1996), 106–11.

105. Eldridge, J., Dilley, A., Austin, H. *et al.* The role of protein C, protein S, and resistance to activated protein C in Legg-Perthes disease. *Pediatrics* 107 (2001), 1329–34.

106. Cote, H. C., Brumme, Z. L., Craib, K. J. *et al.* Changes in mitochondrial DNA as a marker of nucleoside toxicity in HIV-infected patients. *New Engl. J. Med.* **346** (2002), 811–20.

107. Glesby, M. J. Overview of mitochondrial toxicity of nucleoside reverse transcriptase inhibitors. *Topics in HIV Med.* **10** (2002), 42–6.

108. The Perinatal Safety Review Working Group. Nucleoside exposure in the children of HIV-infected women receiving antiretroviral drugs: absence of clear evidence for mitochondrial disease in children who died before 5 years of age in five United States cohorts. *J. AIDS* **25** (2000), 261–8.

109. Moyle, G. Clinical manifestations and management of antiretroviral nucleoside analog-related mitochondrial toxicity. *Clin. Ther.* **22** (2000), 911–36.

110. Falco, V., Rodriguez, D., Ribera, E. *et al.* Severe nucleoside-associated lactic acidosis in human immunodeficiency virus-infected patients: report of 12 cases and review of the literature. *Clin. Infect. Dis.* **34** (2002), 838–46.

111. McComsey, G. A. & Lederman, M. M. High doses of riboflavin and thiamine may help in secondary prevention of hyperlactatemia. *AIDS Reader* **12** (2002), 222–4.

112. Arrigoni-Martelli, E. & Caso, V. Carnitine protects mitochondria and removes toxic acyls from xenobiotics. *Drugs Exp. Clin. Res.* **27** (2001), 27–49.

113. Fawzi, W. W., Mbise, R. L., Hertzmark, E. *et al.* A randomized trial of vitamin A supplements in relation to mortality among human immunodeficiency virus-infected and uninfected children in Tanzania. *Pediatr. Infect. Dis. J.* **18** (1999), 127–33.

114. Filteau, S. M., Rollins, N. C., Coutsoudis, A., Sullivan, K. R., Willumsen, J. F. & Tomkins, A. N. The effect of antenatal vitamin A and beta-carotene supplementation on gut integrity of infants of HIV-infected South African women. *J. Pediatr. Gastroenterol. Nutr.* **32** (2001), 464–70.

115. Fawzi, W. W., Msamanga, G. I., Spiegelman, D. *et al.* Randomised trial of effects of vitamin supplements on pregnancy outcomes and T cell counts in HIV-1 infected women in Tanzania. *Lancet* **351** (1998), 1477–82.

116. Amadi, B., Kelly, P., Mwiya, M. *et al.* Intestinal and systemic infection, HIV, and mortality in Zambian children with persistent diarrhea and malnutrition. *J. Pediatr. Gastroenterol. Nutr.* **32** (2001), 550–4.

17

Neurobehavioral function and assessment of children and adolescents with HIV-1 infection

Pamela L. Wolters, Ph.D.[1] and Pim Brouwers, Ph.D.[2]

[1]HIV and AIDS Malignancy Branch, National Cancer Institute and Medical Illness Counseling Center, Bethesda, MD
[2]Texas Children's Cancer & Sickle Cell Centers, Baylor College of Medicine, Houston, TX

Infants and children infected with human immunodeficiency virus-type 1 (HIV-1) are at increased risk for developing central nervous system (CNS) disease characterized by cognitive, language, motor, and behavioral impairments. The severity of HIV-related CNS manifestations in children range on a continuum from subtle impairments in selective domains to severe deterioration of global developmental skills.

HIV-related CNS dysfunction in children is primarily the result of HIV-1 infection in the brain [1, 2]. HIV-1 has been isolated from the CNS tissue of fetuses [3] and the cerebral spinal fluid (CSF) of adults soon after infection [4, 5] suggesting early CNS invasion. The timing of CNS infection for infants is variable and likely influences neuropathology and neurodevelopmental effects [3, 6–8]. Astrocytes, macrophages, and microglia may be infected with HIV-1, while neurons seem to remain largely uninfected. Various neurotoxic factors released by the virus and host cells are postulated as the main cause of neurologic damage [2, 9]. Secondary CNS complications due to immune deficiency, such as brain tumors, other infections, or cerebrovascular diseases, also may cause CNS manifestations but are less common and usually occur in older children [10].

Early in the epidemic, approximately 50–90% of children with HIV-1 infection exhibited severe CNS manifestations [11, 12] termed HIV encephalopathy. More recent studies, however, report that the prevalence of encephalopathy in HIV-infected children is approximately 13–23% [13–16]. Children exhibit CNS disease more frequently than adults (16% vs 5%) [16] with new pediatric cases of encephalopathy occurring primarily during the first 2 years after birth [16] and often as the initial AIDS-defining symptom [16, 17]. Adults, as well as older children and adolescents, may develop CNS complications several years after infection during more advanced stages of the disease [17, 18].

This decline in the prevalence of severe HIV-related CNS manifestations may be related in part to the earlier and more generalized use of combination antiretroviral treatment (ART), including highly active antiretroviral therapy (HAART) that combines various agents with at least one protease inhibitor (PI) or non-nucleoside reverse transcriptase inhibitor (NNRTI) [19–22]. Highly active antiretroviral therapy is effective in suppressing systemic viral replication [23], which in turn may reduce the number of HIV-infected cells entering the CNS. However, the CNS is a separate compartment from the rest of the body and it may serve as a reservoir for persistent HIV-1 infection [24]. Many antiretroviral agents, including PIs, do not penetrate well into the CNS [25, 26]. Since HAART has become available, a proportional increase in AIDS dementia complex compared with other AIDS defining illnesses has occurred in adults with HIV-1 disease [27]. Thus, combination ART may provide systemic benefits but not be as effective in treating the CNS [28] so that HIV-infected patients with well-controlled systemic disease may still be at risk for developing CNS manifestations.

In addition to the effects of HIV-1 on the developing brain, infected children also may have other medical and environmental risk factors that can contribute to neurobehavioral abnormalities. Thus, assessment of neurobehavioral functioning throughout childhood and adolescence is important for identifying and monitoring the effects of HIV-1 on the CNS over time, evaluating response to antiretroviral therapy, making treatment decisions, and planning educational and rehabilitative interventions. Neuropsychological test scores also can provide information, beyond that obtained from medical surrogate markers of HIV status, that is predictive of later disease progression [29, 30].

17.1 Clinical presentation of HIV-related CNS disease in children

Pediatric HIV-related encephalopathy has characteristic features and distinct patterns, although the clinical presentation varies in onset, severity, and prevalence in different subgroups. Factors associated with variations in the presentation of HIV-related CNS manifestations include age at infection, route and timing of transmission, maternal and child disease status, genetic factors, treatment history, and other medical and environmental conditions.

Infants and young children tend to exhibit the highest rates of HIV-related CNS disease (66–75%) and the most severe neurodevelopmental impairments [31–33] while older children and adolescents tend to have the lowest rates and less severe manifestations of CNS disease (33%) [13, 33, 34]. The greatest risk for encephalopathy occurs during the first year of life, when it is often the initial AIDS-defining symptom [14–17]. Children with early onset of HIV encephalopathy, before the age of 1 year, have smaller head circumference and lower body weight at birth, suggesting a different pathophysiology compared with later-occurring encephalopathy [16].

Vertically infected children with in utero transmission (positive HIV-1 cultures at birth or DNA PCR at birth) display more severe HIV disease [35] and poorer neurodevelopmental function [8] compared with children with presumed intrapartum infection. Children with vertically acquired infection tend to have more severe CNS manifestations than children who were infected via blood or blood products, even in the perinatal period [17]. Adolescents infected with HIV, often through sexual transmission, also appear to have fewer CNS symptoms, with a clinical presentation resembling that seen in adults [18].

The risk of encephalopathy is higher in HIV-infected children born to mothers with more advanced disease as measured by CD4$^+$ cell count and viral load at the time of delivery [36]. In addition, high plasma viral loads [15, 16, 37, 38], more severe immunodeficiency early in life [14–16, 35], and genetic factors in the child [39, 40] are associated with more rapid HIV disease progression, including encephalopathy. HIV-infected children who are naïve to ART [33] or who might be on monotherapy [34] appear to be at greater risk of developing CNS manifestations than children on combination ART, such as HAART [22]. However, children with HIV-1 infection exposed to ZDV in utero and for 6 weeks after birth did not differ in the incidence of encephalopathy or cognitive function compared with children who had not been treated [16, 41].

Finally, other medical and environmental conditions, such as maternal substance abuse during pregnancy, low birthweight, preterm birth, exposure to toxic substances (i.e. lead), other CNS infections, impoverished socioeconomic and environmental background, and psychosocial difficulties, also may negatively influence the development of children with HIV-1 infection. As vertically infected children live longer, such conditions will have a greater impact on neurobehavioral function and need to be considered when assessing the effects of HIV-1 on the developing CNS.

17.1.1 Patterns of HIV-related CNS disease in children

Despite variations in the presentation of CNS disease among different subgroups of children with HIV-1 infection, three main patterns have been described: encephalopathy, CNS compromise, and apparently not affected [42, 43].

HIV-related encephalopathy is characterized by pervasive and severe CNS dysfunction. Children with HIV-related encephalopathy exhibit global impairments in cognitive, language, motor, and social skills as well as significant neurologic impairments that affect their day-to-day functioning. Although overall functioning generally is impaired in encephalopathic children, differential deficits may be observed in selective functions. For example, expressive language is often more severely impaired or may deteriorate more quickly than receptive language. HIV-related encephalopathy can be progressive (subacute or plateau subtypes) or static [44–46]. *Subacute progressive encephalopathy*, the most severe subtype, is characterized by progressive, global deterioration and loss of previously acquired abilities and skills. In the *plateau course of progressive encephalopathy*, the acquisition of new skills becomes slower compared with their previous rate of development or may stop, but previously acquired milestones are not lost. Both subacute and plateau subtypes result in a significant decline in standardized scores on repeated neurodevelopmental testing. Children with *static encephalopathy* continue to consistently gain new skills and abilities but at a slower rate than their normally developing peers. Thus, their scores on standardized tests are below average but remain stable over time. The prevalence of encephalopathy appears to be declining in pediatric HIV disease, most likely due to earlier treatment and improved therapeutic options. New cases of encephalopathy are seen most often in infants and young children [13, 14, 16], particularly those naïve to ART [33], and older children in advanced stages of disease [18]. In the revised Centers for Disease Control and

Prevention (CDC) classification system for HIV infection in children less than 13 years of age, encephalopathy is a condition listed in Category C [47].

HIV-related CNS compromise is characterized by overall cognitive functioning that is within normal limits but with either significant decline in psychometric test scores in one or more areas of neurobehavioral functioning, which remains above the low average range, or significant impairments in selective neurodevelopmental functions [43, 48]. Patients who were functioning within normal limits but exhibited significant improvements after initiation or change in ART also are included in this category. Children with HIV-related CNS compromise continue to have adequate functioning in school and activities of daily living. With the widespread availability of HAART, children displaying CNS disease are more likely to exhibit this more subtle form of CNS compromise rather than the more severe and pervasive encephalopathy that was frequently seen during the first decade of the AIDS epidemic. Central nervous system compromise is not yet a condition listed in the revised CDC classification system for HIV infection in children [47].

The CNS of children is considered to be *apparently not affected* by HIV when their cognitive functioning is at least within the normal range and without evidence of HIV-associated significant deficits, decline in functioning, neurological abnormalities that affect day-to-day functioning, or therapy-related improvements.

Children infected with HIV-1 also may have *non-HIV-related CNS impairments*. Some HIV-1-infected children may be at greater risk for these non-HIV-related CNS impairments because of their complicated medical histories and/or difficult social situations. It is possible for children to exhibit both HIV and non-HIV-related impairments. Determining whether developmental deficits are related to HIV-1 disease or other etiologies is complex but important for making treatment decisions.

The specific criteria used by the neurobehavioral team at the HIV and AIDS Malignancy Branch of the National Cancer Institute to classify the above patterns of CNS disease in children with HIV-1 infection is presented in Table 17.1. These criteria were developed to determine a child's CNS classification in a consistent and objective manner to help standardize neurobehavioral research efforts in pediatric AIDS.

17.1.2 Domains of neuropsychological impairment

General cognitive function

In children with frank HIV encephalopathy, the effects of the disease on the CNS tends to be generalized with cognitive function and brain structures severely and globally affected [43, 49, 50], although some domains (i.e. receptive/expressive language, gross/fine motor) may be differentially impaired. Furthermore, measures of general cognitive functioning are sensitive to HIV-related changes in CNS function and correlate well with information obtained through other studies, such as brain imaging [49, 51], cerebrospinal fluid analysis [1, 52] and virological and immunological parameters [53]. However, in children with less severe CNS manifestations, mild cortical atrophy on CT brain scans tends to be more anterior than posterior [7]. Thus, selective functions may be differentially affected by HIV while general cognitive ability is preserved, particularly in the less advanced stages of the disease. Neuropsychological features characteristic of pediatric HIV disease are described below by various domains of functioning.

Language

Children with symptomatic HIV-1 infection frequently exhibit speech and language abnormalities [12, 54–56], which may appear prior to declines in general cognitive function [54, 57] and even when receiving ART [57]. Expressive language is significantly more impaired than receptive language in pediatric HIV disease. Although children with HIV-1 encephalopathy exhibit more deficient overall language skills than non-encephalopathic children, the degree of discrepancy between receptive and expressive language is similar for both these groups [56]. Furthermore, uninfected siblings score higher than their HIV-infected siblings on tests of both expressive and receptive language and do not show a discrepancy between these two language components [56] suggesting that the deficit is related to HIV disease and not environmental factors. Such language deficits may be due in part to an impoverished representation of words and objects likely related to reduced neural networks in the brain [58]. The differential deficit in expressive language also may reflect a more general HIV-associated impairment of expressive behavior [59], including motor function and emotional language [60].

Attention

Attention deficits have been frequently noted in children with HIV-1 infection, however, it is unclear whether an increased prevalence of attentional problems exists in these children and whether these problems are directly attributable to HIV [61, 62]. Attention has many components, such as divided, focused, and sustained attention, which may be differentially affected in pediatric HIV disease. Several studies found increased rates of attentional

Table 17.1 Specific criteria for classification of HIV-related CNS disease in children used at the HIV and AIDS Malignancy Branch of the National Cancer Institute

HIV-related encephalopathy

One or more of the following criteria must be met:

Loss of previously-acquired skills

Significant drop in cognitive test scores, generally to the borderline/delayed range with functional deficits (deficits in day-to-day functioning)

Cognitive test scores are in the borderline/delayed range with functional deficits (and no history of significant drop or previous testing available)

Significantly abnormal neurologic exam with functional deficits (i.e. significant tone, reflex, cerebellar, gait, or movement abnormalities)

Significant improvement in cognitive test scores over approximately a 6-month period associated with a new treatment when baseline scores are in the borderline to delayed range (no history of previous testing) with or without significant brain imaging or neurologic abnormalities (retrospective classification).

Subtypes of HIV encephalopathy

Progressive:

Subacute: Children exhibit a loss of previously acquired skills, resulting in a significant decline in raw and standard score on psychometric tests, and new neurologic abnormalities

Plateau: Children either do not gain further skills or exhibit a slowed rate of development compared with their previous rate of development, resulting in a significant drop in standard scores on psychometric tests

Static: Children exhibit consistent but slower than normal development in the delayed range or their neuropsychological functioning remains stable for at least 1 year after a significant decline (IQ scores remain below average and without significant decline for at least 1 year).

HIV-related CNS compromise

One or more of the following criteria must be met:

Significant drop in cognitive test scores, but generally still above the delayed range, with or without mild brain imaging abnormalities, with no loss of previously acquired skills and no apparent functional deficits (adaptive behavior and school performance stable) or

Cognitive test scores in the borderline range, with no significant functional deficits (and no history of significant drop or previous testing)

Cognitive test scores within normal limits (low average range or above) with no significant functional deficits and moderate to severe brain imaging abnormalities consistent with HIV-related changes

Abnormal neurologic findings but not significantly affecting function

Significant improvement in cognitive test scores over approximately a 6-month period associated with a new treatment when baseline scores are in the low average to average range (no history of previous testing) and no neurologic or brain-imaging abnormalities (retrospective classification)

Non-HIV-related CNS condition

Overall cognitive test scores or selective areas of deficits below the Low Average range, but careful review of medical and family history suggests factors other than HIV disease most likely explain the low scores

Considerations for classification of HIV encephalopathy or CNS compromise

No other factors can reasonably explain the drop in cognitive test scores, compromised/delayed cognitive functioning, and/or abnormal neurologic exam (such as myopathy, neuropathy, cord lesions, CNS opportunistic infections, neoplasms, or vascular diseases, non-HIV-related developmental or learning disabilities, behavioral problems, or psychosocial/environmental circumstances), and the impairments are considered most likely due to HIV, classify as either HIV-related encephalopathy or CNS compromise (depending on the criteria met)

If other factors (i.e. behavioral, acute illness, other infection, etc.) may *possibly* explain the drop in scores or low cognitive functioning, do *not* classify as HIV-related CNS compromise or encephalopathy and re-evaluate at a later time

Table 17.1 (*cont.*)

Definitions used in the criteria

Significant decline in cognitive function:

For infants from birth to 42 months (on the Bayley Scales)[a,b]

A decline of 2 standard deviations (30 points) in the Mental Developmental Index (MDI) on the Bayley Scales, or

A decline of 1 standard deviation (15 points) in the MDI to the mildly delayed range or below on the Bayley Scales (< 85), maintained over two assessments (separated by at least 1 month), or

A loss of raw score over any period greater/equal to 2 months

For children > 30 months (on IQ tests)[a,b]

A loss of ≥ 1 standard deviation in McCarthy GCI (16 points) or Wechsler Full Scale IQ (15 points) *and* at least 15%, or

A loss of ≥ 20 IQ points in *either* the Verbal or Performance Composite Scores,

[a]The significant drop in scores occurs within approximately 1 year.

[b]Cannot attribute the decline in cognitive functioning to other factors (such as change in test, behavioral/emotional factors, lack of appropriate schooling, acute illness, medication effects, other diseases of the CNS, etc.)

Significant improvement in cognitive function:

For infants from birth to 42 months (on the Bayley Scales)[c]

An increase of 1 to 2 standard deviations in the MDI (15 to 30 points) maintained over at least 2 assessments, dependent in part on the age of the child.

For children > 30 months (on IQ tests)[c]

The same degree of change as with a significant decline, except test scores increase rather than decrease.

[c]Occurs within approximately 6-months of starting a new antiretroviral treatment.

[d]Cannot be attributed to other factors, such as a change in environment of caregivers, effect of other medications, improvement in test behavior, etc.

Ranges used in the criteria:		
Cognitive functioning:		Brain Imaging:
Average range	90–110	Degree of cortical atrophy (mild = 1, moderate = 2, severe = 3)
Low average range	80–89	Absence = 0/presence = 1 of basal ganglia calcifications
Borderline range	70–79	
Delayed range	< 70	*Rating of severity:*
		Mild = 1
		Moderate = 2
		Severe = 3 +

* This pediatric HIV CNS classification system was developed by Wolters, Brouwers, and Civitello

problems in HIV-positive children, but also in various uninfected control groups [61–63], suggesting an etiology other than HIV. On the other hand, studies assessing attention using continuous performance tasks suggest that children and adults with HIV-1 infection exhibit deficits in sustained attention [64, 65] that appear related to HIV disease since these deficits are not found in uninfected control groups. Attention deficits in children with HIV-1 may contribute to school and learning problems and may respond to stimulant medication.

Memory

In general, studies of children with vertically acquired HIV-1 infection have documented memory impairments [66–68] while studies of children with transfusion-acquired HIV infection, either for hemophilia or neonatal problems, have not found deficits in memory function [62, 63, 69, 70]. More recently, however, declines in memory functioning over time were found in HIV-infected hemophiliacs with low CD4[+] counts [71]. In addition, children with evidence of HIV CNS compromise exhibited significantly poorer performance on verbal learning and recall trials compared with children without CNS compromise, while these two groups performed similarly on a recognition task [72, 73]. Such a pattern suggests a retrieval deficit, which is similar to findings from studies of memory in HIV-infected adults, and may indicate subcortical pathology [74–76]. Since the memory deficits are more frequent and severe in children with neurologic abnormalities [68, 72, 73] and poorer immune function [71], the etiology is likely related to HIV infection rather than other factors.

Behavioral functioning

In addition to cognitive deficits, children with HIV-1 infection also may display behavioral abnormalities. Behavioral functioning may be negatively influenced by the effects of HIV disease on the CNS, the psychological stresses of living with a chronic illness, and other familial genetic factors. As assessed by a standardized parent report scale, children with encephalopathy exhibited more severe impairments in everyday behaviors, such as daily living skills and socialization skills, compared with children without encephalopathy [77]. Futhermore, deficits in adaptive behavior were associated with CT brain scan abnormalities [51] and immune status [78], and improved with ART [77], suggesting that impairments in adaptive functioning are related to the effects of HIV-1 on the CNS. In contrast, several studies found similar levels of emotional and behavioral problems, including hyperactivity, when comparing HIV-infected children with HIV-exposed but uninfected children [61, 79] and/or with a demographically matched non-HIV-exposed control group [61, 80] as assessed on behavior checklists completed by the primary caregiver. These findings suggest that some behavior problems are not related to the effects of HIV on the CNS but rather to other etiologies, such as environmental conditions, biological factors, or psychosocial difficulties.

Motor functioning

Children with HIV-1 CNS disease frequently exhibit motor impairments, which often co-exist with cognitive deficits [33, 81, 82]. In a large multicenter clinical trial, approximately 23% of symptomatic children who were naïve to antiretroviral therapy exhibited some type of motor dysfunction [33]. Infants less than 1 year of age developed motor impairments more frequently than school-age children (45% vs 9%, respectively) [33]. Children with encephalopathy exhibit the most severe motor involvement and may lose previously attained motor milestones [44]. Gross motor function, particularly running speed and agility, tends to be more impaired than fine motor skills [83]. Oral-motor functioning also may be

affected, resulting in articulation problems, expressive language deficits, and feeding and swallowing difficulties [55]. Motor deficits may interfere with developmental progress and the performance of everyday living skills. Furthermore, motor dysfunction is highly predictive of later disease progression [30]. Thus, the evaluation of motor skills is an important part of the neurobehavioral assessment. Please see Chapter 26 for more information on motor dysfunction in pediatric AIDS.

17.2 Neurobehavioral assessment of children and adolescents with HIV-1 infection

17.2.1 Purposes of neurobehavioral assessment

Psychological assessment is a critical component of the comprehensive multidisciplinary evaluation of children and adolescents with HIV-1 disease and serves three main purposes: (1) to determine whether neurobehavioral deficits may be attributed to HIV associated factors, which is important when considering therapeutic options; (2) to monitor neurobehavioral growth over time to assess the longitudinal effects of HIV on the CNS and evaluate the effectiveness and possible toxicities of antiretroviral therapies; and (3) to identify strengths and weaknesses in neurobehavioral functioning to assist the multidisciplinary team with planning for rehabilitative, educational, and psychosocial interventions [84]. Furthermore, deficient scores on neuropsychological tests and motor dysfunction predict later disease progression, independently from virological and immunological markers [29, 30], and thus, may be useful to predict long-term outcomes in children with HIV infection.

17.2.2 Methodological issues in longitudinal neurobehavioral assessment

Repeated assessments are necessary to monitor neurobehavioral development over time. When conducting longitudinal assessments of children and adolescents with HIV-1 disease the following methodological issues need to be considered: (1) Selection of domains for assessment; (2) evaluation of developmental change over time; (3) frequency of repeated testing and practice effects; (4) special test administration procedures; and (5) interpretation of test results, specifically the attribution of observed impairments or changes to HIV, its treatments, or other factors.

Selection of domains for assessment
Many abilities may be affected by HIV and should be evaluated in the neurobehavioral assessment or by professionals

Table 17.2 List of the neurobehavioral functions to be assessed and psychometric tests that can be used as part of a comprehensive psychological assessment of children with HIV infection

Function	Psychometric test	Age range*
General intelligence	Bayley Scales of Infant Development (Mental)-2nd edn. [116]	1–3.5
	Mullen Scales of Early Learning [117]	0–5.8
	Differential Abilities Scale – Preschool and School Age Levels [118]	2.6–17.11
	McCarthy Scales of Children's Abilities [119]	2.4–8.6
	Wechsler Preschool and Primary Scale of Intelligence-III [120]	2.6–7.3
	Wechsler Intelligence Scale for Children-4th edn. [121]	6–16.11
	Wechsler Adult Intelligence Scale-III [122]	16–74
Language	Peabody Picture Vocabulary Test-III [123]	2.5–90
	Expressive Vocabulary Test [124]	2.6–90
	Verbal Fluency [125]	> 2.5
	Preschool Language Scale [126]	0–6
	Clinical Evaluation of Language Fundamentals – III [127]	6–21
Visuospatial	Developmental Test of Visual-Motor Integration-4R [128]	3–17.11
Memory and learning	Children's Memory Scale [129]	5–16.11
	California Verbal Learning Test-Children's Version [130]	5–16.11
	McCarthy Memory Scale [119]	2.4–8.6
	Stanford-Binet Memory Scale-5th edn. [131]	2–90
Attention	Digit Span Subtest [121, 122]	≥ 6
	Trail Making Test [132]	≥ 6
	Connors' Continous Performance Task II [133]	≥ 6
Concept formation	Ravens Progressive Matrices [134]	≥ 5.5
Motor function	Bayley Scales of Infant Development (Motor)-2nd edn. [116]	0–2 1/2
	Peabody Developmental Motor Scales [135]	0.5–6
	Bruininks–Oseretsky Test of Motor Proficiency [136]	> 5.5
	Grooved Pegboard [137]	> 5
Behavior	Vineland Adaptive Behavior Scales [138]	0–19
	Achenbach Child Behavior Checklist [139]	2–16
	Connors' Rating Scales [140]	3–17
	Behavior Assessment System for Children [141]	2.6–18
	Behavior Rating Inventory of Executive Function [142]	5–18

* Age range in years, for which the test is standardized.

from other disciplines, including neurology, neuroradiology, and rehabilitation medicine.

Neurobehavioral assessment

The neurobehavioral assessment battery should include an age-appropriate measure of general mental abilities such as an intelligence test. In addition, one should include tests that evaluate specific abilities such as language (receptive, expressive), attention (sustain, shift), visuospatial function, motor (fine, gross), memory (visual, verbal), and

executive function, which may identify the more subtle effects of HIV on the CNS that may not be found when using an overall general cognitive measure [57]. In addition to evaluating neurocognitive functioning, measures of the child's relevant everyday behaviors and quality of life in the home environment should be obtained, such as a measure of adaptive behavior. Assessment of socio-emotional functioning and academic achievement are also recommended particularly when the child or adolescent is exhibiting difficulties in these domains. Table 17.2 lists the neurobehavioral functions to be assessed and representative tests to be used as part of a comprehensive psychological assessment for different ages of children and adolescents with HIV-1 infection.

Referral for assessment by other disciplines

Deterioration in gait or speech, a slowed rate of development, or decline in neurobehavioral test scores, may suggest HIV-related CNS disease and a child with any of these symptoms should be referred to a neurologist for further evaluation. Focal neurobehavioral deficits or abrupt changes in mental status, even in those with pre-existing HIV-related CNS disease, may indicate secondary CNS complications, including opportunistic infections, stroke, and neoplastic processes [48]. Such changes in functioning should prompt immediate and thorough medical, neuroimaging, and neurologic evaluations. In addition, children who exhibit oral-motor or speech deficits should be referred to a speech pathologist while children with motor dysfunction should be referred to a physical and occupational therapist for further evaluation and rehabilitation services [55, 85].

Assessing developmental change over time

When longitudinally assessing children it is imperative to use standardized tests with reliable age norms. Most children will show developmental growth over time but the critical factor is to determine whether the rate of this growth is the same, greater, or smaller than the normative group. Differences in the growth rate of neurobehavioral functions, reflected by changes in the standardized test scores of children with HIV-1 infection, may be related to the CNS effects of HIV disease or antiretroviral treatment. However, the impact of socio-environmental, psychosocial, and educational factors should also be taken into consideration. Studies of children with other disorders have indicated that environmental, socio-demographic, and family factors (family distress, family functioning, family resources, parent adjustment, and family interactions) may modify neurodevelopmental course and affect outcome following an insult to the CNS [86, 87].

As the child grows older, test instruments need to be changed to utilize age-appropriate measures and norms, since most standardized psychometric tests for children have restricted age ranges [88]. If the child is part of a longitudinal study, it is best to continue using the same test administered at baseline for as long as possible so congruent comparisons can be made over time. Age overlap exists between most commonly used tests, allowing for some flexibility in changing to the next age-appropriate measure. It is often difficult to interpret the meaning of interval change when a new test is administered. Therefore, the change to a new instrument should be done when the child is considered healthy with no new developmental concerns. When transitioning from the child to the adult version of the Wechsler intelligence test, often used in longitudinal HIV studies, minimal effects have been found [89]. Therefore, if the scores decline significantly when changing between these tests, the drop may be due to HIV-related CNS disease. In this situation, re-administering the new test or the one that was previously given should be done as soon as repeat testing is considered valid for a chronically ill population (i.e. in 6 months) to continue monitoring the child's CNS status.

Frequency of repeated testing and practice effects

When planning for a follow-up neurobehavioral evaluation, several factors need to be considered including the child's potential risk of developing CNS disease, the rate of disease progression, possible treatment effects, and potential practice effects. For example, infants and young children with HIV-1 infection have a higher risk of developing severe CNS disease than older children or adults and practice effects are less of a concern for this young age group. Therefore, shorter intervals between testing are recommended for infants and young children. On the other hand, school-age children and adolescents with HIV-1 infection have a lower probability of developing CNS disease, tend to exhibit more subtle neurocognitive changes, and are more likely to demonstrate practice effects. Thus, test-retest intervals need to be longer in older children and adolescents, particularly in those without evidence of HIV-related CNS disease or those with higher IQs who may show more benefit from repeated assessments [89]. However, IQ scores from the Wechsler Intelligence Scales in children and adolescents were found to be highly reliable and free of significant practice effects over several years, supporting their use in longitudinal studies [89]. In consideration of these assessment issues, the recommended neurobehavioral testing schedule for children with HIV-1 is presented in Table 17.3.

Special test administration procedures

Some children with HIV-1 infection may exhibit special needs that require modification of the psychological test battery or procedures to obtain a valid assessment of their cognitive function. For example, children with HIV-related CNS disease may have impaired gross and/or fine motor skills, sensory defects, or diminished expressive language. Some children may exhibit high activity levels, short attention spans, and uncooperative behaviors, or become fatigued during the test session, which can make the

Table 17.3 Recommended neurodevelopmental serial assessment schedule for children with HIV-1 infection at various ages

Age of child	Serial assessment schedule
< 2 year	Evaluate every 6 months due to a higher risk of developing CNS disease
2–8 years	Evaluate every year unless they exhibit neurodevelopmental deficits, in which case they should be assessed every 6 months*
> 8 years	Evaluate every 2 years if child exhibits stable functioning in the average range; otherwise, evaluate every year*

* Shorter batteries of individual subtests and specific function tests can be administered between the major evaluations to further decrease the testing burden on children while still monitoring the effects of the disease.

evaluation process difficult to complete. Finally, some children may not be fluent in English.

For children who cannot be assessed with the standard assessment battery due to visual, hearing, or physical impairments, alternative tests that are designed specifically for children with these disabilities or non-standard assessment procedures (i.e. use of interpreters or eye gaze instead of a pointing response) should be used. For a child who is easily fatigued or exhibits behavioral difficulties, the examiner may need to use behavior management techniques or multiple test sessions. Testing should be conducted when the child is in an optimal state. Thus, the child should not be febrile, hungry or sleep deprived, and testing after certain medical procedures, such as sedation, eye dilation, or those that are upsetting to the child, should be avoided.

Differential diagnosis

The determination of whether a child's neurobehavioral deficits or change in functioning is related to HIV disease as opposed to other medical, environmental, or social factors is critical for the formulation of an effective treatment plan. If a change in neurobehavioral function is abrupt, or the manifestations are focal or lateralized, the etiology may be due to non-HIV-related medical causes, such as opportunistic infections, stroke, or neoplastic processes [48]. In such cases, immediate referral for a neurologic evaluation, neuroimaging studies, and examination of CSF is critical for determining the appropriate diagnosis and treatment. If a change in neurobehavioral functioning is attributed to HIV-1 infection, then the selection of a treatment regimen

that may be relatively more effective at inhibiting viral replication within the CNS is important. If the changes or the deficits are more consistent with other non-HIV associated factors, such as birth trauma, or are considered a static expression of earlier HIV-associated CNS insult, then specific treatments targeting CNS viral replication are less of a concern. Determining the etiology of CNS manifestations in children with HIV infection is challenging due to the wide range of functions that may be affected, the progressive nature of the disease, and the pre-existing medical conditions or environmental factors that may confound the effects of HIV on the CNS. Following is a brief description of information to be considered when interpreting neurobehavioral test results and changes in CNS function.

(a) Birth and medical history. Birth trauma, hypoxia, severe prematurity, low birth weight, maternal substance abuse, exposure to toxic substances (i.e. lead), CNS infections other than HIV, head injuries, and chronic illnesses may alter neurobehavioral development, resulting in delays and deficits. Thus, such factors need to be considered when determining whether CNS manifestations are related to HIV.

(b) Developmental and educational history. A loss or no substantial gain over previously acquired developmental milestones in young children or declining school performance in older children may indicate HIV-related CNS effects. Lack of appropriate environmental stimulation or schooling, however, also may result in a gradual decline in psychometric test scores over time [90]. Thus, the child's caregiver should be carefully interviewed about these issues.

(c) Psychometric test results. Comparing current test scores with previous results is important for evaluating whether changing neurobehavioral functioning may be related to HIV-1 infection and its treatment. Obtaining test results from assessments done at the child's school also may facilitate the interpretation of current neurobehavioral scores. A significant decline in test scores may indicate a progression in HIV-related CNS disease [32], suggesting the need for a possible adjustment of antiretroviral treatment, while a significant improvement may suggest a reversal of deficits related to treatment effects.

Inspection of the neuropsychological profile also is useful to identify patterns of deficits that have been related to HIV disease. For example, patients in the milder stages of CNS compromise tend to exhibit somewhat more pronounced patterns of strengths and weaknesses in selective domains such as language, memory, psychomotor speed, and attention, compared with children with encephalopathy who display a more global pattern of severe impairment. Deviations from such profiles may require a more in-depth assessment to rule out alternative explanations.

(d) Environment and family factors. Various environmental factors, such as culture, education, and socioeconomic status can influence the development of a child's cognitive abilities [90, 91] as well as their response to brain injury [86, 87]. The general cognitive ability of children and their parents and siblings are strongly correlated [92] and some behavioral and learning problems are hereditary [93]. When previous test results are not available for comparison, consideration of the environment and family can help to grossly estimate whether delays or deficits may be associated with HIV disease. Such interpretations should be done with extreme caution since many other factors may influence cognitive development, including lack of regular school attendance and lengthy hospitalizations.

(e) Neuroimaging findings. Children with HIV-related CNS disease often exhibit neuroimaging abnormalities that may be correlated with their level of neurocognitive functioning [7, 49]. Brain imaging studies together with the psychometric test results can help determine whether neurobehavioral deficits may be related to HIV. In particular, the presence and severity of cortical atrophy may be a good indicator of the degree of HIV-related CNS compromise in children [45, 94]. As assessed by computed tomography (CT) brain scans, intra-cerebral calcifications in young vertically infected children have been associated with poor prognosis and encephalopathy, particularly when moderate to severe cortical atrophy is also noted. These calcifications tend to progress despite treatment, even when improvements in neurocognitive functioning or other imaging measures are observed [94]. This pattern suggests that cerebral calcifications, once present, do not reflect disease progression. Minor white matter abnormalities detected on MRI have not been associated with altered cognitive function [95]. More extensive white matter changes, i.e. when they become evident on CT scans, have been associated with cognitive impairments [51].

Proton magnetic resonance spectroscopy (^{1}HMRS) allows for non-invasive measurement of brain metabolites associated with different aspects of cell function [96], which may provide early markers of HIV infection in the brain that are detectable prior to changes in cognitive function or structural neuroimaging [97, 98]. Studies in children with symptomatic HIV infection, particularly those with HIV-associated CNS disease, have commonly found a decrease in N-acetyl aspartate (NAA) signal or the NAA/Cr (creatine) ratio, which both suggest a decrease in neuronal density, and an increase in the lactate signal, which may indicate active inflammation or severe tissue damage causing impaired blood perfusion and resulting ischemia [98–101]. In one study, initiation of antiretroviral therapy in two children with progressive encephalopathy resulted in an increase in the NAA/Cr ratio and a decrease in the lactate peak [101]. Magnetic resonance spectroscopy is not a standard component of the clinical evaluation of children with HIV but clearly offers possibilities to further monitor HIV-associated CNS disease, evaluate the effects of therapy, and investigate the neuropathogenesis of neurobehavioral manifestations.

(f) Neurological findings. Motor and cognitive deficits are each frequent indicators of HIV-related CNS disease but may be found independent of one another [44]. Tone abnormalities, such as spastic diplegia and central hypotonia, and movement disorders, such as rigidity, bradykinesia, and dystonia that affect day-to-day functioning suggest HIV-related encephalopathy. Neuropathies as potential side effects of treatment or manifestations of HIV disease also need to be evaluated. As stated earlier, if changes in neurobehavioral function are acute, focal, or lateralized, the patient should be referred immediately for further medical and neurological evaluations to investigate non-HIV-related etiologies. See Chapter 26 for more details.

(g) Behavioral observations. Direct observation by the examiner of the child's behavior during the interview and testing, including affect, attention, activity level, response style, dealing with difficulties and failures on various subtests, and parent–child interaction is critical for interpreting neuropsychological test results. Behavioral ratings of the child's functioning in the home and school environment obtained from parent, teacher, and self-report questionnaires, provide additional information. In conjunction with the neurocognitive test scores, such behavioral information can help determine whether some behaviors are attributable to HIV or other factors.

(h) Immunological and virological testing. Low CD4$^+$ T lymphocyte counts and high plasma HIV-1 RNA concentrations strongly predict HIV disease progression [102, 103] and have been associated with more severe cognitive impairments and brain imaging abnormalities [38, 53]. Furthermore, a decrease in the fraction of lymphocytes that are CD4$^+$ T cells have been associated with increases in cognitive dysfunction and brain-imaging abnormalities [45]. The concentrations of HIV-1 RNA in the CSF were higher and detected more often in encephalopathic children than those without encephalopathy [1, 104] and were associated with the degree of cortical atrophy [94]. However, the level of HIV-1 RNA in the plasma is not consistently correlated with such levels in the CSF and may not be a good indicator of the effects of HIV on the CNS in children [1, 94].

These data seem to suggest that the CNS may be a distinct compartment with regard to viral replication. Immune and plasma virologic measures can thus be utilized to evaluate the significance of neurobehavioral test data but should be used with caution due to inter- and intra-patient variability, compartmentalization of the CNS, and the modifying factor of treatment, which may act differently on the markers of the immunologic, virologic [105], and neurologic domains. This potential CNS compartmentalization of HIV-1 replication may have important implications for the evolution of resistant virus during ART, particularly considering the inefficient penetration of many antiretroviral agents into the CNS.

(i) Other evaluations. Children with HIV-1 infection are at risk for opportunistic infections that may impair vision and hearing, which in turn can negatively affect developmental and psychological test performance. Thus, audiological and ophthalmological evaluations are very important for interpreting psychometric test results. Physical, occupational, and speech therapy evaluations provide additional valuable data regarding the child's neurobehavioral functioning. Social workers can supply useful information regarding the child's family history and current home environment. All members of the multidisciplinary team contribute data that can be useful for determining if the child's neurobehavioral functioning has been affected by HIV or other factors.

17.3 Effects of antiretroviral treatment on cognitive function

Antiretroviral treatment may be preventative and/or therapeutic for HIV-associated CNS disease. With the availability of effective HAART, the prevention of CNS disease appears to be related to the suppression of systemic viral replication, which reduces or eliminates the invasion of HIV-carrying cells into the CNS. However, the CNS is a separate compartment from the rest of the body and it may serve as a reservoir for persistent HIV-1 infection [24]. Some antiretroviral agents have been found to penetrate the blood–brain barrier [26, 106, 107], inhibit viral replication in the CNS [108, 109], and reduce the neurotoxic effects of the virus on the brain [9, 110]. In children with evidence of HIV-associated CNS manifestations, treatment studies have shown that some antiretroviral drugs, particularly used in combination [28], may improve neurobehavioral functioning [111–113] as well as cortical atrophy [114]. These improvements in CNS functioning are likely due to treatment-related decreases in viral replication in the brain [109, 115]. Thus, children with HIV-related neurobehavioral deficits should be given antiretroviral therapy that includes at least one agent that has adequate CNS penetration, such as ZDV or stavudine (d4T). Therapy for HIV disease is discussed in more detail in Chapters 18 and 22.

17.4 Summary

Neurobehavioral deficits can be a significant morbidity of pediatric HIV-1 infection. Since no current measure can predict which children may develop HIV-related CNS disease, regular psychometric testing can identify early neurobehavioral changes in functioning. The development of HIV-related neurobehavioral deficits indicates the need for antiretroviral therapy that is active within the CNS. Longitudinal neurobehavioral assessments are important for evaluating response to treatment. Findings from psychometric testing also are useful for planning appropriate individual educational, rehabilitative, and psychosocial interventions. In addition, as older children and adolescents with HIV infection become increasingly responsible for taking their medications, adherence to complex treatment regimens may be negatively affected by neurobehavioral deficits, which should be monitored and taken into consideration when instructing these patients about their medications. Periodic monitoring of neurobehavioral functioning is critical for the appropriate management of HIV-1 infection in children and adolescents and should be used in conjunction with other data to plan an effective treatment strategy for the child or adolescent and their family.

ACKNOWLEDGMENTS

Support for this chapter was provided to Pam Wolters by HIV and AIDS Malignancy Branch, National Cancer Institute Research Contract #NO1-SC-07006 awarded to the Medical Illness Counseling Center, Chevy Chase, MD and to Pim Brouwers by National Institute of Health grants U01-A127551-15 and U01-JD41983 awarded to Baylor College of Medicine, Houston, TX.

REFERENCES

1. Sei, S., Stewart, S. K., Farley, M. *et al.* Evaluation of human immunodeficiency virus (HIV) type 1 RNA levels in cerebrospinal fluid and viral resistance to zidovudine in children with HIV encephalopathy. *J. Infect. Dis.* **174** : **6** (1996), 1200–6.
2. Zheng, J. & Gendelman, H. E. The HIV-1 associated dementia complex: a metabolic encephalopathy fueled by viral

replication in mononuclear phagocytes. *Curr. Opin. Neurol.* **10** : 4 (1997), 319–25.

3. Lyman, W. D., Kress, Y., Kure, K., Rashbaum, W., Rubinstein, A. & Soeiro, R. Detection of HIV in fetal central nervous system tissue. *AIDS* **4** (1990), 917–20.

4. Ho, D., Rota, T., Schooley, R. *et al.* Isolation of HTLV-III from cerebrospinal fluid and neural tissues of patients with neurologic syndromes related to the acquired immunodeficiency syndrome. *New Engl. J. Med.* **313** : 24 (1985), 1493–7.

5. Davis, L., Hjelle, B. L., Miller, V. E. *et al.* Early viral brain invasion in iatrogenic human immunodeficiency virus infection. *Neurology* **42** (1992), 1736–9.

6. Civitello, L., Brouwers, P., DeCarli, C. & Pizzo, P. Calcification of the basal ganglia in children with HIV infection. *Ann. Neurol.* **36** (1994), 506.

7. DeCarli, C., Civitello, L. A., Brouwers, P. & Pizzo, P. A. The prevalence of computed axial tomographic abnormalities of the cerebrum in 100 consecutive children symptomatic with the human immune deficiency virus. *Ann. Neurol.* **34** : 2 (1993), 198–205.

8. Smith, R., Malee, K., Charurat, M. *et al.* Timing of perinatal human immunodeficiency virus type 1 infection and rate of neurodevelopment. *Pediatr. Infect. Dis. J.* **19** (2000), 862–71.

9. Gendelman, H. E., Zheng, J., Coulter, C. L. *et al.* Suppression of inflammatory neurotoxins by highly active antiretroviral therapy in Human Immunodeficiency Virus-associated dementia. *J. Infect. Dis.* **178** (1998), 1000–7.

10. Sharer, L. R. & Mintz, M. Neuropathology of AIDS in children. In F. Scaravilli (ed.), *AIDS : the Pathology of the Nervous System.* Berlin : Springer Verlag (1993), pp. 201–14.

11. Belman, A. L., Diamond, G., Dickson, D. *et al.* Pediatric acquired immunodeficiency syndrome : neurologic syndromes. *Am. J. Dis. Child.* **142** : 1 (1988), 29–35.

12. Epstein, L. G. Neurologic manifestations of HIV infection in children. *Pediatrics* **78** : 4 (1986), 678–87.

13. Blanche, S., Newell, M., Mayaux, M. *et al.* Morbidity and mortality in European children vertically infected by HIV-1. *J. AIDS Hum. Retrovirol.* **14** (1997), 442–50.

14. Lobato, M. N., Caldwell, M. B., Ng, P. & Oxtoby, M. J. Encephalopathy in children with perinatally acquired human immunodeficiency virus infection. *J. Pediatrics* **126** : 5 (1995), 710–5.

15. Cooper, E. R., Hanson, C., Diaz, C. *et al.* Encephalopathy and progression of human immunodeficiency virus disease in a cohort of children with perinatally acquired human immunodeficiency virus infection. Women and Infants Transmission Study Group. *J. Pediatr.* **132** : 5 (1998), 808–12.

16. Tardieu, M., Chenadec, J. L., Persoz, A., Meyer, L., Blanche, S. & Mayaux, M. J. HIV-1-related encephalopathy in infants compared with children and adults. *Neurology* **54** (2000), 1089–95.

17. Mintz, M. Clinical comparison of adult and pediatric NeuroAIDS. *Adv. Neuroimmunol.* **4** (1994), 207–21.

18. Mitchell, W. Neurological and developmental effects of HIV and AIDS in children and adolescents. *Mental Retard. Develop. Disabilities Res. Rev.* **7** (2001), 211–16.

19. Brodt, H. R., Kamps, B. S., Gute, P., Knupp, B., Staszewski, S. & Helm, E. B. Changing incidence of AIDS-defining illnesses in the era of antiretroviral combination therapy. *AIDS* **11** (1997), 1731–8.

20. d'Arminio Monforte, A., Duca, P. G., Vago, L., Grassi, M. P. & Moroni, M. Decreasing incidence of CNS AIDS-defining events associated with antiretroviral therapy. *Neurology* **54** (2000), 1856–9.

21. Palella, F. J., Delaney, K. M., Moorman, A. C. *et al.* Declining morbidity and mortality among patients with advanced human immunodeficiency virus infection. *New Engl. J. Med.* **338** : 13 (1998), 853–60.

22. Tardieu, M. & Boutet, A. HIV-1 and the central nervous system. In *Current Topics in Microbiology and Immunology.* Berlin : Springer Verlag (2002), pp. 183–95.

23. Deeks, S. G., Smith, M., Holodniy, M. & Kahn, J. O. HIV-1 Protease Inhibitors. *J. Am. Med. Assoc.* **277** : 2 (1997), 145–53.

24. Sonza, S. & Crowe, S. Reservoirs for HIV infection and their persistence in the face of undetectable viral load. *AIDS Patient Care and STDs* **15** : 10 (2001), 511–18.

25. Aweeka, F., Jayewaardene, A., Staprana, S. *et al.* Failure to detect nelfinaavir in the cerebrospinal fluid of HIV-1-infected patients with and without AIDS dementia complex. *J. AIDS Hum. Retroviol.* **20** (1999), 39–43.

26. Swindells, S. *Therapy of HIV-1 Infection : A Practical Guide for Providers.* New York, NY : Chapman & Hall (1998).

27. Dore, G. J., Correll, P. K., Li, Y., Kaldor, J. M., Coopera, D. A. & Brew, B. J. Changes to AIDS dementia complex in the era of highly active antiretroviral therapy. *AIDS* **13** (1999), 1249–53.

28. Raskino, C., Pearson, D. A., Baker, C. J. *et al.* Neurologic, neurocognitive, and brain growth outcomes in human immunodeficiency virus-infected children receiving different nucleoside antiretroviral regimens. *Pediatrics* **104** : 3 (1999), e32.

29. Llorente, A. M., Brouwers, P., Charurat, M. *et al.* Early neurodevelopmental markers predictive of morbidity and mortality in infants infected with HIV-1. *Dev. Med. Child Neurol.* **45** : 2 (2003), 76–84.

30. Pearson, D. A., McGrath, N. M., Nozyce, M. *et al.* Predicting HIV disease progression in children using measures of neuropsychological and neurological functioning. Pediatric AIDS clinical trials 152 study team. *Pediatrics* **106** : 6 (2000), E76.

31. Chase, C., Vibbert, M., Pelton, S., Coulter, D. & Cabral, H. Early neurodevelopmental growth in children with vertically transmitted human immunodeficiency virus infection. *Arch. Pediatr. Adolesc. Med.* **149** (1995), 850–5.

32. Chase, C., Ware, J., Hittelman, J. *et al.* Early cognitive and motor development among infants born to women infected with human immunodeficiency virus. *Pediatrics* **106** : 2 (2000), E25.

33. Englund, J. A., Baker, C. J., Raskino, C. *et al.* Clinical and laboratory characteristics of a large cohort of symptomatic, human immunodeficiency virus-infected infants and children. *Pediatr. Infect. Dis. J.* **15** (1996), 1025–36.

34. McKinney, R. E., Johnson, G. M., Stanley, K. *et al.* A randomized study of combined zidovudine-lamivudine versus didanosine

monotherapy in children with symptomatic therapy-naive HIV-1 infection. *J. Pediatr.* **133** : **4** (1998), 500–8.

35. Mayaux, M. J., Burgard, M., Teglas, J.-P. *et al.* Neonatal characteristics in rapidly progressive perinatally acquired HIV-1 disease. *J. Am. Med. Assoc.* **275** : **8** (1996), 606–10.

36. Blanche, S., Mayaux, M. J., Rouzioux, C. *et al.* Relation of the course of HIV infection in children to the severity of the disease in their mothers at delivery. *New Engl. J. Med.* **330** : **5** (1994), 308–12.

37. Lindsey, J. C., Hughes, M. D., McKinney, R. E. *et al.* Treatment-mediated changes in human immunodeficiency virus (HIV) Type I RNA and CD4 cell counts as predictors of weight growth failure, cognitive decline, and survival in HIV-infected children. *J. Infect. Dis.* **182** (2000), 1385–93.

38. Pollack, H., Kuchuk, A., Cowan, L. *et al.* Neurodevelopment, growth, and viral load in HIV-infected infants. *Brain, Behav. Immunity* **10** (1996), 298–312.

39. Just, J., Abrams, E., Louie, L. *et al.* Influence of host genotype on progression to acquired immunodeficiency syndrome among children infected with human immunodeficiency virus type 1. *J. Pediatrics* **127** (1995), 544–9.

40. Sei, S., Boler, A. M., Nguyen, G. T. *et al.* Protective effect of CCR5 delta32 heterozygosity is restricted by SDF-1 genotype in children with HIV-1 infection. *AIDS* **15** (2001), 1343–52.

41. Culnane, M., Fowler, M., Lee, S. *et al.* Lack of long-term effects of in utero exposure to zidovudine among uninfected children born to HIV-infected women. *J. Am. Med. Assoc.* **281** : **2** (1999), 151–7.

42. Working Group of the American Academy of Neurology AIDS Task Force. Nomenclature and research case definitions for neurologic manifestations of human immunodeficiency virus-type 1 infection. *Neurology* **41** (1991), 778–85.

43. Wolters, P. L. & Brouwers, P. Evaluation of neurodevelopmental deficits in children with HIV infection. In H. E. Gendelman, S. A. Lipton, L. Epstein & S. Swindells (eds.), *The Neurology of AIDS*. New York, NY : Chapman & Hall (1998), pp. 425–42.

44. Belman, A. L. HIV-1 associated CNS disease in infants and children. In R. W. Price & S. W. Perry (eds.), *HIV, AIDS and the Brain*. New York, NY : Raven Press (1994), pp. 289–310.

45. Brouwers, P., DeCarli, C., Tudor-Williams, G., Civitello, L., Moss, H. A. & Pizzo, P. A. Interrelations among patterns of change in neurocognitive, CT brain imaging, and CD4 measures associated with antiretroviral therapy in children with symptomatic HIV infection. *Adv. Neuroimmunol.* **4** (1994), 223–31.

46. Epstein, L., Sharer, L. R., Joshi, V. V., Fojas, M. M., Koenigsberger, M. R. & Oleske, J. Progressive encephalopathy in children with acquired immune deficiency syndrome. *Ann. Neurol.* **17** (1985), 488–96.

47. Centers for Disease Control. 1994 Revised classification system for human immunodeficiency virus infection in children less than 13 years of age; Official authorized addenda: Human immunodeficiency virus infection codes and official guidelines for coding and reporting ICD-9-CM. *MMWR*: Centers for Disease Control (1994).

48. Brouwers, P., Wolters, P. & Civitello, L. Central nervous system manifestations and assessment. In P. A. Pizzo & C. M. Wilfert (eds.), Pediatric AIDS: *The Challenge of HIV Infection in Infants, Children and Adolescents*, 3rd edn. Philadelphia, PA : Williams & Wilkins (1998), pp. 293–308.

49. Brouwers, P., DeCarli, C., Civitello, L., Moss, H. A., Wolters, P. L. & Pizzo, P. A. Correlation between computed tomographic brain scan abnormalities and neuropsychological function in children with symptomatic human immunodeficiency virus disease. *Arch. Neurol.* **52** (1995), 39–44.

50. Brouwers, P., Belman, A. L. & Epstein, L. Central nervous system involvement: manifestations, evaluation, and pathogenesis. In P. A. Pizzo & C. M. Wilfert (eds.), Pediatric AIDS: *The Challenge of HIV Infection in Infants, Children and Adolescents*, 2nd edn. Baltimore, MD: Williams & Wilkins (1994), pp. 433–55.

51. Brouwers, P., van der Vlugt, H., Moss, H. A., Wolters, P. L. & Pizzo, P. A. White matter changes on CT brain scan are associated with neurobehavioral dysfunction in children with symptomatic HIV disease. *Child Neuropsychol.* **1** : **2** (1995), 93–105.

52. Brouwers, P., Heyes, M. P., Moss, H. A. *et al.* Quinolinic acid in the cerebrospinal fluid of children with symptomatic human immunodeficiency virus type 1 disease : relationship to clinical status and therapeutic response. *J. Infect. Dis.* **168** (1993), 1380–6.

53. Brouwers, P., Tudor-Williams, G., DeCarli, C. *et al.* Relation between stage of disease and neurobehavioral measures in children with symptomatic HIV disease. *AIDS* **9** (1995), 713–20.

54. Coplan, J., Contello, K. A., Cunningham, C. K. *et al.* Early language development in children exposed to or infected with Human Immunodeficiency Virus. *Pediatrics* **102** : **1** (1998), E8.

55. Pressman, H. Communication disorders and dysphagia in pediatric AIDS. *ASHA* **34** (1992), 45–7.

56. Wolters, P. L., Brouwers, P., Moss, H. A. & Pizzo, P. A. Differential receptive and expressive language functioning of children with symptomatic HIV disease and relation to CT scan brain abnormalities. *Pediatrics* **95** (1995), 112–19.

57. Wolters, P. L., Brouwers, P., Civitello, L. & Moss, H. A. Receptive and expressive language function of children with symptomatic HIV infection and relationship with disease parameters: a longitudinal 24 month follow-up study. *AIDS* **11** : **9** (1997), 1135–44.

58. Brouwers, P., Van Engelen, M., Lalonde, F. *et al.* Abnormally increased semantic priming in children with symptomatic HIV-1 disease : evidence for impaired development of semantics? *J. Int. Neuropsychol. Soc.* **7** (2001), 491–501.

59. Moss, H. A., Wolters, P. L., Brouwers, P., Hendricks, M. L. & Pizzo, P. A. Impairment of expressive behavior in pediatric HIV-infected patients with evidence of CNS disease. *J. Pediatr. Psychol.* **21** : **3** (1996), 379–400.

60. Roelofs, K., Wolters, P. L., Fernandez-Carol C, van der Vlugt, H., Moss, H. A. & Brouwers, P. Impairments in expressive emotional language in children with symptomatic HIV infection : relation with brain abnormalities and immune function. *J. Int. Neuropsychol. Soc.* **2** (1996), 193.

61. Havens, J., Whitaker, A., Feldman, J. & Ehrhardt, A. Psychiatric morbidity in school-age children with congenital human immunodeficiency virus infection: A pilot study. *Dev. Behav. Pediatr.* **15** : 3 (1994), S18–25.

62. Whitt, J. K., Hooper, S. R, Tennison, M. B. *et al.* Neuropsychologic functioning of human immunodeficiency virus-infected children with hemophilia. *J. Pediatr.* **122** (1993), 52–9.

63. Loveland, K. A., Stehbens, J., Contant, C. *et al.* Hemophilia growth and development study: Baseline neurodevelopmental findings. *J. Pediatr. Psychol.* **19** : 2 (1994), 223–39.

64. Law, W. A., Mapou, R. L., Roller, T. L., Martin, A., Nannis, E. D. & Temoshok, L. R. Reaction time slowing in HIV-1 infected individuals: role of the preparatory interval. *J. Clin. Exp. Neuropsychol.* **17** : 1 (1995), 122–33.

65. Watkins, J. M., Cool, V. A., Usner, D. *et al.* Attention in HIV-infected children : results from the Hemophilia Growth and Development Study. *J. Int. Neuropsychol. Soc.* **6** : 4 (2000), 443–54.

66. Boivin, M., Green, S., Davies, A., Giordani, B., Mokili, J. & Cutting, W. A preliminary evaluation of the cognitive and motor effects of pediatric HIV infection in Zairian children. *Health Psychol.* **14** : 1 (1995), 13–21.

67. Fundaro, C., Miccinesi, N., Baldieri, N., Genovese, O., Rendeli, C. & Segni, G. Cognitive impairment in school-age children with asymptomatic HIV infection. *AIDS Patient Care STDs* **12** : 2 (1998), 135–40.

68. Levenson, R., Mellins, C., Zawadzki, R., Kairam, R. & Stein, Z. Cognitive assessment of human immunodeficiency virus-exposed children. *Am. J. Dis. Child.* **146** (1992), 1479–83.

69. Cohen, S. E., Mundy, T., Kaarassik, B., Lieb, L., Ludwig, D. D. & Ward, J. Neuropsychological functioning in children with HIV-1 infection through neonatal blood transfusion. *Pediatrics* **88** : 1 (1991), 58–68.

70. Smith, M. L., Minden, D., Netley, C., Read, S., King, S. & Blanchette, V. Longitudinal investigation of neuropsychological functioning in children and adolescents with hemophilia and HIV infection. *Dev. Neuropsychol.* **13** : 1 (1997), 69–85.

71. Loveland, K., Stehbens, J., Mahoney, E. *et al.* Declining immune function in children and adolescents with hemophilia and HIV infection : effects on neuropsychological performance. *J. Pediatr. Psychol.* **25** : 5 (2000), 309–22.

72. Klaas, P., Wolters, P. L., Martin, S., Civitello, L. & Zeichner, S. Verbal learning and memory in children with HIV [Abstract]. *J. Int. Neuropsychol. Soc.* **8** (2002), 187.

73. Perez, L. A., Wolters, P. L., Moss, H. A., Civitello, L. A. & Brouwers, P. Verbal learning and memory in children with HIV infection [Abstract]. *J. Neurovirol.* **4** (1998), 362.

74. Brouwers, P., Mohr, E., Hildebrand, K. *et al.* A novel approach to the determination and characterization of HIV dementia. *Can. J. Neurolog. Sci.* **23** : 2 (1996), 104–9.

75. Stout, J. C., Salmon, D. P., Butters, N. *et al.* Decline in working memory associated with HIV infection. *Psychol. Med.* **25** (1995), 1221–32.

76. White, D., Taylor, M., Butters, N. *et al.* Memory for verbal information in individuals with HIV-associated dementia complex. *J. Clin. Exp. Neuropsychol.* **19** : 3 (1997), 357–66.

77. Wolters, P., Brouwers, P., Moss, H. & Pizzo, P. Adaptive behavior of children with symptomatic HIV infection before and after Zidovudine therapy. *J. Pediatr. Psychol.* **19** : 1 (1994), 47–61.

78. Nichols, S., Mahoney, E., Sirois, P. *et al.* HIV-associated changes in adaptive, emotional, and behavioral functioning in children and adolescents with hemophilia : results from the hemophilia growth and development study. *J. Pediatr. Psychol.* **25** : 8 (2000), 545–56.

79. Mellins, C. A., Smith, R., O'Driscoll, P. *et al.* High rates of behavioral problems in perinatally HIV-infected children are not linked to HIV disease. *Pediatrics* **111** : 2 (2003), 384–93.

80. Bachanas, P., Kullgren, K., Schwartz, K. *et al.* Predictors of psychological adjustment in school-age children infected with HIV. *J. Pediatr. Psychol.* **26** : 6 (2001), 343–52.

81. Aylward, E. H., Butz, A. M., Hutton, N., Joyner, M. L. & Vogelhut, J. W. Cognitive and motor development in infants at risk for human immunodeficiency virus. *Am. J. Dis. Child.* **146** (1992), 218–22.

82. Gay, C. L., Armstrong, F. D., Cohen, D. *et al.* The effects of HIV on cognitive and motor development in children born to HIV-seropositive women with no reported drug use : Birth to 24 months. *Pediatrics* **96** (1995), 1078–82.

83. Parks, R. A. & Danoff, J. V. Motor performance changes in children testing positive for HIV over 2 years. *Am. J. Occup. Ther.* **53** : 5 (1999), 524–8.

84. Wolters, P. L., Brouwers, P. & Moss, H. A. Pediatric HIV disease : effect on cognition, learning, and behavior. *School Psychol. Quart.* **10** : 4 (1995), 305–28.

85. Lord, D., Danoff, J. & Smith, M. Motor assessment of infants with human immunodeficiency virus infection: a retrospective review of multiple cases. *Pediatr. Phys. Ther.* **7** (1995), 9–13.

86. Yeates, K. O., Taylor, H. G., Drotar, D. *et al.* Preinjury family environment as a determinant of recovery from traumatic brain injuries in school-age children. *J. Int. Neuropsychol. Soc.* **3** : 6 (1997), 617–30.

87. Wade, S. L., Drotar, D., Taylor, H. G. & Stancin, T. Assessing the effects of traumatic brain injury on family functioning: conceptual and methodological issues. *J. Pediatr. Psychol.* **20** : 6 (1995), 737–52.

88. Lindsey, J. C., O'Donnell, K. & Brouwers, P. Methodological issues in analyzing psychological test scores in pediatric clinical trials. *J. Dev. Behav. Pediatr.* **21** (2000), 141–51.

89. Sirois, P. A., Posner, M., Stehbens, J. A. *et al.* Quantifying practice effects in longitudinal research with the WISC-R and WAIS-R : a study of children and adolescents with hemophilia and male siblings without hemophilia. *J. Pediatr. Psychol.* **27** : 2 (2002), 121–31.

90. Burchinal, M. R., Campbell, F. A., Bryant, D. M., Wasik, B. H. & Ramey, C. T. Early intervention and mediating processes in cognitive performance of children of low-income African-American families. *Child Dev.* **68** (1997), 935–54.

91. Neisser, U., Boodoo, G., Bouchard, T. J. *et al.* Intelligence: Knowns and unknowns. *Am. Psychol.* **51** (1996), 77–101.

92. Erlenmeyer-Kimling, L & Jarvik, L. F. Genetics and intelligence : A review. *Science* **142** (1963), 1477–9.

93. Pennington, B. F. & Smith, S. D. Genetic influences on learning disabilities and speech and language disorders. *Child Dev.* **54** (1983), 369–87.

94. Brouwers, P., Civitello, L., DeCarli, C., Wolters, P. & Sei, S. Cerebrospinal fluid viral load is related to cortical atrophy and not to intracerebral calcifications in children with symptomatic HIV disease. *J. Neurovirol.* **6 : 5** (2000), 390–6.

95. Tardieu, M., Blanche, S. & Brunelle, F. Cerebral magnetic resonance imaging studies in HIV-1 infected children born to seropositive mothers. Neuroscience of HIV-1 Infection. In *Satellite Conference of Seventh International Conference on AIDS*, Padova, Italy (1991), p. 60.

96. Kauppinen, R. A. & Willimas, S. R. Nuclear magnetic resonance spectroscopy studies of the brain. *Prog. Neurobiol.* **44** (1994), 87–118.

97. McConnell, J. R., Swindells, S., Ong, C. S. *et al.* Prospective utility of cerebral proton magnetic resonance spectroscopy in monitoring HIV infection and its associated neurological impairment. *AIDS Res. Hum. Retrovirus.* **10 : 8** (1994), 977–82.

98. Salvan, A. M., Lamoureux, S., Michel, G. *et al.* Localized proton magnetic resonance spectroscopy of the brain in children infected with human immunodeficiency virus with and without encephalopathy. *Pediatr. Res.* **44** (1998), 755–62.

99. Lu, D., Pavlakis, S. G., Frank, Y., *et al.* Proton MR spectroscopy of the basal ganglia in healthy children and children with AIDS. *Radiology* **199** (1996), 423–8.

100. Pavlakis, S., Dongfeng, L., Frank, Y. *et al.* Magnetic resonance spectroscopy in childhood AIDS encephalopathy. *Pediatr. Neurol.* **12 : 4** (1995), 277–82.

101. Pavlakis, S. G., Lu, D., Frank, Y. *et al.* Brain lactate and N-acetylaspartate in pediatric AIDS encephalopathy. *Am. J. Neuroradiol.* **19** (1998), 383–5.

102. Mellors, J. W., Munoz, A., Giorgi, J. V. *et al.* Plasma viral load and CD4$^+$ lymphocytes as prognostic markers of HIV-1 infection. *Ann. Intern. Med.* **126** (1997), 946–54.

103. Mofenson, L., Korelitz, J., Meyer, W. A. *et al.* The relationship between serum human immunodeficiency virus type 1 (HIV-1) RNA level, CD4 lymphocyte percent, and long-term mortality risk in HIV-1-infected children. *J. Infect. Dis.* **175** (1997), 1029–38.

104. Pratt, R. D., Nichols, S., McKinney, N., Kwok, S., Dankner, W. & Spector, S. Virologic markers of human immunodeficiency virus type 1 in cerebrospinal fluid of infected children. *J. Infect. Dis.* **174** (1996), 288–93.

105. Jacobson, L. P., Li, R., Phair, J. *et al.* Evaluation of the effectiveness of highly active antiretroviral therapy in persons with human immunodeficiency virus using Biomarker-based equivalence of disease progression. *Am. J. Epidemiol.* **155 : 8** (2002), 760–70.

106. Haas, D. W., Clough, L. A., Johnson, B. W. *et al.* Evidence of a source of HIV type 1 within the central nervous system by ultraintensive sampling of cerebrospinal fluid and plasma. *AIDS Res. Hum. Retrovirus.* **16** (2000), 1491–502.

107. Haworth, S. J., Christofalo, B., Anderson, R. D. & Dunkle, L. M. A single dose study to assess the penetration of stavudine into human cerebrospinal fluid in adults. *J. AIDS and Hum. Retrovirol* **17** (1998), 235–8.

108. Foudraine, N. A., Hoetelmans, R. M. W., Lange, J. M. A. *et al.* Cerebrospinal-fluid HIV-1 RNA and drug concentrations after treatment with lamivudine plus zidovudine or stavudine. *Lancet* **351** (1998), 1547–51.

109. McCoig, C., Castrejon, M. M., Castano, E. *et al.* Effect of combination antiretroviral therapy on cerebrospinal fluid HIV RNA, HIV resistance, and clinical manifestations of encephalopathy. *J. Pediatr.* **141** (2002), 36–44.

110. Mueller, B. U. & Pizzo, P. A. Antiretroviral therapy for HIV infection of the central nervous system in children. In H. E. Gendelman, S. A. Lipton, L. Epstein & S. Swindells (eds.), *The Neurology of AIDS.* New York, NY : Chapman & Hall (1998), pp. 486–95.

111. McKinney, R. E., Maha, M. A., Connor, E. M. *et al.* A multicenter trial of oral zidovudine in children with advanced human immunodeficiency virus disease. *New Engl. J. Med.* **324 : 15** (1991), 1018–25.

112. Brouwers, P., Moss, H., Wolters, P. *et al.* Effect of continuous-infusion Zidovudine therapy on neuropsychologic functioning in children with symptomatic human immunodeficiency virus infection. *J. Pediatr.* **117 : 6** (1990), 980–5.

113. Pizzo, P., Eddy, J., Falloon, J. *et al.* Effect of continuous intravenous infusion of zidovudine (AZT) in children with symptomatic HIV infection. *New Engl. J. Med.* **319 : 14** (1988), 889–96.

114. DeCarli, C., Fugate, L., Falloon, J. *et al.* Brain growth and cognitive improvement in children with human immune deficiency virus-induced encephalopathy after six months of continuous infusion zidovudine therapy. *J. AIDS* **4** (1991), 585–92.

115. Yarchoan, R., Berg, G., Brouwers, P. *et al.* Preliminary observations in the response of HTLV-III/LAV (Human Immunodeficiency Virus) – associated neurological disease to the administration of 3-azido-3-deoxythymidine. *Lancet* **i** (1987), 131–5.

116. Bayley, N. *Bayley Scales of Infant Development*, 2nd edn. San Antonio, TX : Psychological Corporation (1993).

117. Mullen, E. *Mullen Scales of Early Learning.* Circle Pines, MN : American Guidance Service (1995).

118. Elliott, C. *Differential Ability Scales.* San Antonio, TX : Psychological Corporation (1990).

119. McCarthy, D. *McCarthy Scales of Children's Abilities.* San Antonio, TX : Psychological Corporation (1972).

120. Wechsler, D. *Wechsler Preschool and Primary Scale of Intelligence*, 3rd edn. San Antonio, TX: Psychological Corporation (2002).

121. Wechsler, D. *Wechsler Intelligence Scale for Children*, 4th edn. San Antonio, TX : Psychological Corporation (2003).

122. Wechsler, D. *Wechsler Adult Intelligence Scale*, 3rd edn. San Antonio, TX : Psychological Corporation (1997).

123. Dunn, L. M. & Dunn L. M. *Peabody Picture Vocabulary Test*, 3rd edn. Circle Pines, MN: American Guidance Service (1997).

124. Williams, K. *Expressive Vocabulary Test*. Circle Pines, MN: American Guidance Service, Inc. (1997).

125. Spreen, O. & Strauss, E. A. A compendium of neuropsychological tests: administration, norms, and commentary. New York, NY: Oxford University Press (1991).

126. Zimmerman, I., Steiner, V. & Pond, R. *Preschool Language Scale*, 3rd edn. San Antonio, TX: Psychological Corporation (1992).

127. Semel, E., Wiig, E. H. & Secord, W. *Clinical Evaluation of Language Fundamentals*, 3rd edn. San Antonio, TX : Psychological Corporation (1995).

128. Beery, K. The developmental test of visual-motor integration, 4th edn. Cleveland, OH : Modern Curriculum Press (1997).

129. Cohen, M. *Children's Memory Scale*. San Antonio, TX : Psychological Corporation (1997).

130. Delis, D., Kramer, J. & Kaplan, E. *California Verbal Learning Test, Children's Version*. San Antonio, TX : Psychological Corporation (1994).

131. Roid, G. H. *Stanford-Binet Intelligence Scale*, 5th edn. Itasca, IL : Riverside Publishing Company (2003).

132. Reitan, R. & Davidson, L. Clinical neuropsychology : current status and applications. New York, NY: Winston/Wiley (1974).

133. Conners, C. K. & Staff, M. H. S. *Conners' Continuous Performance Test II for Windows*. North Tonawanda, NY: MHS, Inc. (2000).

134. Raven, J., Summers, B., Birchfield, M. *et al. Manual for the Raven's Progressive Matrices and Vocabulary Scales. Research Supplement No. 3: A Compendium of North American Normative and Validity Studies*. London : HK Lewis (1984).

135. Folio, M. & Fewell, R. *Peabody Developmental Motor Scales and Activity Cards*. Chicago, IL: Riverside (1983).

136. Bruininks, R. *Bruininks-Oseretsky Test of Motor Proficiency*. Circle Pines, MN: American Guidance Service (1978).

137. Klove, H. Clinical neuropsychology. *Med. Clin. N. Am.* **26** (1963), 592–600.

138. Sparrow, S., Balla, D. & Cicchetti, D. *Vineland Adaptive Behavior Scales*. Circle Pines, MN: American Guidance Service (1984).

139. Achenbach, T. & Edelbrock, C. *Manual for the Child Behavior Checklist and Revised Child Behavior Profile*. Burlington, VT: University of Vermont (1983).

140. Conners, C. *Conners' Rating Scales*. North Tonawanda, NY: Multi-Health Systems (1989).

141. Reynolds, C. & Kamphaus, R. *Behavior Assessment System for Children*. Circle Pines, MN: American Guidance Service, Inc. (1998).

142. Gioia, G., Isquith, P., Guy, S. & Kenworthy, L. *Behavior Rating Inventory of Executive Function*. Lutz, FL: Psychological Assessment Resources, Inc. (1996).

PART III

Antiretroviral therapy

Antiretroviral therapy

Ross McKinney, Jr, M.D.

Department of Pediatrics, Duke University School of Medicine, Durham, NC

18.1 Introduction

The ultimate goal of antiretroviral therapy for HIV is to cure the patient of infection. Since this objective is not yet achievable, the second target is to provide a simple, inexpensive, well-tolerated regimen that is able to control the infection for a long period of time, even indefinitely. Unfortunately, even this objective is elusive, and current therapies are generally complex, rigid, and burdened by toxicities. They are time-limited in their efficacy, but the length of time the therapies remain effective has been steadily improving, particularly for patients who adhere to their regimens. Much of the recent progress has been attributable to a better understanding of HIV biology, which has made drug selection and use more rational. This chapter will summarize the currently available antiretroviral drugs and outline some basic strategies for their use.

18.2 The biology of HIV and antiretroviral therapy

Chapter 2 describes the HIV life cycle and outlines the steps in the life cycle targeted by antiretroviral drugs, including drugs currently in clinical use, those under development, and those which did not prove to be clinically useful. The viral targets of antiretroviral agents are outlined in Chapter 2, Figures 2.2 and 2.4, and Table 2.1. The antiretroviral drugs in current clinical use inhibit either the viral reverse transcriptase, which makes a cDNA copy of the viral genomic RNA; the viral protease, which cleaves the viral Gag and Gag-Pol polyprotein into the subunits required to make a fully mature, infectious virion; or block the fusion of the viral envelope with the plasma membrane of its would-be future host cell. Additional viral targets are the subject of drug development efforts, but there are no currently approved antiviral drugs directed at these other targets (e.g. the viral integrase or chemokine receptors).

There are two classes of reverse transcriptase inhibitors (RTIs), the nucleoside analogue RTIs (NRTIs) and the nonnucleoside RTIs (NNRTIs). Nucleoside-analogue reverse transcriptase inhibitors (NRTIs) are modified nucleosides that are designed to lack a 3′OH group (see Chapter 2, Figure 2.4). They are phosphorylated by host cell kinases and then incorporated into the elongating polynucleotide chain. Their incorporation produces a prematurely terminated cDNA molecule because another nucleotide cannot add to the chain due to the absent 3′ OH. The viral reverse transcriptase has a greater relative affinity for the modified nucleosides than does the human DNA polymerase, which is the reason nucleoside analogues have a tolerable therapeutic index. The non-nucleoside RT inhibitors, NNRTIs, act through a different mechanism than the NRTIs. The NNRTIs interfere with binding at the active site of the reverse transcriptase. The NNRTIs have no effect on cellular DNA polymerases and are so specific they have no effect on the reverse transcriptase of HIV-2. Non-nucleoside RTIs and NRTIs have very different side-effect profiles. Nonnucleoside RTIs can be used in combination with NRTIs, often with synergistic activity (see also Chapter 21).

HIV's Gag virion structural proteins and the Pol proteins are synthesized as a long polyprotein. The polyprotein must be cleaved into many smaller proteins by the viral protease in order to produce a fully mature and infectious virion. The HIV protease is an aspartyl protease with some similarities to cellular aspartyl proteases, but several relatively specific inhibitors of the HIV protease have been developed. Several of these protease inhibitors (PIs) have excellent antiviral activity.

The fusion inhibitors (like enfuvirtide, also known as T-20, and its related follow-on compound, T-1249) bind to the gp41 envelope glycoprotein and inhibit the formation of the gp41 structure required for insertion of the gp41 fusion peptide into the host cell plasma membrane, inhibiting the fusion of the lipid bilayer of the virus and that of the host cell membrane. These drugs are peptides, and require parenteral, rather than oral, administration.

Sub-optimal antiretroviral dosing or lack of adherence can permit continued viral replication in the presence of low concentrations of drug, promoting the development of resistance to the agents. The development of resistant viruses can have important implications for the long-term efficacy of antiretroviral therapeutic regimens (see Chapter 21).

The doses of antiretroviral agents are summarized in the formulary section of the Appendices. The formulary includes doses both for FDA-approved drugs for children and, so that readers may have some appreciation of drugs currently under development, the doses for antiretroviral drugs that are in advanced stages of pediatric clinical development. Some of the drugs are not specifically approved for use in pediatrics and dosing recommendations for those drugs represent estimates that are based on the available literature and clinical experience, and may not be correct. Dosing and indications may change. New side-effects and drug interactions may become known. Clinicians should take care to consult a current version of the package insert when prescribing antiretroviral agents, particularly newer agents. Many antiretroviral drugs have serious side-effects and potentially harmful interactions with other drugs. Patients must be carefully monitored for these potential problems. Antiretroviral therapy should be managed by or in close consultation with an expert in the care of pediatric HIV disease.

18.3 Antiretroviral agents

18.3.1 Nucleoside analogue reverse transcriptase inhibitors

The NRTIs were the first class of antiretroviral drugs to be used in HIV disease. They can be divided into two categories: the thymidine derivatives and non-thymidine NRTIs. The two thymidine derivatives are zidovudine (ZDV) and stavudine (d4T). These two agents are antagonistic, probably because the two compete with each other for

a cellular kinase. In general, most combination regimens include at least two RTIs, beginning with either ZDV or d4T. The second agent is generally selected from among lamivudine (3TC), didanosine (ddI), and zalcitabine (ddC). The role of nucleotide analogues like tenofovir (Gilead Sciences), which has assumed an increasingly important role in HIV therapy for adults, has yet to be established in pediatrics. More details concerning the choice of antiretroviral agents, and the recommended criteria for starting and changing antiviral therapy, can be found in Chapter 22.

The effective pharmacokinetic properties of the NRTIs are determined by the pharmacokinetic properties of the intracellular tri-phosphate form of the drug. The serum half-life of the unphosphorylated native drugs is relatively short, and most are rapidly excreted, some after hepatic glucuronidation. However, within the cell, the phosphorylated forms of the drugs may have a prolonged half-life, which allows for less frequent dosing intervals than the serum half-life would suggest.

Zidovudine (ZDV)

Overview

Zidovudine, (AZT or ZDV, Retrovir – GlaxoSmithKline; Combivir, as a fixed dose combination with lamivudine – GlaxoSmithKline; Trizivir, as a fixed dose combination with lamivudine and abacavir – GlaxoSmithKline), was the first FDA-approved antiretroviral drug. It is a chain terminating, thymidine-derived NRTI. The drug has substantial, although tolerable, side-effects, and demonstrated clinical efficacy in children. However, while ZDV monotherapy has clinical benefits, resistance develops over time, so the drug is now used only in combination regimens, except in the setting of regimens designed to interrupt vertical transmission (see Chapters 8 and 22). Zidovudine is available as both liquid and capsules.

Antiviral activity

As monotherapy, ZDV typically produces a 0.5 to 0.7 log decline in RNA copy number. The effect lasts for several months to years. In children, ZDV monotherapy produces only mild improvements in CD4$^+$ lymphocyte counts [1]. It improves weight growth, at least in the short term, and can improve cognitive function in children with HIV encephalopathy [1].

The primary resistance mutations to ZDV are at codons 41, 67, 70, 210, 215, and 219. The first to appear is at codon 70, while the most important site is 215. Both contribute to multidrug resistance against NRTIs. A complex of mutations including codon 151 may also produce multinucleoside resistance.

Pharmacokinetics

Zidovudine has a short serum half-life (roughly 1 hour) in children beyond the first few months of life. The drug is first glucuronidated in the liver, then renally excreted. In young infants, the half life is prolonged, both because of limited glucuronidation capability, and because of immature renal function. The active form of ZDV is zidovudine triphosphate. The drug is phosphorylated by cellular kinases. The intra-cellular half-life is approximately 3 hours, explaining why ZDV can be given as infrequently as twice per day.

Clinical trials

The first placebo-controlled trial of ZDV in adults demonstrated the efficacy of ZDV, and the study was halted early in 1986 [2]. Two hundred and eighty-two patients with AIDS or advanced AIDS-related symptoms were treated with ZDV or placebo. Of the 145 ZDV-treated patients, only 1/145 died. In comparison, 16/137 patients in the placebo group died. The outcome was highly significant. While this result unequivocally showed the short-term clinical benefit of ZDV, many questions were left unanswered, including issues such as when to start therapy, how long the treatment would last, and what role resistance would eventually play.

The first pediatric trial of ZDV was performed from 1986–87. It demonstrated that ZDV could be used in children in a manner very similar to adults, although children may have had fewer adverse events [3]. Benefits of ZDV treatment included faster than anticipated weight gain, decreased hepato-splenomegaly, and lowering of IgG and IgM concentrations toward more normal values. The first large Phase II trial of ZDV in children had very similar results, confirming the positive effects of ZDV treatment on growth [1].

Pediatric AIDS Clinical Trials Group Protocol (PACTG) 152 demonstrated that ZDV plus ddI, or ddI alone were clinically superior to ZDV monotherapy [4]. Similarly, PACTG Trial 300 demonstrated that either combination ZDV/ddI or ZDV/3TC were superior to ddI monotherapy. Pediatric ACTG protocol 338 demonstrated that combination regimens containing ritonavir (RTV) and ZDV/3TC or d4T, produced better short-term virus suppression than ZDV/3TC alone.

Pediatric ACTG protocol 076 established that ZDV monotherapy had a role in the prevention of vertical HIV transmission (mother-to-infant) [5]. For details, see Chapter 8. Zidovudine also has been used in post-exposure prophylaxis regimens aimed at blocking infection following occupational exposures. This is discussed in more detail in Chapter 24. Zidovudine has been used in combination regimens during pregnancy that have reduced the transmission rate to < 2%. Whether ZDV should be used as monotherapy after delivery when a combination regimen was used during pregnancy remains an open question (see Chapter 8).

Adverse effects

Alone or in combination, ZDV has a significant adverse event profile [1]. The most common problems are hematologic: anemia and neutropenia. These may respond to dose adjustment, although care should be taken to remain in a therapeutic range. Some physicians use erythropoietin or filgrastim (g-CSF) to combat these side-effects. Thrombocytopenia is rarely produced by ZDV. Zidovudine reliably produces an increase in red cell volume (MCV), and can lead to an erythrocytic macrocytosis, with MCVs >100 fl. Indeed, the absence of an increase in MCV in patients for whom ZDV has been prescribed can be a clinically useful indication of poor compliance. Zidovudine has been associated with myopathy and cardiomyopathy, probably through a toxic effect on mitochondrial polymerases. The mitochondrial problems can also manifest through lactic acidosis, sometimes associated with hepatic steatosis. Zidovudine can also produce restlessness, mild headaches, nausea, and fatigue, particularly in older children. There are some theoretical concerns regarding potential long-term and transplacental carcinogenicity of ZDV, and presumably other NRTIs, and while ZDV has mutagenic and carcinogenic potential in certain animal models, there are no human data to support these concerns. Long-term follow-up studies of children exposed to ZDV in utero and as newborns as a component of strategies to prevent mother-to-infant transmission have not exhibited any significant long-term toxicities [6].

Didanosine (ddI)

Overview

Didanosine (ddI, Videx – Bristol Myers Squibb) is an NRTI that is metabolized from di-deoxyinosine (ddI) to its active form, di-deoxyadenosine (ddA). It has a good side-effect profile in children; its use in young children is limited primarily by inconvenient dosage regimens, principally caused by its chemical instability in acid conditions such as those found in the stomach and its consequent requirement for oral co-administration of substantial buffering, and by taste problems [7, 8]. Didanosine is available as a liquid mixed in antacid (usually Maalox), as a chewable/dispersible tablet, and as an extended release, enteric-coated capsule (Videx EC). The last formulation is the most practical for patients because of its superior palatability and convenience.

Antiviral effects

Didanosine monotherapy has antiviral effects similar to ZDV, as measured by surrogate markers. It has somewhat better durability as a monotherapy than ZDV, but it is now almost always given in combinations [4, 9].

The resistance mutations most often associated with ddI are at codons 65 and 74, although it is difficult to demonstrate antiviral resistance to ddI in vitro. Since the drug's beneficial effects can be exhausted (as demonstrated by surrogate marker changes), clinical resistance occurs despite the failure to show resistance in vitro.

Pharmacokinetics

Didanosine is acid labile, but to a lesser degree than ddA. Acid in the stomach will inactivate ddI, but the drug can be adequately absorbed if it is administered simultaneously with an antacid. Didanosine is typically given to young children as a pre-mixed suspension in flavored antacid. The intracellular half-life of ddA-triphosphate is quite long (more than 24 hours), so that it may be possible to administer ddI once daily, a considerable advantage given the complexity of many antiretroviral regimens. The concept of once-daily dosing has yet to be demonstrated to be effective in children, although adult trials appear promising.

Didanosine should be given, when possible, on an empty stomach, ideally 1 hour before or 2 hours after a meal. However, with small children who eat often this may not be possible, and the importance of the daily schedule for compliance should be weighed against a relatively small loss in absorption due to food.

Didanosine liquid is not stable at ambient temperatures. It needs to be stored under refrigerated conditions, and some clinics give patients ice chests to use in transporting ddI suspension home from the pharmacy. The shelf-life, even refrigerated, is only 30 days. The chewable tablets are somewhat more convenient, but the taste can be challenging for children. If tablets are used, the minimum dose is two tablets at a time, since the tablets contain an antacid and two tablets are needed to supply enough antacid to provide adequate buffering capacity. The enteric coated preparation is by far the most convenient, but young children may not be large enough for the minimum size capsule (and may not be able to swallow capsules in any case). The enteric coating protects the ddI during its transport through the stomach, then allows the drug to be absorbed in the more basic environment of the intestinal tract.

Clinical trials

Pediatric ACTG protocol 152 demonstrated that ddI monotherapy was more effective than ZDV alone, and perhaps as effective as combination ZDV/ddI [4]. However, PACTG protocol 300 then found that both ZDV/3TC and ZDV/ddI were more effective than ddI monotherapy, both clinically and with regard to surrogate markers [10]. Didanosine monotherapy should only be used infrequently, if at all, and then only in families with marginal medication adherence as a stopgap approach. However, children who received ddI monotherapy did better clinically than those who were given ZDV, confirming the drug's beneficial clinical effects.

Adverse effects

Didanosine is generally well tolerated, although some patients have difficulty taking the drug because of its taste. The most common adverse events are peripheral neuropathy and pancreatitis. The neuropathy usually presents as paresthesias, most often of the feet, and may appear as a gait disturbance in younger children. Pancreatitis typically presents as abdominal pain, nausea, and vomiting. As opposed to other causes of abdominal pain, pancreatitis is usually associated with a rise in amylase and lipase levels, and may be confirmed in some instances through the use of ultrasonography. There is, however, no utility in routinely monitoring serum amylase levels for patients on ddI, since most episodes of pancreatitis are relatively acute and signaled first by pain. In addition, high amylase concentrations are often released by the salivary glands in children with HIV. In order to determine whether an elevated serum amylase is attributable to pancreatitis or parotitis, a fractionated amylase can be performed. This assay can distinguish between pancreatic and salivary isoenzymes. However, the isoenzyme assays have some overlap, so that a very high salivary amylase will give a falsely elevated pancreatic fraction. To improve the predictive value of amylase measurements, a serum lipase can be obtained. In most instances where both enzyme concentrations are high, pancreatitis should be suspected.

Some children experience abdominal symptoms such as diarrhea, pain, or nausea during treatment with ddI. Some of the effects may be from the antacid.

Stavudine (d4T)

Clinical overview

Stavudine (d4T, Zerit – Bristol Myers Squibb) is a thymidine-derived nucleotide with clinical potency roughly equivalent to ZDV. The advantages of d4T are that it can be given on a twice-daily dosing schedule, side-effects are relatively uncommon in children, and timing around food is not an issue. Stavudine is available in an FDA-approved liquid preparation, as well as capsules. An extended release form of d4T has recently been FDA approved, and offers larger children the option of once-daily dosing.

Antiviral effects

Stavudine is similar to ZDV in effect, producing a 0.7–0.8 $\log_{10}$ decrease in viral RNA concentration when used as monotherapy. Resistance to d4T involves mutations at essentially the same reverse transcriptase amino acid residues as ZDV, although mutations at amino acid 75 can also contribute to resistance. As with ddI, in vitro resistance is hard to document, although clinical exhaustion of potency is clearly demonstrable using surrogate markers.

Pharmacokinetics

Stavudine has a relatively long intracellular half life (3–4 hours) and can be given on a twice-daily schedule. No special arrangements for mealtime are required since it is well absorbed on a full or empty stomach. Because d4T is renally excreted, dosage adjustment may be required in patients with renal problems. As with all of the nucleoside analogue drugs, d4T is phosphorylated intracellularly to the active triphosphate form. Zidovudine competes with d4T for the kinase that accomplishes the phosphorylations, so ZDV inhibits D4T phosphorylation. Therefore, ZDV and D4T should not be used simultaneously.

Clinical trials

Trials with d4T in children have demonstrated a good safety profile. It has been studied as monotherapy [11] and in combination with ddI [9] and 3TC (Adult ACTG Trial 306). The clinical effects of combination therapy with ddI or 3TC are similar to those seen with ZDV in combination with both those drugs. Stavudine can also be combined with PIs or NNRTIs. It should not be co-administered with ZDV.

Adverse effects

Stavudine is generally well tolerated by children. In adults, d4T is associated with peripheral neuropathy in a high proportion of patients. However, neuropathy appears to be less common in children. Stavudine is also associated rarely with anemia, pancreatitis, headache, and gastrointestinal disturbances. A major concern with d4T has been an interaction with ddI. There appears to be an increased rate of lactic acidosis, at times with fatal outcome, in all patients, although the incidence is still uncommon. In pregnant women, however, the incidence of lactic acidosis appears to be markedly elevated, which has meant the combination of d4T with ddI in pregnant women is now contraindicated. Some anecdotal evidence also suggests that the risks of pancreatitis may be worse when d4T and ddI are used together.

Lamivudine

Overview

Lamivudine (3TC, Epivir – GlaxoSmithKline; Combivir, as a fixed dose combination with zidovudine – GlaxoSmithKline; Trizivir, as a fixed dose combination with zidovudine and abacavir – GlaxoSmithKline) is a well-tolerated cytosine analogue and is a relatively potent NRTI in the absence of resistance, but a single nucleotide substitution in RT dramatically increases resistance to the drug. The drug is well tolerated, and frequently is used together with ZDV and d4T as the 'nucleoside backbone' component of combination regimens. Liquid and tablet preparations are available.

Antiviral effect

As monotherapy, 3TC can produce up to one $\log_{10}$ decreases in plasma concentrations of HIV RNA. However, resistance to 3TC monotherapy occurs quickly and requires only a single point mutation at amino acid 184 in the RT gene. Lamivudine is virtually always used in combination with another NRTI, particularly d4T or ZDV (the two thymidine-analogue NRTIs). The benefits of 3TC were confirmed in Pediatric ACTG protocol 300, where ZDV/3TC was clinically superior to monotherapy ddI [10]. Lamivudine also appears to make tenofovir more effective, particularly when the M184V mutation is present. In order to maintain the M184V mutation and its tenofovir hypersensitizing effect, 3TC should be continued even when resistance appears to be present. Resensitization and hypersusceptibility are discussed in more detail in Chapter 21. Lamivudine, even considering the potential problems with resistance, is widely used as one of the NRTI components in HAART regimens.

Pharmacokinetics

Lamivudine has a relatively long half-life and is renally excreted. It may be given every 12 hours, and has recently been approved in adults for once-daily dosing. There are no food-related interactions. The dosage should be reduced in patients with renal impairment.

Clinical trials

Pediatric ACTG Trial 300 compared ZDV/3TC with ddI monotherapy. The combination was superior in regard to clinical outcomes and surrogate markers. In adult trials, lamivudine has been demonstrated to be a potent agent when added to the regimen of patients who were already on ZDV. Lamivudine has also been shown to potentiate the therapeutic effects of tenofovir in adult trials, particularly when the 184V mutation is present.

Adverse effects

Lamivudine is a well-tolerated compound. The only major side-effect has been pancreatitis, which was primarily seen in a very ill, multiply-antiretroviral treated group of children at the National Cancer Institute. Subsequent studies have demonstrated that pancreatitis is quite rare. For example, there were no instances of 3TC-associated pancreatitis in PACTG protocol 300 (patients followed a median of 11 months), while there were eight cases of pancreatitis in patients treated with DDI-containing regimens. Lamivudine can occasionally cause headaches, gastrointestinal upset, fatigue, and elevated hepatic transaminases. None of these is a common reason for dosage adjustment.

Zalcitabine

Overview

Zalcitabine (ddC, Hivid – Roche) has been used relatively sparingly in children, because there is no liquid formulation, because of its side effects profile, and because there is extensive cross resistance between ddC and other NRTIs, notably ddI and 3TC (see below). The available capsule formulation is geared toward adult dosing.

Antiviral effects

Zalcitabine is roughly comparable to ddI in activity, and HIV exhibits a considerable degree of cross-resistance between ddI and ddC, and between 3TC and ddC. In general, once a patient has had ddI experience, there will be little benefit from a shift to ddC. The most important resistance mutations occur at RT amino acid residues 65, 69, 74, and 184. The 184 methionine to valine mutation that confers high-level resistance against 3TC also confers resistance against ddC, making ddC generally not useful for patients who have failed 3TC therapy.

Pharmacokinetics

Zalcitabine is given every 8 hours. There are some medications which affect ddC's renal clearance (cimetidine, amphotericin, foscarnet, and aminoglycosides). Antacids may decrease absorption.

Clinical trials

Two large trials of ddC have been completed in children, PACTG studies 138 [12] and 190 [13]. The first was a phase II/III trial of two dosage regimens of ddC monotherapy for children who had progressed while receiving ZDV or were intolerant of it. In that study, ddC was generally well tolerated. More than half the children had stabilization of growth and a decline in p24 antigen concentrations. Thirty percent of the children had an increase in CD4 counts and gained weight. In PACTG protocol 190, ddC (0.03 mg/kg/day) or placebo was added to ZDV in patients who were clinically stable. There were relatively few differences in the two arms, although children who received ZDV/ddC had a slower decline in CD4 cell counts.

Adverse effects

Zalcitabine has been associated with a peripheral neuropathy that most frequently affects the distal extremities, especially the feet. While the symptoms of neuropathy usually begin with numbness or paresthesias, it can be quite painful, and may persist for several weeks after discontinuation of the ddC. Zalcitabine is rarely associated with pancreatitis or painful oral ulcerations. Headache and fatigue can sometimes occur.

Abacavir

Overview

Abacavir (ABC, Ziagen – GlaxoSmithKline; Trizivir, as a fixed dose combination with zidovudine and lamivudine – GlaxoSmithKline) is a relatively potent novel carbocyclic guanosine analogue nucleoside that has excellent activity when used as initial antiviral therapy. Both capsule and liquid preparations are available. Its major drawback has been a hypersensitivity syndrome, generally seen in the first few weeks of dosing. Those patients who have rash, fever, and abdominal pain during their first few weeks on ABC should, in most cases, have it stopped immediately. They should not be re-challenged, since profound hypotension has been seen in some patients on re-institution of ABC after interruption.

Antiviral effects

Abacavir is probably the most potent of current NRTI compounds as initial therapy, but resistance to it has been observed even when patients have not been exposed to ABC, presumably due to cross-resistance with other NRTIs (see below). Most studies have evaluated abacavir in combination with other antiretroviral agents. When used with PIs in therapy-naïve adults, ABC produced two $\log_{10}$ decreases in RNA copy number.

There is substantial cross-resistance between ABC and other nucleosides, particularly the thymidine analogues. Resistance sites also include the ddI resistance codons like 65, 74, and 115, and the 3TC resistance codon 184, although the relative importance of each remains to be determined.

Pharmacokinetics

Abacavir is administered on an every 12-hour schedule. The drug is cleared by glucuronidation and by the alcohol dehydrogenase system, which produces a carboxylic acid metabolite. The serum half-life is approximately one hour. There is no food effect on absorption. ABC crosses the blood–brain barrier in a manner similar to ZDV, with a CSF/plasma ratio of approximately 0.2.

Clinical trials

The first pediatric study to use ABC, PACTG protocol 330, evaluated monotherapy ABC in a cohort of very therapy-experienced children [14]. Unfortunately, in that setting, the drug had little virologic effect. The study had a phase where a second NRTI was added to the ABC monotherapy, but again little benefit was seen, probably due to already established antiviral resistance. Studies of ABC in adults have demonstrated good antiviral activity, comparable with PIs and NNRTIs, with average decreases in viral load of 1.5–2.1 logs. Penta 5 was a European evaluation of initial ABC/3TC vs ZDV/3TC vs ABC/ZDV as the nucleoside component in an initial treatment regimen for therapy-naïve patients. Combination ABC/3TC was the most effective regimen and continued to be through 160 weeks, both in terms of viral load and patient growth [15]. There has been considerable interest in the trizivir fixed dose combination as an all NRTI regimen, particularly in adolescents, but recent results suggest that this combination may be inferior to combination regimens that include a PI or NNRTI (see below).

Adverse effects

The main concern with ABC is an idiosyncratic allergic reaction manifested by rash, fever, abdominal pain, nausea, and vomiting. This reaction seems to occur most often in the first 3 weeks of therapy, and if it occurs there should be no ABC re-challenge. Patients have progressed to shock and even death as a result of re-challenge after an episode of hypersensitivity. This reaction can be difficult to distinguish from the rash syndrome of nevirapine and even from some infectious conditions (adenovirus, scarlet fever). There appears to be a definable genetic pre-disposition to the reaction in that patients with certain HLA subtypes may have an increased risk of developing the hypersensitivity reaction.

Tenofovir

Overview

Tenofovir disoproxil fumarate (TDF, Viread – Gilead Sciences) is a nucleo*tide* analogue reverse transcriptase inhibitor, unlike the other members of the class, which are nucleo*side* analogues. A nucleotide is a phosphorylated nucleoside, which means that TDF, as administered, is already monophosphorylated. Both the nucleoside analogue reverse transcriptase inhibitors and TDF must be phosphorylated by cellular kinases to the triphosate form before they can function as substrates for reverse transcriptase, but TDF bypasses the first phosphorylation step. (Thus, as a nucleotide analogue the active form of the drug is tenofovir diphosphate.) Since the kinases that catalyze phosphorylation to the monophosphate may be less active in resting cells, TDF may offer some advantages in that it may have greater activity in resting cells.

Antiviral effects

Tenofovir is similar to ZDV in potency. As monotherapy, it produces a 0.6–1.5 $\log_{10}$ decrease in plasma virus RNA concentration [16]. Resistance is conferred by mutations at RT codon K65R, although there are probably contributions from M41L and L210W. Virus with several nucleoside analogue-associated mutations (NAMS; see also Chapter 21) appears to be relatively resistant. Codon T69D may also play a role in resistance, although data are still preliminary. The 69 insertion mutation complex that confers high-level resistance to the NRTIs also confers high level resistance to tenofovir.

Tenofovir is also active against hepatitis B, although studies in pediatric patients are limited.

Pharmacokinetics

Tenofovir disoproxil fumarate is a pro-drug which is converted to tenofovir in the gastrointestinal tract. Oral bioavailability in adults is roughly 25% (fasted), and the drug is better absorbed when taken with food. Tenofovir is cleared renally, with no involvement of the cytochrome P450 system. Its long intracellular half-life means the drug can be administered once a day.

Tenofovir interacts with ddI, causing increased ddI exposure. When the drugs are used in combination, a reduced ddI dose is probably indicated. TDF causes decreases in atazanavir levels (see below) and the combination of atazanavir and TDF should either be avoided or atazanavir should be boosted with ritonavir.

Clinical trials

Clinical information on TDF in children is still preliminary. A pediatric Phase I/II trial is underway to evaluate TDF at the National Cancer Institute using a dose of 175 mg/m^2, and further phase II/III studies are in development. In adult phase III trials, TDF is comparable to d4T as first line treatment in naïve patients (when combined with 3TC and EFV), and has been used successfully as part of second and third-line regimens for patients treated previously with other antiretroviral drugs.

Adverse effects

Gastrointestinal problems (diarrhea, nausea, vomiting) can occur, but are not frequent. Liver transaminase elevations have been reported. Nephrotoxicity may rarely occur. As with the nucleoside RT inhibitors, lactic acidosis has been reported with TDF. In studies of young animals, higher doses of TDF have caused decreases in bone mineral density, a finding that suggests that if the drug is used in children there should be careful consideration given to this potential toxicity.

Emtricitabine (FTC)

Overview

Emtricitabine (FTC, Emtriva – Gilead Sciences) is a NRTI very similar in its resistance profile to 3TC. Studies are in progress in children (for example, PATCG protocol 1021), and while it appears to have predictable pharmacokinetics and activity, it is not yet approved.

Antiviral effects

Emtricitabine is similar to ZDV in potency. Resistance is conferred by mutations at RT codon M184V/I, as it is for 3TC. Cross resistance with 3TC and zalcitabine is present in most FTC resistant isolates.

Pharmacokinetics

While studies in children are still preliminary, FTC pharmacokinetics appear to be relatively predictable in children. Food does not affect absorption, and the oral bioavailability of capsule FTC is 93% in adult studies (according to the Emtriva package insert). The half-life is approximately 10 hours, and clearance is renal (a mix of filtration and active tubular secretion). Dosage should be downwardly adjusted in renal failure. Drug interactions have been minimal to date. A dose of 6 mg/kg/day gave an AUC comparable with the standard adult dose of 200 mg/day [17].

Clinical trials

Clinical information on FTC in children is still preliminary. A pediatric Phase I/II trial is underway to evaluate FTC in combination with DDI and Efavirenz in a once-daily dosing scheme. In a comparable adult study, 78% of therapy-naïve patients maintained a viral load of less than 50 RNA copies/mL at 48 weeks.

Adverse effects

Adverse effects of FTC have been relatively uncommon. The most notable adverse effect has been hyperpigmentation of the palms and/or soles. The mechanism is unknown. Lactic acidosis and severe hepatomegaly with steatosis is a rare but severe problem for all NRTIs.

18.3.2 Non-nucleoside Reverse Transcriptase Inhibitors

There are three licensed NNRTIs, nevirapine (NVP), delavirdine (DLV), and efavirenz (EFV), which are similar in their activity. Efavirenz is the most widely used NNRTI, but there are few data on its use in children under age 3 years. Nevirapine is the most widely used NNRTI in young children, since there is a liquid formulation of NVP. Efavirenz has a liquid formulation, but that formulation is not approved in the USA, and pediatric dosing is based on giving multiples of small capsules. Because it lacks a liquid preparation and is probably less potent, DLV is the least used and studied of the three. Single amino acid change mutations, for example mutations at codon 103, confer high level resistance to all the available NNRTIs. Cross resistance among these three agents is almost complete, so if a patient becomes unresponsive to one NNRTI another NNRTI should not be substituted.

Nevirapine

Overview

Nevirapine (NVP, Viramune – Roxane/Boehringer Ingelheim) is a benzodiazepine NNRTI that was developed simultaneously in children and adults, although the adult preparation was FDA-approved substantially before the pediatric. The drug is quite potent, even as monotherapy, but rapidly selects for resistant virus.

Antiviral effects

A single point mutation, at codon 103 or at codon 181 of the RT, leads to high level NVP resistance [18] (see Chapter 21). Codons Y188L and V106A can also decrease NVP sensitivity. Used as monotherapy, almost complete drug resistance can be seen consistently after as little as 4–6 weeks, and appreciable resistance can be found in some patients following even a single dose. When NVP is part of a combination, the drug has activity similar to PIs, although clinically the rapid development of resistance can still be significant.

Pharmacokinetics

The pharmacokinetics of NVP are complex. The drug is lipophilic and distributes into body tissues well. Nevirapine administration auto-induces its metabolism, so that the same dose given over time leads to a decreasing serum concentration. The change in clearance is approximately 1.5–2-fold. Because the induction of metabolism plateaus over time, NVP is given once per day for the 14 days, then twice daily dosing is initiated. The adult serum half-life is approximately 25 hours. In neonates, hepatic immaturity means NVP metabolism is very slow, and a single oral dose can produce several days at a therapeutic concentration. This effect of NVP, combined with its potency, low cost, and the fact that NVP crosses the placenta well, are the reasons a two-dose NVP regimen (one maternal dose plus one newborn dose) was evaluated for perinatal prophylaxis.

Clinical trials

Nevirapine was used in combination with ZDV and ddI in PACTG protocol 180, an attempt to aggressively treat newborn infants [19]. It was also included as part of a salvage regimen in PACTG protocol 245, a study in advanced HIV disease [20]. In the former case, most children appeared to have some benefit from the combination of ZDV/ddI/NVP, and two children had nearly complete virus suppression. Pediatric ACTG protocol 180 was not, however, a comparative study. Pediatric ACTG protocol 245 compared ZDV/ddI, ddI/NVP, and ZDV/ddI/NVP. The last approach appeared to be the most effective.

Adverse effects

Nevirapine is associated with two primary adverse effects. First, early after initiation of therapy, hepatitis and/or elevated hepatic transaminases can develop. The other major side effect is rash, which occurs in approximately 8% of children. Nevirapine rash begins as a macular-papular eruption, most often within 5 weeks of starting therapy. In most cases the rash evolves to include fever and malaise. Nevirapine should be stopped if rash occurs because the exanthem can evolve to severe Stevens–Johnson syndrome.

Delavirdine

Overview

Delavirdine (DLV, Rescriptor – Pfizer) is the second FDA-approved NNRTI. It has no liquid formulation, and there are almost no data about its use in children. It is dosed three times per day and there is a high-level of cross-resistance with NVP. The major side-effect, rash, is less severe than that of NVP. Since there is no liquid formulation and since it offers no apparent benefit over the other available NNRTIs it is not widely used in pediatrics.

Antiviral effects

Delavirdine is similar to other NNRTIs in potency. The resistance pattern varies slightly, although the key sites appear to be RT amino acid mutations K103N and Y181C (in common with other NNRTIs), along with Y188L, P236L, and V106A. Delavirdine has been evaluated in combination with NRTIs, which can delay the development of DLV resistance. However, some investigators feel the benefits of DLV are less than the other NNRTIs.

Pharmacokinetics

Delavirdine has not been studied in children. Dosing in adults is every 8 hours. The drug is hepatically excreted. Delavirdine inhibits the cytochrome P450 system, in contrast to NVP, and so tends to increase PI concentrations. Systemic exposure to ritonavir, for example, is increased by 70%.

Clinical trials

Data on DLV are quite limited. An adult trial compared DLV/ZDV/3TC to ZDV/3TC and ZDV/DLV in a group of largely antiretroviral naïve adults. The triple therapy group had a larger drop in RNA copy number than the ZDV/3TC group, which was in turn better than the ZDV/DLV cohort (mean decreases in HIV plasma RNA concentrations at week 24: -2.25 $\log_{10}$/mL, -1.32 $\log_{10}$/mL, and -0.55 $\log_{10}$/mL, respectively) [21].

Adverse effects

The main adverse effect of DLV is rash. The rash is milder than that seen with NVP, and most cases occur within the first month of treatment. The rash is generalized, maculopapular, and can be pruritic.

Efavirenz

Overview

Efavirenz (EFV, Sustiva – Bristol Myers Squibb; outside the USA: Stocrin – Merck) was FDA approved for adults and children older than 3 years in September 1998. Solid and liquid formulations exist, but only the solid formulation has been approved and is available in the USA. Efavirenz (Stocrin) liquid is available in certain countries outside the USA. Efavirenz has a long half-life, which allows once a day administration. Because of its activity and because of concerns about the metabolic side-effects of the PIs, efavirenz has become an increasingly widely used component of initial highly active antiretroviral therapy (HAART) regimens.

Antiviral effects

Efavirenz has activity similar to other NNRTIs. The resistance pattern is also similar to other NNRTIs, since mutation K103N in the RT gene produces a nearly 20-fold decrease in susceptibility. Studies indicate that efavirenz may sometimes retain effectiveness in the face of the Y181C RT mutation that affects most NNRTIs, as well as the P236L delavirdine-associated mutation, but the spectrum of other mutations in RT apparently influences the degree of resistance when the Y181C mutation is present. Other resistance substitutions have been seen at codons L100I, V108I, Y181C, Y188L, G190S, and P225H.

Pharmacokinetics

Efavirenz is hepatically excreted. The drug induces cytochrome P450 isoform CYP 3A4, which may decrease PI concentrations. The half-life is long, 40–55 hours, allowing daily dosing. There is good CNS penetration. Efavirenz decreases the levels of saquinavir, to a degree that the drugs should generally not be used together, although it may be possible to use SQV boosted by ritonavir.

Clinical trials

Efavirenz, in combination with nelfinavir and one or more nucleoside RT inhibitor, was demonstrated in PACTG protocol 382 to be effective in children who were naïve to NNRTIs and protease inhibitors [22]. Seventy-six percent of the children had a viral load less than 400 copies/mL at week 48. Studies have also used EFV in combination with emtricitabine (FTC) and ddI in a once-daily regimen with good preliminary efficacy, although the FTC component is not yet FDA approved [23]. In studies in adults, initial highly active antiretroviral therapy regimens utilizing efavirenz in combination with two NRTIs are as effective as regimens employing a PI with two NNRTIs.

Adverse effects

The most common EFV-related problems are rash, dizziness, and other minor central nervous system (CNS) abnormalities. Patients also sometimes report CNS side-effects, including dizziness, impaired concentration, somnolence, hallucinations, and vivid dreams. The impact of these side-effects may be less when the drug is given at bedtime, as recommended. Rash, most often a maculopapular eruption, occurred in 30–40% of children, with 7% reporting severe rash. The rash usually resolves with continued treatment. However, the most problematic toxicity concern is in pregnant women. While efavirenz has not yet been documented to cause birth defects in humans, 3 of 20 pregnant monkeys dosed with efavirenz gave birth to infants with significant birth defects. The three had cleft palate, microphthalmia, and anencephaly with unilateral anophthalmia. It is recommended that women not use EFV during pregnancy, particularly early in gestation, and that birth control be used while a woman is on efavirenz.

18.3.3 HIV-protease inhibitors

The HIV structural proteins are initially translated as long poly-proteins that must be proteolytically cleaved by the viral protease into their viral mature form for infectious virus to be produced (see Chapter 2). The HIV PIs are effective because they can specifically inhibit the HIV protease while not affecting host proteases. The most closely related human proteases are in the renin-angiotensin converting enzyme family. Most of the current protease inhibitors are peptitidomimetic: they emulate the substrate of the enzyme; they bind the HIV protease enzyme active site in ways similar to the normal HIV polyprotein substrate, but inhibit the enzyme rather than being cleaved by it. Unfortunately, the protease inhibitors can be difficult to use in children. They are relatively hydrophobic and so are not readily made into suspensions or water-based solutions, and require agents such as ethanol, propylene glycol, or vitamin E to help solubilize them in liquid preparations. The PIs taste bad, and they interact with the liver's P450 cytochromes in complex ways. Some protease inhibitors induce certain P450 isoforms, while inhibiting others. Ritonavir, as an example, is a relatively broad inhibitor of the P450 enzyme system and it induces its own metabolism. Ritonavir's complicated pharmacokinetic interactions complicate the use of many other drugs.

Multi-protease inhibitor resistance has been demonstrated as mutations accumulate at L10F/I/R/V, M46I/L, I54V/M/L, V82A/F/T/S, I84V, and L90M. In addition, each PI has specific, associated mutations. Use of any PI begins the progression toward multi-drug resistance, although some like nelfinavir seem less likely to induce multi-drug resistance.

Amprenavir

Overview

Amprenavir (APV, Agenerase – GlaxoSmithKline) has a relatively unique resistance pattern, which makes it a candidate for use in combination with other protease inhibitors. There are both capsule and liquid formulations. The drug is approved by the FDA for adults and children 4 years old and older.

Antiviral effects

Amprenavir has a potent antiviral effect, similar to other protease inhibitors. When used as monotherapy, the predominant resistance mutation selected is I50V. In standard combination therapy, mutations are selected that include V32I, M46I/L, I47V, I54L/M, and I84V. Amprenavir has been evaluated in combination with other PIs, and there appear to be enough differences in its resistance pattern so that using APV with other PIs can sometimes be beneficial. Interactions with IND and NLV appeared to be particularly favorable in vitro [24].

Pharmacokinetics

Amprenavir is cleared by the cytochrome P450 system, which it also inhibits. However, APV does not appear to induce or inhibit its own metabolism. Specifically, APV inhibits the CYP3A4 isoform of the cytochrome P450 system, the most common isoform. The plasma half-life is somewhat variable, but is approximately 7 hours, which is very suitable for twice-daily dosing. The liquid form of APV currently contains propylene glycol and large quantities of vitamin E and is not suitable for children under the age of 4 years.

Clinical trials

Published clinical experience with APV is still relatively limited in children. It has good virological effect when used in combination with NRTIs, producing undetectable viral loads in most treatment-naïve patients. In combination with 2 NRTIs, the median HIV viral load decreased $1.41 \log_{10}$ in protease inhibitor-naïve children [25].

Adverse effects

The most common adverse effects with APV are gastrointestinal. Some patients have headache, malaise, or fatigue. There may be some cutaneous reactions. Amprenavir is related to sulfonamides, so should be used with caution in patients with severe sulfa allergy.

Indinavir

Clinical overview

Indinavir (IDV, Crixivan – Merck) is widely used to treat adult patients, but pediatric experience is very limited to date. Indinavir is potent, has a similar resistance pattern to ritonavir, and produces several adverse effects. Although pediatric studies are not complete, it appears IDV will be administered every 8 hours in children, and should be given on an empty stomach. The medication is only soluble at an acid pH, so food in the stomach buffers the pH and makes the IDV less available. The every 8-hour dosing, the need for an empty stomach, and the lack of an approved liquid formulation make the drug relatively unappealing for pediatric use, especially in young children.

Like the other protease inhibitors, IDV has interactions with numerous other medications (see Chapter 19). The extent of these interactions is somewhat less than with RTV, which makes drug interactions somewhat easier to manage.

Antiviral effects

Indinavir is a potent agent, comparable with RTV. The pattern of mutations seen is almost identical to that of RTV, and there is a high degree of cross-resistance. It was in the initial trials of IDV that it was learned that low doses of the agent allowed the evolution of PI-resistant quasi-species. When patients were subsequently switched to higher doses of IDV, no antiviral effect was seen due to the existence of

mutations which had evolved at the lower dose. Thus, subtherapeutic dosing, either by mis-prescription or erratic compliance, will allow permanent PI resistance to occur.

Pharmacokinetics

Indinavir is only soluble at low pH. As a result, it needs to be taken on an empty stomach. Once absorbed, it is carried on plasma proteins and metabolized by glucuronidation and the cytochrome P450 system. Some IDV is excreted through the kidneys. Because of urine's neutral pH, the IDV can precipitate and produce kidney stones. Indinavir has interactions in both directions with drugs that affect the cytochrome P450 system. It inhibits the metabolism of many drugs, and its many interactions are reviewed in Chapter 19.

Clinical trials

Pediatric experience with IDV is somewhat limited. A phase I/II study was performed at the National Cancer Institute and collaborating centers. Patients received monotherapy for the first 16 weeks, then combination therapy with ZDV/3TC. Several patients had hematuria, some with flank pain. In adults, when IDV and 3TC were added to patients who had been on long-term ZDV, the effects were striking. Twenty-eight of the 31 patients treated with three drugs reached < 500 RNA copies/mL by week 24, compared with none of the patients who received only 3TC in addition to ZDV, and 12/28 who added only IDV [26].

Adverse effects

Because of its solubility characteristics, IDV can form crystals in the kidney after filtration through the glomerulus. These crystals can agglomerate into small kidney stones. In order to minimize the formation of IDV stones, patients treated with IDV should drink large amounts of water or other fluids. The proportion of children who will have stones is not yet known, although some studies have suggested a higher peak IDV plasma level after oral dosing in children, which might lead to more stone formation.

Other side-effects of IDV include: hyperbilirubinemia, which occurs in 5–10% of patients; nausea; abdominal pain; headache; and rarely, diabetes. As with the other protease inhibitors, some adult and pediatric patients exhibit a pattern of fat re-distribution and dyslipidemias in association with IDV.

Lopinavir plus ritonavir

Clinical Overview

Lopinavir (LPV, – Abbott) is available only in a fixed-ratio combination with ritonavir (LPV/r, Kaletra). LPV/r is probably the most potent of the PIs. Lopinavir by itself has a very short half-life, so the ritonavir (RTV) is co-administered to inhibit LPV metabolism by the cytochrome P450 enzyme system. The combination can be given every 12 hours. Liquid Kaletra is, like liquid ritonavir, a bad-tasting solution with 42% ethanol. There is significant debate among clinicians concerning LPV/r's optimal role in antiretroviral therapy. Some studies suggest that it is more potent and produces a more durable virologic response than other available PIs, leading some clinicians to suggest that it be used for initial therapy. Other clinicians note that LPV resistance is associated with a somewhat different spectrum of resistance mutations than the other PIs, so that LPV/r can often be used to good effect in a second line "salvage" treatment regimen, and thus suggest that other PIs be used for initial treatment and that LPV/r be held in reserve. Lopinavir plus ritonavir is FDA approved for children 6 months of age and older.

Antiviral effects

Kaletra is probably the most potent PI currently licensed. There are 11 mutations which have been linked to LPV resistance: L10F/I/R/V, K20M/R, L24I, M46I/L, F53L, I54V/L, L63P, A71V/T, V82A/F/T/S, I84V, and L90M. The presence of 6–8 mutations produce high level resistance and is associated with clinical failure.

Pharmacokinetics

Lopinavir plus ritonavir can be dosed every 12 hours, and is available as either a capsule or liquid. Attention must be paid to drug–drug interactions, because the ritonavir component, in particular, inhibits the cytochrome P450 system resulting in extensive drug interactions. In addition, Kaletra liquid is 42% ethanol. Lopinavir plus ritonavir should be taken with food, both to enhance absorption and improve tolerability.

Clinical trials

One Abbott-sponsored trial, Study 940, assessed the clinical efficacy of LPV/r in 100 children, 44 antiretroviral naïve and 56 experienced. After 48 weeks of the study, 80% of the 44 naïve patients had plasma HIV RNA levels below 400 copies per mL, while 71% of the antiretroviral-treatment experienced patients had plasma HIV RNA levels below 400 copies per mL. The mean CD4+ lymphocyte count increases were 404 and 284 cells/μL for the naïve and experienced patients, respectively [27].

Adverse effects

The most common adverse experiences are gastrointestinal upset and diarrhea. As with other PIs, triglyceride levels and elevated cholesterol are fairly common. Pancreatitis

has been rarely reported in association with LPV/r. Exacerbation or new onset of diabetes mellitus has also been associated with LPV/r.

Nelfinavir

Clinical overview

Nelfinavir (NLV, Viracept, – Agouron/Pfizer) is a less convenient drug to administer than ritonavir, but has fewer adverse reactions. The medication is available in tablets and a granular powder. The powder is somewhat bulky and there are sufficient questions about its bioavailability that many centers prefer to use the caps dispersed in a solution like milk or formula.

Antiviral effects

Nelfinavir is similar to other PIs in its antiviral effect. It requires a different set of resistance mutations than ritonavir or indinavir. The most important mutation is D30N, which was found in 56% of patients who received NLV monotherapy by 12 to 16 weeks. There is marked cross-resistance between NLV and the other PIs, although patients who fail NLV and have only low-level resistance may respond to other PIs or PI combinations. HIV with high level NLV resistance is also resistant to other PIs. For these HIVs with high level resistance, 65–80% of isolates with more than 10-fold resistance to NLV also had more than a four-fold increase in resistance to other PIs [28]. HIV that is resistant to other PIs usually has significant resistance to NLV, so treatment with NLV offers little benefit if a patient has failed therapy with another PI.

Pharmacokinetics

Nelfinavir is hepatically metabolized by multiple cytochrome P450 isoforms, including CYP3A. The adult plasma half-life is 3.5–5 hours. The drug is highly protein bound, and relatively little is cleared through the kidneys. Most of the drug is excreted through the gastrointestinal tract and feces. The standard dosage interval is every 8–12 hours. The granular powder is difficult for most children to take, and many centers use a dispersed capsule if the correct dosage can be achieved.

Clinical trials

The phase I/II trial of NLV in children demonstrated a potent antiviral effect when NLV was given in combination with NRTIs. The best effect was seen in children who received at least one new NRTI when NLV was started. In those children, 8/11 followed to 34 weeks had undetectable virus loads [29]. Nelfinavir may be somewhat less effective in children who have already been treated with multiple agents, although several centers have noted CD4+

lymphocyte counts improve even after the level of virus suppression becomes marginal.

In adults, NLV combined with ZDV/3TC in treatment-naïve patients was very effective. Eighty-one percent of adults treated with 750 mg NLV plus ZDV/3TC were able to achieve plasma HIV RNA concentrations below the limits of detection, compared with 18% of subjects assigned ZDV-3TC alone.

Adverse effects

Nelfinavir has a tolerable level of adverse drug effects. The most common adverse effect is diarrhea, which is generally manageable with symptomatic measures. Some children may, however, be unable to tolerate NLV due to diarrhea. Less common problems include tiredness, abdominal pains, and rashes. Diabetes can occur rarely, as it does with all PIs.

Ritonavir

Clinical overview

Ritonavir (RTV, Norvir, – Abbott) was the first protease inhibitor FDA approved for children. It is available in both a liquid formulation and gel-caps. The liquid has a bad taste and contains 43% ethanol. Ritonavir is potent, but because of significant side-effects and drug interactions, needs to be used with care.

Antiviral effects

Ritonavir is very potent and has a relatively complex pattern of resistance mutations. The mutations conferring resistance to RTV are, however, almost identical with those conferring resistance to IDV, so patients who are failing therapy with one drug are unlikely to benefit from a switch to the other. The main mutations associated with RTV resistance have been at protease codons 82, 84, and 90. Some patients with high-level resistance to NLV will also be refractory to RTV, although it depends on which anti-NLV mutations are present.

Pharmacokinetics

The pharmacokinetics of RTV are complicated by its effect on hepatic enzymes. Ritonavir is hepatically metabolized by the cytochrome P450 system. Complicating its clearance, RTV generally inhibits P450, but induces its own metabolism. Ritonavir is begun at half the normal dose, then increased after a period of induction. Because of the induction of metabolism, this strategy of a low dose moving to a higher one will yield drug concentrations that are fairly constant. Ritonavir metabolism appears to be saturable, so that increasing doses beyond some threshold level may produce higher than expected levels.

Ritonavir is well absorbed orally, regardless of food. The half-life is 3–4 hours. There are many interactions with other medications that can affect the metabolism of the RTV as well as the other compounds. These important interactions are reviewed in Chapter 19.

Ritonavir as a boosting agent

Because of RTV's effect on cytochrome P450 enzymes, it is often used to prolong the half life of other drugs, particularly other PIs. This aspect of RTV was exploited in the formulation of LPV/r (Kaletra), but will be used to improve the pharmacokinetic properties of many of the PIs. The aspect of RTV is still being developed, but recommendations will be forthcoming regarding optimum use of other drugs in combination with RTV.

Clinical trials

The pediatric benefits of RTV have been demonstrated by PACTG protocol 338. Ritonavir-containing regimens (ZDV/3TC/RTV or D4T/RTV) had a larger suppression of viral load and a better CD4 cell response than did a ZDV/3TC containing regimen when given to stable, therapy-experienced children. The study was not powered to answer clinical efficacy questions [30, 31].

Adverse effects

Ritonavir is associated with many problematic side-effects. Nausea and vomiting are produced both by the RTV itself, and by the ethanol solvent. In some children the nausea becomes chronic and does not decrease with time. Ritonavir can also produce diarrhea, anorexia, headaches, circumoral paresthesias, and elevated hepatic transaminases. In rare circumstances, it may produce diabetes. Hypercholesterolemia and hypertriglyceridemia are both common.

Care should be taken in co-administering any drug with RTV. There is a long list of absolute and relative contraindications, including many drugs commonly used in HIV disease (see Chapter 19). The common thread is clearance by the cytochrome P450 enzyme system.

Saquinavir

Clinical overview

There is less information about pediatric use of saquinavir (SQV, Invirase [hard gel capsule] or Fortivase [soft-gel capsule – see below], Roche) than other PIs, primarily because the only approved formulation is adult-sized capsules. Saquinavir is most often used in combination with ritonavir. This combination is rational both because SQV has a distinct resistance pattern, and because RTV increases serum SQV levels. Some patients who have failed NLV may respond to the combination of RTV and SQV, although they will do best if new NRTIs are introduced at the same time.

Although there is no pediatric dose for SQV yet, it seems probable the dosing interval will be every 8 hours. In most cases it will be given in combination with RTV. The adult capsules are relatively large and several must be taken at each dosing interval. The drug interactions of SQV are very much like the other PIs, although are less significant than those of RTV.

Antiviral effects

While some mutations that confer resistance to the other PIs also confer resistance to SQV, for example L10R/V, V82A, I84V, and L90M, the SQV resistance pattern also has some unique features. The key mutations conferring resistance to SQV are G48V and L90M. In its soft-gel preparation, it is probably similar to other PIs in potency.

Pharmacokinetics

Saquinavir is administered as a soft-gel capsule (Fortivase). The previous formulation (Invirase) was not adequately bioavailable (less than 5% absorbed). The soft-gel capsule is enjoying wider use than the hard-gel capsule. However, the levels of SQV and the clinical effects are much improved when the hard-gel capsule is administered together with ritonavir. While absorption of the soft gel capsules in children is similar to adults, children appear to clear oral SQV somewhat more rapidly, and a higher mg/kg dose is required [31]. Food increases SQV absorption in the soft-gel formulation. Saquinavir is cleared almost entirely by cytochrome P450 CYP3A4. The plasma half-life is 1.6 hours, and the standard dosing interval is every 8 hours. Concomitant NLV, IND, or RTV therapy increase SQV levels by inhibiting hepatic metabolism (approximately 4-fold, 6-fold, and 20-fold, respectively). Ritonavir can, in fact, increase the serum half-life of SQV so that only twice-daily dosing is required. Saquinavir does not penetrate well into the CSF.

Clinical trials

There is very little clinical information on SQV in children. The new soft-gel capsules improved the clinical effects seen in adults. The first large study of SQV, ACTG 229, used the original SQV preparation in a three-way comparison of SQV/ZDV, ZDV/DDC, and SQV/ZDV/DDC in treatment-experienced patients. The SQV/ZDV combination produced the least improvements in CD4+ lymphocyte counts and plasma HIV RNA concentrations. The triple combination was better, but the positive effects of the combination were relatively short-lived. The new soft-gel capsule combined with ZDV/3TC is more potent. In antiretroviral naïve-patients, SQV/ZDV/3TC was able to decrease the plasma HIV RNA concentrations in 61% of the patients to below the level of detection (20 copies/mL) [32].

Adverse effects

Saquinavir is generally well tolerated. The most common adverse experiences are diarrhea, abdominal pain, headache, and nausea. Diabetes may rarely occur. Photosensitivity can occur with SQV, so sunscreen and protective clothing are suggested.

Atazanavir

Clinical overview

Atazanavir is a protease inhibitor which has been FDA approved for adults. It has two advantages in adults: (1) once daily dosing; (2) minimal changes in lipid concentrations, unlike most of the other protease inhibitors. However, ATZ appears to have a shorter half-life in children and adolescents, which means that to achieve once-daily dosing, RTV boosting is required. The RTV boosting may then negate atazanavir's decreased likelihood of causing dyslipidemia. Cross resistance between ATZ and other PIs is common, so the drug does not offer much promise in second-line or salvage regimens.

Antiviral effects

The primary mutation isolated from patients failing ATZ therapy has been I50L, often in combination with A71V. Resistance is also associated with I84V, L90M, A71V/T, N88S/D, and M46I (according to the Reyataz package insert).

Pharmacokinetics

Pharmacokinetic studies of ATZ in children are ongoing. Determining a correct dose has not been as easy as simply extrapolating from adult regimens, and to obtain a once-daily regimen in children has required RTV boosting. Atazanavir has many pharmacokinetic interactions because it is an inhibitor of CYP3A and UGT1A1, a pattern typical of PIs. It interacts with antacids, including proton pump inhibitors like omeprazole, leading to decreased absorption of ATZ. Stomach acid neutralizing agents should not be used with ATZ. Concomitant administration of ATZ and TDF lead to significant decreases in ATZ concentrations (a ~40% in Cmin and a ~25% in AUC). If for some special reason this combination must be used, then ATZ should be boosted with ritonavir.

Clinical trials

There is very little clinical information on ATZ in children. Pediatric ACTG protocol 1020A, a study of ATZ in therapy-naïve and experienced patients is ongoing.

Adverse effects

Atazanavir produces total hyperbilirubinemia in 35–50% of patients. In roughly 10% of patients, this effect will be severe enough to produce jaundice and scleral icterus. As a result, because of concerns about kernicterus, ATZ is contraindicated in children less than 3 months old. Other adverse effects are similar to other PIs and NNRTIs.

18.3.4 Fusion inhibitors

Enfuvirtide
Overview

Enfuvirtide (ENF, Fuzeon – Trimeris/Roche) is the first in a novel category of antiretroviral drugs, the fusion inhibitors. Enfuvirtide is a 36 amino acid peptide that is homologous to a portion of the viral gp41 envelope glycoprotein. It acts by mimicking the native viral portion of gp41, complexing with the virus gp41 and blocking the conformational changes in that molecule that allow fusion of the virus's lipid bilayer and the cell membrane (see Chapter 2). The limitations to ENF include its expense and the fact that it must be administered through injection. Although the drug has been licensed, its availability will likely be limited for some time because it is difficult and expensive to produce.

Antiviral effects

Enfuvirtide acts to block viral fusion with the host cell membrane. Resistance mutations occur in the gp41 envelope gene, primarily in the region of the first heptide repeat (HR-1). Several candidate resistance mutations have been noted: G36D/S, I37V, V38A/M, Q39R, N42T, and N43D. Resistance appears to develop relatively rapidly if ENF is used as monotherapy.

Pharmacokinetics

Enfuvirtide is a synthetic peptide, and administration of the active form requires subcutaneous injection on an every 12-hour schedule. It does not interact with or alter the metabolism of most other antiretroviral drugs.

Clinical trials

In adults, the benefits of ENF were demonstrated by comparing ENF plus a combination of other antiretroviral drugs selected using knowledge of the patient's antiretroviral history and an assessment of the resistance profile of the patient's virus (an "optimized background regimen")

versus the optimized background regimen alone in highly antiretroviral-experienced patients. In the ENF group, 32.7% of patients achieved plasma HIV RNA concentrations below 400 copies/mL, while 15% of the control group achieved plasma HIV RNA concentrations below 400 copies/mL [33]. There is one pediatric phase I study, which demonstrated pharmacokinetics and safety similar to adults, but only limited efficacy data are available.

Adverse effects

By far the most common adverse effect is the generation of injection site reactions. Whether there are other drug-associated adverse reactions is not yet established.

18.3.5 Combination antiretroviral regimens

Antiretroviral drugs are virtually always given in combinations. While monotherapy with several drugs in clinical trials has demonstrated significant clinical benefit, single-drug regimens yield only limited decreases in plasma HIV RNA, modest increases in CD4+ lymphocyte numbers, and lead to rapid emergence of drug resistance. As a result, multi-drug regimens, HAART, are standard. Virtually all first-line combination regimens begin with an NRTI "backbone." One of the greatest limitations in current therapeutic strategies is that there are a limited number of NRTIs, and cross resistance is probably more of a problem than was originally believed. For example, there are currently only two thymidine-derived NRTIs, ZDV and d4T, and one or the other will form a component of most regimens. However, these two drugs have a considerable degree of cross-resistance. Tenofovir may eventually be another option, but experience is currently limited, and it may present particular problems for pediatrics. Zidovudine and d4t should not be used simultaneously in the same regimen, since both drugs require phosphorylation by the same kinase and will compete with each other for the first phosphorylation step.

After starting with a thymidine-derived NRTI, most combinations add 3TC or ddI. The combination of ddI and d4T has a higher rate of adverse side-effects than other combinations, including metabolic problems such as lactic acidosis, and pancreatitis, and so is a combination currently viewed with disfavor. The problems with lactic acidosis are particularly frequent in pregnant women; the combination of d4T and ddI is clearly contraindicated during pregnancy.

The other available nucleoside, abacavir, can be used in combination with both ZDV and 3TC, or simply with 3TC. It appears to be the most potent of the nucleosides, particularly when used in a first-line regimen. Abacavir is less effective as second-line therapy.

The convenience of fixed-dose combination tablets makes some combinations more appealing in children large enough to take the tablets. The fixed dose combination of ZDV and 3TC as Combivir (Glaxo SmithKline), and ABC, ZDV, and 3TC as trizivir (Glaxo SmithKline), both of which are dosed twice a day, offer some advantages in decreasing pill burden and potentially improving adherence. Trizivir used alone, in particular, has garnered considerable interest from clinicians caring for adolescents because of its low pill burden and the increased potential for adherence. However, recent results indicate that Trizivir alone is less effective than Trizivir plus a PI, or Combivir plus a PI, so Trizivir used alone will probably be less-favored approach in the future.

After the nucleoside backbone has been chosen, a third and sometimes a fourth drug will be added, depending on the patient's clinical details, prior antiretroviral therapy, resistance testing, if available, the patient's age, and adherence considerations. Among the protease inhibitors, there is no clear choice for first-line therapy. Nelfinavir is often given because of its relatively good tolerability, and because second-line PI regimens are somewhat easier to construct after NLV failure than after other PIs. Lopinavir plus ritonavir is probably the most potent option, but its taste and the ethanol content of the liquid preparation are obstacles for many children. The NNRTIs, either NVP (for young children) or EFV (in older children), are convenient and viable options for components of first-line therapy, as long as the family appears to be likely to be medication-adherent. Because high-level resistance develops rapidly when the currently available NNRTIs are used alone, many clinicians would not construct an antiretroviral combination therapeutic regimen using the NNRTIs if there are doubts about the ability of the family to be strictly adherent.

The decisions regarding initial therapy cannot be made casually. Many factors, particularly a family's ability to adhere to complex medical regimens, need to be considered. Erratic compliance with any antiretroviral drug is likely to select resistant virus that limits the future effectiveness of other drugs in the same class. Thus, care must be taken in selecting the regimen, including information like the family's daily schedule, their history of medical compliance, school attendance, and whether the school system knows the child's diagnosis. These issues will be considered further in Chapter 22.

In selecting a salvage therapy for children failing their initial regimen, the choice will usually include the other thymidine-derived NRTI (ZDV or d4T) or possibly TDF, an alternate non-thymidine NRTI (3TC or ddI), and one or two drugs from among the PIs and NNRTIs. As discussed above, even if the patient had been previously treated with 3TC, many clinicians would continue to treat with 3TC because of its ability to hypersensitize to other NNRTIs (e.g. AZT, TDF). The choice will depend on the patient's prior experience and resistance testing. Once a patient has documented resistance to an antiretroviral, they will maintain 'archived' reservoirs of virus resistant to that agent for life, and the resistant species will rapidly reappear if therapy with that antiretroviral is reinstituted (see also Chapters 4 and 5). However, antiretroviral-resistant virus is less "fit" and in some ways less pathogenic than the wild-type virus, so even after viral breakthrough has occurred there continues to be an advantage to using an antiretroviral regimen. This advantage must be weighed against the ongoing selection of resistance while drugs are used in the face of ongoing replication.

There are relatively limited therapeutic options currently available for children. As a result, there is a finite number of effective changes in antiretroviral regimens available, probably no more than three regimens in toto, using currently available drugs. Other regimens will have limited benefit, with either incomplete suppression or a short period of complete suppression. Regimen switches should not be made casually, and careful consideration should be given for the clinical need to change, taking into account factors like adherence, symptoms, CD4$^+$ lymphocyte count changes, and viral load. Hopefully, the number of options and potential switches will increase as progress is made in pediatric antiretroviral research.

REFERENCES

1. McKinney, R. E., Jr., Maha, M. A., Connor, E. M. *et al.* A multicenter trial of oral zidovudine in children with advanced human immunodeficiency virus disease. The Protocol 043 Study Group. *New Engl. J. Med.* **324** : **15** (1991), 1018–25.

2. Fischl, M. A., Richman, D. D., Grieco, M. H. *et al.* The efficacy of azidothymidine (AZT) in the treatment of patients with AIDS and AIDS-related complex. A double-blind, placebo-controlled trial. *New Engl. J. Med.* **317** : **4** (1987), 185–91.

3. McKinney, R. E., Jr., Pizzo, P. A., Scott, G. B. *et al.* Safety and tolerance of intermittent intravenous and oral zidovudine therapy in human immunodeficiency virus-infected pediatric patients. Pediatric Zidovudine Phase I Study Group. *J. Pediatr.* **116** : **4** (1990), 640–7.

4. Englund, J. A., Baker, C. J., Raskino, C. *et al.* Zidovudine, didanosine, or both as the initial treatment for symptomatic HIV-infected children. AIDS Clinical Trials Group (ACTG) Study 152 Team. *New Engl. J. Med.* **336** : **24** (1997), 1704–12.

5. Connor, E. M., Sperling, R. S., Gelber, R. *et al.* Reduction of maternal-infant transmission of human immunodeficiency virus type 1 with zidovudine treatment. Pediatric AIDS Clinical

Trials Group Protocol 076 Study Group. *New Engl. J. Med.* **331** : **18** (1994), 1173–80.

6. Maha, M. A. Nucleoside exposure in the children of HIV-infected women receiving antiretroviral drugs: absence of clear evidence for mitochondrial disease in children who died before 5 years of age in five United States cohorts. *J. Acquir. Immune. Defic. Syndr.* **25** : **3** (2000), 261–8.

7. Butler, K. M., Husson, R. N., Balis, F. M. *et al.* Dideoxy-inosine in children with symptomatic human immunodeficiency virus infection. *New Engl. J. Med.* **324** : **3** (1991), 137–44.

8. Mueller, B. U., Butler, K. M., Stocker, V. L. *et al.* Clinical and pharmacokinetic evaluation of long-term therapy with didanosine in children with HIV infection. *Pediatrics* **94** : **5** (1994), 724–31.

9. Kline, M. W., Fletcher, C. V., Federici, M. E. *et al.* Combination therapy with stavudine and didanosine in children with advanced human immunodeficiency virus infection: pharmacokinetic properties, safety, and immunologic and virologic effects. *Pediatrics* **97** : **6** (1996), 886–90.

10. McKinney, R. E., Jr., Johnson, G. M., Stanley, K. *et al.* A randomized study of combined zidovudine-lamivudine versus didanosine monotherapy in children with symptomatic therapy-naive HIV-1 infection. The Pediatric AIDS Clinical Trials Group Protocol 300 Study Team. *J. Pediatr.* **133** : **4** (1998), 500–8.

11. Kline, M. W., Van Dyke, R. B., Lindsey, J. C. *et al.* A randomized comparative trial of stavudine (d4T) versus zidovudine (ZDV, AZT) in children with human immunodeficiency virus infection. AIDS Clinical Trials Group 240 Team. *Pediatrics* **101** : **2** (1998), 214–20.

12. Spector, S. A., Blanchard, S., Wara, D. W. *et al.* Comparative trial of two dosages of zalcitabine in zidovudine-experienced children with advanced human immunodeficiency virus disease. Pediatric AIDS Clinical Trials Group. *Pediatr. Infect. Dis. J.* **16** : **6** (1997), 623–6.

13. Bakshi, S. S., Britto, P., Capparelli, E. *et al.* Evaluation of pharmacokinetics, safety, tolerance, and activity of combination of zalcitabine and zidovudine in stable, zidovudine-treated pediatric patients with human immunodeficiency virus infection. AIDS Clinical Trials Group Protocol 190 Team. *J. Infect. Dis.* **175** : **5** (1997), 1039–50.

14. Kline, M. W., Blanchard, S., Fletcher, C. V. *et al.* A phase I study of abacavir (1592U89) alone and in combination with other antiretroviral agents in infants and children with human immunodeficiency virus infection. AIDS Clinical Trials Group 330 Team. *Pediatrics* **103** : **4** (1999), e47.

15. Gibb, D., Giaquinto, C., Walker, A. *et al.* Three year follow-up of the PENTA 5 trial. (Abstract 874). In *10th Annual Conference on Retroviruses and Opportunistic Infections*, Boston, MA (2003).

16. Barditch-Crovo, P., Deeks, S. G., Collier, A. *et al.* Phase I/II trial of the pharmacokinetics, safety, and antiretroviral activity of tenofovir disoproxil fumarate in human immunodeficiency virus-infected adults. *Antimicrob. Agents. Chemother.* **45** : **10** (2001), 2733–9.

17. Saez-Llorens, X., Violari, A., Ndiweni, D. *et al.* Once-daily emtricitabine in HIV-infected pediatric patients with other antiretroviral agents. In *10th Conference on Retroviruses and Opportunistic Infections*, Boston, MA (2003).

18. de Jong, M. D., Vella, S., Carr, A. *et al.* High-dose nevirapine in previously untreated human immunodeficiency virus type 1-infected persons does not result in sustained suppression of viral replication. *J. Infect. Dis.* **175** : **4** (1997), 966–70.

19. Luzuriaga, K., Bryson, Y., Krogstad, P. *et al.* Combination treatment with zidovudine, didanosine, and nevirapine in infants with human immunodeficiency virus type 1 infection. *New Engl. J. Med.* **336** : **19** (1997), 1343–9.

20. Burchett, S., Carey, V., Yong, F. *et al.* Virologic activity of didanosine (ddI), zidovudine (ZDV), and nevirapine (NVP) combinations in pediatric subjects with advanced HIV disease (ACTG 245). [Abstract 245]. In *5th Annual Conference on Retroviruses and Opportunistic Infections*, Chicago, IL (1998).

21. Wathen, L., Freimuth, W. & Getchel, L. Use of HIV-1 RNA PCR in patients on Rescriptor (DLV)+Retrovir (ZDV)+Epivir (3TC), ZDV+3TC, or DLV+ZDV allowed early differentiation between treatment arms. [Abstract 694]. In *5th Annual Conference on Retroviruses and Opportunistic Infections*, Chicago, IL (1998).

22. Starr, S. E., Fletcher, C. V., Spector, S. A. *et al.* Combination therapy with efavirenz, nelfinavir, and nucleoside reverse-transcriptase inhibitors in children infected with human immunodeficiency virus type 1. Pediatric AIDS Clinical Trials Group 382 Team. *New Engl. J. Med.* **341** : **25** (1999), 1874–81.

23. McKinney, R. E., Rathore, M. & Jankelevich, S. PACTG 1021: An ongoing phase I/II study of once-daily emtricitabine, didanosine, and efavirenz in therapy-naive or minimally treated patients. [Abstract 373]. In *10th Annual Conference on Retroviruses and Opportunistic Infections*, Boston, MA (2003).

24. Sadler, B. M., Gillotin, C., Lou, Y. *et al.* Pharmacokinetic study of human immunodeficiency virus protease inhibitors used in combination with amprenavir. *Antimicrob. Agents. Chemother.* **45** : **12** (2001), 3663–8.

25. Yogev, R., Church, J., Flynn, P. M. *et al.* Pediatric trial of combination therapy including the protease inhibitor amprenavir (APV). [Abstract 430]. In *6th Conference on Retroviruses and Opportunistic Infections*, Chicago, IL (1999).

26. Gulick, R. M., Mellors, J. W., Havlir, D. *et al.* Treatment with indinavir, zidovudine, and lamivudine in adults with human immunodeficiency virus infection and prior antiretroviral therapy. *New Engl. J. Med.* **337** : **11** (1997), 734–9.

27. Abbott Laboratories. Kaletra (lopinavir/r) package insert (2002).

28. Hertogs, K., Mellors, J. W., Schel, P. *et al.* Patterns of cross-resistance among protease inhibitors in 483 HIV-1 isolates. [Abstract 395]. In *5th Annual Conference on Retroviruses and Opportunistic Infections*, Chicago, IL (1998).

29. Krogstad, P., Wiznia, A., Luzuriaga, K. *et al.* Treatment of human immunodeficiency virus 1-infected infants and children with the protease inhibitor nelfinavir mesylate. *Clin. Infect. Dis.* **28** : **5** (1999), 1109–18.

30. Nachman, S. A., Stanley, K., Yogev, R. *et al.* Nucleoside analogs plus ritonavir in stable antiretroviral therapy-experienced HIV-infected children: a randomized controlled trial. Pediatric AIDS Clinical Trials Group 338 Study Team. *J. Am. Med. Assoc.* **283** : 4 (2000), 492–8.

31. Kline, M. W., Brundage, R. C., Fletcher, C. V. *et al.* Combination therapy with saquinavir soft gelatin capsules in children with human immunodeficiency virus infection. *Pediatr. Infect. Dis. J.* **20** : 7 (2001), 666–71.

32. Sension, M., Farthing, C., Pattison, T. P., Pilson, R. & Siemon-Hryczyk, P. Fortovase (Saquinavir soft gel capsule: SQV-SGC) in combination with AZT and 3TC in antiretroviral naive HIV-1 infected patients. [Abstract 369]. In *5th Annual Conference on Retroviruses and Opportunistic Infections*, Chicago, IL (1998).

33. Delfraissy, J., Montaner, J., Eron, J. J. *et al.* Summary of pooled efficacy and safety analyses of enfuvirtide (ENF) treatment for 24 weeks in TORO 1 and TORO 2 phase III trials in highly antiretroviral (ARV) treatment-experienced patients. In *10th Conference on Retroviruses and Opportunistic Infections*, Boston, MA; February 10–14, 2003. [Abstract 568].

19

Antiretroviral drug interactions

Thomas N. Kakuda, Pharm.D.[1] and Courtney V. Fletcher, Pharm.D.[2]

[1]Associate Clinical Research Scientist, Abbott Laboratories
[2]Professor, University of Colorado Health Sciences Center, Denver, CO

Treatment of HIV-infected patients requires unavoidable polypharmacy, during which drug interactions can occur. Pharmacokinetic interactions are those that affect the absorption, distribution, metabolism, or excretion of a drug. Interactions that produce antagonistic, additive, or synergistic effects are considered pharmacodynamic interactions. Not all interactions are clinically adverse and in some cases, interactions can be beneficial. The objective of this chapter is to provide the clinician with a framework for understanding drug interactions by applying the principles of pharmacology in the context of HIV medicine.

19.1 Pharmacokinetic drug interactions

19.1.1 Absorption

The absorption of oral drugs is affected by several conditions such as fasting, gastric pH, and enteric P-glycoprotein (PGP) expression. Drug–food interactions are delineated in Table 19.1; also listed are antiretroviral drugs that may be administered without regard to food. Drugs that increase gastric pH include antacids (including the buffer in older formulations of didanosine), H_2-receptor antagonists, and proton pump inhibitors. These drugs can impair the bioavailability of drugs that require a low pH for optimal absorption such as delavirdine, indinavir, itraconazole, and ketoconazole. This interaction can usually be avoided by administrating the gastric pH-raising agent 1–2 hours later [1–3]. Didanosine is an example of a drug much better absorbed in an alkaline environment because it is acid labile. The original formulation of didanosine included a buffer (calcium carbonate and magnesium hydroxide in tablets or citrate-phosphate in sachets) or had to be reconstituted in antacid. Contrary to previous reports, the buffer in didanosine does not affect dapsone absorption but has been shown to significantly decrease ciprofloxacin absorption [4, 5]. The latter interaction occurs because di- and trivalent cations in the buffer can chelate fluoroquinolones – it is not related to didanosine per se. Didanosine or antacids do not interfere with nevirapine. The new formulation of didanosine (Videx® EC) does not have significant interactions with ciprofloxacin, indinavir, or azole antifungals [6, 7]. Lastly, drug absorption may also be affected by transporters in the gut. P-glycoprotein expression in the gastrointestinal tract, for example, may account for the poor bioavailability of saquinavir and perhaps other protease inhibitors (PIs) [8].

19.1.2 Distribution

The space to which a drug distributes in the body is a function of binding to plasma proteins and tissues. Albumin or α_1-acid glycoprotein (α_1-AGP, orosomucoid) are the two plasma proteins that bind most drugs. For example, PIs bind preferentially to α_1-AGP. It is the free or unbound fraction of drug that is typically available to exert a pharmacologic effect. Most of the PIs are highly protein bound (90–99%) with the exception of indinavir (~60%) [9]. Enfuvirtide (T-20), a fusion inhibitor, is also highly protein bound. Among the non-nucleoside reverse transcriptase inhibitors (NNRTIs), efavirenz and delavirdine are highly protein bound (98–99%) with nevirapine only moderately (~60%) protein bound [10]. Nucleoside and nucleotide reverse transcriptase inhibitors (NRTIs) have negligible protein binding (< 50%). When two or more drugs exhibiting extensive protein binding are given concomitantly,

Table 19.1 Drug–food interactions

Drugs best administered with food

    albendazole

    amiodarone

    atazanavir

    atovaquone

    carbamazepine

    erythromycin ethylsuccinate

    hydralazine

    hydrochlorothiazide

    itraconazole capsules[a]

    lithium citrate

    lopinavir/ritonavir

    nelfinavir[a]

    para-aminosalicylic acid[b]

    propranolol

    rifabutin

    ritonavir

    saquinavir[a]

    tenofovir

Drugs best administered on an empty stomach (1 hour prior to the meal or 2 hours after)

    ampicillin

    azithromycin

    didanosine (all formulations)

    efavirenz[c]

    indinavir (without ritonavir)

    itraconazole solution

    penicillin VK

    rifampin

Antiretroviral drugs that may be administered without regard to food

    abacavir

    amprenavir

    delavirdine

    enfuvirtide

    fosamprenavir

    indinavir/ritonavir

    lamivudine

    nevirapine

    stavudine

    zidovudine

Drugs appearing in bold are those likely to be prescribed to an HIV-infected patient.

[a] Absorption is better with a fatty meal.

[b] Absorption is better when sprinkled on acidic food (apple sauce or yogurt) or mixed with juice.

[c] Coadministration with food may increase efavirenz plasma concentrations and incidence of central nervous system side-effects.

there is a potential for one drug to displace the other drug from the binding site; consequently, the unbound drug may exert a larger pharmacological effect. This interaction can go in both directions. In general, protein-binding displacement is a clinically insignificant interaction since there is a dynamic equilibrium between unbound drug in the plasma and the extravascular region. Highly protein-bound drugs ($>70\%$), however, may exhibit a significant displacement interaction if the drug is given intravenously, eliminated primarily by hepatic metabolism (i.e. has a high extraction ratio) and has a narrow therapeutic index. Such drugs include alfentanil, buprenorphine, fentanyl, hydralazine, lidocaine, midazolam, or verapamil. In these instances, close monitoring of the patient is warranted if the situation cannot be avoided [11]. None of the current antiretroviral drugs including enfuvirtide appear to have significant protein-binding interactions.

19.1.3 Metabolism

The liver is the primary organ for biotransformation of both endogenous and exogenous chemicals. The purpose of this process is to convert lipophilic substances to more water-soluble metabolites, thereby facilitating their elimination. Biotransformation often involves two sequential steps: phase I reactions (oxidation, reduction, or hydrolysis) and phase II reactions (conjugation). Phase I reactions are primarily mediated by the cytochrome P-450 (CYP450) enzyme system. The CYP450 consists of several isozymes, six of which are involved in the majority of drug metabolism: CYP 1A2, 2C9/10, 2C19, 2D6, 2E1, and 3A. These isozymes are present to varying degrees based on age, ethnicity, and other factors [12–14]. Table 19.2 summarizes selected CYP450 substrates, inhibitors, and inducers; information regarding population polymorphisms and age-specific issues is included where known. This table provides a method for clinicians to predict relevant drug interactions by determining which drugs decrease or increase CYP450 activity (inhibitors or inducers, respectively) and drugs that might be affected by these changes (substrates). Enfuvirtide and NRTIs do not significantly affect CYP450 activity, therefore metabolic drug interactions are less likely to occur with these agents. Delavirdine and the PIs with the exception of tipranavir inhibit CYP 3A to varying degrees with ritonavir having the most potent effect [15, 16]. Because many drugs are substrates of the CYP3A isozyme, concomitant administration with a PI or delavirdine may increase plasma concentrations of the substrate. Depending on the drug, increased concentrations can lead to toxicity (in which case the combination should be avoided or an alternative medication used) or it can be therapeutically useful. Ritonavir boosted regimens (e.g. lopinavir/ritonavir)

Table 19.2 Select cytochrome P-450 subfamily substrates, inhibitors, and inducers

CYP1A2

Substrates

  acetaminophen, alprazolam, amitriptyline, clomipramine, desipramine, exogenous steroids, haloperidol, imipramine, propranolol, **tenofovir**, theophylline, thioridazine

Inhibitors

  azithromycin, **erythromycin**, fluoroquinolones, grapefruit juice, **isoniazid**, **ketoconazole**

Inducers

  charcoal in food, cigarette smoke, phenobarbital, phenytoin, **rifampin**, **ritonavir**

Note: Activity in neonates is very low but matures to adult activity approximately 120 days after birth. Expression of this gene may be polymorphic.

CYP2C9/10

Substrates

  diazepam, ibuprofen, naproxen, phenytoin

Inhibitors

  amiodarone, chloramphenicol, cimetidine, **fluconazole**, **isoniazid**, **metronidazole**, **miconazole**, omeprazole, **ritonavir**, **sulfamethoxazole**

Inducers

  rifampin

Note: Infants between the age of 1–6 months have activity comparable with adults. Children 3–6 years old have significantly greater activity but become comparable with adult activity after puberty.

CYP2C19

Substrates

  diazepam, imipramine, S-mephenytoin, propranolol

Inhibitors

  ketoconazole

Note: 3–5% of whites, and 20% of Asians have reduced expression of this gene (poor metabolizers).

CYP2D6 (debrisoquine/sparteine hydroxylase)

Substrates

  amitriptyline, chlorpromazine, clomipramine, codeine, desipramine, dextromethorphan, haloperidol[a], hydrocodone, imipramine, **indinavir**, meperidine, metoprolol, morphine, nortriptyline, oxycodone, propranolol, **ritonavir**, **saquinavir**, thioridazine[a], timolol, tramadol, trazodone

Inhibitors

  amiodarone, cimetidine, clomipramine, desipramine, haloperidol, quinidine, **ritonavir**

Note: Pregnancy increases CYP2D6 activity. Infants less than 28 days old have at most 20% of adult activity and therefore should be considered poor metabolizers. Activity comparable with adults occurs by 10 years of age or sooner. 5–10% of whites, 2% of blacks, and 1–2% of Asians have reduced expression of this gene (poor metabolizers).

CYP2E1

Substrates

  acetaminophen, ethanol, halothane, isoflurane, **isoniazid**, theophylline

Inhibitors

  Isoniazid

Inducers

  Ethanol

CYP3A

Substrates

  acetaminophen, alfentanil, alprazolam, amitriptyline[a], **amprenavir**, astemizole, benzphetamine, cannabinoids, carbamazepine, chlorpromazine, cisapride, **clarithromycin**, clindamycin, clonazepam, clorazepate, cocaine, corticosteroids, cyclophosphamide, cyclosporine, **dapsone**, desipramine, dextromethorphan, diazepam, diltiazem, docetaxol, dronabinol, **efavirenz**, ergotamine, erythromycin, estazolam, estrogens, ethosuximide, etoposide, fentanyl, fexofenadine, flurazepam, ifosfamide, imipramine, **indinavir**, itraconazole, ketoconazole, lansoprazole, lidocaine, **lopinavir**, meperidine, miconazole, midazolam, nefazodone, **nevirapine**, nifedipine, nortriptyline, ondansetron, oral contraceptives, paclitaxel, phenobarbital, phenytoin, quinidine, quinine, **rifabutin**, **rifampin**, **ritonavir**, **saquinavir**, tacrolimus, terfenadine, testosterone, triazolam, trimethoprim, verapamil, zileuton

Inhibitors

  amiodarone, **amprenavir**, **azithromycin**, cimetidine, **clarithromycin**, clotrimazole, cyclosporine, **delavirdine**, diltiazem, econazole, **erythromycin**, **fluconazole**, grapefruit juice, **indinavir**, **isoniazid**, **itraconazole**, **ketoconazole**, **metronidazole**, miconazole, norfloxacin, propoxyphene, quinine, **ritonavir**, **saquinavir**, troleandomycin, verapamil, zafirlukast

Inducers

  carbamazepine, dexamethasone, **efavirenz**, ethosuximide, **nevirapine**, **rifabutin**, **rifampin**, phenobarbital, phenytoin, **tipranavir**, troglitazone

Note: High levels of CYP3A are present during embryogenesis. CYP3A4 activity is greater in infants and children compared with adults. Expression of this gene may be polymorphic.

Drugs appearing in bold are those likely to be prescribed to an HIV-infected patient.

[a] indicates a minor metabolic pathway for this drug.

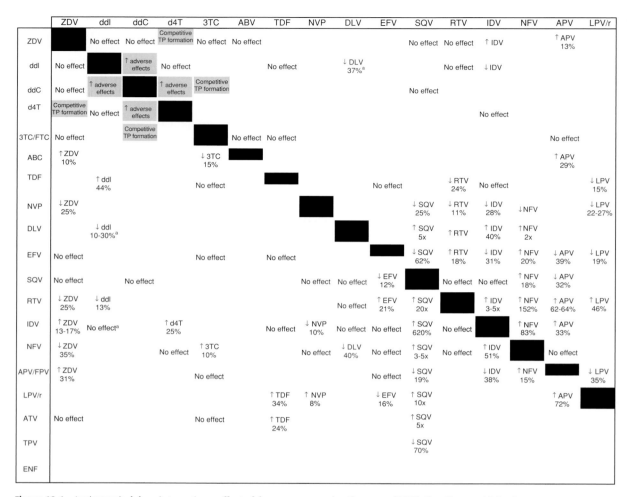

Figure 19.1. Antiretroviral drug interactions: effect of drug on area-under-the-curve (AUC). See Chapter 19 for drug names.

represent examples of using the interaction advantageously [9, 15].

Instead of inhibition, some drugs can induce drug metabolism. Rifampin is a potent inducer of CYP3A and 2C9/10 and increases the metabolism of PIs and delavirdine, among other drugs. Deferment of PI treatment for the duration of rifampin therapy or substitution with rifabutin (if treating *Mycobacterium avium* complex) is recommended due to this interaction [17]. Efavirenz, nevirapine, tipranavir (an investigational PI) and certain anti-convulsants are also CYP3A inducers. Decreases in the plasma concentrations of some PIs have been noted with concomitant efavirenz or nevirapine therapy [10]. Dose adjustment of the PI or adding ritonavir may be required to compensate for cytochrome induction. Lastly, some drugs may exhibit both inhibition and induction properties. Figure 19.1 represents the pharmacokinetic interactions among currently available antiretroviral drugs.

Conjugation (phase II) reactions increase the water solubility of a metabolite, thereby facilitating its excretion. Phase II reactions are mediated by transferases including uridine diphosphoglucuronyltransferase (UDPGT) and N-acetyl transferase (NAT); UDPGT is responsible for conjugation of glucurinic acid with bilirubin, zidovudine, and its metabolite 3′-amino-3′deoxythymidine. Atovaquone and fluconazole (doses > 200 mg/day) inhibit UDPGT causing decreased zidovudine clearance [3, 18]. Inhibition of UDPGT by atazanavir and indinavir may also be responsible for the hyperbilirubinemia seen with these drugs [19]. Inhibition of glucuronidation may be more serious in infants than adolescents and adults since adult activity of UDPGT is not achieved until 6–18 months of age [14].

19.1.4 Excretion

Renal elimination can be affected by two processes: inhibition of tubular secretion or alterations in glomerular

Table 19.3 Drugs with overlapping toxicities

Crystalluria	Hematologic	Hyperglycemia	Pancreatitis
acyclovir[a]	α-interferon	corticosteroids	alcohol
ganciclovir	amphotericin	**didanosine**	aminosalicylates
indinavir	cidofovir	megesterol	calcium
Sulfonamides	dapsone	pentamidine	**didanosine**
	doxorubicin	***protease inhibitors***	**lamivudine**[b]
Dermatologic	flucytosine		pentamidine
α-interferon	ganciclovir	Hyperlipidemia	valproic acid
abacavir	interleukin-2	α-interferon	
amprenavir	pentamidine	β-antagonists	Peripheral neuropathy
bleomycin	pyrimethamine	corticosteroids	cidofovir
delavirdine	sulfadiazine	cyclosporine	dapsone
efavirenz	TMP-SMX	**efavirenz**	**didanosine**
indinavir	**zidovudine**	***protease inhibitors***	ethambutol
interleukin-2		thiazide diuretics	ethionamide
nevirapine	Hyperbilirubinemia		isoniazid
TMP-SMX	**atazanavir**	Hyperuricemia	metronidazole
	cyclosporine	cyclosporine	phenytoin
Gastrointestinal (N/V)	dapsone	**didanosine**	**stavudine**
adefovir	**indinavir**	**ritonavir**	thalidomide
α-interferon	interleukin-2		TMP-SMX
doxorubicin	interleukin-6		**zalcitabine**
foscarnet	lithium	Nephrotoxicity	
ganciclovir	methotrexate[a]	adefovir	Uveitis
interleukin-2	octreotide	aminoglycosides	ethambutol
probenecid	pancuronium	amphotericin	**indinavir**
ritonavir		cidofovir	rifabutin
tipranavir		foscarnet	sulfonamides
zidovudine		ganciclovir	terbenafine
		interleukin-2	
		pentamidine	
		tenofovir	

Abbreviations: N/V, nausea and vomiting; TMP-SMX, trimethoprim-sulfamethoxazole.
Drugs appearing in **bold** are those likely to be prescribed to an HIV-infected patient. *Italics* represent pharmacological classes.
[a] At higher doses.
[b] Primarily in children.

filtration. Cimetidine, probenecid, and trimethoprim are known inhibitors of renal tubular secretion and may lead to increased plasma concentrations of drugs primarily eliminated by this route. For example, trimethoprim-sulfamethoxazole increases the exposure of lamivudine by 44% but has no effect on indinavir [20, 21]. Probenecid is used with cidofovir to reduce the incidence of nephrotoxicity. However, probenecid can interact negatively with zidovudine; zidovudine should be discontinued or dose-reduced 50% on the day of cidofovir administration.

Ganciclovir competes for renal tubular secretion with didanosine and zidovudine and increases their plasma concentrations; this interaction may be more clinically significant for didanosine [22].

Alterations in kidney function can occur from renal disease or may be drug-induced. All NRTIs with the exception of zidovudine have significant renal elimination. Concomitant use with a nephrotoxic drug may require a dosage adjustment of the NRTI, as would administration to a patient with renal insufficiency [23].

Table 19.4 Clinically significant drug interactions with commonly prescribed HIV/AIDS medications

HIV/AIDS drug	Interaction with	Comments
Antiretroviral drugs		
Zidovudine	atovaquone	Zidovudine AUC ↑ 31.
	cidofovir	Hold zidovudine on day of infusion (see probenecid)
	fluconazole	Zidovudine AUC ↑74%; may require dose adjustment
	ganciclovir	Consider holding zidovudine during induction therapy to avoid neutropenia
	nelfinavir	Zidovudine AUC ↓ 35%; may require dose adjustment
	probenecid	Zidovudine AUC ↑ 106%; discontinue zidovudine or reduce dose 50%
	rifampin	Zidovudine AUC ↓ 47%; may require dose adjustment
	stavudine	Contraindicated due to competitive phosphorylation (see text)
	valproic acid	Zidovudine AUC ↑ 80%; may require dose adjustment
	Miscellaneous	See Table 19.3, drugs that may cause gastrointestinal or hematologic side-effects
Didanosine	allopurinol	Didanosine AUC ↑ ~4-fold; co-administration is not recommended
	delavirdine	Separate administration by at least 1–2 hours if using Videx or consider Videx EC (see text)
	fluoroquinolones	Separate administration by at least 1–2 hours if using Videx or consider Videx EC (see text)
	ganciclovir	Didanosine AUC ↑ 111%; may require dose adjustment
	hydroxyurea	↑ risk of adverse effects
	indinavir	Separate administration by at least 1–2 hours if using Videx or consider Videx EC (see text)
	itraconazole[a]	Separate administration by at least 1–2 hours if using Videx or consider Videx EC (see text)
	ketoconazole	Separate administration by at least 1–2 hours if using Videx or consider Videx EC (see text)
	ribavirin	Phosphorylation increased in vitro >50%, ↑ risk of adverse effects
	tetracycline	Separate administration by at least 1–2 hours if using Videx or consider Videx EC (see text), doxycycline, or minocycline
	tenofovir	Didanosine AUC ↑ 44%; may require dose adjustment
	Miscellaneous	See Table 19.3, drugs that may cause hyperglycemia, hyperuricemia, pancreatitis, and peripheral neuropathy
Zalcitabine	*aminoglycosides*	↑ risk of peripheral neuropathy due to ↑ concentrations from renal impairment
	amphotericin	↑ risk of peripheral neuropathy from renal impairment
	antacids[e]	↓ zalcitabine absorption; separate administration by at least 2 hours
	cimetidine	Zalcitabine AUC ↑ 36%; may require dose adjustment
	doxorubicin	Phosphorylation inhibited in vitro >50%, clinical significance unknown
	foscarnet	↑ risk of peripheral neuropathy from renal impairment
	lamivudine	Contraindicated due to competitive phosphorylation (see text)
	probenecid	↑ zalcitabine plasma conc.; may require dose adjustment
	Miscellaneous	See Table 19.3, drugs that may cause peripheral neuropathy
Stavudine	indinavir	Stavudine AUC ↑ 25%
	zidovudine	Contraindicated due to competitive phosphorylation (see text)
	Miscellaneous	See Table 19.3, drugs that may cause peripheral neuropathy
Lamivudine	zalcitabine	Contraindicated due to competitive phosphorylation (see text)
	TMP-SMX	Lamivudine AUC ↑ 44%
	Miscellaneous	See Table 19.3, drugs that may cause pancreatitis
Abacavir	amdoxovir	Potential contraindication due to competitive phosphorylation
	amprenavir	Amprenavir AUC ↑ 29%; no dose adjustment recommended
	Miscellaneous	See Table 19.3, drugs that may cause dermatologic side effects

19.2 Pharmacodynamic drug interactions

Pharmacodynamic interactions occur when two drugs share similar mechanisms of action. These interactions may be additive, synergistic, or antagonistic. The NRTIs are often used in combination because of their additive or synergistic interaction. However, not all combinations of NRTIs are feasible. For example, stavudine and zidovudine are antagonistic because they are both thymidine analogues and share a common activation pathway. In contrast, lamivudine is a cytosine analogue, and its initial phosphorylation is governed by a different set of kinases; thus lamivudine can be co-administered with either zidovudine or stavudine. Lamivudine, however, should not be given with emtricitabine or zalcitabine, both cytosine analogues, because of the potential for intracellular phosphorylation competition [24]. Other potential interactions of this nature include amdoxovir and abacavir, both guanosine derivatives, and tenofovir and didanosine, both adenosine analogues. Further studies of these and other intracellular NRTI interactions are needed. Tenofovir does increase plasma didanosine concentrations by approximately 44%, which may be sufficient to increase the likelihood of adverse reactions.

A pharmacodynamic interaction can also occur when drugs produce similar side-effects. Common side effects of antiretroviral drugs are categorized in Table 19.3; drugs that produce similar side-effects are also presented. The use of two or more drugs with common adverse effects is likely to increase the probability of or the intensity with which the side-effect occurs. Clinically significant interactions with commonly prescribed HIV medications are summarized in Table 19.4. Suggestions for avoiding select interactions are provided; many of the strategies rely on using an alternative non-interacting drug or dose adjustment.

19.3 Conclusion

Pharmacokinetic interactions can result in a change in systemic concentrations and may occur at the level of absorption, distribution, metabolism, or excretion. An alteration in systemic concentrations can result in beneficial or undesired therapeutic responses. The effects produced by a drug can also be affected by pharmacodynamic drug interactions, which can manifest as additive, antagonistic, or synergistic effects. Knowledge of the pharmacologic profile of the agents involved will provide the clinician with an ability to predict whether two drugs may interact and the likely outcome of that interaction.

ACKNOWLEDGMENTS

Grant Support: RO1 AI33835, UO1 AI41089, and UO1 AI38858 from the National Institute of Allergy and Infectious Diseases.

REFERENCES

1. Morse, G. D., Fischl, M. A., Shelton, M. J. et al. Single-dose pharmacokinetics of delavirdine mesylate and didanosine in patients with human immunodeficiency virus infection. Antimicrob. Agents Chemother. **41** : **1** (1997), 169–74.
2. Shelton, M. J., Mei, H., Hewitt, R. G. & DeFrancesco, R. If taken 1 hour before indinavir (IDV), didanosine does not affect IDV exposure, despite persistent buffering effects. Antimicrob. Agents Chemother. **45** : **1** (2001), 298–300.
3. Lomaestro, B. M. & Piatek, M. A. Update on drug interactions with azole antifungal agents. Ann. Pharmacother. **32** (1998), 915–28.
4. Sahai, J., Garber, G., Gallicano, K., Oliveras, L. & Cameron D. W. Effects of the antacids in didanosine tablets on dapsone pharmacokinetics. Ann. Intern. Med. **123** : **8** (1995), 584–7.
5. Knupp, C. A. & Barbhaiya, R. H. A multiple-dose pharmacokinetic interaction study between didanosine (Videx) and ciprofloxacin (Cipro) in male subjects seropositive for HIV but asymptomatic. Biopharm. Drug Dispos. **18** : **1** (1997), 65–77.
6. Damle, B. D., Mummaneni, V., Kaul, S. & Knupp, C. Lack of effect of simultaneously administered didanosine encapsulated enteric bead formulation (Videx EC) on oral absorption of indinavir, ketaconazole, or ciprofloxacin. Antimicrob. Agents Chemother. **46** : **2** (2002), 385–91.
7. Damle, B. D., Hess, H., Kaul, S. & Knupp, C. Absence of clinically relevant drug interactions following simultaneous administration of didanosine-encapsulated, enteric-coated bead formulation with either itraconazole or fluconazole. Biopharm. Drug Dispos. **23** : **2** (2002), 59–66.
8. Huisman, M. T., Smit, J. W. & Schinkel, A. H. Significance of P-glycoprotein for the pharmacology and clinical use of HIV protease inhibitors. AIDS **14** (2000), 237–42.
9. Acosta, E. P. Pharmacokinetic enhancement of protease inhibitors. J. Acquir. Immune Defic. Syndr. **29** (2002), S11–18.
10. Smith, P. F., DiCenzo, R. & Morse, G. D. Clinical pharmacokinetics of non-nucleoside reverse transcriptase inhibitors. Clin. Pharmacokinet. **40** : **12** (2001), 893–906.
11. Sansom, L. & Evans, A. M. What is the true clinical significance of plasma protein binding displacement interactions? Drug Safety **12** : **4** (1995), 227–33.
12. Leeder, J. S. & Kearns, G. L. Pharmacogenetics in pediatrics: implications for practice. Ped. Clin. N. Amer. **44** (1997), 55–77.
13. de Wildt, S. N., Kearns, G. L., Leeder, J. S. & van den Anker, J. N. Cytochrome P450 3A: ontogeny and drug disposition. Clin. Pharmacokinet. **37** : **6** (1999), 485–505.
14. de Wildt, S. N., Kearns, G. L., Leeder, J. S. & van den Anker, J. N. Glucuronidation in humans: pharmacogenetic and

developmental aspects. *Clin. Pharmacokinet.* **36** : **6** (1999), 439–52.

15. Rathbun, R. C. & Rossi, D. R. Low-dose ritonavir for protease inhibitor pharmacokinetic enhancement. *Ann. Pharmacother.* **36** (2002), 702–6.

16. Tran, J. Q., Gerber, J. G. & Kerr, B. M. Delavirdine: clinical pharmacokinetics and drug interactions. *Clin. Pharmacokinet.* **40** : **3** (2001), 207–26.

17. Burman, W. J., Gallicano, K. & Peloquin, C. Therapeutic implications of drug interactions in the treatment of human immunodeficiency virus-related tuberculosis. *Clin. Infect. Dis.* **28** (1999), 419–30.

18. Lee, B. L., Tauber, M. G., Sadler, B., Goldstein, D. & Chambers, H. F. Atovaquone inhibits the glucuronidation and increases the plasma concentrations of zidovudine. *Clin. Pharmacol. Ther.* **59** (1996), 14–21.

19. Zucker, S. D., Qin, X., Rouster, S. D. *et al.* Mechanism of indinavir-induced hyperbilirubinemia. *Proc. Natl. Acad. Sci.* **98** : **22** (2001), 12671–6.

20. Moore, K. H. P, Yuen, G. J., Raasch, R. H. *et al.* Pharmacokinetics of lamivudine administered alone and with trimethoprim-sulfamethoxazole. *Clin. Pharmacol. Ther.* **59** (1996), 550–8.

21. Sturgill, M. G., Seibold, J. R., Boruchoff, S. E., Yeh, K. C., Haddix, H. & Deutsch, P. Trimethoprim/sulfamethoxazole does not affect the steady-state disposition of indinavir. *J. Clin. Pharmacol.* **39** (1999), 1077–84.

22. Cimoch, P. J., Lavelle, J., Pollard, R., *et al.* Pharmacokinetics of oral ganciclovir alone and in combination with zidovudine, didanosine, and probenecid in HIV-infected subjects. *J. AIDS* **17** (1998), 227–34.

23. Jayasekara, D., Aweeka, F. T., Rodriguez, R., Kalayjian R. C., Humphreys, M. H. & Gambertoglio, J. G. Antiviral therapy for HIV patients with renal insufficiency. *J. Acquir. Immune. Defic. Syndr.* **21** (1999), 384–95.

24. Stein, D. S. & Moore, K. H .P. Phosphorylation of nucleoside analog antiretrovirals: a review for clinicians. *Pharmacotherapy* **21** : **1** (2001), 11–34.

Metabolic complications of antiretroviral therapy in children

Carol J. Worrell, M.D.

HIV and AIDS Malignancy Branch, National Cancer Institute, Bethesda, MD 20892

20.1 Introduction

The introduction of highly active antiretroviral therapy (HAART) has revolutionized the care of HIV-1 infected children and adults in the developed world. As the morbidity and mortality attributable to the complications of HIV infection itself have decreased, the recognition of unforeseen toxicities attributable to HAART has increased. Pediatricians who care for HIV-infected children and adolescents increasingly face a population that has had extensive and prolonged exposure to HAART. There is mounting evidence in the adult literature that the magnitude and breadth of toxicities associated with HAART can be substantial, yet there remains considerable uncertainty with respect to the definitions of particular syndromes, their etiology, their prevalence, the appropriate diagnostic criteria to be used in identifying them, and their management. Further, the consequences of these changes for the overall health of the patients remain unclear. The pediatric data are quite limited, and the available information suggests that the manifestations of such toxicities in HIV-infected children can be subtle and may vary with developmental stage, with different patterns manifesting in younger children than have been described in adults. Metabolic complications have been reported in association with the use of nucleoside reverse transcriptase inhibitors (NRTIs) and protease inhibitors (PIs). Nonnucleoside reverse transcriptase inhibitors (NNRTIs) have not been directly implicated. There may be significant intra-class variability, with individual drugs within a given class associated more strongly than others with specific complications. The complications discussed in this chapter will include the fat redistribution syndrome, abnormalities in lipid and glucose metabolism, and hyperlactatemia and lactic acidosis.

20.2 Fat redistribution syndrome, lipid abnormalities, and insulin resistance

20.2.1 Background

While this constellation of clinical and laboratory abnormalities is often referred to as the lipodystrophy syndrome, a widely used case definition of lipodystrophy in the context of HIV infection does not yet exist. Although originally associated with the introduction of protease inhibitors, it appears that host, disease, and drug-related factors may all contribute to the development of these abnormalities. The relative contribution of each factor remains obscure.

Host-related factors that have consistently been associated with these changes include older age and white race, each of which is associated with an increased risk of subcutaneous fat wasting [1–4]. Non-white race and female gender may be associated with an increased tendency to develop central obesity as opposed to peripheral fat wasting [1, 5]. There is also some evidence to suggest that dysregulation of inflammatory responses, particularly when they lead to elevated levels of tumor necrosis factor alpha (TNF-α), may contribute to the altered fat distribution and metabolic abnormalities associated with HAART [6–8].

Alterations in body fat distribution have been shown to predate the HAART era and may be associated with HIV infection itself. Kotler et al. documented alterations in the distribution of fat in HIV-infected patients consisting of increased visceral and decreased subcutaneous fat content regardless of treatment status (i.e. untreated, treated with a non-PI-containing antiretroviral regimen, or treated with a PI-containing antiretroviral regimen) [9]. Alterations in lipid metabolism during HIV infection have also been well documented prior to HAART. AIDS itself is associated with elevated levels of plasma triglycerides and very low density lipoprotein (VLDL) and free fatty acids (FFA), and decreased levels of cholesterol, high density lipoproteins (HDL), and low density lipoproteins (LDL) [10]. Duration of HIV infection, HIV RNA at baseline, and HIV RNA response to HAART have all been associated with the development of lipodystrophy [2–4, 11]. CD4 count at baseline and CD4 response to therapy have been less consistently associated with these changes.

Although the first reports of lipodystrophy occurred with the introduction of PI therapy, several studies have documented the occurrence of fat redistribution in patients treated with NRTIs alone [2–4, 11–16]. PIs and NRTIs are believed to exert their effects on fat distribution and lipid metabolism by different mechanisms, and may act synergistically when used in combination [17]. In an open-label, randomized study comparing therapy with ritonavir/saquinavir vs therapy with stavudine/ritonavir/saquinavir in patients who were naïve to both stavudine and PIs and were followed for 96 weeks, lipodystrophy occurred in 8% of patients treated with the dual PI regimen vs 25% of patients treated with the dual PI plus stavudine regimen, a difference which was statistically significant ($P = 0.003$). Both groups were similar with respect to the percentage of patients with prior antiretroviral (NRTI) experience (49 % vs 43 % respectively). When the analysis was limited to patients who were antiretroviral naïve at the start of the study, the results remained significant (5 % vs 24 % respectively, $P = 0.008$) [18]. The diagnosis of lipodystrophy, however, included fat redistribution only and was based solely on physician report without any supporting objective standards or measurements. Other studies have also suggested that the addition of PI therapy to NRTI therapy may accelerate the progression of symptoms already present in patients who had been receiving therapy with NRTIs alone [2, 19, 20]. Drug-related factors will be discussed in more detail below.

Many of the descriptions of HIV-associated lipodystrophy were compiled using suboptimal study designs. It appears that lipodystrophy in the setting of HIV infection is likely to be a progressive, cumulative process with multiple factors contributing to its pathogenesis. Most studies have been cross-sectional in design with the result that the relative contribution of drugs in use at the time of study may be overestimated and associated with outcomes that actually

represent cumulative effects [1]. Stavudine, for example, has often been associated with an increased risk of lipodystrophy, yet given that it became available after several other NRTIs had been in use and was widely used with PIs when that class first became available stavudine usage may, at least in part, be a surrogate marker for previous prolonged NRTI therapy [1].

The lack of widely used case definitions has created significant heterogeneity in the way different investigators characterize lipodystrophy, and therefore significant variability in the characteristics of the patients chosen for study. Lipodystrophy has been defined in some studies as a syndrome that includes dyslipidemia and/or altered glucose metabolism, and in others as a syndrome that consists of fat redistribution (also not consistently defined) without other associated metabolic changes. In addition, there are no widely used criteria to assess the severity of the changes.

Wide variations exist in the use of terminology and diagnostic methodology among studies. Diverse criteria have been used for diagnosis and have included one or more of the following: self-report; physician report; anthropometric measurements (skin-fold thickness, waist to hip ratio, etc.); bioelectrical impedance analysis (BIA); dual-energy x-ray absorptiometry (DEXA); computed tomography (CT); and magnetic resonance imaging (MRI). Some studies have relied solely on self-report and/or physician report, thereby drawing conclusions from data which can be highly subjective [18, 21–24]. Some techniques, most notably anthropometrical measurements and BIA, require a high degree of technical expertise and are particularly subject to inter-observer variability. One result of the heterogeneity in definitions and methodologies is the wide variation in estimates of the prevalence and cumulative incidence of lipodystrophy among antiretroviral users between cross-sectional studies, which range from 3–83% [4, 21, 25, 26].

20.2.2 Fat redistribution syndrome

Fat redistribution syndrome (FRS) is characterized by altered body habitus due to lipoatrophy, lipohypertrophy, or a combination of both [27]. The hallmarks of the alterations in body shape associated with antiretroviral use are the loss of subcutaneous fat from the face, limbs, or buttocks (lipoatrophy) and the increase of fat deposition centrally, with increased abdominal girth due to visceral fat accumulation, breast enlargement, dorsocervical fat accumulation ("buffalo hump"), and the development of lipomas (lipohypertrophy) [20, 27–29]. The overall appearance is of peripheral wasting and central obesity; it is not always associated with a change in weight. These phenotypic changes can occur independently of dyslipidemia and altered glucose metabolism [4, 11, 30].

Other disease processes are associated with alterations in body fat distribution, including Cushing's syndrome, growth hormone deficiency, hypothyroidism, and testosterone deficiency. Most studies have not demonstrated an association between FRS and these other disease processes. In general, abnormal serum levels of hormones including cortisol, ACTH, prolactin, testosterone, follicle stimulating hormone (FSH), luteinizing hormone (LH), thyroid hormones, and growth hormone have not been demonstrated [2, 4, 11, 13, 14, 25, 31–35]. Two groups of investigators have, however, found correlations between serum hormone levels and FRS. Hadigan *et al.* found significantly increased levels of free testosterone and a significantly elevated LH/FSH ratio (hyperandrogenemia) in a small cross-sectional study of treatment-experienced, HIV-infected women with lipodystrophy (defined as FRS and abnormalities in lipid and glucose metabolism) [36]. Christeff *et al.* found low dihydroepiandrosterone (DHEA) levels and an increased cortisol/DHEA ratio in men receiving HAART who had lipodystrophy (defined as FRS and abnormalities in lipid, but not glucose, metabolism)[37]. Finally, Kotler *et al.* described a subset of patients with HIV infection and altered fat distribution with normal serum levels of cortisol but elevated 24-hour urinary free cortisol excretion [9].

Several trials have documented the occurrence of FRS in HIV-infected pediatric patients, and estimates of the incidence of FRS in HIV-infected children on antiretroviral therapy range from 18–33% [35, 38–41]. All three forms of FRS (lipoatrophy, lipohypertrophy, and the combined form) have been described in HIV-infected children. In a cross-sectional study of 39 HIV-infected children, Jaquet *et al.* observed an overall incidence of FRS of 33.3% [35]. The presence of lipoatrophy and/or lipohypertrophy was determined by clinical characteristics and anthropometric measurements. Twenty percent of the children with FRS had truncal lipohypertrophy, 8% had peripheral lipoatrophy, and 5% had the combined form of FRS. The combined form of FRS was observed only in adolescents and the changes were more severe than those seen in pre-pubertal children. Ninety percent of the children had been on a stable antiretroviral regimen for more than 12 months. Two children were not receiving antiretroviral therapy, one was receiving dual NRTI therapy, 29 were receiving two NRTIs plus one PI, one was receiving triple NRTI therapy, and four were receiving two NRTIs and an NNRTI. The PIs used included nelfinavir (n = 18), ritonavir (n = 9), saquinavir (n = 2), indinavir (n = 1), and amprenavir (n = 1). Nucleoside analogue RTIs used included stavudine (n = 36), didanosine (n = 21), lamivudine (n = 16), and zidovudine

(n = 1). Age, gender, duration of HIV infection, $CD4^+$ cell count, and plasma HIV RNA level did not differ significantly between the groups with and without FRS [35].

Fat redistribution may not always be clinically apparent in pre-pubertal children. Arpadi *et al.* followed 28 HIV-infected children in a longitudinal observational study of body composition, and found that eight children (29%) had lipodystrophy, defined as the combined form (truncal fat accumulation plus extremity lipoatrophy) by DEXA scanning. Only one of these children had been identified clinically [39]. In this study, a significantly higher proportion of children with FRS than children without FRS were being treated with PIs and stavudine ($P = 0.04$ and $P = 0.03$ respectively), but duration of therapy with PIs and stavudine did not differ between children with and without FRS. Children with FRS had significantly lower $CD4^+$ lymphocyte counts and significantly higher viral loads at baseline than children without FRS. Immune response to therapy, manifested as an increase in $CD4^+$ lymphocyte count of ≥ 200 cells/μL, was not associated with the development of FRS, nor was race, sex, body mass index or body mass percentage.

In a study by Meneilly *et al.* body composition changes were observed in younger children. In this cross-sectional study of 29 HIV-infected children with a median age of 6.88 years (range 2–12.9), FRS was documented in 28% of patients. All three forms of FRS (lipoatrophy, lipohypertrophy, and combined) were observed. The presence of FRS was determined by anthropometrics and clinical examination. Information with respect to Tanner staging was not reported. There was no significant difference in the duration of therapy with PIs, NNRTIs, or stavudine between children with abnormalities and those without. The children with body composition changes were more likely to have ever received stavudine ($P = 0.033$) [40].

In another study of 34 HIV-infected children on a stable HAART regimen with good immunologic and virologic responses, 6 children (18%) had clinical evidence of peripheral lipoatrophy and truncal lipohypertrophy [41]. Lipodystrophy was defined as the combined form of FRS, and fat distribution was assessed using a combination of DEXA scanning and MRI. All children were receiving HAART regimens which consisted of stavudine, lamivudine, and one PI (indinavir, nelfinavir, or ritonavir). While 85% of the patients studied were in Tanner stages II–V of development, the distribution of cases according to Tanner stage is not provided by the authors. Abnormalities in fat distribution were again detected in patients without clinical evidence of FRS. The ratio of limb fat/trunk fat (measured by DEXA) was significantly decreased in all 34 HIV-infected children when compared with healthy controls ($P < 0.0001$). The ratio of trunk fat/total fat was increased in both the children with clinical FRS and in those without when compared with healthy controls ($P = 0.001$ and $P < 0.0001$ respectively), as was the ratio of limb fat/total fat ($P < 0.0001$ and $P = 0.009$, respectively). Finally, children with clinical FRS had a higher content of intra-abdominal adipose tissue (measured by MRI) than either HIV-infected children without FRS ($P < 0.0003$) or healthy controls ($P < 0.0001$). No significant differences were demonstrated between any of the groups with respect to CDC clinical or immunological classification, duration of prior exposure to NRTIs, duration of current HAART regimen, or type of PI currently in use.

Finally, a recent study by Amaya *et al.*, demonstrated FRS by physical examination and parental questionnaire in 18% of 40 HIV-infected children ranging in age from 2–16 years who had been on stable antiretroviral regimens for at least 12 months [38]. Fat redistribution syndrome was defined as lipoatrophy, lipohypertrophy, or a combination of both. The mean age of the children with FRS was significantly higher than that of the unaffected children ($P = 0.006$). There were no significant associations between the presence of FRS and/or metabolic changes and HIV RNA levels, exposure to specific antiretrovirals, or duration of either PI or NRTI therapy. Of interest was the finding of a significant association between the development of "lipodystrophy features" (defined here as FRS, hyperlipidemia, and insulin resistance) and the dosing levels of antiretrovirals. Children receiving pediatric dosing regimens as opposed to adult dosing regimens were less likely to develop lipodystrophy ($P = 0.003$), however, this finding may be partially confounded by age, as children receiving adult doses of drugs tend to be older.

20.2.3 Abnormalities in lipid and glucose metabolism

Lipoatrophy and lipohypertrophy can contribute to disorders of carbohydrate and lipid metabolism in several ways. Adipocytes function both as storage depots for fat and as endocrine cells which secrete several molecules that influence insulin sensitivity and energy balance, blood pressure control, and coagulation. These molecules include leptin and Acrp30 (adiponectin), which are insulin sensitizers, as well as TNF-α and IL-6, which are insulin antagonists [42]. Other substances secreted by adipocytes include complement factors, prothrombotic agents, and angiotensinogen, some or all of which may play a role in mediating the complications associated with obesity [43]. When lipoatrophy is predominant, such as in lipodystrophic syndromes not associated with HIV, the loss of "adequate adipocyte capacity" leads to excess calories being diverted away from

their normal storage areas, resulting in dyslipidemia and lipid accumulation (in the form of triglycerides) in tissues such as the liver, muscle, and pancreatic β cells [42].

The anatomic distribution of adipose tissue into visceral (as opposed to subcutaneous) depots also contributes to disturbances of lipid and glucose metabolism, and is known to be a strong and independent predictor of adverse outcomes such as coronary artery disease and diabetes in the non-HIV-infected population [44]. Enlargement of visceral abdominal adipose tissue depots is a major component of the lipohypertrophy that is seen in HIV-infected patients. Accumulation of visceral abdominal adipose tissue has been associated with glucose intolerance, hyperinsulinemia, and hypertriglyceridemia, although the mechanisms behind these associations remain unclear. The similarities between HIV-associated lipodystrophy and Syndrome X – a syndrome consisting of abdominal obesity, insulin resistance, mild hypertension, elevated levels of VLDL and small, dense LDL, and decreased HDL levels which is associated with a very high rate of premature coronary artery disease – have justifiably raised tremendous concern among HIV clinicians and researchers [42–44].

Although dyslipidemia and insulin resistance have most often been reported in association with PI therapy, Hadigan *et al.* have also demonstrated significant fasting hyperinsulinemia and hypertriglyceridemia associated with truncal adiposity in HIV-infected women who had not been treated with PIs [5]. HIV infection itself is associated with a reduction of HDL levels early in the disease followed by increases in triglyceride levels due to increases in VLDL levels, increased levels of FFA, and decreased levels of total cholesterol, HDL, and LDL as the disease progresses [10, 27]. Mild to moderate elevations in triglyceride levels have been documented in other studies of PI-naïve, NRTI-treated patients [5, 27]. Protease inhibitor therapy has been associated with increases in LDL cholesterol and triglyceride levels, and decreases in HDL cholesterol levels [27].

With respect to glucose metabolism, PI therapy has been associated with the following spectrum of abnormalities in the adult literature: hyperglycemia (usually asymptomatic), impaired glucose tolerance, insulin resistance, new onset non-insulin dependent diabetes mellitus, increases in insulin requirements of patients with pre-existing insulin-dependent diabetes mellitus, and, rarely, diabetic ketoacidosis [21, 27, 45, 46]. While insulin resistance may occur in as many as 40% of patients treated with PIs, rates of hyperglycemia and diabetes are considerably lower (3–17% and 1–6%, respectively) [47, 48].

The occurrence of dyslipidemia and abnormalities of glucose metabolism have been demonstrated in pediatric patients receiving antiretroviral therapy [38, 40, 49–52]. A retrospective analysis of patients treated with regimens containing one or two NRTIs plus either ritonavir or nelfinavir demonstrated an increase in total serum cholesterol levels in both groups, which was significantly more pronounced in the group receiving ritonavir [50]. Triglyceride levels were also significantly increased, but only in the ritonavir group. In a cross-sectional study of 29 HIV-infected children described earlier, hypertriglyceridemia was documented in 41%, hypercholesterolemia in 41%, and a combination of both in 24% [40]. None of the patients had abnormal fasting glucose levels. Insulin and C-peptide levels were not measured in this study.

Melvin *et al.* were able to demonstrate significant ($P <$ 0.0001) elevations in levels of total cholesterol, LDL cholesterol, and apolipoprotein B in PI vs non-PI treated children in a cross-sectional study of 35 HIV-infected children [49]. Twenty-three children were treated with PIs, including indinavir [1], nelfinavir [8], ritonavir [7], ritonavir/saquinavir [5], and nelfinavir/saquinavir [2]. Sixty-five percent of the children on PIs were also receiving nevirapine. Of the remaining children, two were untreated and the others were receiving therapy with NRTIs as follows: didanosine alone [5], stavudine/lamivudine [2], and stavudine/didanosine [2]. No differences were seen in triglyceride, fasting glucose, or insulin levels. Interestingly, there were also no significant differences detected between the two groups with respect to body composition as evaluated by DEXA and anthropometry. The differences remained nonsignificant when controlled for age, however, the majority of patients in both groups were in Tanner stages I–II (79% in the PI-treated group and 67% in the non PI-treated group). A significant difference was demonstrated between the two groups with respect to HIV RNA levels, which were lower in the PI-treated group ($P < 0.001$). CD4$^+$ cell counts also tended to be higher in the PI-treated group ($P = 0.09$).

In the cross-sectional study of 39 HIV-infected children by Jaquet *et al.*, mentioned above, abnormalities in glucose metabolism as well as dyslipidemia were observed (35). Hypercholesterolemia was observed in 23% of patients with FRS and in 15.4% of patients without FRS. Hypertriglyceridemia was observed in 15.4% of patients with FRS and in 11.5% of patients without it. There was no difference between the groups with and without FRS with respect to mean fasting blood glucose and all children had normal glucose tolerance. However, the children with FRS demonstrated higher plasma insulin levels and higher fasting insulin: glucose ratios than the children without FRS, although these differences did not reach statistical significance ($P = 0.07$ for both comparisons).

A cross-sectional evaluation of 40 HIV-infected children by Amaya *et al.* (see above) revealed hypercholesterolemia

in 68%, hypertriglyceridemia in 28%, and insulin resistance in 8% [38]. Insulin resistance was defined as an abnormally elevated fasting insulin or C-peptide level with a normal serum glucose level. Fasting serum glucose levels were normal for children. The mean age of the children with insulin resistance was significantly higher than that of the unaffected group ($P = 0.007$).

20.2.4 Proposed mechanisms of PI-associated effects

As discussed above, PI use is associated with dyslipidemia and insulin resistance. Additional evidence supporting a contribution of PI therapy to the development of dyslipidemia was provided by the observation of elevated triglyceride levels in HIV-seronegative individuals undergoing short-term therapy that included indinavir for postexposure prophylaxis, and the observation that short-term ritonavir in healthy (HIV-uninfected) volunteers results in significant increases in triglyceride and VLDL levels as well as reductions in HDL levels [53]. The effects of individual PIs on lipid metabolism are fairly similar with the exception of ritonavir, which appears to cause a higher degree of hypertriglyceridemia than other PIs [22, 50].

Protease inhibitor therapy has also been associated with changes in body habitus [4, 18, 21, 25, 26, 37, 54]. Both the risk of fat wasting and the probability of intra-abdominal fat accumulation increase with the duration of PI therapy [1, 2, 21, 26, 48, 55]. While all PIs have been implicated in the development of FRS, few prospective studies have been carried out to determine the relative effects of individual PIs [20]. Carr *et al.* reported that patients receiving a combination of ritonavir and saquinavir had less body fat, higher lipids, and a shorter time to lipoatrophy than patients receiving indinavir [21]. In another study, patients receiving amprenavir had a significantly lower incidence of fat redistribution than patients treated with indinavir (3% vs 12%, respectively) [56].

The pathogenesis of PI-associated metabolic changes is unknown. Several hypotheses have been proposed that involve the interaction of PIs with various proteins involved in adipocyte function and differentiation, lipid handling, and glucose transport. In vitro and in vivo studies investigating the mechanisms underlying the adverse effects associated with PIs are currently underway.

20.2.5 Proposed mechanisms of NRTI-associated effects

Nucleoside analogue RTI use has been independently associated with the development of FRS and, in particular, to the development of lipoatrophy [2–4, 11–16]. The probability of developing lipoatrophy increases with the duration of NRTI therapy [2]. Among the NRTIs, stavudine has been the most widely implicated in the development of FRS. As mentioned above, stavudine use, at least in part, serves as a surrogate marker for previous NRTI exposure. Nevertheless, randomized trials comparing regimens containing stavudine with regimens containing zidovudine have also demonstrated a higher prevalence of FRS in patients receiving stavudine-containing regimens when controlled for prior NRTI exposure [3, 57].

Nucleoside analogue RTI-associated fat redistribution is believed to occur as a result of tissue-specific mitochondrial toxicity. Clinical manifestations that have been attributed to NRTI-related mitochondrial toxicity include lipoatrophy, myopathy, cardiomyopathy, peripheral neuropathy, pancreatitis, hepatic steatosis and lactic acidosis, anemia, and proximal renal tubular dysfunction (associated with adefovir therapy). Nucleoside analogues such as the NRTIs are known to inhibit DNA polymerase γ, the polymerase responsible for mitochondrial DNA replication [2, 32, 47, 58–61]. In late 1998 Brinkman *et al.* proposed a mechanism for the mitochondrial toxicity of NRTIs based on the action of nucleoside analogues on DNA polymerases and its effect on mitochondrial function [59]. DNA polymerases are enzymes that catalyze the formation of new DNA strands using an original DNA strand as a template and triphosphorylated nucleosides (dNTPs) as substrates. The reverse transcriptase enzyme (RT) that is encoded by HIV and targeted by the NRTIs is a type of DNA polymerase; it initially functions as an RNA-dependent DNA polymerase when it uses the viral RNA genome brought into the host cell with the virion as a template for the synthesis of the first strand of complementary DNA. For the synthesis of the second strand, to make the complete, double-stranded cDNA copy of the viral genome, RT uses the first strand of cDNA as a template and functions as a DNA-dependent DNA polymerase. The NRTIs are nucleoside analogues, which become phosphorylated to become NRTI-triphosphates, analogues of nucleotide triphosphates (dNTPs). The NRTI-triphosphates inhibit the HIV RT, but they can also inhibit other DNA polymerases, including various cellular DNA polymerases. The NRTI-triphosphates act as competitive inhibitors of the polymerases and also inhibit DNA synthesis by causing premature termination of the newly synthesized DNA strand; they are, to varying extents, known to be more potent inhibitors of DNA polymerase γ than of the other human DNA polymerases in vitro. DNA polymerase γ is the only DNA polymerase that mediates the replication of mitochondrial DNA, and its inhibition leads

to impairment of mitochondrial replication and function. Mitochondrial DNA is particularly vulnerable to mutation because it has no protective histones and is exposed to oxygen radicals generated by the respiratory chain. The main function of mitochondria is to generate energy for the cell in the form of adenosine triphosphate (ATP). Agents that are toxic to mitochondria lead to impaired ATP synthesis. The oxidative phosphorylation system generates energy by using intracellular fatty acids and glucose as fuel. Impairment of the system leads to the intracellular accumulation of fat (in the form of free fatty acids and triglycerides) and lactate [59, 61].

20.2.6 Diagnosis

Fat redistribution

Anthropometric measurements

Measurements of simple body circumferences over time (i.e. abdominal circumference, waist to hip ratios, limb circumference) can be useful by indicating that a significant change may be occurring, but cannot accurately determine its nature (i.e. loss of fat mass versus loss of lean body mass). Skinfold measurements using calipers can be imprecise and are very operator-dependent. They should be collected under highly standardized conditions [1].

Dual energy x-ray absorptiometry

Dual energy x-ray absorptiometry gives a two-dimensional image that is very reliable for measuring limb fat and total body fat, but cannot distinguish subcutaneous abdominal fat from visceral fat. Therefore, visceral abdominal adipose tissue can not be quantified with this technique [20]. It can be used to assess regional changes in fat distribution using ratios of limb to truncal fat, limb fat to total fat, etc. There are two caveats to remember when using DEXA in this manner. The first is that fat loss or gain may not occur simultaneously in different areas measured in the same patient, potentially skewing the ratios [1]. The second is that fat loss or gain can occur simultaneously in a single area (e.g. subcutaneous fat loss and visceral fat gain in the abdomen) which may also lead to misleading results [20]. Comparisons between different machines within the same or at different institutions require standardization of calibration.

Single cut CT or MRI

Single cut CT or MRI produces three-dimensional images that can distinguish between subcutaneous and visceral fat compartments. Single cut CT or MRI scans at L4 can be used to analyze abdominal fat, and can be used in combination with DEXA scans to more fully characterize changes in fat distribution [1, 20, 27, 29]. Single cut scans of the mid-thigh and/or the arm have been used to characterize peripheral fat content. Standardization of calibration is required when comparing results from different machines.

Whole body CT or MRI
Whole body CT or MRI can also be utilized but are impractical due to their cost and the lack of standardization of measures for whole body fat changes.

Dyslipidemia
Dyslipidemia is diagnosed by a fasting lipid profile. This should include total cholesterol, HDL cholesterol, and triglycerides. Low density lipoprotein cholesterol is calculated from these values, except when the triglyceride level exceeds 400 mg/dL, at which point the calculated value becomes unreliable [62]. In this event, decisions may be based on the direct measurement of LDL (not uniformly available and generally expensive), or on the calculation of non-HDL cholesterol using the formula: non-HDL cholesterol = total cholesterol − HDL cholesterol [63].

There are currently no recommendations for the monitoring of either dyslipidemia or abnormalities in glucose metabolism (discussed below) for pediatric patients with HIV infection. The Adult AIDS Clinical Trials Group recommends obtaining fasting lipid profiles before the initiation of HAART; this should be repeated after 3 months of therapy and if normal, once yearly or with any change in antiretroviral regimen [29, 63].

Abnormalities of glucose metabolism
Monitoring for abnormalities of glucose metabolism essentially involves monitoring for changes associated with non-insulin dependent diabetes mellitus. These include evidence of insulin resistance (high fasting plasma insulin and C-peptide levels), suggestive evidence of insulin resistance such as impaired fasting glucose (a level of 110–125 mg/dL), impaired glucose tolerance (a serum glucose level between 140–199 mg/dL 2 hours after a 75 g oral glucose load), or evidence of frank diabetes mellitus (fasting glucose ≥ 126 mg/dL or 2-hour glucose level after a glucose challenge of ≥200 mg/dL) [20, 63].

It should be kept in mind that fasting glucose can be normal in the setting of insulin resistance, so that this test alone may not be sufficient to determine the presence of abnormalities in glucose metabolism. An evaluation should probably be performed of all children who are starting PI-based HAART, as well as those with significant dyslipidemia and/or body habitus changes. A 2-hour oral glucose tolerance test should be obtained when evidence of a significant disturbance of glucose homeostasis is observed.

20.2.7 Management

There are currently no recommendations for the management of FRS, dyslipidemia, or abnormalities of glucose metabolism for pediatric patients with HIV infection. Recommendations for the management of dyslipidemia in otherwise healthy children (i.e. those without a history of familial hypercholesterolemia) consist primarily of dietary and lifestyle interventions; pharmacologic agents are used very conservatively and bile acid sequestrants are considered the first line of therapy. However, these drugs may potentially interfere with absorption of antiretroviral drugs and are generally quite unpalatable [64, 65]. Pilot studies in HIV-infected adults with metabolic changes and/or FRS have shown improvement in lipid profiles, insulin sensitivity, and body habitus after the institution of dietary changes and exercise regimens [66–69]. Lipid-lowering agents such as 3-hydroxy-3-methyl-glutaryl coenzyme A reductase inhibitors (statins) and fibrates (e.g. gemfibrozil, fenofibrate) have been used in HIV-infected adults with dyslipidemia, but there are significant safety concerns with respect to potential interactions with PIs via the cytochrome P-450 system (statins and fibrates) and hepatotoxicity (fibrates) [29].

Insulin-sensitizing agents such as metformin and thiazolidinediones (the glitazones) may not be ideal choices because of potential toxicities. Metformin has been associated with lactic acidosis and must be used with caution in patients with underlying renal or hepatic disease. The glitazones are inducers of CYP3A4 and may lower plasma levels of PIs; they can also cause severe hepatotoxicity. Interestingly, both classes of drugs have been associated with reductions in visceral adipose tissue in addition to improvements in insulin sensitivity, and the thiazolidinediones have been associated with increases in subcutaneous fat [29, 63].

Finally, treatment with recombinant human growth hormone has been associated with reductions in total and visceral fat in adult patients with FRS; however, many patients developed glucose intolerance on therapy and the benefits appear to be short-lived, with recurrence of fat accumulation when therapy is stopped [27, 63, 70].

The potential for changes in antiretroviral therapy to reverse metabolic and body habitus changes associated with HAART has been examined in adults in several small studies that have yielded mixed results [71–77].

The substitution of nevirapine for a PI in HAART regimens in NNRTI-naïve patients appears to be associated with improvement of the lipid profile (and with maintenance of virologic and immunologic gains from PI-based HAART), and may also lead to some improvement in morphologic changes, but the evidence for the latter effect is less compelling [72–74]. Studies of regimens containing efavirenz have not shown a consistent benefit. Other strategies have focused on abacavir as either a substitute for a PI in HAART regimens on which patients have achieved virologic suppression, or as an NRTI substitute in regimens containing stavudine or zidovudine. Small but significant improvements have been seen after abacavir substitution in both settings with respect to lipoatrophy, lipid abnormalities, and insulin sensitivity [75–77]. The ability to maintain virologic suppression and immunologic gains in the long term with a triple NRTI regimen remains a concern, as does the effectiveness of abacavir in the setting of the NRTI-experienced patient [62, 78]. The preliminary results of a large, randomized trial in which patients on PI-based HAART with viral loads <200 copies/mL were randomly assigned to switch to either abacavir, nevirapine, or efavirenz suggested a significant advantage after 6 months in the abacavir arm with respect to reductions in LDL and total cholesterol levels and discontinuations due to adverse events. However, greater improvements in HDL and triglyceride levels were seen in the nevirapine group [79]. In the overall cohort, significant reductions in plasma insulin levels, insulin resistance, LDL, and total cholesterol, as well as increases in HDL, were seen with respect to the values obtained at baseline on PI therapy.

20.3 Hyperlactatemia and lactic acidosis

Another proposed consequence of mitochondrial toxicity related to treatment with NRTIs is a spectrum of abnormalities characterized by disturbances in lactate homeostasis. The spectrum of disease ranges from asymptomatic hyperlactatemia to lactic acidosis with hepatic steatosis and its accompanying high mortality rate. This latter complication fortunately appears to be quite rare, perhaps occurring in less than 1% of patients; however, its precise incidence is difficult to ascertain as most cases have been reported as isolated events rather than in the context of whole populations of patients [27, 80].

In the adult population, reports of this type of toxicity have been confined exclusively to patients with current NRTI exposure; signs and symptoms can sometimes improve when therapy is withdrawn. The pediatric experience has been somewhat different and has focused on mitochondrial dysfunction primarily as a late after-effect of NRTI exposure. Studies in children have centered around the perinatal period and early infancy after reports emerged of severe, sometimes fatal, instances of mitochondrial toxicity in HIV-uninfected children who had been exposed to NRTIs for prophylaxis of vertical transmission. This will be discussed in more detail below. The pediatric data in this area are even more limited than the data available regarding fat redistribution and abnormalities of lipid and glucose metabolism and primarily consists of uncontrolled case series and isolated case reports.

20.3.1 Background

The proposed mechanism of mitochondrial damage by NRTIs is outlined above. Impairment of oxidative phosphorylation leads to the synthesis of ATP via anaerobic glycolysis, resulting in an excess production of lactate in the cell that eventually enters the systemic circulation. Normally, lactate homeostasis is very precise and serum concentrations are maintained within a very narrow range (0.3–1.0 mmol/L in arterial blood and 0.8–2.0 mmol/L in venous blood). The liver, and, to a lesser extent, the kidneys have the ability to markedly increase their level of lactate clearance under conditions of lactate excess [80]. The pathways that lead to lactic acidosis from a state of increased production of lactate are not completely understood. A combination of increased production in many tissues and decreased clearance may be required for a patient to develop fulminant lactic acidosis. Sustained production of ATP by anaerobic glycolysis results in the production of organic acids and is believed to lead to a drop in pH, thereby compromising hepatic and renal function and diminishing clearance of lactate from the systemic circulation [63].

Mitochondrial dysfunction can result in a broad spectrum of abnormalities, and multi-organ system dysfunction with broad phenotypic variation is characteristic. Findings can include varying combinations of hyperlactatemia, myopathy, cardiomyopathy, hepatopathy, encephalopathy, peripheral neuropathy, and pancreatitis [81, 82].

20.3.2 Asymptomatic (compensated) hyperlactatemia

This type of clinical (or sub-clinical) presentation consists of mild to moderate elevations of venous lactate levels which can occur on a chronic or an intermittent basis and may be common in adult patients treated with HAART regimens that include NRTIs [80, 83]. A prospective, longitudinal study of 349 HIV-infected adults in which venous lactate measurements were obtained over a period of 18 months revealed that 65% of patients had an elevated lactate concentration on at least one occasion when samples were collected under highly standardized conditions [83]. Importantly, the presence of mild to moderate elevations in lactate was not associated with progression to symptomatic hyperlactatemia or fulminant lactic acidosis. Other studies in adults have estimated the incidence of mild to moderate hyperlactatemia at between 8 and 35% [84–86].

A small prospective study by Giaquinto *et al.* reported elevated venous lactate levels (defined here as > 2.5 mmol/L) on at least one occasion in 17 (85%) of 20 infants who had been exposed to NRTIs in utero and to zidovudine during delivery and for 6 weeks after birth [87]. Nucleoside analogue RTI exposure in utero consisted of zidovudine [2], stavudine/lamivudine [1], and zidovudine/lamivudine [7]; seven mothers were on PI-containing regimens which presumably also contained NRTIs, but these are not specified. All lactate levels subsequently returned to normal. None of the infants were symptomatic. In the same report, lactate levels were also examined in a cross-sectional manner in 36 HIV-infected children with an average age of 9 years (range 5 months to 17 years). Twenty-nine children (81%) were being treated with at least one NRTI including 24 (66.6%) who were receiving triple therapy with PI-containing regimens. Specific NRTI exposure was not clarified further. Of the 29 children receiving treatment, 3 (8%) had mildly elevated lactate levels (mean 2.9 mmol/L). None of the children were symptomatic.

A second small, prospective study by Alimenti *et al.* [88] followed plasma lactate levels in 25 infants who were exposed to HAART in utero and to zidovudine in the neonatal period. Lactate levels were found to be above the normal limit (2.1 mmol/L in this study) on at least one occasion in 92% of the infants. Lactate levels of $\geq$ 5 mmol/L were documented in 36%. The number of infants with persistent hyperlactatemia is not specified, but most experienced resolution of this finding by 6 months of age. The mothers' HAART regimens consisted of 2 NRTIs (zidovudine and lamivudine 'most often') with nevirapine (20/25) or a PI (5/25). The mean duration of in utero exposure to HAART was 17 weeks (range 3.5–38 weeks), and 50% of the infants were also exposed to heroin, cocaine, or methadone. Maternal lactate levels at the end of pregnancy were normal in the 17 mothers who were tested. No associations were found between peak lactate levels in the infants and maternal substance use, duration of in utero exposure to HAART, or exposure to specific drugs including stavudine, nevirapine,

and PIs. One infant reportedly had symptoms "consistent with those of adult lactic acidemia," but no further detail is given.

20.3.3 Symptomatic hyperlactatemia

This syndrome has not yet been described in children. The presentation described in adults consists of hyperlactatemia in the setting of non-specific symptoms – abdominal pain, nausea, abdominal distention, fatigue, exercise-induced dyspnea, and abnormal liver function tests – which may ultimately progress to fulminant lactic acidosis [80, 89, 90]. Tachycardia, weight loss, or peripheral neuropathy may also be present [89]. Most patients show symptomatic improvement after cessation of antiretroviral therapy. Lactate levels may increase initially after cessation of antiretrovirals and may take weeks to months to normalize. Hepatic steatosis is usually present and micro- and macrovesicular steatosis may be seen on liver biopsy [90]. Some patients may tolerate re-challenge with an NRTI [80].

20.3.4 Decompensated lactic acidosis

The presentation of lactic acidosis associated with NRTI therapy is much more severe than that of symptomatic hyperlactatemia. The predominant presenting symptoms are again gastrointestinal and non-specific, and may consist of nausea, vomiting, abdominal pain and distention, tender hepatomegaly, fatigue, malaise, and prostration [80]. There may be concurrent pancreatitis, neuropathy, and elevated creatine kinase. Fulminant metabolic acidosis develops rapidly, leading to arrhythmias and organ failure [80]. In adults, this syndrome appears to be significantly associated with age, female gender, obesity, pre-existing liver disease (e.g. chronic hepatitis B or C), and the use of stavudine [63, 80, 89, 90].

This syndrome has been described in HIV-infected pediatric patients in isolated case reports [91–93]. Miller *et al.* describe a 16-year-old girl being treated with stavudine, didanosine, and nelfinavir for 3 months who presented with a 3-day history of nausea, vomiting, and abdominal pain, and who was noted to have severe metabolic acidosis, elevated lactate levels, hepatic steatosis, pancreatitis, and myopathy [92]. Diffuse fatty infiltration of the liver and pancreatic inflammation and necrosis were seen on abdominal CT. A muscle biopsy revealed increased fat droplets in the myocytes with occasional 'ragged-red' fibers. Antiretroviral drugs were discontinued. The patient ultimately recovered and was placed on zidovudine, nevirapine, and nelfinavir without recurrence of her symptoms.

Church *et al.* describe a vertically infected toddler who had not received NRTI prophylaxis perinatally and was placed on zidovudine, didanosine, and nelfinavir at approximately 3 months of age [93]. The child subsequently developed neurologic symptoms consisting of developmental regression, progressive leg stiffness, and a spastic gait at 18–19 months of age. An MRI of the brain (t_2-weighted) revealed patchy foci of increased signal in the peripheral and deep cerebral white matter. By 23 months of age he had profound motor delay, generalized areflexia, lactic acidosis, and marked organic aciduria. Antiretroviral therapy was discontinued. The child's condition deteriorated markedly and he required prolonged and intensive cardiorespiratory support. Eventually, his cardiopulmonary status improved as did the sensory and motor abnormalities. A repeat MRI at 29 months revealed improvement of the white matter densities and by 33 months he remained developmentally delayed but continued to show improvement.

Scalfaro *et al.* [94] describe a case of severe lactic acidosis occurring in a neonate who was receiving zidovudine as perinatal prophylaxis and had been exposed to zidovudine in utero, intrapartum, and postpartum. After an initially difficult course due to severe persistent fetal circulation (PFC) requiring mechanical ventilation and anemia, the infant improved dramatically within the first week of life. Zidovudine was continued during this period and a single lactate level of 1.9 mmol/L was documented on the sixth day of life. The infant did well until the ninth day of life when she developed sudden, severe respiratory distress, mild hepatomegaly, and abdominal petechiae. Her lactate level had risen to 14 mmol/L; her aspartate aminotransferase (AST) was also elevated two-fold. The infant was re-intubated and responded to treatment with bicarbonate, fluid support, and cessation of zidovudine. Lactate and AST values returned to normal quickly and the metabolic acidosis resolved over 24 hours. The patient was extubated after 18 hours. Zidovudine was not re-introduced. The infant subsequently did well, and was without evidence of metabolic acidosis or HIV infection after 11 months of follow-up.

20.3.5 Delayed manifestations of mitochondrial toxicity

The presentations described above all involve patients who were receiving therapy with NRTIs at the time abnormalities were detected, and all of the patients responded to withdrawal of NRTI therapy. Another presentation of fulminant disease believed to be due to NRTI-related mitochondrial dysfunction has been described in HIV-uninfected, NRTI-exposed children that manifests itself months after the exposure has ceased. Blanche *et al.* described eight children with persistent mitochondrial dysfunction after perinatal exposure to NRTIs [95, 96]. The mothers had received either zidovudine alone or, as part of a separate study, zidovudine plus lamivudine, beginning at 32 weeks gestation and continuing through delivery. The infants then continued the same regimen their mothers had received for the first 6 weeks of life. Two children were identified via investigations of serious adverse events; six were identified retrospectively. None of the children were identified while still receiving NRTI prohylaxis, with the earliest signs and symptoms beginning at 4 months of age. There was considerable phenotypic variation among the affected children, who ranged from asymptomatic with persistent biochemical abnormalities to floridly symptomatic with signs and symptoms consistent with what has been described in inherited mitochondrial disorders. Two of the children, one whose disease course resembled that of Leigh's syndrome and another whose course resembled that of ALPERS syndrome, died. Five of the children had persistently elevated blood lactate concentrations. Upon examination of enzyme activity in skeletal muscle mitochondria, all of the children were found to have decreased activity in respiratory-chain complexes I, IV, or both. Partial defects in complex IV were believed to be present in the three asymptomatic patients. No substantial decrease in mitochondrial DNA content was observed in the two patients who were most severely affected or in the one other patient in which this was examined. Large deletions or duplications of mitochondrial DNA were not seen in any patient, and none of the mutations associated with the currently characterized mitochondrial diseases was found.

This level of mitochondrial disease (8/1754) far exceeds the estimated background prevalence of mitochondrial disease of 1/3000–1/4000 in the general population [81]. The ethnic make-up of the affected children was diverse. Four women were of African origin (not further specified), one was from North Africa, and three were European. One mother was co-infected with hepatitis C; her child's hepatitis C status is not reported. Only one mother was receiving any medication other than the prescribed NRTI prophylaxis, iron, and vitamins; this was trimethoprim/sulfamethoxazole. Zidovudine dosing was 500 mg per day for the mothers, and 8 mg/kg/day for the infants. Lamivudine was given at doses of 300 mg per day for the mothers, and 4 mg/kg/day for the infants. In the zidovudine/lamivudine group, mean prenatal exposure to NRTIs was 17.2 weeks (range 0–40) and mean postnatal exposure was 5.2 weeks (range 2–6 weeks).

As a result of these observations, several large databases including over 23 000 children with perinatal exposure to

HIV who were uninfected or of indeterminate status have been examined retrospectively for evidence of mitochondrial diseases [96–100]. None have found evidence suggestive of mitochondrial dysfunction or metabolic disease; however, the majority of the reviews focused on causes of death and may have missed less severe presentations [97, 99, 100]. Nevertheless, two large studies have looked specifically for signs and symptoms that could be associated with mitochondrial/metabolic complications and not found evidence of them [95, 96].

20.3.6 Diagnosis and management

Diagnosis is based on clinical signs and symptoms and requires a high index of suspicion. Routine monitoring of lactate levels has not been shown to be of benefit and is not recommended [63, 83, 86]. Lactate levels should always be obtained under standardized conditions and with the patient at rest, and should be confirmed if abnormal. When lactate levels are obtained based on clinical suspicion, levels of 2–5 mmol/L are considered mild–moderate, and levels > 5 mmol/L are considered indicative of severe acidemia [27, 86]. Antiretrovirals should be held for lactate levels > 5 mmol/L and other causes of associated clinical findings (e.g. myopathy, neuropathy, transaminitis) should be excluded while a diagnosis of NRTI-related mitochondrial toxicity is pursued.

Multi-system disease is almost always present in the symptomatic forms of hyperlactatemia. Specific diagnostic studies (e.g. electrocardiogram, echocardiography, abdominal CT, MRI of the brain, liver biopsy, muscle biopsy, etc.) should be obtained according to the presenting symptoms. Biochemical studies specifically looking for mitochondrial failure should be obtained in consultation with a neurologist and include: blood and CSF lactate; skin biopsy for fibroblast culture and biochemical studies; muscle biopsy for histology, mitochondrial DNA studies, respiratory-chain enzyme activity, and electron microscopy [81].

In addition to early detection and discontinuation of antiretrovirals in severe cases, further treatment is supportive. Treatment options that are based on the treatment of inherited mitochondrial disease and whose use has been reported anecdotally in NRTI-related lactic acidosis include respiratory chain co-factors, antioxidants, and nutrients: riboflavin, thiamine, L-carnitine, coenzyme Q10, vitamins C, E, and A, and idebenone (an analogue of coenzyme Q10) [27, 63]. No firm dosing recommendations exist for any of these agents in this setting.

20.4 Conclusion

Metabolic complications due to antiretroviral therapy occur in children as well as in adults. Developmental stage appears to play a significant role in determining their presentations, which in younger children can be quite distinct from that seen in adults. Nucleoside analogue RTIs and PIs can contribute to changes in fat distribution and alterations of lipid and glucose metabolism independently, however, the greatest impact appears to occur when they are used in combination. Current data do not suggest that PIs contribute to mitochondrial toxicity and the development of hyperlactatemia and lactic acidosis. The effects described are cumulative and progressive, yet both the pediatric and the adult literature consist largely of cross-sectional studies, uncontrolled case series, and isolated case reports. The overall effect is that a reading of the literature raises as many questions as it answers. Well-designed prospective, longitudinal studies are needed but will remain difficult to design as long as consensus regarding the definitions of particular syndromes remains elusive.

REFERENCES

1. John, M., Nolan, D. & Mallal, S. Antiretroviral therapy and the lipodystrophy syndrome. *Antivir. Ther.* **6** : **1** (2001), 9–20.
2. Mallal, S. A., John, M., Moore, C. B., James, I. R. & McKinnon, E. J. Contribution of nucleoside analogue reverse transcriptase inhibitors to subcutaneous fat wasting in patients with HIV infection. *AIDS* **14** : **10** (2000), 1309–16.
3. Chene, G., Angelini, E., Cotte, L., *et al.* Role of long-term nucleoside-analogue therapy in lipodystrophy and metabolic disorders in human immunodeficiency virus-infected patients. *Clin. Infect. Dis.* **34** : **5** (2002), 649–57.
4. Gervasoni, C., Ridolfo, A. L., Trifiro, G. *et al.* Redistribution of body fat in HIV-infected women undergoing combined antiretroviral therapy. *AIDS* **13** : **4** (1999), 465–71.
5. Hadigan, C., Miller, K., Corcoran, C., Anderson, E., Basgoz, N. & Grinspoon, S. Fasting hyperinsulinemia and changes in regional body composition in human immunodeficiency virus-infected women. *J. Clin. Endocrinol. Metab.* **84** : **6** (1999), 1932–7.
6. Mynarcik, D. C., McNurlan, M. A., Steigbigel, R. T., Fuhrer, J. & Gelato, M. C. Association of severe insulin resistance with both loss of limb fat and elevated serum tumor necrosis factor receptor levels in HIV lipodystrophy. *J. AIDS* **25** : **4** (2000), 312–21.
7. Ledru, E., Christeff, N., Patey, O., de Truchis, P., Melchior, J. C. & Gougeon, M. L. Alteration of tumor necrosis factor-alpha T-cell homeostasis following potent antiretroviral therapy: contribution to the development of human immunodeficiency

virus-associated lipodystrophy syndrome. *Blood* **95**:**10** (2000), 3191–8.

8. Duong, M., Petit, J. M., Piroth, L. *et al.* Association between insulin resistance and hepatitis C virus chronic infection in HIV-hepatitis C virus-coinfected patients undergoing antiretroviral therapy. *J. AIDS* **27**:**3** (2001), 245–50.

9. Kotler, D. P., Rosenbaum, K., Wang, J. & Pierson, R. N. Studies of body composition and fat distribution in HIV-infected and control subjects. *J. AIDS Hum. Retrovirol.* **20**:**3** (1999), 228–37.

10. Grunfeld, C., Pang, M., Doerrler, W., Shigenaga, J. K., Jensen, P. & Feingold, K. R. Lipids, lipoproteins, triglyceride clearance, and cytokines in human immunodeficiency virus infection and the acquired immunodeficiency syndrome. *J. Clin. Endocrinol. Metab.* **74**:**5** (1992), 1045–52.

11. Lo, J. C., Mulligan, K., Tai, V. W., Algren, H. & Schambelan, M. "Buffalo hump" in men with HIV-1 infection. *Lancet* **351**:**9106** (1998), 867–70.

12. Carr, A., Miller, J., Law, M. & Cooper, D. A. A syndrome of lipoatrophy, lactic acidaemia and liver dysfunction associated with HIV nucleoside analogue therapy: contribution to protease inhibitor-related lipodystrophy syndrome. *AIDS* **14**:**3** (2000), F25–32.

13. Saint-Marc, T., Partisani, M., Poizot-Martin, I. *et al.* A syndrome of peripheral fat wasting (lipodystrophy) in patients receiving long-term nucleoside analogue therapy. *AIDS* **13**:**13** (1999), 1659–67.

14. Saint-Marc, T., Partisani, M., Poizot-Martin, I., *et al.* Fat distribution evaluated by computed tomography and metabolic abnormalities in patients undergoing antiretroviral therapy: preliminary results of the LIPOCO study. *AIDS* **14**:**1** (2000), 37–49.

15. Galli, M., Ridolfo, A. L., Adorni, F. *et al.* Body habitus changes and metabolic alterations in protease inhibitor-naive HIV-1-infected patients treated with two nucleoside reverse transcriptase inhibitors. *J. AIDS* **29**:**1** (2002), 21–31.

16. Mulligan, K., Tai, V. W., Algren, H., *et al.* Altered fat distribution in HIV-positive men on nucleoside analog reverse transcriptase inhibitor therapy. *J. AIDS* **26**:**5** (2001), 443–8.

17. Mallon, P. W., Cooper, D. A. & Carr, A. HIV-associated lipodystrophy. *HIV Med* **2**:**3** (2001), 166–73.

18. van der Valk, M., Gisolf, E. H., Reiss, P. *et al.* Increased risk of lipodystrophy when nucleoside analogue reverse transcriptase inhibitors are included with protease inhibitors in the treatment of HIV-1 infection. *AIDS* **15**:**7** (2001), 847–55.

19. Hadigan, C., Corcoran, C., Stanley, T., Piecuch, S., Klibanski, A. & Grinspoon, S. Fasting hyperinsulinemia in human immunodeficiency virus-infected men: relationship to body composition, gonadal function, and protease inhibitor use. *J. Clin. Endocrinol. Metab.* **85**:**1** (2000), 35–41.

20. Jain, R. G., Furfine, E. S., Pedneault, L., White, A. J. & Lenhard, J. M. Metabolic complications associated with antiretroviral therapy. *Antiviral. Res.* **51**:**3** (2001), 151–77.

21. Carr, A., Samaras, K., Burton, S. *et al.* A syndrome of peripheral lipodystrophy, hyperlipidaemia and insulin resistance in patients receiving HIV protease inhibitors. *AIDS* **12**:**7** (1998), F51–8.

22. Tsiodras, S., Mantzoros, C., Hammer, S. & Samore, M. Effects of protease inhibitors on hyperglycemia, hyperlipidemia, and lipodystrophy: a 5-year cohort study. *Arch. Intern. Med.* **160**:**13** (2000), 2050–6.

23. Heath, K. V., Hogg, R. S., Chan, K. J. *et al.* Lipodystrophy-associated morphological, cholesterol and triglyceride abnormalities in a population-based HIV/AIDS treatment database. *AIDS* **15**:**2** (2001), 231–9.

24. Struble, K. & Piscitelli, S. C. Syndromes of abnormal fat redistribution and metabolic complications in HIV-infected patients. *Am. J. Health Syst. Pharm.* **56**:**22** (1999), 2343–8.

25. Dong, K. L., Bausserman, L. L., Flynn, M. M. *et al.* Changes in body habitus and serum lipid abnormalities in HIV-positive women on highly active antiretroviral therapy (HAART). *J. AIDS* **21**:**2** (1999), 107–13.

26. Carr, A., Samaras, K., Thorisdottir, A., Kaufmann, G. R., Chisholm, D. J. & Cooper, D. A. Diagnosis, prediction, and natural course of HIV-1 protease-inhibitor-associated lipodystrophy, hyperlipidaemia, and diabetes mellitus: a cohort study. *Lancet* **353**:**9170** (1999), 2093–9.

27. Herman, J. & Easterbrook, P. The metabolic toxicities of antiretroviral therapy. *Int. J. STD AIDS* **12** (2001), 555–64.

28. Qaqish, R., Rublein, J. & Wohl, D. HIV-associated lipodystrophy syndrome. *Pharmacotherapy* **20**:**1** (2000), 13–22.

29. Wanke, C. A., Falutz, J. M., Shevitz, A., Phair, J. P. & Kotler, D. P. Clinical evaluation and management of metabolic and morphologic abnormalities associated with human immunodeficiency virus. *Clin. Infect. Dis.* **34**:**2** (2002), 248–59.

30. Saint-Marc, T. & Touraine, J. L. "Buffalo hump" in HIV-1 infection. *Lancet* **352**:**9124** (1998), 319–20.

31. Shikuma, C. M., Waslien, C., McKeague, J. *et al.* Fasting hyperinsulinemia and increased waist-to-hip ratios in non-wasting individuals with AIDS. *AIDS* **13**:**11** (1999), 1359–65.

32. Carr, A. & Cooper, D. A. Adverse effects of antiretroviral therapy. *Lancet* **356**:**9239** (2000), 1423–30.

33. Estrada, V., Serrano-Rios, M., Martinez Larrad, M. T. *et al.* Leptin and adipose tissue maldistribution in HIV-infected male patients with predominant fat loss treated with antiretroviral therapy. *J. AIDS* **29**:**1** (2002), 32–40.

34. Herry, I., Bernard, L., de Truchis, P. & Perronne, C. Hypertrophy of the breasts in a patient treated with indinavir. *Clin. Infect. Dis.* **25**:**4** (1997), 937–8.

35. Jaquet, D., Levine, M., Ortega-Rodriguez, E. *et al.* Clinical and metabolic presentation of the lipodystrophic syndrome in HIV-infected children. *AIDS* **14**:**14** (2000), 2123–8.

36. Hadigan, C., Corcoran, C., Piecuch, S., Rodriguez, W. & Grinspoon, S. Hyperandrogenemia in human immunodeficiency virus-infected women with the lipodystrophy syndrome. *J. Clin. Endocrinol. Metab.* **85**:**10** (2000), 3544–50.

37. Christeff, N., Melchior, J. C., Mammes, O., Gherbi, N., Dalle, M. T. & Nunez, E. A. Correlation between increased cortisol:DHEA ratio and malnutrition in HIV-positive men. *Nutrition* **15**:**7–8** (1999), 534–9.

38. Amaya, R., Kozinetz, C., McMeans, A., Schwarzwald, H. & Kline, M. Lipodystrophy syndrome in human immunodeficiency virus-infected children. *Pediatr. Infect. Dis. J.* **21** : **5** (2002), 405–10.

39. Arpadi, S. M., Cuff, P. A., Horlick, M., Wang, J. & Kotler, D. P. Lipodystrophy in HIV-infected children is associated with high viral load and low CD4+ -lymphocyte count and CD4+ -lymphocyte percentage at baseline and use of protease inhibitors and stavudine. *J. AIDS* **27** : **1** (2001), 30–4.

40. Meneilly, G., Forbes, J., Peabody, D., Remple, V. & Burdge, D. Metabolic and body composition changes in HIV-infected children on antiretroviral therapy. In *8th Conference on Retroviruses and Opportunistic Infections*, February 4–8, 2001, Chicago, IL (2001).

41. Brambilla, P., Bricalli, D., Sala, N. *et al.* Highly active antiretroviral-treated HIV-infected children show fat distribution changes even in absence of lipodystrophy. *AIDS* **15** : **18** (2001), 2415–22.

42. Savage, D. B. & O'Rahilly, S. Leptin: a novel therapeutic role in lipodystrophy. *J. Clin. Invest.* **109** (2002), 1285–6.

43. Flier, J. Obesity. In E. Braunwald, *et al.*, (eds.), *Harrison's Principles of Internal Medicine*, 15th edn. New York McGraw-Hill Companies (2001).

44. Montague, C. T. & O'Rahilly, S. The perils of portliness: causes and consequences of visceral adiposity. *Diabetes* **49** : **6** (2000), 883–8.

45. Carr, A. HIV protease inhibitor-related lipodystrophy syndrome. *Clin. Infect. Dis.* **30** (Suppl. 2) (2000), S135–42.

46. Behrens, G., Dejam, A., Schmidt, H. *et al.* Impaired glucose tolerance, beta cell function and lipid metabolism in HIV patients under treatment with protease inhibitors. *AIDS* **13** : **10** (1999), F63–70.

47. Powderly, W. G. Long-term exposure to lifelong therapies. *J. AIDS* **29** (Suppl. 1) (2002), S28–40.

48. Mulligan, K., Grunfeld, C., Tai, V. W. *et al.* Hyperlipidemia and insulin resistance are induced by protease inhibitors independent of changes in body composition in patients with HIV infection. *J. AIDS* **23** : **1** (2000), 35–43.

49. Melvin, A. J., Lennon, S., Mohan, K. M. & Purnell, J. Q. Metabolic abnormalities in HIV type 1-infected children treated and not treated with protease inhibitors. *AIDS Res. Hum. Retrovir.* **17** : **12** (2001), 1117–23.

50. Cheseaux, J. J., Jotterand, V., Aebi, C. *et al.* Hyperlipidemia in HIV-infected children treated with protease inhibitors: relevance for cardiovascular diseases. *J. AIDS* **30** : **3** (2002), 288–93.

51. Bitnun, A., Sochett, E., Babyn, P. *et al.* Glucose homeostasis, serum lipids and abdominal adipose tissue distribution in protease inhibitor-treated and protease inhibitor-naive HIV-infected children. In *9th Conference on Retroviruses and Opportunistic Infections*, Seattle, WA (2002).

52. Arpadi, S. M., Cuff, P. A., Horlick, M. & Kotler, D. P. Visceral obesity, hypertriglyceridemia and hypercortisolism in a boy with perinatally acquired HIV infection receiving protease inhibitor-containing antiviral treatment. *AIDS* **13** : **16** (1999), 2312–3.

53. Purnell, J. Q., Zambon, A., Knopp, R. H. *et al.* Effect of ritonavir on lipids and post-heparin lipase activities in normal subjects. *AIDS* **14** : **1** (2000), 51–7.

54. Carr, A., Samaras, K., Chisholm, D. J. & Cooper, D. A. Pathogenesis of HIV-1-protease inhibitor-associated peripheral lipodystrophy, hyperlipidaemia, and insulin resistance. *Lancet* **351** : **9119** (1998), 1881–3.

55. Miller, K. D., Jones, E., Yanovski, J. A., Shankar, R., Feuerstein, I. & Falloon, J. Visceral abdominal-fat accumulation associated with use of indinavir. *Lancet* **351** : **9106** (1998), 871–5.

56. Fetter, A., Nacci, P., Lenhard, J. *et al.* Fat distribution and retinoid-like symptoms are infrequent in NRTI-experienced subjects treated with amprenavir. In *7th Conference on Retroviruses and Opportunistic Infections*, San Francisco, CA (2000).

57. Joly, V., Flandre, P., Meiffredy, V. *et al.* Assessment of lipodystrophy in patients previously exposed to AZT, ddI, or ddC, but naive for d4T and protease inhibitors (PI), and randomized between d4T/3TC/Indinavir and AZT/3TC/Indinavir (NOVAVIR trial). In *8th Conference on Retroviruses and Opportunistic Infections*, February 4–8, 2001. Chicago, IL (2001).

58. Brinkman, K., Smeitink, J. A., Romijn, J. A. & Reiss, P. Mitochondrial toxicity induced by nucleoside-analogue reverse-transcriptase inhibitors is a key factor in the pathogenesis of antiretroviral-therapy-related lipodystrophy. *Lancet* **354** : **9184** (1999), 1112–5.

59. Brinkman, K., ter Hofstede, H. J., Burger, D. M., Smeitink, J. A. & Koopmans, P. P. Adverse effects of reverse transcriptase inhibitors: mitochondrial toxicity as common pathway. *AIDS* **12** : **14** (1998), 1735–44.

60. Cote, H. C., Brumme, Z. L., Craib, K. J. *et al.* Changes in mitochondrial DNA as a marker of nucleoside toxicity in HIV-infected patients. *New Engl. J. Med.* **346** : **11** (2002), 811–20.

61. Kakuda, T. N. Pharmacology of nucleoside and nucleotide reverse transcriptase inhibitor-induced mitochondrial toxicity. *Clin. Ther.* **22** : **6** (2000), 685–708.

62. Dube, M. P., Sprecher, D., Henry, W. K. *et al.* Preliminary guidelines for the evaluation and management of dyslipidemia in adults infected with human immunodeficiency virus and receiving antiretroviral therapy. Recommendations of the Adult AIDS Clinical Trial Group Cardiovascular Disease Focus Group. *Clin. Infect. Dis.* **31** : **5** (2000), 1216–24.

63. The Adult AIDS Clinical Trials Group. AACTG Metabolic Complications Guides. In *Adult AIDS Clinical Trials Group* (2002).

64. American Academy of Pediatrics. Committee on Nutrition. "Cholesterol in childhood". *Pediatrics* **101** : **1** (1998), 141–7.

65. Wedekind, C. A. & Pugatch, D. Lipodystrophy syndrome in children infected with human immunodeficiency virus. *Pharmacotherapy* **21** : **7** (2001), 861–6.

66. Roubenoff, R., Weiss, L., McDermott, A. *et al.* A pilot study of exercise training to reduce trunk fat in adults with HIV-associated fat redistribution. *AIDS* **13** : **11** (1999), 1373–5.

67. Jones, S. P., Doran, D. A., Leatt, P. B., Maher, B. & Pirmohamed, M. Short-term exercise training improves body composition

and hyperlipidaemia in HIV-positive individuals with lipodystrophy. *AIDS* **15**:**15** (2001), 2049–51.

68. Moyle, G., Baldwin, C. & Phillpot, M. Managing metabolic disturbances and lipodystrophy: diet, exercise, and smoking advice. *AIDS Read* **11**:**12** (2001), 589–92.

69. Hadigan, C., Jeste, S., Anderson, E. J., Tsay, R., Cyr, H. & Grinspoon, S. Modifiable dietary habits and their relation to metabolic abnormalities in men and women with human immunodeficiency virus infection and fat redistribution. *Clin. Infect. Dis.* **33**:**5** (2001), 710–7.

70. Mauss, S., Wolf, E. & Jaeger, H. Reversal of protease inhibitor-related visceral abdominal fat accumulation with recombinant human growth hormone. *Ann. Intern. Med.* **131**:**4** (1999), 313–4.

71. Estrada, V., De Villar, N. G., Larrad, M. T., Lopez, A. G., Fernandez, C. & Serrano-Rios, M. Long-term metabolic consequences of switching from protease inhibitors to efavirenz in therapy for human immunodeficiency virus-infected patients with lipoatrophy. *Clin. Infect. Dis.* **35**:**1** (2002), 69–76.

72. Barreiro, P., Soriano, V., Blanco, F., Casimiro, C., de la Cruz, J. J. & Gonzalez-Lahoz, J. Risks and benefits of replacing protease inhibitors by nevirapine in HIV-infected subjects under long-term successful triple combination therapy. *AIDS* **14**:**7** (2000), 807–12.

73. Martinez, E., Conget, I., Lozano, L., Casamitjana, R. & Gatell, J. M. Reversion of metabolic abnormalities after switching from HIV-1 protease inhibitors to nevirapine. *AIDS* **13**:**7** (1999), 805–10.

74. van der Valk, M., Kastelein, J. J., Murphy, R. L. *et al.* Nevirapine-containing antiretroviral therapy in HIV-1 infected patients results in an anti-atherogenic lipid profile. *AIDS* **15**:**18** (2001), 2407–14.

75. Carr, A., Workman, C., Smith, D. E. *et al.* Abacavir substitution for nucleoside analogs in patients with HIV lipoatrophy: a randomized trial. *J. Am. Med. Assoc.* **288**:**2** (2002), 207–15.

76. McComsey, G., Lonergan, T., Fisher, R., Sension, M., Hoppel, C. & Hessenthaler, S. Improvements in lipoatrophy are observed after 24 weeks when stavudine is replaced by either abacavir or zidovudine. In *9th Conference on Retroviruses and Opportunistic Infections*, February 2002. Seattle, WA (2002).

77. Walli, R., Huster, K., Bogner, J. & Goebel, F. Switching from PI to ABC improves insulin sensitivity and fasting lipids – 12-month follow-up. In *8th Conference on Retroviruses and Opportunistic Infections*, February, 2001. Chicago, IL (2001).

78. Currier, J. S. Metabolic complications of antiretroviral therapy and HIV infection. In *Medscape HIV/AIDS Annual Update 2001*. Medscape (2001).

79. Fisac, C., Fumero, E., Crespo, M. *et al.* A randomized trial of metabolic and body composition changes in patients switching from PI-containing regimens to abacavir, efavirenz, or nevirapine. In *9th Conference on Retroviruses and Opportunistic Infections*, February, 2002. Seattle, WA (2002).

80. John, M. & Mallal, S. A. Hyperlactatemia syndromes in people with HIV infection. *Curr. Opin. Infect. Dis.* **15** (2002), 23–9.

81. Haas, R. H. A comparison of genetic mitochondrial disease and nucleoside analogue toxicity. Does fetal nucleoside toxicity underlie reports of mitochondrial disease in infants born to women treated for HIV infection? *Ann. N. Y. Acad. Sci.* **918** (2000), 247–61.

82. Vu, T. H., Sciacco, M., Tanji, K. *et al.* Clinical manifestations of mitochondrial DNA depletion. *Neurology* **50**:**6** (1998), 1783–90.

83. John, M., Moore, C. B., James, I. R. *et al.* Chronic hyperlactatemia in HIV-infected patients taking antiretroviral therapy. *AIDS* **15**:**6** (2001), 717–23.

84. Boubaker, K., Flepp, M., Sudre, P. *et al.* Hyperlactatemia and antiretroviral therapy: the Swiss HIV Cohort Study. *Clin. Infect. Dis.* **33**:**11** (2001), 1931–7.

85. Vrouenraets, S. M. E., Treskes, M., Regez, R. M. *et al.* Hyperlactatemia in HIV-infected patients: the role of NRTI treatment. In *8th Conference on Retroviruses and Opportunistic Infections*, Chicago, IL (2001).

86. Brinkman, K. Management of hyperlactatemia: no need for routine lactate measurements. *AIDS* **15**:**6** (2001), 795–7.

87. Giaquinto, C., De Romeo, A., Giacomet, V. *et al.* Lactic acid levels in children perinatally treated with antiretroviral agents to prevent HIV transmission. *AIDS* **15**:**8** (2001), 1074–5.

88. Alimenti, A., Burdge, D. R., Oglivie, G. S., Money, D. M. & Forbes, J. C. Lactic acidemia in human immunodeficiency virus-uninfected infants exposed to perinatal antirectroviral therapy. *Pediatr. Infect. Dis. J.* **22**:**9** (2003), 782–9.

89. Gerard, Y., Maulin, L., Yazdanpanah, Y. *et al.* Symptomatic hyperlactataemia: an emerging complication of antiretroviral therapy. *AIDS* **14**:**17** (2000), 2723–30.

90. Lonergan, J. T., Behling, C., Pfander, H., Hassanein, T. I. & Mathews, W. C. Hyperlactatemia and hepatic abnormalities in 10 human immunodeficiency virus-infected patients receiving nucleoside analogue combination regimens. *Clin. Infect. Dis.* **31**:**1** (2000), 162–6.

91. Scalfaro, P., Chesaux, J. J., Buchwalder, P. A., Biollaz, J. & Micheli, J. L. Severe transient neonatal lactic acidosis during prophylactic zidovudine treatment. *Intens. Care Med.* **24**:**3** (1998), 247–50.

92. Miller, K. D., Cameron, M., Wood, L. V., Dalakas, M. C. & Kovacs, J. A. Lactic acidosis and hepatic steatosis associated with use of stavudine: report of four cases. *Ann. Intern. Med.* **133**:**3** (2000), 192–6.

93. Church, J. A., Mitchell, W. G., Gonzalez-Gomez, I. *et al.* Mitochondrial DNA depletion, near-fatal metabolic acidosis, and liver failure in an HIV-infected child treated with combination antiretroviral therapy. *J. Pediatr.* **138**:**5** (2001), 748–51.

94. Scalfaro, P., Chesaux, J. J., Buchwalder, P. A., Biollaz, J. & Mitcheli, J. L. Severe transient neonated lactic acidosis during prophylactic zidovudine treatment. *Intensive Care Med.* **24**:**3** (1998), 247–50.

95. Blanche, S., Tardieu, M., Rustin, P. *et al.* Persistent mitochondrial dysfunction and perinatal exposure to antiretroviral nucleoside analogues. *Lancet* **354**:**9184** (1999), 1084–9.

96. Culnane, M., Fowler, M., Lee, S. S. *et al.* Lack of long-term effects of in utero exposure to zidovudine among uninfected children born to HIV-infected women. Pediatric AIDS Clinical Trials Group Protocol 219/076 Teams. *J. Am. Med. Assoc.* **281** : **2** (1999), 151–7.

97. Lindegren, M. L., Rhodes, P., Gordon, L. & Fleming, P. Drug safety during pregnancy and in infants. Lack of mortality related to mitochondrial dysfunction among perinatally HIV-exposed children in pediatric HIV surveillance. *Ann. N. Y. Acad. Sci.* **918** (2000), 222–35.

98. Bulterys, M., Nesheim, S., Abrams, E. J. *et al.* Lack of evidence of mitochondrial dysfunction in the offspring of HIV-infected women. Retrospective review of perinatal expo-sure to antiretroviral drugs in the Perinatal AIDS Collabora-tive Transmission Study. *Ann. N. Y. Acad. Sci.* **918** (2000), 212–21.

99. Dominguez, K., Bertolli, J., Fowler, M. *et al.* Lack of definitive severe mitochondrial signs and symptoms among deceased HIV-uninfected and HIV-indeterminate children less than or 5 years of age. Pediatric Spectrum of HIV Disease project (PSD), USA. *Ann. N. Y. Acad. Sci.* **918** (2000), 236–46.

100. The Perinatal Safety Review Working Group. Nucleoside exposure in the children of HIV-infected women receiving antiretroviral drugs: abscence of clear evidence for mitochon-drial disease in children who died before 5 years of age in five United States cohorts. *J. AIDS* **25** (2000), 261–8.

HIV drug resistance

Frank Maldarelli, M.D., Ph.D

HIV Drug Resistance Program, National Cancer Institute, Bethesda, MD

21.1 Introduction

One of the most challenging limitations of antiretroviral therapy is the emergence of drug-resistant mutants of HIV, which occurs in 30–40% of treated patients. This chapter outlines the virologic, pharmacologic, and host factors involved in the development of HIV drug resistance, the clinical rationale for resistance testing, the various commercially available testing modalities, and the role of testing algorithms in clinical management. Several excellent reviews on HIV drug resistance testing have recently been published [1–8].

21.2 Virologic factors contributing to development of drug resistance

Several points regarding HIV replication (see also Chapters 2, 4, and 5) are essential for understanding the development of HIV drug resistance and are reviewed here. Retrovirus replication (Figure 21.1) is rapid [9–12], and error prone [13, 14]. During reverse transcription, error rates have been estimated at 1 error per 1–300 000 incorporated bases [15, 16]. As a result, it is likely that drug-resistance mutants are present prior to initiation of drug therapy [17]. Retrovirus replication proceeds with frequent recombination between different viruses, sometimes with potentially significant genetic differences [18], and recent epidemiologic studies provide strong evidence of frequent recombination within patients [19–22]. HIV recombination was described in a premature infant multiply transfused with blood from two different HIV-infected donors [23], and other in vitro and animal in vivo experiments [18, 24, 25] support this observation. Under conditions of drug selection pressure, recombination may represent a potent mechanism responsible for facilitating the spread of drug-resistance mutations [21, 22]. Although antiretroviral drugs used in combination can decrease circulating amounts of virus to below the limits of detection, currently available antiretroviral therapy cannot eradicate virus from an infected person [26–30]; presumably viral replication continuing at some low level, even during antiretroviral therapy, can allow for the selection of drug-resistant virus and the consequent evolution of drug resistance. Persaud and co-workers [31–33], noted that HIV genes amplified from patients with viral loads suppressed to less than 50 copies/mL plasma could contain drug-resistance mutations.

Other critical factors contribute to the development of HIV drug resistance, including the pharmacology of the antiretroviral agents, and host factors.

21.3 Identification and characterization of HIV drug-resistance mutations

When a new antiretroviral agent is characterized, one important set of studies involves the characterization of the mutations that confer resistance to the drug. HIV can evolve resistance to every known antiretroviral agent; resistance mutations may emerge rapidly and easily – for some drugs the result of single amino acid changes conferring high-level resistance or for other drugs the result of the

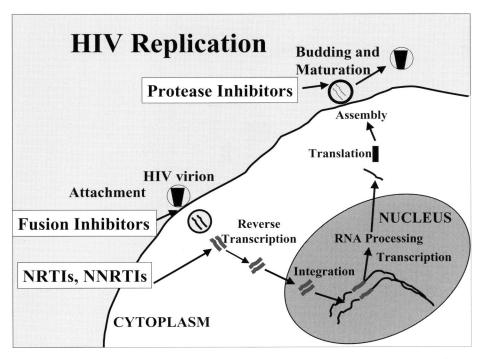

Figure 21.1. Steps in HIV replication. HIV infection can be interrupted during spreading HIV replication at stages of fusion, reverse transcription, or maturation. Cells with incorporated proviruses are not sensitive to inhibition by current inhibitors. NRTI, nucleoside analogue reverse transcription inhibitors; NNRTI, non-nucleoside RTIs.

accumulation of many different mutations each conferring a small degree of resistance to the virus. Drug resistance mutations have traditionally been identified using a combination of in vitro experiments and in vivo observations. In vitro identification of resistance mutations typically involves tissue culture infections using a molecular clone of HIV incubated in the presence of antiretrovirals for prolonged periods. These prolonged experiments begin with the virus being exposed to low levels of drug, followed by exposure to progressively escalating drug concentrations. Some mutations emerging in these experiments may confer resistance to antiretrovirals, but mutations observed in such circumstances may also represent random changes that do not confer resistance that were randomly fixed in the population. Further confirmatory studies using recombinant viruses, constructed to contain the mutations observed to develop during the prolonged incubations and tested both singly and in combination are essential to ensure that the identified mutations are involved in drug resistance.

Drug-resistance mutations are also identified by comparing the sequence of HIV obtained from patients undergoing therapy with a given antiretroviral to that of wild-type virus. Confirmation that specific residues are responsible for drug resistance requires that the mutations observed in vivo subsequently confer resistance when introduced into recombinant viruses studied in tissue culture infections.

Results of in vivo and in vitro experiments often concur, although disparate results may be obtained. For instance, in vitro studies of stavudine (d4T) resistance often demonstrate the emergence of a resistant virus encoding a valine to threonine change at amino acid position 75 [34], yet this mutation is infrequent in patients with persistent viremia on d4T-containing regimens. Similarly, mutations at position 74 emerge in vitro after exposure to didanosine (ddI); such mutations occur, but are not invariably present in patients failing ddI, and more complex patterns are often present [35].

Collections of drug-resistance mutations are often depicted in tables (see Figures 21.2 and 21.3); such tables, although useful, do not depict degrees of resistance or complexities of interactions among mutations. Online compendia of mutations, frequently updated (e.g. hivdb. stanford.edu, hiv-web.lanl.gov (a sequence compendium

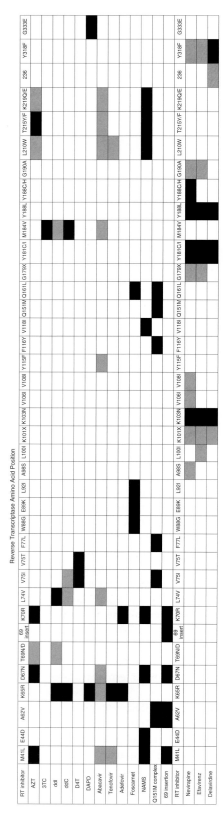

Figure 21.2. The figure lists the principal amino acids conferring resistance to the HIV reverse transcriptase inhibitors, and shows the mutations that are included in the nucleoside analogue (NAMS) group of mutations, and the 69 insertion and Q151M multiple resistance complexes. Mutations that confer high-level resistance are indicated by black boxes. "Secondary" mutations are shown in gray. They do not confer significant resistance themselves, but further decrease sensitivity to the drugs when primary mutations are present. See text for details.

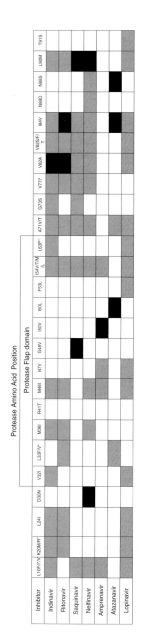

Figure 21.3. The figure lists the principal amino acids conferring resistance to the HIV protease inhibitors. Mutations that confer high level resistance (decreased sensitivity to the drug by three- to five-fold or more) are indicated by black boxes. "Secondary" mutations are shown in gray. They do not confer significant resistance themselves, but further decrease sensitivity to the drugs when primary mutations are present. See text for details.

HIV-1 Reverse Transcriptase

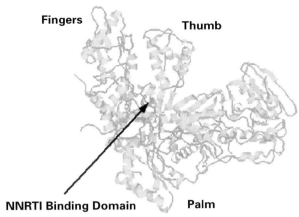

Figure 21.4. HIV reverse transcriptase X-ray crystal structure of HIV RT heterodimer demonstrating typical fingers, palm, and thumb domains; crystallographic data [147] were displayed using RASMOL and the NCBI Entrez suite of structural information at www.ncbi.nlm.nih.gov.

of utility for researchers), www.hivresistanceweb.com, www.iasusa.org/resistance/mutations/index.html, provide additional information concerning antiretroviral resistance mutations.

21.4 Mechanisms of drug resistance

21.4.1 Nucleoside and nucleotide reverse transcriptase inhibitors

Reverse transcriptase (RT), the viral enzyme that catalyzes the synthesis of the cDNA copy of the viral RNA genome, is structurally similar to a variety of DNA polymerases with a "right hand" configuration, including a palm domain that carries out catalytic polymerization, as well as fingers and thumb domains that ensure correct positioning of dNTP and template positioning (Figure 21.4). Reverse transcriptase synthesizes a full length DNA copy (provirus) from virion-encapsidated RNA (Figure 21.5). To produce proviral DNA, RT must carry out a series of reactions, including RNA-dependent DNA polymerization, the synthesis of a cDNA copy of the viral RNA genome using the RNA as a template; RNase H activity, the degradation of the RNA in the RNA–DNA hybrid molecule created during the first step of reverse transcription; and DNA-dependent DNA polymerization, the synthesis of a complementary DNA strand to make a double-stranded provirus. HIV RT can catalyze

the removal of an incorporated nucleotide in an excision mechanism, which can remove nucleotides at the end of the growing DNA chain, but it does have the same kind of "proof-reading" activity that some DNA polymerases have that can specifically eliminate misincorporated bases during DNA synthesis.

Nucleoside reverse transcriptase inhibitors (NRTIs) act as chain terminators of reverse transcription. They are incorporated into growing DNA strands, but prevent incorporation of additional nucleosides. Two general mechanisms confer drug resistance to NRTIs: excision and steric hindrance. HIV RT can catalyze the removal of an incorporated nucleotide in an excision mechanism. Mutations that enhance this function cause resistance by enabling the RT to remove the otherwise lethal chain-terminating nucleotide analogues more efficiently. Resistance mutations that act through steric mechanisms block the drugs from binding to RT. For NNRTIs, mutations inhibit binding of drug to the enzyme. The convention for denoting resistance mutations uses the single letter amino acid code that occurs in the wild type enzyme followed by the amino acid position of the mutation, followed by the single letter amino acid code for the mutant, e.g. M184V refers to a methionine (M) in the wild type changed to valine (V) in the mutant at amino acid position 184 of reverse transcriptase. If alternative amino acids are present a forward slash is utilized: T215Y/F indicates that either tyrosine or phenylalanine resistance mutation occurs at position 215.

Nucleoside analogue RTI resistance due to excision mechanisms

Nucleoside associated mutations (NAMs)
Therapy with a number of NRTIs results in emergence of a suite of mutations in RT (nucleoside-associated mutations, NAMS) conferring a variable degree of resistance to the NRTIs. These RT NAMS are sometimes called "thymidine analogue mutations" (or TAMS) because they were initially noted to confer resistance to the thymidine analogue RTIs, such as zidovudine. Nucleoside-associated mutations include M41L, D67N, K70R, L210W, T215Y/F, and K219Q/E. The mechanism through which NAMs confer resistance has been unclear, as these mutants do not appear to affect NRTI-triphosphate incorporation, as would be expected for a mutation that altered the ability of the NRTIs to interact with RT and be incorporated into the growing cDNA. Instead, several groups demonstrated that RT containing NAMS could remove zidovudine (AZT or ZDV) incorporated into cDNA at higher than wild-type

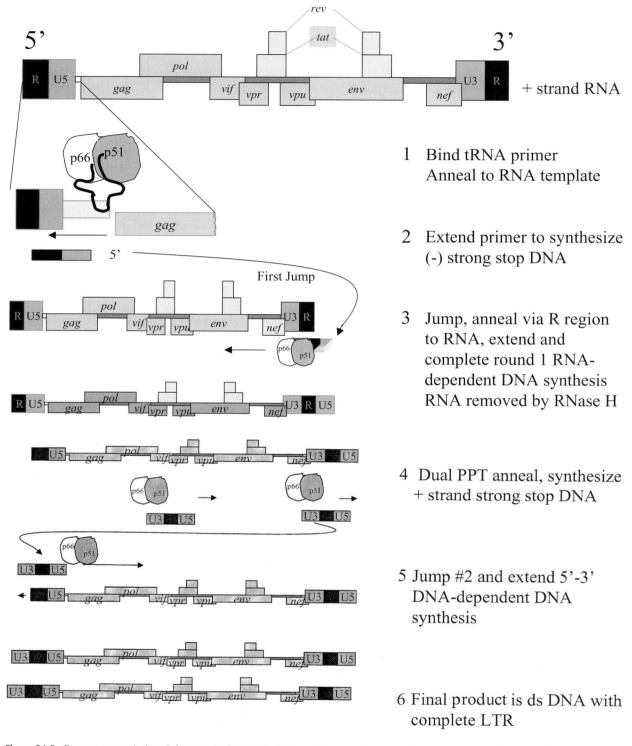

Figure 21.5. Reverse transcription. Substrate single-stranded HIV mRNA consisting of coding sequences and distinct end structures (unique 5' (U5) regions, unique 3' regions (U3), and common repeat (R) sequences) is converted into double-stranded proviral DNA with identical long terminal repeat (U3-R-U5) structures at 5' and 3' ends. Stages 1–6 indicate sequential steps in the reverse transcription process.

levels via an excision mechanism. Excision is an energy-requiring reaction, with either pyrophosphate alone or ATP representing the energy donor. Intracellularly, it is likely that ATP functions as the pyrophosphate donor. Interestingly, the putative ATP binding domain within RT is in close proximity to amino acids 67, 70, 210, 215, and 219. The mutant RT can thus excise the NRTI from the cDNA at increased levels, so that the NRTI no longer terminates the growing cDNA chain and synthesis of the cDNA can continue, producing a functional provirus. One suggestion is that NAMS facilitate binding of ATP to RT, which results in more effective excision of NRTIs incorporated into the cDNA. While this mechanism appears to help explain resistance to AZT, stavudine (d4T) and perhaps abacavir, the role of excision to didanosine (ddI) and tenofovir resistance remains less certain.

69/70 insertion mutation

A group of mutations consisting of an insertion of a variable number of amino acids between amino acids 69 and 70, and additional associated mutations (M41L, A62V, D67N, and K70R) confer high-level resistance to all NRTIs [36, 37]. The insertion mutants appear to act through excision mechanisms [38–40]. The presence of these mutations in a patient's virus severely limits the clinical utility of the NRTIs. Mutations that involve the deletion of amino acids may also occur in this region [41], with similar high-level NRTI-cross resistance; deletion of amino acid 69 has reported to confer high-level NNRTI resistance [42].

T215Y/F mutation

Of the different NAMs, mutations at position 215 are probably the most important, conferring high-level resistance to AZT. T215Y/F was a marker for disease progression in the ACTG 175 AZT monotherapy study and is a marker for clinical disease progression in adults [43] and children, where T215 mutations were associated with clinical deterioration [44] and with the emergence of a more cytopathic, syncytium-inducing virus phenotype [45].

Nucleoside analogue RTI resistance due to steric and positional effects

A number of HIV drug-resistance mutations are localized near the active site of the enzyme. Analysis of certain mutations conferring drug resistance revealed that these mutations lead to changes in the structure of RT that hinder the triphosphophosphorylated drugs from interacting with RT and being incorporated into the cDNA while permitting incorporation of the natural dNTP. Mutations may act directly by altering the shape of RT's active site or the region surrounding the active site, or by changing the orientation of the incoming nucleotide with respect to the template.

M184V

M184V confers strong resistance to lamivudine (3TC) and zalcitabine (ddC), and is observed within weeks after 3TC monotherapy. A combination of crystallographic and enzymatic studies have suggested that replacement of methionine with valine at position 184 results in steric hindrance, preventing the dideoxy analogues 3TC and ddC from gaining access to the enzyme active site [46, 47]. A second 184 mutant, M184I, appears to act in similar fashion [47]. M184I emerges after 3TC therapy, often prior to M184V, but is quickly replaced by M184V. It has been suggested that both mutants exist prior to the initiation of 3TC therapy within the large numbers of viruses present within a patient (see Chapter 5). M184I is likely more prevalent than M184V among the viral population prior to the start of treatment, but M184V confers greater resistance to 3TC, becoming the dominant mutant upon prolonged therapy [48].

K65R

K65R is a key mutation conferring resistance to ddI, tenofovir, adefovir, and abacavir. Crystallographic studies suggest that the "fingers" domain, including amino acid 65, lies in close proximity to the incoming dNTP; the amino group on the lysine side chain at amino acid position 65 in the wild-type enzyme contacts the gamma phosphate of the incoming triphosphate via a salt bridge [49, 50]. Apparently, the guanido group supplied by arginine in the resistant mutant affects interactions with ddATP such that it is no longer an efficient dNTP donor for RT. Although K65R is a characteristic mutation that is often seen when the virus is exposed to drug in vitro, it does not appear commonly in clinical specimens [51]; K65R increases sensitivity to AZT [52] in the presence of NAMs, and so may not be selected in the presence of pre-existing NAMs.

Q151M complex

Mutations characterized by the presence of Q151M and including A62V, V75I, F77L, and F116Y emerged in early studies of alternating AZT/ddI monotherapy. Q151 lies in the part of RT near the incoming nucleotide, and steric interference of incoming dideoxy NRTIs has been suggested as the mechanism by which this suite of mutations results in high-level resistance to all NRTIs [49, 53]. The additional mutations are thought to affect the region surrounding Q151M to accommodate the methionine residue [49]. Fortunately, the Q151 complex comprises a relatively small proportion of resistant viruses [54].

L74V

The position of L74 is also near the incoming nucleotide [49, 53], and lies near the RT amino acids that stabilize the position of the incoming base as it recognizes and interacts with the template RNA. The L74V mutation thus may affect binding of the dNTP directly and indirectly. L74V is typically associated with ddI exposure [35].

21.4.2 Non-nucleoside reverse transcriptase inhibitors

The non-nucleoside reverse transcriptase inhibitors (NNRTIs) are chemically diverse compounds that inhibit cDNA synthesis but, unlike the NRTIs, do not directly compete with the native dNTPs. Incubation of an NNRTI with RT results in spatial rearrangement of a series of RT residues into a hydrophobic domain or "pocket" that binds NNRTI molecules within the palm at the base of the thumb domain (Figure 21.4). Non-nucleoside RTI binding results in disruption of the configuration of the polymerase active site, blocking further dNTP incorporation. Mutations in RT that change the spatial characteristics of NNRTI binding region, or entry to the pocket to which the NNRTIs bind, effectively exclude NNRTIs and result in drug resistance. Such mutations cluster in specific domains within the reverse transcriptase (amino acids 100–110, 180–190, 225–235), corresponding to the boundaries of the pocket that forms upon incubation with NNRTIs. Even though the approved NNRTIs have different chemical structures, they all bind to the same site in RT, so mutations that confer resistance to one NNRTI also confer resistance to the others. One potent mutation conferring cross resistance to NNRTIs is the lysine to arginine mutation at position 103, a mutation that prevents effective drug binding [55]. In the presence of some known NNRTI mutations, but in the absence of K103N, some in vitro studies suggest efavirenz retains a significant degree of antiretroviral activity; this observation may not have durable clinical applicability [56, 57]. As recently reported, results of the ACTG 398 study [58] suggested that even relatively small phenotypic changes in NNRTI resistance was associated with virologic failure with efavirenz-containing regimens. Other mutations conferring resistance to NNRTIs, including Y181C and multiple amino acid changes at position Y188 confer a significant degree of NNRTI cross resistance.

The known set of mutations in RT that confer or contribute to resistance is not limited to the prinicipal mutations listed in Figure 21.2. Additional mutations and polymorphisms that may play a role in HIV drug resistance continue to be identified.

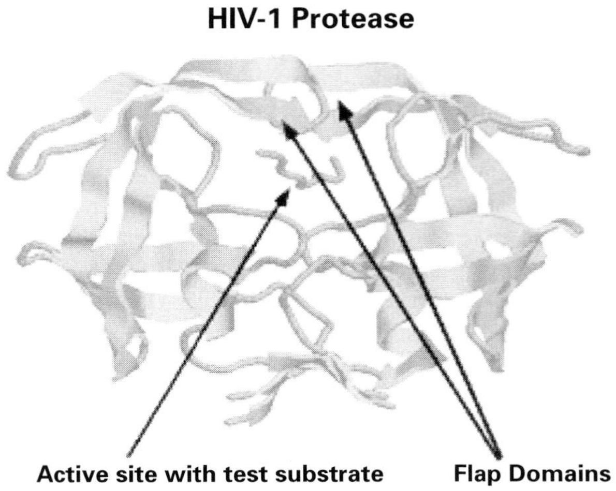

HIV-1 Protease

Active site with test substrate   Flap Domains

Figure 21.6. HIV protease. Crystallographic data of protease homodimer. Active site location of Asp25 and position of flap domains are indicated. Data [61] were displayed using RASMOL and the NCBI Entrez suite of structural information at www.ncbi.nlm.nih.gov.

21.4.3 Protease inhibitors

The HIV protease is a 99 amino acid aspartyl protease that processes the HIV Gag and Gag/Pol polyprotein precursor, an essential maturational step in the HIV life cycle [59] (see Figure 2.2; Chapter 2); protease is part of the *gag/pol* polyprotein, and so the initial processing events take place while protease is still part of the precursor. In the absence of protease activity, when the enzyme is inhibited by protease inhibitors (PIs), the polyprotein precursors are not processed and the virion does not assume its mature, infectious form.

Protease is active as a homodimer and has two-fold symmetry (Figure 21.6); at least nine distinct cleavage sites within Gag and Gag/Pol are processed by protease, albeit with 400-fold differences in catalytic efficiency (Figure 21.7). Analyses of crystallographic data have identified critical adjacent "flap" domains, in addition to the active site itself [60, 61]. The flap domains appear to permit substrates to gain access to the active site [60]; they may also bind an essential water molecule that participates in catalysis [59]. Peptidomimetic inhibitors with structural resemblance to authentic cleavage sites were designed using the symmetrical aspects of the molecule and with knowledge of the cleavage sites. Resistance to protease inhibitors occurs with mutations both in regions of the molecule that bind the drug and in adjacent "flap" domain (amino acids 47–52) overlying the active site that may affect substrate binding and proteolysis [62]. Resistance-conferring mutations may

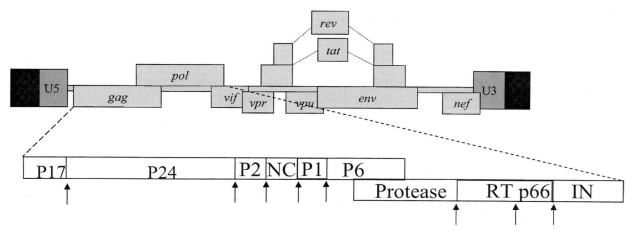

Figure 21.7. HIV genomic organization with *gag/pol* detail. Arrows indicate sites of cleavage by HIV protease.

have effects on the stability of protease, its ability to dimerize, and enzymatic activities [63]; a unified theory of the precise structural changes occurring after specific mutations continues to be elucidated using the combination of structural enzymatic and mutational studies.

Mutation patterns that confer resistance to the protease inhibitors are often complex. Certain "primary" resistance mutations decrease sensitivity to individual PIs (Figures 21.2 and 21.3, in black) by a modest amount, –3 to 5-fold. Other, "secondary" mutations (Figures 21.2 and 21.3, in gray) do not confer resistance to the PIs when present by themselves, but further decrease sensitivity to the drugs when primary mutations are present. Primary mutations are relatively specific for individual protease inhibitors, but secondary mutations can confer resistance to many protease inhibitors. HIV that is significantly resistant to one PI is often broadly cross-resistant to others [64–66].

Beyond a few characteristic mutations, simple genotyping may not clearly predict protease resistance. As an example, mutations in 11–14 different amino acid substitutions can contribute to lopinavir resistance [67]. Difficulties in precisely quantitating the relative contributions of different PI mutations has resulted in attempts to quantitate PI resistance as a function of total number of PI resistance mutations.

Several important primary PI mutations include:

D30N. D30 appears to lie close to the protease active site and specifically interacts with the P2′ amino acid (the amino acid two residues distal to the peptide bond undergoing cleavage). D30N is a specific primary mutation conferring resistance to nelfinavir; interestingly, the presence of D30N does not appear to significantly compromise sensitivity to

indinavir, saquinanvir, ritonavir, or lopinavir/ritonavir (Kaletra)[68].

M46I/L/V. M36 is an amino acid in the flap region that interacts on the solvent exposed face of the molecule away from the substrate [62], and contributes to resistance to nelfinavir, indinavir, saquinanvir, ritonavir, and lopinavir/ritonavir.

G48V/L. This is a mutation in the flap domain that may affect binding of inhibitors, conferring resistance to saquinavir, perhaps by steric repulsion [69] that contributes prominently to SQV resistance.

I50V/L. I50 is a key amino acid residue in the flap domain that may have hydrophobic interactions with the substrate (or inhibitor). I50V mutation may permit a degree of flexibility that decreases binding of small molecules such as inhibitors, while permitting binding of large substrates. I50V confers resistance to amprenavir [70]; I50L appears to be a critical mutation for atazanavir, but may sensitize to amprenavir, indinavir, and saquinavir.

V82A. V82A is a primary resistance mutation involved in substrate binding. V82A may cause rearrangements in hydrogen bonding that effectively exclude PI binding while permitting substrate binding [61], or may result in active site expansion, reducing protease inhibitor binding [71]. V82A was the most frequent mutation identified in children with viremia after failing their first PI-containing regimen [72].

L90M. L90M is a mutation reported to interact with catalytic amino acid E25; the L90M mutation may destabilize the protease dimmer and affect stability of the enzyme [63, 73]. L90M is associated with resistance to a variety of PIs, and contributes significantly to resistance to nelfinavir and saquinavir.

21.4.4 Cleavage site mutations

In addition to resistance mutations occurring within the protease gene proper, additional mutations emerge at protease cleavage sites within gag and Gag/Pol polyproteins. In vitro enzymatic evidence indicates that mutant protease cleaves the mutant sites at greater efficiency than wild-type cleavage sites; similarly, recombinant viruses encoding mutant protease and mutant cleavage sites grow faster than mutant protease with wild-type cleavage sites [74–77]. As compared with data for the protease itself, there are fewer data regarding the number and type of cleavage site mutations and association with PI therapy, although A431V and L449F have been consistently observed, and recently linked to mutations at position 46 and 50 within protease [78, 79]. The regions of Gag and Gag/Pol polyproteins affected by the cleavage site mutations are typically not sequenced in viral genotyping assays and so would not be identified outside of a research setting.

21.4.5 Fusion inhibitors

Several novel peptide agents have been developed to inhibit early steps in HIV replication. Following attachment via CD4 and coreceptor binding, conformational changes in the HIV envelope glycoprotein complex result in transient exposure of a fusion domain that mediates membrane fusion via a spring-loaded mechanism (See Chapter 2). Two recent inhibitors, enfuvirtide (T-20, Fuzeon) and T-1249 are inhibitors of the fusion process and have been tested in clinical trials [80, 81]. Enfuvirtide and T-1249 are peptides that include a short part of the gp41 amino acid sequence. They bind to gp41 and prevent it from forming the "six helix" bundle required for insertion of the gp41 fusion domain into the host-cell plasma membrane. Enfuvirtide has been recently approved by the U.S. Food and Drug Administration. Prior to therapy, wild-type HIV exhibits wide (> 10-fold) range of susceptibility to inhibition by T-20. Following exposure to fusion inhibitors, resistant viruses emerge within 2 weeks in monotherapy situations, and mutations in at least three amino acids have been associated with resistance [82]. A single amino acid change was associated with an eight-fold decrease in drug sensitivity, and combinations of mutations further decreased sensitivity. Sequences outside the enfuvirtide binding region, including the highly variable V3 region, are reported to influence inhibition, perhaps contributing to the wide baseline variation in inhibition.

21.4.6 Duration of HIV drug-resistance mutations

Duration of HIV drug-resistance mutations following drug interruption is variable. Certain drug-resistance mutations, including M184V and certain PI-resistance mutations, appear to be subject to severe negative selection, presumably because of reductions in replication capacity; interruption of drug suppression may lead to re-emergence of wild-type virus within weeks. In contrast, other resistance mutations may persist for several years [83].

21.4.7 Resensitization and hypersusceptibility

During early phenotypic studies of HIV from drug-treated individuals, several investigators noticed that the presence of certain mutations conferring resistance to one antiretroviral rendered the virus more sensitive to other antiretrovirals [70, 84–86]. Examples include mutations conferring resistance to foscarnet that resulted in increased sensitivity to AZT [84], an NNRTI mutation (Y181C) decreased resistance to AZT, and ddI resistance mutation L74V decreased resistance to AZT [85]. In protease, the mutation at N88S, which contributes to resistance to nelfinavir and perhaps atazanivir sensitizes to amprenavir [87]. Sensitization to NNRTIs may also occur, although mutations responsible for this phenomenon have not been well characterized.

Perhaps the most significant example of NRTI resensitization is the mutation M184V. Although the M184V mutation confers resistance by steric mechanisms, this mutation has additional effects on RT sensitivity to other antiretrovirals. Combination of M184V with the RT NAMS results in increased sensitivity to AZT or D4T compared with RT with NAMs alone. The reasons for this resensitization remain uncertain, although it has been suggested that M184V inhibits excisions. The presence of M184V is likely to confer benefit in the presence of TAMS in AZT-, d4T- and perhaps tenofovir-containing regimens.

Hypersusceptibility may have useful clinical implications: NRTI-experienced, NNRTI-naïve patients beginning NNRTI-containing regimens have a greater reduction in plasma viral RNA when the hypersusceptibility mutations are present [88]. In patients with complicated resistance patterns and few antiretroviral therapy options, clinicians sometimes elect to continue treatment with 3TC, together with ZDV, d4T, or tenofovir, even when a patient's virus has the M184V mutation, hoping to maintain the higher sensitivity to the other NRTIs. Drug-experienced, NNRTI-naïve individuals starting EFV have a better virologic response when their virus is hypersusceptible to EFV [58]. These studies raise questions regarding timing and sequencing of antiretrovirals, especially EFV, and future investigations may reveal useful practical correlates of hypersusceptibility.

21.5 HIV drug-resistance assays

A variety of HIV drug-resistance assays are available for clinical use, but are generally divided into assays that determine either genotypic or phenotypic resistance. All commercial resistance assays use plasma as starting material.

21.5.1 Genotyping assays

Genotyping assays determine the nucleic acid sequence of portions of the HIV genome relevant to drug resistance, generally using HIV RNA from plasma samples. The methodology for determining the sequence of RNA directly is exceedingly cumbersome and expensive. As an alternative, HIV RNA is reverse transcribed in vitro into cDNA using exogenously added reverse transcriptase, and the cDNA is then sequenced. DNA sequencing has become highly automated, fast, and relatively inexpensive. In order to obtain sufficient material to determine the presence of HIV drug-resistance mutations, the cDNA product must be amplified using polymerase chain reaction (PCR) techniques. The presence of drug-resistance mutations in the PCR product may be determined by a variety of techniques. The most straightforward method involves direct nucleic acid sequencing, and comparing the sequence to standard wild-type HIV to identify changes corresponding to drug resistance. In general, the regions responsible for drug resistance available for sequencing include protease and a portion of reverse transcriptase. Reverse transcriptase is a relatively large gene and studies demonstrated that mutations conferring resistance are confined to a region encompassed by amino acids 1–400. As outlined above, resistance to protease inhibitors may be affected by mutations at Gag/Pol polyprotein cleavage sites that are outside the protease and RT domains, and as such are not reported by typical resistance sequencing. Using the genetic code, the inferred amino acid sequence is deduced from the nucleic acid sequence, and an interpretation concerning resistance is rendered based on the known qualities of the different mutants (see below). Because the assays examine the bulk properties of all the genetically diverse virus present in a sample of plasma, these assays do not provide sequence information about individual viral genomes. They only provide average sequence information about viral species present in relatively large numbers of circulating viruses; only variants composing 20–25% of the population or more will be represented in the final analysis. This has significant clinical implications because minority resistant viral species may exist within a patient and these resistant species may not be detected through viral genotypic assays. This is particularly true for highly experienced patients who are no longer receiving certain antiretrovirals. These patients may harbor minority resistant "archived" viral species that are not detected by viral genotyping, but which can re-emerge when treatment with certain drugs is resumed.

Several assays are commercially available, either as a service (Virco/Johnson and Johnson, Virologic) or as kits (TrueGene/Visible Genetics). All assays require some minimum viral load for determination of the genotype. The viral load necessary to detect mutations is a function of the ability to synthesize cDNA; 1000 copies HIV RNA/mL are generally required. Samples with between 1000–5000 RNA copies/mL are occasionally difficult to amplify, and amplification sometimes succeeds with lower viral loads. The TrueGene kit has been used with pediatric samples [89]; genotypic results were obtained from samples with viral loads < 1000 and with small volumes (< 0.5 mL) and genotypes were obtained on 98% of samples. Turnaround time for the commercial services is in the order of 1–2 weeks.

Several methods are available that detect genotypic changes in HIV without direct nucleic acid sequencing of large regions of HIV RT or protease. Assays for individual HIV mutations have been investigated using hybridization technologies (line probe (LIPA) assays, microarray (GeneChip, Affymetrix) assays, mutation-specific PCR assays, and oligonucleotide ligation assays (OLA) that utilize either probe array techniques or single mutation detection methods. These assays that detect single point mutations may be more sensitive than population-based sequencing or phenotyping assays in detecting minority mutant species [54], but natural sequence variability near the mutation itself can significantly affect hybridization [90, 91].

21.5.2 Phenotyping

Assessing resistance from a series of complex mutational patterns is often difficult. Phenotyping provides a functional evaluation of drug susceptibility. The use of recombinant DNA technology [92–95] to construct chimeric plasmids consisting of gag/pol sequences from patient isolates cloned into laboratory-adapted HIV strains has permitted reliable and reproducible measurement of in vitro resistance. Two assays are commercially available [96, 97]

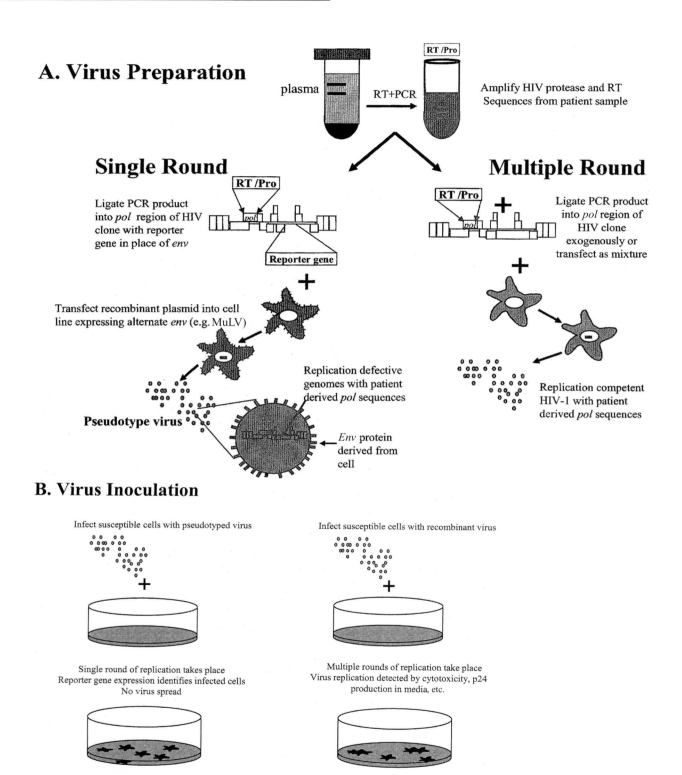

Figure 21.8. Comparison of HIV single round and multiple round phenotyping assays. See text for details.

C. Quantitating resistance

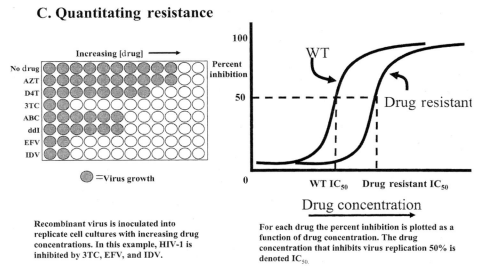

Recombinant virus is inoculated into replicate cell cultures with increasing drug concentrations. In this example, HIV-1 is inhibited by 3TC, EFV, and IDV.

For each drug the percent inhibition is plotted as a function of drug concentration. The drug concentration that inhibits virus replication 50% is denoted IC_{50}.

Figure 21.8. *(cont.)*

(Figure 21.8). HIV protease and RT sequences are amplified from patient material via reverse transcription and PCR. The PCR product is introduced into a recombinant molecular clone of HIV [98]. The recombinant HIV clone containing the patient RT or protease genes are transfected into cells capable of producing HIV virions. The virions have the patient RT or protease gene and are subsequently used to inoculate cultures of susceptible cells. Parallel cultures are inoculated with wild type HIV. Infections are carried out in the presence or absence of increasing concentrations of antiviral agents, and the growth of these permits an estimate of the degree of resistance for individual mutations. Resistance is characterized using the linear portion of the dose-response curve (see Figure 21.8C); results are typically reported as the concentration of drug that inhibits virus replication by 50% (IC_{50}). Comparison of this value to the IC_{50} obtained for a standard laboratory strain shows by what fold a patient's virus is resistant to a particular drug compared with a wild-type virus.

Commercially available phenotyping assays evaluate only a portion of the HIV *gag/pol* gene, without inclusion of all protease cleavage sites; as described above, cleavage sites may vary after drug resistance emerges, and effects on drug susceptibility may occur [74]. Commercially, phenotyping is performed with multiple round infections (Virco) or in single round assays (Virologic) using vectors which are capable of only a single round of infection. These defective viruses encode a reporter gene to identify infected cells, allowing for easy quantitation. Conceptually, the two commercial assays appear to offer different advantages. Single round assays eliminate the possibility that resistance

may spontaneously arise during the cultivation of wild type virus in the presence of the drug [99]. Multi-round cultivation assays may detect low level resistance that may not manifest in a single round assay. In practice, however, the two commercial phenotyping assays have remarkably concordant results [100]. Improvements in interpretation algorithms and additions to the databases will undoubtedly continue to improve interpretation and consistency.

Increases in IC_{50} are associated with drug resistance, but the degree of virologic resistance associated with clinical drug failure are not clear in all circumstances. Establishment of effective cutoffs has been a major aspect of phenotyping assay development. For some antiretrovirals, such as efavirenz or 3TC, where single amino acid changes produce high level resistance, large increases in IC_{50} are noted. In these examples, 50–1000-fold changes may occur, and identifying resistance is straightforward. For some newer agents, such as abacavir [101], or lopinavir/ritonavir [102], phenotypic sensitivity has been prospectively studied in clinical trials, and useful estimates of clinical sensitivity were obtained. Drugs such as ddI or d4T have been noted to have a more restricted dynamic range in phenotyping assays and cutoffs are relatively difficult to assign. Retrospective analyses of virologic responses to d4T-containing salvage regimens [103] that revealed only minor increases in phenotypic resistance (1.4–1.8-fold greater than wild type) were associated with clinical failure [104]. One approach has been to evaluate the distribution of drug resistance in isolates from drug-naïve individuals and assigning cutoffs at IC_{50} levels several standard deviations beyond the mean drug-naïve level [105].

21.5.3 Interpretation of genotypic and phenotypic data

In general, patient viral genotypes tend to be complex, and often require sophisticated algorithms to arrive at useful interpretations. Summaries of resistance mutations are available (see Figures 21.2 and 21.3 for examples). Although such tables offer some useful perspective, they are limited by the volume and detail of data; they cannot be both comprehensive and comprehensible, and additional explanations are often necessary [106]. Genotype algorithms are under continuous review and improvements continue to be made. Several rules-based algorithms are available in which individual mutations are assigned a score based on clinical or in vitro data, a sum of all mutations generated for the sample, and the level of resistance (susceptible, low-level, high-level resistance, etc.) is assessed based on the score [6, 106]. Alternatively, several companies, including Virologic and Virco, have established large relational databases correlating genotypic and phenotypic information on individual samples that yield assessments of resistance based on proprietary methods of interpretation. The database can then be queried with new genotypic information and the average phenotype of matching genotypes determined. In some cases the database is supplemented with additional information regarding individual mutations, improving the utility of the interpretation [107]. The two principal commercially available phenotypic interpretation services are the Virtual Phenotype (Virco) and Phenosense GT (Virologic). The utility of any genotyping determination may be limited when considering newly introduced drugs with new resistance profiles, or with complex genotypes where there may be few matching genotypes present in the database. In such cases, rules-based interpretations may be employed. Results of genotyping and phenotyping assays have been directly compared [108] with generally good concordance; 81% agreement for NRTIs and 90–91% agreement for NNRTIs and PIs.

New bioinformatics approaches have been successfully utilized to predict resistance phenotypes based on genotypic information [109]. One algorithm that detects resistance due to characteristic mutation patterns and appears to be relatively sensitive to subtle mutational effects has been incorporated into an online prediction system, geno2pheno (http://www.genafor.org/). Future validation studies will be necessary to assess the clinical utility of this and other programs.

Several studies have integrated the use of resistance testing with parallel drug-level monitoring to derive an estimate of the "inhibitory quotient" using the drug level at trough and the fold resistance to individual antivirals [110, 111] or to antiviral regimen [112] (see also Chapter 23).

Viral replication capacity and viral fitness assays

Patients who have experienced virologic failure with multiple antiretroviral regimens develop virus that is resistant to all available antiretroviral agents. In such patients, genotypic and phenotypic information often provides little practical data, and often only shows that the virus is broadly resistant. There may be no clear optimal antiretroviral regimens for these patients and it may be clinically advantageous to give therapy not with the aim of decreasing viral replication to below the limits of detection, but instead to try to maintain the least pathogenic resistant variant. Some drug-resistant virus appears to be less "fit," or pathogenic, than the wild-type virus. Recently, methods to measure viral replication have become available; although these methods do not provide "fitness" information per se and are generally referred to as "relative replication assays" to emphasize this distinction. Several reviews of replication capacity have recently summarized these studies [113–116].

Replication assays are already currently available from one company (Virologic), as part of the routine phenotyping assay results. Relative replication capacity is reported as a percent of wild type, with 95% confidence intervals. At present, the utility of replication assays has not been demonstrated in controlled clinical trials.

21.6 Evidence base for the use of drug-resistance assays in clinical management of HIV infection

Several randomized, prospective studies have investigated the utility of resistance testing in the management of antiretroviral therapy [111, 117–120]. Details of the trial design are critical to interpreting the results of these studies, including disease stage and treatment experience of the enrolled patients, prior NNRTI experience, the type of resistance assay used (genotype or phenotype), the algorithm used to determine resistance from the genotype or phenotype, how the resistance testing information was utilized to guide treatment decisions (as recommendations or "expert" panel decisions), the duration of follow-up, and specific outcome measures. VIRADAPT [110] and GART [112] were two early prospective genotyping studies that randomized patients to two arms: genotyping and standard of care. Genotyping results were provided to clinicians with suggestions concerning the choice of antiretrovirals, but clinicians were not bound to follow the advice. GART patients with genotyping were prescribed significantly more antiretrovirals, and more hydroxyurea, although analyses suggested that the advantage of genotyping was present even after controlling for the administration of additional antiretrovirals. The benefit in both of these trials appeared to be the ability of genotyping to identify a greater number of active antiretrovirals.

VIRA3001 [120] was a randomized study comparing phenotyping with standard of care in 272 viremic patients. At week 16 the phenotyping arm demonstrated a greater effect on reducing HIV viremia measured by proportion of patients with HIV RNA concentrations <400 copies/mL. In the secondary analysis, phenotyping was also superior to standard of care in reducing viremia.

The benefit of "expert" advice was investigated in HAVANA [117], which examined the utility of genotyping and expert advice. Genotyping was superior to no genotyping, even in the absence of expert advice, using only an algorithm to interpret the genotype. In addition, expert advice was beneficial even in the absence of genotyping.

ARGENTA compared the efficacy of genotyping and standard of care in reducing viral loads [119]. Although the proportion of patients with viral loads < 500 copies/mL was significantly greater in the genotyping arm after 12 weeks, the effect was not sustained and no benefit of genotyping was detected at 24 weeks. The durability of clinical benefit from resistance testing beyond 1 year has not yet been studied prospectively. Many of the studies were performed prior to widespread use of ultra-sensitive assays capable of detecting viral loads down to 50 copies/mL, and used the reduction in viral load to < 400 copies/mL or < 500 copies/mL as the measure of success; it is not clear whether all successful treatments reached the more stringent measure of suppression.

Several trials have failed to demonstrate a clinical benefit from resistance testing. NARVAL, a randomized study comparing phenotyping, genotyping, and standard of care [118], showed no benefit of resistance testing in the entire cohort, but in a subanalysis, patients with limited prior antiretroviral experience including only a single PI did appear to benefit from resistance testing. Some studies may have failed to show a benefit due to resistance testing because some patients in these studies may have had such extensive prior experience with antiretroviral therapy, and had virus that was so resistant, that few would be expected to have an excellent response to a new therapy.

None of these studies specifically studied pediatric patients; a randomized trial of resistance testing in pediatric patients (PERA, PENTA-8) using genotyping has been initiated (www.ctu.mrc.ac.uk/penta/pera.htm).

21.7 Use of resistance testing in clinical practice

21.7.1 Guidelines for the use of resistance testing

Several sets of guidelines recommend the use of resistance testing in defined circumstances, including the DHHS/Kaiser Guidelines (www.aidsinfo.nih.gov), and the IAS and Euro Guidelines Group for HIV Resistance [121, 122]. Resistance testing has been recommended: in evaluation of patients following single or multiple regimen failures, and in primary HIV infection in geographic areas with high resistance. Resistance testing for newly diagnosed patients has been recommended or considered but cannot be considered standard of care; specific testing of pregnant women has been recommended by IAS but not by DHHS.

21.7.2 Pregnancy and maternal fetal transmission of drug-resistant HIV

Among the studies examining maternal–fetal transmission of drug-resistant HIV, two principal questions have emerged: what is the genetic relationship between virus infecting the mother and the infant, and whether drug-resistant mutations in the mother constitute a risk factor for maternal–infant transmission. In general maternal–fetal transmission results in infection with a subset of maternal HIV. In cases where maternal virus has detectable drug-resistance mutations, HIV in infected offspring may or may not contain the identical complement of resistance mutations identified in the mother [123–126]. Analyses of HIV from participants in the landmark HIVNET 012 study of single-dose nevirapine revealed the development of resistance mutations after single-dose therapy [127–129]. Several retrospective studies have investigated whether drug-resistance mutations are preferentially transmitted or excluded during maternal–fetal transmission, but no consensus has emerged. The presence of AZT-resistance mutations was a risk factor for maternal–infant transmission in a Women and Infants Transmission Study (WITS) independent of viral load [130]; in contrast, analysis of women followed in the Swiss HIV and Pregnancy Study revealed none of the few women with virus encoding T215Y/F mutation transmitted HIV to offspring [131].

HIV may be transmitted via breastfeeding [132] but factors facilitating transmission of wild-type or drug-resistant virus by this mode of transmission are poorly understood.

21.7.3 Resistance testing – practical considerations

Practitioners contemplating the use of resistance testing must choose among the available assays. Genotyping is less expensive, but genotyping and phenotyping may provide complementary information [133]. Resistance testing is a single aspect of the clinical evaluation of HIV-infected individuals, and can only supplement an accurate and comprehensive history. Graphs detailing drug history and adherence, viral load, and CD4$^+$ lymphocyte counts over time are extremely useful in understanding the results of any drug-resistance testing. Several points regarding interpretation of resistance testing in clinical settings bear enumerating:

- Genotyping results report the presence of drug-resistance mutations, sensitivity is inferred but not guaranteed.
- Phenotyping results may indicate sensitivity, but the utility of cutoffs has not been clinically determined for all antiretrovirals. Increases in IC$_{50}$ values of 1.8-fold or more have been associated with resistance.
- Phenotyping cutoffs for certain drugs have been adjusted (ddI, d4T) since the assays were introduced; results of phenotypic assays prior to adjustment may suggest drug sensitivity when resistance is present.
- A patient's virus may continue to evolve, particularly when treatment continues with high viral loads. Resistance results obtained at one time may not reflect the viral genotype or phenotype at subsequent times.
- Additional mutations may be present but not evident because the patient is not currently taking a particular drug at the time the test was performed. In a patient, resistance mutations may only be apparent when virus is subject to the selective pressure produced by the drug.
- As outlined above, mutations conferring resistance continue to accumulate as viremia persists in the presence of continued antiretroviral therapy to PIs, increasing the degree of resistance.
- The presence of mutations conferring resistance to NNRTIs generally precludes their use in any future regimen. High-level resistance resulting from K103N suggests there is little utility to continuing NNRTI therapy.
- The presence of Q151M complex or 69 insertion mutants results in high-level cross-resistance to NRTIs. Construction of salvage regimens should be adjusted accordingly, anticipating little or no antiviral contribution from NRTIs.
- The presence of M184V confers high-level resistance to lamivudine, but increases activity of AZT, d4T, and perhaps tenofovir in the presence of NAMs. Continued therapy with lamivudine maintains M184V and may help preserve some degree of activity in complex resistance profiles including NAMs. Lamivudine has a favorable toxicity and drug interaction profile; including this agent in salvage regimens carries little negative consequence and may provide a degree of indirect antiviral activity.
- Results of HIV drug-resistance tests represent one aspect of the evaluation of the patient with drug-resistant HIV. The successful construction of salvage regimens cannot be dictated simply by genotypes or phenotypes, but must include consideration of prior therapy, patient tolerability, etc. In a final analysis, the best drug regimens are those constructed in cooperation with the patient and the healthcare team.

21.7.4 Special considerations

Resistance in non B HIV-1 subtypes and in HIV-2
HIV-2

HIV-2 is a human immunodeficiency virus with a relatively restricted geographic distribution [134]. Cases of HIV-2 remain highest in West Africa, where the virus was originally described; spread to countries with traditional or colonial ties to West African countries have reported cases [134, 135]. Few cases of HIV-2 have been reported in the U.S.A., but HIV-1 and HIV-2 co-infections are possible, presenting certain therapeutic difficulties. Although NRTIs and PIs inhibit HIV-2 in vitro, NNRTIs, including efavirenz, do not. The first crystal structure of the HIV-2 RT was recently published with several significant differences in the NNRTI binding pocket noted [136], perhaps explaining the resistance of HIV-2 RT to NNRTIs. As therapy with NNRTIs is likely to be ineffective for HIV-2, it is important to evaluate the possibility of HIV-2 co-infection in HIV-1-infected patients originating from HIV-2 endemic areas undergoing therapy.

Evidence of drug resistance has recently been reported in HIV-2-infected individuals undergoing antiretroviral therapy. Several typical NRTI resistance mutations were noted; of concern, the Q151M complex was detected in numbers higher than observed in HIV-1 [137, 138]).

Non-B HIV-1 subtypes

HIV-1 is divided into a series of subtypes (see Chapter 2). Commercial genotyping and phenotyping assays were developed using subtype B HIV, the predominant strain circulating in North America and Western Europe. Several studies have addressed the subtype-specific differences in HIV. No substantial differences in therapeutic efficacy have been reported in HIV therapy in other subtypes, suggesting antiretroviral therapy is effective in non-B clades, although the numbers of patients in individual subtypes ware relatively small [139, 140]. Drug susceptibilities of non-B subtypes [141–143], including isolates from children [144], are reported to be similar to standard B strains.

21.7.5 Cross-resistance to antiviral agents for infections due to other viruses

Adefovir, tenofovir, and 3TC all inhibit hepatitis B virus; adefovir and 3TC are approved for therapy of hepatitis B infection. In certain circumstances, patients may be treated for hepatitis B, but not HIV. Clearly, the use of mono- or dual therapy for HBV in the absence of specific antiretroviral therapy for HIV will result in emergence of mutations in HIV, which may limit subsequent HIV therapy. It is possible that the lower dose of adefovir used to treat hepatitis B does not represent sufficient drug-selective pressure and does not result in emergence of new mutations in HIV, but clinical data are lacking. In a small study of 13 patients, no emergence of K655R or the NAM K70E in patients with persistent HIV viremia was apparent after 12 months of therapy with adefovir [145].

Future directions

Future directions in HIV resistance will include investigations of mechanisms of resistance to protease and reverse transcriptase, and delineation of resistance mechanisms to new antiviral agents, such as fusion inhibitors and integrase inhibitors. Resistance testing will continue to be refined as more sequences are analyzed. New antivirals will require extensive resistance analysis; it has been an all too common observation that all new antivirals are introduced with many attempts, but little success, at identifying mutations conferring resistance. It has been an equally common observation that high-level resistance is soon identified for all antiretrovirals. One indication of the potency of an antiretroviral agent is the presence and prevalence of resistance mutations to that agent in the population.

Understanding HIV replication capacity and hypersusceptibility may become useful in management of highly experienced patients. Resistance testing has been reported useful in relatively short-term studies, but the duration of response remains an issue, as does the role of resistance testing in highly experienced patients with few available drug options. The use of resistance information to predict therapeutic outcomes is currently in its infancy, although algorithms to predict viral load responses are under study [146]. Expansion of resistance-testing methods and algorithms to accurately detect resistance mutations in alternative HIV subtypes will be especially important as antiretroviral therapy is increasingly used in areas where non-B subtypes are prevalent.

REFERENCES

1. Van Houtte, M. Update on resistance testing. *J. HIV Ther.* **6**:**3** (2001), 61–4.
2. Geretti, A. M. & Easterbrook, P. Antiretroviral resistance in clinical practice. *Int. J. STD AIDS* **12**:**3** (2001), 145–53.
3. Hanna, G. J. & D'Aquila, R. T. Clinical use of genotypic and phenotypic drug resistance testing to monitor antiretroviral chemotherapy. *Clin. Infect. Dis.* **32**:**5** (2001), 774–82.
4. Rice, H. L. & Zolopa, A. R. HIV drug resistance testing: an update for the clinician. *AIDS Clin. Care* **13**:**10** (2001), 89–91, 94–6, 100.
5. Schmidt, B., Walter, H., Zeitler, N. & Korn, K. Genotypic drug resistance interpretation systems – the cutting edge of antiretroviral therapy. *AIDS Rev.* **4**:**3** (2002), 148–56.
6. Shafer, R. W. Genotypic testing for human immunodeficiency virus type 1 drug resistance. *Clin. Microbiol. Rev.* **15**:**2** (2002), 247–77.
7. Haubrich, R. & Demeter, L. International perspectives on antiretroviral resistance. Clinical utility of resistance testing: retrospective and prospective data supporting use and current recommendations. *J. AIDS* **26** (Suppl. 1) (2001), S51–9.
8. Lerma, J. G. & Heneine, W. Resistance of human immunodeficiency virus type 1 to reverse transcriptase and protease inhibitors: genotypic and phenotypic testing. *J. Clin. Virol.* **21**:**3** (2001), 197–212.
9. Ho, D. D., Neumann, A. U., Perelson, A. S., Chen, W., Leonard, J. M. & Markowitz, M. Rapid turnover of plasma virions and CD4 lymphocytes in HIV-1 infection. *Nature* **373**:**6510** (1995), 123–6.
10. Sato, H., Orenstein, J., Dimitrov, D. & Martin, M. Cell-to-cell spread of HIV-1 occurs within minutes and may not involve the participation of virus particles. *Virology* **186**:**2** (1992), 712–24.
11. Perelson, A. S., Essunger, P., Cao, Y. *et al.* Decay characteristics of HIV-1-infected compartments during combination therapy. *Nature* **387**:**6629** (1997), 188–91.
12. Mittler, J. E., Markowitz, M., Ho, D. D. & Perelson, A. S. Improved estimates for HIV-1 clearance rate and intracellular delay. *AIDS* **13**:**11** (1999), 1415–17.
13. O'Neil, P. K., Sun, G., Yu, H., Ron, Y., Dougherty, J. P. & Preston, B. D. Mutational analysis of HIV-1 long terminal repeats to explore the relative contribution of reverse transcriptase and RNA polymerase II to viral mutagenesis. *J. Biol. Chem.* **277**:**41** (2002), 38053–61.
14. Paoloni-Giacobino, A., Rossier, C., Papasavvas, M. P. & Antonarakis, S. E. Frequency of replication/transcription errors in (A)/(T) runs of human genes. *Hum. Genet.* **109**:**1** (2001), 40–7.
15. Mansky, L. M. & Temin, H. M. Lower in vivo mutation rate of human immunodeficiency virus type 1 than that predicted from the fidelity of purified reverse transcriptase. *J. Virol.* **69**:**8** (1995), 5087–94.
16. Vartanian, J. P., Sala, M., Henry, M., Wain-Hobson, S. & Meyerhans, A. Manganese cations increase the mutation rate of human immunodeficiency virus type 1 ex vivo. *J. Gen. Virol.* **80**:**8** (1999), 1983–6.
17. Coffin, J. M. HIV viral dynamics. *AIDS* **10** (Suppl. 3) (1996), S75–84.
18. Hu, W. S., Rhodes, T., Dang, Q. & Pathak, V. Retroviral recombination: review of genetic analyses. *Front Biosci.* **8** (2003), D143–55.
19. Gomez Carrillo, M., Avila, M. & Hierholzer, J. *et al.* Mother-to-child HIV type 1 transmission in Argentina: BF recombinants

have predominated in infected children since the mid-1980s. *AIDS Res. Hum. Retrovirus.* **18** : **7** (2002), 477–83.

20. McCutchan, F. E. Understanding the genetic diversity of HIV-1. *AIDS* **14** (Suppl. 3) (2000), S31–44.

21. Kellam, P. & Larder, B. A. Retroviral recombination can lead to linkage of reverse transcriptase mutations that confer increased zidovudine resistance. *J. Virol.* **69** : **2** (1995), 669–74.

22. Morris, A., Marsden, M., Halcrow, K. *et al.* Mosaic structure of the human immunodeficiency virus type 1 genome infecting lymphoid cells and the brain: evidence for frequent in vivo recombination events in the evolution of regional populations. *J. Virol.* **73** : **10** (1999), 8720–31.

23. Diaz, R. S., Sabino, E. C., Mayer, A., Mosley, J. W. & Busch, M. P. Dual human immunodeficiency virus type 1 infection and recombination in a dually exposed transfusion recipient. The Transfusion Safety Study Group. *J. Virol.* **69** : **6** (1995), 3273–81.

24. Wooley, D. P., Smith, R. A., Czajak, S. & Desrosiers, R. C. Direct demonstration of retroviral recombination in a rhesus monkey. *J. Virol.* **71** : **12** (1997), 9650–3.

25. Iglesias-Sanchez, M. J., López, G. & Galíndez, C. Analysis, quantification, and evolutionary consequences of HIV-1 in vitro recombination. *Virology* **304** : **2** (2002), 392–402.

26. Reinhart, T. A., Rogan, M. J., Viglianti, G. A., Rausch, D. M., Eiden, L. E. & Haase, A. T. A new approach to investigating the relationship between productive infection and cytopathicity in vivo. *Nat. Med.* **3** : **2** (1997), 218–21.

27. Orenstein, J. M., Feinberg, M., Yoder, C. *et al.* Lymph node architecture preceding and following 6 months of potent antiviral therapy: follicular hyperplasia persists in parallel with p24 antigen restoration after involution and CD4 cell depletion in an AIDS patient. *AIDS* **13** : **16** (1999), 2219–29.

28. Orenstein, J. M., Bhat, N., Yoder, C. *et al.* Rapid activation of lymph nodes and mononuclear cell HIV expression upon interrupting highly active antiretroviral therapy in patients after prolonged viral suppression. *AIDS* **14** : **12** (2000), 1709–15.

29. Dyrhol-Riise, A. M., Voltersvik, P., Berg, O. G., Olofsson, J., Kleivbo, S. & Asjo, B. Residual human immunodeficiency virus type 1 infection in lymphoid tissue during highly active antiretroviral therapy: quantitation and virus characterization. *AIDS Res. Hum. Retrovirus.* **17** : **7** (2001), 577–86.

30. Lafeuillade, A., Khiri, H., Chadapaud, S., Hittinger, G. & Halfon, P. Persistence of HIV-1 resistance in lymph node mononuclear cell RNA despite effective HAART. *AIDS* **15** : **15** (2001), 1965–9.

31. Persaud, D., Pierson, T., Ruff, C. *et al.* A stable latent reservoir for HIV-1 in resting CD4(+) T lymphocytes in infected children. *J. Clin. Invest.* **105** : **7** (2000), 995–1003.

32. Hermankova, M., Ray, S. C., Ruff, C. *et al.* HIV-1 drug resistance profiles in children and adults with viral load of <50 copies/ml receiving combination therapy. *J. Am. Med. Assoc.* **286** : **2** (2001), 196–207.

33. Ruff, C. T., Ray, S. C., Kwon, P. *et al.* Persistence of wild-type virus and lack of temporal structure in the latent reservoir for

human immunodeficiency virus type 1 in pediatric patients with extensive antiretroviral exposure. *J. Virol.* **76** : **18** (2002), 9481–92.

34. Lacey, S. F. & Larder, B. A. Novel mutation (V75T) in human immunodeficiency virus type 1 reverse transcriptase confers resistance to 2′,3′-didehydro-2′,3′-dideoxythymidine in cell culture. *Antimicrob. Agents Chemother.* **38** : **6** (1994), 1428–32.

35. Winters, M. A., Shafer, R. W., Jellinger, R. A., Mamtora, G., Gingeras, T. & Merigan, T. C. Human immunodeficiency virus type 1 reverse transcriptase genotype and drug susceptibility changes in infected individuals receiving dideoxyinosine monotherapy for 1 to 2 years. *Antimicrob. Agents Chemother.* **41** : **4** (1997), 757–62.

36. Larder, B. A., Bloor, S., Kemp, S. D. *et al.* A family of insertion mutations between codons 67 and 70 of human immunodeficiency virus type 1 reverse transcriptase confer multinucleoside analog resistance. *Antimicrob. Agents Chemother.* **43** : **8** (1999), 1961–7.

37. Lobato, R. L., Kim, E. Y., Kagan, R. M. & Merigan, T. C. Genotypic and phenotypic analysis of a novel 15-base insertion occurring between codons 69 and 70 of HIV type 1 reverse transcriptase. *AIDS Res. Hum. Retrovirus.* **18** : **10** (2002), 733–6.

38. Lennerstrand, J., Stammers, D. K. & Larder, B. A. Biochemical mechanism of human immunodeficiency virus type 1 reverse transcriptase resistance to stavudine. *Antimicrob. Agents Chemother.* **45** : **7** (2001), 2144–6.

39. Mas, A., Parera, M., Briones, C. *et al.* Role of a dipeptide insertion between codons 69 and 70 of HIV-1 reverse transcriptase in the mechanism of AZT resistance. *EMBO J.* **19** : **21** (2000), 5752–61.

40. Boyer, P. L., Sarafianos, S. G., Arnold, E. & Hughes, S. H. Nucleoside analog resistance caused by insertions in the fingers of human immunodeficiency virus type 1 reverse transcriptase involves ATP-mediated excision. *J. Virol.* **76** : **18** (2002), 9143–51.

41. Ross, L., Johnson, M., Ferris, R. G. *et al.* Deletions in the beta3-beta4 hairpin loop of HIV-1 reverse transcriptase are observed in HIV-1 isolated from subjects during long-term antiretroviral therapy. *J. Hum. Virol.* **3** : **3** (2000), 144–9.

42. Suzuki, K., Kaufmann, G. R., Mukaide, M. *et al.* Novel deletion of HIV type 1 reverse transcriptase residue 69 conferring selective high-level resistance to nevirapine. *AIDS Res. Hum. Retrovirus.* **17** : **13** (2001), 1293–6.

43. Rey, D., Hughes, M., Pi, J. T., Winters, M., Merigan, T. C. & Katzenstein, D. A. HIV-1 reverse transcriptase codon 215 mutation in plasma RNA: immunologic and virologic responses to zidovudine. The AIDS Clinical Trials Group Study 175 Virology Team. *J. AIDS Hum. Retrovirol.* **17** : **3** (1998), 203–8.

44. Principi, N., Marchisio, P., De Pasquale M. P., Massironi, E., Tornaghi, R. & Vago, T. HIV-1 reverse transcriptase codon 215 mutation and clinical outcome in children treated with zidovudine. *AIDS Res. Hum. Retrovirus.* **10** : **6** (1994), 721–6.

45. Mellado, M. J., Cilleruelo, M. J., Ortiz, M. & *et al.* Viral phenotype, antiretroviral resistance and clinical evolution in human

immunodeficiency virus-infected children. *Pediatr. Infect Dis. J.* **16** : **11** (1997), 1032–7.

46. Gao, H. Q., Boyer, P. L., Sarafianos, S. G., Arnold, E. & Hughes, S. H. The role of steric hindrance in 3TC resistance of human immunodeficiency virus type-1 reverse transcriptase. *J. Mol. Biol.* **300** : **2** (2000), 403–18.

47. Sarafianos, S. G., Das, K., Clark, A. D., Jr. *et al.* Lamivudine (3TC) resistance in HIV-1 reverse transcriptase involves steric hindrance with beta-branched amino acids. *Proc. Natl. Acad. Sci. U.S.A.* **96** : **18** (1999), 10027–32.

48. Frost, S. D., Nijhuis, M., Schuurman, R., Boucher, C. A. & Brown, A. J. Evolution of lamivudine resistance in human immuno-deficiency virus type 1-infected individuals: the relative roles of drift and selection. *J. Virol.* **74** : **14** (2000), 6262–8.

49. Huang, H., Chopra, R., Verdine, G. L. & Harrison, S. C. Structure of a covalently trapped catalytic complex of HIV-1 reverse transcriptase: implications for drug resistance. *Science* **282** : **5394** (1998), 1669–75.

50. Sluis-Cremer N., Arion, D., Kaushik, N., Lim, H. & Parniak, M. A. Mutational analysis of Lys65 of HIV-1 reverse transcriptase. *Biochem. J.* **348** : **1** (2000), 77–82.

51. Winston, A., Mandalia, S., Pillay, D., Gazzard, B. & Pozniak, A. The prevalence and determinants of the K65R mutation in HIV-1 reverse transcriptase in tenofovir-naive patients. *AIDS* **16** : **15** (2002), 2087–9.

52. Bazmi, H. Z., Hammond, J. L., Cavalcanti, S. C., Chu, C. K., Schinazi, R. F. & Mellors, J. W. In vitro selection of mutations in the human immunodeficiency virus type 1 reverse transcriptase that decrease susceptibility to (-)-beta- D-dioxolane-guanosine and suppress resistance to 3′-azido-3′-deoxythymidine. *Antimicrob. Agents Chemother.* **44** : **7** (2000), 1783–8.

53. Ray, A. S., Basavapathruni, A. & Anderson, K. S. Mechanistic studies to understand the progressive development of resistance in human immunodeficiency virus type 1 reverse transcriptase to abacavir. *J. Biol. Chem.* **277** : **43** (2002), 40479–90.

54. Schmit, J. C., Ruiz, L., Stuyver, L. *et al.* Comparison of the LiPA HIV-1 RT test, selective PCR and direct solid phase sequencing for the detection of HIV-1 drug resistance mutations. *J. Virol. Methods* **73** : **1** (1998), 77–82.

55. Hsiou, Y., Ding, J., Das, K. *et al.* The Lys103Asn mutation of HIV-1 RT: a novel mechanism of drug resistance. *J. Mol. Biol.* **309** : **2** (2001), 437–45.

56. Casado, J. L., Moreno, A., Hertogs, K., Dronda, F. & Moreno, S. Extent and importance of cross-resistance to efavirenz after nevirapine failure. *AIDS Res. Hum. Retrovirus.* **18** : **11** (2002), 771–5.

57. Antinori, A., Zaccarelli, M., Cingolani, A. *et al.* Cross-resistance among nonnucleoside reverse transcriptase inhibitors limits recycling efavirenz after nevirapine failure. *AIDS Res. Hum. Retrovirus.* **18** : **12** (2002), 835–8.

58. Mellors, J., Vaida, F., Bennett, K., Hellmann, N. S., DeGruttola, V. & Hammer, S. for the ACTG 398 Study Team. Efavirenz hypersusceptibility improves virologic response to multidrug salvage regimens in ACTG 398. In *9th Conference on Retroviruses and Opportunistic Infections* (2002), Abstract 45.

59. Swanstrom, R. & Erona, J. Human immunodeficiency virus type-1 protease inhibitors: therapeutic successes and failures, suppression and resistance. *Pharmacol. Ther.* **86** : **2** (2000), 145–70.

60. Scott, W. R. & Schiffer, C. A. Curling of flap tips in HIV-1 protease as a mechanism for substrate entry and tolerance of drug resistance. *Structure Fold Des.* **8** : **12** (2000), 1259–65.

61. Prabu-Jeyabalan, M., Nalivaika, E. & Schiffer, C. A. Substrate shape determines specificity of recognition for HIV-1 protease: analysis of crystal structures of six substrate complexes. *Structure (Camb)* **10** : **3** (2002), 369–81.

62. Shao, W., Everitt, L., Manchester, M., Loeb, D. D. Hutchison, C. A., 3rd & Swanstrom, R. Sequence requirements of the HIV-1 protease flap region determined by saturation mutagenesis and kinetic analysis of flap mutants. *Proc. Natl. Acad. Sci. U.S.A.* **94** : **6** (1997), 2243–8.

63. Mahalingam, B., Louis, J. M., Reed, C. C. *et al.* Structural and kinetic analysis of drug resistant mutants of HIV-1 protease. *Eur. J. Biochem.* **263** : **1** (1999), 238–45.

64. Hertogs, K., Bloor, S., Kemp, S. D. *et al.* Phenotypic and geno-typic analysis of clinical HIV-1 isolates reveals extensive pro-tease inhibitor cross-resistance: a survey of over 6000 samples. *AIDS* **14** : **9** (2000), 1203–10.

65. Shafer, R. W., Winters, M. A., Palmer, S. & Merigan, T. C. Multiple concurrent reverse transcriptase and protease mutations and multidrug resistance of HIV-1 isolates from heavily treated patients. *Ann. Intern. Med.* **128** : **11** (1998), 906–11.

66. Harrigan, P. R. & Larder, B. A. Extent of cross-resistance between agents used to treat human immunodeficiency virus type 1 infection in clinically derived isolates. *Antimicrob. Agents Chemother.* **46** : **3** (2002), 909–12.

67. Kempf, D. J., Isaacson, J. D., King, M. S. *et al.* Identification of genotypic changes in human immunodeficiency virus pro-tease that correlate with reduced susceptibility to the pro-tease inhibitor lopinavir among viral isolates from protease inhibitor-experienced patients. *J. Virol.* **75** : **16** (2001), 7462–9.

68. Kemper, C. A., Witt, M. D., Keiser, P. H. *et al.* Sequencing of protease inhibitor therapy: insights from an analysis of HIV phenotypic resistance in patients failing protease inhibitors. *AIDS* **15** : **5** (2001), 609–15.

69. Markland, W., Rao, B. G., Parsons, J. D. *et al.* Structural and kinetic analyses of the protease from an amprenavir-resistant human immunodeficiency virus type 1 mutant rendered resistant to saquinavir and resensitized to amprenavir. *J. Virol.* **74** : **16** (2000), 7636–41.

70. Tisdale, M., Myers, R. E., Maschera, B., Parry, N. R., Oliver, N. M. & Blair, E. D. Cross-resistance analysis of human immuno-deficiency virus type 1 variants individually selected for resis-tance to five different protease inhibitors. *Antimicrob. Agents Chemother.* **39** : **8** (1995), 1704–10.

71. Kovari, L. C., Vickery, J. F., Logsdon, B., Proteasa, G., Winters, M. & Winters, T. C. Expansion of the HIV-1 protease active site correlates with clinical progression to multidrug resistance. In

XXI International HIV Drug Resistance Workshop: Basic Principles and Clinical Implications, Seville, Spain (2002).

72. Servais, J., Hainaut, M., Schmitz, V. *et al*. Resistance testing in children changing human immunodeficiency virus type 1 protease inhibitor. *Pediatr. Infect. Dis. J.* **21** : **3** (2002), 214–20.

73. Mahalingam, B., Louis, J. M., Hung, J., Harrison, R. W. & Weber, I. T. Structural implications of drug-resistant mutants of HIV-1 protease: high-resolution crystal structures of the mutant protease/substrate analogue complexes. *Proteins* **43** : **4** (2001), 455–64.

74. Robinson, L. H., Myers, R. E., Snowden, B. W., Tisdale, M. & Blair, E. D. HIV type 1 protease cleavage site mutations and viral fitness: implications for drug susceptibility phenotyping assays. *AIDS Res. Hum. Retrovirus.* **16** : **12** (2000), 1149–56.

75. Doyon, L., Croteau, G., Thibeault, D., Poulin, F., Pilote, L. & Lamarre, D. Second locus involved in human immunodeficiency virus type 1 resistance to protease inhibitors. *J. Virol.* **70** : **6** (1996), 3763–9.

76. Croteau, G., Doyon, L., Thibeault, D., McKercher, G., Pilote, L. & Lamarre, D. Impaired fitness of human immunodeficiency virus type 1 variants with high-level resistance to protease inhibitors. *J. Virol.* **71** : **2** (1997), 1089–96.

77. Zhang, Y. M., Imamichi, H., Imamichi, T. *et al*. Drug resistance during indinavir therapy is caused by mutations in the protease gene and in its Gag substrate cleavage sites. *J. Virol.* **71** : **9** (1997), 6662–70.

78. Bally, F., Martinez, R., Peters, S., Sudre, P. & Telenti, A. Polymorphism of HIV type 1 gag p7/p1 and p1/p6 cleavage sites: clinical significance and implications for resistance to protease inhibitors. *AIDS Res. Hum. Retrovirus.* **16** : **13** (2000), 1209–13.

79. Maguire, M. F., Guinea, R., Griffin, P. *et al*. Changes in human immunodeficiency virus type 1 Gag at positions L449 and P453 are linked to I50V protease mutants in vivo and cause reduction of sensitivity to amprenavir and improved viral fitness in vitro. *J. Virol.* **76** : **15** (2002), 7398–406.

80. Kilby, J. M., Lalezari, J. P., Eron, J. J. *et al*. The safety, plasma pharmacokinetics, and antiviral activity of subcutaneous enfuvirtide (T-20), a peptide inhibitor of gp41-mediated virus fusion, in HIV-infected adults. *AIDS Res. Hum. Retrovirus.* **18** : **10** (2002), 685–93.

81. Starr-Spires, L. D. & Collman, R. G. HIV-1 entry and entry inhibitors as therapeutic agents. *Clin. Lab. Med.* **22** : **3** (2002), 681–701.

82. Wei, X., Decker, J. M., Liu, H. *et al*. Emergence of resistant human immunodeficiency virus type 1 in patients receiving fusion inhibitor (T-20) monotherapy. *Antimicrob. Agents Chemother.* **46** : **6** (2002), 1896–905.

83. Boucher, C. A., van Leeuwen, R., Kellam, P. *et al*. Effects of discontinuation of zidovudine treatment on zidovudine sensitivity of human immunodeficiency virus type 1 isolates. *Antimicrob. Agents Chemother.* **37** : **7** (1993), 1525–30.

84. Tachedjian, G., Mellors, J., Bazmi, H., Birch, C. & Mills, J. Zidovudine resistance is suppressed by mutations conferring resistance of human immunodeficiency virus type 1 to foscarnet. *J. Virol.* **70** : **10** (1996), 7171–81.

85. Larder, B. A. 3'-Azido-3'-deoxythymidine resistance suppressed by a mutation conferring human immunodeficiency virus type 1 resistance to nonnucleoside reverse transcriptase inhibitors. *Antimicrob. Agents Chemother.* **36** : **12** (1992), 2664–9.

86. St Clair, M. H., Martin, J. L., Tudor-Williams, G. *et al*. Resistance to ddI and sensitivity to AZT induced by a mutation in HIV-1 reverse transcriptase. *Science* **253** : **5027** (1991), 1557–9.

87. Ziermann, R., Limoli, K., Das, K., Arnold, E., Petropoulos, C. J. & Parkin, N. T. A mutation in human immunodeficiency virus type 1 protease, N88S, that causes in vitro hypersensitivity to amprenavir. *J. Virol.* **74** : **9** (2000), 4414–9.

88. Haubrich, R. H., Kemper, C. A., Hellmann, N. S. *et al*. The clinical relevance of non-nucleoside reverse transcriptase inhibitor hypersusceptibility: a prospective cohort analysis. *AIDS* **16** : **15** (2002), F33–40.

89. Cunningham, S., Ank, B., Lewis, D. *et al*. Performance of the applied biosystems ViroSeq human immunodeficiency virus type 1 (HIV-1) genotyping system for sequence-based analysis of HIV-1 in pediatric plasma samples. *J. Clin. Microbiol.* **39** : **4** (2001), 1254–7.

90. Sturmer, M., Morgenstern, B., Staszewski, S. & Doerr, H. W. Evaluation of the LiPA HIV-1 RT assay version 1: comparison of sequence and hybridization based genotyping systems. *J. Clin. Virol.* **25** (Suppl. 3) (2002), 65–72.

91. Reinis, M., Vandasova, J., Stankova, M., Linka, M. & Bruckova, M. Human immunodeficiency virus 1 strains resistant to nucleoside inhibitors of reverse transcriptase in isolates from the Czech Republic as monitored by line probe assay and nucleotide sequencing. *Acta Virol.* **45** : **5–6** (2001), 279–86.

92. Shi, C. & Mellors, J. W. A recombinant retroviral system for rapid in vivo analysis of human immunodeficiency virus type 1 susceptibility to reverse transcriptase inhibitors. *Antimicrob. Agents Chemother.* **41** : **12** (1997), 2781–5.

93. Martinez-Picado, J., Sutton, L., De Pasquale, M. P., Savara, A. V. & D'Aquila, R. T. Human immunodeficiency virus type 1 cloning vectors for antiretroviral resistance testing. *J. Clin. Microbiol.* **37** : **9** (1999), 2943–51.

94. Race, E., Dam, E., Obry, V., Paulous, S. & Clavel, F. Analysis of HIV cross-resistance to protease inhibitors using a rapid single-cycle recombinant virus assay for patients failing on combination therapies. *AIDS* **13** : **15** (1999), 2061–8.

95. Walter, H., Schmidt, B., Korn, K., Vandamme, A. M., Harrer, T. & Uberla, K. Rapid, phenotypic HIV-1 drug sensitivity assay for protease and reverse transcriptase inhibitors. *J. Clin. Virol.* **13** : **1–2** (1999), 71–80.

96. Hertogs, K., de Bethune, M. P., Miller, V. *et al*. A rapid method for simultaneous detection of phenotypic resistance to inhibitors of protease and reverse transcriptase in recombinant human immunodeficiency virus type 1 isolates from patients treated with antiretroviral drugs. *Antimicrob. Agents Chemother.* **42** : **2** (1998), 269–76.

97. Petropoulos, C. J., Parkin, N. T., Limoli, K. L., *et al*. A novel phenotypic drug susceptibility assay for human

immunodeficiency virus type 1. *Antimicrob. Agents Chemother.* **44**:**4** (2000), 920–8.

98. Kellam, P. & Larder, B. A. Recombinant virus assay: a rapid, phenotypic assay for assessment of drug susceptibility of human immunodeficiency virus type 1 isolates. *Antimicrob. Agents. Chemother.* **38**:**1** (1994), 23–30.

99. Debiaggi, M., Bruno, R., Sacchi, P., Achilli, G., Romero, E. & Filice, G. Distinct mutational drug resistance profiles of HIV-1 RNA in plasma and culture isolates of patients receiving antiretroviral therapy. *Intervirology* **45**:**1** (2002), 52–5.

100. Qari, S. H., Respess, R., Weinstock, H. *et al.* Comparative analysis of two commercial phenotypic assays for drug susceptibility testing of human immunodeficiency virus type 1. *J. Clin. Microbiol.* **40**:**1** (2002), 31–5.

101. Falloon, J., Ait-Khaled, M., Thomas, D. A. *et al.* HIV-1 genotype and phenotype correlate with virological response to abacavir, amprenavir and efavirenz in treatment-experienced patients. *AIDS* **16**:**3** (2002), 387–96.

102. Kempf, D. J., Isaacson, J. D., King, M. S. *et al.* Analysis of the virological response with respect to baseline viral phenotype and genotype in protease inhibitor-experienced HIV-1-infected patients receiving lopinavir/ritonavir therapy. *Antivir. Ther.* **7**:**3** (2002), 165–74.

103. Calvez, V., Costagliola, D., Descamps, D. *et al.* Impact of stavudine phenotype and thymidine analogues mutations on viral response to stavudine plus lamivudine in ALTIS 2 ANRS trial. *Antivir. Ther.* **7**:**3** (2002), 211–18.

104. Shulman, N. S., Hughes, M. D., Winters, M. A. *et al.* Subtle decreases in stavudine phenotypic susceptibility predict poor virologic response to stavudine monotherapy in zidovudine-experienced patients. *J. AIDS* **31**:**2** (2002), 121–7.

105. Harrigan, P. R., Montaner, J. S., Wegner, S. A. *et al.* World-wide variation in HIV-1 phenotypic susceptibility in untreated individuals: biologically relevant values for resistance testing. *AIDS* **15**:**13** (2001), 1671–7.

106. Rhee, S. Y., Gonzales, M. J., Kantor, R., Betts, B. J., Ravela, J. & Shafer, R. W. Human immunodeficiency virus reverse transcriptase and protease sequence database. *Nucleic. Acids Res.* **31**:**1** (2003), 298–303.

107. Petropoulos, C. 15,000 viruses can't be wrong: a clearer picture of HIV drug resistance. In *Third Annual HIV DRP Symposium Antiviral Drug Resistance* (2002).

108. Dunne, A. L., Mitchell, F. M., Coberly, S. K. *et al.* Comparison of genotyping and phenotyping methods for determining susceptibility of HIV-1 to antiretroviral drugs. *AIDS* **15**:**12** (2001), 1471–5.

109. Beerenwinkel, N., Schmidt, B., Walter, H. *et al.* Diversity and complexity of HIV-1 drug resistance: a bioinformatics approach to predicting phenotype from genotype. *Proc. Natl. Acad. Sci. U.S.A.* **99**:**12** (2002), 8271–6.

110. Durant, J., Clevenbergh, P., Garraffo, R. *et al.* Importance of protease inhibitor plasma levels in HIV-infected patients treated with genotypic-guided therapy: pharmacological data from the Viradapt Study. *AIDS* **14**:**10** (2000), 1333–9.

111. Durant, J., Clevenbergh, P., Halgon, P. *et al.* Drug-resistance genotyping in HIV-1 therapy: the VIRADAPT randomised controlled trial. *Lancet* **353**:**9171** (1999), 2195–9.

112. Baxter, J. D., Merigan, T. C., Wentworth, D. N. *et al.* Both baseline HIV-1 drug resistance and antiretroviral drug levels are associated with short-term virologic responses to salvage therapy. *AIDS* **16**:**8** (2002), 1131–8.

113. Nijhuis, M., Deeks, S. & Boucher, C. Implications of antiretroviral resistance on viral fitness. *Curr. Opin. Infect. Dis.* **14**:**1** (2001), 23–8.

114. Clavel, F., Race, E. & Mammano, F. HIV drug resistance and viral fitness. *Adv. Pharmacol.* **49** (2000), 41–66.

115. Quiñones-Mateu, M. A. & Arts, E. J. HIV-1 Fitness: implications for drug resistance, disease progression, and global epidemic evolution. In *HIV-1 Sequence Compendium 2001*. Los Alamos, NM: Theoretical Biology and Biophysics Group, Los Alamos National Laboratory (2001).

116. Maldarelli, F. HIV-1 fitness and replication capacity – what are they and can they help in patient management. *Curr. Infect. Dis. Rep.* **5**:**1** (2003), 77–84.

117. Tural, C., Ruiz, L., Holtzer, C. *et al.* Clinical utility of HIV-1 genotyping and expert advice: the Havana trial. *AIDS* **16**:**2** (2002), 209–18.

118. Meynard, J. L., Vray, M., Morand-Joubert, L. *et al.* Phenotypic or genotypic resistance testing for choosing antiretroviral therapy after treatment failure: a randomized trial. *AIDS* **16**:**5** (2002), 727–36.

119. Cingolani, A., Antinori, A., Rizzo, M. G. *et al.* Usefulness of monitoring HIV drug resistance and adherence in individuals failing highly active antiretroviral therapy: a randomized study (ARGENTA). *AIDS* **16**:**3** (2002), 369–79.

120. Cohen, C. J., Hunt, S., Sension, M. *et al.* A randomized trial assessing the impact of phenotypic resistance testing on antiretroviral therapy. *AIDS* **16**:**4** (2002), 579–88.

121. Vandamme, A. M., Houyez, F., Banhegyi, D. *et al.* Laboratory guidelines for the practical use of HIV drug resistance tests in patient follow-up. *Antivir. Ther.* **6**:**1** (2001), 21–39.

122. Hirsch, M. S., Brun-Vezinet, F., D'Aquila, R. T. *et al.* Antiretroviral drug resistance testing in adult HIV-1 infection: recommendations of an International AIDS Society-USA Panel. *J. Am. Med. Assoc.* **283**:**18** (2000), 2417–26.

123. Palumbo, P., Holland, B., Dobbs, T. *et al.* Antiretroviral resistance mutations among pregnant human immunodeficiency virus type 1-infected women and their newborns in the United States: vertical transmission and clades. *J. Infect. Dis.* **184**:**9** (2001), 1120–6.

124. Johnson, V. A., Petropoulos, C. J., Woods, C. R. *et al.* Vertical transmission of multidrug-resistant human immunodeficiency virus type 1 (HIV-1) and continued evolution of drug resistance in an HIV-1-infected infant. *J. Infect. Dis.* **183**:**11** (2001), 1688–93.

125. Clarke, J. R., Braganza, R., Mirza, A. *et al.* Rapid development of genotypic resistance to lamivudine when combined with zidovudine in pregnancy. *J. Med. Virol.* **59**:**3** (1999), 364–8.

126. Niehues, T., Walter, H., Homeff, G., Wahn, V. & Schmidt, B. Selective vertical transmission of HIV: lamivudine-resistant maternal clone undetectable by conventional resistance testing. *AIDS* **13 : 17** (1999), 2482–4.

127. Eshleman, S. H., Mracna, M., Guay, L. A. *et al.* Selection and fading of resistance mutations in women and infants receiving nevirapine to prevent HIV-1 vertical transmission (HIVNET 012). *AIDS* **15 : 15** (2001), 1951–7.

128. Eshleman, S. H. & Jackson, J. B. Nevirapine resistance after single dose prophylaxis. *AIDS Rev.* **4 : 2** (2002), 59–63.

129. Jackson, J. B., Becker-Pergola, G., Guay, L. A. *et al.* Identification of the K103N resistance mutation in Ugandan women receiving nevirapine to prevent HIV-1 vertical transmission. *AIDS* **14 : 11** (2000), F111–15.

130. Welles, S. L., Pitt, J., Colgrove, R. *et al.* HIV-1 genotypic zidovudine drug resistance and the risk of maternal–infant transmission in the women and infants transmission study. The Women and Infants Transmission Study Group. *AIDS* **14 : 3** (2000), 263–71.

131. Kully, C., Yerly, S., Erb, P. *et al.* Codon 215 mutations in human immunodeficiency virus-infected pregnant women. Swiss Collaborative 'HIV and Pregnancy' Study. *J. Infect. Dis.* **179 : 3** (1999), 705–8.

132. Coutsoudis, A., Kuhn, L., Pillay, K. & Coovadia, H. M. Exclusive breast-feeding and HIV transmission. *AIDS* **16 : 3** (2002), 498–9.

133. Parkin, N., Chappey, C., Maroldo, L., Bates, M., Hellmann, N. S. & Petropoulos, C. J. Phenotypic and genotypic HIV-1 drug resistance assays provide complementary information. *J. AIDS* **31 : 2** (2002), 128–36.

134. Clavel, F. HIV-2, the West African AIDS virus. *AIDS* **1 : 3** (1987), 135–40.

135. Toro, C., Soriano, V., Tuset, C. *et al.* Infection with retroviruses other than HIV-1 in Spain: a retrospective analysis for HIV-2, HTLV-I, and/or HTLV-II. *HIV Clin. Trials* **3 : 5** (2002), 397–402.

136. Ren, J., Bird, L. E., Chamberlain, P. P., Stewart-Jones, G. B., Stuart, D. I. & Stammers, D. K. Structure of HIV-2 reverse transcriptase at 2.35-A resolution and the mechanism of resistance to non-nucleoside inhibitors. *Proc. Natl. Acad. Sci. U.S.A.* **99 : 22** (2002), 14410–15.

137. Rodes, B., Holguin, A., Soriano, V. *et al.* Emergence of drug resistance mutations in human immunodeficiency virus type 2-infected subjects undergoing antiretroviral therapy. *J. Clin. Microbiol.* **38 : 4** (2000), 1370–4.

138. van der Ende, M. E., Guillon, C., Boers, P. H. *et al.* Antiviral resistance of biologic HIV-2 clones obtained from individuals on nucleoside reverse transcriptase inhibitor therapy. *J. AIDS* **25 : 1** (2000), 11–18.

139. Pillay, D., Walker, A. S., Gibb, D. M. *et al.* Impact of human immunodeficiency virus type 1 subtypes on virologic response and emergence of drug resistance among children in the Paediatric European Network for Treatment of AIDS (PENTA) 5 trial. *J. Infect. Dis.* **186 : 5** (2002), 617–25.

140. Frater, A. J., Beardall, A., Ariyoshi, K. *et al.* Impact of baseline polymorphisms in RT and protease on outcome of highly active antiretroviral therapy in HIV-1-infected African patients. *AIDS* **15 : 12** (2001), 1493–502.

141. Palmer, S., Alaeus, A., Albert, J. & Cox, S. Drug susceptibility of subtypes A, B, C, D, and E human immunodeficiency virus type 1 primary isolates. *AIDS Res. Hum. Retrovirus.* **14 : 2** (1998), 157–62.

142. Caride, E., Brindeiro, R., Hertogs, K. *et al.* Drug-resistant reverse transcriptase genotyping and phenotyping of B and non-B subtypes (F and A) of human immunodeficiency virus type I found in Brazilian patients failing HAART. *Virology* **275 : 1** (2000), 107–15.

143. Weidle, P. J., Kityo, C. M., Mugyenyi, P. *et al.* Resistance to antiretroviral therapy among patients in Uganda. *J. AIDS* **26 : 5** (2001), 495–500.

144. Brindeiro, P. A., Brindeiro, R. M., Mortensen, C. *et al.* Testing genotypic and phenotypic resistance in human immunodeficiency virus type 1 isolates of clade B and other clades from children failing antiretroviral therapy. *J Clin. Microbiol.* **40 : 12** (2002), 4512–19.

145. Delaugerre, C., Marcelin, A. G., Thibault, V. *et al.* Human immunodeficiency virus (HIV) Type 1 reverse transcriptase resistance mutations in hepatitis B virus (HBV)-HIV-coinfected patients treated for HBV chronic infection once daily with 10 milligrams of adefovir dipivoxil combined with lamivudine. *Antimicrob. Agents Chemother.* **46 : 5** (2002), 1586–8.

146. Foulkes, A. S. & De, G. V. Characterizing the relationship between HIV-1 genotype and phenotype: prediction-based classification. *Biometrics* **58 : 1** (2002), 145–56.

147. Ding, J., Das, K., Hsiou, Y. *et al.* Structure and functional implications of the polymerase active site region in a complex of HIV-1 RT with a double-stranded DNA template-primer and an antibody Fab fragment at 2.8 A resolution. *J. Mol. Biol.* **284 : 4** (1998), 1095–111.

Initiating and changing antiretroviral therapy

Lynne M. Mofenson, M.D.[1] and Leslie K. Serchuck, M.D.[2]

[1]Chief, Pediatric, Adolescent and Maternal AIDS Branch, Center for Research for Mothers and Children, NIH, Rockville, MD
[2]Medical Officer, Pediatric, Adolescent and Maternal AIDS Branch, Center for Research for Mothers and Children, NIH Rockville, MD

22.1 Introduction

Guidelines for antiretroviral therapy in children must incorporate considerations unique to pediatric HIV infection. Such considerations include: age-related changes in drug pharmacokinetics; issues related to diagnosis of perinatal infection (early diagnosis permits therapy to be initiated during primary HIV infection); normal age-related changes in immunologic parameters; differences between children and adults in the natural history of HIV infection (i.e. differences in virologic parameters during primary infection, in the rapidity of disease progression, and in the frequency of central nervous system (CNS) and growth abnormalities); prior antiretroviral exposure of newly infected infants (in utero and neonatal exposure to drugs used for maternal treatment and transmission prophylaxis); and pediatric-specific adherence issues (i.e. availability and palatability of drug formulations; relationship of drug administration to food intake in young infants; dependence on caregiver for administration of drugs).

Prospective, randomized, controlled clinical trials offer the best evidence for formulation of guidelines. However, most antiretroviral drugs are approved for use in pediatric patients based on efficacy data from clinical trials in adults, with supporting pharmacokinetic and safety data from phase I/II trials in children; additionally, efficacy in most adult trials has been based on surrogate marker data, as opposed to clinical endpoints. Thus, guidelines for treatment of HIV-infected children often have to rely on data regarding virologic/immunologic response to drug regimens in adult clinical trials, taking into account the specific considerations in pediatric HIV infection delineated above, and with attention to data from pediatric populations when available.

Management of HIV infection is complex and evolving rapidly. Guidelines for pediatric antiretroviral therapy have been developed in the USA and Europe, and by the World Health Organization (WHO). The US pediatric guidelines are available from the HIV/AIDS Treatment Information Service internet site at http:/AIDSInfo.nih.gov. These pediatric guidelines complement the antiretroviral guidelines for adults (also available at http://AIDSInfo.nih.gov) that are applicable to post-pubertal adolescents [1, 2]. European pediatric treatment guidelines were developed by the Pediatric European Network for the Treatment of AIDS (PENTA) (http://www.ctu.mrc.ac.uk/PENTA) [3]. The European guidelines are similar to the US guidelines, with the exception that the PENTA guidelines are somewhat more conservative concerning therapy initiation. Finally, guidelines for antiretroviral therapy of children in resource-poor countries have been developed by the World Health Organization (WHO) (http://www.who.int/3by5/publications/documents/arv_guidelines/en). The US pediatric guidelines for antiretroviral therapy are the focus of this chapter, and the other guidelines are addressed only briefly. None of these guidelines are intended to supplant the clinical judgment of experienced clinicians. Whenever possible, HIV-infected children should be managed by, or in consultation with, a pediatric HIV specialist.

22.2 When should antiretroviral therapy be started?

Initiation of highly active antiretroviral therapy (HAART) in HIV-infected adults and children has been shown to delay

Table 22.1 Factors to consider in decisions regarding initiation of antiretroviral therapy in HIV-infected infants, children, and adolescents

The severity of HIV disease and risk of progression as determined by presence or history of HIV-related serious or AIDS-defining illnesses, and the child's CD4$^+$ cell count and plasma HIV RNA level

Availability of appropriate and palatable drug formulations for the child and pharmacokinetic information on appropriate dosing in the child's age group

Potency, complexity (e.g. dosing frequency, food and fluid requirements), and potential short- and long-term adverse effects of the antiretroviral regimen

Effect of initial regimen choice on later therapeutic options

Presence of co-morbidity that could affect drug choice, such as tuberculosis, hepatitis B or C infection, or chronic renal or liver disease (for example, co-administration of rifampin can significantly reduce drug levels of nevirapine and most protease inhibitors; viral hepatitis can predispose to hepatic toxicity of nucleoside and non-nucleoside antiretroviral drugs; and, depending upon the route of metabolism/excretion for individual drugs, dose modification may be required for individuals with significant renal/liver disease)

Potential antiretroviral drug interactions with other medications required by the child

The ability of the caregiver and child to adhere to the regimen

HIV disease progression and improve survival [4–6]. However, debate continues as to the most beneficial time to begin HAART. A number of factors, shown in Table 22.1, need to be considered in making decisions about initiating antiretroviral therapy in HIV-infected children.

22.2.1 Adults and post-pubertal adolescents

The benefits of starting therapy in symptomatic adults with advanced HIV disease have been well established in randomized clinical trials, where initiation of HAART when CD4$^+$ cell counts were below 200 cells/mm^3 clearly improved morbidity and mortality [7–9], but the optimal time for starting HAART in asymptomatic infected adults with CD4$^+$ cell counts above 200 cells/mm^3 is unknown. Studies of early vs delayed zidovudine (ZDV) monotherapy in asymptomatic HIV-infected adults and children have not demonstrated a long-term benefit from early initiation of ZDV [10–12]. However, studies to address early vs deferred initiation of the much more potent therapies now available are lacking.

Arguments in favor of early initiation of HAART include the recognition that HIV disease is progressive; control of viral replication is easier to achieve and maintain in persons with lower viral load at the time therapy is started; control of replication prior to extensive viral genetic evolution may decrease the likelihood and delay the development of antiretroviral drug resistance; and early treatment may preserve or prevent immune system destruction. Arguments for delaying therapy in adults are based on the

relatively low risk of clinical progression in adults with early HIV infection (allowing preservation of the maximum number of treatment options); the lack of curative therapy and the unknown duration of virologic response to current therapies; difficulties with adherence to HAART which can lead to development of drug-resistant virus; and an increasing recognition of drug-related toxicities.

Current guidelines for initiation of antiretroviral therapy in adults, also relevant for infected postpubertal adolescents (Tanner Stage V), recommend initiation of HAART in all adults with symptomatic HIV infection (AIDS or severe symptoms) (Table 22.2). In asymptomatic or mild-to-moderately symptomatic adults, HAART is recommended for all patients with CD4$^+$ cell count below 200 cells/mm^3.

For asymptomatic adults with CD4$^+$ cell count between 200 and 350 cells/mm^3, many experts would offer treatment (Table 22.2), although this is still controversial. Data from the Multicenter AIDS Cohort Study indicate that although the 3-year risk of progression to AIDS in untreated adults with CD4$^+$ cell counts between 200 and 350 cells/mm^3 was 39%, this risk was related to plasma HIV RNA levels, and was relatively low (4%) for HIV RNA < 20 000 copies/mL [2]. Therefore, some clinicians choose to defer therapy in patients in this CD4$^+$ cell count category and to carefully monitor CD4$^+$ cell counts and plasma HIV RNA levels.

For asymptomatic adults with CD4$^+$ cell counts above 350 cells/mm^3, both an aggressive and a conservative approach are outlined (Table 22.2). In the aggressive approach, therapy is recommended for those with CD4$^+$

Table 22.2 United States Public Health Service guidelines for HIV-infected postpubertal adolescents and adults: indications for initiation of antiretroviral therapy

Clinical category	CD4+ Cell Count	Plasma HIV RNA	Recommendation
Chronic infection			
Symptomatic	Any value	Any value	Treat
Asymptomatic	CD4+ T cells < 200/mm^3	Any value	Treat
Asymptomatic	CD4+ T cells >200 but < 350/mm^3	Any value	Treatment should be offered, although it is recognized this is controversial
Asymptomatic	CD4+ T cells > 350/mm^3	> 55 000 copies/mL	*Aggressive approach*: Treat *Conservative approach*: Defer therapy but increase frequency of monitoring of CD4+ cell count and HIV RNA levels
Asymptomatic	CD4+ T cells > 350/mm^3	< 55 000 copies/mL	Defer and monitor CD4+ cell count
Acute infection[a]	Any value	Any value	Consider therapy (discuss potential benefits/risks with patient)

Modified from [2].

[a] Acute primary infection or documented seroconversion within the previous 6 months.

cell counts above 350 cells/mm^3 if plasma HIV RNA is > 55 000 copies/mL. In the conservative approach, patients with plasma HIV RNA > 55 000 copies/mL would be monitored frequently, but not treated.

Therapy for adults with acute HIV infection should be considered, although treatment in such circumstances is based on theoretical considerations and not definitive clinical trial data. During acute HIV infection there are very high levels of viral replication with widespread viral dissemination, and early deletions in the T-cell repertoire have been observed. The rationale for early treatment of primary infection is to decrease the number of infected cells, maintain or restore HIV-specific immune responses, preserve immune function, and to possibly lower the viral "set point" to improve the subsequent course of disease.

22.2.2 Infants, children, and pre-pubertal adolescents

Adherence is especially important to consider when initiating therapy in children. Antiretroviral therapy is most effective in patients naïve to therapy prior to the development of antiretroviral-resistant virus. Resistance can develop rapidly when drug concentrations fall below therapeutic levels (either due to inadequate dosage or incomplete adherence). Adherence to antiretroviral therapy has been firmly linked to virologic, immunologic, and clinical response to therapy, and adherence levels of ≥ 90–95% have been required to maintain viral suppression in some studies, including a study in children [13–16].

Achievement of such high levels of adherence is difficult even for adults, and in children is especially problematic. Barriers to adherence specific to the pediatric population include the fact that infants and young children are dependent upon their caregivers to administer their medication; the lack of palatability of most of the liquid drug formulations, which can affect the child's willingness to accept and retain the medication; timing of drug administration around food for drugs that require administration on a full or empty stomach can be difficult, particularly for infants who require frequent feeding; and many psychosocial issues related to administration of drugs in the school or day-care setting or specific to adolescents (including issues related to privacy and disclosure). Therefore, it is essential to fully assess and discuss potential adherence problems with the family and to address potential barriers to adherence prior to initiating therapy [17]. Participation by the child and the family in the decision-making process is important, particularly in situations for which definitive efficacy data are not available. Continued assessment and reinforcement of the need for adherence to the prescribed regimen at each follow-up visit is critical to maintain good adherence (see Chapter 13).

Table 22.3 United States Public Health Service guidelines for HIV-infected infants, children and young adolescents: indications for initiation of antiretroviral therapy

Clinical category		CD4$^+$ cell percentage		Plasma HIV RNA copy number	Recommendation
Children < 1 year of age					
Symptomatic (Clinical category A, B, or C)	*or*	<25% (Immune category 2 or 3)		Any value^a	Treat
Asymptomatic (Clinical category N)	*and*	≥25% (Immune category 1)		Any value^a	Consider treatment^b
Children ≥ 1 year of age					
AIDS (Clinical category C)	*or*	<15% (Immune category 3)		Any value	Treat
Mild-moderate symptoms (Clinical category A or B)	*or*	15–25%^{c} (Immune category 2)	*or*	≥ 100 000 copies/mL^d	Consider treatment
Asymptomatic (Clinical category N)	*and*	>25% (Immune category 1)	*and*	< 100 000 copies/mL^d	Many experts would defer therapy and closely monitor clinical, immune, and viral parameters

Modified from [1].

^{a} Plasma HIV RNA levels are higher in HIV-infected infants than older children and adults, and may be difficult to interpret in infants < 12 months of age because overall HIV RNA levels are high and there is overlap in RNA levels between infants who have and those who do not have rapid disease progression.

^{b} Because HIV infection progresses more rapidly in infants than older children or adults, some experts would treat all HIV-infected infants < 6 months or < 12 months of age, regardless of clinical, immunologic, or virologic parameters.

^{c} Many experts would initiate therapy if CD4$^+$ cell percentage is between 15–20%, and defer therapy with increased monitoring frequency in children with CD4$^+$ cell percentage 21%–25%.

^{d} There is controversy among pediatric HIV experts regarding the plasma HIV RNA threshold warranting consideration of therapy in children in the absence of clinical or immune abnormalities; some experts would consider initiation of therapy in asymptomatic children if plasma HIV RNA levels were between 50 000 to 100 000 copies/mL.

Similar to the adult treatment guidelines, antiretroviral therapy is recommended for HIV-infected children who have AIDS or severe symptoms, or who have evidence of significant immune suppression (Table 22.3). Clinical trial data in children as well as adults have demonstrated that antiretroviral therapy in symptomatic patients slows clinical and immunologic disease progression and reduces mortality [18, 19]. Additionally, trials in adults have shown that antiretroviral therapy slows disease progression in those who are immunosuppressed and at least mildly symptomatic [20, 21]. While placebo-controlled trials have not been conducted in pediatric patients, improvements in neurologic and neurodevelopmental status, growth, immunologic and/or virologic parameters have been demonstrated in clinical tri-

als of single drug or combination antiretroviral therapy in previously untreated, symptomatic pediatric patients [18, 19, 22–26].

However, recommendations for initiation of antiretroviral therapy in children with less severe symptoms or who are asymptomatic and who have only mild or moderate immune suppression are complicated by differences between HIV-infected children and adults in the rapidity of disease progression; the high viral loads seen in perinatally acquired infection; and age-related changes in CD4$^+$ counts (see Chapter 5). Because HIV-infected infants under 12 months of age are at particularly high risk for disease progression [27], and surrogate markers such as CD4$^+$ cell count and plasma HIV RNA levels are less predictive of progression risk in this age group [28], recommendations for

Table 22.4 European guidelines for HIV-infected infants, children and young adolescents: indications for initiation of antiretroviral therapy

Age	Symptoms		CD4+ cell count		HIV RNA level	Recommendation
<12 months	Clinical category C (AIDS)	or	<15%	or	Any	Treat
	Clinical category B (Moderate symptoms)	or	15–20%	or	>1 000 000 copies/mL	Consider
	Clinical category N or A (No or mild symptoms)	and	>20%	and	<1 000 000 copies/mL	Defer
≥12 months	Clinical category C (AIDS)	or	<15%	or	Any	Treat
	Clinical category B (Moderate symptoms)	or	15–20%	or	>100 000 copies/mL	Consider
	Clinical category N or A (No or mild symptoms)	and	>20%	and	<100 000 copies/mL	Defer

Modified from [2].

initiation of therapy in infants are more aggressive than those for older children.

HIV-infected infants under 12 months of age
The US guidelines recommend initiation of therapy for infants under the age of 12 months who have HIV-related clinical (CDC Pediatric Clinical Category A, B, or C) or immunologic (CDC Pediatric Immune Category 2 or 3) symptoms, regardless of HIV RNA level (Table 22.3). Therapy should be considered for HIV-infected infants under the age of 12 months who are asymptomatic and have normal immune parameters. Because of the high risk for rapid progression of HIV disease, many experts would treat all HIV-infected infants < 12 months old, regardless of clinical, immunologic, or virologic parameters. Other experts would treat all infected infants < 6 months old, and would rely on clinical and immunologic parameters and assessment of adherence issues for decisions regarding initiation of therapy in infants 6–12 months of age. European pediatric treatment guidelines have been more conservative than those in the USA, and currently suggest initiation of therapy could be deferred in infants who are asymptomatic or have mild symptoms, have CD4+ cell percentages > 20%, and HIV RNA levels < 1 000 000 copies/mL (Table 22.4) [3].

The risks and benefits of early initiation of therapy in infants should be discussed with the caregiver and issues of adherence should be addressed prior to initiation of therapy. Administration of antiretroviral therapy during infancy permits initiation of therapy during the period of primary infection, and is consistent with recommendations in guidelines for treatment of adults with acute HIV infection. Early initiation of therapy could theoreti-

cally diminish viral dissemination, lead to prolonged virologic suppression, and preserve thymic function, resulting in immune preservation, clinical stability, and normal growth and cognitive development. Some limited data are available to address the efficacy of aggressive therapy for HIV-infected infants. In an epidemiologic cohort that evaluated factors associated with disease progression in HIV-infected children under 2 years of age, children who received early treatment with HAART regimens were significantly less likely to progress to AIDS or death than those who received no antiretroviral therapy [29]. Several additional small studies have demonstrated that early initiation of HAART in HIV-infected infants can result in durable viral suppression and normalization of immunologic responses to non-HIV antigens in some infants, despite the very high levels of viral replication observed in infants with perinatal infection [30–34]. The proportion of children in these studies with viral levels remaining below quantification after 12–24 months of therapy ranged from 18–62%. Control of plasma viremia to levels below the detection limits, along with the lack of detection of extra-chromosomal replication intermediates, suggest good control of viral replication in some of these infants. Although some infants have become HIV seronegative and have lost HIV-specific immune responses, therapy is not curative. Proviral HIV-1 DNA continues to be detectable in peripheral blood lymphocytes and viral replication resumes if therapy is discontinued. The lack of persistent HIV specific immune responses in these infants contrasts with the persistent HIV specific immune responses reported in adults who receive combination antiretroviral therapy within 3–4 months of acquisition of infection [35, 36].

There are potential problems with early initiation of therapy for infants. Accurate antiretroviral pharmacokinetic data may not be available for infants, and it may be difficult for families of infants to assure adherence to a complicated regimen. Resistance to antiretroviral drugs can develop rapidly (particularly in the setting of high viral replication as observed in infected infants) when drug concentrations are sub-therapeutic, either because of incomplete adherence or inadequate dosage. The possibility of toxicities such as lipodystrophy, dyslipidemia, glucose intolerance, osteopenia, and mitochondrial dysfunction is a concern [37–42].

HIV-infected children over 12 months of age
Since the risk of disease progression slows in children over the age of 12 months, the option of deferring treatment can be considered for older children. The degree of clinical symptoms that suggest a need for therapy in children over 1 year old who do not have AIDS is unclear. It is clear that children with clinical AIDS (Clinical category C) or severe immune suppression (Immune category 3) are at high risk of progression and death, and treatment is recommended for all such children, regardless of virologic status (Table 22.3).

However, children over age 12 months with mild–moderate clinical symptoms (Clinical category A or B) or moderate immune suppression (Immune category 2) are at lower risk for progression than those with severe clinical and immunologic findings [43]. Plasma HIV RNA levels can provide adjunctive information about prognosis in children with mild–moderate clinical symptoms or immune suppression. HIV RNA levels have a better predictive value for disease progression in children over 12 months of age compared with infants; use of HIV RNA in combination with $CD4^+$ lymphocyte count improves prognostic value over use of either alone [44–46]. In one study of primarily untreated young children, high HIV RNA levels (>100 000 copies/mL) were shown to be associated with elevated mortality risk, particularly if $CD4^+$ lymphocyte percentage was <15%; however, mortality rates did not significantly differ by HIV RNA level in children with <100 000 copies/mL [44]. Similar data regarding predictive value of this HIV RNA threshold in older children was observed in a meta-analysis in nearly 4000 HIV-infected children from eight cohort studies and nine clinical trials in the USA and Europe [28].

The US guidelines therefore recommend that treatment should be started for all children over the age of 12 months with AIDS (Clinical category C) or severe immune suppression (Immune category 3), and be considered for children who have mild–moderate clinical symptoms (Clinical categories A or B), moderate immuno-logic suppression (Immune category 2), and/or confirmed plasma HIV RNA levels ≥100 000 copies/mL (Table 22.3). Many experts would defer treatment in asymptomatic children aged ≥1 year with normal immune status in situations in which the risk for clinical disease progression is low (e.g. HIV RNA <100 000 copies/mL) and when other factors (i.e. concern for adherence, safety, and persistence of antiretroviral response) favor postponing treatment. These recommendations are similar to the approach favored by many pediatric HIV specialists in Europe (Table 22.4) [3, 47].

If therapy is deferred, the clinician should carefully monitor virologic, immunologic, and clinical status. Factors that should be considered in deciding when to initiate therapy include: development of clinical symptoms; high or increasing HIV RNA levels; rapidly declining $CD4^+$ lymphocyte count or percentage to values approaching those indicative of severe immune suppression (CDC Pediatric immune category 3); and the ability of the caregiver and child to adhere to the prescribed regimen.

There is controversy among pediatric HIV experts regarding the exact plasma HIV RNA threshold that would warrant consideration of therapy in asymptomatic infected children with normal immune status. While the US guidelines suggest that an HIV RNA level >100 000 copies/mL indicates the need to initiate therapy, some experts would consider initiation of therapy in asymptomatic children if plasma HIV RNA levels were between 50 000 to 100 000 copies/mL. Similarly, some experts would not wait until immune suppression is severe (<15%) to start therapy in an asymptomatic child, but would initiate therapy if $CD4^+$ cell percentage is between 15–20%, and continue to defer therapy with increased monitoring frequency in children with $CD4^+$ cell percentage between 21–25%.

22.2.3 Differences between US and European PENTA guidelines for children

The primary difference between the US and European guidelines relates to when to initiate therapy in HIV-infected infants under the age of 12 months. The difficulties of long-term adherence, problems with data on optimal dosing for infants, and an increasing recognition of the potential for drug toxicity has led to a more cautious and less aggressive approach to initiation of therapy in this age group in the PENTA guidelines (Table 22.4) [3]. Treatment is recommended for infants <12 months of age only in the case of AIDS-related symptoms or $CD4^+$ cell percentage <15% indicating severe immune suppression. Treatment is considered for infants if they have moderate symptoms (CDC Clinical Stage B), $CD4^+$ percentage 15–20%, or HIV

RNA levels >1 000 000 copies/mL; treatment is deferred for infants with no or mild symptoms and CD4$^+$ percentage >20% and HIV RNA levels <1 000 000 copies/mL. For children aged >12 months, the recommendations are similar to those in the USA.

22.2.4 World Health Organization interim guidelines for resource-limited settings

Guidelines for antiretroviral therapy have generally been developed for application in high- and middle-income countries and extrapolated to resource-limited settings. However, in April 2002 (and revised in December 2003), the WHO released interim guidelines for antiretroviral use in resource-limited settings, with the intent of facilitating the dramatic scale-up that is needed in countries with limited infrastructures and significant resource limitations in order to provide care to millions of infected people. These guidelines can be accessed on the WHO website (http://www.who.int/3by5/publications/documents/arv_guidelines/en). Recognizing that the availability of affordable and accurate laboratory testing is severely constrained in many resource-limited countries, these guidelines reflect decision-making in situations in which virologic assays and CD4$^+$ cell counts may not be available.

In children, the WHO recommends offering combination antiretroviral therapy to HIV-infected children under the age of 18 months with WHO Pediatric stage III HIV disease (i.e. clinical AIDS) or advanced symptomatic HIV disease regardless of CD4$^+$ percentage, or with WHO Pediatric stage I or II disease and a CD4$^+$ percentage <20% (Table 22.5). If CD4$^+$ assays are not available, treatment should be considered for children under 18 months of age with WHO Pediatric stage III disease (regardless of total lymphocyte count), or with WHO Pediatric stage II disease and total lymphocyte count < 2500 cells/mm^3.

It was recognized that viral diagnostic assays are not available in some resource-limited settings, and therefore a definitive diagnosis of HIV infection would not be possible until 18 months of age, at which time the child may have developed significant symptoms. Therefore, the guidelines recommend that, if CD4$^+$ assays are available, children who are HIV-seropositive, have had an AIDS-defining illness (WHO Pediatric stage III disease), and who also have CD4$^+$ cell percentage <20%, may be considered for therapy even if virologic testing is not available. HIV antibody testing must be repeated at 18 months of age to confirm the diagnosis of HIV infection; therapy would be continued only in those children who remain HIV-seropositive. If CD4$^+$ cell assays are not available, HIV-exposed children under the age of 18 months

without a definitive diagnosis of HIV infection should not be considered for treatment, regardless of clinical symptoms.

For children over the age of 18 months who are HIV-seropositive, WHO recommends therapy if they have WHO stage III HIV disease (i.e. clinical AIDS) regardless of CD4$^+$ percentage. For those older children with WHO stage I or II HIV disease (i.e. asymptomatic or moderate symptoms), antiretroviral therapy is recommended if the CD4$^+$ percentage is < 15%. If CD4$^+$ assays are not available, treatment should be considered for children 18 months of age or older with WHO Pediatric stage III disease (regardless of total lymphocyte count), or with WHO Pediatric stage II disease and total lymphocyte count < 1500 cells/mm^3.

22.3 What is the recommended initial antiretroviral regimen?

Early clinical trials in adults and children evaluated antiretroviral treatment consisting of a single nucleoside analogue reverse transcriptase inhibitor (NRTI), which provided substantial clinical benefit despite the limited potency of monotherapy [19, 22–26]. Subsequent comparative clinical trials in symptomatic infected adults and children demonstrated that initial therapy with dual NRTI combination antiretroviral regimens was better than NRTI monotherapy [18, 19, 48, 49]. However, it was the development of new classes of antiretroviral drugs, the non-nucleoside reverse transcriptase inhibitors (NNRTIs) and protease inhibitors (PI), and use of these drugs in combination with NRTIs, that dramatically changed the course of HIV disease in adults and children, resulting in substantial decreases in overall morbidity and mortality in resource-rich countries since 1996 [5, 6]. Studies in adults and children have demonstrated that combination therapy that includes a PI (generally with two NRTIs) is superior to dual NRTI therapy [50–52].

Based on these pediatric and adult clinical trial data, combination therapy is now recommended for all infected children and adults treated with antiretroviral drugs (Tables 22.6 and 22.7). Compared with monotherapy with the currently available antiretroviral drugs, combination therapy yields significantly lower rates of disease progression, a greater and more sustained virologic and immunologic response, and less frequent development of drug resistance. Therefore, with the exception of the use of ZDV as perinatal transmission prophylaxis in infants of indeterminate infection status during the first 6 weeks of life, monotherapy with currently available antiretroviral drugs is no longer recommended

Table 22.5 World Health Organization guidelines for HIV-infected infants, children, and young adolescents: indications for initiation of antiretroviral therapy in resource-poor settings

CD4$^+$ Testing	Age	HIV diagnostic testing	Treatment recommendation
If CD4$^+$ testing is available	<18 months	Positive HIV virologic test[a]	WHO Pediatric stage III disease (AIDS), irrespective of CD4$^+$ cell percentage[b] WHO Pediatric stage I disease (asymptomatic) or stage II disease with CD4$^+$ percentage <20%[c]
		HIV virologic testing not available but infant HIV seropositive or born to known HIV-infected mother (Note: HIV antibody test *must* be repeated at age 18 months to obtain definitive diagnosis of HIV infection)	WHO Pediatric stage III disease (AIDS) with CD4$^+$ cell percentage <20%
	≥18 months	HIV seropositive	WHO Pediatric stage III disease (AIDS) irrespective of CD4$^+$ cell percentage[b] WHO Pediatric stage I disease (asymptomatic) or stage II disease with CD4$^+$ percentage <15%[c]
If CD4$^+$ testing is not available	<18 months	Positive HIV virologic test	WHO Pediatric stage III[b] WHO Pediatric stage II disease with total lymphocyte count 2500 cells/mm^3
		HIV virologic testing not available but infant HIV seropositive or born to known HIV-infected mother	Treatment not recommended[d]
	≥18 months	HIV seropositive	WHO Pediatric stage III disease[b] WHO Pediatric stage II disease with total lymphocyte count 1150 cells/mm^3

[a] HIV DNA PCR or HIV RNA or immune complex dissociated p24 antigen assays.

[b] Initiation of antiretroviral therapy (ARV) can also be considered for children who have advanced WHO Pediatric stage II disease including such events as severe recurrent or persistent oral candidiasis outside the neonatal period, weight loss, fevers, or recurrent severe bacterial infections, irrespective of CD4$^+$ count.

[c] The rate of decline in CD4$^+$ percentage (if measurement available) should be factored into the decision-making.

[d] Many of the clinical symptoms in the WHO Pediatric stage II and III disease classification are not specific for HIV infection and significantly overlap those seen in children without HIV infection in resource-limited settings; thus, in the absence of virologic testing and CD4$^+$ cell assay availability, HIV-exposed children <18 months of age should generally not be considered for ART regardless of symptoms except in unusual circumstances (e.g., a child with a classic AIDS-defining event such as *Pneumocystis jiroveci* pneumonia (PCP) or crytococcal meningitis.

[e] Total lymphocyte count (<2500 cells/mm^3 for children <18 months old or <1500 cells/mm^3 for children ≥18 months old) can be substituted for CD4$^+$ when the latter is not available and when the child has HIV-related symptoms. Its utility among asymptomatic children is unknown. Therefore, in the absence of CD4$^+$ assays, asymptomatic HIV-infected children (WHO Pediatric stage I) should not be treated.

Table 22.6 United States Public Health Service guidelines for HIV-infected infants, children, and young adolescents: recommended antiretroviral options for initial therapy

Protease inhibitor-based regimens

Strongly recommended:	Two NRTIs[a] *plus* lopinavir/ritonavir *or* nelfinavir *or* ritonavir
Alternative recommendation:	Two NRTIs[a] *plus* amprenavir (children ≥4 years old)[b] *or* indinavir

Non-nucleoside reverse transcriptase inhibitor-based regimens

Strongly recommended:	Children > 3 years: Two NRTIs[a] *plus* efavirenz[c] (with or without nelfinavir)
	Children ≤ 3 years or who cannot swallow capsules: Two NRTIs[1] *plus* nevirapine[c]
Alternative recommendation:	Two NRTIs[1] *plus* nevirapine[c] (children >3 years)

Nucleoside analogue-based regimens

Strongly recommended:	None
Alternative recommendation:	Zidovudine *plus* lamivudine *plus* abacavir
Use in special circumstances:	Two NRTIs[a]

Regimens that are not recommended

Monotherapy[d]

Certain two NRTI combinations[a]

Two NRTIs *plus* saquinavir soft or hard gel capsule as a sole protease inhibitor[e]

Insufficient data to recommend

Two NRTIs[a] *plus* delavirdine

Dual protease inhibitors, including saquinavir soft or hard gel capsule with low dose ritonavir, with the exception of lopinavir/ritonavir[d]

NRTI *plus* NNRTI *plus* protease inhibitor[f]

Tenofovir-containing regimens

Enfuvirtide (T-20)-containing regimens

Emtricitabine (FTC)-containing regimens

Atazanavir-containing regimens

Fosamprenavir-containing regimens

Modified from [1].

[a] Dual NRTI combination recommendations:

Strongly recommended choices: zidovudine plus didanosine or lamivudine; or stavudine plus lamivudine.

Alternative choices: abacavir plus zidovudine or lamivudine; or didanosine plus lamivudine.

Use in special circumstances: stavudine plus didanosine; or zalcitabine plus zidovudine.

Not recommended: zalcitabine plus didanosine, stavudine, or lamivudine; or zidovudine plus stavudine.

Insufficient data: tenofovir- or emtricitabine-containing regimens.

[b] Amprenavir should not be administered to children under age 4 years due to the propylene glycol and vitamin E content of the oral liquid preparation and lack of pharmacokinetic data in this age group.

[c] Efavirenz is currently available only in capsule form, although a liquid formulation is currently under study to determine appropriate dosage in HIV-infected children under age 3 years; nevirapine would be the preferred NNRTI for children under age 3 years or require a liquid formulation.

[d] Except for zidovudine chemoprophylaxis administered to HIV-exposed infants during the first 6 weeks of life to prevent perinatal HIV transmission; if an infant is confirmed as HIV-infected while receiving zidovudine prophylaxis, antiretroviral therapy should either be discontinued or changed to a combination antiretroviral drug regimen.

[e] With the exception of lopinavir/ritonavir, data on the pharmacokinetics and safety of dual protease inhibitor combinations (e.g. low dose ritonavir pharmacologic boosting of saquinavir, indinavir, or nelfinavir) are limited, use of dual protease inhibitors as a component of initial therapy is not recommended, although such regimens may have utility as secondary treatment regimens for children who have failed initial therapy. Saquinavir soft and hard gel capsule require low dose ritonavir boosting to achieve adequate levels in children, but pharmacokinetic data on appropriate dosing not yet available.

[f] With the exception of efavirenz plus nelfinavir plus one or two NRTIs, which has been studied in HIV-infected children and shown to have virologic and immunologic efficacy in a clinical trial.

NRTI: Nucleoside analogue reverse transcriptase inhibitor.

NnRTI: Non-nucleoside analogue reverse transcriptase inhibitor.

Table 22.7 United States Public Health Service Guidelines for HIV-infected postpubertal adolescents and adults: recommended antiretroviral options for initial therapy

Non-nucleoside reverse transcriptase inhibitor-based regimens

Preferred regimens	Efavirenz *plus* (lamivudine *or* emtricitabine[a]) *plus* (zidovudine *or* tenofovir DF *or* stavudine[b]) – except for pregnant women or women with pregnancy potential
Alternative regimens	Efavirenz *plus* (lamivudine *or* emtricitabine[a]) *plus* didanosine or abacivir – except for pregnant women or women with pregnancy potential
	Nevirapine *plus* (lamivudine *or* emtricitabine[a]) *plus* (zidovudine *or* stavudine[b] *or* didanosine or abacivir)

Protease inhibitor-based regimens

Preferred regimens	Lopinavir/ritonavir *plus* (lamivudine[b]) *plus* (zidovudine *or* stavudine[b])
Alternative regimens	Fosamprenavir[c] *plus* (lamivudine *or* emtricitabine[a]) *plus* (zidovudine *or* stavudine[b] or abacavir)
	Fosamprenavir/ritonavir *plus* (lamivudine or emtricitabine) *plus* (zidovudine or stavudine[b] or abacavir)
	Atazanavir *plus* (lamivudine *or* emtricitabine[a]) *plus* (zidovudine *or* stavudine[b])
	Lopinavir/ritonavir *plus* (emtricitabine[a]) *plus* (zidovudine or stavudine[b] or abacavir)
	Indinavir/ritonavir[c] *plus* (lamivudine or emtricitabine[a]) *plus* (zidovudine or stavudine[b] or abacavir)
	Nelfinavir[d] *plus* (lamivudine *or* emtricitabine[a]) *plus* (zidovudine *or* stavudine[b] or abacavir)
	Saquinavir (sgc *or* hcg)[e] /ritonavir[c] *plus* (lamivudine *or* emtricitabine[b]) *plus* (zidovudine *or* stavudine[b] or abacavir)

Nucleoside analogue-based regimen – only when a PI- or NNRTI-based regimen cannot or should not be used as first-line therapy

Only as alternative to PI- or NNRTI-based regimen

Abacavir *plus* lamivudine *plus* zidovudine (*or* stavudine[b])

Modified from [1].

[a] Long-term efficacy data on emtricitabine used in combination with these regimens is limited or not available.

[b] Higher incidence of lipoatrophy, hyperlipidemia, and mitochondrial toxicities reported with stavudine than with other NRTIs.

[c] Low-dose (100–400 mg) ritonavir.

[d] Nelfinavir available in 250 mg or 625 mg tablet.

[e] sgc = soft gel capsule; hgc = hard gel capsule.

NNRTI: Non-nucleoside analogue reverse transcriptase inhibitor.

NRTI: Nucleoside analogue reverse transcriptase inhibitor.

PI: Protease inhibitor.

for treatment of HIV infection. Infants confirmed as HIV-infected while receiving ZDV chemoprophylaxis during the first 6 weeks of life should have ZDV discontinued pending decisions regarding initiation of antiretroviral therapy.

When using combination therapy, all drugs should be started at the same time or within 1–2 days of each other. Sequential initiation of drugs increases the possibility that antiretroviral resistance will develop due to incomplete viral suppression during the initial stages of therapy.

22.3.1 Children and pre-pubertal adolescents

The initial antiretroviral regimen chosen for infected infants theoretically could be influenced by the antiretroviral regimen their mother may have received during pregnancy. Current data do not suggest that the antiretroviral regimen for infected infants should routinely be chosen on the basis of maternal antiretroviral use [53, 54]. However, it will be important to continue to monitor the frequency of perinatal transmission of antiretroviral-resistant HIV isolates because maternal therapy with multiple antiretroviral agents is becoming increasingly common and the prevalence of resistant viral strains in the HIV-infected population may increase over time [55]. Current US guidelines suggest consideration of resistance testing prior to initiation of therapy in newly diagnosed infants under the age of 12 months, particularly if the mother has known or suspected infection with drug-resistant virus [1]. However, there are no definitive data at this time that demonstrate that resistance testing in this setting correlates with greater success of initial antiretroviral therapy.

There are few randomized, phase III clinical trials in children that provide direct comparison of different treatment regimens. Recommendations for initial therapy in children have been based upon clinical trials demonstrating durable viral suppression and immunologic and clinical improvement (when such data are available), preferably in children as well as adults; the incidence and types of drug toxicity with the regimen; availability and palatability of formulations appropriate for pediatric use; dosing frequency, and food and fluid requirements; and potential for drug interactions.

Antiretroviral drug regimens are classified as follows: strongly recommended; recommended as alternative; use in special circumstances; not recommended; or insufficient data to make a recommendation [1]. Recommendations on the optimal initial therapy for children are continually being modified as new data become available, new therapies or drug formulations are developed, and late toxicities become recognized. The most up-to-date pediatric guidelines can be accessed at: http://www.AIDSInfo.nih.gov.

As of July 2004, there are 20 antiretroviral drugs approved for use in HIV-infected adults and adolescents; 12 of these have an approved pediatric treatment indication. These drugs fall into several major classes: nucleoside analogue or nucleotide reverse transcriptase inhibitors (NRTIs, NtRTIs), non-nucleoside reverse transcriptase inhibitors (NNRTIs), PIs, and fusion inhibitors. A dual NRTI combination forms the backbone of recommended regimens, and is given with a protease inhibitor, an NNRTI, or a third NRTI.

Each class-based regimen has advantages and disadvantages. Protease inhibitor-based regimens are highly potent, but have a high pill burden and the liquid formulations are often unpalatable to children. NNRTI-based regimens are palatable and effective, but have a low genetic barrier to resistance that can lead to rapid development of genetic mutations in the virus that confer resistance to all drugs in the NNRTI class if therapy does not fully suppress viral replication. Triple NRTI-based regimens spare other drug classes, but appear to have lower potency than other regimens. Within each drug class, some drugs may be preferred over others for children, based on the extent of pediatric experience, drug formulation (including taste and volume of liquid formulations and pill size and number), storage and food requirements, and short- and long-term toxicity.

Choice of dual NRTI backbone

The dual NRTI combinations with the most experience in children are ZDV/lamivudine (3TC), ZDV/didanosine (ddI), and stavudine (d4T)/3TC, which are the strongly recommended dual NRTI combinations for inclusion in initial therapy regimens in children. Alternative dual NRTI combinations include ZDV/abacavir (ABC), 3TC/ABC, and ddI/3TC. Although some studies have shown that dual NRTI backbone regimens containing ABC may have similar potency to ZDV/3TC [56], ABC has the potential for ABC-associated life-threatening hypersensitivity reactions in about 5% of patients [57, 58], and therefore ABC-containing regimens are viewed as alternative rather than recommended in children. Because there is less pediatric experience with ddI/3TC than the recommended dual NRTIs, it is also recommended as an alternative. The dual NRTI combinations d4T/ddI and ZDV/zalcitabine (ddC) are recommended for use only in special circumstances; d4T/ddI-based combination regimens are associated with greater rates of neurotoxicity, hyperlactatemia, and lipodystrophy than ZDV/3TC-based therapies [59, 60], and ddC is less potent than the other NRTI drugs and has greater toxicity, and thus would not be first choice for inclusion in an initial therapy regimen. Certain dual NRTI drug combinations should not be given. These include ZDV and d4T, due to pharmacologic and 3TC and ddC due to pharmacologic, interactions that can result in potential virologic antagonism, and dual regimens combining ddC with ddI or d4T or 3TC, as pediatric experience with these combinations is limited and there is overlapping neurotoxicity between the drugs. Emtricitabine (FTC) is approved for use in adults aged 18 years or older; while under study in children, pharmacokinetic, safety, and efficacy data in pediatric patients are not yet available and no pediatric formulation is commercially available [1]. Therefore, there are insufficient data to recommend use of FTC for initial therapy in children.

Strongly recommended regimens for initial therapy

Based on clinical trials in infected adults and children, the antiretroviral regimens that are strongly recommended for initial therapy in children include the combination of two NRTIs plus one of the recommended PIs, or the combination of two NRTIs plus the NNRTI efavirenz for children over the age of 3 years or nevirapine for children under the age of 3 years or who cannot take capsules (Table 22.6). Choice of a dual NRTI backbone is discussed above.

Lopinavir, nelfinavir, and ritonavir are the recommended PIs for use in PI-based regimens in young children because they are available in appropriate formulations (nelfinavir is available in a powder which can be mixed with water or food; lopinavir and ritonavir are available as liquids) and there is experience with these drugs in pediatric populations, with relatively low rates of toxicity [52, 61–65]. In adult clinical trials, combination therapy with two NRTIs and a potent PI can produce sustained suppression of viral replication to undetectable levels; similar pediatric data indicate such therapy also can reduce HIV RNA to undetectable levels in a substantial proportion of children, although the rate of response may be somewhat less than in adults, particularly for younger children [32–34, 62–64]. Additionally, longer-term clinical and immunologic benefits have been reported in children receiving these regimens, including improvements in growth, an important measure of response to therapy in children [66–69].

Efavirenz, in combination with two NRTIs with or without nelfinavir, is the strongly recommended NNRTI for NNRTI-based initial therapy of children over the age of 3 years who can take capsules, based on clinical trial experience in children and because higher rates of toxicity have been observed in clinical trials in adults with nevirapine. In a pediatric clinical trial, efavirenz in combination with one or two NRTIs and the PI nelfinavir reduced viral load to < 400 copies/mL in 76% of treated children and to < 50 copies/mL in 63% [70]. The regimen was well-tolerated and virologic response sustained through 48 weeks. However, this regimen contains drugs from all three available drug classes and therefore there is the potential for development of resistance to all three classes if virologic failure occurs. In clinical trials in adults, a PI-sparing regimen of efavirenz in combination with dual NRTIs was associated with an excellent virologic and immunologic response comparable to PI-containing regimens, with similar or better tolerability [71, 72]. While there have not been clinical trials of efavirenz as part of a PI sparing regimen as initial therapy in pediatric patients, it seems reasonable to extrapolate efficacy from the adult data. A liquid formulation of efavirenz is under study in children under the age of 3 years and is available by expanded access and in a few countries outside the USA [73]. Because efavirenz is only commercially available in a capsule in the USA and nevirapine is available in a liquid formulation, nevirapine is the strongly recommended NNRTI for children who require a liquid formulation or who are under the age of 3 years.

Alternative regimens for initial therapy

Antiretroviral regimens recommended as alternatives for initial therapy of children include two NRTIs with the PIs indinavir or amprenavir (the latter only for children over 4 years of age); the combination of two NRTIs with nevirapine (for children aged 3 years or older); or the triple NRTI combination of ZDV/3TC/ABC (Table 22.6). Each of these alternative regimens has demonstrated evidence of virologic suppression in some children [69, 74, 75]. However, either experience in the pediatric population is more limited than for the strongly recommended regimens or the extent and durability of suppression less well defined in children. Additionally, for some drugs, although clinical trials in children have demonstrated reasonable virologic response in combination regimens, the potential for serious adverse effects (3–5% rate of hypersensitivity reactions with ABC; 6–9% rate of severe rash and/or hepatitis with nevirapine; and 9–13% rate of nephrolithiasis with indinavir) make them less favorable choices for initial therapy at this time.

There is no liquid formulation of indinavir, and therefore it can only be used in children who can swallow capsules. Additionally, there has been a high rate of hematuria, sterile leukocytouria, and nephrolithiasis reported in pediatric patients receiving indinavir [69, 76]. Amprenavir liquid formulation cannot be administered to children under the age of 4 years due to the high concentration of propylene glycol and vitamin E in the liquid preparation. Thus, initial PI-based regimens containing either of these drugs are viewed as alternative as opposed to strongly recommended regimens.

Clinical trials in adults are conflicting in terms of comparative efficacy of nevirapine and efavirenz, with some studies showing more virologic failures with nevirapine and others showing equivalent efficacy of the two drugs [77–79]. However, serious hepatobiliary toxicity appears more frequent in adult studies with use of nevirapine than efavirenz (79, 80). No comparative trials of nevirapine and efavirenz have been conducted in children. Because of the potential for higher rates of hepatic toxicity, a nevirapine-based regimen is viewed as an alternative rather than as recommended for NNRTI-based regimens, with the exception of children under the age of 3 years (for whom no data are available on appropriate dose for efavirenz, the recommended NNRTI) or those who require a liquid formulation (which is not yet available for efavirenz).

Triple NRTI regimens can be considered as alternative regimens as initial therapy when PI- or NNRTI-based regimens cannot be given (for example, due to potential important drug interactions). Data on the efficacy of triple NRTI regimens for treatment of antiretroviral-naïve children are limited; in small observational studies, response rates of 47–50% have been reported [81–83]. A European study found that the dual NRTI backbone of ABC/ZDV or ABC/3TC had greater virologic efficacy than combination ZDV/3TC when studied alone or in combination with nelfinavir in treatment-naïve children [83]. A triple-NRTI regimen spares the initial use of PIs and NNRTIs and can be administered twice a day in children, which may facilitate adherence. However, a clinical trial (ACTG 5095) in antiretroviral-naïve adults that compared initial therapy with ABC/ZDV/3TC, efavirenz/ZDV/3TC, or efavirenz/ZDV/3TC/ABC found that the triple NRTI regimen was inferior to the efavirenz-based regimens, with a higher incidence of and an earlier time to virologic failure (National Institute of Allergy and Infectious Diseases. Physician letter, AACTG protocol 5095, March 13, 2003. Available at: http://www.nlm.nih.gov/databases/alerts/hiv.html.). After 48 weeks of therapy, 74% of adults receiving ABC/ZDV/3TC had HIV RNA < 200 copies/mL compared with 89% of patients receiving efavirenz-based regimens. Therefore, because of the uncertain long-term durability of viral load suppression with this triple NRTI regimen, the recent adult data suggesting an inferior virologic response with ABC/ZDV/3TC compared with efavirenz-based regimens, and the potentially life-threatening hypersensitivity syndrome associated with ABC in 5% of recipients [57, 58], the use of this triple NRTI drug combination is recommended as an alternative for initial therapy.

Use in special circumstances for initial therapy

Dual NRTI therapy alone is recommended for initial therapy only in special circumstances (Table 22.6). Therapy with two NRTIs alone has been shown to provide clinical, virologic, and immunologic benefit in pediatric studies, but the extent and durability of virologic suppression is less than with PI-containing combination regimens [18, 19, 52]. Use of a regimen consisting of two NRTIs alone might be considered when the healthcare provider or guardian/patient has concerns regarding the feasibility of adherence to a more complex drug regimen. It is important to note that drug regimens that do not result in sustained viral suppression, such as a dual NRTI regimen, may result

in the development of viral resistance to the drugs being used and cross-resistance to other drugs within the same drug class. Thus, a dual NRTI regimen would be chosen for initial therapy only under very limited circumstances.

Not recommended for initial therapy

Antiretroviral regimens not recommended for initial treatment of antiretroviral-naïve children include monotherapy, certain dual NRTI combinations (ZDV and d4T; and ddC and ddI, d4T or 3TC), and saquinavir-soft gel capsule or saquinavir-hard gel capsule as sole PIs (Table 22.6). These combinations are not recommended either because of pharmacological antagonism, potential overlapping toxicities, or inferior virologic response. There are only limited data on saquinavir in children, and pharmacokinetic studies have found lower than expected plasma drug concentrations [85, 86]. Combining saquinavir with another PI, either nelfinavir or ritonavir, is required in children to increase saquinavir exposure to acceptable levels; however, these regimens have been principally studied in small numbers of antiretroviral-experienced population of children, as opposed to initial therapy, and appropriate dosing of dual PI regimens in pediatric patients is not yet established [84–86].

Insufficient data to recommend for initial therapy

There are a number of antiretroviral drugs or regimens for which there are insufficient data to recommend for use as initial therapy of antiretroviral-naïve children, although they may be of use in children who have failed other antiretroviral drug regimens (Table 22.6). The NNRTI delavirdine has not been studied in HIV-infected children and is not available in a liquid formulation. Dual PI-based regimens (with the exception of lopinavir-ritonavir, a co-formulated preparation) have only limited data on appropriate dosing and safety in children; these regimens often use one PI, often ritonavir, to "boost" levels of the other PI to a therapeutic range [88]. There are also minimal pediatric data on regimens containing agents from three drug classes (e.g. NRTI plus NNRTI plus a PI), with the exception of efavirenz plus nelfinavir and one or two NRTIs, which has been shown to be effective in HIV-infected children [71]. The reverse transcriptase inhibitors tenofovir and emtricitabine (FTC), and the PIs atazanavir and fosamprenavir do not have pediatric pharmacokinetic and safety data currently available and are not available in liquid formulations. Finally, the fusion inhibitor T-20 has been approved for children over the age of 6 years [88], but requires administration by subcutaneous injection and has only been studied in treatment-experienced children; thus, more data are needed before it would be considered for use as initial therapy.

22.3.2 Adults and post-pubertal adolescents

Regimens recommended for initial therapy for infected adults and adolescents include some antiretroviral drug combinations or agents not yet recommended for initial therapy in children (Table 22.7). Use of drugs that inhibit the liver cytochrome P450 metabolic enzyme system can produce substantial increases in drug levels of PIs, which are metabolized by this system. Low, non-therapeutic doses of ritonavir, a potent P450 inhibitor, can act as a pharmacologic "enhancer" when administered with other protease inhibitors, resulting in elevated plasma concentrations of the second drug at a lower dosage and longer elimination kinetics than if the drug was administered alone [88]. This approach exploits pharmacokinetic interactions to allow reduced dosing frequency as well as reduced dose of the second drug; potentially can provide additive or synergistic antiviral effects; may delay the appearance of drug-resistance mutations raising the genetic barrier for resistance by using drugs with non-overlapping resistance profiles; and overcome low-level reduced sensitivity to this drug class. In infected adults, low-dose ritonavir in combination with saquinavir, indinavir, nelfinavir, fosamprenavir, and amprenavir, either as dual PI therapy alone or combined with one or two NRTIs, has been well tolerated and shown substantial antiretroviral activity [88]. Most of these studies have been conducted in treatment-experienced patients, and it is unclear whether dual PIs offer any substantial benefit compared to single PI regimens for initial therapy. A few dual PI regimens have been studied in a small number of children [66, 89]. However, because data on the pharmacokinetics, safety, and efficacy of dual PI combinations in children are limited, use of such regimens for initial therapy is not recommended in children, with the exception of lopinavir/ritonavir. The NRTI emtricitabine, the PI atazanavir, and the nucleotide reverse transcriptase inhibitor tenofovir have been approved for treatment of adults; however, studies to define appropriate dosage and safety in children are still in initial phases. Additional new antiretroviral drugs and combinations are under study, and it is highly likely that other drug combinations capable of suppressing viral replication will become available in the future and will increase treatment options for children.

22.4 When should a change in antiretroviral therapy be considered?

The reasons to consider changing an antiretroviral regimen include: (1) evidence of disease progression based on virologic, immunologic, or clinical parameters indicating therapeutic failure of the current regimen; (2) toxicity or intolerance to the current regimen; and (3) consideration of new data demonstrating that a drug or regimen is superior to the current regimen.

Failure of an antiretroviral regimen can occur for many reasons, including problems with absorption or metabolism of a drug due to inherent characteristics of the individual or pharmacokinetic interactions with concomitant medications leading to sub-therapeutic drug levels; pre-existing or acquired drug resistance; and/or problems with patient adherence to the regimen. Adherence can be a special problem in pediatrics and innovative techniques may be needed to ensure compliance. Close family and medical follow-up are essential to ensure adherence with new therapeutic regimens. If inconsistent adherence to therapy is identified as a problem, renewed efforts to educate the caregivers and patient, and closer follow-up from supportive members of a multi-disciplinary care team, may improve adherence.

22.5 Virologic considerations for changing therapy

HIV RNA parameters for adults that warrant consideration of changing antiretroviral therapy are shown in Table 22.8. These recommendations are also appropriate for infected post-pubertal adolescents (Tanner Stage V). However, because the natural history of HIV RNA in perinatal infection differs from what is observed in infected adults, these recommendations are modified for pediatrics; specific virologic findings that should prompt consideration of a change in the initial therapeutic regimen for children are shown in Table 22.9.

The timeline used to judge virologic therapeutic response may differ in children. Virologic response should be assessed 4 weeks after initiating or changing therapy. However, the time to achieve a maximal virologic response to therapy will vary depending on the baseline HIV RNA value at the time therapy is started. Because HIV RNA levels in perinatal infection are extremely high compared with most infected adults, the initial response of infected infants and young children to initiation of antiretroviral therapy may be slower than that observed in adults. If baseline HIV RNA levels are very high (e.g. $>1\,000\,000$ copies/mL), virologic response may not be observed until after 8–12 weeks or more of therapy. However, if baseline HIV RNA levels were similar to those observed in infected adults, a response time more consistent with that of adults would be expected.

The suppression of plasma HIV RNA to undetectable levels may be achieved less often in children despite potent combination therapy due to the high level of viral

Table 22.8 United States Public Health Service guidelines for HIV-infected postpubertal adolescents and adults: considerations for changing antiretroviral therapy

Virologic considerations	1. Incomplete virologic response (not achieving HIV RNA < 400 copies/mL by 24 weeks or < 50 copies/mL by 48 weeks in a treatment-naïve patient starting therapy)[a]
	2. Virologic rebound (repeated detection of viremia after achieved virologic suppression)[b]
Immunologic considerations	1. Failure to increase 25–50 CD4$^+$ cells/μL over the first year of therapy
	2. Experiencing a decrease in CD4$^+$ cell count below the baseline CD4$^+$ cell count on therapy
Clinical considerations	1. Occurrence or recurrence of HIV-related events (after at least 3 months on an antiretroviral regimen), excluding immune reconstitution syndromes

Modified from [2].

[a] Baseline HIV RNA may impact the time course of response, and some patients may take longer than others to suppress viremia.

[b] The degree of plasma HIV RNA increase should be considered, and the healthcare provider may consider short-term observation in a patient whose plasma HIV RNA increases from undetectable to low-level detectability (e.g., 500–5000 copies/mL) at 4 months. In this situation, the patient should be followed very closely.

replication. However, significant clinical benefit may be seen with decrements in HIV RNA that do not result in undetectable levels; in one pediatric trial, there was a 54% reduction in the relative risk of disease progression for every $1.0 \log_{10}$ decrease in HIV RNA from baseline [45, 46]. Therefore, the initial HIV RNA level of the child at the start of therapy should be taken into consideration when contemplating potential drug changes, as well as the nadir achieved with therapy. For example, an immediate change in therapy may not necessarily be warranted if there is a sustained $1.5–2.0 \log_{10}$ fall in HIV RNA copy number, even if RNA remains detectable at relatively low levels. Given the observation that HIV-infected infants often have much higher viral loads than adults and the fact that even the most effective current combination antiretroviral therapies only decrease viral loads by factors of 10–100 (1–2 logs), it may be difficult to decrease the viral loads of many infants to below detectable limits. Rapid modifications of antiretroviral therapy might not achieve this goal and could unnecessarily and prematurely exhaust the patient's therapeutic options. However, it should also be recognized that failure to maximally suppress viral replication might be associated with increased risk for viral mutations and selection for drug-resistant viral variants. Resistance testing is recommended in children, as in adults, in the setting of persistent or increasing HIV RNA levels [1].

Following achievement of a maximal virologic response, HIV RNA levels should be measured at least every 3 months as a means of monitoring continued response to therapy. At least two measurements taken at least a week apart should be performed before considering a change. Intra-patient biologic variation in HIV RNA levels may be greater in young children than adults, making it somewhat more difficult to define a significant change in HIV RNA copy number in children. Repeated measurement of HIV RNA levels in a clinically stable, infected adult can vary by as much as 3-fold (0.5 $\log_{10}$) in either direction over the course of a day or on different days; this inherent biologic variability must be considered when interpreting changes in HIV RNA levels over time. In the natural history of perinatal HIV infection, the most rapid decline in plasma HIV RNA levels in untreated infected children occurs in the first 15–24 months of life (average decline, 0.6 $\log_{10}$ per year), with a slower decline until approximately 4–5 years of age (average decline, 0.3 $\log_{10}$ per year) [44, 90, 91]. Therefore, the definition of a significant plasma HIV RNA change for pediatric patients differs by age (see Chapter 5). For children < 2 years old, a change should be > 5-fold (0.7 $\log_{10}$) on repeated testing to be viewed as significant, whereas for children >2 years old, a change >3-fold (0.5 $\log_{10}$) is significant.

22.6 Immunologic considerations for changing therapy

In HIV-infected adults, disease progression risk has been shown to increase directly with baseline plasma HIV RNA concentration and inversely with baseline CD4$^+$ lymphocyte number; at any given HIV RNA level, patients with lower CD4$^+$ counts have poorer prognosis.

Table 22.9 United States Public Health Service guidelines for HIV-infected infants, children, and young adolescents: considerations for changing antiretroviral therapy

Virologic considerations[a]	1. Less than a minimally acceptable virologic response after 8–12 weeks of therapy. For children receiving aggressive antiretroviral therapy, such a response is defined as a less than 10-fold ($1.0 \log_{10}$) decrease from baseline HIV RNA levels.
	2. HIV RNA not suppressed to undetectable levels after 4–6 months of antiretroviral therapy.[b]
	3. Repeated detection of HIV RNA in children who initially had undetectable levels in response to antiretroviral therapy.[c]
	4. Substantial reproducible increase[c] in plasma viremia from the nadir of suppression, defined as:
	• For children < 2 years old, an increase of >5-fold (>$0.7 \log_{10}$) copies/mL.
	• For children ≥2 years old, an increase of >3-fold (>$0.5 \log_{10}$) copies/mL.
Immunologic considerations[a]	1. Change in pediatric CDC immune category.[d]
	2. For children with $CD4^+$ percentage <15% (pediatric CDC immune category 3), a persistent decline of 5% or more in $CD4^+$ cell percentage (e.g. from 15% to 10%).
	3. A rapid and substantial decrease in absolute $CD4^+$ lymphocyte count (e.g. >30% decline <6 months).
Clinical considerations	1. Progressive neurodevelopmental deterioration.
	2. Growth failure defined as persistent decline in weight growth velocity despite adequate nutritional support and without other explanation.
	3. Disease progression, as defined by advancement from one pediatric CDC clinical category to another.[e]

Modified from [1].

[a] At least two measurements (at least 1 week apart) should be performed before considering a change.

[b] The initial HIV RNA level of the child at the start of therapy as well as the level achieved with therapy should be considered when contemplating potential drug changes.

[c] Continued observation with more frequent evaluation of HIV RNA levels should be considered if the HIV RNA increase is limited (i.e. less than 5000 copies/mL). The presence of repeatedly detectable or increasing RNA levels suggests the development of resistance mutations.

[d] Minimal changes in $CD4^+$ percentile that may result in CDC immune category change (e.g. from 26% to 24%, or 16% to 14%) may not be as concerning as a major rapid substantial change in $CD4^+$ percentile within the same immune category (e.g. a drop from 35% to 25% in a short period of time).

[e] In patients with stable immunologic and virologic parameters, progression from one clinical category to another may not in itself represent an indication to change therapy.

Treatment-mediated changes in $CD4^+$ count after 6 months of therapy predict prognosis in adult clinical trials [92]. $CD4^+$ lymphocyte count and plasma HIV RNA also predict disease progression and mortality in children [44–46]. In one pediatric study, there was a 1.3-fold increase in mortality risk, independent of HIV RNA level, for every 5% decline in $CD4^+$ percent [44].

Interpretation of $CD4^+$ lymphocyte changes in pediatric patients is complicated by the normal age-related changes in absolute number; $CD4^+$ lymphocyte percent is more stable and less affected by age (see Chapter 5). Antiretroviral therapy should not be changed due to an apparent decline in $CD4^+$ lymphocyte values unless the change is validated by at least two repeated measurements obtained at least a week apart. Specific immunologic findings that should prompt consideration of a change in therapy for children are shown in Table 22.9.

22.7 Clinical considerations for changing therapy

In infected adults and children, clinical deterioration, defined as a new AIDS-defining diagnosis acquired after treatment is initiated, is an indication for a change in therapy (Tables 22.8 and 22.9). However, if the patient has had a good virologic response to therapy, the appearance of a new opportunistic infection may not reflect a failure of therapy, but persistence of severe immunocompromise. Defects in T cell phenotype (e.g. continued depletion of naive CD4$^+$ cells) and repertoire (e.g. disruption of T cell beta-chain family expression) may persist despite significant increases in CD4$^+$ counts during therapy [93].

As in infected adults, prognosis is poorer in children with more advanced CDC clinical categories [94]. However, in children with stable immunologic and virologic parameters, development of HIV-related infectious complications may not in itself represent an indication to change therapy. In children, involvement of the CNS and growth failure are common manifestations of HIV infection and have been shown to improve with therapy [18, 19, 67]. Thus, deterioration in these latter parameters may be more useful than development of opportunistic infections in determining therapeutic failure in children (Table 22.9). Central nervous system disease is monitored clinically (physical examination and standard neurodevelopmental testing (see Chapter 17), and radiographically (e.g. computerized tomography [CT] or magnetic resonance imaging [MRI]). Persistent or progressive neurologic deterioration is defined as the presence of two or more of the following: impairment in brain growth (e.g. assessed by serial head circumference measurements or neuroimaging); decline of cognitive function documented by psychometric testing; or clinical motor dysfunction. Clinical findings that should prompt consideration of a change in therapeutic regimen in children are shown in Table 22.9.

22.8 Choosing a new antiretroviral regimen

Recommendations for choice of a new antiretroviral regimen differ according to the reason for the change. Reasons for a change in antiretroviral regimen include toxicity or intolerance, and disease progression (virologic, immunologic, or clinical).

22.8.1 When a change is due to toxicity or intolerance

The nature and severity of the toxicity or intolerance are important considerations in decisions about alterations in therapy. In determining the relationship of clinical or laboratory toxicity to antiretroviral therapy, alternative explanations such as HIV-related disease progression, intercurrent infections, or toxicity secondary to concomitant medications must be considered. Severe and potentially fatal toxicities such as pancreatitis, hepatic failure, lactic acidosis, or

severe skin rash or Stevens–Johnson syndrome require discontinuation of therapy. If a child develops an ABC hypersensitivity reaction, ABC should never be restarted since hypotension, renal and respiratory insufficiency, and death have occurred within hours of rechallenge. Similarly, nevirapine should not be restarted in children who experience a severe skin rash; who develop cutaneous bullae or target lesions, mucosal involvement, or symptoms consistent with hypersensitivity; or who have had nevirapine-associated hepatitis. When therapy requires discontinuation, all drugs should be stopped temporarily to avoid development of drug resistance. In such cases, following resolution of the toxicity, restarting the drug regimen with change of a single drug is permissible. The substituted drug should ideally be in a similar class (e.g. substitute one NRTI for another NRTI) but have different toxicity or tolerance characteristics.

However, in the presence of non-life-threatening toxicities in a patient in whom virologic, immunologic, and clinical response are adequate, all efforts should be made to continue the current therapeutic regimen. This should include use of adjunctive therapies that are directed at the observed toxicity, such as erythropoietin and/or transfusions for treatment of anemia, or granulocyte-stimulating factor for neutropenia. Some toxicity may be transient in nature, and therapy may be safely continued with close monitoring (e.g. nausea secondary to therapy with certain PIs), while other toxicities may require only a temporary or permanent reduction in dose. Due to concerns about the development of resistance in the presence of subtherapeutic drug levels, antiretroviral drugs should only be reduced to the lower end of their therapeutic range, and adequacy of continued antiretroviral activity should be confirmed by monitoring HIV RNA levels.

The toxicities of antiretroviral drugs can occur at different frequencies in children and adults and/or have different implications for children. Chapters 18 and 19 detail toxicities observed in pediatric patients with the currently available antiretroviral drugs.

22.8.2 When a change is due to virologic, immunologic, or clinical disease progression

An assessment of adherence problems is important in choosing a new therapeutic regimen. For example, certain drug combinations may be difficult for young infants to take because of requirements regarding food intake. Therefore, other regimens might be preferable (e.g. ddI cannot be given with food due to decreased drug absorption, whereas ritonavir must be taken with food to increase absorption).

When changing therapy, all medications taken by the patient should be reviewed for possible drug interactions with the new regimen. Alterations in drug absorption, distribution, metabolism, or elimination induced by one drug can result in altered pharmacokinetics of one or more other drugs; pharmacodynamic synergy or antagonism between antiretroviral agents could affect toxicity or efficacy. Drugs metabolized by cytochrome P450, such as NNRTIs and protease inhibitors, have particularly significant interactions with many drugs (see Chapter 19).

Antiretroviral history and the impact of change on future treatment are important when choosing a new regimen. Replacement with a regimen containing drugs the child has not previously received would be ideal. However, the number of available drug options may be restricted due to prior antiretroviral drug experience and limited data on pharmacokinetics and safety of some combination regimens in children (e.g. low-dose ritonavir boosted dual PI regimens), and it may not be possible to provide a completely new regimen. In that case, the failing regimen should be changed to incorporate at least two new drugs. Change in or addition of a single drug to a failing regimen is suboptimal and not recommended, as it promotes development of resistance to the new agent. For children failing initial therapy, change in dual NRTI backbone and of the drug class of the third drug (e.g. change of PI to NNRTI, or vice versa) should be feasible. However, there is no consensus about the best approach to salvage therapy for children with more antiretroviral experience. Interchange of NNRTI drugs should be avoided due to cross-resistance. The mutation patterns associated with PI resistance overlap; resistance to one may result in reduced susceptibility to some or all of the other currently available PIs; for example, high-level cross-resistance exists between ritonavir and indinavir.

Data from some but not all studies in adults experiencing virologic failure have demonstrated a modest short-term virologic benefit with use of genotypic or phenotypic resistance testing to guide choice of a new therapeutic regimen compared with clinical judgment alone [96–99]. Resistance testing should be considered in children when changing a failing regimen [1]. However, interpretation of the results can be difficult because the mutations that lead to resistance are not fully understood and there is a potential for cross-resistance to other drugs to be conferred by certain mutations. Additionally, while the presence of viral resistance to a particular drug suggests that the drug is unlikely to successfully suppress viral replication, the absence of resistance to a drug does not ensure that its use will be successful. Consultation with an HIV specialist is advised for interpretation of test results. Resistance assays should be performed while the patient is receiving the drug regimen, because in the absence of drug pressure, wild-type virus is likely to replace resistant strains and mask the presence of resistant virus (see Chapter 21).

For children with extensive prior treatment with all three antiretroviral drug classes, approaches have included the following: continuing the current regimen if partial virologic suppression was achieved and the patient is immunologically and clinically stable; use of "mega-HAART" (treatment with 4–6 antiretroviral drugs in an attempt to overcome resistance and suppress viral replication, often including two NRTIs, an NNRTI and 2–3 PIs); use of "drug holidays" to see if wild-type virus will again predominate (although, since all prior species are archived and can rapidly re-emerge, many would argue that this approach should not be considered); recycling previously tolerated medications; or discontinuing therapy. Data suggest that HIV with multi-drug resistance mutations has reduced replication capacity and pathogenicity compared with wild-type virus. Some patients who have failed multiple antiretroviral drug regimens and have actively replicating, drug-resistant virus have had low rates of clinical progression and stabilization of $CD4^+$ cell numbers if viral load is sustained 0.5 logs below the patient's pretreatment value [99].

22.9 Conclusions

Although the pathogenesis of HIV infection and the general virologic and immunologic principles underlying the use of antiretroviral therapy are similar for all HIV-infected individuals, there are unique considerations for HIV-infected infants, children, and adolescents. Most children acquire HIV infection through perinatal exposure, which raises the possibility of initiating therapy during the period of primary infection if sensitive diagnostic tests are used to determine infection status early in life. Because perinatal infection occurs during the development of the infant immune system, both the clinical manifestations and course of immunologic and virologic markers of infection differ from those in adults. These differences must be taken into consideration when using immunologic and virologic markers for therapeutic decision-making in children. Additionally, changes in drug pharmacokinetics during the transition from the newborn period to adulthood require specific evaluation of drug dosing and toxicities in infants and children. Finally, unique issues related to compliance exist for pediatric patients that need to be addressed to achieve optimal response to therapy.

Guidelines for antiretroviral therapy in children have evolved over time. The initial years of the HIV epidemic, prior to the availability of antiretroviral drugs for children, were characterized by a focus on prevention of opportunistic infections and palliative care. In the early 1990s, antiretroviral drugs were approved for use in children, and monotherapy was shown to provide clinical benefit. As the results of clinical trials became available, dual antiretroviral therapy was shown to further improve clinical outcome. Currently, more complex, multidrug regimens, often including several antiretroviral drug classes, have been shown to provide potent suppression of viral replication, significant immunologic reconstitution, and are associated with dramatic decreases in HIV-related morbidity and mortality in infected children and adults.

What constitutes the most appropriate therapy for an individual child will depend on multiple factors, including potency, complexity, and toxicity of the drug combination, interactions with other drugs the child is taking, the ability of the child and family to adhere to the regimen, and prior antiretroviral treatment. Current US treatment guidelines recommend that antiretroviral therapy be initiated in infected infants under the age of 12 months who have any clinical symptoms of HIV disease or immune suppression, even if these are mild, while therapy could be deferred in children over 12 months with no or mild symptoms and mild immune suppression. Combination therapy, preferably with a potent PI or the NNRTI efavirenz in combination with two NRTIs, is the treatment regimen of choice. In Europe, although guidelines for older children are similar to those in the US, guidelines for infants are more conservative, deferring therapy in infants under the age of 12 months with no or mild symptoms until significant clinical, immunologic, and/or virologic progression is identified. Due to concerns regarding drug resistance, if modification of therapy is required due to clinical, immunologic, or virologic progression, the failing regimen should be changed to include at least two new antiretroviral drugs. Resistance testing prior to changing therapy should be considered to assist in selection of a new regimen in children who have virologic failure. Because treatment recommendations are expected to continually change over time, the healthcare provider is advised to review updated guidelines as they become available.

REFERENCES

1. Centers for Disease Control and Prevention. Guidelines for the use of antiretroviral agents in pediatric HIV infection. *MMWR* **47**: **RR–4**, (1998), 1–43 (updates available at http://AIDSInfo.nih.gov).

2. Centers for Disease Control and Prevention. Guidelines for the use of antiretroviral agents in HIV-infected adults and adolescents. *MMWR* **47**: **RR-5** (1998), 43–82 (updates available at http://AIDSInfo.nih.gov).

3. Sharland, M., Castelli, G., Ramos, J. T., Blanche, S. & Gibb, D. M. PENTA guidelines for the use of antiretroviral therapy in paediatric HIV infection – 2001. Updates available at http://www.ctu.mrc.ac.uk/PENTA.

4. Patella, F. J. Jr., Delaney, K. M., Moorman, A. C. *et al.* Declining morbidity and mortality among patients with advanced human immunodeficiency virus infection. *New Engl. J. Med.* **338** (1998), 853–60.

5. Gortmaker, S. L., Hughes, M., Cervia, J. *et al.* Effect of combination therapy including protease inhibitors on mortality among children and adolescents infected with HIV-1. *New Engl. J. Med.* **345** (2001), 1522–8.

6. De Martino, M., Tovo, P. -A., Balducci, M. *et al.* Reduction in mortality with availability of antiretroviral therapy for children with perinatal HIV-1 infection. *J. Am. Med. Assoc.* **284** (2000), 190–7.

7. Hammer, S. M., Squires, K. E., Hughes, M. D. *et al.* Controlled trial of two nucleoside analogues plus indinavir in persons with human immunodeficiency virus infection and CD4 cell counts of 200 per cubic millimeter or less. AIDS Clinical Trials Group 320 Study Team. *New Engl. J. Med.* **337** (1997), 725–33.

8. Fischl, M. A., Richman, D. D., Grieco, M. H. *et al.* The efficacy of azidothymidine (AZT) in the treatment of patients with AIDS & AIDS-related complex. *New Engl. J. Med.* **317** (1987), 185–91.

9. Idemyor, V. Commentary: Continuing debate over HIV therapy initiation. *HIV Clin. Trials* **3** (2002), 173–6.

10. Volberding, P. A., Lagakos, S. W., Koch, M. A. *et al.* Zidovudine in asymptomatic human immunodeficiency virus infection – a controlled trial in persons with fewer than 500 CD4-positive cells per cubic millimeter. *New Engl. J. Med.* **322** (1990), 941–9.

11. Concorde Coordinating Committee. Concorde: MRC/ANRS randomized, double-blind controlled trial of immediate and deferred zidovudine in symptom-free HIV infection. *Lancet* **343** (1994), 871–81.

12. Pediatric European Network for Treatment of AIDS (PENTA). Five year follow-up of vertically HIV infected children in a randomised double blind controlled trial of immediate verus deferred zidovudine: the PENTA 1 trial. *Arch. Dis. Child.* **84** (2001), 230–6.

13. Mannheimer, S., Friedland, G., Matts, J. *et al.* The consistency of adherence to antiretroviral therapy predicts biologic outcomes for human immunodeficiency virus-infected persons in clinical trials. *Clin. Infect. Dis.* **34** (2002), 1115–21.

14. Paterson, D., Swindells, S., Mohr, J. *et al.* Adherence to protease inhibitor therapy and outcomes in patients with HIV infection. *Ann. Intern. Med.* **133** (2000), 21–30.

15. Bartlett, J. A. Addressing the challenges of adherence. *J. Acquir. Immune Defic. Syndr.* **29** (2002), S2-S10.

16. Van Dyke, R. B., Lee, S., Johnson, G. M. *et al.* Reported adherence as a determinant of response to highly active antiretroviral therapy in children who have human immunodeficiency virus infection. *Pediatrics* **109**: 4 (2002), URL: http://www.pediatrics.org/cgi/content/full/109/e61.

17. Pontali, E., Feasi, M., Toscanini, F. *et al.* Adherence to combination antiretroviral treatment in children. *HIV Clin. Trials* **2** (2001), 466–73.

18. McKinney, R. E., Johnson, G. M., Stanley, K. *et al.* A randomized study of combined zidovudine-lamivudine versus didanosine monotherapy in children with symptomatic therapy-naïve HIV-1 infection. *J. Pediatr.* **133** (1998), 500–8.

19. Englund, J., Baker, C., Raskino, C. *et al.* Zidovudine, didanosine or both as initial treatment for symptomatic HIV-infected children. *New Engl. J. Med.* **336** (1997), 1704–12.

20. Fischl, M. A., Richman, D. D., Hansen, N. *et al.* The safety and efficacy of zidovudine in the treatment of subjects with mildly symptomatic HIV infection: a double-blind, placebo-controlled trial. *Ann. Intern. Med.* **112** (1990), 727–37.

21. Volberding, P. A., Lagakos, S. W., Grimes, J. M. *et al.* The duration of zidovudine benefit in persons with asymptomatic HIV infection – prolonged evaluation of protocol 019 of the AIDS Clinical Trials Group. *J. Am. Med. Assoc.* **272** (1994), 437–42.

22. Pizzo, P. A., Eddy, J., Falloon, J. *et al.* Effect of continuous intravenous infusion of zidovudine (AZT) in children with symptomatic HIV infection. *New Engl. J. Med.* **319** (1988), 889–96.

23. McKinney, R. E., Maha, M. A., Connor, E. M. *et al.* A multicenter trial of oral zidovudine in children with advanced human immunodeficiency virus disease. *New Engl. J. Med.* **324** (1991), 1018–25.

24. Butler, K. M., Husson, R. N., Balis, F. M. *et al.* Dideoxyinosine in children with symptomatic human immunodeficiency virus infection. *New Engl. J. Med.* **324** (1991), 137–44.

25. Lewis, L. L., Venzon, D., Church, J. *et al.* Lamivudine in children with human immunodeficiency virus infection: a phase I/II study. *J. Infect. Dis.* **174** (1996), 16–25.

26. Kline, M. W., Dunkle, L. M., Church, J. A. *et al.* A phase I/II evaluation of stavudine (d4T) in children with human immunodeficiency virus infection. *Pediatrics* **96** (1995), 247–52.

27. Gray, L., Newell, M. L., Thorne, C. *et al.* Fluctuations in symptoms in human immunodeficiency virus-infected children: the first 10 years of life. *Pediatrics*, **108** (2001), 116–22.

28. HIV Paediatric Prognostic Markers Collaborative Study Group. Short-term risk of disease progression in HIV-1-infected children receiving no antiretroviral therapy or zidovudine monotherapy: estimates according to CD4 percent, viral load, and age. *Lancet* **362** (2003), 1605–11.

29. Abrams, E. J., Wiener, J., Carter, R. *et al.* Maternal health factors and early pediatric antiretroviral therapy influence the rate of perinatal HIV-1 disease progression in children. *AIDS* **17** (2003), 867–77.

30. Luzuriaga, K., Bryson, Y., Krogstad, P. *et al.* Combination treatment with zidovudine, didanosine and nevirapine in infants with human immunodeficiency virus type 1 infection. *New Engl. J. Med.* **336** (1997), 1343–9.

31. Luzuriaga, K., McManus, M., Catalina, M. *et al.* Early therapy of vertical HIV-1 Infection: Control of viral replication and absence of persistent HIV-1 specific immune responses. *J. Virol.* **74** (2000), 6984–91.

32. Luzuriaga, K., McManus, M., Mofenson, L. *et al.* A trial of three antiretroviral regimens in HIV-1-infected children. *N. Engl. J. Med.* **350** (2004), 2471–80.

33. Hainault, M., Peltier, C. A., Gerard, M. *et al.* Effectiveness of antiretroviral therapy initiated before the age of 2 months in infants vertically infected with human immunodeficiency virus type 1. *Eur. J. Pediatr.* **159** (2000), 778–82.

34. Faye, A., Bertone, C., Teglas, J. P. *et al.* Early multitherapy including a protease inhibitor for human immunodeficiency virus type 1-infected infants. *Pediatr. Infect. Dis. J.* **21** (2002), 518–25.

35. Altfeld, M., Rosenberg, E. S., Shankarappa, R. *et al.* Cellular immune responses and viral diversity in individuals treated during acute and early HIV-1 infection. *J. Exp. Med.* **193** (2001), 169–80.

36. Markowitz, M., Vesanen, M., Tenner-Racz, K. *et al.* The effect of commencing combination antiretroviral therapy soon after human immunodeficiency virus type 1 infection on viral replication and antiviral immune responses. *J. Infect. Dis.* **179** (1999), 525–37.

37. Carr, A. & Cooper, D. A. Adverse effects of antiretroviral therapy. *Lancet* **356** (2000), 1423–30.

38. Melvin, A. J., Lennon, S., Mohan, K. M. & Purnell, J. Q. Metabolic abnormalities in HIV type 1-infected children treated and not treated with protease inhibitors. *AIDS Res. Hum. Retrovirus.* **17** (2001), 1117–23.

39. Arpadi, S. M., Cuff, P. A., Horlick, M., Wang, J. & Kotler, D. P. Lipodystrophy in HIV-infected children is associated with high viral load and low CD4+-lymphocyte count and CD4+-lymphocyte percentage at baseline and use of protease inhibitors and stavudine. *J. AIDS Hum. Retrovirol.* **27** (2001), 30–4.

40. Mora, S., Sala, N., Bricalli, D., Zuin, G., Chiumello, G., & Vigano, A. Bone mineral loss through increased bone turnover in HIV-infected children treated with highly active antiretroviral therapy. *AIDS* **15** (2001), 1823–9.

41. Cossarizza, A., Pinti, M., Moretti, L. *et al.* Mitochondrial functionality and mitochondrial DNA content in lymphocytes of vertically infected human immunodeficiency virus-positive children with highly active antiretroviral therapy-related lipodystrophy. *J. Infect. Dis.* **185** (2002), 299–305.

42. Brambilla, P., Bricalli, D., Sala, N. *et al.* Highly active antiretroviral-treated HIV-infected children show fat distribution changes even in absence of lipodystrophy. *AIDS* **15** (2001), 2415–22.

43. Galli, L., de Martino, M., Tovo, P. A. *et al.* Predictive value of the HIV paediatric classification system for the long-term course of perinatally infected children. *Int. J. Epidemiol.* **29** (2000), 573–8.

44. Mofenson, L. M., Korelitz, J., Meyer, W. A. *et al.* The relationship between serum human immunodeficiency virus type 1 (HIV-1) RNA level, CD4 lymphocyte percent, and long-term mortality risk in HIV-1-infected children. *J. Infect. Dis.* **175** (1997), 1029–38.

45. Palumbo, P. E., Raskino, C., Fiscus, S. *et al.* Virologic and immunologic response to nucleoside reverse-transcriptase

inhibitor therapy among human immunodeficiency virus-infected infants and children. *J. Infect. Dis.* **179** (1999), 576–83.

46. Palumbo, P. E., Raskino, C., Fiscus, S. *et al.* Predictive value of quantitative plasma HIV RNA and CD4+ lymphocyte count in HIV-infected infants and children. *J. Am. Med. Assoc.* **279** (1998), 756–61.

47. Sharland, M., Gibb, D. & Giaquinto, C. on behalf of the PENTA Steering Committee. Current evidence for the use of paediatric antiretroviral therapy – a PENTA analysis. *Eur. J. Pediatr.* **159** (2000), 649–56.

48. Delta Coordinating Committee. Delta: a randomized, double-blind controlled trial comparing combinations of zidovudine plus didanosine or zalcitabine with zidovudine alone in HIV-infected individuals. *Lancet* **348** (1996), 283–91.

49. Hammer, S. M., Katzenstein, D. A., Hughes, M. D. *et al.* A trial comparing nucleoside monotherapy with combination therapy in HIV-infected adults with CD4 cell counts from 200 to 500 per cubic millimeter. *New Engl. J. Med.* **335** (1996), 1081–90.

50. Hammer, S. M., Squires, K. E., Hughes, M. D. *et al.* A controlled trial of two nucleoside analogues plus indinavir in persons with human immunodeficiency virus infection and CD4 counts of 200 per cubic millimeter or less. *New Engl. J. Med.* **337** (1997), 725–33.

51. Collier, A. C., Coombs, R. W., Schoenfeld, D. A. *et al.* Treatment of human immunodeficiency virus infection with saquinavir, zidovudine and zalcitabine. *New Engl. J. Med.* **334** (1996), 1011–17.

52. Nachman, S. A., Stanley, K., Yogev, R. *et al.* Nucleoside analogs plus ritonavir in s antiretroviral-experienced HIV-infected children – a randomized controlled trial. *J. Am. Med. Assoc.* **283** (2000), 492–8.

53. Eastman, P. S., Shapiro, D. E., Coombs, R. W. *et al.* Maternal viral genotypic zidovudine resistance and infrequent failure of zidovudine therapy to prevent perinatal transmission of human immunodeficiency virus type 1 in pediatric AIDS Clinical Trials Group Protocol 076. *J. Infect. Dis.* **177** : 3 (1998), 557–64.

54. McSherry, G. D., Shapiro, D. E., Coombs, R. W. *et al.* The effects of zidovudine in the subset of infants infected with human immunodeficiency virus type-1 (Pediatric AIDS Clinical Trials Group Protocol 076). *J. Pediatr.*, **134** : 6 (1999), 717–24.

55. Parker, M. M., Wade, N., Lloyd, R. M. Jr. *et al.* Prevalence of genotypic drug resistance among a cohort of HIV-infected newborns. *J. AIDS* **32** : 3 (2003), 292–7.

56. Paediatric European Network for Treatment of AIDS (PENTA). Comparison of dual nucleoside-analogue reverse-transcriptase inhibitor regimens with and without nelfinavir in children with HIV-1 who have not previously been treated: the PENTA 5 randomised trial. *Lancet*, **359** : 9308 (2002), 733–40.

57. Hetherington, S. Understanding drug hypersensitivity: what to look for when prescribing abacavir. *AIDS Reader* **11** (2001), 620–2.

58. Hewitt, R. G. Abacavir hypersensitivity reaction. *Clin. Infect. Dis.* **34** (2001), 1137–42.

59. Carr, A. & Cooper, D. A. Adverse effects of antiretroviral therapy. *Lancet* **356** (2000), 1423–30.

60. Coghlan, M. E., Sommadossi, J.-P., Jhala, N. C. *et al.* Symptomatic lactic acidosis in hospitalized antiretroviral-treated patients with human immunodeficiency virus infection: a report of 12 cases. *Clin. Infect. Dis.* **33** (2001), 1914–21.

61. Saez-Llorens, X., Violari, A., Deetz, C. O. *et al.* Forty-eight-week evaluation of lopinavir/ritonavir, a new protease inhibitor, in human immunodeficiency virus-infected children. *Pediatr. Infect. Dis. J.* **22** : 3 (2003), 216–24.

62. Saez-Llorens, X., Violari, A., Deetz, C. O. *et al.* Forty-eight-week evaluation of lopinavir/ritonavir, a new protease inhibitor, in human immunodeficiency virus-infected children. *Pediatr. Infect. Dis. J.* **22**(3) (2003), 216–24.

63. Krogstad, P., Lee, S., Johnson, G. *et al.* Nucleoside-analogue reverse transcriptase inhibitors plus nevirapine, nelfinavir, or ritonavir for pretreated children infected with human immunodeficiency virus type 1. *Clin. Infect. Dis.* **34** (2002), 991–1001.

64. Wiznia, A., Stanley, K., Krogstad, P. *et al.* Combination nucleoside-analogue reverse transcriptase inhibitor(s) plus nevirapine, nelfinavir, or ritonavir in stable, antiretroviral-experienced HIV-infected children: week 24 results of a randomized controlled trial – PACTG 377. *AIDS Res. Hum. Retrovirus.* **16** (2000), 1113–21.

65. Floren, L. C., Wiznia, A., Hayashi, S. *et al.* Nelfinavir pharmacokinetics in stable human immunodeficiency virus-positive children: Pediatric AIDS Clinical Trials Group protocol 377. *Pediatrics* **112** (2003), e220–227. URL: http://www.pediatrics.org/cgi/content/full/112/3/e220.

66. Van Rossum, A. M. C., Geelen, S. P. M., Hartwig, N. G., *et al.* Results of 2 years of treatment with protease inhibitor-containing antiretroviral therapy in Dutch children infected with human immunodeficiency virus type 1. *Clin. Infect. Dis.* **34** (2002), 1008–16.

67. Verweel, G., van Rossum, A. M. C., Hartwig, N. *et al.* Treatment with highly active antiretroviral therapy in human immunodeficiency virus type 1-infected children is associated with a sustained effect on growth. *Pediatrics* **109** : 2 (2002), E25 URL: http://www.pediatrics.org/cgi/content/full/109/2/e25.

68. Miller, T. L., Mawn, B. E., Orav, E. J. *et al.* The effect of protease inhibitor therapy on growth and body composition in human immunodeficiency virus type 1-infected children. *Pediatrics* **107** : 5) (2001), E77. URL: http://www.pediatrics.org/cgi/content/full/107/5/e77.

69. Jankelevich, S., Mueller, B. U., Mackall, C. L. *et al.* Long-term virologic and immunologic responses in human immunodeficiency virus type 1-infected children treated with indinavir, zidovudine and lamivudine. *J. Infect. Dis.* **183** (2001), 1116–20.

70. Starr, S. E., Fletcher, C. V., Spector, S. A. *et al.* Combination therapy with efavirenz, nelfinavir, and nucleoside reverse transcriptase inhibitors in children infected with human immunodeficiency virus type 1. *New Engl. J. Med.* **341** (1999), 1874–81.

71. Staszewski, S., Morales-Ramirez, J., Tashima, K. *et al.* Efavirnez plus zidovudine and lamivudine, efavirenz plus indinavir, and indinavir plus zidovudine and lamivudine in the treatment of HIV-1 infection in adults. *New Engl. J. Med.* **341** (1999), 1865–73.

72. Friedl, A. C., Ledergerber, B., Flepp, M. *et al.* Response to first protease inhibitor- and efavirenz-containing antiretroviral combination therapy – the Swiss HIV Cohort Study. *AIDS* **15** (2001), 1793–800.

73. Starr, S. E., Fletcher, C. V., Spector, S. A. *et al.* Efavirenz liquid formulation in human immunodeficiency virus-infected children. *Pediatr. Infect. Dis. J.* **21** : 7 (2002) 659–63.

74. Verweel, G., Sharland, M., Lyall, H. *et al.* Nevirapine use in HIV-1-infected children. *AIDS* **17** (2003), 1639–47.

75. Saez-Llorens, X., Nelson, R. P., Emmanuel, P. *et al.* A randomized, double-blind study of triple nucleoside therapy of abacavir, lamivudine, and zidovudine versus lamivudine and zidovudine in previously treated human immunodeficiency virus type 1-infected children. *Pediatrics* **107** (2001), e4. URL: http://www.pediatric.org/cgi/content/full/107/1/e4.

76. Van Rossum, A. M., Dieleman, J. P., Fraaij, P. L. *et al.* Persistent sterile leukocyturia is associated with impaired renal function in human immunodeficiency virus type 1-infected children treated with indinavir. *Pediatrics* **110** : 2 (2002), e19.

77. Cozzi-Lepri, A., Phillips, A. N., d'Arminio Monforte, A. *et al.* Virologic and immunologic response to regimens containing nevirapine or efavirenz in combination with 2 nucleoside analogues in the Italian Cohort Naïve Antiretrovirals (I.Co.N.A.) study. *J. Infect. Dis.* **185** : 8 (2002), 1062–9.

78. Nunez, M., Soriano, V., Martin-Carbonero, L. *et al.* SENC (Spanish efavirenz vs. nevirapine comparison) trial: a randomized, open-label study in HIV-infected naïve individuals. *HIV Clin. Trials* **3**(3) (2002), 186–94.

79. van Leth, F., Phanuphak, P., Ruxrungtham, K. *et al.* Comparison of first-line antiretroviral therapy with regimens including nevirapine, efavirenz, or both drugs, plus stavudine and lamivudine, a randomised open-label trial, the 2NN Study. *Lancet* **363**(9417) (2004), 1253–63.

80. Sulkowski, M. S., Thomas, D. L., Mehta, S. H. *et al.* Hepatotoxicity associated with nevirapine or efavirenz-containing antiretroviral therapy: role of hepatitis C and B infections. *Hepatology* **35** : 1 (2002), 182–9.

81. Saavedra, J., McCoig, C., Mallory, M. *et al.* Clinical experience with triple nucleoside (NRTI) combination ZDV/3TC/abacavir (ABC) as initial therapy in HIV-infected children. In *41st Interscience Conference on Antimicrobial Agents and Chemotherapy.* (September 22–25, 2001, Chicago, IL [Abstract 1941].

82. Wells, C. J., Sharland, M., Smith, C. J. *et al.* Triple nucleoside analogue therapy with zidovudine (AZT), lamivudine (3TC), and abacavir (ABC) in the paediatric HIV London South Network (PHILS-NET) cohort. In *XIV International AIDS Conference.* July 7–12, 2002, Barcelona, Spain [Abstract TuPeB4625].

83. Paediatric European Network for Treatment of AIDS (PENTA). Comparison of dual nucleoside analogue reverse transcriptase inhibitor regimens with and without nelfinavir in children with HIV-1 who have not previously been treated: the PENTA 5 randomised trial. *Lancet* **359** (2002), 733–40.

84. Kline, M. W., Brundage, R. C., Fletcher, C. V. *et al.* Combination therapy with saquinavir soft gelatin capsules in children with human immunodeficiency virus infection. *Pediatr. Infect. Dis. J.* **20** (2001), 666–71.

85. Grub, S., DeLora, P., Ludin, E. *et al.* Pharmacokinetics and pharmacodynamics of saquinavir in pediatric patients with human immunodeficiency virus infection. *Clin. Pharmacol. Ther.* **71** (2002), 122–30.

86. Hoffmann, F., Notheis, G., Wintergerst, U. *et al.* Comparison of ritonavir plus saquinavir- and nelfinavir plus saquinavir-containing regimens as salvage therapy in children with human immunodeficiency virus type 1 infection. *Pediatr. Infect. Dis. J.* **19** (2000), 47–51.

87. Moyle, G. Use of HIV protease inhibitors as pharmacoenhancers. *AIDS Reader* February (2001), 87–98.

88. Church, J. A., Cunningham, C., Hughes, M. *et al.* Safety and antiretroviral activity of chronic subcutaneous administration of T-20 in human immunodeficiency virus 1-infected children. *Pediatr. Infect. Dis. J.* **21** (2002), 653–9.

89. van Rossum, A. M. C., de Groot, R., Hartwig, N. G. *et al.* Pharmacokinetics of indinavir and low-dose ritonavir in children with HIV-1 infection. *AIDS* **14** (2000), 2209–19.

90. Shearer, W. T., Quinn, T. C., LaRussa, P. *et al.* Viral load and disease progression in infants infected with human immunodeficiency virus type 1. *New Engl. J. Med.* **336** (1997), 1337–42.

91. McIntosh, K., Shevitz, A., Zaknun, D. *et al.* Age- and time-related changes in extracellular viral load in children vertically infected by human immunodeficiency virus. *Pediatr. Infect. Dis. J.* **15** (1996), 1087–91.

92. Marschner, I. C., Collier, A. C., Coombs, R. W. *et al.* Use of changes in plasma levels of human immunodeficiency virus type 1 RNA to assess the clinical benefit of antiretroviral therapy. *J. Infect. Dis.* **177** (1998), 40–7.

93. Connors, M., Kovacs, J. A., Krevat, S. *et al.* HIV infection induces changes in CD4+ T-cell phenotype and depletions within the CD4+ T cell repertoire that are not immediately restored by antiviral or immune-based therapies. *Nat. Med.* **3** (1997), 533–40.

94. Barnhart, H. X., Caldwell, M. B., Thomas, P. *et al.* Natural history of human immunodeficiency virus disease in perinatally infected children: an analysis from the Pediatric Spectrum of Disease Project. *Pediatrics* **97** (1996), 710–6.

95. Durant, J., Clevenbergh, P., Halfon, P. *et al.* Drug-resistance genotyping in HIV-1 therapy: the VIRADAPT randomised controlled trial. *Lancet* **353** (1999), 2195–9.

96. Cohen, C. J., Hunt, S., Sension, M. *et al.* A randomized trial assessing the impact of phenotypic resistance testing on antiretroviral therapy. *AIDS* **16** (2002), 579–88.

97. Cingolani, A., Antinori, A., Rizzo, M. G. *et al.* Usefulness of monitoring HIV drug resistance and adherence in individuals failing highly active antiretroviral therapy: a randomized study (ARGENTA). *AIDS* **16** (2002), 369–79.

98. Meynard, J.-L., Vray, M., Morand-Joubert, L. *et al.* Phenotypic or genotypic resistance testing for choosing antitretroviral therapy after treatment failure: a randomized trial. *AIDS* **16** (2002), 727–36.

99. Yeni, P. G., Hammer, S. M., Carpenter, C. C. J. *et al.* Antiretroviral treatment for adult HIV infection in 2002: updated recommendations of the International AIDS Society-USA Panel. *J. Am. Med. Assoc.* **288** (2002), 222–35.

23

Therapeutic drug monitoring

Stephen C. Piscitelli, Pharm.D.

Discovery Medicine – Antivirals, GlaxoSmithKline, Research Triangle Park, NC 27709

Therapeutic drug monitoring (TDM) refers to the adjustment of drug doses based on measured plasma concentrations to attain values within a "therapeutic window." Clinicians have used these principles for years to adjust doses of drugs including theophylline, aminoglycosides, digoxin, and anticonvulsants. However, TDM has not generally been used for monitoring the treatment of chronic infectious diseases. There is growing evidence that TDM may be useful in some circumstances to insure HIV-infected patients have adequate blood concentrations for efficacy without producing toxicity. This may be especially true for children where there is wide variability in plasma concentrations. A number of critical questions remain to be addressed before TDM is used routinely in HIV infection. To this end, several large clinical trials have recently been initiated that may help to define its role.

A number of retrospective studies have demonstrated that plasma concentrations of antiretroviral drugs correlate with antiviral activity [1–4]. It is clear that drug concentrations are an important predictor of response to HIV treatment. However, these findings are quite different than assessing the value of using TDM in the clinic to guide antiretroviral therapy for an individual. This chapter will review the available data, describe which drugs can be monitored, indicate when samples should be collected, and address practical concerns and issues for the clinician.

23.1 Drugs as TDM candidates

Some antiretrovirals share many of the characteristics of drugs that require monitoring of plasma levels, including variable inter-subject pharmacokinetics, serious consequences if there is a lack of effect or drug toxicity, documented relationships between drug concentration and effect or toxicity, identification of a therapeutic range, and the availability of rapid and accurate assays.

Plasma concentrations of protease inhibitors (PIs) may vary by more than 10-fold between individuals receiving the same dose [5]. This is especially true for children who have been shown to have wide inter-patient variability in pharmacokinetic parameters of PIs [6]. There is also a common misconception that boosting with ritonavir (RTV) decreases the inter-patient variability. While the mean concentration has been shown to increase with RTV added, the overall variability remains high [7]. Thus, even with RTV boosting, there will likely be some patients with suboptimal plasma concentrations.

There are obvious serious consequences for patients if plasma concentrations are above or below the optimal range. Sustained low plasma concentrations will invariably lead to the development of resistance and high concentrations may result in toxicity. Since HIV disease is lifelong, it makes sense to use every tool possible to achieve a durable response and avoid adverse effects.

The identification of a therapeutic range remains problematic. Treatment-experienced patients, infected with virus that has high, but not insurmountable levels of resistance to antiretrovirals, are likely to need much higher concentrations for an antiviral response compared with treatment naïve patients. In addition, target concentrations may be different between patients due to demographic factors such as weight and gender. Several laboratories and companies possess large databases of plasma concentrations that could also be used to define a therapeutic range, or at least an expected range of concentrations. There have been attempts to establish "normal ranges" for antiretrovirals based on large data sets but further refinement is warranted.

23.2 Which antiretrovirals are candidates for TDM?

Protease inhibitors and non-nucleoside reverse transcriptase inhibitors (NNRTIs) meet many of the conditions for TDM and could be monitored during therapy. There are many retrospective studies demonstrating that PI concentrations correlate with antiviral activity [1–4]. More recent data also suggest that NNRTI concentrations correlate with effect [8]. The long half-life of NNRTIs combined with their generally high concentrations ensure that most patients with wild-type virus will have therapeutic concentrations even if their adherence is less than perfect. However, TDM for NNRTIs is important because the small percentage of patients with suboptimal levels are at clear risk for the rapid development of resistance and treatment failure, since a single amino acid substitution in reverse transcriptase is sufficient to render the virus highly resistant to currently available NNRTIs. This raises the dilemma of whether all patients should receive TDM to identify the small percentage who will benefit the most.

Nucleoside reverse transcriptase inhibitors (NRTIs) are actually pro-drugs that must be converted intracellularly to their active forms. Thus, the concentration in the plasma does not accurately reflect the concentration of the active moiety at the site of action. While some studies have shown relationships between plasma levels and antiviral effect for NRTIs, findings are generally inconsistent and monitoring of NRTIs is not recommended [9, 10]. However, there may be certain instances such as evaluation of toxicity or adherence when assessment of plasma concentrations would be helpful.

23.3 Unique TDM issues for children

The rapid development and maturation of liver enzyme activity and renal function, combined with changes in body fat and protein, complicate the dosing of HIV-infected children and make plasma concentrations difficult to predict. There may also be differences in drug absorption between children and adults due to changes in gastric pH, gastric emptying time, or other factors. Attempts to dose children by applying pharmacokinetic data from adults have consistently shown poor results. Similarly, dosages based on pharmacokinetic data from older children may not apply

to young children and infants. Clinical trials with nelfinavir and efavirenz using mg/kg doses based on adults have shown that adequate concentrations are often not achieved [11, 12]. In some cases, dosing based on BSA may be more consistent than dosing based on weight. Indinavir has also been shown to require increased doses or shorter dosing intervals in children compared with adults to achieve similar concentrations [13]. For these reasons, a consensus panel on TDM in HIV infection agreed that children represent a population that may benefit the most from TDM [14].

23.4 Clinical trials of TDM

The beneficial role of TDM in HIV clinical practice remains to be demonstrated. Over the past 5 years, a number of studies have described relationships between antiretroviral drug concentrations and antiviral effect. Results from four prospective, randomized trials of TDM in HIV-infected patients have been reported. ATHENA is an ongoing study of 600 patients randomized to TDM or no TDM [15, 16]. In treatment-naïve patients, indinavir and nelfinavir doses were adjusted based on the "concentration ratio," a measure of the patient's drug level compared with the mean expected drug level in the population at any time during the dosage interval. Blood samples were collected at each clinic visit and concentrations were reported back to the physician within 4 weeks. Fifty-five patients receiving indinavir (2/3 boosted with RTU) and 92 patients receiving nelfinavir were randomized to concentration-targeted therapy or standard dosing. Data were analyzed using a non-completer equals failure approach. For indinavir, 75% of patients in the TDM group achieved viral loads < 500 copies/mL at 12 months compared with 48% in the standard dose group (P < 0.05). Improved outcome with TDM for indinavir was primarily driven by reduced toxicity leading to fewer discontinuations while on TDM. For nelfinavir, the TDM group had a higher percentage of patients < 500 copies/mL compared with standard dosing (81% vs 59%; $P < 0.05$), a result primarily due to fewer virological failures in the TDM group. Results in treatment-experienced patients are not yet available.

Conversely, PHARMADAPT, which used trough plasma PI concentrations to modify salvage therapy, did not show a significant improvement in virologic outcomes at 12 weeks [17]. Patients failing therapy with a viral load of > 2000 copies/mL were genotyped and a new regimen was selected. They were then randomized to TDM or standard dosing. Samples were collected at week 4 of the new regimen and reported back at week 8. At week 12, the percentage of patients achieving a viral load < 200 copies/mL was 52% in the standard group and 45% in the TDM group. The lack of a difference may have occurred because only 22% of patients receiving TDM had a modification of PI therapy and because dosage modifications did not occur until 8 weeks into therapy. This may have been too late for an effective intervention; a patient's virus may have developed resistance by that time. In addition, the concentration that inhibits 50% of replication (IC_{50}) for wild-type virus was used as target concentrations in PHARMADAPT, and this target may have been too low in this antiretroviral-experienced population.

A prospective trial in HIV-infected patients evaluated TDM of all drugs in a three-drug regimen [18]. Forty treatment-naïve patients were randomized to receive indinavir, zidovudine, and lamivudine by concentration-guided therapy or per standard fixed doses. Of 33 evaluable patients, 15 of 16 in the TDM arm and 9 of 17 in the standard dose arm had HIV RNA levels < 50 copies/mL at week 52 ($P = 0.017$). Those patients in the TDM arm also reached undetectable viral loads in a significantly shorter period of time. Adverse effects were not different between study groups.

The GENOPHAR study randomized patients failing therapy with viral load > 1000 RNA copies/mL to either treatment based on genotyping or treatment based on genotyping and TDM [19]. An expert committee selected the drug regimen based on the genotype results for both groups, and patients in the TDM arm could have their doses adjusted during the trial. At week 24, the genotype alone group had 34/59 (58%) patients with viral load < 200 copies/mL while 40/61 (66%) of the genotype with TDM patients were undetectable ($P = $ NS).

These clinical trials demonstrate that TDM may be useful in some settings and not others. It is understandable that TDM alone could be useful in treatment-naïve patients where standard doses can achieve high enough concentrations to block replication of wild-type virus. However, in treatment-experienced patients, it is likely that some measurement of the sensitivity of the virus must be used in conjunction with drug levels for optimal treatment. The concept of a monitoring tool that incorporates both plasma concentrations and resistance testing is described below.

23.5 The IQ ratio

Recent studies have evaluated the phenotype or "virtual" phenotype used along with the plasma concentration as a potential tool to optimize drug therapy. The ratio of the Cmin (trough level) to the protein binding-adjusted IC_{50} is

often called the Inhibitory Quotient or IQ. A number of variations in calculating the IQ have been described including the "Virtual IQ" and the "Normalized IQ" [20]. Both of these variations use the fold-change in the sensitivity of the virus compared with wild type from the Virtual Phenotype™ (Virco) test in their equations and attempt to correct for protein binding.

Regardless of the specific equation, a number of small trials have demonstrated relationships between IQ and clinical outcome. Retrospective studies with lopinavir and indinavir have shown a correlation between the Virtual IQ and clinical outcome after 24–48 weeks [21, 22]. These studies identified breakpoints of 2 for indinavir and 15 for lopinavir that were associated with improved clinical outcome. The Virtual IQ has also been shown to be predictive of outcome in PI-experienced patients receiving regimens containing lopinavir, ritonavir, and amprenavir [23–25]. In these studies, resistance testing or drug level measurement alone was not associated with improved outcome, while IQ was predictive. These trials suggest that integration of the drug level and virus susceptibility to the drug may provide more complete information than either measurement used alone. Two large multicenter IQ trials initiated by the AIDS Clinical Trials Group (ACTG) will further evaluate the clinical utility of the IQ ratio in HIV-infected patients and help define which patients will receive the most benefit.

23.6 Plasma levels and toxicity

In contrast to the large number of studies demonstrating relationships between plasma drug concentrations and antiviral activity, there is limited information linking drug levels with toxicity. Indinavir concentrations have been examined in patients experiencing urological complaints compared with a group with no urological adverse events. The indinavir concentration in 14/15 patients with urological complaints was higher than the mean in the control group (n = 14) [26]. A study in subjects receiving a regimen of stavudine, lamivudine, saquinavir, and nelfinavir reported that abdominal pain was associated with higher plasma levels of saquinavir and nelfinavir [27]. Increased concentrations of ritonavir have also been reported to be associated with gastrointestinal complaints [28]. While these data may be intriguing, it remains difficult to use plasma concentrations to predict, avoid, or reduce toxicity. Some clinicians are willing to increase doses based on low drug levels but may be reluctant to decrease the dose if levels are high, for fear of compromising efficacy. It is also important to note that some toxicities, such as hyperlipidemia and fat redistribution, are unlikely to

Table 23.1 Proposed target trough concentrations in treatment-naïve patients

Drug	Concentration (ng/ml)
Protease inhibitors	
Amprenavir	150–400
Indinavir	80–120
Lopinavir/ritonavir	1000–2000
Nelfinavir	700–1000
Ritonavir	1500–2100 (full dose)
Saquinavir	100–250
Non-nucleoside reverse transcriptase inhibitors	
Efavirenz	1000–1100
Nevirapine	3400

Source: Reference [29].

have a definitive dose–response relationship with plasma levels.

23.7 Target concentrations and plasma sampling

Retrospective studies have provided some target concentrations for treatment-naïve patients [29]. Table 23.1 shows general therapeutic ranges that the clinician can use for TDM in treatment-naïve patients. For treatment-experienced patients, these concentrations are likely too low. In the experienced population, plasma concentrations should be used along with resistance testing. A simple method on using drug levels with phenotyping to guide therapy has been described previously [29].

The specific parameter to monitor, whether it be peak, trough, or area under the curve (AUC), has not been adequately defined. There appears to be general agreement that trough concentrations correlate best with antiviral effect. This seems reasonable from a biologic rationale in keeping concentrations of the antiretroviral above a threshold level throughout the dosage interval to avoid any breakthrough replication. The trough is also the easiest to collect from a practical and feasibility standpoint. However, collection of a trough sample relies upon the patient to accurately recall the time of their last dose. Without directly observed dosing, the use of patient-recorded dosing times may lead to a trough concentration that was drawn several hours away from the true trough. Such errors clearly complicate interpretation of drug levels. A definitive study to address this question has not been performed. Data to support the use of the trough concentration for modeling also include in vivo modeling of protease inhibitors and a clinical trial of BID vs TID indinavir [30, 31]. In this study, the BID regimen was inferior in antiviral activity and had lower trough values although the AUCs were similar between the regimens.

Another approach to TDM sampling is the concentration ratio [14]. This method compares the plasma concentration of an individual patient at any time during the dosing interval to a mean value that was determined in subjects who had extensive pharmacokinetic sampling after a directly observed dose. From this control group, a reference concentration-time curve is constructed that can be compared with a patient sample at any time after administration. For example, an individual's sample collected at 4 hours after their last dose would be compared with the mean 4-hour value from the reference group. The patient's dose might be adjusted if the concentration was above or below some predetermined confidence interval of the reference value at 4 hours.

Pharmacokinetic modeling is another method for TDM sampling where one or more concentrations are collected at random times after a dose (i.e. 2 and 4 hours after dosing) [14]. Using a mathematical model and previous information on the drug's pharmacokinetics, the trough concentration can be estimated. This approach has an advantage in that other parameters (AUC, maximum concentration [Cmax], plasma clearance) can also be estimated and used to guide therapy. This method can be very accurate if more than one sample is obtained. The model does require validation and pharmacokinetics expertise for calculation and interpretation. Collection of multiple samples may also be inconvenient for patients and medical staff in a busy clinic.

23.8 Problems, concerns, and unresolved issues

A number of practical and logistical challenges may limit the widespread use of TDM for antiretroviral therapy. A primary limitation of TDM is that it does not provide information on long-term adherence. A patient could not have taken their drugs correctly for weeks, but may do so for the 2 or 3 days immediately before their clinic appointment if they know a TDM sample will be taken. The drug concentration in such a patient would appear to be adequate although the patient may be failing therapy due to non-adherence. Another problem could be the upward adjustment of a dose in a patient who was non-adherent based on low levels and subsequent toxicity when the patient starts to adhere to the new dose. Clearly, a successful TDM program needs to be coupled with adherence monitoring so that plasma concentrations can be accurately interpreted.

Intra-patient variability for key pharmacokinetic parameters also appears to be large for some antiretrovirals, particularly in pediatric populations, suggesting that

Table 23.2 Commercial laboratories that measure antiretroviral concentrations for individual patients

Consolidated Laboratories, Van Nuys, CA
Mayo Clinic, Rochester, MN
National Jewish Hospital, Denver, CO
Specialty Labs, Santa Monica, CA
TDM Service, University of Liverpool, UK

Table 23.3 Clinical situations for therapeutic drug monitoring in HIV-infected patients

Experimental regimens (i.e. Once Daily Dosing)
Confirm adequate concentrations in children
Confirm adequate concentrations in pregnant women
Document levels in patients with organ dysfunction
In conjunction with resistance testing in patients failing therapy (IQ ratio)
Provide additional information in patients experiencing drug toxicity
Evaluation for unknown drug interactions (mega-HAART, enzyme inducers, herbal remedies, etc.)

Table 23.4 Questions to ask before altering a dose based on a TDM result

Did the patient follow the drug's dietary restrictions?
Was the sample collected at the correct time (trough value)?
Has the patient been adherent with his/her therapy?
Was the dose observed or was the dose taken at the correct time?
Is the pill burden of the new regimen reasonable?

clinical decisions should be made only after two or more trough levels are collected and not after a single determination. Intra-patient variability may be large because concentrations can be affected by small changes in diet, time of administration, concomitant illnesses, or other unknown factors. However, intra-patient variability has been reported to be modest when these factors are controlled for, and most importantly, is smaller than inter-patient variability [32].

Logistical issues cannot be ignored in the use of TDM. Currently, there are no rapid tests for antiretroviral drug levels that can be performed in the hospital or clinic. Samples must be shipped to a reference laboratory for measurement. Table 23.2 shows a number of commercial laboratories that measure concentrations of antiretrovirals for a fee. Several academic centers also perform these tests for research purposes. Accurate sample collection, timely processing, storage and shipping of plasma, and rapid turnaround times for assay results must be assured. A more important factor is the quality of the reference laboratory. Since there is no common assay method among laboratories, the clinician needs some assurance that the results being reported back are accurate. An international quality assurance program has been developed whereby participating laboratories received samples with spiked amounts of various PIs and NNRTIs [33]. Laboratories send their results back to a central site and are given a report of how well their method compared with the actual concentrations. A similar program exists for laboratories participating in ACTG trials. Clinicians should select a laboratory that participates in such a program and has demonstrated that it can produce accurate results.

23.9 Practical issues for the clinician

Adjustment of drug doses should only be performed in a thoughtful and methodical manner. The clinician should first identify the reason for the measurement. This could be an inadequate response, dose-limiting toxicity, potential drug interaction, starting a new regimen in a special population (children, pregnant women, patients with organ dysfunction), or others (Table 23.3). In general, TDM should not be used for adherence testing as the concentration only describes the patient's drug administration in the past 1–2 days.

If TDM is to be performed, the sample should be collected at steady-state which generally is at least 2 weeks into a new regimen. The time of the patient's last dose should be recorded and a trough sample should be collected. The sample should be sent to a TDM laboratory following the processing and shipping instructions of the specific facility.

When the patient's concentration is reported, clinicians should carefully consider several factors before adjusting the dose (Table 23.4). These include an understanding of the patient's adherence, the current pill burden, and the quality of the sample collection. The dosage change should not be dramatic and limited to a 15–20% increase in the dose of the drug or the addition a second drug such as low-dose ritonavir to optimize the pharmacokinetics. The drug level should be repeated in 2–4 weeks to evaluate the change. It is important to note that TDM in clinical practice is mainly focused on PIs, however, concentrations of NNRTIs have also been reported to correlate with outcome [8].

23.10 Conclusion

There is increasing interest in TDM as a tool for improving therapy for HIV-infected patients. A number of trials have shown that TDM is both feasible and can improve outcomes, however, large randomized trials are ongoing and will provide more definitive answers. The treatment of HIV-infected patients is complicated. It is critical to understand that successful TDM programs cannot exist by themselves but must be used in conjunction with other interventions such as adherence counseling, management of adverse effects, resistance testing, and treatment of concomitant illnesses.

REFERENCES

1. Burger, D. M., Hoetelmans, R. M. W., Hugen, P. W. H. et al. Low plasma concentrations of indinavir are related to virological treatment failure in HIV-1 infected patients on indinavir-containing triple therapy. Antiviral. Ther. 3 (1998), 315–20.

2. Durant, J., Clevenbergh, P., Garraffo, R. et al. Importance of protease inhibitor plasma levels in HIV-infected patients treated with genotypic-guided therapy: pharmacological data from the Viradapt study. AIDS 14 (2000), 1333–9.

3. Hoetelmans, R. M. W., Reijers, M. H., Weverling, G. J. et al. The effect of plasma drug concentrations on HIV-1 clearance rate during quadruple drug therapy. AIDS 12 (1998), F111–15.

4. Schapiro, J. M., Winters, M. A., Stewart, F. et al. The effect of high-dose saquinavir on viral load and CD4+ T-cell counts in HIV-infected patients. Ann. Intern. Med. 124 (1996), 1039–50.

5. Acosta, E. P., Henry, K., Weller, D. et al. Indinavir concentrations and antiviral effect. Pharmacotherapy 19 (1999), 708–12.

6. Acosta, E. P., Nachman, S., Wiznia, A., et al. Pharmacokinetic evaluation of nelfinavir in combination with nevirapine or ritonavir in HIV infected children. In 40th Interscience Conference on Antimicrobial Agents and Chemotherapy, September 17–20, 2000, Toronto, Canada [Abstract 1642].

7. Gibbons, E. S., Reynolds, H. E., Tija, J. F. et al. The Liverpool therapeutic drug monitoring service – a summary of the service and examples of use in clinical practice. 5th International Congress on Drug Therapy in HIV infection. AIDS 14 (Suppl. 4) (2000), S89.

8. Marzolini, C., Telenti, A., Decosterd, L. A. et al. Efavirenz plasma levels can predict treatment failure and central nervous system side effects in HIV-1-infected patients. AIDS 15 (2001), 71–5.

9. Drusano, G. L., Yuen, G. J., Lambert, J. S., Seidlin, M., Dolin, R. & Valentine, F. T. Relationship between dideoxyinosine exposure, CD4 counts, and p24 antigen levels in human immunodeficiency virus infection. A phase I trial. Ann. Intern. Med. 116 (1992), 562–6.

10. Hoetelmans, R. M., Burger, D. M., Meenhorst, P. L. & Beijnen, J. H. Pharmacokinetic individualisation of zidovudine therapy. Current state of pharmacokinetic-pharmacodynamic relationships. Clin. Pharmacokinet. 30 (1996), 314–27.

11. Brundage, R. C., Fletcher, C. V., Fenton, T. et al. Efavirenz and nelfinavir pharmacokinetics in HIV infected children under 2 years of age. In 7th Conference on Retroviruses and Opportunistic Infections. February 2000, San Francisco, CA [Abstract 719].

12. Rongkavilit, C., Van Heeswijk, R. P. G., Risuwanna, P. et al. The safety and pharmacokinetics of nelfinavir in a dose escalating study in HIV-1 exposed newborn infants. HIV-NAT 007. In 2nd International Workshop on Clinical Pharmacology of HIV Therapy. April 2001, Nordwijk, the Netherlands [Abstract 3.1].

13. Fletcher, C. V., Brundage, R. C., Remmel, R. P. et al. Pharmacological characteristics of indinavir, didanosine, and stavudine in human immunodeficiency infected children receiving combination therapy. Antimicrob. Agents Chemother. 44 (2000), 1029–34.

14. Back, D., Gatti, G., Fletcher, C. et al. Therapeutic drug monitoring in HIV infection: current status and future directions. AIDS 16 (Suppl. 1) (2002), S5-37.

15. Burger, D. M., Hugen, P. W. H., Droste, J. et al. Therapeutic drug monitoring of indinavir in treatment naïve patients improves therapeutic outcome after 1 year: results from ATHENA. In 2nd International Workshop on Clinical Pharmacology of HIV Therapy, April 2–4, 2001, Noordwijk, the Netherlands [Abstract 6.2a].

16. Burger, D. M., Hugen, P. W. H., Droste, J. et al. Therapeutic drug monitoring of nelfinavir 1250 bid in treatment naïve patients improves therapeutic outcome after 1 year: results from ATHENA. In 2nd International Workshop on Clinical Pharmacology of HIV Therapy, April 2–4, 2001, Noordwijk, the Netherlands [Abstract 6.2b].

17. Clevenbergh, P., Durant, J., Garraffo, R. et al. Usefulness of protease inhibitor therapeutic drug monitoring? PharmAdapt: A prospective multicentric randomized controlled trial: 12 week results. In 8th Conference on Retroviruses and Opportunistic Infections Feb 4–8, 2001, Chicago, IL, [Abstract 260B].

18. Fletcher, C. V., Anderson, P. L., Kakuda, T. N. et al. Concentration-controlled compared with conventional antiretroviral therapy for HIV infection. AIDS 16 (2002), 551–60.

19. Bossi, P., Peytavin, G., Delaugerre, C. et al. GENOPHAR: A randomized study of plasmatic drug measurements associated with genotypic resistance testing in patients failing antiretroviral therapy. In 9th Conference on Retroviruses and Opportunistic Infections. February 24–27, 2002, Seattle, WA [Abstract 585-T].

20. Piscitelli, S. C. The role of therapeutic drug monitoring in the management of HIV-infected patients. Curr. Infect. Dis. Rep. 4 (2002), 353–8.

21. Kempf, D., Hsu, A., Isaacson, J. et al. Evaluation of the inhibitory quotient as a pharmacodynamic predictor of the virological response to protease inhibitor therapy. In 2nd International Workshop on Clinical Pharmacology of HIV Infection. April 2–4, 2001, Noordwijk, the Netherlands [Abstract 7.3].

22. Kempf, D., Hsu, A., Jiang, P. *et al.* Response to ritonavir intensification in indinavir recipients is highly correlated with inhibitory quotient. In *8th Conference on Retroviruses and Opportunistic Infections*, February 4–8, 2001, Chicago, IL [Abstract 523].

23. Phillips, E., Tseng, A., Walker, S. *et al.* The use of virtual inhibitory quotient in antiretroviral experienced patients taking amprenavir/lopinavir combinations. In *9th Conference on Retroviruses and Opportunistic Infections*, February 24–28, 2002, Seattle, WA [Abstract 130].

24. Piscitelli, S. C., Metcalf, J. A., Hoetelmans, R. H. *et al.* Relative inhibitory quotient is a significant predictor of outcome for salvage therapy with amprenavir plus either ritonavir or nelfinavir plus amprenavir. In *8th ECAAC*, Athens, Greece (2002).

25. Castagna, A., Danise, A., Hasson, H. *et al.* The normalized inhibitory quotient of lopinavir is predictive of viral load response over 48 weeks in a cohort of highly experienced HIV-1 infected individuals. In *9th Conference on Retroviruses and Opportunistic Infections* February 24–28, 2002 Seattle, WA [Abstract 128].

26. Dieleman, J. P., Gyssens, I. C., van der Ende, M. E., de Marie, S. & Burger, D. M. Urological complaints in relation to indinavir plasma concentrations in HIV-infected patients. *AIDS* **13** (1999), 473–8.

27. Reijers, M. H., Weigel, H. M., Hart, A. A. *et al.* Toxicity and drug exposure in a quadruple drug regimen in HIV-1 infected patients participating in the ADAM study. *AIDS* **14** (2000), 59–67.

28. Gatti, G., Di Biagio, A., Casazza, R. *et al.* The relationship between ritonavir plasma levels and side-effects: implications for therapeutic drug monitoring. *AIDS* **13** (1999), 2083–9.

29. Acosta, E. P. & Gerber, J. G. Position paper on therapeutic drug monitoring of antiretroviral agents. *AIDS Res. Hum. Retrovirus.* **18** (2002), 825–34.

30. Drusano, G., D'Aregenio, D., Preston, S. *et al.* Use of drug effect interaction modelling with Monte Carlo Simulation to examine the impact of dosing interval on the projected antiviral activity of the combination abacavir and amprenavir. *Antimicrob. Agents Chemother.* **44** (2000), 1655–9.

31. Haas, D. W., Arathoon, E., Thompson, M. A. *et al.* Comparative studies of two-times daily versus three times daily indinavir in combination with zidovudine and lamivudine. *AIDS* **14** (2000), 1973–8.

32. Acosta, E. P., Kakuda, T. N., Brundage, R. C. *et al.* Pharmacodynamics of human immunodeficiency virus type 1 protease inhibitors. *Clin. Infect. Dis.* **30** (Suppl. 2) (2000), S151–9.

33. Aarnouste, R., Burger, D., Verweij-Van Wissen, C. *et al.* An international interlaboratory quality control program for therapeutic drug monitoring in HIV infection. In *8th Conference on Retroviruses and Opportunistic Infections*. February 4–8, 2001, Chicago, IL [Abstract 734].

HIV postexposure prophylaxis for pediatric patients

Kenneth L. Dominguez, M.D., M.P.H.

Division of HIV/AIDS Prevention, Centers for Disease Control and Prevention, Atlanta, GA

24.1 Background

Postexposure prophylaxis (PEP) refers to the timely administration of antiretroviral (ARV) chemoprophylaxis to reduce the probability of becoming infected with HIV after an acute well-defined exposure. PEP can be categorized as occupational (oPEP) or non-occupational (nPEP). This chapter summarizes the epidemiology of various types of HIV exposures, including strategies for preventing these exposures and recent findings from animal and human studies which lend support for the use of oPEP and nPEP, reviews current United States Public Health Service (USPHS) recommendations for oPEP and nPEP, and addresses special considerations regarding nPEP for pediatric patients. Prevention of mother-to-child transmission (MTCT) of HIV is addressed in Chapter 8. The USPHS oPEP recommendations continue to recommend a two-tiered system of three ARVs vs two ARVs, depending on level of risk. The chapter highlights a change in the USPHS nPEP recommendations, which now emphasize the importance of using three-drug regimens, when feasible, for all exposures that warrant PEP in order to be consistent with the current standard of care regarding treatment of established HIV infection.

24.1.1 Occupational postexposure prophylaxis

For the purposes of this chapter, healthcare personnel (HCP) are defined as persons whose activities involve contact with patients or with patients' blood or other body fluids in a healthcare, laboratory, or public-safety setting [1]. Occupational exposures that could place HCP at risk for HIV infection include: (a) percutaneous injury (e.g. a needlestick or cut with a sharp object); or (b) contact of mucous membrane or non-intact skin (e.g. exposed skin that is chapped, abraded, or afflicted with dermatitis) with blood, tissue, or other body fluids that are potentially infectious. Non-intact skin exposures with potentially infectious body materials are not considered to be of risk except for direct contact (i.e. without barrier protection) with concentrated HIV in a research laboratory or production facility. Other body fluids include: (a) semen, vaginal secretions, or other body fluids contaminated with visible blood that have been implicated in the transmission of HIV infection; and (b) fluids with an undetermined risk of HIV transmission, i.e. cerebrospinal, synovial, pleural, peritoneal, pericardial, and amniotic fluids [1]. In the absence of visible blood in the fluid or substance, exposure to saliva, tears, sweat, urine, or feces is not considered to pose a risk for HIV transmission and does not require postexposure follow-up. Although mother-to-child transmission (MTCT) of HIV can occur through breastfeeding [2], exposure to breast milk has not been implicated in occupational transmission of HIV.

24.1.2 Non-occupational postexposure prophylaxis

Examples of non-occupational exposures to HIV include exposure to HIV through unprotected sex or through sharing needles with HIV-infected persons. More common pediatric consultations for nPEP involve sexual abuse or exposure to discarded needles.

24.1.3 Studies of the biologic plausibility of PEP

In 1990, the USPHS published the first statement on oPEP [3]. Because of lack of convincing data on the efficacy of

PEP at the time, this statement did not recommend or discourage PEP, but rather outlined considerations surrounding the possible use of zidovudine (ZDV) for PEP. Since then, additional data provide a rationale for HIV PEP in both occupational and non-occupational settings, including information regarding primary HIV pathogenesis, the biological plausibility of the effectiveness of ARV drug administration for the PEP, and the effectiveness of ARV drugs for PEP in animal and human studies [1].

Primary HIV pathogenesis and biological plausibility of PEP effectiveness

In a primate model of simian immunodeficiency virus (SIV), SIV infection was limited to dendritic-like cells at the site of SIV inoculation during the first 24 hours, moved to regional lymph nodes over the next 24–48 hours, and reached the peripheral blood within 5 days [4]. It seems biologically plausible that PEP, if started within hours after HIV exposure, could prevent spread of infection beyond the initially infected cells or lymph nodes.

Effectiveness of PEP in animal and human studies

Animal and human data support the biological plausibility of the effectiveness of HIV nPEP, and suggest nPEP can be justified as an intervention to reduce the probability of becoming infected with HIV after an acute, well-defined exposure. Animal models of the effectiveness of PEP vary by: type of animal, type of virus, route and strength of inoculation, drug used for PEP, and the number, timing, and duration of doses of PEP (Table 24.1). Most studies inoculated macaque primate models with SIV either intravenously or orally. All studies initiated PEP between 24 hours pre-exposure and 72 hours postexposure, and most used more than one dose of a single ARV drug such as ZDV or (R)-9-(2-phosphonylmethoxypropyl) adenine (PMPA or tenofovir) at varying time points of up to 28 days after exposure. All studies exhibited a range of effectiveness in preventing infection, or decreasing the severity of the initial infection, depending on the specific characteristics of the model. For example, two studies that did not demonstrate effectiveness of PEP in preventing infection were associated with decreased severity of infection (as evidenced by decreased initial viremia, decreased antigenemia, and/or preservation of CD4$^+$ cell counts) if PEP was started within a few hours of exposure [7, 13]. Other studies have shown similar responses as evidenced by slower disease progression after infection or less severe initial infection despite the presence of drug-resistant viral strains [12, 16]. In general, early initiation of PEP within a few hours of exposure was associated with the highest effectiveness.

Human studies have been primarily observational. A case control study evaluated HIV seroconversion in HCP in the USA, France, and the UK with percutaneous exposure (i.e. needlestick or cut with a sharp object) to HIV-infected blood [17, 18]. Cases had HIV seroconversion temporally associated with the exposure and no other concurrent exposure to HIV. Controls had a documented occupational percutaneous exposure to HIV-infected blood and were HIV seronegative through at least 6 months after exposure. Postexposure prophylaxis (consisting of 1000 mg/day of ZDV for 3–4 weeks) was received by 9 of 33 (27%) cases, and 247 of 679 (36%) of controls. Risk factors for HIV transmission included characteristics of both the exposures (e.g. those involving large quantities of blood) and of the source patient (e.g. having terminal HIV-related illness) (Table 24.2). After controlling for other factors, the likelihood of HIV infection among HCP who received PEP with ZDV was approximately 81% lower than among those who did not receive such PEP. Observational studies and registries designed to collect information about nPEP are being conducted and established. Among registries in the USA, France, Switzerland, and Australia, no seroconversions have been reported among 350 individuals who received nPEP after exposure to HIV. Such results could be attributable to the low risk for seroconversion associated with nonoccupational exposures (Centers for Disease Control and Prevention (CDC), unpublished data). Limited data regarding PEP of infants to prevent MTCT exist (see Chapter 8).

24.1.4 Studies of nPEP in pediatric practice

Few data exist regarding PEP in pediatric patients. In 1998, a nPEP survey of pediatric infectious disease and pediatric emergency medicine departments was conducted [19]. Less than 20% of physicians reported institutional policies for HIV nPEP and 33% had ever initiated HIV nPEP in their patients. In another study, eight of ten pediatric and adolescent patients offered HIV nPEP in an urban academic pediatric emergency department were started on nPEP. Only two patients (40%) completed the full course of 4 weeks of nPEP and only five of the ten (50%) returned for follow-up testing between 4–28 weeks after exposure [20]. Financial concerns, side-effects, additional psychiatric and substance abuse issues as well as the degree of parental involvement influenced whether PEP and HIV follow-up testing was completed. The authors conclude that any successful PEP program should include psychosocial support, HIV-related community resources, early follow-up with a physician knowledgeable about pediatric ARV therapy to

Table 24.1 Selected animal models of postexposure prophylaxis (PEP)

Authors	Animal	Virus	Route of inoculation	PEP regimen	Time of initiation of PEP		Percent effectiveness by time of initiation	Duration of PEP	Percent effectiveness by duration	Decrease in severity of infection
					Pre-exposure	Postexposure				
McClure et al. [5]	Macaque	SIV	IV	ZDV	None	1 hour 24–72 hour	33% 0%	14 days		Yes, death delayed
Shih et al. [6]	Mouse	HIV/SCID	IV	ZDV	None	30 min, 1–2 hours 8, 24, 36 hours 48 hours	100% <100% 0%	14 days		
Martin et al. [7]	Macaque	SIV	IV	ZDV	None	1, 8,24,72 hours	0%			
Bottiger et al. [8]	Macaque	SIV	IV	BEA-005	None	8 hours 24 hours 3–6 days	100% 50% 0%	3 days		
Tsai et al. [9]	Macaque	SIV	IV	PMPA	None	4, 24 hours 48, 72 hours	100% <100%	3, 10 days 28 days	<100% 100%	
Van Rompay et al. [10]	Macaque	SIV	Oral	PMPA	2 hours	Immediate	0% 75%	13 days		
Van Rompay et al. [11]	Macaque	SIV	Oral	PMPA	4 hours	20 hours	40%	28 days		Yes, 60% delayed viremia
Van Rompay et al. [12]	Macaque	SIV	Oral	PMPA	24 hours	Every day (first 2 days) Every day (≥ 3rd day)	100% <100%	28 days		
Le Grand et al. [13]	Macaque	SHIV	IV	ZDV+3TC+IDV	None	4 hours	0%	28 days		Yes, decreased viral load and preserved CD4+ cells
Otten et al. [14]	Macaque	HIV-2	Intra-vaginal	PMPA	None	12, 36 hours 72 hours	100% 75%	28 days		Yes, decreased viral load
Van Rompay et al. [15]	Macaque	SIV	Oral	PMPA	4 hours 1 hour	20 hours 25 hours 1 hour	75% 50% 100%			

Table 24.2 Logistic regression analysis of risk factors for HIV transmission after percutaneous exposure to HIV-infected blood[a]

Risk factor	Adjusted odds ratio	(95% confidence interval)
Deep injury	15	(6.0–41)
Visible blood on device	6.2	(2.2–21)
Procedure involving needle in a vein or artery	4.3	(1.7–12)
Terminal illness in source patient	5.6	(2.0–16)
Postexposure use of zidovudine	0.19	(0.06–0.52)

[a] *Source*: Reference [18].

assess compliance, and a written institutional protocol to provide a co-ordinated and standardized approach.

In a similar study at another urban academic pediatric medical center, seven pediatric and adolescent patients were offered nPEP with ZDV and 3TC after sexual assault, three (47%) had 98% compliance with total days of therapy, and four of seven returned for testing through 6 months postexposure and were HIV-uninfected [21]. The side-effects reported included abdominal pain and transient anemia. The authors recommend a well-structured specialized program to manage sexual assault nPEP and the associated follow-up.

24.2 Epidemiology of exposures to HIV

24.2.1 Exposures among HCP

The average risk for HIV infection for HCP exposed to HIV-infected blood has been estimated at 0.3% for percutaneous exposures [22], and 0.09% for mucous membrane exposures [23]. The risk is unknown for skin exposures, but is thought to be less than that for mucous membrane exposures [24]. As of December 31, 2002, the CDC has received reports of 57 USA. HCP with documented HIV seroconversion temporally associated with occupational HIV exposure and has been informed of an additional 139 HCP who report occupationally acquired HIV infection without such documentation [25].

The risk of HIV transmission from exposures that involve a larger volume of blood, especially when the source patient's viral load is probably high, is estimated to exceed the average risk of 0.3% [26].

There are very limited epidemiological data on the most common exposures to blood for HCP in pediatric health-care settings. One study in a pediatric healthcare facility reported 113 sharp object injuries (SOIs) (six injuries/100 employees/year) [27]. Most SOIs involved needles (71%) and contamination with blood or body fluid (88%). Nurses and physicians experienced the highest percentage of SOIs (46% and 23%, respectively), and phlebotomists experienced the highest rate of SOIs at 25.5 injuries per 100 full-time equivalent employees per year. Of 88 known source patients, one tested positive for hepatitis B virus (HBV) surface antigen, two for hepatitis C virus (HCV), and none for HIV. A study involving 74 hospitals between 1993 and 1995 documented 50 human bite exposures among HCP per 41 677 occupied hospital beds for a rate of 12 human bite exposures per 10 000 occupied hospitals beds per year [28]. Ten of 28 incidents in which descriptions of bites were available involved children. None of the injuries involving blood resulted in HIV seroconversion.

Prevention

Measures to prevent occupational HIV exposures include strict adherence to standard precautions [29] and Office of Safety and Health (OSHA) guidelines [30]. Examples include the use of safer medical devices where appropriate [31], properly restraining patients when drawing lab samples, being well trained in doing procedures involving sharps, and using gloves when managing patients who might be combative, or when manipulating the oral cavity [28]. The use of gloves for handling breast milk is not necessary except in situations where exposures to breast milk might be frequent, as in breast milk banking [32], or if the HCP has non-intact skin.

24.2.2 Exposures among children in healthcare settings

Children are present in hospitals either as patients or visitors and are subject to situations that could place them at risk for HIV infection. There have been case reports of children that were probably exposed inadvertently to blood from an HIV infected person in the hospital or during in-home healthcare [33, 34]. One child suffered laceration to the inside of oral mucosa after biting through a glass blood sample tube filled with blood from an adult patient with a history of injecting drug use but unknown HIV-infection status [35]. Newborns have been inadvertently fed the expressed breast milk intended for another infant [35–36]. An infant was inadvertently taken to the wrong mother to be breast fed while in the hospital [37]. Such exposures to breast milk would generally be considered to carry a low risk for HIV exposure unless the hospital is located in a geographic area with a high seroprevalence in women of child-bearing age.

Prevention

Measures to prevent pediatric exposures to HIV in health-care settings include rapid disposal of used needles in sharps containers located out of the reach of children but readily accessible to HCP [38], and use of standard procedures for labeling and dispensing bottles of expressed breast milk. Healthcare institutions may consider adapting existing recommendations related to bottles of expressed breast milk designed for day-care centers to hospital settings (Box 24.1) [39]. A bottle of expressed breast milk which has been properly labeled with the mother's and infant's hospital identifiers should always be checked against the infant's identification bracelet prior to bottle feedings of expressed breast milk. In addition, healthcare institutions which allow feeding of infants with human donor milk should use donor milk banks that adhere to existing state laws or regulations or national guidelines that insure proper screening of donors and sterilization of milk [40–42].

24.2.3 Exposures among children outside of the healthcare setting

Children can be exposed to HIV outside of the hospital setting. Examples of such exposures include sexual abuse involving oral, anal, or vaginal penetration by an HIV-infected perpetrator, needlesticks in the home or public areas with recently discarded syringes containing HIV-infected blood, exposures to HIV-containing breast milk, and human bites that compromise the skin's integrity and involve an exchange of HIV-infected blood.

Sexual abuse

There were 88 238 cases of various types of sexual abuse in children less than 18 years of age reported in the USA during 1999 [43], including 26 cases of sexual abuse (17 confirmed, 9 suspected) among children with AIDS [44]. These cases probably represent an underestimate due to the under-reporting of such abuse.

Among adults, the probability of HIV transmission associated with a single act of unprotected receptive anal intercourse has been estimated to be between 0.008 to 0.032 [45] and associated with vaginal intercourse to be between 0.0005 and 0.0015 [46–48]. The medical literature suggests that child sexual abuse may be a more efficient means of transmitting HIV than adult sexual abuse because of differences in thickness of vaginal epithelium [49], higher frequency of repeated molestations, particularly by a

---

Box 24.1. Preventing and managing bottle switches in day-care centers

[adapted from Ref. 39]

1. Make sure that parents label each child's bottle of formula or breast milk with the child's name and the date
   - Only use a bottle labeled for that child on that date
   - Never accept an unlabeled bottle from a parent
   - Do not use any unlabeled bottles that have been accidentally accepted
2. In the event that a child has mistakenly been given another child's bottle of expressed breast milk, do the following:
   - Inform the parents of the child who was given the wrong bottle that:
     - Their child was given another child's bottle of expressed breast milk
     - The risk of transmission of HIV is very small (see discussion below)
     - They should notify the child's physician of the exposure
     - The child should have a baseline test for HIV
   - Inform the mother who expressed the breast milk of the bottle switch, and ask:
     - If she has ever had an HIV test and, if so, if she would be willing to share the results with the parents
     - If she does not know if she has ever had an HIV test, if she would be willing to contact her obstetrician and find out and, if she has, share the results with the parents
     - If she has never had an HIV test, if she would be willing to have one and share the results with the parents and
     - When the breast milk was expressed and how it was handled prior to being brought to the facility
   - Provide the exposed child's physician with information on when the milk was expressed and how the milk was handled prior to being brought to the facility.
3. Risk of HIV transmission from expressed breast milk drunk by another child is believed to be low because:
   - In the USA, women who are HIV-infected and aware of that fact are advised not to breast feed their infants
   - Chemicals present in breast milk act, together with time and cold temperatures, to destroy the HIV present in expressed breast milk

parent [50] or multiple perpetrators [51], and longer-term abuse in children [52].

Any child that has been sexually assaulted should be assessed within 72 hours of sexual assault [53]. The clinician should: (a) review the local HIV/AIDS epidemiology and assess risk for HIV infection in the assailant; (b) evaluate circumstances of the assault that may affect risk for HIV transmission; (c) consult with an HIV specialist if considering PEP; (d) discuss PEP, including its toxicity and unknown efficacy with the caregiver; (e) if indicated, provide enough medication to last until the return visit 3–7 days later at which time the child can be re-evaluated, including his/her tolerance of the medication (if PEP is prescribed); and (f) perform HIV testing at baseline and then at 6 weeks, 3 months, and 6 months later.

The following situations are associated with a high risk of transmission of sexually transmitted infections (STIs), and HIV testing should be performed if: (a) one or more children in a household has signs or symptoms of an STI; (b) the suspected assailant is known to have a STI, or to be at high risk for STIs (e.g. the individual has multiple sexual partners or a history of STIs); (c) the patient or his/her parent(s) requests testing; (d) there is a high prevalence of STIs in the community; (e) there is evidence of genital, oral, or anal penetration or ejaculation; or (f) the assault involved traumatic mucosal injuries of the anus or vagina, associated with bleeding and contact with the semen of a known HIV-infected assailant. An example of a lower risk exposure is the sexual abuse of a child by a perpetrator with unknown HIV infection status in an area with low HIV seroprevalence.

Prevention

Examples of strategies to prevent the sexual abuse of children include: (1) educating caretakers about teaching children to refuse to engage in abusive situations, to avoid keeping secrets related to abuse, and to disclose abusive situations to someone who is trusted; and (2) educating parents to select day-care centers with licensed day-care workers, open and visible play areas, and policies that allow parental visitation and do not allow for individual instruction in isolated settings [54].

Breast milk exposures

Globally, breast-milk transmission of HIV represents an important mode of MTCT of HIV. In the USA, exposure to breast milk from an unknown or unscreened source is unlikely to result in HIV transmission but each exposure must be considered on a case-by-case basis. Such exposures may occur through the switching or mislabeling of bottles containing expressed breast milk (e.g. in day-care settings), or allowing an infant to breastfeed from a wet nurse with unknown HIV infection status, or using expressed, unpasteurized human milk that has not been screened for HIV. The likelihood that HIV is present in the breast milk of an unknown or unscreened source is low in the USA because the seroprevalence of HIV among pregnant women has been estimated at less than 2 per 1000 [55]. The USPHS guidelines recommended that pregnant woman undergo HIV testing and that HIV-infected women should not breast feed their infants [56]. The risk of such an exposure would increase if the source individual is determined to have a history of behaviors that put her at risk for HIV transmission or comes from a community with a high HIV seroprevalence.

Prevention

Based on the 2001 CDC guidelines, prenatal HIV testing should be offered to all pregnant women and routine rapid HIV testing should be offered to all pregnant women whose HIV status is still unknown at the time of delivery [57]. HIV-infected mothers in resource-rich settings should be counseled to avoid breastfeeding, and clinicians should provide education to HIV-infected mothers regarding feeding options. Every effort should be made to avoid exposure to HIV-contaminated breast milk. Other prevention strategies are listed in the section on pediatric exposures in healthcare settings.

Discarded needles or syringes

The risk of HIV transmission from discarded needles in public places is thought to be low [58]. It is estimated that the probability of HIV transmission associated with a puncture wound involving a known HIV-contaminated needle in a healthcare setting is 0.0032 [59–60]. It is likely that discarded needles in outdoor public settings have a lower risk for transmission due to the effect of environmental factors and the length of time between injection drug use and a subsequent, accidental puncture wound. The stability of HIV under various environmental conditions has been shown to decrease over time [61]. HIV RNA was detected in 3.8% of needles used for intramuscular or subcutaneous infections in HIV-infected persons [62]. At room temperature, survival of HIV in syringes was halved when the volume of blood was decreased 10-fold [63]. Less than 1% of syringes had viable HIV detected when left at room temperature for more than a week [63]. The following factors are likely to increase the risk or are required for HIV transmission in needlestick injuries: presence of blood in a needle or syringe emptying into the wound; large needle bore size; deep puncture wounds; a needlestick injury directly into a vein or artery; a short lag time from time of discarding the needle or syringe to time of injury; positive HIV infection status of source individual; and a high sero-prevalence among persons frequenting the geographic area where the needle was discarded [64]. For example, a child injured by picking up a freshly discarded syringe from a known HIV-infected injection drug user would be at high risk of acquiring HIV infection. However, most pediatric needlestick injuries do not occur under such circumstances and would be considered to have a very low risk for transmission.

Prevention

Children should be educated to avoid playing in areas known to be frequented by injecting drug users and to avoid playing with discarded needles and syringes [65]. Needle exchange programs may play a role in decreasing the number of discarded needles in public places [65].

Human bites

It has been estimated that 250 000 human bites occur annually in the USA [66]. Fifty percent of children at one day-care center were bitten at least once in a year [67]. There is currently no evidence that human bites without the presence of blood-tinged saliva in the wound pose an HIV infection risk to the victim. Although biting has been cited as a possible mode of transmission in several case reports, in all of the well-documented reports, the bites were by adults and involved severe biting with blood exchange [68]. One documented seroconversion occurred in a man bitten by an HIV-infected sex worker with blood-tinged saliva [69].

Management of bite wounds should include an evaluation for breaks or abrasions in the skin of the bite victim. Should such breaks or abrasions occur, the person who inflicted the bite should be evaluated for the presence of blood in the mouth or oral lesions which may cause the wound to be contaminated with blood. Proper wound care includes irrigation, debridement, immobilization and elevation of the affected body part and antimicrobial prophylaxis [70].

Prevention

Biting in day-care centers may be deterred by setting limits for a child's behavior, teaching and reinforcing coping skills, and providing other acceptable avenues or activities for children to release or redirect their anger [68].

Sports-related and day-care related bleeding injuries

The risk of transmitting HIV or other blood-borne pathogens through sports-related injuries during athletic activities is considered to be low [71, 72]. In order to transmit a blood-borne pathogen during an athletic activity,

blood from a bleeding wound or exudative skin lesion of an HIV-infected athlete would have to contaminate the skin lesion or exposed mucous membranes of another athlete. In the US National Football League, an average of 3.5 players per team per game experience bleeding injuries for an estimated risk of HIV transmission of one per 85 million physical contacts between two randomly chosen professional football players in one game [72]. The likelihood of transmission of blood-borne pathogens in contact sports is estimated at 1 in 4 million/player/game for HIV and 1 in 20 000/player/game for HBV [73] because of HBV's higher concentration in the blood and higher stability in the environment. There have been no substantiated cases of HIV transmission and two cases of HBV transmission between athletes during an athletic event [74–75].

Similar to sports-related injuries, the incidence of injuries in day-care centers is low, the overall reported incidence of injuries in day-care settings has ranged from 0.25 to 2.50 per 100 000 child-hours in various studies [76–79]. In a survey of 133 day-care sites in Washington State, with an incidence rate of 1.99 injuries/100 000 child-hours, 39% of injuries required sutures.

Prevention

Guidelines to prevent blood-borne pathogen transmission during athletic activities [80–83] or at day-care facilities [84] have been described. Once a child or athlete has suffered a bleeding injury the physical activity associated with the injury should be stopped until the wound has been cleaned and dressed, the bleeding has stopped, blood-contaminated skin has been washed with soap and water, and blood-contaminated mucous membranes have been flushed with ample water. Gloves should be made available to staff in charge of cleaning wounds or surfaces contaminated with blood. Blood-contaminated surfaces should be cleaned with bleach solution (1 part bleach/100 parts water, or 1 tablespoon bleach/1 quart water, or $1/4$ cup of bleach/1 gallon of water) and allowed to dry before reusing [80, 85].

24.3 United States PHS occupational postexposure prophylaxis recommendations

The USPHS oPEP recommendations [1] underscore the need to balance the risk for infection against the potential toxicity or ARV agents. Because PEP is potentially toxic and side-effects are common, its use is not justified for exposures that pose a negligible risk for transmission. For exposures that represent an increased risk for transmission, aggressive treatment using a highly active expanded

Table 24.3 Basic and expanded postexposure prophylaxis regimens for occupational exposures

Regimen Category/Application	Suggested 28-day PEP drug regimens[a]
Basic 2-drug Occupational HIV exposures for which there is recognized transmission risk (see Table 24.1)	Select one of the following dual regimens: ZDV + 3TC 3TC + d4T d4T + ddI
Expanded 3-drug Occupational HIV exposures that pose an increased risk for transmission (e.g. larger volume of blood and/or higher virus titer) (see Table 24.1)	Basic 2-drug regimen + one of the following: *Recommended:* Indinavir (IDV) Nelfinavir (NFV) Efavirenz (EFV) Abacavir (ABC) *Use as PEP with expert consultation:* Ritonavir (RTV) Saquinavir (SQV) Amprenavir (AMP) Delaviridine (DLV) Lopinavir/Ritonavir Generally not recommended for use as PEP: Nevirapine (NVP)

[a] See doses in Table 24.4.

regimen that includes three ARV drugs is recommended. However, most exposures do not represent an increased transmission risk and, for these exposures, CDC recommends a basic two-drug regimen (Tables 24.3 and 24.4). In addition, the 2001 HIV oPEP recommendations also address oPEP for HBV and HCV.

24.3.1 First steps in management of exposures and considerations for determining the level of risk in occupational exposures and the appropriateness of offering PEP

Care of the exposure site
Wound and skin sites exposed to blood or body fluids should be washed with soap and water. Mucous membranes should be flushed with water. Postexposure prophylaxis may be instituted immediately and discontinued at a later time should the detailed evaluation determine that the exposure does not warrant continued PEP.

The occupational exposure report and considerations for determining level of risk
For the purposes of PEP, how does one determine whether the exposed person should be given PEP, and if so, whether the basic or expanded regimen should be given and how

should this be documented? Box 24.2 contains a list of the details regarding the occupational exposure and the postexposure management which should be noted in the exposed person's medical record, in addition to any other local, state, or federal requirements.

Tables 24.5a and 24.5b take into account both the details of the exposure and the HIV infection status of the occupational exposure source to determine the appropriate level of risk and recommendations for follow-up [1]. In general, the following types of injuries or exposures require further evaluation: (1) percutaneous injuries, mucous membrane exposures, or skin exposures with compromised skin integrity (e.g. dermatitis, abrasion, or open wound) to blood, fluids that contain blood, or potentially infectious fluids; (2) exposures to blood-filled hollow needle or visibly bloody devices; (3) direct contact with concentrated virus in a research laboratory or production facility; and (4) bites with blood exposure to either person involved.

Evaluation of the source and exposed individuals for evidence of blood-borne infections, including HIV, HBV, and HCV
The source individual should be informed of the exposure, and once informed consent is obtained, should be tested for HbsAg, anti-HCV, and HIV antibody [1]. In addition, the

Table 24.4 Doses of antiretrovirals used for occupational postexposure prophylaxis

Drug preparations	Adult dose
Nucleoside analogue reverse transcriptase inhibitors (NRTIs)	
Zidovudine (AZT, ZDV)	200 mg tid; 300 mg bid
Lamivudine (3TC)	150 mg bid
	40 mg bid (weight ≥ 60 kg)
	30 mg bid (weight < 60 kg)
Didanosine (ddI)	200 mg bid (weight ≥ 60 kg) on empty stomach
	125 mg bid (weight < 60 kg) on empty stomach
	200 mg bid (weight ≥ 60 kg) on empty stomach
	125 mg bid (weight < 60 kg) on empty stomach
	250 mg bid (weight ≥ 60 kg) on empty stomach
	125 mg bid (weight < 60 kg) on empty stomach
	400 mg qd (weight ≥ 60 kg)
	250 mg qd (weight < 60 kg)
Abacavir (ABC)	300 mg bid
Non-nucleoside reverse transcriptase inhibitors (NNRTIs)	
Efavirenz (EFV; DMP-266)	600 mg once daily
Protease inhibitors (PIs)	
Indinavir (IDV)	800 mg q 8 hour, on empty stomach
Nelfinavir (NFV)	1250 mg bid, with meals or snack
	750 mg tid, with meals or snack
Lopinavir/ritonavir (ABT 378, LPV/RTV)	see formulary
Amprenavir (APV)	1200 mg (eight 150 mg capsules) bid; see adult treatment guidelines for APV/RTV combination bid or qd treatment regimen

a Dose is under study in clinical trials.

Box 24.2. Recommendations for Contents of Occupational Exposure Report

(Adapted from [1])

- Date and time of exposure
- The procedure being performed
  - how and where exposure occurred and if sharps device involved, type of device
- The exposure
  - type of exposure: percutaneous injury (e.g. needlestick or other penetrating sharps, etc.), mucous membrane exposure (e.g. splash in eye, etc.), nonintact skin exposure (e.g. broken or abraded skin, etc.), bites resulting in blood exposure to either person involved
  - type and amount of fluid/tissue: blood, fluids containing blood, or potentially infectious fluid or tissue (semen; vaginal, cerebrospinal, synovial, pleural, peritoneal, pericardial, and amniotic fluids)
  - severity of exposure, depth of wound, duration of contact, condition of skin
  - likelihood of presence of HIV, HBV, or HCV in source material
- The source of exposure:
  - infection status of person
    - HIV: presence of HIV antibody
    - HBV: presence of HbsAg
    - HCV: presence of HCV antibody
    - or other infectious disease
    - stage of disease, history of antiretroviral therapy, antiretroviral resistance information, viral load, CD4$^+$ T cell count, liver enzymes (e.g. ALT)
  - If infectious status unknown, determine risk for HIV, HBV, or HCV infection
    - Known sources: consider medical diagnoses, clinical symptoms (e.g. acute syndrome suggestive of primary HIV infection), history of risk behaviors
    - Unknown sources: consider likelihood of bloodborne pathogen infection among patients in the exposure setting
- Susceptibility of exposed person
  - hepatitis B vaccination and vaccine-response status
  - HIV, HBV, and HIV immune status
- Details about care of exposed site: washing of wound, flushing of mucous membranes
- Details about counseling, postexposure management, and follow-up
- Current medication history of exposed person and ability to swallow pills

Table 24.5a Recommended HIV postexposure prophylaxis for percutaneous injuries

Exposure type	Infection status of source				
	HIV-infected Class 1[a]	HIV-infected Class 2[a]	Source of unknown HIV infection status[b]	Unknown source[c]	HIV-uninfected
Less severe[d]	Recommend basic 2-drug PEP	Recommend expanded 3-drug PEP	Generally, no PEP warranted; however, consider basic 2-drug PEP[e] for source with HIV risk factors[b]	Generally, no PEP warranted; however, consider 2-drug PEP[e] in settings where exposure to HIV-infected persons is likely	No PEP warranted
More severe[f]	Recommend expanded 3-drug PEP	Recommend expanded 3-drug PEP	Generally, no PEP warranted; however, consider basic 2-drug PEP[e] for source with HIV risk factors[b]	Generally, no PEP warranted; however, consider 2-drug PEP[e] in settings where exposure to HIV-infected persons is likely	No PEP warranted

[a] HIV-infected, Class 1 – asymptomatic HIV infection or known low viral load; HIV-infected, Class 2 – symptomatic infection, AIDS, acute seroconversion, or known high viral load. If drug resistance is a concern, obtain expert consultation. Initiation of PEP should not be delayed pending expert consultation, and, because expert consultation alone cannot substitute for face-to-face counseling, resources should be available to provide immediate evaluation and follow-up care for all exposures.

[b] If PEP is offered and taken and the source is later determined to be HIV-uninfected, PEP should be discontinued.

[c] Unknown source (e.g. a needle from a sharps disposal container).

[d] Less severe (e.g. solid needle and superficial injury).

[e] The designation 'consider PEP' indicates that PEP is optional and should be based on an individualized decision between the exposed person and the treating clinician.

[f] More severe (e.g. large-bore hollow needle, deep puncture, visible blood on device, or needle used in patient's artery or vein).

Table 24.5b Recommended HIV postexposure prophylaxis for mucous membrane exposures and non-intact skin[a] exposures (Reprinted from Ref.[1])

Exposure type	HIV-infected Class 1[b]	HIV-infected Class 2[b]	Unknown HIV infection status of the source patient[c]	Unknown source[d]	HIV-uninfected
			Infection status of source		
Less severe[e]	Consider basic 2-drug PEP	Recommend expanded 3-drug PEP[f]	Generally, no PEP warranted; however, consider basic 2-drug PEP[f] for source with HIV risk factors[g]	Generally, no PEP warranted; however, consider 2-drug PEP[f] in settings where exposure to HIV-infected persons is likely	No PEP warranted
Large volume[h]	Recommend basic 2-drug PEP	Recommend expanded 3-drug PEP	Generally, no PEP warranted; however, consider basic 2-drug PEP[f] for source with HIV risk factors[g]	Generally, no PEP warranted; however, consider 2-drug PEP[f] in settings where exposure to HIV-infected persons is likely	No PEP warranted

[a] For skin exposures, follow-up is indicated only if there is evidence of compromised skin integrity (e.g. dermatitis, abrasion, or open wound).

[b] HIV-infected, Class 1 – asymptomatic HIV infection or known low viral load. HIV-infected, Class 2 – symptomatic infection, AIDS, acute seroconversion, or known high viral load. If drug resistance is a concern, obtain expert consultation. Initiation of PEP should not be delayed pending expert consultation, and, because expert consultation alone cannot substitute for face-to-face counseling, resources should be available to provide immediate evaluation and follow-up care for all exposures.

[c] HIV infection status of the source patient is unknown (e.g. deceased individual with no samples available for HIV testing).

[d] Unknown source (e.g. splash from inappropriately disposed blood).

[e] Small volume (i.e. a few drops).

[f] The designation 'consider PEP' indicates that PEP is optional and should be based on an individualized decision between the exposed person and the treating clinician.

[g] If PEP is offered and taken and the source is later determined to be HIV-uninfected, PEP should be discontinued.

[h] Large volume (i.e. major blood splash).

source person's medical record information available at the time of exposure (e.g. previous medical history, laboratory test results and diagnoses) may help confirm or exclude blood-borne virus infection [1]. An FDA-approved rapid HIV antibody test such as the Ora-quick test [86] should be considered for use. The newly revised draft CDC nPEP guidelines that are currently under review recommend that such rapid testing should be conducted within an hour after exposure [87]. Repeatedly reactive HIV EIA (non-p24 antigen type) or rapid HIV antibody tests are suggestive of infection and can be used to make initial decisions on PEP management. Additional information on HIV rapid tests can be found at www.cdc.gov/hiv/pubs/rt.htm. Confirmation by HIV Western blot of a reactive result should be conducted before notifying the source patient of the final results. A negative HIV EIA or rapid HIV antibody test is an excellent indicator of the absence of HIV antibody. Direct virus assays such as HIV RNA viral load tests or HIV p24 antigen EIA tests for routine screening of source patients are not recommended due to concerns about high false positive rates in this setting [88, 89]. Because source testing can take some time to complete, and given that PEP may not be effective if not given soon after exposure, clinicians may have to make a decision about PEP based on incomplete information (e.g. prior to initiating HIV testing or obtaining HIV testing results). A baseline evaluation of HIV-exposed HCP should include testing for HIV within hours after their exposure unless the source person is known to be HIV seronegative, and obtaining information about current medication history and any medical conditions or circumstances which might influence drug selection (e.g. pregnancy, breast-feeding, hepatic, or renal disease). The HIV-exposed HCP should be counseled about the signs and symptoms of acute retroviral syndrome and to return quickly for evaluation should an acute HIV infection be suspected. The exposed person should be re-evaluated within 72 hours postexposure to determine whether additional information about the exposure or source person has become available. If the source person is found to be definitively HIV-uninfected and has no symptoms of HIV infection or AIDS, the exposed person no longer needs to be followed up (e.g. no need for baseline HIV testing or PEP). If the source individual is found to be HIV-infected, the exposed HCP should be retested periodically for a minimum of 6 months after exposure (e.g. 6 weeks, 12 weeks, and 6 months after exposure). If the exposed individual is not on oPEP and is within the window period for initiating it, oPEP should be offered. A 12-month follow-up HIV test is indicated in exposed HCP if they become HCV-infected following exposure to an HIV-HCV co-infected source individual. Similarly, any exposed HCP who develops an illness compatible with an acute retroviral syndrome should undergo HIV testing regardless of the interval since exposure. Confidentiality of the source and exposed individuals should be maintained. If the HIV infection status of the source patient is unknown or cannot be determined, decisions about PEP should be made on a case-by-case basis, considering the risk of transmission from the exposure and the likelihood that the source patient is HIV-infected. Information about seroprevalence rates of HIV, HBV, or HCV in the community or institution from which the source material or source person originates may be helpful in evaluating the risk for exposure. The reliability and interpretation of tests of needles or other sharp instruments implicated in exposures is unknown and not recommended. The possible need for prophylaxis against hepatitis B virus should also be considered. Additional guidelines on the management of occupational exposures to HBV and HBC can be accessed at the following website: http://www.cdc.gov/mmwr/PDF/RR/RR5011.pdf.

24.3.2 HIV treatment principles used in developing oPEP recommendations

The selection of the regimens recommended for oPEP reflects the consideration of efficacy data, site of activity in the HIV replication cycle, and drug side-effects. The USPHS emphasizes, however, that the determination of which agents, number of agents to use, and when to alter a PEP regimen is empiric [1]. Selected drugs from three classes of ARV agents are recommended for use for oPEP: nucleoside analogue reverse transcriptase inhibitors (NRTIs), non-nucleoside reverse transcriptase inhibitors (NNRTIs) and protease inhibitors (PIs).

Combination regimens have been shown to be more effective than monotherapy in reducing viral load and are therefore recommended for oPEP. Dual and triple combination regimens have been shown to be superior to monotherapy in reducing viral load. Highly active antiretroviral therapy (HAART) regimens containing, for example, NRTIs with a PI and/or an NNRTI, have been shown to be superior to dual therapy alone in reducing HIV viral load [90]. Although there are no studies to support the idea that using other ARV drugs in addition to ZDV will enhance the effectiveness of PEP, it is felt that the same factors which improve the efficacy of HIV treatment might similarly improve PEP efficacy. Because ARVs have associated adverse effects, the USPHS oPEP guidelines reserve the use of triple-drug HAART regimens for more severe exposures. These guidelines describe a two-tiered paradigm of "basic" or "expanded" prophylaxis for less severe and more severe exposures, respectively. Although

Table 24.6 Two-drug and three-drug pediatric nPEP regimens[a]

	A. 2-drug PEP regimens
Strongly recommended	ZDV + [3TC[b] or ddI]
	d4T + 3TC
Alternative recommendation with expert consultation	ABC + [ZDV or 3TC]
	ddI + 3TC
Use in special circumstances	d4T + ddI or ZDV + ddC
Not recommended	ddC + [ddI or d4T or 3TC]
	ZDV + d4T

	B. Three-drug HAART Pediatric nPEP drug regimens[a]	
Strongly recommended	Recommended two drug regimen from above	+ Nelfinavir or Lopinavir/Ritonavir
	Recommended two drug regimen from above	+ Efavirenz[c]
Alternative recommendation	Recommended two drug regimen from above	+ Amprenavir[d] or IDV[e]
	ZDV + 3TC	+ ABC[f]
Not recommended	Two drug regimen from above	+ Nevirapine
	Two drug regimen from above	+ Saquinavir

[a] Adapted from [87].

[b] ZDV + 3TC available as a combination formulation, use of which would decrease pill burden and may improve adherence.

[c] Efavirenz recommended for children > 3 years of age. Contraindicated during pregnancy due to teratogenicity in animal studies.

[d] Amprenavir recommended for children ≥ 3 years of age.

[e] IDV recommended for older children who can tolerate swallowing solid tablets or caplets.

[f] ABC + ZDV + 3TC available as a combination formulation, use of which would decrease pill burden and may improve adherence – but potential side effects should be considered.

some treatment regimens include HAART combinations of more than three drugs, current oPEP guidelines recommend the use of triple drug regimens for more severe exposures to maximize adherence and reduce the likelihood of side-effects. In addition, the emergence of resistance to ARV drugs and development of new ARV drugs has prompted some changes in the list of drugs recommended for oPEP.

Basic and expanded oPEP regimens

The USPHS has developed guidelines for dual and triple-drug oPEP regimens, known as basic and expanded regimens, respectively, based on the level of HIV transmission risk (Table 24.3). For lower risk exposures, the USPHS has recommended that a basic or dual drug regimen be considered. Zidovudine/3TC was considered the basic combination of choice. A combination formulation of ZDV/3TC is available, and is convenient (thereby likely to improve adherence). However, recent data suggest that ZDV and 3TC resistance mutations may be common in certain locales [91]. Therefore, clinicians may choose other NRTIs or ARV combinations based on local clinical expe-

rience and knowledge. Table 24.6 lists other dual regimens aside from ZDV/3TC to be considered for basic oPEP regimens.

The addition of a third drug, a PI or an NNRTI, to the basic dual drug regimen is recommended to create the expanded, triple-drug PEP regimen, thereby enhancing the ARV activity of the basic regimen in higher risk exposures. In addition, if the patient becomes HIV-infected, inclusion of a third drug should increase the effectiveness of treatment during this early phase of infection after seroconversion. Table 24.6 lists selected three-drug combinations in three categories: (1) recommended; (2) use as PEP with expert consultation; and (3) generally not recommended for use as PEP. The drugs recommended for use with expert consultation are those which might be used in cases of development of drug resistance to those drugs included in the recommended list and which may require special monitoring due to the potential for adverse events (e.g. hypersensitivity reactions with abacavir). Although nevirapine (NVP) is recognized as a highly potent ARV, it is not generally recommended for PEP due to case reports of serious adverse events related to multi-dose NVP taken for PEP, including

Table 24.7 Main adverse events associated with antiretrovirals (Reprinted from [1])

Antiretroviral class/agent	Primary side-effects and toxicities
Nucleoside reverse transcriptase inhibitors (NRTIs)	Mainly nausea or diarrhea
Zidovudine (ZDV; AZT)	Anemia, neutropenia, nausea, headache, insomnia, muscle pain, and weakness
Lamivudine (3TC)	Abdominal pain, nausea, diarrhea, rash, and pancreatitis
Stavudine (d4T)	Peripheral neuropathy, headache, diarrhea, nausea, insomnia, anorexia, pancreatitis, increased liver function tests (LFT), anemia, and neutropenia
Didanosine (ddI)	Pancreatitis^a, lactic acidosis, neuropathy, diarrhea, abdominal pain, and nausea
Abacavir (ABC)	Nausea, diarrhea, anorexia, abdominal pain, fatigue, headache, insomnia, and hypersensitivity reactions
Nonnucleoside reverse transcriptase inhibitors (NNRTIs)	Severe skin reactions (Stevens–Johnson syndrome, toxic epidermal necrolysis)
Nevirapine (NVP)	Rash (including cases of Stevens–Johnson syndrome), fever, nausea, headache, hepatitis, increased LFTs, rarely fatal hepatic necrosis
Delaviridine (DLV)	Rash (including cases of Stevens–Johnson syndrome), nausea, diarrhea, headache, fatigue, and increased LFTs
Efavirenz (EFV)^b	Rash (including cases of Stevens–Johnson syndrome), insomnia, somnolence, dizziness, trouble concentrating, and abnormal dreaming
Protease inhibitors (PIs)	New onset diabetes mellitus, hyperglycemia, diabetic ketoacidosis, exacerbation of pre-existing diabetes mellitus, and dyslipidemia
Indivinavir (IDV)	Nausea, abdominal pain, nephrolithiasis^c, and indirect hyperbilirubinemia
Nelfinavir (NFV)	Diarrhea^d, nausea, abdominal pain, weakness, and rash
Ritonavir (RTV)	Weakness, diarrhea, nausea, circumoral paresthesia, taste alteration, and increased cholesterol and triglycerides
Saquinavir (SQV)	Diarrhea, abdominal pain, nausea, hyperglycemia, and increased LFTs
Amprenavir (AMP)	Nausea, diarrhea, rash, circumoral paresthesia, taste alteration, and depression
Lopinavir/ritonavir	Diarrhea, fatigue, headache, nausea, and increased cholesterol and triglycerides

^{a} Fatal and nonfatal pancreatitis in patients treated > 4 weeks.
^{b} See text regarding use of EFV, d4T + ddI, IDV, ZDV + 3TC in pregnant women.
^{c} Nephrolithiasis less of a problem with good hydration (see text).
^{d} Diarrhea may be controlled with antimotility agents.

hepatotoxicity and fulminant liver failure requiring liver transplantation, hypersensitivity syndrome, skin reactions, and rhabdomyolysis [1, 92] (Table 24.7). It is important to distinguish this recommendation to avoid multi-dose NVP for PEP from separate recommendations concerning the use of the two-dose NVP regimen (one dose to the mother at labor, one dose to the infant shortly after birth) for prevention of MTCT of HIV [93].

In general, clinical experience or judgment may influence an individual practitioner to use alternate drug combinations for either the basic or expanded PEP regimens. When possible, persons with expertise in the management of HIV-infected patients should be consulted in the selection and implementation of PEP regimens.

Timing of initiation and duration of PEP after exposure

Postexposure prophylaxis should be implemented as soon as possible after an occupational exposure, preferably within hours. Postexposure prophylaxis is less effective when initiated after 24–36 hours, but since the interval after which no benefit is derived from PEP is unknown, PEP may be considered even after 36 hours [1]. Some experts suggest postexposure prophylaxis for non-occupational exposures should be initiated as soon as feasible within 72 hours after exposure, although clinicians may consider administering nPEP for patients seeking care more than 72 hours after a significant exposure if they believe the benefits outweigh the risks. Although the appropriate duration of PEP is not known, based on the CDC case control study and animal data [9], a 28-day regimen is recommended.

Postexposure prophylaxis drug toxicity monitoring

Among HCP on PEP enrolled in a national surveillance system and registry, 50% experienced adverse symptoms and nearly 33% stopped taking PEP because of adverse signs and symptoms [94–97]. Such side-effects and discontinuation of PEP were more common among HCP taking three-drug versus two-drug combination regimens in two studies [95–97]. The most common side-effects associated with ARV agents and methods used to lessen certain of these side-effects are well described (Table 24.7).

Nevirapine toxicity deserves special mention as severe toxicity has been reported in 22 patients taking NVP-containing ARV regimens including two cases of life-threatening liver failure, one of which required liver transplantation, and other cases of hepatotoxicity, skin reaction (including one documented and two possible cases of Stevens–Johnson syndrome), and rhabdomyolysis [92, 98]. Of the 22 cases, 16 adults received oPEP, five adults received nPEP, and one child who had suffered a needlestick exposure received PEP. Most regimens contained three drugs (range: one to five). Onset of symptoms occurred between 3–36 days with the median onset at 14 days. Because of severity and rapidity of onset of these severe toxicities, NVP is not recommended for use as PEP.

Toxicity monitoring should include a complete blood count and renal and hepatic chemical function tests at baseline and 2 weeks after starting PEP (Table 24.8). Potential toxicities and measures to minimize these effects, drug interactions [1], and methods for monitoring these side-effects should be discussed with patients to maximize adherence to PEP regimens. The following side-effects should be reported immediately to the clinician: rash, fever, back or abdominal pain, pain on urination or blood in the urine, and symptoms of hyperglycemia (e.g. increased thirst and/or frequent urination). The US Food and Drug Administration [Telephone (800) 332–1088 in the USA] and/or the manufacturer should be informed of unusual, serious, or unexpected toxicity associated with receipt of ARV drugs. In addition, pregnant HCP who are exposed to ARVs through PEP should be reported to the Antiretroviral Pregnancy Registry [Telephone (800) 258–4263 in the USA, or write to the Antiretroviral Pregnancy Registry, 1011 Research Park, 1011 Ashes Drive, Wilmington, NC 28405].

Finally, HCP receiving PEP who become HIV-infected should be encouraged to contact the CDC [Telephone: 800-893-0485 or 404-639-1250] regarding enrollment into a clinical protocol to evaluate such events.

Considerations involving pregnant HCP

Certain ARV drugs or combinations of drugs either are not recommended, or should be used with caution, in pregnant women. Efavirenz (EFV) is associated with teratogenic effects in primate studies [99]. Stavudine (d4T) in combination with didanosine (ddI) have been associated with fatal and non-fatal lactic acidosis in pregnant women [100]. Indinavir (IDV) may lead to hyperbilirubinemia in newborns; therefore, it should not be administered to women shortly before delivery [101]. Finally, the combination of ZDV and 3TC has been reported as possibly related to two cases of mitochondrial toxicity and death in HIV-uninfected infants exposed to the drugs perinatally in France [102]. However, no similar deaths have been found in an exhaustive review of 20 000 infants in the major US perinatal cohorts [103].

Resistance to ARV agents

Despite the documentation of resistance mutations in source patients [91, 104, 105] and the transmission of resistant HIV strains after occupational exposure [104], the relevance of such exposures to resistant virus is not fully understood. Although it is recommended that resistance testing information on the source be collected at the time of the initial exposure and taken into account in the selection of the PEP regimen, resistance testing of all source patients is not recommended because it is unlikely that results would arrive in time to make adjustments in the 28-day PEP regimen and there are no data to support such an approach.

HIV postexposure counseling and education

HIV-exposed HCP should be counseled regarding the prevention of secondary transmission, particularly during the initial 6–12 weeks after exposure when seroconversion might occur. Specifically, sexual abstinence and the use of condoms should be encouraged, while breast-feeding and the donation of blood, plasma, organs, tissue, or semen should be discouraged. Exposed persons should also be encouraged to seek medical advice should the following signs and symptoms of acute HIV infection or viremia appear: fever, rash, myalgia, fatigue, malaise, or lymphadenopathy. Early initiation of HAART relative to HIV seroconversion may improve the immune system's long-term ability to combat HIV infection [106]. Information about adherence to the PEP regimen and management of side-effects should emphasize the need to complete the full course of the regimen, the potential

Table 24.8 Summary of management and follow-up of postexposure prophylaxis

	Time between HIV exposure and initiation of PEP	Time from onset of PEP					
		2 weeks	4 weeks	6 weeks	12 weeks	6 months	12 months
PEP	1. Clean exposure site and determine if PEP is indicated. 2. Choose PEP regimen: consider exposed person's medication history/medical conditions or circumstances (i.e. pregnancy, breast-feeding, renal or hepatic disease). See Tables 24.3–24.7, 24.9. 3. If indicated, start PEP within hours, but no more than 72 hours after HIV exposure. May consider initiating PEP before all work-up completed if HIV results delayed >1 hour		Stop PEP after 28 days or sooner if source determined to be HIV seronegative.				
HIV testing	Baseline HIV test of source: If source is HIV seronegative, do not start PEP or provide further PEP follow-up to exposed person. If source's HIV infection status is unknown, determine if PEP indicated on a case-by-case basis. Re-evaluate within 72 hours if more information about source becomes available. If source is HIV seropositive, conduct baseline testing of exposed person			repeat	repeat	repeat	repeat if exposed person becomes HCV-infected following exposure to source co-infected with HCV-HIV
Monitor for ARV toxicity	Baseline tests: At a minimum: CBC; renal and hepatic function tests. If PI given: Monitor for hyperglycemia If IDV given: Monitor for crystalluria, hematuria, hemolytic anemia, and hepatitis. If toxicity noted, consider modifying regimen and other diagnostic procedures	Repeat					
Counsel exposed person	Counsel exposed person: 1. To use precautions to prevent secondary HIV transmission during follow-up. 2. If PEP is prescribed inform patient about possible drug toxicities and the need for monitoring and possible drug interactions.		Period of time during which exposed person most likely to transmit if recently HIV-infected and experiencing HIV viremia: person on PEP should use precautions to prevent secondary HIV transmission *especially* during this time period: • Exercise sexual abstinence or use condoms • Refrain from donating blood, plasma, organs, tissue, or semen • Refrain from breast-feeding				

side-effects and drug interactions, and ways in which these can be minimized and monitored. The following side-effects should be reported immediately to the healthcare provider: rash, fever, back or abdominal pain, pain on urination or blood in the urine, and symptoms of hyperglycemia (e.g. increased thirst and/or frequent urination). The potential toxicities, laboratory tests for monitoring toxicities, and drug interactions to consider with ARV therapy or prophylaxis is described in detail in Chapters 18 and Chapter 19. Patients should also be told how to prevent and manage side-effects including drinking at least 48 ounces of fluid per 24-hour period to limit the incidence of nephrolithiasis associated with indinavir, and the use of prescription antimotility agents to limit the diarrhea associated with nelfinavir, saquinavir, and ritonavir. When recommending or offering PEP, exposed persons should also be informed that knowledge about the efficacy and toxicity of PEP is limited. A summary of recent human and animal PEP efficacy data also may be provided.

24.4 HIV nPEP for exposures in children and adolescents

Since 1999, at least four states have published either nPEP guidelines [107–109] or clinical advisories [110]. The American Academy of Pediatrics has released its own guidelines [111]. The USPHS guidelines for nPEP are undergoing revision [87]. The recommendations for nPEP in children and adolescents in this chapter are based on oPEP guidelines [1], nPEP guidelines [87, 112], and treatment guidelines for pediatric [113] and adult [90] guidelines.

24.4.1 New policy recommendations pertinent to pediatric nPEP

The CDC's stance in 1998 as a result of its initial consultation with the USPHS on nPEP was that it was a clinical intervention of unproven efficacy, but did not recommend or discourage its use and did not make specific ARV drug recommendations [112]. Recent data from animal models was presented earlier in this chapter that supports the use of nPEP as late as 72 hours after an exposure to reduce the likelihood of HIV transmission. In the draft revised USPHS nPEP guidelines [87], it is noted that data from animal models, perinatal clinical trials, studies of healthcare workers receiving oPEP and observational nPEP studies suggest that nPEP may be effective in reducing the risk of HIV acquisition and recommend that specific ARV drug regimens be used based on the most current USPHS adult ARV treatment

guidelines [90]. Individuals who present for care within 72 hours of exposure to an HIV-infected person with a significant risk for HIV transmission would be eligible to receive an nPEP ARV regimen based on the most current ARV HIV treatment recommendations, with the caveat that those individuals presenting after 72 hours of exposure with a significant risk could be offered nPEP if the caregiver believed the benefits of nPEP outweighed the risks [87].

Current UPSHS oPEP guidelines [1] recommend three-drug regimens for more severe or increased risk exposures, and two-drug regimens for less severe exposures because there is insufficient evidence to support three-drug regimens for both levels of exposure. Based on the assumption that HAART's ability to maximally suppress viral replication translates into a higher likelihood of preventing the establishment of HIV infection in an exposed individual, the revised nPEP guidelines recommend a 28-day course of a three-drug HAART regimen for all persons presenting for care within 72 hours of nonoccupational exposures that represents a significant risk of HIV transmission with a known HIV-infected source [87]. In addition, because there is no evidence to suggest that a three-drug HAART regimen is more effective than a two-drug regimen, the revised nPEP guidelines suggest that a two-drug regimen could be considered when there is a concern regarding potential difficulties with adherence or adverse events requiring immediate medical attention.

A list of selected nPEP recommendations by selected states or national organizations are noted in Box 24.3. Most recommend offering PEP within 72 hours and using two-drug or three-drug regimens. The New York State Department of Health AIDS Institute generally recommends three drugs, but their Committee could not reach a consensus on number of drugs to be used because of the issues of better adherence with two-drug regimens versus the superiority of three-drug regimens for HIV treatment purposes. The American Academy of Pediatrics acknowledges that many clinicians would use three drugs but that two drugs may be considered in certain situations including issues related to toxicity and ease of adherence [111].

24.4.2 Principles for pediatric PEP

The PEP recommendations for children in this chapter are based on both the oPEP recommendations for HCP with occupational exposures [1] and for persons with non-occupational exposures [87, 112], and the most current guidelines on HIV ARV therapy in children [113] and adults [90]. However, nPEP for exposed children should always be initiated in close consultation with a physician expert in the care of HIV-infected children. Based on a review

Box 24.3. Comparison of selected nPEP policies

Policy State/Date of release	Offer PEP within how many hours?	No. of PEP drugs	Pediatric recommendations
New York State Department of Health AIDS Institute: March, 2002 [107]	36 hours	"In general three drugs," but no consensus reached between two or three drugs Notes common use of AZT/3TC/Nelfinavir	Detailed recommendations
State of California: 2001 [109]	72 hours	Two or three drugs depending on level of risk	Consult pediatric HIV specialist
Massachusetts Dept. Health Clinical Advisory October 20, 2000 [110]	72 hours	Not specified	Not specified
Rhode Island Department of Health, August 1, 2002 [108]	72 hours, but may be given afterwards in special circumstances	Two or three drugs depending on level of risk	Special considerations listed in terms of dosing, support services, informed consent, necessity for caretaker involvement
American Academy of Pediatrics, 2003 [111]	72 hours	Physician choice: many physicians will choose three; some will prefer two	Detailed instructions
Centers for Disease Control and Prevention, 2004 (nPEP Guidelines) [87]	72 hours	Three drugs from list of preferred and alternative regimens. Consider two drugs if concerns regarding potential adherence or toxicity issues	See APP nPEP guidelines [111] and USPHS pediatric ARV guidelines [113]

of the most recent national nPEP guidelines and current data from oPEP and nPEP studies, the following are essential principles to be considered for administering pediatric nPEP.

1. The effectiveness of combination therapy is greater than that of monotherapy to treat HIV infection. Similarly, the effectiveness of combination PEP is assumed to be greater than that of monoprophylaxis to prevent HIV infection.

   Three-drug regimens are recommended for treatment of HIV-infected pediatric patients. Two-drug treatment regimens are recommended only under special circumstances. Triple drug combinations that include a PI are superior to the dual NRTI combination regimens alone

in reducing viral load to undetectable levels and increasing CD4$^+$ lymphoctye number [114].

2. Monotherapy for HIV infection should be avoided based on its poor efficacy relative to HAART and rapid emergence of resistance. Similarly, it is assumed that monoprophylaxis to prevent transmission of HIV should be avoided, except for prevention of MTCT [113].

   Prophylaxis with ZDV is recommended during the first 6 weeks for an HIV-exposed infant after birth to an HIV-infected mother.

3. Because the duration of PEP is only 28 days, drugs which do not require graded dosing schemes, and are maximally effective throughout the entire course, should be considered drugs of choice for PEP.

Ritonavir is an example of a drug which requires a graded dosing scheme of five days when initiating therapy. Although it is appropriate for treatment of HIV, it would not be a first choice nPEP medication because the patient would not be on the maximally inhibitory dose of the medication until 5 days after starting nPEP.

4. Two-drug NRTI combinations are not optimal for and used under special circumstances for treatment of HIV [113] and are considered the basic oPEP regimen for lower risk HIV exposures [1]

The revised USPHS nPEP recommendations are permissive of the use of two-drug regimens in significant exposures when adherence or drug toxicity is a consideration [87].

5. Triple drug combinations are used as part of the expanded oPEP regimen for higher-risk HIV exposures [1] and are considered the first choice regimen for HIV treatment and for nPEP based on the revised nPEP guidelines [87].

The triple drug combination of choice is a highly active PI (nelfinavir) in combination with two NRTIs (ZDV and 3TC). The dual NRTI combination of choice to be used with the PI is ZDV and 3TC. Zidovudine and ddC is a less preferred choice for use in combination with a PI [113]. The PI of choice for PEP is nelfinavir because it has fewer side-effects and does not require step-wise dosing. Lopinavir/ritonavir is the only Pl approved by the US FDA for use in children 6 months of age or older. Although no other PI aside from lopinavir/ritonavir is FDA-approved for children under 2 years of age, the current treatment guidelines recommend the use of pediatric formulations of ritonavir and nelfinavir in infants, with the understanding that optimal dosing of these agents in young infants has not been defined, but is under study in clinical trials [113]. Nelfinavir would be preferable to ritonavir, because of ritonavir's graded dosing schedule.

6. Pill burden, side-effects, potency of, and formulations of medications are important considerations in choosing a PEP regimen.

Because it has been shown that it is difficult for both adults and children to adhere to a full 28-day course of PEP, clinicians should take these factors into account in choosing a PEP regimen.

7. Approved ARV drugs for adults may be used in children despite lack of FDA approval for pediatric formulations.

Some recommended ARV drugs are not yet FDA-approved for use in children or for use in all age groups among children. However, current pediatric ARV treatment guidelines [113] state that the absence of clinical trials addressing pediatric-specific manifestations of HIV infection does not preclude the use of any approved ARV drug in children and that all ARV drugs approved for treatment of HIV infection may be used for children when indicated – irrespective of labeling notations. However, because some physicians may wish to assign priority to particular ARV regimens for PEP purposes based on the FDA-approval status of the drugs, more detailed information about age-specific considerations is provided in the next section.

8. Clinicians faced with a decision regarding PEP should consult with a physician with expertise in pediatric HIV care.

Pediatric ARV therapy is a rapidly evolving field and physicians with expertise in pediatric HIV care should be consulted whenever possible when deciding on PEP regimens (Box 24.4).

24.4.3 Age-specific considerations for PEP in children

The choice of drugs available for treatment of HIV is more limited for children than for adults. Some drugs available for treatment of adults are not FDA-approved, are not recommended for use in children, or lack formulations suitable for small children. However, current pediatric ARV guidelines state that FDA labeling practices should not necessarily limit use of ARVs in children [113]. Pediatric ARV therapy is a rapidly evolving field. Clinicians faced with a decision regarding PEP should consult with a physician with expertise in pediatric HIV care and consider the most current local and national [113] recommendations. No definitive recommendations exist for PEP in older infants and in children. However, a reasonable approach must take into account which pediatric formulations are available in a particular area, which are available through compassionate use programs, which are accessible in the appropriate time frame for PEP, and which have age-appropriate dosing schemes available for the child in question.

Other alternate drugs for nPEP are listed in Table 24.6, as are drugs not recommended for nPEP. The dosing for the ARV drugs used in pediatric PEP is generally the same for that used to treat pediatric HIV infection and the duration of treatment is usually 4 weeks. In addition, although NVP is approved for treatment of HIV infection in children older than 2 months of age, multiple-use NVP is not currently recommended for PEP in the U.S.A. due to its toxicity [98]. Table 24.9 describes the antiretroviral agents approved by the US FDA for the treatment of HIV infection in children by age category.

Box 24.4. PEP management resources (adapted from [1])

National Clinicians' Postexposure Prophylaxis Hotline (PEP line)
Run by University of California-San Francisco/San Francisco General Hospital staff; supported by the Health Resources and Services Administration Ryan White CARE Act, HIV/AIDS Bureau, AIDS Education and Training Centers, and CDC.

Phone: (888) 448-4911
Internet:<http://www.ucsf.edu/hivcntr>

Needlestick!
A website to help clinicians manage and document occupational blood and body fluid exposures. Developed and maintained by the University of California, Los Angeles (UCLA), Emergency Medicine Center, UCLA School of Medicine and funded in part by CDC and the Agency for Healthcare Research and Quality

Internet:<http://www.needlestick.mednet.ucla.edu>

Hepatitis Hotline

Phone: (888) 443-7232
Internet:<http://www.cdc.gov/hepatitis>

Reporting to CDC: Occupationally acquired HIV infections and failures of PEP

Phone: (800) 893-0485

HIV Antiretroviral Pregnancy Registry

Phone: (800) 258-4263
Fax: (800) 800–1052
Internet:<http://www.APRegistry.org>

nPEP Surveillance:
CDC National PEP Registry: Collects information on persons who either receive or are considered for nPEP. It is run for CDC by John Snow, Inc.

Phone: 1-(877) HIV-1PEP (1-877-448-1737)
Internet:<http://www.hivpepregistry.org>

Reporting unusual or severe toxicities: Contact manufacturer directly or FDA

FDA: 1-800-332-1088

Selected nPEP guidelines:

American Academy of Pediatrics

www.aappolicy.aappublications.org/cgi/
content/full/pediatrics;111/6/1475
PEP in Children and Adolescents for nonoccupational exposure to HIV

New York State Dept. of Health
AIDS Institute

www.hivguidelines.org
*HIV PEP for children beyond the perinatal period
HIV PEP following sexual assault*

State of California

www.dhs.cahwnet.gov/ps/ooa/Reports/
PDF/HIVProphylaxisFollowing Sexual Assault.pdf
Offering HIV prophylaxis following sexual assault: recommendations for the State of California

Commonwealth of Massachusetts

http://www.state.ma.us/dph/aids/
guidelines/ca_exposure_nonwork.htm
Clinical advisory:HIV prophylaxis for non-occupational exposures

Rhode Island Dept. Health/Brown University AIDS Program

www.brown.edu/Departments/BRUNA/backnpep.htm
Nonoccupational human immunodeficiency virus postexposure prophylaxis guidelines for Rhode Island healthcare practitioners

Table 24.9 Antiretrovirals approved by the US FDA for treatment of HIV infection in children by age category

Drug	0 to < 3 months	3 months to < 2 years	≥ 2 years
NRTIs			
Abacavir	No	Yes	Yes
Zalcitabine	No	No	Yes, ≥ 13 years of age
Didanosine	Yes, ≥2 weeks	Yes	Yes
Stavudine	Yes	Yes	Yes
Zidovudine	Yes	Yes	Yes
Lamivudine	No[a]	Yes	Yes
NNRTIs			
Delaviridine	No	No	Yes, ≥ 16 years of age
Efavirenz	No	No	Yes, ≥ 3 years of age
Nevirapine	No	Yes (>2 months)	Yes
PIs			
Amprenavir	No	No	Yes, ≥ 4 years of age
Indinavir	No	No	Yes (Adolescents/adults)
Lopinavir/Ritonavir	No	Yes (≥6 months)	Yes
Nelfinavir	No	No	Yes
Ritonavir	No	No	Yes
Saquinavir	No	No	Yes, > 16 years of age

[a] Use of 3TC recommended in children < 3 months of age, despite absence of FDA approval [113].
NRTIs, nucleoside analogue reverse transcriptase inhibitors; NNRTIs, non-nucleoside analogue reverse transcriptase inhibitors; PIs, protease inhibitors.

Term infants, age less than 3 months
Zidovudine is an FDA-approved ARV drug for both HIV therapy and prophylaxis from the time of birth. ddI and d4T are approved for treatment of infants younger than 3 months of age. However, d4T is not recommended in combination with ZDV. In addition, experts feel that enough data exist regarding 3TC dosing for infants younger than 3 months of age to consider it safe to use for therapy of HIV-infected infants [113] (see Table 24.4 for 3TC dose under study for infants younger than 3 months of age). For infants exposed to HIV after birth, prophylaxis with ZDV and 3TC is considered the PEP two-drug regimen of choice in this and other age groups, unless there is a high level of resistance mutations to these drugs in the community. Stavudine (d4T) is also FDA-approved in children 5 weeks of age or older, but is not recommended in combination with ZDV [113]. An expanded regimen for infants using a PI and two NRTIs (including ZDV) might be considered for higher risk exposures using investigational dosing schemes.

Children aged at least 3 months but less than 2 years
Zidovudine, 3TC, ddI, d4T, abacavir, nevirapine, and lopinavir/ritonavir are the only FDA-approved ARVs for HIV therapy in this age group. However liquid formulations of nelfinavir and ritonavir are recommended for use in older infants [121] and nevirapine is not recommended as a PEP agent. The nPEP regimens of choice in this age group include the two-drug nPEP regimen of ZDV/3TC and a three-drug regimen adding nelfinavir or lopinavir/ritonavir. An investigational dose for nelfinavir is noted in Table 24.4. Lopinavir/ritonavir is an approved PI combination in this age group for children 6 months of age and older.

Children aged 2–13 years
Zidovudine, 3TC, ddI, d4T, abacavir, nevirapine, nelfinavir, lopinavir/ritonavir, and ritonavir have been approved by the FDA for therapy of HIV infection for this entire age group. In addition, the following drugs have been approved for the following age groups: amprenavir (>4 years), ddC (≥ 13 years), delaviridine (≥16 years), efavirenz (≥ 3 years), saquinavir (>16 years), and indinavir (adolescent/adults). The nPEP regimens of choice in this age group include the two-drug nPEP regimen of ZDV/3TC and a three-drug regimen adding nelfinavir, lopinavir/ritonavir, or efavirenz as the third drug. Multi-dose NVP is not recommended as a PEP agent.

Adolescent dosing

Adolescent dosages should be prescribed according to Tanner staging of puberty and not by age [113]. Therefore, those in Tanner stages I and II should be dosed according to pediatric schedules and those in Tanner V should be dosed using adult schedules. Youth undergoing growth spurts (Tanner III females and Tanner IV males) should be closely monitored for medication efficacy and toxicity when using adult or pediatric dosing guidelines [113].

24.4.4 Considerations for determining level of risk in non-occupational HIV exposures and the appropriateness of administering PEP

In addition to the considerations for determining level of risk for occupational exposures (Tables 24.5a and 24.5b), and those described earlier in this chapter by type of exposure, the following generic considerations should be taken into account for non-occupational HIV exposures [115]: (a) the likelihood that the source is infected with HIV; (b) the likelihood of transmission, including the many cofactors that might increase or decrease transmission risk; (c) characteristics (e.g. viral load, stage of infection) of an HIV-infected source; (d) isolated versus recurrent HIV exposures; (e) time delay between possible exposure and presentation for medical care; and (f) ability to adhere to the ARV regimen. Factors to consider in determining level of risk in pediatric exposures are described earlier in this chapter. Each case must be evaluated individually taking into account the specifics of each situation. In general, the USPHS guidelines consider significant exposures to be exposures of the vagina, rectum, eye, mouth, or other mucous membranes, non-intact skin, or percutaneous contact with blood, semen, vaginal secretions, rectal secretions, or any body fluid that is visibly contaminated with blood from a source who is known or suspected to be HIV-infected [87]. These guidelines recommend consideration of the use of nPEP in individuals with significant exposures presenting for care within 72 hours after exposure to a source patient known to be HIV-infected. In addition, they suggest that similar exposures to a source patient with unknown HIV infection status be considered for nPEP on a case-by-case basis [87].

24.4.5 Prophylaxis for infectious agents other than HIV after accidental needlesticks with discarded needles and sexual assault

Recommendations for management of percutaneous exposures to other infectious agents other than HIV have been described [58] and guidelines for HBV and HCV exposures have recently been incorporated into the HIV oPEP guidelines [1]. Because HBV may survive on fomites for at least several days, one should check the HBV vaccination status of a child with a percutaneous exposure. For children who have completed their HBV immunization regimen, no further action is needed. Children who have not completed their regimen, should receive an additional HBV vaccination and be scheduled to receive their remaining doses. Experts differ in their opinions on the need to administer Hepatitis B immunoglobulin (HBIG) to children who have not completed the HBV immunization regimen. Healthcare personnel with occupational blood-borne exposures should be screened for HCV in addition to HBV and HIV [1]. Should the clinician elect to test for HCV in a pediatric nPEP exposure, it should be done at time of injury and then 6 months later with a confirmatory test for positive tests [58]. It is thought that the risk for transmission for hepatitis A virus (HAV) and HCV through discarded needles is very low and therefore administration of immune globulin for HAV is not recommended [58]. In addition, tetanus toxoid and tetanus immunoglobulin should be administered based on the vaccination history of the person who has been injured.

Children or adolescents who are victims of sexual abuse should receive a baseline evaluation, and then follow-up evaluations at 2 and 12 weeks afterwards for detection of STDs [53]. Sexual contacts of patients who have acute HBV should receive HBIG and begin the hepatitis B vaccine series within 14 days after the most recent sexual contact.

24.5 Summary

In general, either a basic or expanded combination ARV regimen is recommended for oPEP, depending on level of risk, and should be continued for 4 weeks. The combination of ZDV with 3TC is recommended as the two-drug or basic regimen of choice and the combination of ZDV with 3TC and nelfinavir are recommended as the three-drug or expanded regimen of choice. Alternate regimens also may be considered. Based on animal data and human studies, nPEP should be considered as a means of reducing HIV transmission after significant exposures among patients presenting within 72 hours of exposure. The therapeutic principles established for oPEP [1] and pediatric HIV therapy [113] may be applied to nPEP for children and adolescents with some exceptions. Optimal therapy for most HIV-infected children and adults includes the use of triple combination ARV drug therapy. Recently updated USPHS nPEP recommendations to encourage the use of triple-drug ARV PEP regimens for all exposures that warrant nPEP except for those where adherence or toxicity may be an issue. Although NVP is approved for use in treatment of HIV-infected children, multiple-use NVP is not recommended for use in HIV PEP due to its severe toxicity associated with both oPEP and nPEP. Determining the level of risk in these situations must be done on a case-by-case basis. Table 24.8 summarizes the important points to keep in mind for occupational PEP, however, most are applicable to nPEP as well. In addition to preventing infection in exposures that have already occurred, there needs to be continuing public health and clinical emphasis on preventing these exposures from occurring in the first place in both occupational and non-occupational settings.

ACKNOWLEDGMENT

I would like to acknowledge Drs Mary Glenn Fowler, Dawn Smith, Alan Greenberg, and Allyn Nakashima for their insightful comments and the assistance of Ms Hang Nguyen in the preparation of this manuscript.

DISCLAIMER

The use of trade names is for identification only and does not imply endorsement by the USPHS or the US Department of Health and Human Services.

REFERENCES

1. Centers for Disease Control and Prevention. Updated U.S. Public Health Service Guidelines for the Management of Occupational Exposures to HBV, HCV, and HIV and Recommendations for Post Exposure Prophylaxis. *MMWR* **50**:**RR-11** (2001), 1–52.

2. Nduati, R., John, G., Mbori-Ngacha, D. *et al*. Effect of breast-feeding and formula feeding on transmission of HIV-1: a randomized clinical trial. *J. Am. Med. Assoc.* **283** (2000), 1167–74.

3. Centers for Disease Control and Prevention. Public Health Service statement on management of occupational exposure to human immunodeficiency virus, including considerations regarding zidovudine postexposure use. *MMWR* **39**:**RR-1** (1990), 1–14.

4. Spira, A. I., Marx, P. A., Patterson, B. K. *et al*. Cellular targets of infection and route of viral dissemination after an intravaginal inoculation of simian immunodeficiency virus into rhesus macaques. *J. Exp. Med.* **183**:**1** (1996), 215–225.

5. McClure, H. M., Anderson, D. C., Ansari, A. A., Fultz, P. N., Klumpp, S. A. & Schinazi, R. F. Nonhuman primate models for evaluation of AIDS therapy. *Ann. N. Y. Acad. Sci.* **616** (1990), 287–98.

6. Shih, C. C., Kaneshima, H., Rabin, L. *et al*. Postexposure prophylaxis with zidovudine suppresses human immunodeficiency virus type 1 infection in SCID-hu mice in a time-dependent manner. *J. Infect. Dis.* **163**:**3** (1991), 625–7.

7. Martin, L. N., Murphey-Corb, M., Soike, K. F., Davison-Fairburn B. & Baskin, G. B. Effects of initiation of 3′-azido, 3′-deoxythymidine (zidovudine) treatment at different times after infection of rhesus monkeys with simian immunodeficiency virus. *J. Infect. Dis.* **168**:**4** (1993), 825–35.

8. Böttiger, D., Johansson, N. G., Samuelsson, B. *et al*. Prevention of simian immunodeficiency virus, SIVsm, or HIV-2 infection in cynomolgus monkeys by pre- and postexposure administration of BEA-005. *AIDS* **11**:**2** (1997), 157–62.

9. Tsai, C. C., Emau, P., Follis, K. E. *et al*. Effectiveness of postinoculation (R)-9-(2-phosphonylmethoxypropyl) adenine treatment for prevention of persistent simian immunodeficiency virus SIVmne infection depends critically on timing of initiation and duration of treatment. *J. Virol.* **72**:**5** (1998), 4265–73.

10. Van Rompay, K. K., Marthas, M. L., Lifson, J. D. *et al*. Administration of 9-[2-(phosphonomethoxy)propyl]adenine (PMPA) for prevention of perinatal simian immunodeficiency virus infection in rhesus macaques. *AIDS Res. Hum. Retrovirus.* **14**:**9** (1998), 761–73.

11. Van Rompay, K. K., Berardi, C. J., Aguirre, N. L. *et al*. Two doses of PMPA protect newborn macaques against oral simian immunodeficiency virus infection. *AIDS* **12**:**9** (1998), F79–83.

12. Van Rompay, K. K., Miller, M. D., Marthas, M. L. *et al*. Prophylactic and therapeutic benefits of short-term 9-[2-(R)-(phosphonomethoxy)propyl]adenine (PMPA) administration to newborn macaques following oral inoculation with simian immunodeficiency virus with reduced susceptibility to PMPA. *J. Virol.* **74**:**4** (2000), 1767–74.

13. Le Grand, R., Vaslin, B., Larghero, J. *et al*. Post-exposure prophylaxis with highly active antiretroviral therapy could not protect macaques from infection with SIV/HIV chimera. *AIDS* **14**:**12** (2000), 1864–6.

14. Otten, R. A., Smith, D. K., Adams, D. R. *et al*. Efficacy of post-exposure prophylaxis after intravaginal exposure of pig-tailed macaques to a human-derived retrovirus (human immunodeficiency virus type 2). *J. Virol.* **74**:**20** (2000), 9771–5.

15. Van Rompay, K. K., McChesney, M. B., Aguirre, N. L., Schmidt, K. A., Bischofberger, N. & Marthas, M. L. Two low doses of tenofovir protect newborn macaques against oral simian immunodeficiency virus infection. *J. Infect. Dis.* **184**:**4** (2001), 429–38.

16. Van Rompay, K. K., Cherrington, J. M., Marthas, M. L. *et al*. 9-[2-(Phosphonomethoxy)propyl]adenine (PMPA) therapy prolongs survival of infant macaques inoculated with simian immunodeficiency virus with reduced susceptibility to PMPA. *Antimicrob. Agents Chemother.* **43**:**4** (1999), 802–812.

17. Centers for Disease Control. Case-control study of HIV seroconversion in health-care workers after percutaneous exposure to HIV-infected blood – France, United Kingdom, and United States, January 1988–August 1994. *MMWR* **44**:**50** (1995), 929–33.

18. Cardo, D. M., Culver, D. H., Ciesielski, C. A. *et al.* A case-control study of HIV seroconversion in health care workers after percutaneous exposure. Centers for Disease Control and Prevention Needlestick Surveillance Group. *New Engl. J. Med.* **337** : **21** (1997), 1485–90.

19. Babl, F. E., Cooper, E. R., Kastner, B. & Kharasch, S. Prophylaxis against possible human immunodeficiency virus exposure after nonoccupational needlestick injuries or sexual assaults in children and adolescents. *Arch. Pediatr. Adolesc. Med.* **155** : **6** (2001), 680–2.

20. Babl, F. E., Cooper, E. R., Damon, B., Louie, T., Kharasch, S. & Harris, J. A. HIV postexposure prophylaxis for children and adolescents. *Am. J. Emerg. Med.* **18** : **3** (2000), 282–7.

21. Neu, N., Heffernan, S., Brown, J. & Stimell, M. Pediatric and adolescent HIV prophylaxis after sexual assault [Abstract 491]. In *Program and Abstracts of the 7th Conference on Retroviruses and Opportunistic Infections* (San Francisco, CA; February 2000), 168.

22. Bell, D. M. Occupational risk of human immunodeficiency virus infection in healthcare workers: an overview. *Am. J. Med.* **102** : **5B** (1997), 9–15.

23. Ippolito, G., Puro, V. & De Carli, G. The risk of occupational human immunodeficiency virus infection in health care workers. Italian Multicenter Study. The Italian Study Group on Occupational Risk of HIV infection. *Arch. Intern Med.* **153** : **12** (1993), 1451–8.

24. Fahey, B. J., Koziol, D. E., Banks, S. M. & Henderson, D. K. Frequency of nonparenteral occupational exposures to blood and body fluids before and after universal precautions training. *Am. J. Med.* **90** : **2** (1991), 145–53.

25. Centers for Disease Control and Prevention. Surveillance of Healthcare Personnel with HIV/AIDS, as of December 2002. Available at: http://www.cdc.gov/ncidod/hip/Blood/hivperonnel.htm.

26. Cardo, D. M., Culver, D. H., Ciesielski, C. A. *et al.* A case-control study of HIV seroconversion in health care workers after percutaneous exposure. Centers for Disease Control and Prevention Needlestick Surveillance Group. *New Engl. J. Med.* **337** : **21** (1997), 1485–90.

27. Pettit, L. L., Gee, S. Q. & Begue, R. E. Epidemiology of sharp object injuries in a children's hospital. *Pediatr. Infect. Dis. J.* **16** : **11** (1997), 1019–23.

28. Tereskerz, P. M., Bentley, M. & Jagger, J. Risk of HIV-1 infection after human bites. *Lancet* **348** : **9040** (1996), 1512.

29. Garner, J. S. Guideline for isolation precautions in hospitals. The Hospital Infection Control Practices Advisory Committee. *Infect. Contr. Hosp. Epidemiol.* **17** : **1** (1996), 53–80.

30. US Department of Labor, Occupational Safety and Health Administration. Occupational exposure to blood-borne pathogens; needlesticks and other sharps injuries. *Fed. Regist.* **56** (1991), 64004.

31. Centers for Disease Control and Prevention. Evaluation of safety devices for preventing percutaneous injuries among health-care workers during phlebotomy procedures –

Minneapolis-St Paul, New York City, and San Francisco, 1993–1995. *J. Am. Med. Assoc.* **277** : **6** (1997), 449–50.

32. Centers for Disease Control and Prevention. Update: universal precautions for prevention of transmission of human immunodeficiency virus, hepatitis B virus, and other bloodborne pathogens in health-care settings. *MMWR* **37** : **24** (1988), 377–82.

33. Centers for Disease Control and Prevention. HIV infection in two brothers receiving intravenous therapy for hemophilia. *MMWR* **41** : **14** (1992), 228–31.

34. Blank, S., Simonds, R. J., Weisfuse, I., Rudnick, J., Chiasson, M. A. & Thomas, P. Possible nosocomial transmission of HIV. *Lancet* **344** : **8921** (1994), 512–14.

35. Dominguez, K. Unpublished report from Division of HIV/AIDS, Epidemiology Branch, CDC, Atlanta, GA. March 21, 1997.

36. Dominguez, K. Unpublished Report from Division of HIV/AIDS, Epidemiology Branch, CDC, Atlanta, GA. August 14, 2002.

37. Gambrell, K. Switched baby leads to squabble over HIV testing. Gaithersburg (Maryland) Gazette April 15, (1998), 22.

38. Schuman, A. J. Update: preventing needlesticks and their nasty consequences. *Contemp. Pediatr.* **19** : **7** (2002), 81–99.

39. Hale, C. M. & Polder, J. A. *The ABCs of Safe and Healthy Child Care: A Handbook for Child Care Providers*. Atlanta: Department of Health and Human Service, Centers for Disease Control and Prevention Publication (1996).

40. Centers for Disease Control and Prevention. Guidelines for preventing transmission of human immunodeficiency virus through transplantation of human tissue and organs. Centers for Disease Control and Prevention. *MMWR* **43** : **RR-8** (1994), 1–17.

41. American Association of Blood Banks. *Standards for Blood Banks and Transfusion Services*, 21 edn. Bethesda, Maryland (2002).

42. U.S. Department of Health and Human Services, Administration on Children Youth and Families. *Child Maltreatment 1999*. Washington, DC: US Government Printing Office (2001).

43. U.S. Department of Health and Human Services, Administration on Children Youth and Families. *Child Maltreatment 1999*. Washington, DC: US Government Printing Office (2001).

44. Lindegren, M. L., Hanson, I. C., Hammett, T. A., Beil, J., Fleming, P. L. & Ward, J. W. Sexual abuse of children: intersection with the HIV epidemic. *Pediatrics* **102** : **4** (1998), E46.

45. DeGruttola, V., Seage, G. R., III, Mayer, K. H. & Horsburgh, C. R., Jr. Infectiousness of HIV between male homosexual partners. *J. Clin. Epidemiol.* **42** : **9** (1989), 849–56.

46. Wiley, J. A., Herschkorn, S. J. & Padian, N. S. Heterogeneity in the probability of HIV transmission per sexual contact: the case of male-to-female transmission in penile-vaginal intercourse. *Statist. Med.* **8** : **1** (1989), 93–102.

47. Downs, A. M. & De, V., I. Probability of heterosexual transmission of HIV: relationship to the number of unprotected sexual contacts. European Study Group in Heterosexual Transmission of HIV. *J. AIDS Hum. Retrovirol.* **11** : **4** (1996), 388–95.

48. Peterman, T. A., Stoneburner, R. L., Allen, J. R., Jaffe, H. W. & Curran, J. W. Risk of human immunodeficiency virus transmission from heterosexual adults with transfusion-associated infections. *J. Am. Med. Assoc.* **259**:**1** (1988), 55–8.

49. Gutman, L. T., Herman-Giddens, M. E., McKinney, R. E., Jr. Pediatric acquired immunodeficiency syndrome. Barriers to recognizing the role of child sexual abuse. *Am. J. Dis. Child.* **147**:**7** (1993), 775–80.

50. Abel, G. G., Becker, J. V., Mittelman, M. & Cunningham-Rathner, J. Self-reported sex crimes of nonincarcerated paraphiliacs. *J. Interpers. Violence* **2**:**1** (2003), 3–25.

51. Gutman, L. T., St Claire, K. K., Weedy, C. *et al.* Human immunodeficiency virus transmission by child sexual abuse. *Am. J. Dis. Child.* **145**:**2** (1991), 137–41.

52. Faller, K. *Child Sexual abuse: an Interdisciplinary Manual for Diagnosis, Care, Management, and Treatment.* New York, NY: Columbia University Press (1988).

53. Centers for Disease Control and Prevention. Sexually transmitted diseases treatment guidelines 2002. *MMWR* **51**:**RR-6** (2002), 1–78.

54. Wissow, L. S. Child maltreatment. In C. D. DeAngelis (ed.), *Oski's Pediatrics: Principles and Practice.* Philadelphia: Lippincott Williams & Wilkins (1999), pp. 507–24.

55. Gwinn, M. & Wortley, P. M. Epidemiology of HIV infection in women and newborns. *Clin. Obstetr. Gynecol.* **39**:**2** (1996), 292–304.

56. Centers for Disease Control and Prevention. U.S. Public Health Service recommendations for human immunodeficiency virus counseling and voluntary testing for pregnant women. *MMWR* **44**:**RR-7** (1995), 1–15.

57. Centers for Disease Control and Prevention. Revised Recommendations for HIV Screening of Pregnant Women. *MMWR* **50**:**RR-19** (2001), 59–86.

58. American Academy of Pediatrics. Injuries from discarded needles in the community. In L. K. Pickering (ed.), *Red Book 2003: Report of the Committee on Infectious Diseases.* 26th edn. El Grove Village, IL: American Academy of Pediatrics 2003, 180–2.

59. New York Public Health Law. Sec. 2505 (McKinney, 1999).

60. Gerberding, J. L. Prophylaxis for occupational exposure to HIV. *Ann. Intern. Med.* **125**:**6** (1996), 497–501.

61. Resnick, L., Veren, K., Salahuddin, S. Z., Tondreau, S. & Markham, P. D. Stability and inactivation of HTLV-III/LAV under clinical and laboratory environments. *J. Am. Med. Assoc.* **255**:**14** (1986), 1887–91.

62. Rich, J. D., Dickinson, B. P., Carney, J. M., Fisher, A. & Heimer, R. Detection of HIV-1 nucleic acid and HIV-1 antibodies in needles and syringes used for non-intravenous injection. *AIDS* **12**:**17** (1998), 2345–50.

63. Abdala, N., Reyes, R., Carney, J. M. & Heimer, R. Survival of HIV-1 in syringes: effects of temperature during storage. *Substance Use Misuse* **35**:**10** (2000), 1369–83.

64. Centers for Disease Control and Prevention. Public Health Service guidelines for the management of health-care worker exposures to HIV and recommendations for postexposure prophylaxis. Centers for Disease Control and Prevention. *MMWR* **47**:**RR-7** (1998), 1–33.

65. Bell, T. A. & Hagan, H. C. Management of children with hypodermic needle injuries. *Pediatr. Infect. Dis. J.* **14**:**3** (1995), 254–5.

66. American Academy of Pediatrics Bite wounds. In L. K. Pickering (ed.), *Red Book 2003: Report of the Committee on Infectious Diseases.* 26th edn. Elk Grove Village, IL: American Academy of Pediatrics. 2003, 180–2.

67. Garrard, J., Leland, N. & Smith, D. K. Epidemiology of human bites to children in a day-care center. *Am. J. Dis. Child.* **142**:**6** (1988), 643–50.

68. Chanock, S., Donowitz, L. & Simonds, R. Medical issues related to provision of care for the HIV-infected child in the hospital, home, day care, school, and community. In P. A. Pizzo & C. M. Wilfert (eds.), *Pediatric AIDS: The Challenge of HIV Infection in Infants, Children, and Adolescents.* Baltimore, MD: Williams and Wilkins (1998), pp. 645–61.

69. Liberti, T., Lieb, S. & Scott, R. Blood-to-blood transmission of HIV-1 by human bite. *Int. Conf. AIDS* **11**:**1** (1996), 170.

70. Bunzli, W. F., Wright, D. H., Hoang, A. T., Dahms, R. D., Hass, W. F. & Rotschafer, J. C. Current management of human bites. *Pharmacotherapy* **18**:**2** (1998), 227–34.

71. Seward, H. G., Orchard, J. W., Hazard, H. & Collinson, D. C. Frequency of bleeding in football. *Med. J. Austr.* **159**:**5** (1993), 353.

72. Brown, L. S., Jr., Drotman, D. P., Chu, A., Brown, C. L., Jr. & Knowlan, D. Bleeding injuries in professional football: estimating the risk for HIV transmission. *Ann. Intern. Med.* **122**:**4** (1995), 273–4.

73. Sheridan, J. W. Blood borne infections in sport. *Sport Health* **10** (1992), 1.

74. Kashiwagi, S., Hayashi, J., Ikematsu, H., Nishigori, S., Ishihara, K. & Kaji, M. An outbreak of hepatitis B in members of a high school sumo wrestling club. *J. Am. Med. Assoc.* **248**:**2** (1982), 213–14.

75. Ringertz, O. & Zetterberg, B. Serum hepatitis among Swedish track finders. An epidemiologic study. *New Engl. J. Med.* **276**:**10** (1967), 540–6.

76. Chang, A., Lugg, M. M. & Nebedum, A. Injuries among preschool children enrolled in day-care centers. *Pediatrics* **83**:**2** (1989), 272–7.

77. Sacks, J. J., Smith, J. D., Kaplan, K. M., Lambert, D. A., Sattin, R. W. & Sikes, R. K. The epidemiology of injuries in Atlanta day-care centers. *J. Am. Med. Assoc.* **262**:**12** (1989), 1641–5.

78. Cummings, P., Rivara, F. P., Boase, J. & MacDonald, J. K. Injuries and their relation to potential hazards in child day care. *Injury Prev.* **2**:**2** (1996), 105–8.

79. Gunn, W. J., Pinsky, P. F., Sacks, J. J. & Schonberger, L. B. Injuries and poisonings in out-of-home child care and home care. *Am. J. Dis. Child.* **145**:**7** (1991), 779–81.

80. American Academy of Pediatrics, Committee on Sports Medicine and Fitness. Human immunodeficiency virus

25

Cutaneous diseases

Andrew Blauvelt, M.D.

Department of Dermatology, Oregon Health and Science University, Portland, OR

The skin of HIV-infected individuals, both young and old, is a major target organ for numerous infectious, inflammatory, and neoplastic processes. Thus, dermatologists and other clinicians who are adept at diagnosing and treating skin diseases play an extremely important role in the overall care of these patients. For example, many HIV-infected individuals are unaware of their serologic status and present initially with a dermatologic complaint (e.g. the rash of primary HIV infection or herpes zoster). It is thus the responsibility of the astute clinician to inquire about underlying HIV infection. For children, a pediatrician or dermatologist may be the first to suggest HIV disease when evaluating a baby with a particularly recalcitrant case of diaper dermatitis. A second important role for those evaluating the skin of HIV-infected patients is in the recognition of cutaneous clues that are signs of severe systemic infection or cancer (e.g. cutaneous lesions of cryptococcosis or disseminated candidiasis). Prompt and accurate diagnosis through biopsy and microscopic examination of the skin may be life saving in these types of cases. Lastly, clinicians caring for patients with skin diseases associated with HIV disease may provide tremendous symptomatic relief to their patients by correctly diagnosing and treating particularly severe conditions, such as generalized pruritus, widespread genital warts, or numerous disfiguring lesions of molluscum contagiosum on the face.

As with adults, the majority of the cutaneous manifestations of HIV disease are observed in children with greater degrees of immunosuppression [1–4]. Dermatologic problems occur in greater than 90% of children with AIDS. While no single dermatologic condition is pathognomonic for HIV disease, cutaneous infections predominate. Following a brief section on general principles in the dermatologic care of HIV-infected children, specific features of many of the common dermatoses that affect these patients will be outlined.

25.1 General principles

The approach to evaluating the skin of a child with HIV infection should be standardized. Important general principles for examination of the skin are listed in Table 25.1. Primary care clinicians should maintain a low threshold for formally consulting a dermatologist (if available) to assist in the diagnosis and care of HIV-infected children with skin diseases. When performing the physical examination, an important goal is to determine and accurately describe the type and nature of the primary skin lesion. Primary and secondary skin lesions are listed in Table 25.2, along with examples of diseases that manifest with each particular lesion. In addition to identifying primary and secondary lesions, other important aspects of the lesions should be noted, including the shape of the individual lesions (e.g. annular, linear, arciform), the distribution of the lesions (e.g. localized, generalized, grouped, zosteriform, photodistributed), and the color of the lesions (erythematous, violaceous, brown). The correct characterization of the disease leads to a useful list of differential diagnoses, and allows the clinician to communicate information accurately to other doctors. Although physical examination remains the most important "tool" in assessing the skin of patients, a few basic carefully performed bedside procedures can greatly aid in obtaining correct diagnoses. An outline of the materials used in these procedures and basic guidelines for performing them are provided in

Table 25.1 General guidelines for the proper evaluation of dermatologic diseases in HIV-infected children

Always have a parent or guardian in the exam room to assist

Examine the patient in a well-lit room. The oral cavity and many skin lesions are only seen
 with good lighting

It is not absolutely necessary to wear gloves while doing a skin exam on an HIV-infected child,
 however, gloves should always be worn if there is a potential for transmission of blood or
 body fluids, or when a potentially infectious agent, such as scabies or varicella-zoster
 virus, is suspected

Completely examine all skin and mucous membrane surfaces. A complete skin exam should
 be done regardless of whether the lesions are localized or generalized. In particular, don't
 forget the nails, scalp, oral mucosa, genital area, and feet

So that a particularly focused examination can be done to search for a suspected lesion or
 pathogen, know the history well

Always refer the patient for a consultation with a dermatologist if there is significant doubt as
 to proper diagnosis and/or treatment

Tables 25.3 and 25.4, respectively. Several photographs of bedside preps that demonstrate representative positive findings are shown in the color plate section.

25.2 Infectious diseases that predominantly involve the skin and oral mucosa

25.2.1 Fungal infections

Candidiasis

Mucocutaneous candidiasis is the most common dermatologic manifestation in HIV-infected children [5–7]. *Candida albicans* is the most frequently isolated organism. Oral candidiasis typically presents as friable white plaques on the oral mucosa, which is termed the pseudomembranous form of the disease (Figure 25.1). Less commonly, oral candidiasis presents as erythematous atrophic plaques, papillary hyperplasia, chronic hyperplastic plaques, median rhomboid glossitis, or angular cheilitis. On the skin surface, lesions appear as ill-defined erythematous plaques with surrounding "satellite" pustules; the diaper area and other intertriginous areas are typically affected. In children from ages 2 to 6, chronic candidal paronychia (i.e. nail fold infection) with secondary nail dystrophy may occur. In all clinical types of disease, observing spores and non-septated non-branching pseudohyphae on potassium hydroxide (KOH) examination of superficial scale or roofs of pustules confirms the diagnosis. Importantly, mucocutaneous candidiasis in HIV-infected children, when persistent or recurrent, is a sign of relatively severe immunodeficiency. Hoarseness or trouble swallowing should prompt a search for disease involving the larynx or esophagus.

Depending on the extent and severity of infection, treatment of candidiasis consists of topical (e.g. 2% ketoconazole cream twice daily) or systemic antifungal agents.

Dermatophytosis

Dermatophyte infections occur frequently in HIV-infected children, most often after the age of 2 years [1, 2]. *Trichophyton rubrum* is the most common organism isolated. The scalp (tinea capitis), feet (tinea pedis) and nails (onychomycosis) are often affected. In the scalp, lesions usually appear as non-inflammatory scaly plaques with secondary alopecia (Figure 25.2). Typical kerion formation, as observed in HIV-uninfected children, is not common in children with AIDS. Lesions on the feet and other skin surfaces commonly appear as annular plaques with scales on the advancing borders of the lesions. In the nails, infection may occur beneath the nail plate (subungual onychomycosis) or within the superficial nail plate (white superficial onychomycosis) (Figure 25.3). This latter disease, in particular, is not a specific marker for HIV infection, although it often indicates severe underlying immunodeficiency. Diagnosis can be confirmed by the observation of septated branching hyphae on KOH examination of superficial scale obtained from the advancing borders of lesions (Figure 25.4), or by fungal culture of scales. Therapy consists of topical (e.g. 2% ketoconazole cream twice daily) or oral antifungal agents.

Disseminated fungal infection with skin involvement

Disseminated cryptococcosis and histoplasmosis may involve the skin in approximately 10% of cases. Cutaneous cryptococcosis can present with a variety of lesions, including umbilicated papules and nodules (i.e. molluscum-like),

Table 25.2 Primary and secondary skin lesions

Type of primary or secondary lesion	Representative diseases	Typical distinguishing features
Papule (raised lesion <1 cm in diameter)	Verruca vulgaris	Verrucous surface
	Molluscum contagiosum	Smooth surface with central umbilication
	Scabies	Pruritic, excoriated, with burrows
	Insect bites	Pruritic, grouped, on extremities
	Drug eruption	Small, erythematous, on trunk
	Psoriasis	Erythematous, with thick gray scale
	Viral exanthem	Small, erythematous
	Cryptococcosis	Smooth with necrotic centers
	Histoplasmosis	Acneiform
	Kaposi's sarcoma	Smooth, violaceous
Nodule (raised lesion 1–2.5 cm in diameter)	Kaposi's sarcoma	Smooth, violaceous
	Prurigo nodularis	Pruritic, on extremities
Tumor (raised lesion >2.5 cm in diameter)	Kaposi's sarcoma	Violaceous, associated edema
Macule (flat lesion <1 cm in diameter)	Drug eruption	Erythematous, on trunk
	Kaposi's sarcoma	Violaceous
	Viral exanthem	Erythematous, on trunk
Patch (flat lesion >1 cm in diameter)	Kaposi's sarcoma	
Plaque (raised planar lesion)	Psoriasis	Erythematous, with thick gray scale
	Dermatophytosis	Annular, with peripheral scale
	Kaposi's sarcoma	Violaceous
	Cellulitis	Erythematous, edematous, painful
Vesicle (clear fluid-filled lesion <1 cm in diameter)	Herpes simplex	Grouped, painful
	Varicella	Disseminated, erythematous base
	Herpes zoster	Dermatomal, painful
	Impetigo	Golden crust
Bulla (clear fluid-filled lesion >1 cm in diameter)	Impetigo	Golden crust
Pustule (white fluid-filled lesion)	Candidiasis	Satellite lesions near inflammation
	Bacterial folliculitis	Centered around hair follicles
	Psoriasis	With typical scaly papules and plaques
Wheal (hive)	Idiopathic urticaria	Erythematous, edematous, transient
Burrow (linear array of papules)	Scabies	Pruritic, linear
Scale (superficial layers of epidermis)	Seborrheic dermatitis	Greasy, in scalp and eyebrows
	Psoriasis	Thick, gray
	Dermatophytosis	On periphery of lesion
	Xerosis	Fine, diffuse
Crust (dried exudate)	Impetigo	Golden
	Herpes simplex	Grouped
Erosion (loss of epidermis)	Herpes simplex	Painful
Ulcer (loss of epidermis extending into dermis)	Herpes simplex	Painful, chronic coarse
Scar (collagen deposition in dermis)	Herpes zoster	Dermatomal
Excoriations (scratch marks)	Scabies	Associated burrows
	Insect bites	Grouped, on extremities
	Atopic dermatitis	Associated xerosis, systemic signs of atopy
Lichenification (accentuation of skin lines)	Atopic dermatitis	Associated xerosis, systemic signs of atopy

Table 25.3 Basic materials that are extremely useful as diagnostic aids when evaluating dermatologic diseases in HIV-infected children

Microscope and glass slides
10% potassium hydroxide (KOH) to examine skin and mucous membrane scrapings for fungal
  infection
Gram stain kit to examine bacterial contents of pustules and to examine suspected
  herpesvirus lesions for multinucleated Giant cells (Tzanck preps)
Mineral oil to examine skin scrapings for scabies or Demodex infestation
Materials for tissue culture
  Sterile cups for fungal culture
  Bacterial culture swabs
  Viral culture medium for herpes simplex/varicella-zoster virus
Materials for skin biopsy
  2% lidocaine with epinephrine
  30 gauge needles
  3–4 mm punch biopsy devices
  Suture kit
  Cup with 10% formaldehyde
Dermatology textbook for reference

Table 25.4 Basic guidelines for performing bedside dermatologic procedures

Prep	Candidate Diseases	Ideal Procedure
KOH	Dermatophytosis, candidiasis	1. Choose peripheral scale or roofs of intact pustules 2. Scrape scales or roofs with #15 scalpel blade and place contents onto glass slide containing 10% KOH 3. Place cover slip on slide and gently heat with match 4. Examine at low power for hyphae (dermatophytosis) or pseudohyphae and spores (candidiasis) and confirm at high power if necessary
Gram stain	Bacterial infections	1. Choose intact pustule or abscess 2. Express pus/exudate and smear onto glass 3. Fix and stain slide using Gram stain kit 3. Examine at high power with oil for bacteria
Tzanck	Herpes virus infections	1. Choose newest lesions, preferably intact vesicles 2. Remove roofs and scrape bases of blisters with #15 scalpel blade and smear cellular material onto glass slide 3. Fix and stain slide using Gram stain kit 4. Scan at low power for multinucleated giant cells and confirm at high power
Mineral oil	Scabies	1. Choose intact papules or papulovesicles, preferably at the ends of burrows 2. Superficially shave tops of these lesions with #15 scalpel blade and place contents onto glass slide containing mineral oil 3. Examine at low power for mites, eggs, and feces
	Demodex	1. Scrape superficial scales from affected areas onto glass slide containing mineral oil 2. Examine at low power for mites

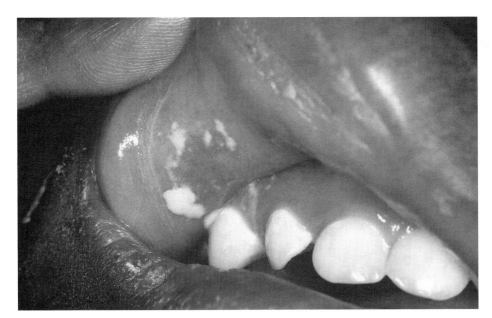

Figure 25.1. Oral candidiasis. The most common mucocutaneous manifestation of HIV disease in children, mucosal candidiasis typically appears as white friable plaques that are easily removed with scraping.

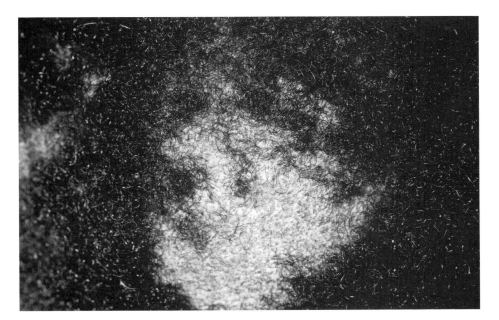

Figure 25.2. Tinea capitis. Classic non-inflammatory scaly plaque associated with secondary alopecia.

cellulitis, abscesses, and ulcers. Cutaneous histoplasmosis can present with acneiform papules and pustules, macules, and plaques, often involving the face. Disseminated coccidiomycosis, aspergillosis, and sporotrichosis may occur as well. Fortunately, these infections have only rarely been reported in children with HIV disease. Nevertheless, it is important to keep in mind these diagnostic possibilities because disseminated fungal infections cause severe dis-

ease with high mortality rates, and because early diagnosis can often lead to life-saving treatment. Diagnosis can be confirmed by skin biopsy in conjunction with special stains to identify organisms, or by fungal culture of affected skin.

Penicillium marneffei is a dimorphic fungus endemic in South-East Asia. Disseminated infections in children with AIDS in this region are not uncommon, with skin

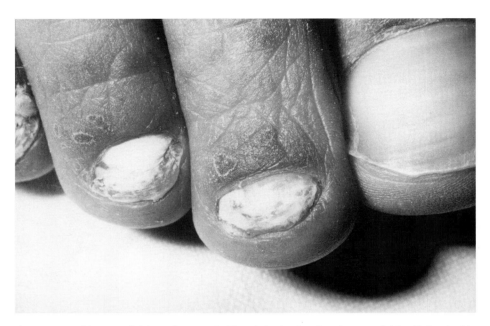

Figure 25.3. White superficial onychomycosis. Tinea infection involves the superficial nail plate in this type of fungal nail infection, and is a harbinger of severe underlying immunodeficiency.

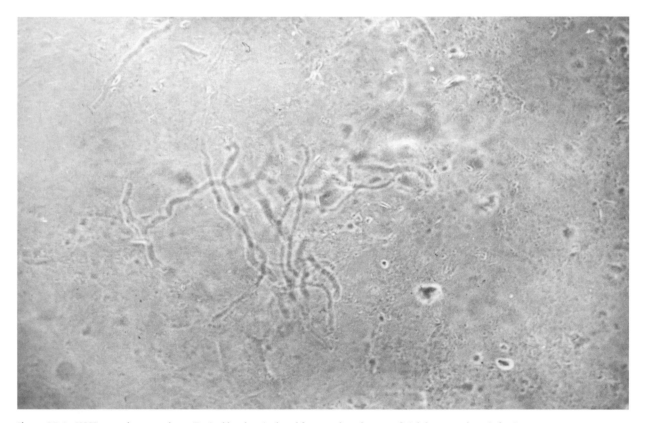

Figure 25.4. KOH prep-dermatophyte. Typical hyphae isolated from scales of a superficial dermatophyte infection.

Figure 25.5. Tzanck prep – herpes simplex infection. Multinucleated giant cells scraped from the floor of an erosion caused by herpes simplex virus. Similar cells are observed from lesions caused by varicella-zoster virus.

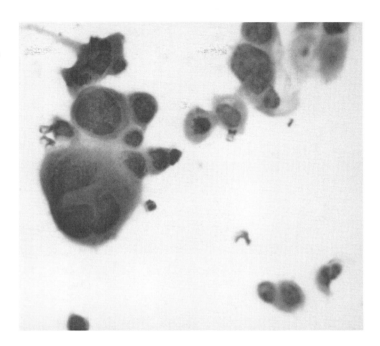

lesions appearing in 67% of cases [8]. Lesions appear as papules with central umbilication (i.e. molluscum-like) on the face and extremities, and are a major clue to the diagnosis. Biopsy of representative skin lesions should be performed to make a definitive diagnosis, especially if a patient appears acutely ill or has symptoms of malaise, fever, or cough.

25.2.2 Viral infections

Herpes simplex virus

Primary herpetic gingivostomatitis is fairly common and may be particularly severe in HIV-infected children [5–7]. Children present with painful ulceration of the lips, tongue, palate, and buccal mucosa. Secondary dehydration may occur when patients avoid eating and drinking because of pain. Diagnosis can be confirmed by observing multinucleated giant cells (scraped from the base of ulcerations) on Tzanck preps (Figure 25.5), or by viral culture. Recurrent herpes simplex virus infection may involve any cutaneous site, regardless of whether disease is caused by herpes simplex 1 or herpes simplex 2. Acute lesions typically present as painful grouped vesicles. As individual lesions age, they become pustular and erosive. Chronic herpes simplex virus infection may not have the classic grouped distribution, and thus may present diagnostic difficulties for the physician. In these cases, lesions often present as chronic painful ulcers and crusted painful erosions (Figure 25.6). Indeed, it is important to always consider herpes simplex

virus infection in any HIV-infected child with these types of lesions. Treatment of herpes simplex infection is outlined in Chapter 41.

Varicella-zoster virus

Varicella (chicken pox) is a primary infection with varicella zoster virus and may be more prolonged and more severe in HIV-infected children compared with disease in HIV-uninfected children [1, 2]. Patients should be closely monitored for systemic disease, including pneumonia, hepatitis, central nervous system (CNS) involvement, pancreatitis, and secondary bacterial infection. Primary lesions of varicella are vesicles with surrounding erythema, usually disseminated, and have been figuratively described as "dew drops on rose petals" (Figure 25.7). Recurrent varicella zoster virus infection (which is rare in healthy children) may present as herpes zoster or chronic disseminated infection. The former occurs as painful vesicles and deep crusted erosions in a dermatomal distribution and often leads to scarring in HIV-infected children. The latter presents as crusted erosions and/or verrucous papules and plaques (Figure 25.8, see color plate) [9], and is not observed in immunocompetent individuals. As with herpes simplex virus infection, diagnosis of varicella-zoster virus infection can be confirmed by observing multinucleated giant cells on Tzanck preps (see Figure 25.5), or by viral culture. Treatment of varicella-zoster virus infections is outlined in Chapter 41.

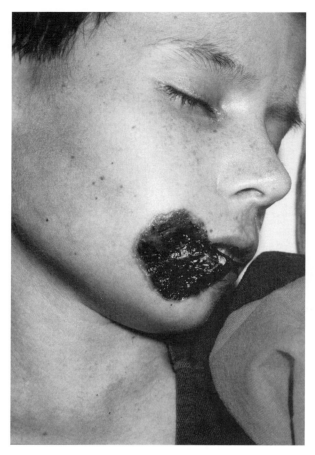

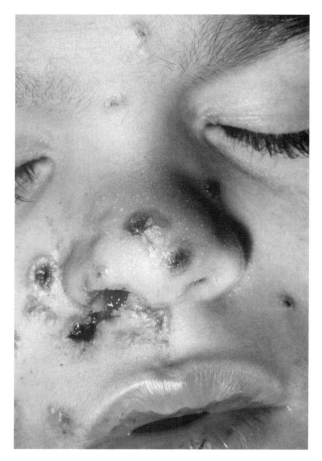

Figure 25.6. Chronic herpes simplex virus infection. Chronic ulcerative lesion in a child with AIDS.

Figure 25.7. Varicella (chicken pox). Varicella may be particularly severe and prolonged in children infected with HIV.

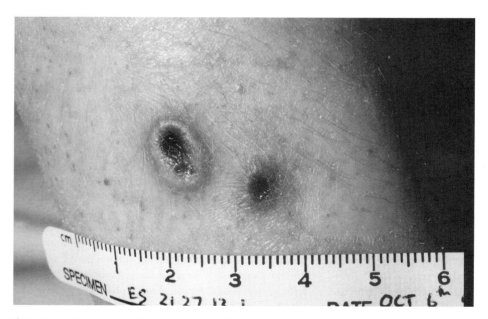

Figure 25.8. Chronic varicella zoster virus infection commonly occurs as scattered crusted erosions and ulcers in children with AIDS.

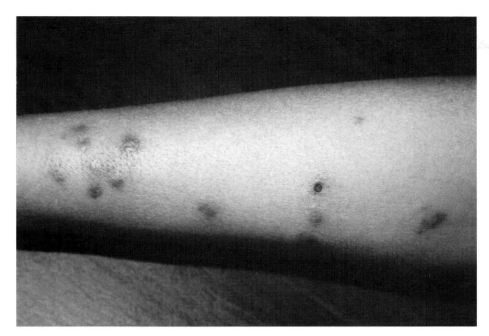

Figure 25.9. Kaposi's sarcoma. Although uncommon in US children with AIDS, Kaposi's sarcoma can occur in children and lesions appear as violaceous patches, plaques, papules, or nodules.

Kaposi's sarcoma-associated herpesvirus

Kaposi's sarcoma-associated herpesvirus (KSHV), also known as human herpesvirus 8 (HHV-8), is a newly described γ-herpesvirus that has been linked to all clinical types of Kaposi's sarcoma (KS) [10]. Infection with KSHV is uncommon in HIV-infected children from the USA and western Europe, and KS is rare in those areas of the world. In sub-Saharan Africa (especially in Uganda, Zimbabwe, and Zambia), however, KSHV infection is endemic and KS is relatively common. In fact, KS is one of the most common pediatric neoplasms in sub-Saharan Africa [11, 12]. Similar to adults, KS in children presents as violaceous patches, plaques, papules, nodules, and tumors (Figure 25.9). Of note, disease in both HIV-infected and HIV-uninfected African children can be particularly aggressive and often involves the lymph nodes, the so-called lymphadenopathic variant of KS. In this form of KS, clinical differentiation from filariasis may be difficult.

Human papillomavirus

Warts are caused by human papillomavirus (HPV) infection within keratinocytes, and are relatively common in HIV-infected children [1, 2]. Lesions appear as multiple verrucous papules (Figure 25.10). At times, lesions are smooth, flat (Figure 25.11), or pedunculated. The hands, feet, and face are commonly involved, although warts may occur on any part of the body. Palmar/plantar warts tend to be caused by HPV type 1, common warts by HPV types 2 and 4, and flat warts by HPV types 3 and 10. Genital warts (also known as condyloma acuminata) in children may or may not be a sign of sexual abuse, and thus this possibility should be considered in a straightforward, but not accusatory manner; condylomas usually contain HPV types 6 or 11. Oncogenic HPV types (e.g. HPV types 16 and 18) are sexually transmitted, and thus are not typically found in children. Treatment of warts in HIV-infected children is often difficult. Individual lesions can be destroyed using cryotherapy (i.e. application of liquid nitrogen) or electrodesiccation, but this is painful and usually requires repeated treatments.

Molluscum contagiosum virus

Molluscum contagiosum is a DNA poxvirus that also infects keratinocytes, and like human papillomavirus, is relatively common in children with HIV disease [1, 2]. Lesions classically appear as multiple dome-shaped umbilicated papules (Figure 25.12), most commonly on the face. If doubt exists as to the correct diagnosis, white material can be expressed from individual lesions, placed onto a slide, and examined for typical molluscum bodies under a microscope (Figure 25.13). Molluscum bodies are large intracytoplasmic viral inclusions that appear as ovoid structures

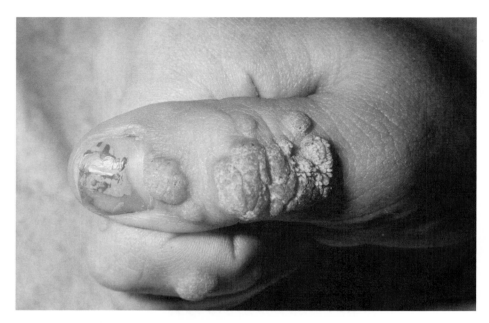

Figure 25.10. Verruca vulgaris. Warts in HIV-infected children are common and are often resistant to treatment.

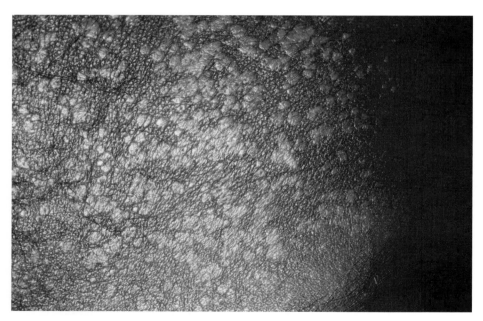

Figure 25.11. Verruca plana (flat warts). Flat warts are relatively common on the face of HIV-infected children and appear as non-inflammatory, smooth, flat-topped papules.

within keratinocytes. Like human papillomavirus, no universally effective topical therapy exists for molluscum. Destructive therapy, using cryosurgery or electrodesiccation, is the most effective treatment for individual lesions. For widespread molluscum contagiosum infection in HIV-infected children, intravenous and topical cidofovir have both been reported to be effective, although cidofovir is not approved by the US Food and Drug administration for use in this disease. As well, improving overall immune function in these children with antiretroviral therapy is likely to lead to resolution of molluscum lesions.

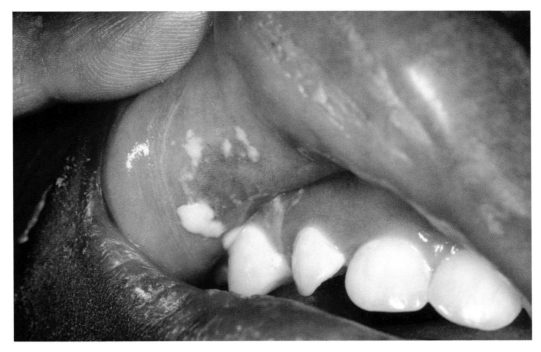

Figure 25.1. Oral candidiasis. The most common mucocutaneous manifestation of HIV disease in children, mucosal candidiasis typically appears as white friable plaques that are easily removed with scraping.

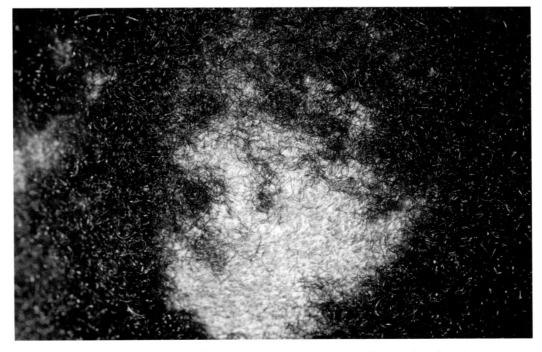

Figure 25.2. Tinea capitis. Classic non-inflammatory scaly plaque associated with secondary alopecia.

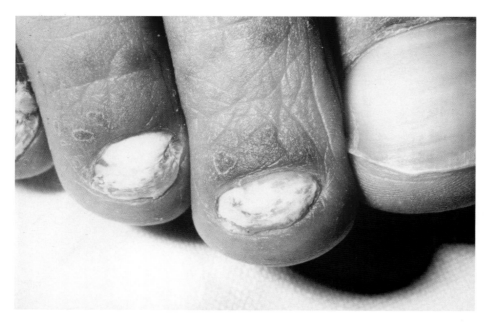

Figure 25.3. White superficial onychomycosis. Tinea infection involves the superficial nail plate in this type of fungal nail infection, and is a harbinger of severe underlying immunodeficiency.

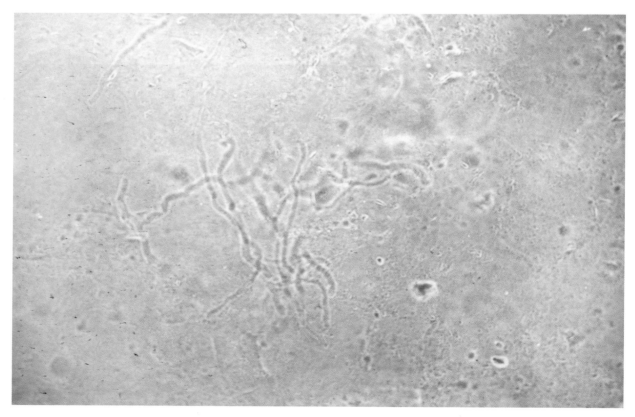

Figure 25.4. KOH prep-dermatophyte. Typical hyphae isolated from scales of a superficial dermatophyte infection.

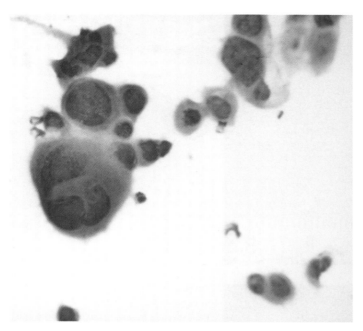

Figure 25.5. Tzanck prep – herpes simplex infection. Multinucleated giant cells scraped from the floor of an erosion caused by herpes simplex virus. Similar cells are observed from lesions caused by varicella zoster virus.

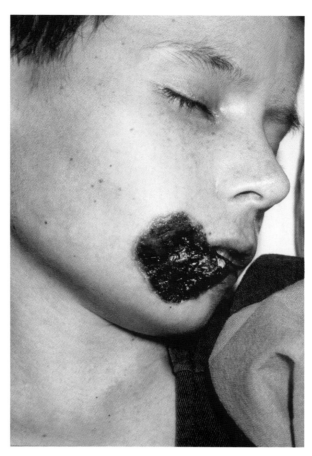

Figure 25.6. Chronic herpes simplex virus infection. Chronic ulcerative lesion in a child with AIDS.

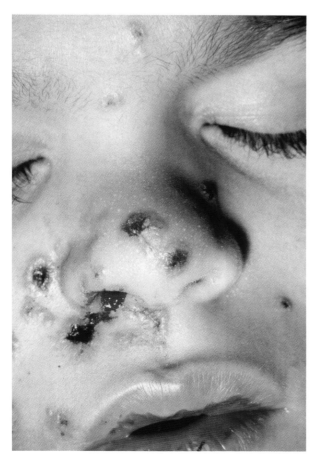

Figure 25.7. Varicella (chicken pox). Varicella may be particularly severe and prolonged in children infected with HIV.

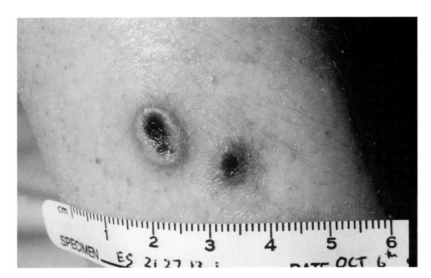

Figure 25.8. Chronic varicella zoster virus infection commonly occurs as scattered crusted erosions and ulcers in children with AIDS.

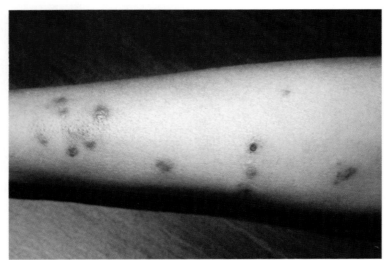

Figure 25.9. Kaposi's sarcoma. Although uncommon in US children with AIDS, Kaposi's sarcoma can occur in children and lesions appear as violaceous patches, plaques, papules, or nodules.

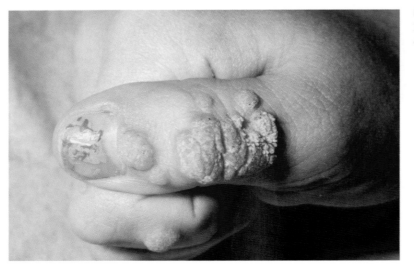

Figure 25.10. Verruca vulgaris. Warts in HIV-infected children are common and are often resistant to treatment.

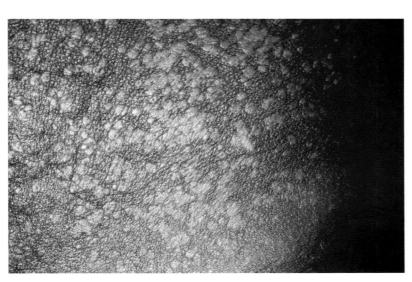

Figure 25.11. Verruca plana (flat warts). Flat warts are relatively common on the face of HIV-infected children and appear as non-inflammatory, smooth, flat-topped papules.

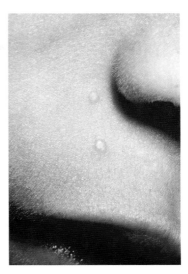

Figure 25.12. Molluscum contagiosum. Smooth dome-shaped papules with central umbilication are classic for molluscum, and are very common in children with HIV disease.

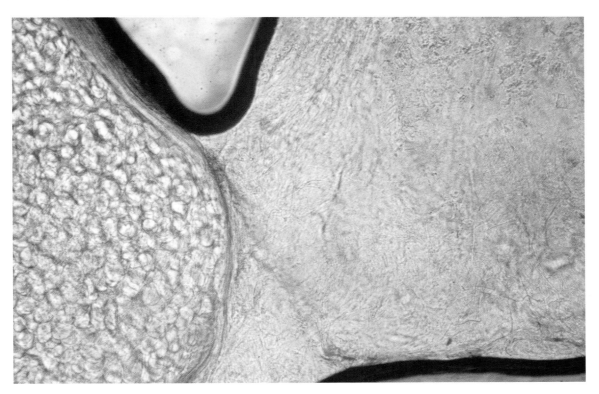

Figure 25.13. Molluscum prep. White material can be expressed from the center of molluscum lesions, placed onto a slide with KOH, and examined for molluscum bodies, which are oval keratinocytes (left side of the picture) infected with molluscum contagiosum virus.

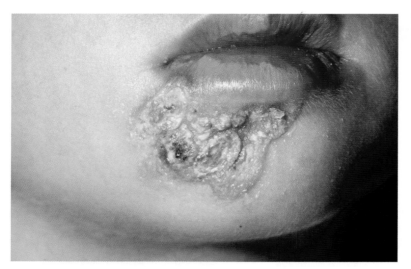

Figure 25.14. Impetigo. Classic presentation of impetigo secondary to *Staphylococcus aureus* infection in a child with HIV disease.

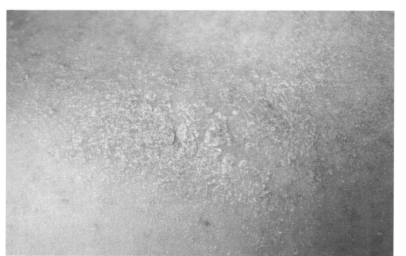

Figure 25.15. Norwegian scabies. Unlike typical scabies, children with Norwegian scabies have prominent scaly non-pruritic lesions, lesions on the scalp, and numerous mites within lesions. Norwegian scabies is a sign of severe underlying immunodeficiency.

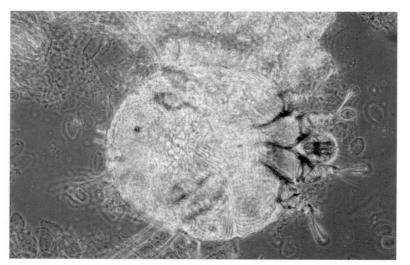

Figure 25.16. Scabies prep-mite. Typical appearance of a scabies mite.

Figure 25.17. Scabies prep-larvae within eggs. Typical appearance of scabies larvae within eggshells.

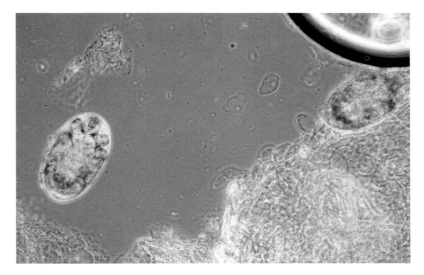

Figure 25.18. Demodicidosis. Prominent scale on the face of a child with AIDS contained numerous Demodex mites and was successfully treated with topical permethrin.

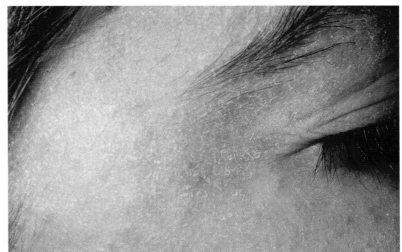

Figure 25.19. Demodex prep. Scales of suspected lesions can be scraped and examined for Demodex mites, which have elongated bodies (compared to scabies mites) and easily recognized legs near the head of the mite.

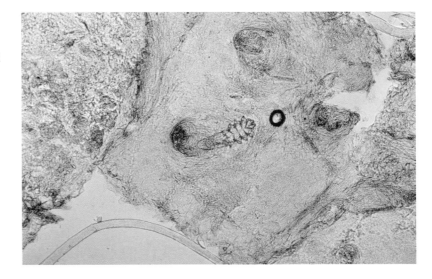

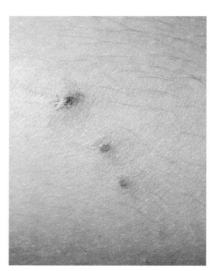

Figure 25.20. Insect bites. To avoid unnecessary treatment, it is important to distinguish insect bites from cutaneous bacterial or viral infection. Lesions are often pruritic, grouped, and located on the distal extremities.

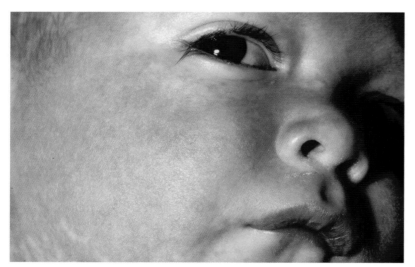

Figure 25.21. Drug eruption secondary to trimethoprim-sulfamethoxazole. Drug eruptions are extremely common in HIV-infected children and often occur 7–14 days following the onset of initial treatment.

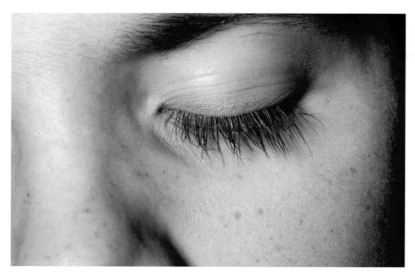

Figure 25.22. Trichomegaly of the eyelashes. A peculiar condition observed in children with AIDS, as well as children with other severe underlying immunodeficiencies.

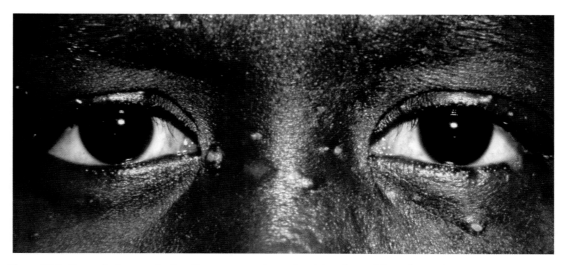

Figure 27.1. External photograph of molluscum contagiosum involving the eyelids. A chronic keratoconjunctivitis can occur with lesions on the eyelid margin.

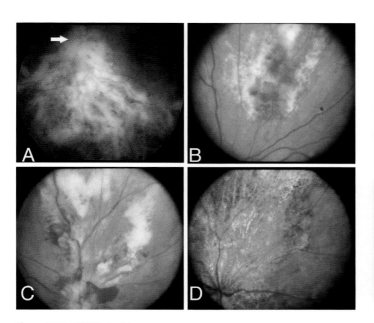

Figure 27.2. CMV retinitis.
A: Retinal photograph of a patient with CMV retinitis involving the optic disc (arrow) with counting fingers vision. The patient was treated with intravenous ganciclovir and the vision improved to 20/40 with residual optic disc pallor.
B: Retinal photograph showing an area of CMV retinitis in the midperiphery. This patient was asymptomatic and was diagnosed during a routine screening examination.
C: Retinal photograph showing CMV retinitis extending from the optic disc to the superior quadrants.
D: Retinal photograph of the patient shown in Figure 27.2C after treatment with intravenous ganciclovir. Note the retinal hemorrhages and necrosis are replaced by an atrophic chorioretinal scar.

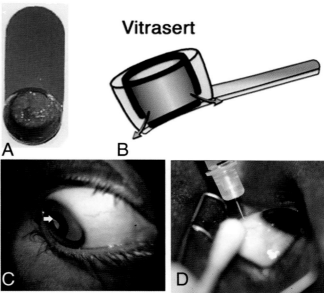

Figure 27.3. Local anti-viral therapy.
A: Vitrasert implant (Bausch and Lomb, Rochester NY) – delivers ganciclovir for the treatment of CMV retinitis for up to 8 months.
B: The release of ganciclovir occurs at the base of the implant and clinical trials have shown the implant to be superior in efficacy to systemic therapy for the treatment of CMV retinitis.
C: External photograph showing the implant through a dilated pupil (arrow). The implant is sutured to the scleral and projects into the vitreous cavity releasing ganciclovir.
D: External photograph showing an intravitreal injection of ganciclovir into the eye in a patient with refractory CMV retinitis. The injections are performed at least weekly under local anesthesia and are not suitable for children under the age of *c.* 15 years without general anesthesia.

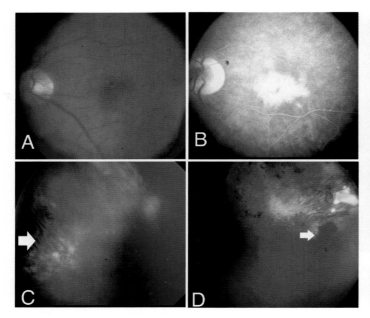

Figure 27.4. Immune recovery uveitis (IRU).

A: Retinal photograph of a patient with IRU. This patient had inactive CMV retinitis in the periphery, a mild vitritis, reduced visual acuity to 20/60 from cystoid macular edema and an epiretinal membrane; all features commonly seen with IRU.

B: A fluorescein angiogram retinal photograph of a patient with IRU and reduced visual acuity. Leakage of fluorescein in the central macula is consistent with cystoid macular edema, a consistent finding in IRU patients with reduced vision.

C: A retinal photograph of a patient with IRU with inactive CMV retinitis (arrow). The remarkable finding in this patient was a moderate vitritis obscuring retinal details.

D: A retinal photograph of a patient with IRU that developed recurrent vitreous hemorrhages. A small area of neovascularization is present at the edge of the healed CMV scar (arrow), a less common finding in patients with IRU. Retinal details inferiorly obscured by overlying vitreous hemorrhage.

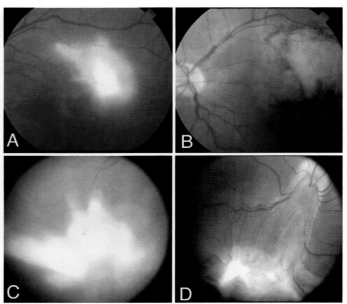

Figure 27.5. Toxoplasmosis chorioretinitis.

A: Retinal photograph of a patient with a presumptive diagnosis of CMV retinitis responding poorly to specific anti-CMV medications. Patient was referred and workup revealed a positive toxoplasmosis titer.

B: Retinal photograph of patient discussed in Figure 27.5A. With a presumptive diagnosis of toxoplasmosis chorioretinitis, following 3 months of treatment with anti-toxoplasmosis medications, the lesion showed resolution with a chorioretinal scar remaining in the posterior pole. Unfortunately, the lesion had extended into the central macula and the vision was reduced to counting fingers.

C: Retinal photograph of a patient who presented to the ER following a seizure. Brain imaging showed a large solitary abscess. Ophthalmologic consultation was requested for complaints of reduced acuity in one eye. Examination showed an exudative subretinal lesion in the macula not typical of CMV retinitis. Further workup revealed a positive toxoplasmosis titer and a brain biopsy confirmed toxoplasmosis.

D: Retinal photograph of patient discussed in Figure 27.5C. Six months following treatment with anti-toxoplasmosis medications, the chorioretinitis resolved with traction of the macula inferiorly.

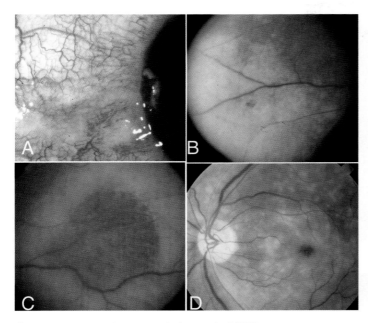

Figure 27.6. Progressive outer retinal necrosis (PORN).

A. External photograph of a patient with zoster ophthalmicus who developed scleral and corneal involvement during the healing phase of the skin disease.

B: Retinal photograph of the patient discussed in Figure 27.6A. He complained of floaters in one eye 3 months after the onset of the zoster ophthalmicus and examination showed a unilateral retinitis involving the deep retinal structures consistent with PORN. Note the relative sparing of the retinal vessels and lack of hemorrhage, typical of this disease.

C: Retinal photograph of a patient with a history of varicella zoster in the T10 dermatome. The patient subsequently developed an outer retinal necrosis in both eyes consistent with PORN.

D: Retinal photograph of the patient discussed in Figure 27.6C. The retinitis progressed rapidly towards the macula and within 2 months, this eye had no light perception despite aggressive use of a combination of anti-HSV, HZV, and CMV medications.

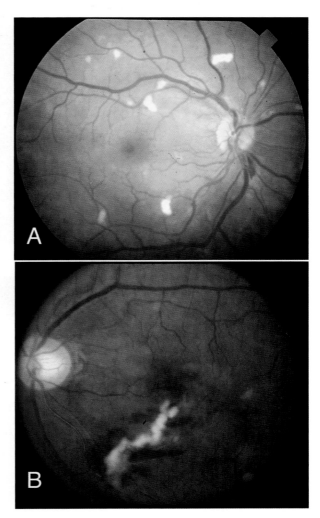

Figure 27.7. HIV microangiopathy.

A: Retinal photograph showing cotton wool spots and a retinal hemorrhage, common findings in patients with CD4+ lymphocyte counts < 100 cells/μL.

B: Retinal photograph showing a branch retinal vein occlusion, an uncommon manifestation of HIV microangioapathy.

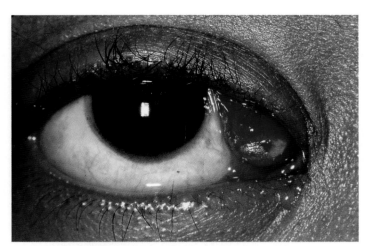

Figure 27.8. External photograph of a Kaposi's sarcoma lesion in the medial orbit extending anteriorly. These lesions can be treated with systemic chemotherapy or radiation.

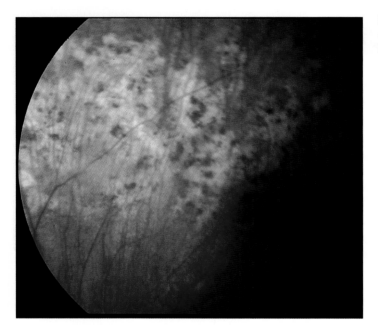

Figure 27.9. Retinal photograph of ddI toxicity associated with didanosine (ddI) therapy. The well-circumscribed depigmented lesions with some hyperpigmented borders are typically observed.

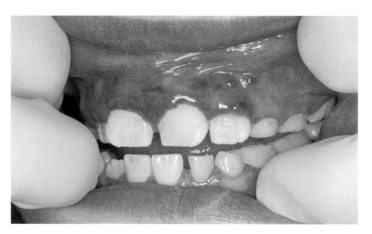

Figure 28.1. Erythematous candidiasis on the gingiva and buccal mucosa of a child with HIV infection.

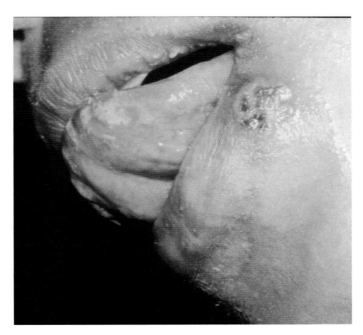

Figure 28.2. A 10-year-old child displays oral features typical of HIV infection: oral candidiasis on the lateral border of the tongue and at the corners of mouth, and a large, recurrent herpetic lesion extraorally.

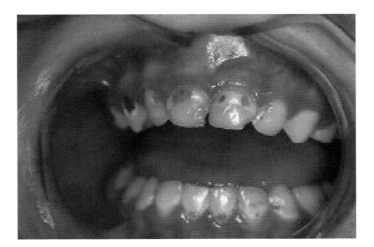

Figure 28.3. Caries of the primary dentition of an HIV-infected child. Caries is evident on the anterior teeth, indicating a very high rate of caries development. These lesions may have been prevented by proper feeding practices and good oral hygiene.

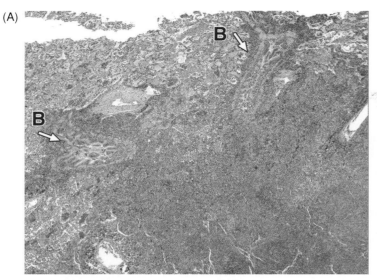

(A)

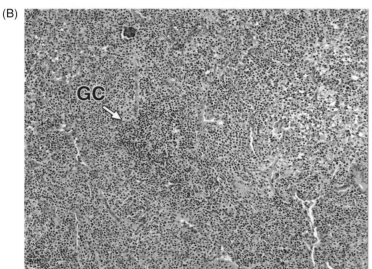

(B)

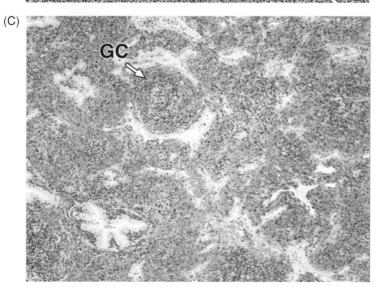

(C)

Figure 31.12. Histopathology of pulmonary MALT (mucosa-associated lymphoid tissue). Panel A. Low power view, hematoxylin and eosin stain. B: bronchiole. Panel B. High power, hematoxylin and eosin stain. GC: germinal center. Panel C. Immunohistochemical staining for the B cell marker. Leu- 22. Histologic findings suggestive of a low-grade lymphoma of MALT: extensive infiltration by a dense lymphoid infiltrate (Panel A) composed of germinal centers (Panel B) with marked plasmacytosis and irregular lymphoid cells characteristic of monocytoid B-lymphocytes. Co-expression of Leu-22 by most of the B cells (Panel C).

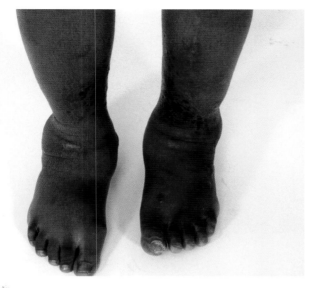

Figure 36.1. Kaposi's sarcoma involving the skin with associated edema.

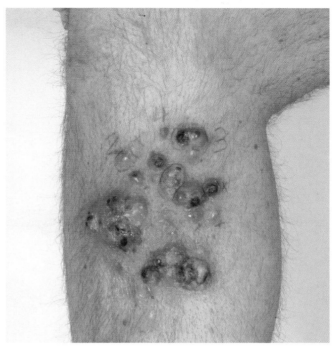

Figure 36.2. Ulcerating nodular lesions in AIDS-Kaposi's sarcoma.

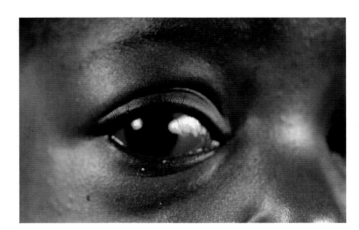

Figure 36.3. Child from Uganda with lymphadenopathic form of Kaposi's sarcoma with conjunctival involvement. (Photo courtesy of Dr. Sam Mbulaiteye, Viral Epidemiology Branch, National Cancer Institute, NIH).

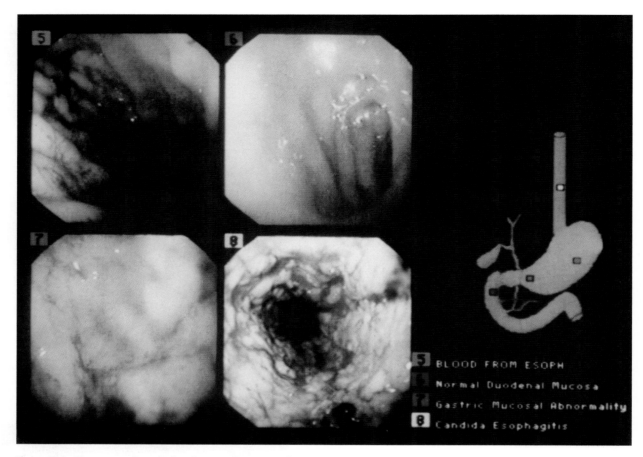

Figure 40.1. Upper gastrointestinal endoscopy showing confluent white-beige plaques on the esophageal mucosa due to *Candida albicans.*

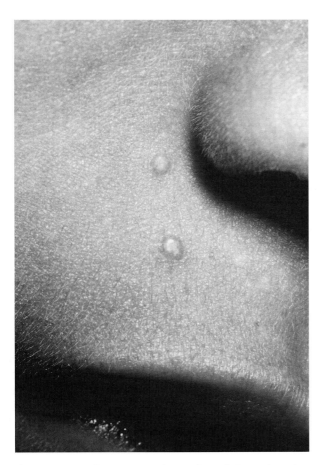

Figure 25.12. Molluscum contagiosum. Smooth dome-shaped papules with central umbilication are classic for molluscum, and are very common in children with HIV disease.

Other viral infections

Oral hairy leukoplakia is caused by chronic active Epstein-Barr virus infection of epithelial cells [5]. Although more common in HIV-infected adults, children may present with typical disease, which includes white verrucous plaques on the lateral aspects of the tongue that cannot be removed with scraping (in contrast to white plaques of pseudomembranous candidiasis that are easily removed with scraping).

In developing countries, measles is often more severe in HIV-infected children compared with those uninfected with HIV [13]. HIV-infected children usually present with a typical morbilliform rash and dramatic signs of acute illness (e.g. malaise, fever, and cough). Mortality, which can be as high as 70% in these cases, is most often secondary to measles giant cell pneumonia.

25.2.3 Bacterial infections

The clinical manifestations of cutaneous bacterial infections are usually similar in HIV-infected and -uninfected children. *Staphylococcus aureus* and *Streptococcus pneumoniae* infection cause impetigo (Figure 25.14), folliculitis, abscesses, wound infection, and cellulitis. Bacterial infection should be suspected when cutaneous erythema, edema, and tenderness are present, and confirmation can be made by bacterial culture if lesions exhibit frank pus or exudate. Treatment consists of oral antibiotics with good activity against *S. aureus*, e.g. dicloxacillin for 10–14 days.

Bacillary angiomatosis, caused by infection with the spirochetes *Bartonella henselae* or *B. quintana*, occurs rarely in HIV-infected children. Lesions appear as erythematous or violaceous exophytic papules or nodules that bleed easily upon minimal trauma. Patients often have a history of exposure to cats. The treatment of choice is oral erythromycin, with the first alternative treatment being oral tetracycline.

Tuberculosis and atypical mycobacterial infections are common in HIV disease, although skin involvement is uncommon. Mycobacterial infection within skin may manifest as reddish-brown papules, nodules, and plaques, as well as abscesses and ulcers. Rarely, BCG vaccination may cause severe disseminated disease in children with AIDS.

25.2.4 Diseases caused by arthropods

Scabies

Scabies is common in HIV-infected children and is caused by the mite *Scabies sarcoptei* [1, 2]. Transmission occurs by contact with an infected individual. Cutaneous manifestations may be relatively mild (e.g. localized pruritus, scattered excoriations, excoriated papules, or areas of dermatitis). Mild infestations may be easily misdiagnosed, since usually less than 10 mites are present on a given individual in a mild infestation. Lesions typically occur on the wrists, axillae, areolae, genitalia, and waist. By contrast, Norwegian, or crusted, scabies often manifests with widespread superficial friable scales (Figure 25.15), less pronounced pruritus, lesions on the scalp, and thousands of mites within lesions. Norwegian scabies is a marker for severe underlying immunodeficiency. Ideally, diagnosis of scabies should be confirmed with a scabies prep, performed by superficially scraping suspicious papules and burrows with a scalpel blade and placing the contents of the scraped material onto a glass slide with a drop of mineral oil. Preps are considered positive if any one following are observed under the microscope: mite (Figure 25.16), mite eggs

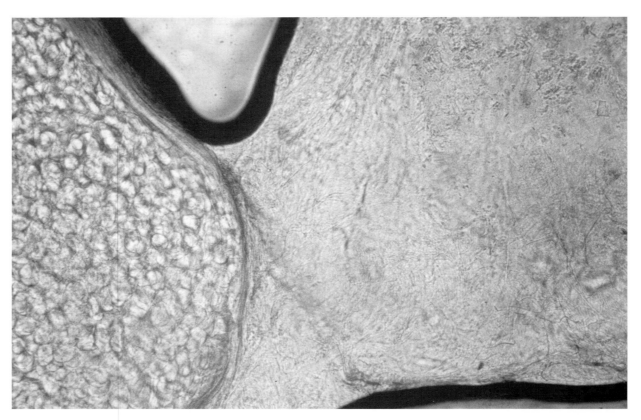

Figure 25.13. Molluscum prep. White material can be expressed from the center of molluscum lesions, placed onto a slide with KOH, and examined for molluscum bodies, which are oval keratinocytes (left side of the picture) infected with molluscum contagiosum virus.

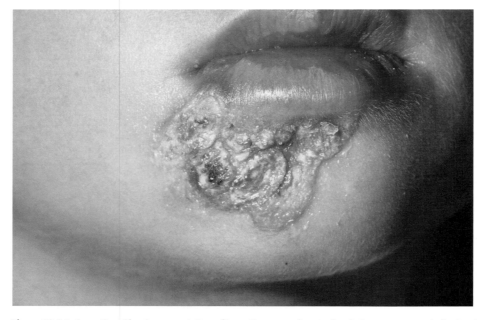

Figure 25.14. Impetigo. Classic presentation of impetigo secondary to *Staphylococcus aureus* infection in a child with HIV disease.

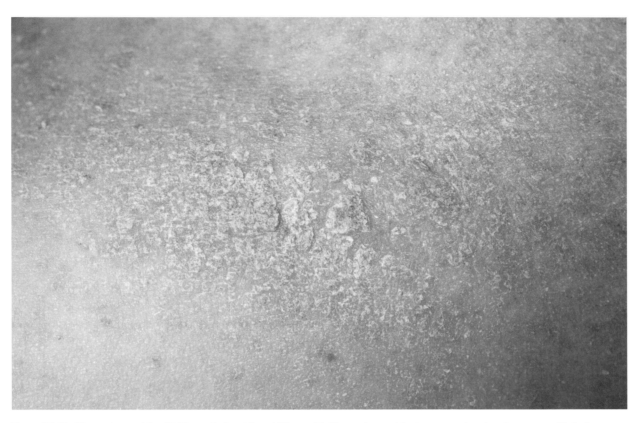

Figure 25.15. Norwegian scabies. Unlike typical scabies, children with Norwegian scabies have prominent scaly non-pruritic lesions, lesions on the scalp, and numerous mites within lesions. Norwegian scabies is a sign of severe underlying immunodeficiency.

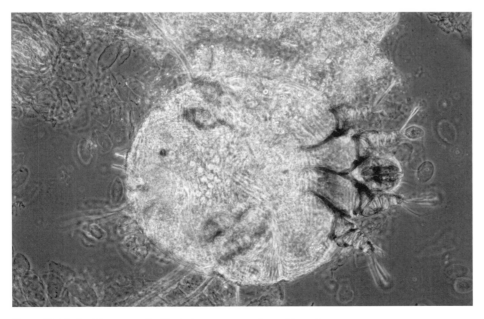

Figure 25.16. Scabies prep-mite. Typical appearance of a scabies mite.

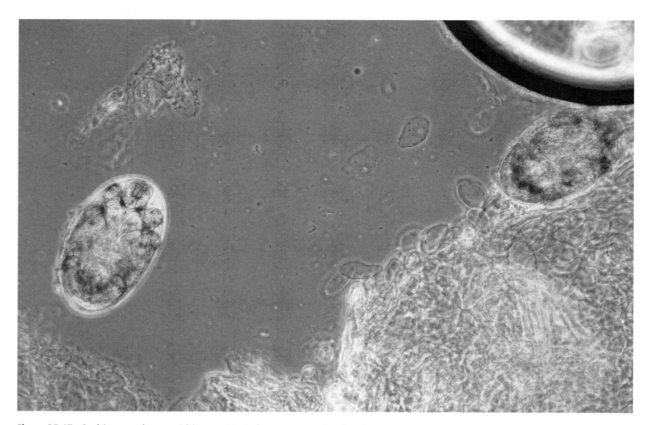

Figure 25.17. Scabies prep-larvae within eggs. Typical appearance of scabies larvae within eggshells.

(Figure 25.17), or mite feces; the latter appear as small circular golden-brown material. The patient and all household contacts should be treated with 5% permethrin cream or lindane, and all bedding should be washed with detergent the morning following treatment. One total body application, followed by an additional application one week later, is curative. Single doses of oral ivermectin are also effective. Because of the potential to cause unnecessary worry among family members, the considerable effort involved in the treatments (i.e. whole body applications and laundering bedding), and the expense of the medications, treatment of individual patients and close contacts for scabies on a presumptive basis (without a positive scabies prep confirmation) is not recommended.

Demodicidosis

Demodex brevis and *Demodex folliculorum* are mites that are part of the normal cutaneous flora. In immunosuppressed children, overgrowth of *Demodex* can at times cause scaly plaques, typically on the face (Figure 25.18). Scraping scales from lesions and observing mites under the microscope confirms the diagnosis (Figure 25.19). In contrast to children with scabies, these patients should not be considered infectious. Treatment with topical permethrin should be considered if patients have observable and/or symptomatic lesions secondary to overgrowth of *Demodex* mites.

Insect bite reactions

Exaggerated responses to bites by mosquitoes and other insects are commonly observed in HIV-infected children. Diagnosis should be suspected when observing grouped erythematous papules (often with prominent excoriations) on the distal extremities (Figure 25.20). The lesions are also commonly secondarily infected with *S. aureus*. Chronic scratching of these lesions may lead to the development of prurigo nodularis. These types of reactions appear to be more prevalent in children who reside in southern US states (particular Florida and Texas) and in Africa.

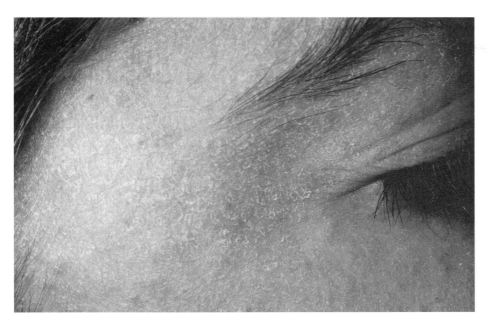

Figure 25.18. Demodicidosis. Prominent scale on the face of a child with AIDS contained numerous Demodex mites and was successfully treated with topical permethrin.

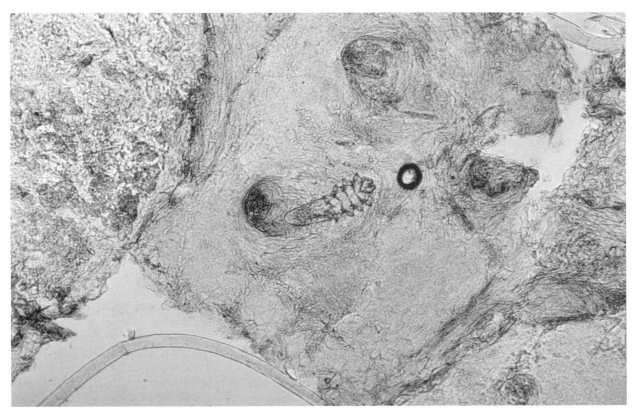

Figure 25.19. Demodex prep. Scales of suspected lesions can be scraped and examined for Demodex mites, which have elongated bodies (compared to scabies mites) and easily recognized legs near the head of the mite.

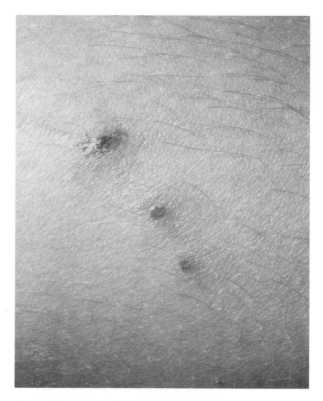

Figure 25.20. Insect bites. To avoid unnecessary treatment, it is important to distinguish insect bites from cutaneous bacterial or viral infection. Lesions are often pruritic, grouped, and located on the distal extremities.

25.3 Non-infectious diseases that predominantly involve the skin and oral mucosa

25.3.1 Drug eruptions

Drug eruptions occur commonly in HIV-infected individuals [1, 2]. Trimethoprim-sulfamethoxizole is particularly notorious, although nearly every medication is capable of causing a widespread erythematous maculopapular eruption (Figure 25.21). Typically, the onset of the rash occurs 7–14 days following initiation of the medication and 1–2 days following re-introducing the medication. Of note, in patients previously sensitized to trimethoprim-sulfamethoxazole, many clinicians are able to successfully re-initiate therapy by systematically administering drugs in incremental doses, beginning with extremely low doses.

Important clinical variants of drug reactions include photosensitive eruptions (which appear to be increasingly common), fixed drug eruptions, erythema multiforme (with classic "targetoid" lesions), Stevens–Johnson syndrome (with mucosal involvement), and toxic epidermal necrolysis. The latter is an extremely severe and dangerous drug reaction that manifests with widespread blistering (and subsequent loss) of skin and mucous membranes, often complicated by fluid and electrolyte imbalance, as well as secondary infection. In particular, non-nucleoside reverse transcriptase inhibitors (e.g. nevirapine) have been implicated in many cases of Stevens–Johnson syndrome. Drugs should be stopped at the first sign of mucosal symptoms, which may include itching or burning sensations prior to the development of visible lesions.

Lipodystrophy associated with protease inhibitor therapy has recently been reported in HIV-infected children [14, 15]. This complication is discussed more fully in Chapter 20.

25.3.2 Dermatitis

Seborrheic dermatitis, a classic cutaneous manifestation in HIV-infected adults, also occurs in HIV-infected children. Disease may occur as scaly plaques involving the scalp and diaper area in infants, or as scaly greasy plaques on the nasolabial folds, eyebrows, and scalp in older children.

Atopic dermatitis may be particularly severe in HIV-infected children, especially in those with AIDS, although it is unclear whether there is an increased incidence of this disease compared with HIV-uninfected children. Severe pruritus and secondary bacterial infections are common complications. Lesions appear as they do in the absence of HIV infection, e.g. poorly demarcated, erythematous, lichenified, scaly plaques in flexural areas.

Diaper dermatitis can often be severe in HIV-infected infants. It is important to rule out and treat candidiasis and dermatophytosis if present. Further evaluation includes properly controlling concomitant diarrhea (which often exacerbates diaper dermatitis) and ruling out underlying nutritional deficiency.

For all types of dermatitis, treatment consists of controlling exacerbating factors and judicious use of topical corticosteroids. Specifically, minor inflammatory skin diseases should be treated with mild corticosteroids, e.g. 2.5% hydrocortisone ointment twice daily, whereas more severe inflammatory skin diseases should be treated with mid-to-high potency topical corticosteroids, e.g. 0.1% triamcinolone acetonide ointment or 0.05% fluocinonide ointment twice daily, respectively. Because disrupted skin is prone to secondary infection with *Staphylococcus aureus*, oral antibiotics are also an important therapeutic component in treating patients with all types of dermatitis.

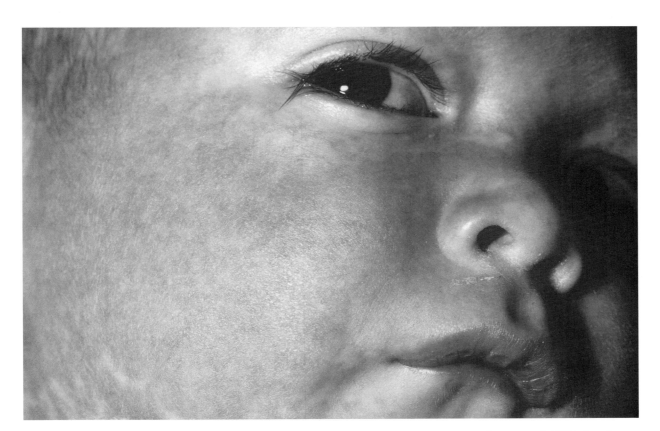

Figure 25.21. Drug eruption secondary to trimethoprim-sulfamethoxazole. Drug eruptions are extremely common in HIV-infected children and often occur 7–14 days following the onset of initial treatment.

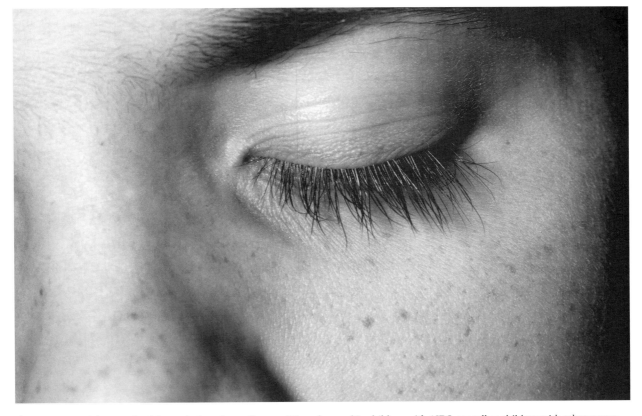

Figure 25.22. Trichomegaly of the eyelashes. A peculiar condition observed in children with AIDS, as well as children with other severe underlying immunodeficiencies.

25.3.3 Miscellaneous disorders

Many other dermatologic diseases have been reported in children infected with HIV. Some of these include psoriasis, xerosis, generalized pruritus, urticaria, vasculitis, vitiligo, dysplastic nevi, aphthous ulcers, alopecia, and trichomegaly of the eyelashes. The latter condition is a peculiar lengthening of the eyelashes (Figure 25.22), with no known cause, associated with severe underlying immunodeficiency. HIV-infected children are also prone to child abuse, and therefore physicians should be aware of cutaneous signs of trauma when examining these individuals. Lastly, in developing countries, nutritional deficiency often exacerbates existing skin conditions or leads to specific cutaneous signs. For examples, protein deficiency (kwashiorkor) is associated with dry scaling skin and thinning of the hair, vitamin C deficiency (scurvy) causes a follicular petechial eruption and bleeding gums, and zinc deficiency (acrodermatitis enteropathica) causes a genital and acral rash with diarrhea.

ACKNOWLEDGMENTS

Special thanks to Dr. Maria Turner for many of the photographs, lively discussions on this topic, and careful reading of the manuscript.

REFERENCES

1. Prose, N. S. Mucocutaneous disease in pediatric human immunodeficiency virus infection. *Pediatr. Clin. N. Am.* **38**:4 (1991), 977–90.
2. Prose, N. S. Cutaneous manifestations of HIV infection in children. *Dermatol. Clin.* **9**:3 (1991), 543–50.
3. Wananukul, S. & Thisyakorn, U. Mucocutaneous manifestations of HIV infection in 91 children born to HIV-seropositive women. *Pediatr. Dermatol.* **16**:5 (1999), 359–63.
4. Stefanaki, C., Stratigos, A. J. & Stratigos, J. D. Skin manifestations of HIV-1 infection in children. *Clin. Dermatol.* **20**:1 (2002), 74–86.
5. Greenspan, D. & Greenspan, J. S. HIV-related oral disease. *Lancet* **348**:9029 (1996), 729–33.
6. Ramos-Gomez, F. J., Petru, A., Hilton, J. F., Canchola, A. J., Wara, D. & Greenspan, J. S. Oral manifestations and dental status in paediatric HIV infection. *Int. J. Paediatr. Dent.* **10**:1 (2000), 3–11.
7. Shiboski, C. H., Wilson, C. M., Greenspan, D., Hilton, J., Greenspan, J. S. & Moscicki, A. B. HIV-related oral manifestations among adolescents in a multicenter cohort study. *J. Adolesc. Health* **29**:3 (Suppl) (2001), 109, 14.
8. Sirisanthana, V. & Sirisanthana, T. Disseminated *Penicillium marneffei* infection in human immunodeficiency virus-infected children. *Pediatr. Infect. Dis. J.* **14**:11 (1995), 935–40.
9. Grossman, M. C. & Grossman, M. E. Chronic hyperkeratotic herpes zoster and human immunodeficiency virus infection. *J. Am. Acad. Dermatol.* **28**:2 (1993), 306–8.
10. Moore, P. S. & Chang, Y. Detection of herpesvirus-like DNA sequences in Kaposi's sarcoma in patients with and without HIV infection. *New Engl. J. Med.* **332**:18 (1995), 1181–5.
11. Ziegler, J. L. & Katongole-Mbidde, E. Kaposi's sarcoma in childhood: an analysis of 100 cases from Uganda and relationship to HIV infection. *Int. J. Cancer* **65**:2 (1996), 200–3.
12. He, J., Bhat, G., Kankasa, C. *et al.* Seroprevalence of human herpesvirus 8 among Zambian women of childbearing age without Kaposi's sarcoma (KS) and mother-child pairs with KS. *J. Infect. Dis.* **178**:6 (1998), 1787–90.
13. Dray-Spira, R., Lepage, P. & Dabis, F. Prevention of infectious complications of paediatric HIV infection in Africa. *AIDS* **14**:9 (2000), 1091–9.
14. Jaquet, D., Levine, M., Ortega-Rodriguez, E, *et al.* Clinical and metabolic presentation of the lipodystrophic syndrome in HIV-infected children. *AIDS* **14**:14 (2000), 2123–8.
15. Arpadi, S. M., Cuff, P. A., Horlick, M., Wang, J. & Kotler, D. P. Lipodystrophy in HIV-infected children is associated with high viral load and low CD4+ -lymphocyte count and CD4+ -lymphocyte percentage at baseline and use of protease inhibitors and stavudine. *J. AIDS* **27**:1 (2001), 30–4.

Neurologic problems

Lucy Civitello, M.D.

Department of Neurology, Children's National Medical Center, Washington, DC, National Institutes of Health, Bethesda, MD

26.1 Introduction

Since the first descriptions of pediatric AIDS in the 1980s, neurodevelopmental abnormalities have been a well-known complication of HIV disease in children, causing significant morbidity and mortality [1–3]. Over the last decade, significant progress has been made in the early diagnosis and treatment of the HIV-infected infant and child. As a result, the prevalence and natural history of neurological illnesses in these patients have changed, with improvement in neurologic outcome in many cases.

The central nervous system (CNS) manifestations of HIV disease can be subdivided into two main groups: (1) those indirectly related to the effects of HIV disease on the brain, such as CNS opportunistic infections (OIs), malignancies, and cerebrovascular disease; and (2) those directly attributable to HIV brain infection.

Peripheral nervous system (PNS) abnormalities occur relatively frequently in adult HIV-infected patients and are usually related to antiretroviral therapy, HIV disease, or OIs [4–7]. Although much less common in infants and children, neuropathies and myopathies do occur, with similar etiologies [8, 9].

26.2 Secondary CNS disorders

26.2.1 Opportunistic infections of the CNS

Children with HIV disease have fewer problems with CNS OIs compared with adults, probably because OIs represent reactivation of previous, relatively asymptomatic infections. Nevertheless, CNS OIs can present significant problems in children, and their incidence may increase because children with HIV disease are living longer. Generally, OIs are seen in patients with severe immunosuppression (CD4+ lymphocyte counts less than 200 cells/μL), and in older children and adolescents. They may also occur in infants and younger children as a result of congenital infection.

The most common CNS OI in children is cytomegalovirus (CMV) infection, which may present as a subacute or chronic encephalitis/ventriculitis, an acute ascending radiculomyelitis or as an acute or subacute neuritis [10–13] (see also Chapter 41). Other viruses (herpes simplex virus [HSV], varicella-zoster virus [VZV]) may also cause an acute or subacute encephalitis [14]. Progressive multifocal leukoencephalopathy (PML), caused by the JC virus (a papova virus), has rarely been reported in the pediatric AIDS population [15].

The second most common CNS OIs in children are fungal infections (*Candida* and *Aspergillus* meningitis and abscess) [10]. Cryptococcal meningitis, although seen in 5–10% of adult AIDS patients, was reported in less than 1% of pediatric AIDS patients followed at the National Cancer Institute over a period of 8 years [16] (see also Chapter 40).

Toxoplasma encephalitis, a protozoan CNS infection, is the most common cause of intracranial mass lesions in adults with AIDS, occurring in 10–50% of patients [17]. However, it has only been reported in about 1% of HIV-infected children [18].

Bacterial CNS infections are also relatively uncommon in children with HIV disease. Initial studies reported a 4–11% incidence of bacterial CNS infections, including *Streptococcus pneumoniae*, *Haemophilus influenzae* type B, *Escherichia coli*, *Staphylococcus aureus* and group B

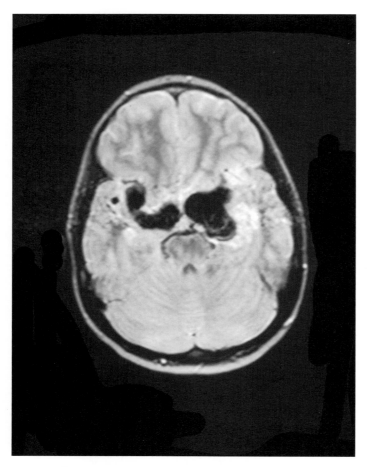

Figure 26.1. Magnetic resonance imaging scan of large aneurysmal dilatations of multiple vessels of the Circle of Willis in an adolescent boy with transfusion-acquired HIV infection. (Image courtesy of Department of Radiology, National Institutes of Health.)

streptococcus [19]. There was only one case of bacterial meningitis in 372 HIV-infected children enrolled in an IVIG trial sponsored by NICHD [20]. Unusual bacterial pathogens need to be considered in these immunocompromised hosts, such as *Mycobacterium tuberculosis*, atypical *Mycobacteria*, syphilis, *Bartonella*, *Listeria monocytogenes* and *Nocardia asteroides* [21].

26.2.2 Neoplasms

Primary CNS lymphoma is the most common cause of CNS mass lesions in pediatric AIDS patients and is the second most common cause of focal neurologic deficits after stroke [22] (see also Chapter 36). These are usually high grade, multifocal B-cell tumors, which present with the subacute onset of change in mental status or behavior, headache, seizures, and new focal neurological signs. The tumors have a predilection for the deep gray matter (basal ganglia and thalamus). On neuroimaging studies, they enhance with contrast and are associated with edema and mass effect. The prognosis is poor [23]. Treatment options include steroids, radiation therapy, and systemic chemotherapy. Metastatic lymphomas tend to cause more peripheral meningeal involvement and are rare in children with HIV disease.

26.2.3 Cerebrovascular disease

Strokes are the most common cause of clinical focal neurologic deficits in children with HIV infection [22, 24]. Strokes may be secondary to hemorrhage (related to coagulopathies), or ischemia. Ischemic strokes may be embolic, or may be related to an infectious vasculitis (for example, VZV) [25]. AIDS patients may also develop a hypercoagulable state related to acquired protein C and/or S deficiencies. In addition, there is a characteristic vasculopathy seen in HIV-infected children resulting in aneurysmal dilatation of vessels of the circle of Willis with or without ischemic infarction or hemorrhage [26, 27]. The etiology of this vasculopathy is unclear but it may be related to direct viral invasion of the vessel walls [28] (Fig. 26.1).

26.3 Primary HIV-related CNS disease

HIV-related CNS disease is a prominent feature in pediatric patients with HIV infection. Even early on in the epidemic, it was recognized that the frequent neurological abnormalities seen in these children were due to the direct effects of HIV infection on the brain and not due to OIs or malignancies [1–3]. HIV was isolated from the brain and cerebrospinal fluid (CSF) in 1985 [29]. Soon after, HIV antigens were detected in the brain, viral particles were visualized in brain macrophages by electron microscopy, HIV nucleic acids were detected in brain tissue by in situ hybridization, and intrathecal anti-HIV antibodies were observed [30–33].

26.3.1 Epidemiology

The prevalence of HIV-related CNS disease in children was estimated at 50–90% in early studies [19, 34, 35]. By the mid 1990s, the prevalence was estimated to be between 20–50% [36–39]. Since the advent of HAART (highly active antiretroviral therapy), the incidence of encephalopathy in children is lower. This decrease in CNS disease has been documented in adults in the Multicenter AIDS Cohort Study [40].

In general, children less than 3 years of age have higher rates of CNS disease than older children and adolescents [36–38]. Patients with more advanced degrees of immune suppression have higher rates of encephalopathy [41]. It is also important to note that HIV-related CNS disease may be the presenting manifestation of HIV infection in as many as 18% of pediatric patients [42]. Early onset of HIV infection (i.e. infection occurring in utero) increases a child's risk for poor neurodevelopmental outcome within the first 30 months of life [43].

Early onset of neurologic symptoms and signs in HIV-infected infants (before the age of 1 year) seems to have a different significance and pathophysiology than those occurring later on in children and adults [44]. When pediatric patients from the French Perinatal Cohort were compared with the French SEROCO Cohort of adults, the cumulative incidence of encephalopathy was higher in children than in adults only during the first year after infection (9.9% vs 0.3%) and during the second year (4.2% vs 0%) but was similar afterward (less than 1% per year in each group). The cumulative incidence at 7 years reached 16% in children and 5% in adults. The early encephalopathy was not prevented by zidovudine (ZDV) use during pregnancy. In addition, the babies who went on to develop early CNS symptoms had significantly smaller head sizes and weights at birth than their counterparts without neurological symptoms. These findings suggest a prenatal onset of HIV brain infection in this subgroup of infants with early onset of neurological disease. It also suggests that the course and pathophysiology of CNS disease in older children and adolescents is more similar to the dementia and motor cognitive dysfunction seen in adults. This may have important therapeutic and preventive implications.

26.3.2 Clinical manifestations

The well-described classic triad of HIV-related encephalopathy identified in the mid-1980s and early 1990s included developmental delays (particularly motor and expressive language), acquired microcephaly and pyramidal tract motor deficits [1–3] (see Chapter 17). In the past, pediatric patients were classified as either having encephalopathy or not. However, it has become increasingly evident that there is a broad spectrum of clinical manifestations and severity of CNS disease in infants and children. These observations have led to the development of a new classification system for pediatric HIV-related CNS disease that is currently used at the HIV and AIDS Malig-

Table 26.1 Clinical manifestations of HIV-related encephalopathy

Progressive encephalopathies
  Subacute Progressive
    Loss of milestones
    Progressive motor dysfunction
    Oromotor dysfunction
    Acquired microcephaly
    Cognitive deterioration
    Apathy
    Progressive long tract signs
    Movement disorders (uncommon)
    Cerebellar signs (uncommon)
    Seizures (uncommon)
    More rapid course (weeks to months)
  Plateau
    No loss of skills
    No or slower acquisition of skills
    Decline in rate of cognitive development
    Motor dysfunction (non-progressive)
    Acquired microcephaly
    More indolent course
  Static encephalopathy
    Fixed deficits
    No loss of skills
    Skills acquired at a stable but slow rate
    Deficient, but stable IQ
    Motor dysfunction (non-progressive)
    Static course
    Many potential etiologies

nancy Branch (HAMB) of the National Cancer Institute (NCI) of the National Institutes of Health (NIH). This system is used to track the CNS status of children on different treatment protocols and natural history studies. Patients are classified based on several clinical observations (see Table 17.1 in Chapter 17).

Patients with encephalopathy have more severe and pervasive CNS dysfunction that affects their day-to-day functioning than patients without encephalopathy. Encephalopathy can be either progressive (subacute – the most severe – or plateau subtypes) or static (Table 26.1). The subacute progressive type is often seen in infants and young children who are naïve to antiretroviral therapy [1–3, 19, 34, 45]. The hallmarks of this disorder are loss of previously acquired milestones, particularly motor and expressive language, with progressive non-focal motor dysfunction (spastic quadriplegia or hypotonia in young infants and spastic diplegia or hypotonia in older infants and children) [46]. The course of this disorder is usually slower, developing over weeks to months, and more insidious than the course observed with OIs, tumor, or stroke. Children with HIV encephalopathy may have prominent oromotor dysfunction, facial diparesis, and abnormal eye movements (particularly nystagmus and impaired upgaze) [34]. Impaired brain growth leads to acquired microcephaly. Progressive cognitive deterioration occurs along with social regression and apathy. Extrapyramidal movement disorders (particularly bradykinesia which can be responsive to L-dopa), cerebellar signs, and symptoms and seizures occur less commonly [47]. Seizures may occur in about 16% of children with HIV-related CNS disease [34]. About half of seizures seen are provoked by febrile illnesses. Recurrent unprovoked seizures (epilepsy) are rarely due to HIV CNS disease; more often they are due to other factors (e.g. complications of prematurity, CNS OIs, etc.). Rarely, infants and toddlers also exhibit generalized subcortical myoclonus that clinically resembles myoclonic seizures (infantile spasms). However EEGs are typically normal and myoclonus resolves with treatment of HIV CNS disease alone.

In the school-aged child, the first complaints may be a decline in academic achievement, change in behavior, and psychomotor slowing. Eventually, progressive cognitive impairment and new pyramidal tract signs (hyperreflexia and gait disturbances) occur.

The course of the plateau type of progressive encephalopathy is more indolent with either the absence of acquisition of new developmental skills or a slower rate of acquisition of skills than previously. The rate of cognitive development declines, as does the rate of brain growth. Motor involvement is common, particularly spastic diplegia.

Children with static encephalopathy tend to have fixed neurodevelopmental deficits with no loss of skills. Development continues at a stable but slow rate. Intelligence quotas are stable but low. Motor dysfunction is common, but not progressive. Whereas the etiology of progressive encephalopathy is related to the direct effects of HIV brain infection, the etiology of static encephalopathy can be varied and can include in utero exposure to drugs, alcohol, and/or infections, prematurity and perinatal difficulties. Other factors to consider include genetic influences, nutritional, endocrinologic, and metabolic factors. Environmental and psychosocial factors may also affect development. Finally, HIV brain infection may play a role as well.

Children with HIV-related CNS compromise have less severe CNS dysfunction and usually function normally (i.e. attend school, interact normally). They typically have normal overall cognitive functioning, but they may have had a significant decline in one or more psychological test (but are still functioning above the delayed range) or they may have significant impairments in selective neurodevelopment functions. Alternatively they may have a mildly abnormal neurological examination (pathologically brisk deep tendon reflexes with extensor plantar responses) without change in their day-to-day functioning. Patients who were functioning in the average cognitive range at baseline and who have shown improvement after institution of or change in antiretroviral therapy are also classified in this category.

The specific domains of neuropsychologic impairment seen in children with HIV disease include expressive (greater than receptive) language, attention, adaptive functioning (socialization, behavior, quality of life), and memory [48–52]. Children are classified as apparently not affected when their cognitive functioning is at least within normal limits and when there has been no evidence of a decline in functioning, or of neurological deficits that affect their day-to-day functioning. In addition, there should be no therapy-related improvements in cognitive or motor functioning.

Psychiatric disturbances have also been described in the pediatric AIDS population, but may be underreported, particularly in the adolescent population [45, 53]. These disturbances may include depression, bipolar disorder, anxiety, and adjustment disorders. In addition, acute psychoses can be seen with varying etiologies (including CNS OIs or tumors, medication side-effects, nutritional deficiencies, and active HIV-related CNS disease).

26.3.3 Neuroradiologic findings

Neuroradiologic studies provide essential information for the evaluation and management of HIV-related CNS disease. The most common abnormalities seen on computed tomography (CT) scans in symptomatic, treatment-naïve, HIV-infected children are ventricular enlargement, cortical atrophy, white matter attenuation and basal ganglia calcifications [54] (Figure 26.2). Calcifications may indicate a selective vulnerability of the basal ganglia of the developing brain to HIV infection. They are seen primarily in vertically infected children or premature babies who were transfused in the neonatal period. They are not seen in adults [55].

In general, greater degrees of CT brain scan abnormalities are seen with more advanced stages of HIV disease [56]. In addition the severity of CT brain abnormalities has been correlated with lower levels of general cognitive abilities and language functioning in children with symptomatic HIV infection [41, 48, 57].

There is also a correlation between cortical atrophy, but not calcifications, on CT scans and CSF RNA viral concentrations [58]. This finding supports the hypothesis that active HIV replication in the CNS is at least in part

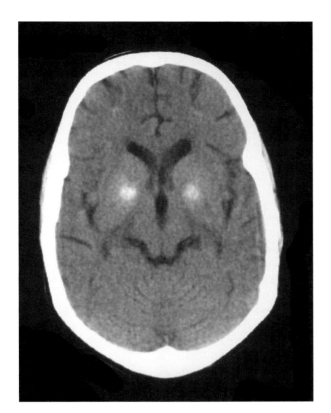

Figure 26.2. Computerized axial tomographic scan depicting cortical atrophy and basal ganglia calcifications in a preschool child with vertically acquired HIV infection. (Image courtesy of Gilbert Vezina, M.D., Children's National Medical Center.)

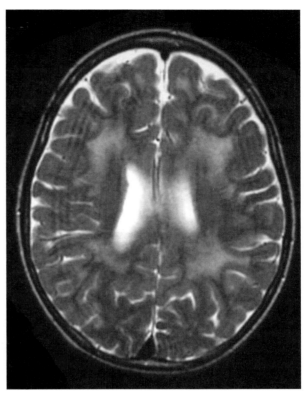

Figure 26.3. Magnetic resonance imaging scan of a school-aged child with vertically acquired HIV infection depicting bright signal in the periventricular white matter. (Image courtesy of Gilbert Vezina, M.D., Children's National Medical Center.)

responsible for the development of cortical atrophy. Calcifications appear to have a different pathophysiologic mechanism and may not be related to active HIV replication, but rather may indicate the timing and location of initial viral entry into the immature brain. A decreased prevalence of CT scan abnormalities has been found in children treated with combination nucleoside analogue antiretroviral therapy, even prior to the availability of protease inhibitors (PIs) [59].

Similar abnormalities are seen on magnetic resonance imaging (MRI) scans although calcifications are not as well seen as on CT scans. White matter abnormalities are more readily seen on MRIs (Figure 26.3). Mild white matter MRI changes in children are not necessarily correlated with cognitive dysfunction, although extensive white matter changes may be associated with cognitive impairments [60, 61].

Proton magnetic-resonance spectroscopy (MRS) studies in adults have revealed decreased levels of N-acetyl aspartate (NAA) (indicating neuronal loss), and increased levels of Choline (Cho) (indicating cell membrane turnover),

and Myo-inositol (MI) (a glial marker), particularly in the white matter [62, 63]. These changes have been correlated with clinical CNS disease. Magnetic-resonance spectroscopy studies in encephalopathic HIV-infected children have shown a decrease in NAA and an increase in MI indicating neuronal loss. Decreased NAA/Cr ratios with lactate peaks (indicative of anaerobic metabolism) were reversed by ZDV in at least two children with HIV-related CNS disease [64, 65]. In general MRS findings in adults and children are consistent with neuronal cell loss and inflammation, some of which can be reversed by antiretroviral treatment.

26.3.4 Cerebrospinal fluid Studies

Routine CSF studies may show non-specific abnormalities, such as a mild pleocytosis or elevated protein level, but are usually normal. In adults, an aseptic meningitis is often seen at the time of seroconversion, but this has seldom been documented in the pediatric population [47].

Children and adults with abnormal brain function have increased levels of HIV RNA in the CSF as compared with those patients with normal brain function [66–69]. As noted above, RNA viral load in the CSF is correlated with cortical atrophy on CT scans in children [58]. Therefore, CSF viral load may be predictive of CNS status. In support of this notion, a study showed that elevated baseline CSF HIV RNA levels in adults significantly predicted progression to neuropsychological impairment at follow-up 1 year later [70].

In addition, markers of immune activation in the CSF (and serum) such as tumor-necrosis factor, beta-2-microglobulin, neopterin, quinolinic acid and certain chemokines have been correlated with CNS disease in both adults and children. These observations may be important in neuropathogenesis [71–75].

26.3.5 Diagnosis of HIV-related CNS disease

The diagnosis of HIV-related CNS disease remains a clinical one, based on history, physical and neurological examinations, and age-appropriate neuropsychological testing, which can be compared with prior testing if available. Other causes of CNS disease should be ruled out, including CNS OIs, malignancies, cerebrovascular disease, and non-HIV related conditions (static encephalopathies due to effects of prematurity, maternal drug use, other congenital infections, genetic, nutritional, and endocrinologic factors, etc.). Neuroimaging should also be part of the work-up to rule out OIs, malignancies and cerebrovascular disease, as well as to identify the characteristic features of HIV-related CNS disease. Cerebrospinal fluid studies should be done primarily to rule out OIs.

26.3.6 Neuropathology

HIV "encephalitis" consists of perivascular, inflammatory cell infiltrates (microglial nodules) composed of microglia, macrophages, and multinucleated giant cells [76, 77]. These infiltrates occur in the subcortical white matter, the deep gray nuclei (putamen, globus pallidus), and pons. The characteristic finding in pediatric CNS disease is a calcific basal ganglia vasculopathy which consists of vascular and perivascular mineralization, sometimes extending into the white matter. This is seen in vertically infected children and in those children who acquired their infection through transfusions early in life. This is not seen in adults.

HIV leukoencephalopathy consists of myelin loss and reactive astrocytosis. In adults, neuronal loss is seen in the hippocampi as well as in the orbitofrontal cortex, along with loss of dendritic arborizations. These features are difficult to appreciate in pediatric patients because there are few standards for neuronal cell counts [78].

26.3.7 Neuropathogenesis

HIV enters the brain early during the course of infection in adults, either as free viral particles or within infected monocytes, which then set up residence in the brain as macrophages [79, 80]. There is evidence that the blood–brain barrier (BBB) is disrupted in HIV CNS disease. Matrix metalloproteinases (which degrade collagen type IV, a component of the BBB) and their inhibitors, both of which are produced and secreted by microglia and macrophages, may be involved in the development of CNS disease [81, 82].

Only two brain cell types, the microglia/macrophage and the astrocyte, have clearly been shown to be infected by HIV [31, 83–87]. In microglia, a productive and cytopathic infection results, but in astrocytes a latent or restricted infection results. However, despite the prominent neuronal cell loss and evidence of neuronal apoptosis, neurons are not thought to be directly infected by HIV.

The above observations lead to several important considerations. First, since glial cells outnumber neurons by 10 : 1 in the CNS, there are potentially a large number of infected cells in the CNS. The brain may act as an important viral reservoir and theoretically may even reseed the periphery. Second, this suggests that products released from HIV-infected glial cells may be responsible for causing neurotoxicity [83, 84, 88]. These products may be derived from the virus or from the host, and can set up a chain of events leading to a significant amount of potentially reversible neuronal dysfunction at sites distant from infected cells.

Infected, activated glial cells release viral proteins (gp120, Tat), as well as a number of host-derived soluble factors, which are toxic to neurons [89, 90]. These factors include the proinflammatory cytokines (TNF alpha, IL-1, IL-6, IFN-gamma and alpha), arachidonic acid and its metabolites, quinolinic acid (an agonist of excitatory amino acid receptors), and nitric oxide [71–74, 91–94]. Chemokines are also released which result in influx of monocytes from peripheral blood into the brain, resulting in an increase in inflammation as well as an increase in the number of target cells for the virus in the brain [95]. The chemokine, monocyte chemoattractant protein-1 (MCP-1) is present in high levels in the CSF and brains of adult patients with HIV dementia. Macrophage inflammatory protein-1 alpha (MIP-1-alpha) and MIP-1-beta may be important in CNS disease as well [69, 75]. In addition, chemokine receptors have been identified as important coreceptors for HIV entry into target cells. Astrocytes express the CXCR4 chemokine receptor and there is evidence that this expression may be related to neuronal damage [96]. Microglia express the CCR5 chemokine receptor [97]. Individuals with defective CCR5 alleles seem to exhibit resistance to HIV-1 infection. This suggests that host factors influencing the host's immune response may be important in the development of CNS HIV disease and that there may be a genetic predisposition to the development of HIV dementia. Alternatively, there may also be other genetic factors that protect the host from developing CNS disease.

This entire process of HIV CNS infection is amplified by cell-to-cell interactions between HIV-infected macrophages and astrocytes, which initiate a self-perpetuating cascade of neurotoxic events in the brain. These events ultimately lead to an increase in the extracellular concentration of the excitatory amino acid glutamate which, through activation of the N-methyl-d-aspartate (NMDA) receptor and non-NMDA excitatory amino acid receptors, leads to increases in intracellular calcium concentrations and eventually disruption of mitochondrial function, generation of nitric oxide and other free radicals and eventual activation of apoptotic and other cellular pathways [83, 84, 88–93, 95, 98–100].

Therapeutic approaches to HIV-related CNS disease should therefore be based on knowledge of the above mechanisms and should target both active HIV replication in the brain as well as the associated indirect neurotoxic events.

26.4 Treatment of HIV-related CNS disease

There are three main types of therapy for HIV CNS disease: (1) antiretroviral, (2) neuroprotective, and (3) symptomatic.

26.4.1 Antiretroviral therapy

There is ample evidence that HIV encephalopathy is at least in part related to active viral replication in the brain [66–68]. There is also evidence that the CNS represents a separate compartment from the rest of the body in HIV disease [101–105]. Plasma viral loads do not necessarily reflect the degree of viral replication in the brain. The brain may also act as a viral reservoir and may theoretically reseed the plasma (103), potentially with species of pathophysiologic significance, for example with drug-resistance mutations. At times of high plasma viral load there may also be virus trafficking into the CNS through a disrupted BBB. If HIV CNS disease is a concern, patients should be treated with drugs able to cross the BBB and reach effective concentrations in the CSF and brain. Some evidence suggests that HIV CNS disease may be worse when the peripheral viral load is high, perhaps due to continued seeding of the CNS from the periphery. Aggressive efforts to decrease the peripheral

viral load may therefore also have beneficial effects upon CNS HIV disease.

The nucleoside analogue reverse transcriptase inhibitors (NRTIs), zidovudine (AZT, ZDV, Retrovir) and stavudine (d4T, Zerit) have relatively good CSF penetration [105, 106]. Both continuous infusion ZDV as well as oral intermittent ZDV have been shown to be clinically beneficial in pediatric patients with HIV-related encephalopathy [107, 108]. Early epidemiologic studies in Europe demonstrated a decreased prevalence of dementia in adult AIDS patients after ZDV was introduced [109]. There are limited studies documenting the clinical efficacy of d4T in CNS disease in pediatric patients [110].

Other NRTIs, didanosine (ddI, Videx), zalcitabine (ddC, Hivid), and lamivudine (3TC, Epivir) have less CSF penetration [105, 106]. One study of pediatric patients suggested clinical benefits of ddI in HIV-related encephalopathy [111]. When either ZDV or ddI were given alone in a recent study of adult HIV-infected patients, motor abnormalities improved [112].

One study, conducted between 1991 and 1995, demonstrated that combination therapy with ZDV and ddI was more effective than either ZDV or ddI alone against HIV encephalopathy in treatment-naïve children. In this study there did not appear to be long-term benefits for ZDV compared with ddI monotherapy [113]. In adults, combinations containing either d4T or ZDV have been found to be equally efficacious in improving motor function [114].

A more recently developed NRTI, abacavir (ABC, Ziagen) crosses the BBB and offers the potential for good CNS coverage in children and adults [105]. However, most studies of the efficacy of abacavir in HIV-related CNS disease have occurred with combinations of other antiretroviral agents.

Of the non-nucleoside reverse transcriptase inhibitors (NNRTIs), nevirapine (NVP, Viramune) has the best potential for treatment of CNS disease. Nevirapine has been studied more extensively than the other NNRTIs in children. It was found to be effective in combination with ZDV and ddI in children with advanced HIV disease [115]. Efavirenz (EFV, Sustiva, Stocrin) and delavirdine (DLV, Rescriptor) have less CSF penetration.

As a rule, PIs have poor CSF penetration, with indinavir (Crixivan) having the best penetration in this group of drugs [105]. Indinavir was shown to be present in the CSF in therapeutic concentrations with a reduction in CSF viral load in 25 adult patients in a Swedish study published in 1999 [116]. Ritonavir (Norvir) and indinavir were the first two PIs used in pediatric clinical trials [117, 118]. Full-scale IQs significantly improved from baseline to 6/7 months and to 18/24 months with either drug (used in combination

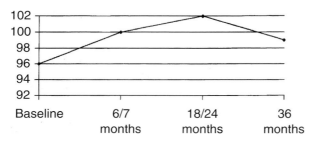

Figure 26.4. Effect of indinavir treatment on full scale IQ from baseline to 6/7 months, to 18/24 months and to 36 months (n = 20). There was a significant improvement in Full-scale IQ over time ($p < 0.02$.) (See [59]).

with two NRTIs), but then appeared to plateau at 36 months, possibly due to the development of drug resistance (Figure 26.4) [59].

HAART has been found to be beneficial in the treatment of HIV CNS disease in many studies in adults. In a recent French study, HAART improved subcortical cognitive functions in adults with HIV-related cognitive dysfunction [119]. These patients demonstrated continued improvement in performance on psychomotor tests with a plateau in improvement on memory tasks, suggesting that sustained HAART therapy may be necessary to produce optimal neurocognitive benefits.

In a large retrospective study in Germany, the prevalence of AIDS dementia and neuropathy, as well as toxoplasma encephalitis, have significantly decreased since the introduction of HAART. CD4$^+$ counts were also significantly higher [120].

In three separate studies, both clinical and proton MRS abnormalities improved in adult HIV-infected patients with mild cognitive impairment who were treated with HAART [121–123]. In the most recent study, both viral loads and CD4$^+$ counts improved at 3 months, but cerebral metabolite concentrations and clinical test measures did not show any improvement until 9 months after the institution of HAART [123].

There have been few reported studies of the effect of HAART on cognitive function in HIV-infected children other than the above-mentioned NCI study [59]. There are two case reports of improvement of HIV-related encephalopathy in children treated with HAART [124, 125].

Since the CSF penetration of PIs is so poor, in vitro models are being used to study transport across the BBB. These studies show that PIs are mainly transported across the BBB in an active process by a plasma membrane localized drug transporter, P-glycoprotein (Pgp). Substances that inhibit Pgp could increase the concentrations of PIs in the brain by decreasing their efflux out of the brain and there-

Table 26.2 Antiretroviral therapy of CNS disease

Nucleoside reverse transcriptase inhibitors (NRTIs)
(In order of potential efficacy in CNS disease)

    ZDV (zidovudine, Retrovir)
    d4T (stavudine, Zerit)
    Abacavir (Ziagen)
    ddI (didanosine, Videx)
    3TC (lamivudine, Epivir)
    ddC (zalcitabine, Hivid)

Non-nucleoside reverse transciptase inhibitors (NNRTIs)
(in order of potential efficacy in CNS disease)

    Nevirapine (Viramune)
    Efavirenz (Sustiva, Stocrin)
    Delavirdine (Rescriptor)

Protease inhibitors
(in order of potential efficacy in CNS disease)

    Indinavir (Crixivan)
    Ritonavir (Norvir)
    Saquinavir (Fortovase, Invirase)
    Nelfinavir (Viracept)
    Amprenavir (Agenerase)

fore might be helpful in treating HIV-related brain injury [126].

Currently, HAART including one NRTI or NNRTI with good CSF penetration is indicated in the treatment of children with HIV-related CNS disease (Table 26.2). Zidovudine, d4T, abacavir and nevirapine have the best CSF penetration among the NRTIs and NNRTIs. The choice of individual drugs would depend on the patient's history of prior antiretroviral use and on drug-resistance patterns. There is not yet clear-cut evidence to suggest that regimens containing multiple CSF-penetrating drugs are superior to those with single CSF-penetrating drugs [114].

26.4.2 Neuroprophylaxis

Once CNS disease is present, antiretroviral regimens may improve neurocognitive dysfunction. However, since there is an improved survival rate for patients with HIV disease who are treated with HAART, it is possible that CNS disease is being delayed and not prevented. Therefore, the prophylactic value of antiretroviral therapy on the CNS is becoming more important. Zidovudine appears to have some beneficial prophylactic effects for HIV CNS disease [109, 127]. The Multicenter AIDS cohort (MAC) study, conducted in the US, has documented the decreasing incidence of CNS disease in adults since the advent of HAART [40].

The prophylactic value of HAART for HIV CNS disease appears to occur in a subgroup of patients with subclinical psychomotor slowing and with clinical motor signs. However, this prophylactic effect appears to be time-limited, which again may be related to the development of drug resistance over time. HAART may not have prophylactic effects for patients with more sustained subclinical psychomotor slowing [128].

26.4.3 Neuroprotection

Neuroprotective strategies (adjunctive therapies) are directed toward blunting the deleterious effects of viral proteins and other potential CNS "toxins," such as cytokines, on neuronal function. These strategies are largely investigational at this time and are not recommended for general use in pediatric patients.

Steroids have the potential to downregulate cytokine production, but no large studies have examined the effects of steroids for HIV-associated dementia [129, 130]. Neither pentoxifylline nor thalidomide, TNF-alpha antagonists, have had beneficial effects in adults with CNS disease [129, 131]. Nimodipine, a calcium channel blocker, may be of benefit in adults who are also receiving ZDV [132]. Memantine is an analogue of the antiviral drug amantadine and acts as an uncompetitive antagonist at the NMDA receptor [133]. Memantine is now being studied as a protective agent [133]. L-deprenyl, an antioxidant and putative antiapoptotic agent, has been shown to reverse in vitro mitochondrial dysfunction in human fetal neurons exposed to CSF from HIV-infected patients with dementia [134]. Clinical trials are in progress. Other antioxidants (thioctic acid (alpha lipoic acid), didox, imidate) are being studied both in vitro and/or in clinical trials [135]. Additional agents under consideration for further study as therapeutic agents for HIV-associated dementia include other antioxidants, other cytokine antagonists, antichemokine agents, other NMDA receptor antagonists, nitric oxide synthase inhibitors, inhibitors of arachidonic acid metabolites, and inhibitors of apoptosis [83].

26.4.4 Symptomatic treatment

Symptomatic treatment includes pharmacologic treatment of pain, movement disorders, seizures, spasticity, attention deficit/hyperactivity disorder (ADHD), and psychiatric/behavioral disorders in children with HIV-related CNS disease. In general, the same agents can be used in the HIV-infected child as in patients without HIV infection. However, one should always keep in mind the bone marrow suppression, liver and pancreatic toxicities of the agents used to treat such neurological and psychiatric disorders, and their effect on metabolism of antiretrovirals, particularly PIs. It is important to note that patients with neurological involvement may be very sensitive to psychotropic medications.

Children with severe neurodevelopmental deficits may benefit from physical, occupational, and speech therapy. Educational remediation is indicated for children with ADHD and/or learning disabilities. Optimal nutrition is extremely important in the care of these children. Other causes of neurodevelopmental disorders, such as endocrinologic and metabolic disturbances, such as hypothyroidism, vitamin and co-factor deficiencies should be carefully sought out and treated. Psychostimulants, such as methylphenidate, have been used in adults with lethargy and progressive slowing [136].

26.5 Other nervous system abnormalities

26.5.1 Myelopathies

Vacuolar myelopathy, seen in up to 30% of adult AIDS patients at autopsy in the past, is rarely seen in children [137]. Spinal corticospinal tract degeneration is one of the characteristic features seen in pediatric AIDS patients at autopsy, but this is not usually a clinical diagnosis [138]. Myelopathies can also be due to OIs (HSV, CMV, VZV) or tumors.

26.5.2 Peripheral neuropathies

Peripheral neuropathies are less common in children than adults with HIV infection. Several patterns of neuropathy, similar to those observed in adult patients, were seen in a retrospective review of 50 children who were referred for nerve conduction velocities [9] due to clinical concerns. The most common pattern was a distal sensory or axonal neuropathy, possibly related to antiretroviral use and/or HIV disease itself. Carpal tunnel syndrome was less common. A subacute demyelinating neuropathy due to HIV infection was seen in one child and a lumbosacral polyradiculopathy related to VZV infection was seen in one adolescent. Paresthesias and pain were the most common presenting complaints, followed by weakness or loss of motor milestones.

Antiretrovirals that have been implicated in peripheral neuropathy include, but are not limited to, the NRTIs ddI, ddC and d4T. Peripheral neuropathies due to these agents can be severe and may require discontinuation of the drug.

26.5.3 Myopathies

Numerous muscle disorders have been described in adults with HIV infection, including HIV myopathy, ZDV and d4T-induced mitochondrial myopathy, and secondary myopathies (due to OIs or lymphoma) [139, 140]. Typically, these patients present with progressive proximal muscle weakness, sometimes with pain and elevated CPK. These muscle disorders can occur in children, but are less common.

26.6 Summary

There is evidence that the incidence of HIV-related CNS disease has declined since the advent of HAART. However, it is possible that CNS disease may become more prevalent in the future as life-expectancy increases and as drug resistance occurs. HAART improves neurocognitive dysfunction in at least a subset of patients with CNS disease. However, nervous system involvement, when it does occur, can have a profound impact on quality of life, and on survival. The accurate diagnosis and management of neurologic disease in pediatric patients remains a challenge.

REFERENCES

1. Belman, A. L., Ultmann, M. H., Horoupian, D. *et al.* Neurological complications in infants and children with AIDS. *Ann. Neurol.* **8** (1985), 560–6.

2. Epstein, L. G., Sharer, L. R., Joshi, V. V. *et al.* Progressive encephalopathy in children with AIDS. *Ann. Neurol.* **17** (1985), 488–96.

3. Epstein, L. G., Sharer, L. R., Oleske, J. M. *et al.* Neurologic manifestations of HIV infection in children. *Pediatrics* **78** (1986), 678–87.

4. Cornblath, D. R. & McArthur, J. C. Predominantly sensory neuropathy in patients with AIDS and AIDS-related complex. *Neurology* **38** (1988), 794–6.

5. So, Y. T., Holtzman, D. M., Abrams, D. I. & Olney, R. K. Peripheral neuropathy associated with acquired immunodeficiency. *Arch. Neurol.* **45** (1988), 945–8.

6. Miller, R. G. Neuromuscular complications of HIV. *West. J. Med.* **160** (1994), 447–54.

7. Simpson, S. M. & Olney, R. K. Peripheral neuropathies associated with HIV infection. *Neurol. Clin.* **10** (1992), 685–711.

8. Raphael, S. A., Price, M. L., Lischner, H. W. *et al.* Inflammatory demyelinating polyneuropathy in a child with symptomatic HIV infection. *J. Pediatr.* **118** (1991), 242–5.

9. Floeter, M. K., Civitello, L. A., Everett, C. R. *et al.* Peripheral neuropathy in children with HIV infection. *Neurology* **49** (1997), 207–12.

10. Kozlowski, P. B., Sher, J. H., Dickson, D. W. *et al.* CNS in pediatric HIV infection: a multicenter study. In P. B. Kozlowski, D. A. Snider, P. M. Vietze & H. M. Wisniewski (eds.), *Brain in Pediatric AIDS*. Basel: Karger (1990), pp. 132–46.

11. Kalayjian, R. C., Cohen, M. L., Bonomo, R. A. *et al.* CMV ventriculoencephalitis in AIDS. *Medicine* **72** (1993), 67–77.

12. Holland, N. R., Power, C. Matthews, V. P. *et al.* CMV encephalitis in AIDS. *Neurology* **44** (1994), 507–14.

13. Fuller, G. N., Guiloff, R. J., Scaravilli, F. *et al.* Combined HIV-CMV encephalitis presenting with brainstem signs. *J. Neurol. Neurosurg. Psychol.* **52** (1989), 975–9.

14. Annunziato, P. W. & Gershon, A. A. Herpesvirus infections in children infected with HIV. In C. M. Wilfert & P. A. Pizzo (eds.), *Pediatric AIDS: The Challenge of HIV Infection in Infants, Children and Adolescents*. Baltimore: Williams and Wilkins (1998), pp. 205–25.

15. Berger, J. R. F., Scott, G., Albrecht, J. *et al.* PML in HIV-l infected children. *AIDS* **6** (1992), 837–42.

16. Walsh, T. J., Muller, F. M., Groll, A. *et al.* Fungal infections in children with HIV. In C. M. Wilfert & P. A. Pizzo (eds.), *Pediatric AIDS: The Challenge of HIV Infection in Infants, Children and Adolescents*. Baltimore: Williams and Wilkins (1998), 183–204.

17. American Academy of Neurology. Evaluation and management of intracranial mass lesions in AIDS. *Neurology* **50** (1998), 21–6.

18. Simonds, R. J. & Gonzalo, O. *Pneumocystis carinii* pneumonia and Toxoplasmosis. In C. M. Wilfert & P. A. Pizzo (eds.), *Pediatric AIDS: The Challenge of HIV Infection in Infants, Childreni and Adolescents*. Baltimore: Williams and Wilkins (1998), pp. 251–65.

19. Belman, A. L., Diamond, G., Dickson, D. *et al.* Pediatric AIDS: neurologic syndromes. *Am. J. Dis. Child.* **142** (1988), 29–35.

20. NICHD IVIG Study Group. IVIG for the prevention of bacterial infections in children with symptomatic HIV infection. *New Engl. J. Med.* **325** (1991), 73–80.

21. Cohen, B. A. & Berger, J. R. Neurologic opportunistic infections in AIDS. In H. E. Gendelman, S. A. Lipton, L. Epstein & S. Swindells (eds.), *The Neurology of AIDS*. New York: Chapman and Hall (1998), 303–32.

22. Dickson, D. W., Llen, A. J. F, Werdenheim, K. M. *et al.* CNS pathology in children with AIDS and focal neurologic signs: stroke and lymphoma. In P. B. Kozlowski, D. A. Snider, P. M. Vietze & H. M. Wisniewski (eds.), *Brain in Pediatric AIDS*. Basel: Karger (1990), 147–57.

23. Epstein, L. G., DiCarlo, F. J., Joshi, V. V. *et al.* Primary lymphoma of the central nervous system in children with AIDS. *Pediatrics* **82** (1988), 355–63.

24. Park, Y. D., Belman, A. L., Kim, T. S. *et al.* Stroke in pediatric AIDS. *Ann. Neurol.* **28** (1990), 303–11.

25. Frank, Y., Lim, W., Kahn, E. *et al.* Multiple ischemic infarcts in a child with AIDS, varicella-zoster infection and cerebral vasculitis. *Pediatric Neurol.* **5** (1989), 64–7.

26. Husson, R. N., Saini, R. & Lewis, L. L. Cerebral artery aneurysms in children infected with HIV. *J. Pediatr.* **121** (1992), 927–30.

Ophthalmic problems

Howard F. Fine, M.D., M.H.Sc.[1], Susan S. Lee, B.S.[2] and Michael R. Robinson, M.D.[2]

[1]Ophthalmology, Wilmer Eye Institute, Johns Hopkins, Baltimore, MD
[2]National Eye Institute, NIH, Bethesda, MD

27.1 Introduction

Ophthalmic disease is common in patients with HIV infection, occurring in up to 75% of patients over the course of their illness [1]. As in other organ systems, a hallmark of the ocular sequelae of HIV infection is the presence of opportunistic infections by bacteria, viruses, fungi, and parasites, which may occur in up to 30% of HIV-positive individuals [2, 3]. HIV-positive children may acquire infections that are also common in immunocompetent patients, although the severity is often greatly increased.

Because children rarely complain of ocular symptoms, eye disease such as cytomegalovirus (CMV) retinitis, is often diagnosed at a more advanced stage. This chapter gives an overview of the ocular manifestations of HIV in children.

27.2 Epidemiology

Ophthalmologic disease in HIV-infected children can involve any part of the eye. The ocular manifestations of HIV infection in children are listed in Table 27.1; few of the disorders occur in more than 5% of children. The most common ophthalmologic disease in HIV-infected children affects the posterior segment (vitreous, retina, and choroid).

27.3 Clinical examination

Routine screening eye examinations are suggested because sight-threatening complications like CMV retinitis can be asymptomatic, and early diagnosis and treatment can prevent loss of sight. Sight-threatening diseases occur most frequently in children with advanced HIV infection and low CD4$^+$ lymphocyte counts. Regular screening examinations should be performed by an experienced ophthalmologist according to Table 27.2 [4].

The complete ophthalmic examination consists of a slit lamp examination for anterior segment disease and a dilated retinal examination primarily to rule out asymptomatic CMV retinitis.

27.4 Lids/conjunctiva

Ocular sequelae of HIV in the lids and conjunctiva of children are not common.

Molluscum contagiosum, a growth of cutaneous papules and nodules with central umbilication, is caused by a pox virus (Figure 27.1). They can occur near the lid margin and be associated with a chronic follicular conjunctivitis [5]. The lesions are usually larger, more numerous, and faster growing in HIV-positive children compared with lesions occurring in normal children [6]. Lesions may be treated with excision, cryotherapy, and/or newer therapeutic agents such as imiquimod [7].

Excessive growth and length of the lashes, termed hypertrichosis or acquired trichomegaly, has been reported in HIV-infected children, especially in end-stage disease. The underlying mechanism is currently unknown [8].

27.5 Cornea/sclera

The HIV virus can damage lacrimal glands, leading to keratoconjunctivitis sicca (dry eye), which is often relieved with

Table 27.1 Ocular manifestations of pediatric HIV infection

Lids/conjunctiva
  Molluscum contagiosum
  Hypertrichosis
  Kaposi's sarcoma
Cornea/sclera
  Keratoconjunctivitis sicca[a]
  Herpes keratitis
  Herpes zoster ophthalmicus
  Corneal microsporidiosis
Vitreous/retina/choroid
  CMV retinitis[a]
  Immune recovery uveitis
  Toxoplasmosis
  Progressive Outer Retinal Necrosis (PORN)
  HIV microangiopathy[a]
  Frosted branch angiitis
Orbit
  Fungi (aspergillosis, mucormycosis)
  Bacteria (*Pseudomonas aeruginosa, Treponema pallidum, Staphylococcus aureus*)
  Parasites (*Toxoplasma gondii*)
  Protozoa (*Pneumocystis carinii*)
Neoplasms
  Burkitt's/Burkitt's-like lymphoma
  Kaposi's sarcoma
Neuro-ophthalmology
  Papilledema
  Optic neuropathy
  Motor neuropathies
  Field defects
  Nystagmus
  Gaze paresis
  Horner's syndrome
Developmental
  AIDS-associated embryopathy
Drug ocular toxicity
  Rifabutin
  Cidofovir
  Didanosine
  Atovaquone

[a] Occurs in more than 5% of patients.

lubrication [9]. This must be distinguished from epithelial keratitis, caused by the herpes viruses including herpes simplex virus (HSV), CMV, and varicella-zoster virus (VZV), which can be associated with significant pain, reduced corneal sensation, dendritic corneal lesions, and secondary glaucoma. Treatment may include topical trifluorothymi-

Table 27.2 Screening examination frequency

Age < 6 years	CD4% < 21	CD4% $\geq$ 21
	q2–3 months	q6 months
Age $\geq$ 6 years	CD4$^+$ cells < 50 cells/μL	CD4$^+$ cells $\geq$ 50 cells/μL
	q2–3 months	q6 months

dine and oral acyclovir or valacyclovir [10]. Varicella-zoster virus keratitis is commonly observed with herpes zoster ophthalmicus, a painful, vesicular dermatitis in the distribution of the ophthalmic division of the trigeminal nerve.

Corneal microsporidiosis causes a bilateral epithelial keratitis associated with blurred vision, photophobia, and foreign body sensation. Treatment with itraconazole, benzomidazoles, fumagilin, or HAART (causing immune reconstitution) has been effective [11].

27.6 Vitreous/retina/choroid

27.6.1 Cytomegalovirus retinitis

Cytomegalovirus retinitis in children with HIV is less common than in adults, yet is still the most common HIV-related ocular infection. The prevalence of CMV retinitis in HIV-positive children in the pre-HAART era was approximately 3–5%. After the introduction of HAART in 1996, the occurrence of CMV retinopathy has been dramatically reduced [2]. The disease is usually associated with low CD4$^+$ counts, < 50 cells/μL. The mean time to development of CMV retinitis is approximately 18 months, once CD4$^+$ counts are low. While older children may complain of floaters and decreased peripheral or central vision, young children often present without subjective visual complaints despite advanced retinitis [12].

Cytomegalovirus retinitis may progress in several ways. Indolent or smoldering CMV is usually peripheral with a granular appearance and progresses slowly, at a rate of 1–3 mm/month without therapy. Fulminant retinitis is marked by a confluent, yellow-white, geographic opacification which follows vascular arcades and may be associated with mild vitritis (Figure 27.2) [13]. Serious sequelae of CMV retinitis include vitreous hemorrhages, often at the edge of advancing retinitis, and retinal detachments, which occurred in almost 40% of adult patients without HAART at 1 year. Risk factors for detachment include the area of retinitis involvement and lower CD4$^+$ T cell counts [14]. Fortunately, with HAART therapy the risk of retinal detachment has decreased by about 60% [15].

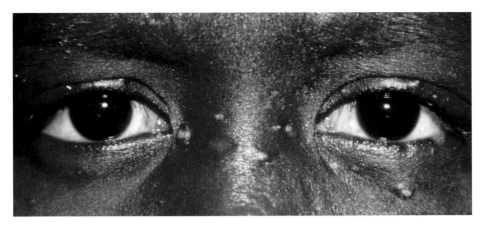

Figure 27.1. External photograph of molluscum contagiosum involving the eyelids. A chronic keratoconjunctivitis can occur with lesions on the eyelid margin.

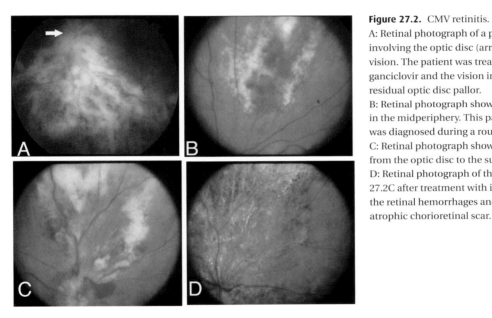

Figure 27.2. CMV retinitis.
A: Retinal photograph of a patient with CMV retinitis involving the optic disc (arrow) with counting fingers vision. The patient was treated with intravenous ganciclovir and the vision improved to 20/40 with residual optic disc pallor.
B: Retinal photograph showing an area of CMV retinitis in the midperiphery. This patient was asymptomatic and was diagnosed during a routine screening examination.
C: Retinal photograph showing CMV retinitis extending from the optic disc to the superior quadrants.
D: Retinal photograph of the patient shown in Figure 27.2C after treatment with intravenous ganciclovir. Note the retinal hemorrhages and necrosis are replaced by an atrophic chorioretinal scar.

Treatment of CMV retinitis is outlined in Table 27.3. Systemic therapy is generally given as an initial induction for 2–3 weeks, followed by maintenance therapy at a lower dosage. Note that maintenance therapy can be safely stopped in those patients with stable retinitis who have recovered CD4+ counts on HAART [16]. Local antiviral therapy is effective and can avoid the serious adverse effects of systemic administration (Figure 27.3). Orally administered valganciclovir has been shown to be as effective as intravenous ganciclovir in adult patients [17], however, clinical trials in a pediatric population have not been reported.

27.6.2 Immune recovery uveitis

Patients with CMV retinitis and depressed CD4+ counts who subsequently regain immune function on HAART therapy can develop inflammation in the eye (uveitis) comprised of vitreous inflammatory cells (vitritis) and edema of the optic disk and macula [18, 19]. This condition, termed immune recovery uveitis, can be sight-threatening, but may be treated with topical, periocular, and/or systemic corticosteroids (Figure 27.4) [19]. Immune recovery uveitis is also associated with a lower risk of retinal detachment, possibly because the inflammation causes chorioretinal

Table 27.3 Treatment of cytomegalovirus retinitis

Systemic therapy:

Systemic agent	Dose	Toxicity
Ganciclovir	Intravenous: 5 mg/kg body weight bid for 14–21 days, then 5 mg/kg maintenance Oral: FDA approved in adults only at 3–6 g/day. Consult pediatric ID specialist	Neutropenia, thrombocytopenia
Foscarnet	Intravenous: 60 or 90 mg/kg body weight bid for 14–21 days, then 90–120 mg/kg maintenance	Nephrotoxicity, electrolyte imbalance (hypocalcemia, hypokalemia, hypomagnesemia)
Cidofovir	Intravenous: 5 mg/kg weekly for 2 weeks, then 5 mg/kg every 2 weeks maintenance	Intravenous: nephrotoxicity, uveitis

Local therapy:

Intraocular agent		
Ganciclovir	Injection: 400–800 μg/0.1 mL 2–3 times/week for 2–3 weeks, then 400–800 μg/0.1 mL 102 times/week maintenance Implant: Releases 1.4 μg/h over 5–8 months, 1–3 week course of intravenous ganciclovir may be used in the perioperative period	Local: vitreous hemorrhage, retinal detachment, endophthalmitis
Foscarnet	Injection: 2.4 mg/0.1 mL 2–3 times/week, then 1.2–2.4 mg/0.05–0.10 mL 1–2 times/week for maintenance	
Cidofovir	Injection: 10–20 μg/0.1 mL every 3–6 weeks	

scarring that firmly secures the retina [15]. The mechanism of immune recovery uveitis may be in part explained because CMV antigens in the eye incite an inflammatory response by a newly reconstituted immune system.

27.6.3 Toxoplasmosis

HIV-infected children are at significant risk for ocular infection with the protozoan *Toxoplasma gondii* [20]. Toxoplasma causes necrotizing retinochoroiditis, which may be unilateral or bilateral; unifocal, multifocal, or diffuse; and is often associated with retinal detachments and marked anterior chamber and vitreal inflammation (Figure 27.5). The supposed route of ocular infection in patients with AIDS, as opposed to immunocompetent patients, is hematogenous, rather than via reactivation of congenital ocular cysts. Diagnosis is made clinically. Serologies can be unreliable in patients with AIDS or with congenital infection. Clinical differentiation of toxoplasmosis from CMV retinitis can be difficult, although marked inflammation favors toxoplasmosis [21]. Standard treatment for HIV-positive children consists of pyrimethamine, sulfadiazine (or clindamycin), and folinic acid [22]. Relapse is common after therapy cessation; the appropriate length of maintenance therapy has yet to be defined. Accurate and early diagnosis of ocular toxoplasmosis is essential to preserve vision and prevent life-threatening intracranial spread or systemic dissemination [21].

Figure 27.3. Local anti-viral therapy.

A: Vitrasert implant (Bausch and Lomb, Rochester NY) – delivers ganciclovir for the treatment of CMV retinitis for up to 8 months.

B: The release of ganciclovir occurs at the base of the implant and clinical trials have shown the implant to be superior in efficacy to systemic therapy for the treatment of CMV retinitis.

C: External photograph showing the implant through a dilated pupil (arrow). The implant is sutured to the sclera and projects into the vitreous cavity releasing ganciclovir.

D: External photograph showing an intravitreal injection of ganciclovir into the eye in a patient with refractory CMV retinitis. The injections are performed at least weekly under local anesthesia and are not suitable for children under the age of about 15 years without general anesthesia.

Figure 27.4. Immune recovery uveitis (IRU).

A: Retinal photograph of a patient with IRU. This patient had inactive CMV retinitis in the periphery, a mild vitritis, reduced visual acuity to 20/60 from cystoid macular edema and an epiretinal membrane; all features commonly seen with IRU.

B: A fluorescein angiogram retinal photograph of a patient with IRU and reduced visual acuity. Leakage of fluorescein in the central macula is consistent with cystoid macular edema, a consistent finding in IRU patients with reduced vision.

C: A retinal photograph of a patient with IRU with inactive CMV retinitis (arrow). The remarkable finding in this patient was a moderate vitritis obscuring retinal details.

D: A retinal photograph of a patient with IRU that developed recurrent vitreous hemorrhages. A small area of neovascularization is present at the edge of the healed CMV scar (arrow), a less common finding in patients with IRU. Retinal details inferiorly obscured by overlying vitreous hemorrhage.

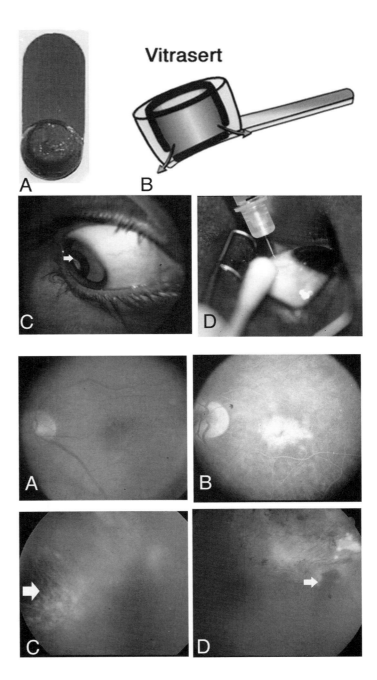

27.6.4 Progressive outer retinal necrosis

Children with HIV are at risk for acquiring progressive outer retinal necrosis (PORN) [23], a rapidly progressive necrotizing retinopathy. The infection is due to either varicella zoster or herpes simplex, and clinically appears as ill-defined, posterior retinal lesions that rapidly progress to full-thickness retinal necrosis (Figure 27.6). Progressive outer retinal necrosis is associated with rapid involvement of the macula and a lack of inflammation and end-stage disease is associated with opaque retinal scarring and detachments. Patients experience rapid, painless vision loss, occasionally after an episode of cutaneous zoster. The visual prognosis is extremely poor, despite aggressive treatment with antivirals (acyclovir, foscarnet) to halt progression and photocoagulation to prevent retinal detachment.

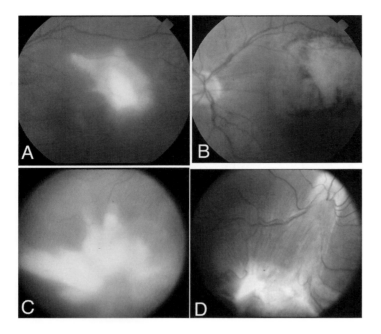

Figure 27.5. Toxoplasmosis chorioretinitis.
A: Retinal photograph of a patient with a presumptive diagnosis of CMV retinitis responding poorly to specific anti-CMV medications. Patient was referred and workup revealed a positive toxoplasmosis titer.
B: Retinal photograph of patient discussed in Figure 27.5A. With a presumptive diagnosis of toxoplasmosis chorioretinitis, following 3 months of treatment with anti-toxoplasmosis medications, the lesion showed resolution with a chorioretinal scar remaining in the posterior pole. Unfortunately, the lesion had extended into the central macula and the vision was reduced to counting fingers.
C: Retinal photograph of a patient who presented to the ER following a seizure. Brain imaging showed a large solitary abscess. Ophthalmologic consultation was requested for complaints of reduced acuity in one eye. Examination showed an exudative subretinal lesion in the macula not typical of CMV retinitis. Further workup revealed a positive toxoplasmosis titer and a brain biopsy confirmed toxoplasmosis.
D: Retinal photograph of patient discussed in Figure 27.5C. Six months following treatment with anti-toxoplasmosis medications, the chorioretinitis resolved with traction of the macula inferiorly.

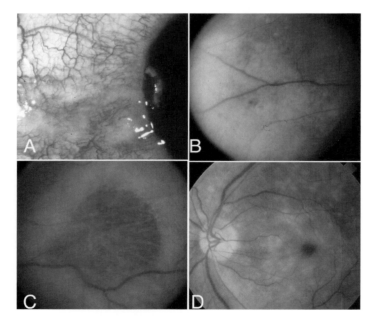

Figure 27.6. Progressive outer retinal necrosis (PORN).
A. External photograph of a patient with zoster ophthalmicus who developed scleral and corneal involvement during the healing phase of the skin disease.
B: Retinal photograph of the patient discussed in Figure 27.6A. He complained of floaters in one eye 3 months after the onset of the zoster ophthalmicus and examination showed a unilateral retinitis involving the deep retinal structures consistent with PORN. Note the relative sparing of the retinal vessels and lack of hemorrhage, typical of this disease.
C: Retinal photograph of a patient with a history of varicella zoster in the T10 dermatome. The patient subsequently developed an outer retinal necrosis in both eyes consistent with PORN.
D: Retinal photograph of the patient discussed in Figure 27.6C. The retinitis progressed rapidly towards the macula and within 2 months, this eye had no light perception despite aggressive use of a combination of anti-HSV, HZV, and CMV medications.

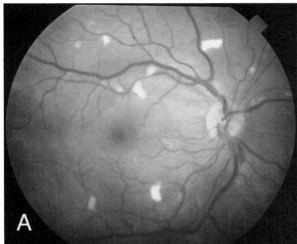
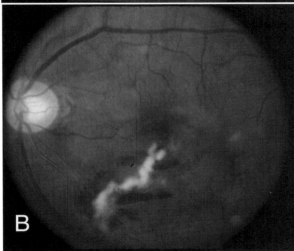

Figure 27.7. HIV microangiopathy.
A: Retinal photograph showing cotton wool spots and a retinal hemorrhage, common findings in patients with CD4+ lymphocyte counts < 100 cells/μL.
B: Retinal photograph showing a branch retinal vein occlusion, an uncommon manifestation of HIV microangioapathy.

27.6.5 HIV microangiopathy

HIV microangiopathy, a microvascular retinal ischemia evidenced by cotton wool spots (nerve fiber layer infarcts) and hemorrhages, is seen much less commonly in HIV-positive children than adults. Retinal venous occlusive disease has also been reported with HIV infection (Figure 27.7). Additionally, children with HIV can exhibit a peripheral perivasculitis, believed to represent an HIV-related infiltrative lymphocytosis [24].

27.6.6 Frosted branch angiitis

Frosted branch angiitis, a white perivascular retinal sheathing associated with decreased visual acuity, has been reported in HIV-positive children and adults and can be associated with CMV retinitis. Initial treatment should be the same as for CMV retinitis. Systemic corticosteroids may be given concurrently, or reserved for refractory disease [25].

27.7 Orbit

Orbital infections in HIV-positive patients include: fungi (aspergillosis, mucormycosis) often invading from the sinuses/orbits to the brain; bacteria (*Pseudomonas aeruginosa, Rhizopus arrhizus, Treponema pallidum, Staphylococcus aureus*) causing orbital cellulitis; parasites (*Toxoplasma gondii*) engendering cysts, panophthalmitis, and orbital cellulitis; and protozoa (*Pneumocystis carinii*) inducing granulomatous orbital inflammation [3].

Although orbital infections are relatively rare, the most common and life-threatening are due to invasive fungi. Pediatric patients with prolonged neutropenia, especially with CD4+ T lymphocyte counts less than 50 cells/μL, are at risk for sino-orbital-cerebral fungal invasion. Additional risk factors for invasion include previous sinus surgery and *Aspergillus* (typically *A. fumigatus*) infection. In the setting of irreversible immunosuppression, the mortality rate is high despite aggressive surgical debridement, including orbital exenteration, and antifungal therapies [26].

27.8 Neoplasms

Some ocular neoplasms in children with HIV are life threatening. Diagnosis can be difficult and delayed when neoplasms masquerade as more common ophthalmic conditions.

Burkitt's/Burkitt's-like lymphoma in children with AIDS has been reported to masquerade as acute bacterial sinusitis and orbital cellulitis. If aggressive antimicrobial therapy is ineffective, prompt imaging and/or biopsy to rule out malignancy is essential so that the appropriate and often curative systemic/intrathecal chemotherapy may be initiated [27].

Kaposi's sarcoma (KS), a common neoplasm in AIDS, may be mistaken for other ocular conditions. On the eyelid, KS may resemble a chalazion. On the conjunctiva, KS can mimic a foreign body granuloma, subconjunctival

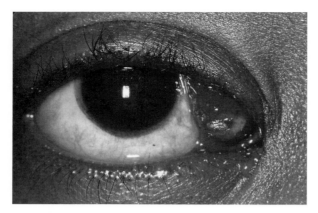

Figure 27.8. External photograph of a Kaposi's sarcoma lesion in the medial orbit extending anteriorly. These lesions can be treated with systemic chemotherapy or radiation.

hemorrhage, or cavernous hemangioma (Figure 27.8). Conjunctival lesions are usually located in the inferior fornix. Since ophthalmic KS is slowly progressive, treatment usually consists of observation alone or focal irradiation for entropion prevention or cosmesis [28].

27.9 Neuro-ophthalmology

Neuro-ophthalmic signs are present in 2–12% of patients with AIDS [4, 24, 29]. Findings include: meningeal involvement (papilledema, optic neuropathy, motor neuropathies); thalalmic-midbrain masses (cranial nerve III involvement); pontine tegmental lesions (pontine gaze paresis, internuclear ophthalmoplegia, nystagmus); cerebellar masses (abnormal spontaneous eye movements); cerebral masses (homonymous hemianopia, papilledema); and pupillary abnormalities (Horner's syndrome). Etiologies include lymphoma, cryptococcus, toxoplasmosis, neurosyphilis, progressive multifocal leukoencephalopathy (PML), CMV, herpes viruses, and HIV infection itself [29, 30]. Cryptococcal meningitis is prevalent in adult HIV patients and can be associated with an optic neuropathy that can lead to blindness [31].

27.10 Developmental manifestations

A developmental AIDS-associated embryopathy has been described which can be associated with growth failure, microcephaly, and other craniofacial abnormalities. In addition, ophthalmic manifestations include prominent palpebral fissures, and hypertelorism [9, 32].

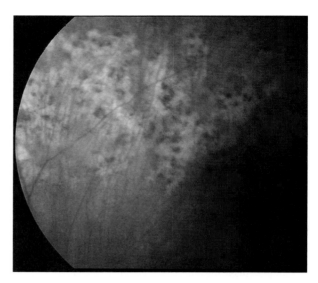

Figure 27.9. Retinal photograph of ddI toxicity associated with didanosine (ddI) therapy. The well-circumscribed depigmented lesions with some hyperpigmented borders are typically observed.

27.11 Drug ocular toxicity

Several of the commonly used antimicrobials in HIV-positive patients are associated with ocular toxicity.

In children, rifabutin can induce bilateral corneal endothelial deposits, which are initially peripheral and stellate in nature [33]. Rifabutin can also cause a mild to severe uveitis that may be associated with hypopyon, vitritis, and/or retinal vasculitis [34]. This reaction may be linked with plasma levels of the drug, which can be increased with concurrent fluconazole therapy [35].

Didanosine (ddI) has been shown to induce retinal lesions and decrease retinal function in approximately 7% of children. The medication adversely affects the retinal pigment epithelium (RPE), causing initial peripheral atrophy and secondary RPE hypertrophy and neurosensory retinal loss (Figure 27.9). The toxicity is likely associated with both cumulative and peak dosing [36].

Cidofovir, both intravenously and intravitreally administered, has been associated with intraocular inflammation in adults, causing iritis, vitritis, and/or hypotony. Concurrent treatment with probenecid may reduce the incidence of toxicity. Treatment of the inflammation with topical corticosteroids is often effective [37].

Atovaquone can cause vortex keratopathy, a swirling pattern of corneal subepithelial deposits. This toxicity is reversible with withdrawal of the drug [38]. Lastly, intravenous ganciclovir and acyclovir may be associated with corneal epithelial inclusions, but studies are inconclusive [9, 39].

27.12 Summary

Understanding the diseases of the eye that occur with HIV infection is crucial to properly diagnose and promptly treat potentially blinding disorders. Diseases such as CMV retinitis can be especially difficult to diagnose in the pediatric population because they are largely asymptomatic. Routine screening eye exams and aggressive therapy are mandatory to save vision.

REFERENCES

1. Mines, J. A. & Kaplan, H. J. Acquired immunodeficiency syndrome (AIDS): the disease and its ocular manifestations. *Int. Ophthalmol. Clin.* **26**:2 (1986), 73–115.

2. Robinson, M. R., Ross, M. L. & Whitcup, S. M. Ocular manifestations of HIV infection. *Curr. Opin. Ophthalmol* **10**:6 (1999), 431–7.

3. Kronish, J. W., Johnson, T. E., Gilberg, S. M., Corrent, G. F., McLeish, W. M. & Scott, K. R. Orbital infections in patients with human immunodeficiency virus infection. *Ophthalmology* **103**:9 (1996), 1483–92.

4. Pizzo, P. A. & Wilfert, C. A (eds.). *Ocular Manifestations of HIV in the Pediatric Population*, 3 edn. Baltimore: Williams & Wilkins (1998).

5. Robinson, M. R., Udell, I. J., Garber, P. F., Perry, H. D., & Streeten, B. W. Molluscum contagiosum of the eyelids in patients with acquired immune deficiency syndrome. *Ophthalmology* **99**:11 (1992), 1745–7.

6. Pelaez, C. A., Gurbindo, M. D., Cortes, C. & Munoz-Fernandez, M. A. Molluscum contagiosum, involving the upper eyelids, in a child infected with HIV-1. *Pediatr. AIDS HIV Infect.* **7**:1 (1996), 43–6.

7. Strauss, R. M., Doyle, E. L., Mohsen, A. H. & Green, S. T. Successful treatment of molluscum contagiosum with topical imiquimod in a severely immunocompromised HIV-positive patient. *Int. J. STD AIDS* **12**:4 (2001), 264–6.

8. Patrizi, A., Neri, I., Trestini, D., Landi, C., Ricci, G. & Masi, M. Acquired trichomegaly of the eyelashes in a child with human immunodeficiency virus infection. *J. Eur. Acad. Dermatol. Venereol.* **11**:1 (1998), 89–91.

9. Cunningham, E. T., Jr. & Margolis, T. P. Ocular manifestations of HIV infection. *New Engl. J. Med.* **339**:4 (1998), 236–44.

10. Chern, K. C., Conrad, D., Holland, G. N., Holsclaw, D. S., Schwartz, L. K. & Margolis, T. P. Chronic varicella-zoster virus epithelial keratitis in patients with acquired immunodeficiency syndrome. *Arch. Ophthalmol.* **116**:8 (1998), 1011–17.

11. Martins, S. A., Muccioli, C., Belfort, R., Jr. & Castelo, A. Resolution of microsporidial keratoconjunctivitis in an AIDS patient treated with highly active antiretroviral therapy. *Am. J. Ophthalmol.* **131**:3 (2001), 378–9.

12. Du, L. T., Coats, D. K., Kline, M. W. *et al.* Incidence of presumed cytomegalovirus retinitis in HIV-infected pediatric patients. *J AAPoS* **3**:4 (1999), 245–9.

13. Kanski, J. J. *Clinical Ophthalmology: A Systemic Approach.* 4 edn. Boston: Butterworth Heinemann Publishers (1999).

14. Rhegmatogenous retinal detachment in patients with cytomegalovirus retinitis: the Foscarnet–Ganciclovir Cytomegalovirus Retinitis Trial. The Studies of Ocular Complications of AIDS (SOCA) Research Group in Collaboration with the AIDS Clinical Trials Group (ACTG). *Am. J. Ophthalmol.* **124**:1 (1997), 61–70.

15. Kempen, J. H., Jabs, D. A., Dunn, J. P., West, S. K. & Tonascia, J. Retinal detachment risk in cytomegalovirus retinitis related to the acquired immunodeficiency syndrome. *Arch. Ophthalmol.* **119**:1 (2001), 33–40.

16. Whitcup, S. M., Fortin, E., Lindblad, A. S. *et al.* Discontinuation of anticytomegalovirus therapy in patients with HIV infection and cytomegalovirus netinitis. *J. Am. Med. Assoc.* **282**:17 (1999), 1633–7.

17. Martin, D. F., Sierra-Madero, J. Walmsley, S., *et al.* A controlled trial of valganciclovir as induction therapy for cytomegalovirus retinitis. *New Engl. J. Med.* **346**:15 (2002), 1119–26.

18. Jabs, D. A., Van Natta, M. L., Kempen, J. H. *et al.* Characteristics of patients with cytomegalovirus retinitis in the era of highly active antiretroviral therapy. *Am. J. Ophthalmol.* **133**:1 (2002), 48–61.

19. Robinson, M. R., Reed, G., Csaky, K. G., Polis, M. A., & Whitcup, S. M. Immune-recovery uveitis in patients with cytomegalovirus retinitis taking highly active antiretroviral therapy. *Am. J. Ophthalmol.* **130**:1 (2000), 49–56.

20. Girard, B., Prevost-Moravia, G., Courpotin, C. & Lasfargues, G. Ophthalmologic manifestations observed in a pediatric HIV-seropositive population. *J. Fr. Ophtalmol.* **20**:1 (1997), 49–60.

21. Holland, G. N., Engstrom, R. E., Jr., Glasgow, B. J. *et al.* Ocular toxoplasmosis in patients with the acquired immunodeficiency syndrome. *Am. J. Ophthalmol.* **106**:6 (1988), 653–67.

22. Lynfield, R. & Guerina, N. G. Toxoplasmosis. *Pediatr. Rev.* **18**:3 (1997), 75–83.

23. Hammond, C. J., Evans, J. A., Shah, S. M., Acheson, J. F. & Walters, M. D. The spectrum of eye disease in children with AIDS due to vertically transmitted HIV disease: clinical findings, virology and recommendations for surveillance. *Graefes Arch. Clin. Exp. Ophthalmol.* **235**:3 (1997), 125–9.

24. Kestelyn, P., Lepage, P., Karita, E. & Van de Perre, P. Ocular manifestations of infection with the human immunodeficiency virus in an African pediatric population. *Ocul. Immunol. Inflamm.* **8**:4 (2000), 263–73.

25. Fine, H. F., Smith, J. A., Murante, B. L., Nussenblatt, R. B. & Robinson, M. R. Frosted branch angiitis in a child with HIV infection. *Am. J. Ophthalmol.* **131**:3 (2001), 394–6.

26. Robinson, M. R., Fine, H. F., Ross, M. L. *et al.* Sino-orbital-cerebral aspergillosis in immunocompromised pediatric patients. *Pediatr. Infect. Dis. J.* **19**:12 (2000), 1197–203.

27. Robinson, M. R., Salit, R. B., Bryant-Greenwood, P. K. *et al.* Burkitt's/Burkitt's-like lymphoma presenting as bacterial sinusitis in two HIV-infected children. *AIDS Patient Care STDS* **15**:9 (2001), 453–8.

28. Shuler, J. D., Holland, G. N., Miles, S. A., Miller, B. J. & Grossman, I. Kaposi sarcoma of the conjunctiva and eyelids associated with the acquired immunodeficiency syndrome. *Arch. Ophthalmol.* **107**:6 (1989), 858–62.

29. Keane, J. R. Neuro-ophthalmologic signs of AIDS: 50 patients. *Neurology* **41**:6 (1991), 841–5.

30. Smith, D. D., Robinson, M. R., Scheibel, S. F., Valenti, W. M. & Eskin, T. A. Progressive multifocal leukoencephalopathy (PML) in two cases of cortical blindness. *AIDS Patient Care* **8**:3 (1994), 110–13.

31. Kestelyn, P., Taelman, H., Bogaerts, J. *et al.* Ophthalmic manifestations of infections with *Cryptococcus neoformans* in patients with the acquired immunodeficiency syndrome. *Am. J. Ophthalmol.* **116**:6 (1993), 721–7.

32. Marion, R. W., Wiznia, A. A., Hutcheon, R. G. & Rubinstein, A. Fetal AIDS syndrome score. Correlation between severity of dysmorphism and age at diagnosis of immunodeficiency. *Am. J. Dis. Child.* **141**:4 (1987), 429–31.

33. Smith, J. A., Mueller, B. U., Nussenblatt, R. B. & Whitcup, S. M. Corneal endothelial deposits in children positive for human immunodeficiency virus receiving rifabutin prophylaxis for *Mycobacterium avium* complex bacteremia. *Am. J. Ophthalmol.* **127**:2 (1999), 164–9.

34. Arevalo, J. F., Russack, V. & Freeman, W. R. New ophthalmic manifestations of presumed rifabutin-related uveitis. *Ophthalmic Surg. Lasers* **28**:4 (1997), 321–4.

35. Johnson, T. M. & Desroches, G. Panuveitis associated with rifabutin prophylaxis in a pediatric HIV-positive patient. *J. Pediatr. Ophthalmol. Strabismus* **35**:2 (1998), 119–21.

36. Whitcup, S. M., Dastgheib, K., Nussenblatt, R. B., Walton, R. C., Pizzo, P. A. & Chan, C. C. A clinicopathologic report of the retinal lesions associated with didanosine. *Arch. Ophthalmol.* **112**:12 (1994), 1594–8.

37. Davis, J. L., Taskintuna, I., Freeman, W. R., Weinberg, D. V., Feuer, W. J. & Leonard, R. E. Iritis and hypotony after treatment with intravenous cidofovir for cytomegalovirus retinitis. *Arch. Ophthalmol.* **115**:6 (1997), 733–7.

38. Shah, G. K., Cantrill, H. L. & Holland, E. J. Vortex keratopathy associated with atovaquone. *Am. J. Ophthalmol.* **120**:5 (1995), 669–71.

39. Wilhelmus, K. R., Keener, M. J., Jones, D. B. & Font, R. L. Corneal lipidosis in patients with the acquired immunodeficiency syndrome. *Am. J. Ophthalmol.* **119**:1 (1995), 14–19.

Oral health and dental problems

Jane C. Atkinson, D.D.S.[1] and Anne O'Connell, B.D.S., M.S.[2]

[1] University of Maryland Dental School, Baltimore, MD
[2] Department of Public and Child Dental Health, Dublin, Ireland

28.1 Oral health and dental problems in the HIV-infected child

Many children with HIV have oral manifestations of the infection (Table 28.1), including some that are part of the 1994 CDC classification system [1]. Since the introduction of antiretroviral therapy (ART) and highly active antiretroviral therapy (HAART), the prevalence of these oral manifestations has decreased. However, in many countries where therapy is less than ideal, such as Romania, Brazil and Mexico, HIV-associated oral lesions have been identified in 55–61% of infected children [2–4]. Their presence can still be used as markers for progression of disease. Referral to a dentist before 1 year of age is recommended for all children, but this is especially important for the HIV-infected child. Careful examination of the soft tissues and teeth is essential by the primary healthcare provider.

28.2 Oral mucosal lesions

28.2.1 Candidiasis

Oral candidiasis (thrush) is by far the most common oral opportunistic infection in HIV-infected children [3–8]. Prevalence estimates in this group range from 28–67% (Table 28.1), and its presence is associated with low or declining CD4 counts [7, 8]. The diagnosis and treatment of *Candida* infections are discussed in detail in Chapter 40.

Oral candidal infections can appear as a red patch (erythematous, Figure 28.1), a white patch that rubs off (pseudomembranous) or as red patches at the corners of the mouth (angular chelitis). Often patients are asymptomatic,

but they may experience oral burning or soreness. The diagnosis of oral candidiasis is based on clinical appearance and the presence of hyphae on a smear prepared with potassium hydroxide. Smears also may be air-dried and stained by a number of techniques commonly used by clinical laboratories to visualize the organism. *Candida* species are isolated most commonly; however, many other species are recovered from the oral cavity [7]. All laboratory results must be correlated with the clinical presentation since HIV-positive patients have greater numbers of *Candida* species in the oral cavity, even in the absence of clinical infection. Treatment can be with systemic or topical antifungal agents, but treatment is complicated with the emergence of resistant strains (see Chapter 40).

28.2.2 Herpes infections

Oral viral infections are not found as frequently as fungal infections [5–9]. Herpes simplex infection is the most common, with a similar presentation in children with or without HIV. However, the disease can be more severe and debilitating for patients with HIV infection. Primary herpetic stomatitis is characterized by fever, lymphadenopathy, and fluid-filled vesicles on the gingiva and palate, which quickly rupture and ulcerate. The vesicular fluid is the best material for culture. After primary infection, the virus establishes a latent infection in the trigeminal ganglion until reactivation. Typically, intraoral recurrent HSV lesions are found on keratinized tissues of the mouth, but lesions may be more severe and involve any oral mucosal surfaces of children with HIV. Extraoral lesions are found on the lips, and heal in 7–14 days without scarring

Table 28.1 Oral manifestations of HIV-infected children

Diagnosis	Prevalence	Features
Oral mucosal changes		
Candidiasis	28–67%	White patches that rub off, red patches intra-orally or redness at corners of mouth
Herpetic stomatitis	3–5%	Both primary and recurrent forms may be more dramatic in HIV-infected children
Aphthous ulcers	Up to 15%	Ulcers of unknown etiology that can be more severe in HIV-infected children
Human papillomavirus	Up to 2%	Intra-oral elevations of tissue (warts)
Hairy leukoplakia	0–2%	White plaques on the lateral border of the tongue that do not rub off
Other viral infections	Very rare	CMV, VZV can cause oral changes
Tumors	Very rare	Kaposi's sarcoma and non-Hodgkin's lymphoma are very rare in this population
Gingival changes		
Gingivitis	> 80%	Erythematous gingival changes from plaque on teeth
Linear gingival erythema	Up to 25%	Specific to HIV infection
HIV-associated periodontitis	Rare	Rapidly advancing periodontal disease
Tooth changes		
Decay	Common	Tooth breakdown can be obvious. Pain is not normally a presenting complaint
Abscesses	Fairly common	Can cause fever and pain
Delayed exfoliation and eruption	Fairly common	Primary teeth may be retained well into teenage years
Parotid gland enlargement	2–11%	
Lymphocytic-mediated		Painless enlargements; clear saliva can be expressed from glands. MRI can be used to confirm presence of cysts
Bacterial infection		Pain on palpation; often, pus can be expressed from glands. May or may not be accompanied by fever

CMV, cytomegalovirus; VZV, varicella-zoster virus.

(Figure 28.2). Burning and tingling may precede vesicle formation. While coating agents can be used as a rinse to decrease discomfort of small intraoral lesions, viscous xylocaine should be discouraged in young children. Intra-oral herpes zoster occurs rarely in children, but was reported recently in a study of Romanian children [4]. It may present as small, crusted, painful ulcerated areas of keratinized intraoral tissues in a unilateral pattern that follows the distribution of the trigeminal nerve. The systemic therapy of herpes virus infections is discussed in detail in Chapter 41.

Epstein–Barr virus (EBV) is the causative agent of oral hairy leukoplakia (OHL) [10]. It is very rare in children with HIV infection. Clinically, the lesion is a white patch along the lateral borders of the tongue that does not wipe off. Diagnosis requires identification of EBV genome in a biopsy specimen or cytologic smear, and lesions are not typically treated.

28.2.3 Other soft tissue infections

Intraoral histoplasmosis, cryptococcus and other systemic mycotic infections have been identified in adults with HIV infection [11, 12]. In the oral cavity, the deep mycoses can appear as nodules on the gingiva and painful ulcerations of the palate and buccal mucosa. Very rarely, tuberculosis will cause soft tissue ulcerations on the tongue and palate, and could be considered as the etiological agent of a lesion in a child with other symptoms of *Mycobacterium* infection [13, 14]. Cytomegalovirus infection can also cause large ulcers of the tongue and buccal mucosa.

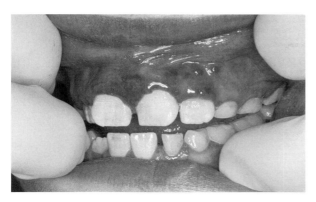

Figure 28.1. Erythematous candidiasis on the gingiva and buccal mucosa of a child with HIV infection.

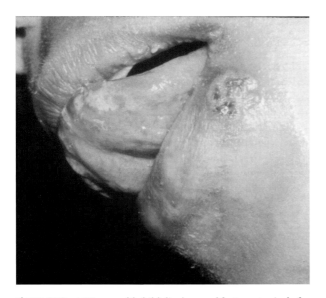

Figure 28.2. A 10-year-old child displays oral features typical of HIV infection: oral candidiasis on the lateral border of the tongue and at the corners of mouth, and a large, recurrent herpetic lesion extraorally.

Human papillomavirus (HPV) causes intraoral warts in adults and children [13, 14]. Both verruca vulgaris and condyloma acuminatum are found intraorally, and are recognized by their characteristic raised or pedunculated appearance. Molluscum contagiosum, caused by a member of the poxvirus family, may involve the lips and face. Inside the mouth, multiple dome-shaped elevations may be present on the soft tissues.

Sometimes, the cause of intraoral ulcerations in both children and adults with HIV infection is not established, despite repeated diagnostic procedures. Treatment of these lesions with topical anesthetics, antimicrobial rinses or topical corticosteroids may be necessary if they persist, are symptomatic, and no etiology is established.

28.3 Neoplasms

In contrast to adults, neoplasms associated with HIV infection are rarely found in the oral cavity of pediatric patients. However, intra-oral Kaposi's sarcoma (KS) and non-Hodgkin's lymphoma have been reported, and intraoral KS will be present in approximately half of affected adults [13, 14]. (See also Chapter 36)

28.4 Salivary gland pathology

Saliva is essential for the maintenance of oral health, having lubricating, physical cleansing, and antibacterial and antiviral properties. Salivary flow may be reduced by the medications used in the treatment of HIV. Medications with potent anticholinergic effects such as diphenhydramine can reduce salivary flow by 50%, which can enhance the development of dental caries or candidal infections.

Although many children with HIV infection may have decreased salivary gland function as a consequence of medication usage, a subset develop enlargement of the salivary glands. Prevalence estimates in controlled studies are 2–14% of children with HIV infection [5–8, 15]. Some enlargements are secondary to a lymphocytic infiltration of the salivary glands; others are the result of bacterial infection. Enlargements from infiltrates can be persistent, uni- or bilateral, and accompanied by xerostomia or pain. The lymphocytic infiltrations may develop cysts containing lymphoid aggregates that can be visualized by magnetic resonance imaging. Clear saliva can be milked from the glands. In contrast, glands infected with bacteria may demonstrate a purulent discharge at the duct openings when massaged (Figure 28.2). Mumps could be considered in a child who has not received the measles–mumps–rubella (MMR) vaccine. Finally, salivary gland tumors do occur in children, regardless of their HIV status. If glands continue to enlarge or a mass is detected on imaging, a fine-needle aspiration or biopsy of the gland must be performed.

The etiology of a salivary gland enlargement will dictate its treatment. Bacterial parotitis usually occurs because of a retrograde infection with oral flora, which usually is sensitive to the penicillins, clindamycin or second-generation cephalosporins. Treatment of lymphocyte-mediated enlargements is rarely indicated. Frequent intake of fluids (preferably water) throughout the day is recommended.

28.5 Periodontal tissues

The severity of periodontal (gum) diseases depends on the presence of certain periodontal pathogens and the immune status of the host. Gingivitis, the most common form of periodontal disease in the general pediatric population, is caused by an accumulation of oral bacteria and food particles at the gum line. Usually, good oral hygiene can reverse the inflammation and return the gingiva to health. Up to 25% [16] of HIV-infected pediatric patients present with linear gingival erythema (LGE), a form of gum disease that is unique to HIV infection. It is characterized by a distinct red band of gingiva that bleeds easily. The inflammation is disproportional to the amount of plaque present, and resolution may not occur with conventional therapy. A more rare form of gingivitis, necrotizing ulcerative gingivitis (NUG), presents with destruction of one or more interdental papilla, tissue sloughing, halitosis, and often pain. Treatment of both conditions includes meticulous oral hygiene, antibacterial mouth rinses (chlorhexidine), antibiotic therapy, and frequent dental cleanings. Very rarely, necrotizing ulcerative periodontitis (NUP), a severe periodontal disease with rapid destruction of periodontal tissues and supporting bone, is found in children with HIV infection [16]. Frequent monitoring by a dentist is essential to prevent progression and ultimate tooth loss. Neutropenia, which sometimes occurs in HIV-infected children, can predispose children to severe pediatric periodontal disease.

28.6 Dental development

Delays in the eruption and exfoliation of primary teeth and eruption of permanent teeth, particularly in symptomatic children, have been noted in HIV-infected children [17–20]. Prevention of dental disease in the primary dentition, therefore, is critical since these teeth will be retained in the mouth for longer than normal.

28.7 Teeth

Dental decay is frequently present in children with HIV-infection and at levels higher than the general population in the primary dentition [19–21]. Many factors have been suggested to explain the unusually high caries incidence in the HIV-infected population, including nutritional supplementation, sweetened pediatric medications, lack of saliva and declining immune system, frequency of fermentable carbohydrates intake, prolonged bottle feeding, and poor

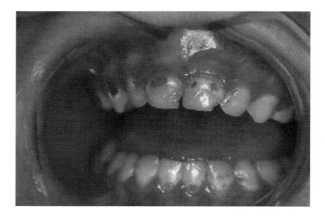

Figure 28.3. Caries of the primary dentition of an HIV-infected child. Caries is evident on the anterior teeth, indicating a very high rate of caries development. These lesions may have been prevented by proper feeding practices and good oral hygiene.

oral hygiene. It may present as nursing or early childhood caries, in which decay occurs on smooth surfaces normally not prone to caries (Figure 28.3). Caries rates of HIV-infected children and their siblings have been compared. While one study reported that HIV-infected children had increases in caries compared with their non-infected siblings [20], others have noted high rates in both groups [19]. Caries are more prevalent in children with advanced HIV disease [21].

28.8 Prevention

All HIV-infected children should have an oral evaluation within the first year to ensure proper treatment. Primary caregivers should be encouraged to:

1. Enroll children in a prevention program that teaches good oral hygiene practices, along with control of dietary sugars. The use of fluorides and the placement of sealants on teeth will minimize the risk of dental caries and the possible dental pain. Prevention is easier than provision of restorative care for the pediatric HIV-infected patient, who often needs intravenous sedation for dental treatments and may have other complications such as neutropenia and thrombocytopenia.

2. Limit the frequency of ingestion of viscous sugar-sweetened liquids or those with low pH (such as sodas, pediatric syrups). Topical treatment of oral candidiasis requires that the antifungal pastilles be retained in the mouth for long periods of time to be effective. These preparations are highly sweetened to disguise the taste and encourage compliance with therapy. Unsweetened

vaginal troches can be used in older children. However, this is not always acceptable to young patients.

3. Limit the use of the bottle to daytime hours. Children should never be put to bed with the bottle. Remind caregivers of the risks of nursing caries when bottles containing juice or high-calorie nutritional supplements are given to children. Administer highly sweetened pediatric medications by syringe to bypass the teeth and minimize the time in the oral cavity.

4. Encourage frequent intake of water to facilitate clearance of food, medicines, and other substances that can initiate tooth decay.

28.9 Conclusion

Children with HIV infection may have inadequate oral health. Soft tissue lesions, especially oral candidiasis, occur frequently in this patient group, and should be treated appropriately. Untreated dental caries is found more often in children from poor families, primarily because they do not have dental insurance or access to a dentist [22]. The HIV-infected child is additionally at risk for periodontal problems. Serious oral sequela can be averted by preventive dental services and regular dental visits.

REFERENCES

1. Centers for Disease Control and Prevention. Revised classification system for HIV in children. *MMWR* **43**: **RR-12** (1994), 1–10.

2. Bretz, W. A., Flaitz, C., Moretti, A., Corby, P., Schneider, L. G. & Nichols, C. M. Medication usage and dental caries outcome-related variables in HIV/AIDS patients. *AIDS Patient Care STDs* **44** (2000), 549–54.

3. Costa, L. R., Villena, R. S., Sucasas, P. S. & Birman, E. G. Oral findings in pediatric AIDS: a case control study in Brazilian children. *ASDC J. Dent. Child.* **65** (1998), 186–90.

4. Flaitz, C., Wullbrandt, B., Sexton, J., Bourdon, T. & Hicks, J. Prevalence of orodental findings in HIV-infected Romanian children. *Pediatr. Dent.* **23** (2001), 44–50.

5. European Collaborative Study. Children born to women with HIV-1 infection: natural history and risk of transmission. *Lancet* **337** (1991), 253–60.

6. Ramos-Gomez, F. J., Hilton, J. F., Canchola, A. J., Greenspan, D., Greenspan, J. S. & Maldonado, Y. A. Risk factors for HIV-related orofacial soft-tissue manifestations in children. *Pediatr. Dent.* **18** (1996), 121–6.

7. Moniaci, D., Cavallari, M., Greco, D. *et al.* Oral lesions in children born to HIV-1 positive women. *J. Oral Pathol. Med.* **22** (1993), 8–11.

8. Barasch, A., Safford, M. M., Catalanotto, F. A., Fine, D. H. & Katz, R. V. Oral soft tissue manifestations in HIV-positive vs. HIV-negative children from an inner city population: a two-year observational study. *Pediatr. Dent.* **22** (2000), 215–20.

9. Eversole, L. R. Viral infections of the head and neck among HIV-seropositive patients. *Oral Surg. Oral Med. Oral Pathol.* **73** (1992), 155–63.

10. Greenspan, J. S., Greenspan, D., Lennette, E. T. *et al.* Replication of Epstein–Barr virus within the epithelial cells of oral hairy leukoplakia, an AIDS-associated lesion. *New Engl. J. Med.* **313** (1985), 1564–71.

11. Economopoulou, P., Laskaris, G. & Kittas, C. Oral histoplasmosis as an indicator of HIV infection. *Oral Surg. Oral Med. Oral Pathol. Oral Radiol. Endod.* **86** (1998), 203–6.

12. Scully, C., de Almeida, O. P. & Sposto, M. R. The deep mycoses in HIV infection. *Oral Dis.* **3, Suppl. 1** (1997), S200–7.

13. Atkinson, J. C., Valdez, I. H. & Childers, E. Oral cavity and associated structures. In C. Moran & F. Mullick (eds.), *Systemic Pathology of HIV Infection and AIDS in Children*. Washington, DC: Armed Forces Institute of Pathology (1997), pp. 55–71.

14. Ramos-Gomez, F. J., Flaitz, C., Catapano, P. *et al.* Classification, diagnostic criteria and treatment recommendations for orofacial manifestations in HIV-infected pediatric patients. *J. Clin. Pediatr. Dent.* **23** (1999), 85–96.

15. Italian Multicentre Study. Epidemiology, clinical features and prognostic factors of paediatric HIV infection. *Lancet* **ii** (1988), 1043–5.

16. Schoen, D. H., Murray, P. A., Nelson, E., Catalanotto, F., Katz, R. V. & Fine, D. H. A comparison of periodontal disease in HIV-infected children and household peers: a two-year report. *Pediatr. Dent.* **22** (2000), 365–9.

17. Valdez, I. H., Pizzo, P. A. & Atkinson, J. C. Oral health of pediatric AIDS patients: a hospital-based study. *ASDC J. Dent. Child.* **61** (1994), 114–18.

18. Hauk, M. J., Moss, M. E., Weinberg, G. A. & Berkowitz, R. J. Delayed tooth eruption: association with severity of HIV infection. *Pediatr. Dent.* **23** (2001), 260–2.

19. Tofsky, N., Nelson, E. M., Lopez, R. N., Catalanotto, F., Fine, D. H. & Katz, R. V. Dental caries in HIV-infected children versus household peers: two-year findings. *Pediatr. Dent.* **22** (2000), 207–14.

20. Madigan, A., Murray, P. A., Houpt, M. I., Catalanotto, F. & Fuerman, M. Caries experience and cariogenic markers in HIV-positive children and their siblings. *Pediatr. Dent.* **18** (1996), 129–36.

21. Hicks, M. J., Flaitz, C. M., Carter, A. B. *et al.* Dental caries in HIV-infected children: a longitudinal study. *Pediatr. Dent.* **22** (2000), 359–64.

22. U.S. Department of Health and Human Services. *Oral Health in America: A report of the Surgeon General*. National Institutes of Health publication 00-4713. Rockville, MD: U.S. Department of Health and Human Services (2000).

Otitis media and sinusitis

Ellen R. Wald, M.D.[1] and Barry Dashefsky, M.D.[2]

[1]University of Pittsburgh School of Medicine; Division of Allergy, Immunology and Infectious Diseases,
Children's Hospital of Pittsburgh, Pittsburgh, PA
[2]Division of Pulmonology, Allergy, Immunology and Infectious Diseases,
UMDNJ – New Jersey Medical School, Newark, NJ

29.1 Introduction and background

Otitis media and sinusitis are among the most common minor bacterial infections affecting children with normal immune function. To date, there has been a paucity of systematic study of these infections in immunocompromised hosts in general. However, substantial experience and a limited literature suggest that, in their acute, chronic, and recurrent forms, they also occur commonly in children who are infected with HIV. Although the causes, manifestations, and clinical courses of most episodes of otitis media and sinusitis in HIV-infected children are indistinguishable from those in immunocompetent children, unusually frequent, prolonged, severe, or otherwise problematic episodes, or those caused by unusual or opportunistic pathogens, can be the sentinel expressions of immunodeficiency that should prompt an assessment for HIV infection.

29.2 Epidemiology of acute otitis media and sinusitis

Acute otitis media (AOM) is a very common occurrence in immunocompetent children with peak frequency during the first 2 years of life. In addition to young age, risk factors for AOM include male gender, a history of severe or recurrent AOM in sibling(s), early age of first AOM, absence of breast feeding, winter season, race (with high rates among Eskimos and other Native Americans, as well as among Australian aborigines), day-care attendance, lower socioeconomic status, and craniofacial anomalies [1].

There are three controlled studies that describe the relative frequency of AOM among HIV-infected children [2–4]. All clearly indicate that, although this common childhood condition does not affect a greater proportion of children infected with HIV than normal children, it does recur significantly more often among children with symptomatic HIV infection.

Acute sinusitis is an extremely common problem among young children with normal immunity. It has been estimated that 5–10% of viral upper respiratory infections (URIs) in young children (which occur 6–8 times annually) are complicated by bacterial sinusitis [5]. There is some evidence that episodes of sinusitis occur more frequently among HIV-infected children than among immunologically normal children [4]. In a trial of intravenous immunoglobulin (IVIG) prophylaxis for serious bacterial infections in HIV-infected children, clinically diagnosed acute sinusitis represented 39% of the episodes of "serious" infection and occurred irrespective of CD4+ count, HIV disease severity classification, and receipt of IVIG [6–7].

29.3 Pathogenesis and natural history OF AOM and sinusitis

In the immunocompetent host, AOM is attributable to dysfunction of the eustachian tube which is responsible for (1) ventilation of the middle-ear cavity; (2) clearance of secretions produced by the mucosa of the middle ear; and (3) protection of the middle ear from nasopharyngeal contents [8]. Viral infection of the upper respiratory tract is the major pathogenetic factor which produces both physiologic and anatomic obstruction of the eustachian tube and effusion within the middle ear. Aspiration of heavily colonized nasopharyngeal contents into the middle ear leads to a suppurative process manifested as AOM.

A similar pathogenesis probably occurs in the immuno-compromised host. Neutropenia, caused by HIV infection or antiretroviral therapy, may also produce mucositis, causing eustachian tube dysfunction. Likewise, nasopharyngeal lymphoid hyperplasia, associated with HIV infection, may obstruct the eustachian tube extrinsically or infiltrate its structure.

In the usual case of sinusitis, either a viral URI or allergy leads to mucositis, resulting in obstruction of the sinus ostia. Colonizing nasopharyngeal flora, which have gained access to the formerly sterile sinuses, proliferate, producing a local inflammatory reaction which damages the mucosa and thereby further impairs ciliary function and local phagocytic activity [5, 9]. Other less common pathogenetic factors include trauma, polyps, gastric or endotracheal tubes or other foreign bodies, septal deviation, dysmotile cilia syndrome, and cystic fibrosis. Exposure to infected siblings or other young children (e.g. at day care), increases the risk of acquiring a viral URI, the usual prelude to bacterial sinusitis.

29.4 Clinical presentation

29.4.1 Otitis media

In both immunocompetent and immunocompromised hosts, AOM usually presents with the abrupt onset of otalgia, fever, or irritability in association with typical otoscopic findings described below. Suppurative complications of AOM include tympanic membrane perforation, cholesteatoma, mastoiditis, and intracranial suppuration including meningitis; brain, subdural or extradural abscess; sinus thrombosis, and phlebitis [10].

29.4.2 Sinusitis

There are two patterns of illness with which acute sinusitis presents in immunocompetent children – either persistent or severe symptoms. Persistent symptoms represent the more common presentation, which is characterized by the presence of unimproving cough and/or rhinorrhea for 10–30 days. Nasal discharge may have any quality (thin, thick, clear, mucoid, or purulent) and cough may be either dry or productive, and, although often worse at night, occurs throughout the day. Breath may be malodorous. Affected

children do not usually appear very ill. If present, fever is usually low-grade. Facial pain and headache are unusual complaints; mild periorbital edema (frequently present upon arising and resolving while upright during the day) may occur. Less commonly, acute sinusitis may present with features of a more severe nature – high fever (> 39 °C) and purulent nasal discharge concurrently for 3–4 consecutive days. Intense headache (supra- or retroorbital), toxicity, or substantial periorbital edema may be features of this presentation.

In immunocompromised hosts, including children with HIV infection, the clinical presentation of sinusitis is most often indistinguishable from that in immunocompetent patients. Unfortunately, the physical examination is usually not helpful in differentiating acute sinusitis from a viral URI. Fungal sinusitis is suggested by the presence of nasal mucosa that are focally pale, gray, or black; have decreased or absent pain sensation; have increased friability; and do not bleed following trauma.

Sinusitis in either the immunocompetent or immuno-compromised host may be complicated by extension of infection to adjacent bone, the orbit, or the central nervous system (CNS) (in the form of an epidural abscess, brain abscess, meningitis, cavernous sinus thrombosis, optic neuritis, or carotid aneurysm). Orbital involvement is signaled by the onset of proptosis, ophthalmoplegia, ocular tenderness, or decreased visual acuity.

29.5 Diagnostic considerations in AOM and sinusitis

29.5.1 Otitis media

The diagnosis of otitis media is based on otoscopic findings. The tympanic membrane is assessed with respect to its contour, color, transparency, architecture, and, most importantly, mobility. Decreased mobility implies the presence of middle ear effusion, which is almost always present in both acute and chronic otitis media. Marked fullness or bulging of a white or yellow, sometimes hyperemic tympanic membrane are typical findings in AOM. Sometimes purulent fluid can be visualized behind an intact tympanic membrane or as it spills through a perforation. Such signs, coupled with the appropriate symptoms, establish a diagnosis of AOM. Opacity of the tympanic membrane, or the presence of clear or mucoid fluid behind it, and decreased mobility, suggest a more chronic, non-suppurative otitis media.

Tympanocentesis should be performed selectively in both immunocompetent and immunocompromised hosts for diagnostic and therapeutic purposes. The major indications for tympanocentesis are failure to respond to medical therapy, suppurative complications such as mastoiditis or CNS abscess, suspicion of an unusual pathogen, otitis media in patients who are seriously ill, or for relief of severe pain [8]. Aspirated fluid should be used for diagnostic purposes as described below with reference to sinus aspiration. Radiographs or computed tomography (CT) scanning may be required occasionally to confirm the presence of inner ear or mastoid involvement, or of intracranial complications.

29.5.2 Sinusitis

The diagnosis of acute bacterial sinusitis is most often made solely on the basis of a clinical presentation with the characteristic persistent symptoms described previously. Physical examination seldom helps distinguish acute bacterial sinusitis from viral rhinosinusitis (a "cold"). In acute sinusitis, radiographic findings include diffuse opacification, mucosal thickening of at least 4–5 mm, or, rarely in children, an air-fluid level. The presence of any of these abnormalities in a child with features of sinusitis of either the persistent or severe variety is associated with a bacterial infection of the maxillary sinuses in 70% of cases [5]. Often, the diagnosis of sinusitis is inferred on the basis of clinical criteria alone. This practice is justified by the strong correlation (88% agreement) between abnormal sinus radiographs and features of persistent sinusitis described above in children less than 6 years of age [5].

Sinus radiographs need not, and therefore should not, routinely be used to confirm the diagnosis of clinically suspected sinusitis in children less than 6 years of age with persistent symptoms; some authorities advocate their selective use in all children older than 6 years suspected of having sinusitis on the basis of presentation with persistent symptoms, and in all children of any age who present with severe symptoms [11]. These recommendations apply to both immunocompetent and immunocompromised hosts.

Computed tomography scans with contrast enhancement are more sensitive than radiographs for detecting sinusitis, but in general should be reserved for evaluation of persistent or recurrent sinusitis not responsive to medical management or associated with suspected complications of the orbit or brain (situations in which surgical intervention is being considered) [11]. Magnetic resonance imaging (MRI) also is useful for diagnosing sinusitis but is less helpful than CT scans. Ultrasonography is not a practically useful diagnostic technique. Transillumination of sinuses is not usually helpful in establishing the diagnosis in children.

Although not routinely used for diagnostic purposes, maxillary sinus aspiration can be safely and effectively performed by a pediatric otolaryngologist as an outpatient procedure using a transnasal approach after careful decontamination and adequate local anesthesia of the area below the inferior turbinate, which the trocar traverses. Aspirated material should be processed promptly for aerobic and anaerobic bacterial cultures as well as for Gram's stain. Recovery of organisms in a density of at least 10^4 cfu/mL is considered indicative of infection [5].

Indications for sinus aspiration and perhaps biopsy include (1) failure to respond to two courses of antibiotics; (2) relief of severe facial pain; (3) orbital or intracranial complications; (4) suspicion of an unusual or opportunistic pathogen; and (5) sinusitis in a severely ill patient. These indications are similar to those for immunocompetent patients. In patients with advanced disease due to HIV, the threshold for an invasive diagnostic procedure should be low. In such cases, in addition to bacterial cultures, aspirated and biopsied material should be processed to facilitate the identification of fungi, viruses, mycobacteria, *Legionella* sp., parasites, protozoa, and possibly *P. jiroveci*, and should be submitted for histologic examination. When fungal infection is suspected on the basis of nasal or facial findings, a biopsy of nasal mucosa should be similarly evaluated for the same diagnostic considerations [12].

29.6 Microbiologic considerations

In immunocompetent children, the bacterial organisms responsible for otitis media vary somewhat with the age of the patient and duration of the infection, but *Streptococcus pneumoniae*, *Haemophilus influenzae*, and *Moraxella catarrhalis* predominate at all ages and in both acute and chronic otitis media [12–13] (see Table 29.1). Respiratory viruses have been isolated from middle ear or nasopharyngeal specimens in approximately 20% of cases of AOM. Their importance in the pathogenesis and etiology of AOM, and as a possible explanation for some apparent antibiotic failures, is now appreciated. Recurrent episodes of AOM, as well as 20–66% of cases of chronic otitis media are caused by the same array of bacterial species as is found in AOM [10]. Chronic suppurative otitis media (CSOM), characterized by persistent otorrhea through a perforated tympanic membrane, is usually attributable to *Pseudomonas aeruginosa*, staphylococci, or *Proteus* spp.; anaerobic organisms have been documented in up to 50% of cases [12]. Occasionally, fungi, especially *Aspergillus* and *Candida* species

Table 29.1 Microbiology of otitis media among immunocompetent and HIV-infected children

	Streptococcus pneumoniae[a]	*Haemophilus influenzae*[b]	*Moraxella catarrhalis*[c]	*Streptococcus pyogenes*	*Staphylococcus aureus*	Anaerobes	Viruses	Other
Otitis media in immunocompetent children	30–40%	15–20%	8–12%	4%	2%	5–6%	20%	
Otitis media in children with HIV	30–40%	15–20%	8–12%	2%	4%[d]	ND	ND	e, f
Sinusitis in immunocompetent children	30–40%	20%	20%	1%			10%	g, h
Sinusitis in children with HIV	30–40%	20%	20%					i, j

[a] 15–38% (average 25%) may be penicillin-nonsusceptible; approximately 50% are highly resistant and 50% intermediately resistant.

[b] 30–50% may be ß-lactamase producing.

[c] 90–100% may be ß-lactamase producing; this bacterial species is less common in adults with AOM.

[d] *S. aureus* is more common in children diagnosed with AOM who are severely immunosuppressed.

[e] *Pseudomonas aeruginosa, Escherichia coli, Proteus mirabilis*, enterococci, and *Candida* species have been isolated from children with HIV.

[f] *Aspergillus, Nocardia, Cryptosporidium* species, and *Pneumocystis* have been recovered from middle ear and external ear canal of adults.

[g] *S. aureus*, anaerobic organisms, and *H. influenzae* are recovered more often from children with chronic sinusitis.

[h] Bacteria found uncommonly in children with acute sinusitis are group C streptococcus, viridans streptococcus, peptostreptococcus, *Moraxella* sp., and *Eikenella corrodens*.

[i] Other organisms recovered from patients with HIV include *S. aureus, P. aeruginosa, S. epidermidis*, group G streptococcus, *Rhizopus arrhizus, Legionella pneumophila*, C. albicans, microsporidium sp., Acanthamoeba sp., Cryptosporidium sp., *A. fumigatus, Mycobacterium avium-intracellulare, Mycobacterium kansasii, Mycobacterium chelonei, Schizophyllum commune, Cryptococcus neoformans*, and cytomegalovirus.

and, rarely, Blastomycosis have been implicated in CSOM, either alone or in combination with bacterial pathogens [12].

In children with HIV who have AOM, the prevalence of the three most common pathogens is similar to that observed in uninfected children [2, 14] (Table 29.1). One study suggests that *S. aureus* is significantly more often associated with AOM in HIV-infected children who are severely immunosuppressed [14].

The microbiology of acute sinusitis is very similar to that of AOM. There have been no systematic studies documenting the microbiology of sinusitis in HIV-infected adults or children. It is likely that they become infected with the same organisms that usually infect immunocompetent hosts, as well as the panoply of uncommon and opportunistic bacterial, viral, fungal, mycobacterial, and protozoal pathogens that have been implicated in a variety of compromised hosts [12].

29.7 Treatment of middle ear and sinus infections

Most episodes of AOM or acute sinusitis in non-toxic children infected with HIV are managed without specific microbiologic data with an orally administered antimicrobial agent that is predictably active against the most likely pathogens. These pathogens include *S. pneumoniae, H. influenzae*, and *M. catarrhalis. H. influenzae* and *M. catarrhalis* are resistant to amoxicillin on the basis of beta-lactamase production approximately 35–50% and 90–100% of the time, respectively [11, 15]. *Streptococcus pneumoniae* are not susceptible to penicillin between 8–38% (average 25%) of the time because of alteration of penicillin-binding proteins. Fifty percent of resistant strains are intermediate in resistance and 50% are highly resistant. Penicillin binding protein-mediated resistance, except for high-level resistance, can often be overcome in vivo by use of high

Table 29.2 Oral antimicrobial therapy for acute otitis media and acute sinusitis in children

Antimicrobial	Daily dosage (mg/kg/day)	Maximum daily dose (mg)	Number of daily doses
Amoxicillin (Many Brands)	45–90	4000	2′
Amoxicillin/clavulanate potassium (Augmentin®)	45–90	4000	2′
Cefdinir (Omnicef®)	14	600	1
Cefpodoxime proxetil (Vantin®)	10	800	2
Cefuroxime axetil (Ceftin®)	30	1000	2
Clarithromycin (Biaxin®)	15	1000	2
Azithromycin (Zithromax®)	10 mg/kg × 1 day* 5 mg/kg × 4 days	500/250	1

*Azithromycin is prescribed at 10 mg/kg as a single daily dose on day 1; the four subsequent daily doses are prescribed at 5 mg/kg/day. The maximum dose for day 1 is 500 mg; the maximum dose for days 2–5 is 250 mg.

doses of penicillins. Risk factors for infection with penicillin-resistant pathogens include attendance at day care, treatment with antimicrobials within the previous 90 days, and age less than 2 years [11]. Candidate antimicrobial agents and dosage recommendations are presented in Table 29.2 [11, 15, 16].

In general, amoxicillin, administered at either a standard dose of 45 mg/kg/day or at a high dose of 90 mg/kg/day, both in two divided doses for 10–14 days, is the agent of choice for empiric treatment of the first episode of AOM or acute sinusitis or the occasional recurrence after at least 3 months in a child with uncomplicated, mildly-to-moderately severe infection who does not attend day care. This permissive dosing range allows the practitioner to individualize therapy to some extent. Early in the respiratory season, lower doses of amoxicillin will suffice in children who are older than 2 years, have not recently received antibiotics, and do not attend day care. For patients with penicillin allergy (provided it is not type 1 hypersensitivity), alternatives to amoxicillin include cefdinir (14 mg/kg/day in a single or two divided doses), cefuroxime (30 mg/kg/day in two divided doses), or cefpodoxime (10 mg/kg/day in two divided doses). Of the three cephalosporins, cefdinir is reputed to be the most palatable. For patients with histories of serious allergic reactions to penicillins, clarithromycin (15 mg/kg/day in two divided doses) or azithromycin

(10 mg/kg/day on day 1 and 5 mg/kg/day on days 2 through 5 as a single daily dose) can be used (notwithstanding the fact that the US Food and Drug Administration has not approved azithromycin for use in sinusitis). Patients known to be infected with penicillin-resistant *S. pneumoniae* can be treated with clindamycin (30–40 mg/kg/day in three divided doses).

For episodes of AOM or acute sinusitis that fail to improve within 48–72 hours of initiation of standard dose amoxicillin, that recur within 90 days of a previous episode treated with antimicrobials, that are moderate or more severe, or that occur in day-care attendees, a broader-spectrum, orally administered antimicrobial should be prescribed. High-dose amoxicillin-clavulanate (90 mg/kg/day of amoxicillin in combination with 6.5 mg/kg/day of clavulanate in divided doses) is an ideal choice. It is important to note that amoxicillin-clavulanate comes in several liquid and tablet formulations that differ in their fixed ratios of amoxicillin to clavulanate (varying from 2 : 1 to 12.9 : 1). Only the new Augmentin ES-600® oral suspension formulation (containing 600 mg of amoxicillin and 42.9 mg of clavulanate per 5 ml) affords an easy means of prescribing amoxicillin at the recommended high dose while avoiding diarrhea associated with the doses of clavulanate that exceed 10 mg/kg/day. (If other formulations are used, it is necessary to prescribe both amoxicillin/clavulanate, each at doses that individually provide 45 mg/kg/day of amoxicillin.) Alternatives include cefdinir, cefuroxime or cefpodoxime. For patients intolerant of oral therapy, treatment may begin with ceftriaxone (50 mg/kg/day) intravenously or intramuscularly until orally administered antimicrobials can be reliably instituted. Because of the emergence of substantial pneumococcal resistance to trimethoprim-sulfamethoxazole and erythromycin-sulfisoxazole, these agents are no longer considered appropriate antimicrobial choices for empiric treatment of AOM and sinusitis.

Decisions about the duration of antimicrobial therapy for AOM and acute sinusitis need to be individualized. Recognizing the demonstrated efficacy of relatively short courses of treatment for uncomplicated AOM in children older than 5 years of age, and being cognizant of the contribution of (prolonged) antibiotic usage to increasing rates of antimicrobial resistance, recent guidelines have endorsed courses of treatment as brief as 5–7 days for clinically responsive episodes of AOM in immunocompetent children of that age [16]. However, children with symptomatic HIV are at significantly increased risk for recurrences of AOM and bacterial sinusitis, as well as for the development of complications and treatment failures, with amoxicillin. In general, we recommend treating recurrent episodes of AOM or acute sinusitis in this population according to the general clinical practice guideline advocated for managing sinusitis in normal hosts [11], i.e. with a broader-spectrum antimicrobial for a duration of 10–21 days (or for at least one week beyond the complete resolution of symptoms). In the case of an HIV-infected child who appears systemically ill or toxic at presentation or during treatment of AOM or acute sinusitis, tympanocentesis or sinus aspiration should be performed, aspirated fluid should be cultured, and a parenterally administered broad-spectrum antimicrobial (e.g. cefotaxime, ceftazidime, ceftriaxone or high-dose ampicillin-sulbactam) should be initiated empirically. (If the tympanic membrane has perforated spontaneously, the canal should be suctioned, cleaned, and a sample of middle ear fluid obtained for culture.) Specific treatment is given as directed by results of cultures and susceptibility testing, and as indicated for specific uncommon or opportunistic organisms that may be implicated.

The duration of antibiotic therapy in patients experiencing recurrent episodes of acute bacterial sinusitis is similar to primary episodes. Most patients with "chronic" sinusitis have an underlying problem such as allergic or non-allergic rhinitis. These patients may benefit from systemic antihistamines or intranasal steroids.

In immunocompetent children, persistence of middle-ear effusion following treatment of AOM despite resolution of signs and symptoms of suppuration is present in up to 50% of cases immediately upon completion of therapy, and gradually resolves in all but 10% over 3 months [17]. Awareness of this natural history and concern for the role of antibiotic usage in promoting antibiotic resistance accounts for the caution to avoid prescribing repeated courses of antimicrobials for otitis media with effusion in the absence of signs and symptoms of recurrent AOM [16]. If the effusion persists for more than 2–3 months and is associated with a significant hearing loss, a second course of treatment with a broader-spectrum antimicrobial may be given, especially before electing a surgical treatment. When middle ear effusion persists unabated for more than 3 months despite treatment with antimicrobials, especially when bilateral, occurring in a young child, or associated with hearing loss, tinnitus, vertigo, or significant changes in the tympanic membrane or middle ear, myringotomy (usually with tympanostomy tube placement) should be considered. These same recommendations apply to children infected with HIV.

To date, *P. jiroveci* has not been reported to cause ear infections in children infected with HIV. The few such adults who have been described appear to have responded to oral trimethoprim-sulfamethoxazole with or without dapsone, or to intravenously administered pentamidine.

Chronic suppurative otitis media should be managed in conjunction with an otolaryngologist who will obtain a specimen for culture, perform daily aural toilet, and undertake serial examinations. Topical therapy with ofloxacin is advised [15]. If the otorrhea does not begin to resolve in 48–72 hours, parenteral antibiotics, initially selected empirically for activity against *P. aeruginosa* and *S. aureus* (e.g. ticarcillin disodium/clavulanate potassium or piperacillin/tazobactam or cefepime), and subsequently chosen according to culture and antimicrobial susceptibility results, may be necessary to effect a cure. Antimicrobial therapy is usually continued for 7 days beyond resolution of the otorrhea. Tympanomastoidectomy is sometimes required if otorrhea persists or recurs despite parenteral therapy.

29.7.1 Sinus infections

In the absence of demonstrated efficacy, routine use of inhaled decongestants is not recommended for patients with sinusitis; however, in selected cases (severe nasal congestion or periorbital swelling) their use for a few days may be helpful. Systemic and local antihistamines, intranasal corticosteroids, and sodium cromolyn appear to help improve symptoms of nasal allergy, but offer minimal if any additional benefit beyond that afforded by antibiotics in the treatment of acute bacterial sinusitis.

Rarely, when patients with acute sinusitis do not respond to parenteral therapy, surgical drainage may be necessary to restore physiologic function to a paranasal sinus. Currently, functional endonasal sinus surgery (endoscopic removal of obstructions in the osteomeatal complex, enlargement of the meatus of the maxillary sinus outflow tract, and anterior ethmoidectomy) represents the most promising surgical option. Limited literature suggests that this procedure produces substantial improvement in carefully selected children with chronic sinusitis [5, 19].

When fungal sinusitis is highly suspected or documented, treatment with amphotericin B should be instituted in an accelerated fashion to quickly achieve a daily dose of 1 mg/kg. Five-fluorocytosine may provide additional benefit as adjunctive therapy. Liposomal amphotericin should be used when use of conventional amphotericin B is either contraindicated or complicated by abnormal renal function. Fluconazole and intraconazole should be reserved for occasions when susceptibility has been demonstrated or can be reliably predicted. Extensive surgical debridement is usually required. Hyperbaric oxygen may be helpful in cases of rhinocerebral mucormycosis [12].

29.8 Prevention of otitis media and sinusitis

The use of chemoprophylaxis to prevent or reduce episodes of recurrent AOM was commonly recommended prior to the advent of extensive antimicrobial resistance (especially penicillin-nonsusceptible *S. pneumoniae*). Current guidelines reserve its use in immunocompetent hosts for highly selected cases that meet stringent criteria of three or more well-documented episodes of AOM within 6 months or four episodes within 12 months [16, 20]. We recommend similarly rigorous criteria for initiating chemoprophylaxis in immunocompromised hosts, including children with HIV infection. Agents for which efficacy had been demonstrated (albeit, prior to the current era of substantial antibiotic resistance) include amoxicillin (at a dose of 20 mg/kg once daily) and sulfisoxazole (at a dose of 50–75 mg/kg/day in two divided doses). At least one publication has reported a failure of prophylaxis with amoxicillin compared with placebo presumably because of the prevalence of resistant middle ear isolates (both beta-lactamase producing *H. influenzae* and *M. catarrhalis* and penicillin-resistant *S. pneumoniae*) [21]. Although concern for its toxicity has led some authorities to caution against the use of trimethoprim-sulfamethoxazole, or sulfisoxazole alone, for

preventing recurrences of otitis media, it has demonstrated efficacy for this purpose when given daily (admittedly, documented at a time of less prevalent antimicrobial resistance). Although its ability to prevent otitis media when administered less frequently (as in thrice-weekly schedules often used in HIV-infected patients for prophylaxis against *P. jiroveci* pneumonia) is unknown, daily administration, if tolerated, is recommended and would provide satisfactory protection for both concerns.

Although antibiotic prophylaxis as a strategy to prevent infection in patients with recurrent episodes of acute bacterial sinusitis has not been systematically studied in either immunocompetent or immunoincompetent hosts, by analogy to its demonstrated effectiveness in reducing episodes of recurrent AOM, it is a potentially effective preventive modality. However, it too should only be prescribed for highly selected patients (including children with HIV infection) who satisfy stringent indications: three or more (clinically) well-diagnosed episodes of acute sinusitis within 6 months, or four episodes within a year [11]. Recommended chemoprophylactic agents are the same as those used for recurrent AOM. In those highly selected instances when prophylaxis is initiated, it should generally be given throughout the respiratory infection season (winter) for those who experience the usual seasonal pattern of otitis media and sinusitis. It should be given for at least 1 year for those whose disease occurs year-round. Myringotomy and tube placement is recommended for patients whose frequency of recurrent AOM is not substantially reduced by chemoprophylaxis and for selected patients with chronic effusion (e.g. those with significant hearing loss).

Heptavalent pneumococcal conjugate vaccine (PCV7) is recommended for universal use in children less than 24 months of age and selectively for others at high risk of invasive pneumococcal disease, including all individuals of any age with HIV infection [22]. A history of frequent otitis media or sinusitis is not currently a formally recommended indication for its administration to children older than 2 years who do not satisfy other "high risk" criteria. However, the impact of immunizing infants with PCV7 on reducing the frequency of: (a) all doctor visits for otitis (by 8.9%); (b) all episodes of otitis media (by 6–7%); (c) episodes of otitis caused by pneumococci of serotypes contained in the vaccine (by 57–66.7%); (d) experiencing three episodes of otitis within 6 months or four within 1 year (by 9.5%); and (e) ventilatory tube placement (by 20.3%) has been well documented in two large studies in the USA [23] and Finland [24]. Although the impact of immunization with PCV7 on rates of sinusitis among hosts with normal immune competence has not been determined, and data relative to its efficacy in reducing both AOM and sinusitis among children with

HIV infection are lacking, routine administration of PCV7 as well as 23-valent pneumococcal polysaccharide vaccine to all HIV-infected children according to published guidelines [22] is strongly recommended.

29.9 Summary

The clinical presentation, diagnosis, microbiology, and management of episodes of AOM and bacterial sinusitis in immunocompetent children and those who are infected with HIV is very similar. In an era of increasing resistance to antimicrobial agents, it is appropriate to obtain samples of middle ear fluid or maxillary sinus aspirates in patients who do not respond to the first or second antibiotic empirically selected for treatment. The recovery of resistant or unusual organisms including uncommon bacteria, or other organisms that occasionally are responsible for AOM or sinusitis in children with HIV infection, will help inform the selection of specific antimicrobial agents.

REFERENCES

1. Teele, D. W., Klein, J. O., Rosner, B., and the Greater Boston Otitis Media Study Group. Epidemiology of otitis media during the first seven years of life in children in Greater Boston: a prospective cohort study. *J. Infect. Dis.* **160** (1989), 83–94.

2. Principi, N., Marchisio, P., Tornaghi, R., Onorato, J., Massironi, E. & Picco, P. Acute otitis media in human immunodeficiency virus-infected children. *Pediatrics* **88** (1991), 566–71.

3. Barnett, E. D., Klein, J. O., Pelton, S. I. & Luginbuhl, L. M. Otitis media in children born to human immunodeficiency virus-infected mothers. *Pediatr. Infect. Dis. J.* **11** (1992), 360–4.

4. Chen, A. Y., Ohlms, L. A., Stewart, M. G. & Kline, M. W. Otolaryngologic disease progression in children with human immunodeficiency virus infection. *Arch. Otolaryngol. Head Neck Surg.* **122** (1996), 1360–3.

5. Wald, E. R. Sinusitis in children. *New Engl. J. Med.* **326** (1992), 319–23.

6. The National Institute of Child Health and Human Development Intravenous Immunoglobulin Study Group. Intravenous immune globulin for the prevention of bacterial infections in children with symptomatic human immunodeficiency virus infection. *New Engl. J. Med.* **325** (1991), 73–80.

7. Mofenson, L. M., Korelitz, J., Pelton, S., Moye, J. Jr., Nugent, R. & Bethel, J. Sinusitis in children infected with human immunodeficiency virus: clinical characteristics, risk factors, and prophylaxis. *Clin. Infect. Dis.* **21** (1995), 1175–81.

8. Bluestone, C. D. & Klein, J. *Otitis Media in Infants and Children,* 2nd edn. Philadelphia: W.B. Saunders Co. (1995).

9. Wald, E. R. Diagnosis and management of sinusitis in children. *Adv. Pediatr. Infect. Dis.* **12** (1996), 1–20.

10. Parsons, D. S. & Wald, E. R. Otitis media and sinusitis: similar diseases. *Otolaryngol. Clin. N. Am.* **29** (1996), 11–25.

11. American Academy of Pediatrics Subcommittee on Management of Sinusitis and Committee on Quality Improvement. Clinical Practice Guideline: Management of Sinusitis. *Pediatrics* **108** (2001), 798–808.

12. Wald, E. R. Infections of the sinuses, ears, and hypopharynx. In J. Shelhamer, P. A. Pizzo, J. E. Parrillo & H. Masur (eds.), *Respiratory Disease in the Immunosuppressed Host.* Philadelphia: J.B. Lippincott Co. (1991), pp. 450–68.

13. Wald, E. R. Haemophilus influenzae as a cause of acute otitis media. *Pediatr. Infect. Dis. J.* **8** (1989), S28-30.

14. Marchisio, P., Principi, N., Sorella, S., Sala, E. & Tornaghi, R. Etiology of acute otitis media in human immunodeficiency virus-infected children. *Pediatr. Infect. Dis. J.* **15** (1996), 58–61.

15. Dowell, S. F., Butler, J. C., Giebink, G. S. *et al.* Acute otitis media: management and surveillance in an era of pneumococcal resistance – a report from the Drug-resistant *Streptococcus pneumoniae* Therapeutic Working Group. *Pediatr. Infect. Dis. J.* **18** (1999), 1–9.

16. Dowell, S. F., Marcy, S. M., Phillips, W. R. *et al.* Otitis media-principles of judicious use of antimicrobial agents. *Pediatrics* **101** (1998), 165–71.

17. Klein, J. O. & Bluestone, C. D. Management of otitis media in the era of managed care. *Adv. Pediatr. Infect. Dis.* **12** (1996), 351–86.

18. Barlow, D., Duckert, L., Kreig, C. & Gates, G. Ototoxicity of topical otomicrobial agents. *Acta. Otolaryngol.* **115** (1995), 231–5.

19. Lusk, R. P. The surgical management of chronic sinusitis in children. *Pediatr. Ann.* **27** (1998), 820–7.

20. Paradise, J. L. Antimicrobial drugs and surgical procedures in the prevention of otitis media. *Pediatr. Infect. Dis. J.* **8** (1989), S35–7.

21. Roark, R. & Berman, S. Continuous twice daily or once daily amoxicillin prophylaxis compared with placebo for children with recurrent acute otitis media. *Pediatr. Infect. Dis. J.* **16** (1997), 376–81.

22. American Academy of Pediatrics. Policy statement: Recommendations for the prevention of pneumococcal infections, including the use of pneumococcal conjugate vaccine (Prevnar), pneumococcal polysaccharide vaccine, and antibiotic prophylaxis. *Pediatrics* **106** (2000), 362–6.

23. Black, S., Shinefield, H., Ray, P. *et al.* Efficacy, safety and immunogenicity of heptavalent pneumococcal conjugate vaccine in children: Northern California Kaiser Permanent Vaccine Study Group. *Pediatr. Infect. Dis. J.* **19** (2000), 187–95.

24. Eskola, J., Kilpi, T., Palmu, A. *et al.* Efficacy of a pneumococcal conjugate vaccine (PncCRM) against acute otitis media. *N. Engl. J. Med.* **344** (2001), 403–9.

Cardiac problems

Gul H. Dadlani[1] and Steven E. Lipshultz, M.D.[1,2]

[1]Divison of Pediatric Cardiology, Golisano Children's Hospital at Strong and University of Rochester Medical Center, Rochester, NY
[2]Department of Pediatrics and Department of Medicine, University of Rochester School of Medicine and Dentistry, Rochester, NY

30.1 Introduction

The cardiovascular complications of HIV infection are increasingly contributing to the overall morbidity and mortality of this pediatric population. The prevalence of cardiovascular disease is estimated to be more than 90% in both symptomatic and asymptomatic HIV-infected children [1]. The spectrum of cardiovascular disorders includes abnormalities in left ventricular (LV) performance, wall thickness, and contractility; dilated cardiomyopathy; myocarditis; pericarditis; and rhythm disturbances. These children may have a wide spectrum of presenting symptoms for their cardiovascular complications, but most are initially asymptomatic. The cardiovascular symptoms may be inadvertently attributed to other causes, such as pulmonary or infectious processes, which may delay treatment. Early detection of and intervention for subclinical cardiovascular abnormalities through routine screening and monitoring will allow the clinician to initiate therapy with the goal of preventing or delaying the onset of clinical cardiovascular complications. Today the survival of pediatric HIV patients has improved and cardiac complications are increasing as the underlying cause of death (Figure 30.1) [2, 3]. Therefore, clinicians need a fundamental understanding of the cardiovascular complications that can arise from HIV infection in pediatric patients.

30.2 Risk factors

Several risk factors for cardiovascular disease among HIV-infected children have been described. The triad of encephalopathy, wasting, and low CD4$^+$ counts in children

with HIV has been shown to be associated with an increased risk of cardiovascular complications and a decreased survival [3]. Encephalopathy can lead to an autonomic neuropathy, which may precipitate arrhythmias or even sudden death [4]. Children with a prior history of a serious cardiac event (Figure 30.2) or who have rapid progression of their disease (an AIDS-defining condition other than lymphoid interstitial pneumonitis/pulmonary hyperplasia or severe immunosuppression in the first year of life) are at increased risk of severe cardiac complications [4]. Co-infection with other viruses has increased cardiac morbidity and mortality in HIV patients [6]. The highest risk of cardiac or noncardiac mortality following a viral co-infection is associated with Epstein–Barr virus (EBV) [4]. Cytomegalovirus (CMV) is a significant predictor of cardiac events, when associated with wasting and a prior history of cardiac abnormalities [6]. Left ventricular dysfunction and increased left ventricular wall thickness as detected by echocardiography (ECHO) are independent risk factors for all-cause mortality in pediatric HIV patients [7]. Cardiotoxic medications used to treat HIV or associated diseases (malignancies) may be another risk factor for the development of cardiovascular complications.

30.3 Types of cardiovascular disease

HIV-infected children are more likely to develop LV dysfunction during the first 2 years of age than uninfected children (Figure 30.3) [7]. This is defined as decreased systolic or diastolic function of the ventricle as identified by ECHO. Left ventricular dysfunction is usually asymptomatic and can occur at any stage of the HIV infection.

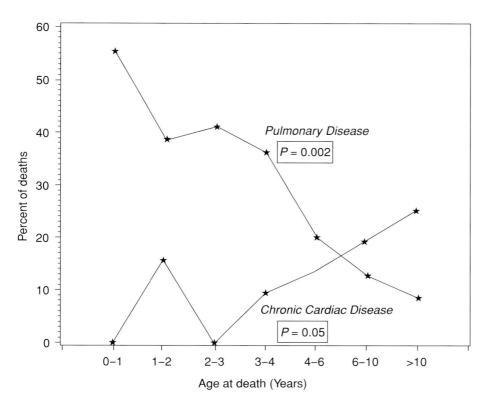

Figure 30.1. Trends in underlying cause of death for 93 HIV-infected children. (From ref [18].)

No. Cases: Cardiac Disease (*n* =11), Pulmonary Disease (*n* = 27)

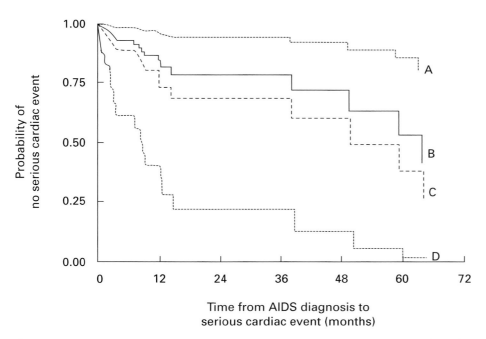

Figure 30.2. Time to occurrence of a serious cardiac event (transient and chronic congestive heart failure, hypotension, severe dysrhythmia, cardiac tamponade, cerebrovascular accident associated with hemodynamic instability, and cardiac arrest) in AIDS patients in 1992. Wasting and prior cardiac events at the time of AIDS diagnosis were significant predictors of subsequent cardiac events in multivariate analyses. Curve A represents AIDS patients with no wasting or prior cardiac events. Curve B represents AIDS patients with no wasting but with a history of prior cardiac events. Curve C represents AIDS patients with wasting and no prior cardiac events. Curve D represents AIDS patients with wasting and a history of prior cardiac events. (From refs. [19, 20].)

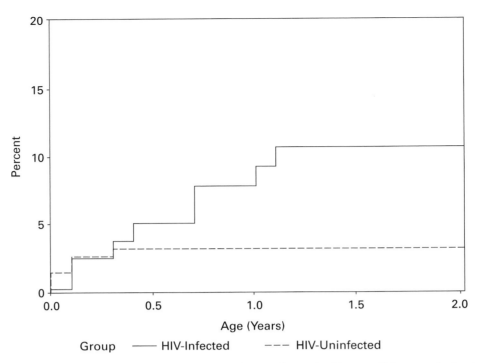

Figure 30.3. Kaplan–Meier cumulative incidence of an initial episode of decreased left ventricular fractional shortening (defined as a shortening fraction of not more than 25%) in HIV-infected and -uninfected children over the first 2 years of life ($P = 0.01$; log-rank test). (From ref [2].)

Increased LV wall thickness can occur with or without LV dysfunction. Both of these echocardiographic findings are useful long-term predictors of mortality in HIV-infected children [6]. The relationship of these changes to LV structure and function remains unknown, but may include any of the risk factors discussed above. Progression of LV dysfunction results in alterations in heart rate, LV preload, LV afterload, and in decreased LV contractility [7].

As LV dysfunction advances, patients develop a cardiomyopathy. A cardiomyopathy is a disease process that affects the structure or function of the myocardium [8]. It can be idiopathic or it can be caused by processes such as ischemia, systemic disease, infection, toxins, or a metabolic process. A dilated cardiomyopathy, which can be caused by HIV infection, occurs when the left or both ventricles become enlarged and poorly contractile. It can present with symptoms of congestive heart failure (CHF), including tachypnea, diaphoresis, pallor, organomegaly, edema, failure to thrive, or wasting.

Myocarditis is a common complication associated with HIV infection. Myocarditis has been defined by the Dallas criteria as "a process characterized by lymphocytic infiltrate of the myocardium with necrosis and/or degeneration of adjacent myocytes not typical of the ischemic

damage associated with coronary artery disease" [9, 10]. This inflammation can be transient or can lead to a cardiomyopathy. Myocarditis can be caused by a variety of agents including: direct HIV infection of the myocyte; viral co-infections with adenovirus, CMV, EBV, coxsackievirus, herpes simplex virus or parvovirus; opportunistic infections with *Toxoplasma gondii*, *Cryptococcus neoformans*, *Mycobacterium tuberculosis*, and *Mycobacterium avium* complex; drug-related toxicities; nutritional deficiencies; or autoimmune reactions [9]. The presentation of myocarditis can range from completely asymptomatic to severe CHF.

Arrhythmias represent a life-threatening cardiovascular complication of HIV infection. HIV encephalopathy can produce an autonomic neuropathy, which has been associated with sinus arrhythmias, bradycardia, hypotension, and cardiac arrest [4]. Many medications used by HIV-infected patients have the potential to provoke arrhythmias by altering the autonomic regulation of the conduction system of the heart. Pentamidine, amphotericin B, ganciclovir, and trimethoprim-sulfamethoxazole have been shown to cause both atrial and ventricular arrhythmias [9]. Pentamidine, especially when given intravenously, can prolong the QT_c interval and induce torsades de pointes, a polymorphic form of ventricular tachycardia [10]. Cardiomyopathies and myocarditis result in myocardial irritability that may induce premature ventricular beats and ventricular arrhythmias. Patients with arrhythmias and conduction disturbances of the heart may present with chest pain, palpitations, syncope, near-syncope, dyspnea, or dizzy spells.

Pericarditis, inflammation of the pericardium, and pericardial effusions, fluid collections within the pericardial space, also occur in HIV patients. The etiological agents are similar to those for myocarditis and include HIV, viral co-infections, opportunistic agents, malignancy, malnutrition, hypothyroidism, autoimmune reactions, and bacterial infections [12]. Children can present with symptoms of chest pain radiating to the neck or shoulder, a pericardial friction rub upon auscultation, pulsus paradoxicus, tachycardia, dyspnea, cough, and ECG changes.

Endocarditis is commonly seen in adult HIV patients with a history of IV drug abuse, but can be encountered in the pediatric population, especially if there is a pre-existing history of congenital heart disease. The most common agents causing endocarditis include *Staphylococcus aureus*, *Streptococcus* Species, *Haemophilus influenzae*, fastidious organisms of the HACEK group (*Haemophilus parainfluenzae*, *H. aphrophilus*, *H. paraphrophilus*, *Actinobacillus actinomycetemcomitans*, *Cardiobacterium hominis*, *Eikenella* species, *Kingella kingae*) and opportunistic agents such as *Cryptococcus* and *Candida* [12]. Patients usually present with persistent fever, fatigue, heart murmur, splenomegaly, signs of systemic micro-emboli (petechiae, Osler nodes, Janeway lesions, and splinter hemorrhages), and a history of congenital heart disease.

Hypertension can affect many pediatric HIV patients. Hypertension is defined as a systolic and/or diastolic blood pressure that is greater than the 95th percentile for age on at least three different occasions. Hypertension can be caused by medications, vasculitis, early or accelerated atherosclerosis, renal disease, autonomic nervous system disturbances, or protease inhibitor-induced insulin resistance with increased sympathetic activity and sodium retention [12]. These affected patients are usually asymptomatic and are diagnosed by routine blood pressure monitoring.

Cardiac malignancies (Kaposi's sarcoma and lymphoma), primary pulmonary hypertension with right ventricular dysfunction, premature coronary artery disease or atherosclerosis, and lipid abnormalities are all cardiac complications that are frequently encountered in adults but less so in the pediatric HIV population. Lipid abnormalities and other metabolic complications of antiretroviral therapy are discussed in Chapter 20. The clinician must keep these other complications in mind as the survival of the pediatric HIV population continues to improve and pediatric patients enter adulthood.

30.4 Evaluation of the pediatric HIV patient for cardiovascular problems

Detecting cardiovascular complications in HIV-infected infants and children can be difficult because symptoms can be masked by involvement of other organ systems. Pulmonary disease, reactive organomegaly, anemia, gastrointestinal disease, renal disease, depression, or neurological abnormalities can overshadow the signs and symptoms of cardiac disease. The clinician should always remember that subclinical cardiac disease may be present before any signs or symptoms manifest themselves.

All evaluations should begin with a comprehensive patient history. This should include: past medical history, past surgical history, birth history, family history, developmental milestones, allergies, diet, medications, and a complete review of systems. The medical provider should focus questions toward the following: previous cardiac events; family history of congenital heart disease or arrhythmias; current medications(s) with potential cardiac toxicity; nutritional status; and, growth and development. The review of systems should try to elicit specific symptoms, which may indicate underlying cardiac problems. The clinician should make a differential diagnosis for each positive symptom. Table 30.1 reviews the cardiac symptoms that should be reviewed during a complete history along with a differential diagnosis for each symptom.

The next step in the evaluation of a pediatric HIV patient for cardiovascular problems should be a complete physical exam. The clinician should remember to check the patient's weight (to rule out wasting syndrome), pulse rate (tachycardia, bradycardia), blood pressure (hypo- or hypertension), and mental status (encephalopathy). Once again, the clinician should make a differential diagnosis related to each physical exam finding. This approach will prevent one from overlooking a subtle cardiovascular finding. Table 30.2 reviews physical examination findings suggestive of cardiovascular disease and their differential diagnosis.

In general, a complete history and physical examination is a reliable way of excluding cardiovascular disease, but HIV patients may have sub-clinical findings many months or years before overt clinical signs and symptoms arise. Therefore, a number of different monitoring modalities have been developed to look for cardiovascular complications in pediatric HIV patients. Early detection of cardiac problems through appropriate screening and monitoring will allow for the identification of patients who could benefit from early intervention or aggressive antiretroviral therapy. Table 30.3 summarizes the diagnosis, detection, and management of cardiovascular problems in HIV patients. In addition, clinicians must review a patient's medications,

Table 30.1 Symptoms suggestive of cardiovascular disease: differential diagnosis

Symptoms	Potential cardiovascular etiology	Other etiologies
Fatigue, dyspnea with exertion	Congestive heart failure	Malnutrition, chronic illness, anemia, depression
Pallor	Congestive heart failure	Malnutrition, chronic illness, anemia
Cyanosis	Structural heart disease	Lung disease, methemyoglobulinemia
Persistent respiratory symptoms: cough, wheezes, tachypnea, dyspnea	Congestive heart failure	Lung disease
Diaphoresis with feedings	Congestive heart failure	Chronic illness, lung disease
Nausea/vomiting	Organomegaly from congestive heart failure	Gastrointestinal disease
Syncope/pre-syncope	Arrhythmia, low cardiac output	Neurologic disease, anemia, hypoglycemia
Failure to thrive	Any form of heart disease	Chronic illness, endocrine, renal, or gastrointestinal disease
Chest pain	Pericarditis, myocarditis, arrhythmia, ischemia	Gastrointestinal or lung disease, costochondritis

Table 30.2 Physical examination findings suggestive of cardiovascular disease: differential diagnosis

Sign	Cardiovascular etiology	Other etiologies
Tachycardia	All forms of heart disease	Anemia, sepsis, fever, dehydration, medications
Bradycardia	All forms of heart disease	Neurologic or pulmonary diseases, medications
Hypertension	Cardiomyopathy	Neurologic or renal diseases, medications
Hypotension	All forms of heart disease	Dehydration, sepsis, or neurologic disease
Jugular venous distention	Congestive heart failure, pericardial tamponade	Liver disease, malnutrition with ascites
Rales, wheezes, rhonchi	Congestive heart failure	Lung disease
Abnormal or displaced precordial impulse	Pericarditis, myocarditis, cardiomyopathy	Sepsis, pneumothorax
Abnormal S2	Structural heart disease, cardiomyopathy	Increased pulmonary pressures
S3/S4	Congestive heart failure	Sepsis, fever, anemia, dehydration
Murmur	Structural heart disease endocarditis, cardiomyopathy	Lung disease, anemia, normal physiology
Organomegaly	Congestive heart failure	Sepsis, liver disease
Poor perfusion	Low cardiac output due to heart disease	Low cardiac output due to sepsis or anemia
Disorientation	Low cardiac output due to heart disease	Low cardiac output due to sepsis, or neurological disease (encephalopathy)
Edema, ascites, decreased urine output	Congestive heart failure	Renal or liver disease, malnutrition, anasarca

Table 30.3 Diagnosis and management of cardiovascular disease

Types of cardiovascular disease	Signs and symptoms	Diagnostic tests	Possible etiologies	Clinical management
Abnormalities of left ventricular structure and dysfunction	May progress to CHF	ECHO will show decreased left ventricular function and increased wall thickness	Unknown; See text (risk factors)	Possibly ACE inhibitor or beta antagonist therapy
Cardiomyopathy	May progress to CHF	CXR may show cardiomegaly, increased pulmonary blood flow. ECHO will show decreased left ventricular function	Unknown; See text (risk factors)	Supportive therapy
Myocarditis	Intercurrent viral-type illness, murmur, CHF, arrhythmia. May present *in extremis* or as sudden death	Same as cardiomyopathy. Laboratory: elevated WBC and other indications of sepsis	Mostly viral etiologies, such as CMV, adenovirus, EBV, parvovirus, herpes virus, coxsackievirus	Treat underlying cause, if possible. IVIG in monthly doses. Steroid therapy unclear
Pericarditis and pericardial effusions	Chest pain, shoulder pain, hacking cough, diaphoresis, pericardial rub, fever, CHF, hemodynamic instability	CXR: enlarged cardiac silhouette without increased intravascular markings. ECHO: pericardial effusion	May be secondary to inflammatory, infectious, malignant, immune, or thyroid abnormalities	Treat the underlying agent if possible. Careful use of diuretics, antiinflammatory and steroids. Pericardiocentesis for diagnostic or if hemo-dynamically compromising
Endocarditis	+/− fever, new murmur, petechiae, CHF	ECHO: valvular abnormalities Labs: blood cultures may be positive	Usually *Staphylococcus aureus*, but also subtypes of *Streptococcus*	Antimicrobial therapy. Surgery if severely hemodynamically compromised.
Premature athero-sclerosis	Asymptomatic	EBCT will detect calcium deposits in coronary arteries	Unknown	Modify traditional risk factors: smoking, diabetes, hypertension, Cholesterol/LDL, physical inactivity, obesity
Hypertension	Asymptomatic	Routine blood pressure monitoring in the office	Medications, vasculitis, unknown	Life style modification, reduced salt intake, anti-hypertensive medications
Arrhythmias or conduction disturbances	Syncope, presyncope, palpitations, chest pain	ECG Holter monitoring	Autonomic neuropathy, medication side-effects, infections irritating the sinus node, AV node or myocardium.	Early referral to a pediatric cardiologist or electrophysiologist and a thorough review of all medication side-effects.
Lipid abnormalities	Asymptomatic	Routine screening of serum lipid panels	Medication side-effects, especially protease inhibitors	Lifestyle modification, initiation of lipid lowering agents to reduce risk of atherosclerosis

CHF, congestive heart failure; ECHO, echocardiography; CXR, chest x-ray; WBC, white blood cells; CMV, cytomegalovirus; EBV, Epstein-Barr virus; ECG, electrocardiogram; EBCT, electron beam computed tomography.

Table 30.4 Cardiovascular interactions of commonly used drugs in HIV patients

Medications	Cardiac Side-Effects
Nucleoside reverse transcriptase inhibitors	Zidovudine – skeletal muscle myopathy, myocarditis, dilated cardiomyopathy Zalcitabine – short-term free radical cardiotoxicity
Non-nucleoside reverse transcriptase inhibitors	Delavirdine and vasoconstrictors can cause ischemia
Protease inhibitors	Implicated in premature atherosclerosis, dyslipidemia, insulin resistance, diabetes mellitus, fat wasting, and redistribution
Antibiotics	Erythromycin: orthostatic hypertension, ventricular tachycardia, bradycardia, torsades (with drug interactions) Rifampin: reduces digoxin therapeutic effect. Clarithromycin: QT prolongation and torsades Trimethoprim/sulfamethoxazole: orthostatic hypertension, anaphylaxis, QT prolongation, torsades, hypokalemia. Sparfloxacin (fluoroquinolones): QT prolongation
Antifungal agents	Amphotericin B: digoxin toxicity (interaction), hypertension, arrhythmia, renal failure, hypokalemia, thrombophlebitis, bradycardia, angioedema, dilated cardiomyopathy. Ketoconazole, fluconazole, itraconazole: QT prolongation and torsades de pointes
Antiviral agents	Foscarnet: reversible cardiac failure, electrolyte imbalances Ganciclovir: Ventricular tachycardia, hypotension
Anti-parasitic agents	Pentamidine: hypotension, QT prolongation, arrhythmias, torsades, ventricular tachycardia, hyperglycemia, hypoglycemia, sudden death. Effects are enhanced by hypomagnesemia and hypokalemia.
Chemotherapeutic agents	Vincristine: arrhythmia, myocardial infarction, cardiomyopathy, cardiac autonomic neuropathy Anthracyclines: myocarditis, cardiomyopathy, cardiac failure
Systemic corticosteroids	Steroids: ventricular hypertrophy, cardiomyopathy, hyperglycemia

because many of the medications used to treat HIV infection have cardiovascular side-effects. Table 30.4 reviews many of the common classes of medications used in HIV therapy and their cardiovascular side-effects. Future research will define which modalities are most sensitive, specific and cost-effective to be used as general screening tools for all HIV patients or restricted to specific subgroups.

Echocardiography is the most important screening tool for the cardiovascular complications of HIV. It is capable of identifying LV systolic dysfunction and increased LV wall thickness. The development of either of these findings has been found to be an independent predictor of all-cause mortality, even when other risk factors are taken into account [6]. These echocardiographic findings are typically asymptomatic, but have been reported to be present more than a year before the patient's death [4]. Early identification of these findings may allow time for preventive or therapeutic interventions. Echocardiography is also useful

for identifying the following: pericardial effusions, valvular heart disease, endocarditis, right ventricular dysfunction which may indicate underlying pulmonary hypertension, endocardial masses or thrombus formation, and LV diastolic dysfunction which may be associated with 30–60% of cases of CHF. Our recommended schedule for echocardiograms is as follows:

- A baseline echocardiogram at the time of HIV diagnosis, then asymptomatic HIV children should have a follow-up echocardiogram every 1–2 years until they become symptomatic [13].
- Once symptomatic with HIV, annual echocardiograms are required [13].
- Any pediatric patient found to have a cardiovascular abnormality should be followed by a pediatric cardiologist.

Electrocardiography and Holter monitoring are used to detect abnormalities in the cardiac conduction system or rhythm disturbances. An electrocardiogram (ECG) should be performed as a baseline study at the time of HIV diagnosis and prior to the introduction of new medications since the potential for prolongation of the QT_c interval exists. Holter monitors provide a 24-hour electrocardiographic recording of a patient's rhythm. Holter monitors are useful if a patient provides a history of symptoms that are consistent with an arrhythmia, such as palpitations, chest pain, syncope, or near-syncope.

Exercise stress testing can assess the degree of cardiac reserve, determine the exercise potential of patients with LV dysfunction, and screen for ischemic changes that can be a marker of premature atherosclerosis [13]. An exercise test is conducted by placing a child on a treadmill or bicycle and following their heart's rate, rhythm, blood pressure, and ECG during exercise. Metabolic exercise stress tests in adults have revealed that individuals with a maximal oxygen uptake (VO_2max) of less than 14 ml/kg/m^2 have significantly reduced survival [13]. The use of exercise or metabolic tests should be considered under the guidance of a pediatric cardiologist in any patient with arrhythmias or significant LV dysfunction.

Cardiac catheterization with endomyocardial biopsy can be a useful invasive diagnostic procedure for HIV patients who have had CHF of an unclear etiology for more than 2 weeks [6]. The biopsy results can lead to a diagnosis of myocarditis from a specific or non-specific etiology. This information may allow the clinician to initiate or redirect the current treatment plan.

Pericardiocentesis can be both a diagnostic and therapeutic invasive procedure for HIV patients with pericardial effusions. Emergent pericardiocentesis may be needed if signs of pericardial tamponade are present.

Non-invasive screening for premature atherosclerosis may be considered in older children as they begin to enter adolescence. New non-invasive technologies are available to image the coronary arteries and assess for premature atherosclerosis without the need for angiography. Electron beam computed tomography is an ultrafast computed tomography scan that is available in many larger cities in the USA. It is capable of imaging 3 mm slices, which can identify calcium deposits within the walls of the coronary arteries. The calcium deposits can be quantitated into a calcium score, which may be predictive of future coronary artery events. Other experimental technologies such as contrast enhanced computed tomography and magnetic resonance angiography can produce non-invasive images of the coronary artery anatomy and identify areas of obstruction.

Serum laboratory tests can also be useful for detecting micronutrient deficiencies, electrolyte abnormalities, myocardial injury, lipid abnormalities, ongoing inflammation and potential thrombotic markers. Selenium and carnitine are two micronutrients that can be screened for as potential causes of a cardiomyopathy. Patients with LV dysfunction should have a cardiac troponin T level measured to evaluate for active myocardial injury secondary to myocarditis [14]. Although we consider a cardiac troponin T level of greater than 0.01 ng/ml as elevated, pediatric standards have yet to be determined. General markers of inflammation, such as highly sensitive C-reactive protein (hsCRP), also are elevated in patients with active myocarditis [13]. Lipid panels should be done routinely on all patients who are on protease inhibitors.

30.5 Management of the pediatric HIV patient with cardiac problems

Prevention of cardiovascular complications is at the cornerstone of the management in HIV-infected children. At the present time, no uniform HIV-specific preventive or therapeutic guidelines have been published. Our recommendations are based on clinical experience and evidence-based results from the general pediatric population. The reduction of traditional coronary artery risk factors for adults may benefit children with HIV since they are at risk for premature atherosclerosis. These include smoking, hypertension, elevated total and LDL cholesterol, low HDL cholesterol, diabetes, and advancing age [15]. Exercise and a healthy diet can decrease cardiovascular risk and also can stimulate the immune system. Good nutritional intake will prevent wasting syndrome and avoid nutritional deficiencies. Routine screening of the blood pressure, lipid panels, and a regular schedule for echocardiograms as other ways of early identification of cardiac problems in HIV patients were discussed previously in this chapter.

30.6 Abnormal left ventricular structure and function, cardiomyopathies, and myocarditis

Immunomodulatory therapy with intravenous immunoglobulin (IVIG) has shown significant promise for two specific sub-groups of pediatric HIV patients with cardiac problems [13]. Pediatric HIV patients without CHF showed less frequent echocardiographic abnormalities of LV structure and function with monthly doses of IVIG (2 g/kg/dose) (Figure 30.4) [13, 16]. HIV-infected children with myocarditis and CHF symptoms that are refractory to traditional anticongestive therapy can achieve resolution of the myocarditis with IVIG therapy [13, 16]. We would consider IVIG use in these situations, although future research is needed to better define more exact guidelines.

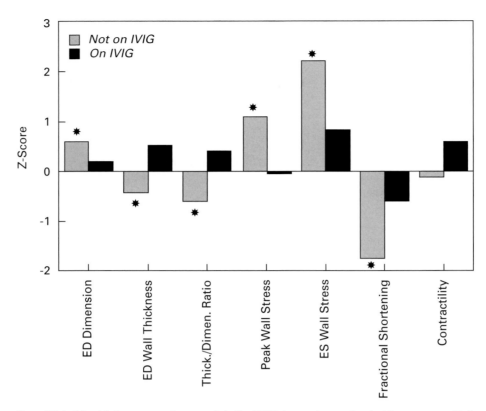

Figure 30.4. Monthly intravenous immunoglobulin (IVIG) therapy is associated with more normal left ventricular structure and function in HIV-infected patients without congestive heart failure. Echocardiographic measurements of left ventricular structure and function in HIV-infected patients without heart failure who received monthly IVIG therapy (black bars) and who did not receive IVIG therapy (shaded bars). Z-scores indicate number of standard deviations above or below normal (z-score = 0) for each parameter. Asterisks indicate that the parameter was significantly different from normal. ED, end-diastolic; ES, end-systolic; thick., left ventricular thickness; dimen., left ventricular dimension. (From ref [13].)

Experimental immunomodulatory therapy is currently being investigated in tumor necrosis factor antagonists and other cytokine modulators [13]. Anti-infective therapy aimed at eradicating co-infections with bacterial, viral, fungal, or other opportunistic agents may improve the symptoms of CHF.

Conventional heart failure therapy can improve the quality of life for many HIV-infected children with CHF. A multi-disciplinary approach including: nutrition, patient counseling, patient education, exercise training, and pharmacotherapy is the best approach to these complex patients [13, 17]. Polypharmacy therapy is used for heart failure and includes digoxin, loop diuretics, ACE inhibitors, aldosterone antagonists, and beta-blockers. Few data are available about the significance of these medications in pediatric HIV patients with heart failure and their use is directed by studies in adult populations.

30.7 Pericardial effusions

Pericardial effusions in HIV patients are usually asymptomatic and well tolerated from a cardiovascular standpoint. The treatment of underlying infections or malignancies that could be causing the pericarditis should be the first priority for the clinician. Highly active antiretroviral therapy (HAART) therapy for HIV infection may also need to be initiated. Effusions may resolve spontaneously in as many as 42% of HIV patients [12]. Traditional therapies such as diuretics and steroids should be used cautiously in this patient population. The steroids may cause further immunosuppression and the diuretics may rapidly reduce intravascular volume. The indications for pericardiocentesis are as follows: pericardial tamponade, diagnostic evaluation of the pericardial fluid, or persistent, poorly tolerated large effusions [12].

30.8 Endocarditis

HIV patients with endocarditis can be very difficult to treat. The causative agent should be identified and treated aggressively (usually with a minimum of 6 weeks of intravenous (IV) antibiotics). The initiation of HAART therapy may improve the patient's immunologic status. Patients should be followed with serial echocardiograms. In larger children or young adults, transesophageal echocardiography may be required to effectively view the heart valves. Early referral to both an infectious disease specialist and a pediatric cardiologist will help direct the treatment plan. Cardiothoracic surgical intervention is only indicated for severe valve dysfunction leading to intractable heart failure that is resistant to medical therapy.

30.9 Arrhythmias

Early referral to a pediatric cardiologist or electrophysiologist is crucial because of the vast array of different arrhythmias an HIV patient can develop. A baseline ECG should always be obtained by the primary provider in any patient with symptoms of arrhythmias or conduction disturbances. A thorough review of the patient's medications and their cardiac side effects should be completed. Any patient with a history of syncope should receive urgent attention.

30.10 Hypertension, lipid abnormalities, and premature atherosclerosis

The clinician caring for HIV-infected pediatric patients must remember that hypertension, lipid abnormalities, and premature atherosclerosis can occur in this population. As antiretroviral therapy improves, children will continue to increase their survival and therefore be susceptible to these traditional adult diseases. Routine office screening of blood pressure should occur at every clinic appointment. Serum lipid panels should be evaluated in all patients as a baseline and then regularly if protease inhibitors are started. Electron beam computed tomography has been able to detect coronary artery calcifications in pediatric patients with coronary artery injuries from Kawasaki disease and may be a useful screening tool for pediatric patients with advanced HIV disease [18]. Future research will need to better define the clinical utility of this technology in HIV patients. Detection of the abnormalities can lead to early initiation of antihypertensive medications or lipid lowering agents, which may improve overall morbidity in the future.

30.11 Referral to a pediatric cardiologist

Referral to a pediatric cardiologist should be considered based upon any of the following:
1. Findings on history:
   Any previous cardiac disease;
   Encephalopathy;
   Severe wasting and malnutrition; or
   Vague chest pain, malaise, fatigue, lethargy, weakness.
2. Findings on physical examination:
   Respiratory symptoms for greater than seven days that are not attributable to a pulmonary or infectious process;
   Signs and symptoms of CHF;
   Evidence of structural or congenital heart disease;
   Frequent arrhythmias or inappropriate tachycardias;
   Episodes of cyanosis, syncope, seizure;
   Pulmonary hypertension with recurrent bronchopulmonary infections; or
   Friction rub, hacking cough, pulsus paradoxicus, poor peripheral perfusion (consistent with pericardial effusion).
3. Findings by echocardiography:
   LV systolic dysfunction;
   LV hypertrophy; or
   Other echocardiographic abnormalities including: pericardial effusions, valvular heart disease, congenital heart disease, regional wall motion abnormalities, and intracardiac thrombi or masses.

30.12 Summary

Cardiovascular complications are common in pediatric HIV patients. Clinicians need to be aware of subtle and asymptomatic cardiac abnormalities such as LV dysfunction, LV hypertrophy, hypertension, and lipid abnormalities, which may be present many years prior to the presentation of overt clinical symptoms. Routine screening with blood pressure monitoring, lipid panels, and echocardiograms may provide early detection of many cardiac problems. In addition, clinicians must be aware of the cardiovascular signs and symptoms that can be obscured by other organ system failure in HIV patients. In the future, early detection and treatment of cardiac disease may prevent a significant amount of the associated morbidity and mortality [21].

REFERENCES

1. Lipshultz, S. E., Chanock, S., Sanders, S. P. *et al.* Cardiovascular manifestations of human immunodeficiency virus in infants and children. *Am. J. Cardiol.* **63** (1989), 1489–97.

2. Starc, T. J., Lipshultz, S. E., Kaplan, S. *et al.* Cardiac complications in children with human immunodeficiency virus infection. *Pediatrics* **104** : 2 (1999), e14.

3. Starc, T. J., Lipshultz, S. E., Easley, K. A. *et al.* Incidence of cardiac abnormalities in children with human immunodeficiency virus infection: the prospective P^2C^2 HIV study. *J. Pediatr.* **141**(3) (2002), 327–34.

4. Luginbuhl, L. M., Orav, E. J., McIntosh, K. & Lipshultz, S. E. Cardiac morbidity and related mortality in children with HIV infection. *J. Am. Med. Assoc.* **269** (1993), 1869–75.

5. Keesler, M. J., Fisher, S. D. & Lipshultz, S. E. Cardiac manifestations of HIV infection in infants and children. *Ann. N. Y. Acad. Sci.* **946** (2001), 169–78.

6. Moorthy, L. N. & Lipshultz, S. E. Cardiovascular monitoring of HIV-infected patients. In S. E. Lipshultz (ed.), *Cardiology in AIDS.* New York: Chapman and Hall (1998) pp. 345–84.

7. Lipshultz, S. E., Easley, K. A., Orav, E. J. *et al.* Cardiac dysfunction and mortality in HIV-infected children. The prospective P^2C^2 HIV multicenter study. *Circulation* **102** (2000), 1542–8.

8. Towbin, J. A. Cardiomyopathies. In J. H. Moller (ed.), *Pediatric Cardiovascular Medicine*, First edn. Philadelphia, PA: Churchill Livingstone (2000), pp. 753–65.

9. Barbaro, G. & Lipshultz, S. Pathogenesis of HIV-associated cardiomyopathy. *Ann. N. Y. Acad. Sci.* **946** (2001), 57–79.

10. Aretz, H. T. Myocarditis: the Dallas criteria. *Hum. Pathol.* **18** (1987), 619–24.

11. Kasten-Sportes, C. & Weinstein, C. Molecular mechanisms of HIV cardiovascular disease. In S. E. Lipshultz (ed.), *Cardiology in AIDS.* New York: Chapman & Hall (1998), pp. 265–82.

12. Barbaro, G., Fisher, S.D. & Lipshultz, S. E. Pathogenesis of HIV-associated cardiovascular complications. *Lancet Infect. Dis.* **1** (2001), 115–24.

13. Lipshultz, S. E., Fisher, S. D., Lai, W. W. & Miller, T. L. Cardiac risk factors, monitoring and therapy for HIV-infected patients. *AIDS* **17** (suppl. 1) (2003), S96–122.

14. Lipshultz, S. E., Rifai, N., Sallan, S. E. *et al.* Predictive value of cardiac troponin T in pediatric patients at risk for myocardial injury. *Circulation* **96** (1997), 2641–8.

15. Pearson, T. New tools for coronary risk assessment. *Circulation* **105** (2002), 886–92.

16. Lipshultz, S. E., Orav, E. J., Sanders, S. P. *et al.* Immunoglobulins and left ventricular structure and function in pediatric HIV infection. *Circulation* **92** (1995), 2220–5.

17. McKelvie, R. Heart failure. *Clin. Evid.* **4** (2000), 34–50.

18. Dadlani, G. H., Gingell, R. L., Orie, J. D. *et al.* Kawasaki patients with coronary artery calcifications detected by ultrafast CT scan: a pediatric population that may be at risk for early atherosclerosis. *Circulation* **104** (Suppl.) (2001), 516.

19. Langston, C., Cooper, E. R., Goldfarb, J. *et al.* HIV-related mortality in infants and children: data from the Pediatric Pulmonary and Cardiovascular Complications of Vertically Transmitted HIV Study. *Pediatrics* **107** : 2 (2001), 328–36.

20. Al-Attar, I., Orav, E. J., Exil, V. *et al.* Predictors of cardiac morbidity and related mortality in children with acquired immune deficiency syndrome. *Pediatr. Res* **37** (1995), 169A.

21. Al-Attar, I., Orav, E. J., Exil, V., Vlach, S. A. & Lipshultz, S. E. Predictors of cardiac morbidity and related mortality in children with acquired immunodeficiency system. *J. Am. Coll. Cardiol.* **41** (2003), 1598–605.

22. Lipshultz, S. E., Easley, K. A., Orav, E. J. *et al.* Cardiovascular status of infants and children of women infected with HIV-1 (P^2C^2 HIV): a cohort study. *Lancet* **360** (2002), 368–73.

Pulmonary problems

Lauren V. Wood, M.D.

HIV and AIDS Malignancy Branch, National Cancer Institute, Bethesda, MD

31.1 Introduction

Despite advances in the treatment of HIV disease and the implementation of highly active antiretroviral therapy (HAART) as the standard of care in resource-rich countries [1], pulmonary diseases continue to cause significant morbidity and mortality in HIV-infected pediatric patients [2, 3]. With the advent of HAART, the incidence of opportunistic infections has declined, although some evidence suggests children may be developing AIDS-defining conditions at higher CD4$^+$ T cell counts than previously [4]. Longitudinal studies have demonstrated that infection remains the most prevalent cause of death for children under 6 years of age, with 32% of deaths caused by pulmonary infection [5]. However, with increasing age, the frequency of HIV-associated pulmonary disease decreases significantly as the underlying cause of death. Common pulmonary diseases seen in pediatric HIV patients include: (1) lympho-proliferative processes that accompany HIV infection, such as lymphoid interstitial pneumonitis (LIP) or pulmonary lymphoid hyperplasia (PLH); (2) conventional infectious processes that may be exacerbated by the immunodeficiency caused by HIV infection; (3) opportunistic infections due to viral, bacterial, and fungal pathogens; and (4) disorders such as asthma/reactive airway disease, that may be associated with pulmonary infection or result from allergies or hypersensitivities which can be worsened by the immune dysregulation accompanying HIV infection.

Pneumocystis carinii pneumonia (PCP) remains the most common pulmonary complication of pediatric HIV infection in the USA [6, 7]. In contrast, pulmonary tuberculosis far exceeds recurrent bacterial infections or PCP as the primary clinical manifestation of pediatric HIV disease in countries where tuberculosis infection is endemic [8, 9]. Improvements in prophylaxis and in the clinical management of HIV disease have led to a substantial decrease in the incidence of PCP [10–12]. Lymphoid interstitial pneumonitis is the second most common pulmonary complication of pediatric HIV infection [7] and historically has been associated with improved survival in affected patients, including those in developing countries [13–15].

Recent advances in understanding the pathogenesis of LIP suggest that it is a cytokine-mediated process that is initiated and perpetuated by immune responses directed against HIV antigens and/or other pathogens such as Epstein–Barr virus (EBV) [16, 17]. Alveolar macrophages act as antigen-presenting cells (APCs) and secrete a variety of pro-inflammatory cytokines including interleukin 1 (IL-1), IL-6, IL-8, IL-15, interferon gamma (IFN-γ), tumor necrosis factor alpha (TNF-α), granulocyte-macrophage colony-stimulating factor (GM-CSF), and macrophage inflammatory protein 1alpha (MIP-1α) [16]. Cytokine recruitment of CD8$^+$ cytotoxic memory T cells (CTLs) results in a virus-specific CTL-mediated immune response that is hypothesized to directly damage the lung and lead to the development of LIP [16, 18]. Further support for the central involvement of cytokines in the pathogenesis of LIP is underscored by recent examination of cytokine and chemokine expression in LIP tissue from HIV-infected pediatric patients demonstrating increased expression of IL-18 and the chemokines RANTES (regulated upon activation, normal T expressed and secreted), MIP1-α and -β, compared with normal lung biopsies from HIV-uninfected controls [19].

Pediatric HIV patients may develop a variety of harmful immune-related pulmonary conditions. These may include a T cell alveolitis due to CD8$^+$ CTLs with both HIV-specific and NK-like cytotoxic activities, an accumulation of activated alveolar macrophages, local hyperproduction of macrophage-derived cytokines, pulmonary neutrophilia in patients with opportunistic infections, and the loss of NK and HIV-specific CTL activities [16, 20]. These conditions impair host responses to pulmonary pathogens, lead to the release of proinflammatory cytokines, and worsen gas exchange, producing a decline in pulmonary function.

The lung contains many cells (e.g. CD4$^+$ T lymphocytes and macrophages) that can be infected by HIV and significant levels of HIV replication may occur in the lung [21]. HIV replication in these cells may result in damage to the lung directly or indirectly through the release of inflammatory mediators by infected cells [18].

31.2 Common respiratory problems

Pediatric HIV patients may present with a variety of relatively non-specific respiratory symptoms, including cough, dyspnea, sputum production, and/or wheezing. These symptoms may result from both pulmonary and non-pulmonary causes. Respiratory symptoms in an HIV-infected child may result from unusual opportunistic infections, lymphoproliferative disorders, immune-mediated conditions, or from processes commonly seen in children without HIV infection. Such common causes of respiratory symptoms may include upper respiratory infections, reactive airway disease, bronchitis, sinusitis, and bacterial pneumonias [22]. Practitioners evaluating pediatric HIV patients with respiratory complaints should consider both the unusual processes associated with HIV infection and the more common disorders prevalent in the general population.

Other primary disease processes may produce respiratory symptoms. Cardiac disease can cause respiratory symptoms, particularly tachypnea, dyspnea, and/or wheezing, with bilateral crepitant rales on auscultation, and bilateral increased interstitial markings and small pleural or lingular effusions on chest radiographs. Pulmonary malignancies may result in respiratory complaints. They include non-Hodgkin's lymphomas, tumors of smooth muscle origin, or mucosa-associated lymphoid tissue (MALT) lesions, and Kaposi's sarcoma, a rare problem in children. Malignancies can present as hilar adenopathy, isolated parenchymal nodules, mediastinal masses or less commonly, diffuse interstitial disease, although they are often incidental findings on routine chest radiographs. Foreign body aspiration is a classic cause of difficult-to-diagnose respiratory distress in children.

Metabolic derangements, particularly systemic acidosis as a consequence of diarrhea and dehydration, can produce hyperventilation characterized by deep, rapid respirations (Kussmaul breathing) as a result of efforts at respiratory compensation.

31.2.1 Lymphoid interstitial pneumonitis

Lymphoid (or lymphocytic) interstitial pneumonitis is the most common lymphoproliferative, non-infectious pulmonary disorder seen among HIV-infected children and its description pre-dated the AIDS era [23]. It occurs in the absence of a detectable opportunistic infection or neoplasm and is characterized histologically by diffuse infiltration with mature, predominately CD8$^+$ T lymphocytes, plasma cells and histiocytes in the alveolar septa and along the lymphatic vessels [24, 25]. Lymphoid interstitial pneumonia is very common in pediatric HIV infection [7, 26] and has been found in up to 30–40% of HIV-infected infants and children with pulmonary disease [13, 27]. Lymphoid interstitial pneumonitis describes a spectrum of disorders that involve pulmonary lymphocytic infiltrates of interstitial lung parenchyma (LIP) and hyperplasia of bronchus-associated lymphoid tissue and the surrounding alveolar spaces or stroma, termed pulmonary lymphoid hyperplasia (PLH) [28]. While the distinction between LIP and PLH is clear histologically, the disorders are indistinguishable clinically, and most clinicians refer to the disorders interchangeably. In the 1994 Revised Classification System for Human Immunodeficiency Virus Infection in Children, LIP is classified as a Category B condition, attributed to and indicative of an HIV-related immunologic deficit [29]. Lymphoid interstitial pneumonitis has been reported in HIV-infected adults [30–32] at a much lower rate than in children, often as part of the diffuse infiltrative lymphocytosis syndrome [33]; it also occurs in HIV-uninfected children and adults as part of the spectrum of interstitial lung disease (ILD), but is uncommon and when present, is associated with autoimmune disorders.

In LIP, as in other forms of ILD, inflammatory cells are recruited into the pulmonary interstitium, alveolar wall, and perialveolar tissues, producing an alveolitis. This may be accompanied by fibroblast proliferation, resulting in interstitial fibrosis with progression to "honeycomb" lung and respiratory failure [34]. The exact etiology of LIP in HIV-infected individuals remains unknown, but appears to involve a multifactorial process, including the direct effects of HIV gene products [35], cytokine hyperproduction, and host responses to HIV and other pathogens. Cytokines from alveolar macrophages may produce localized immune dysregulation, primary lung damage, and clinical disease

[17, 36]. Epstein–Barr virus (EBV) is often found in the lungs of children with LIP and AIDS [37] and an unusually large number of children with LIP have evidence of infection with EBV [31, 38], suggesting a possible role in pathogenesis. Recent studies have investigated the relative contributions of known adhesion pathways in mediating lymphocyte adherence to endothelium and the potential role of human herpesviruses such as EBV in these lesions [39]. Lymphoid interstitial pneumonitis was characterized by infiltration of the pulmonary interstitium with CD8$^+$ T lymphocytes. In some individuals, expansion of the alveolar septae with dense aggregates of B lymphocytes was seen, many of which contained the EBV genome. High levels of vascular cell adhesion molecule-1 (VCAM-1) protein expression were found in venular endothelium from the lungs of children with LIP, but not uninflamed lung from other children with AIDS or lungs from children with non-specific pneumonitis. In addition, CD8$^+$ T cell clones that express very late activation antigen-4 (VLA-4), the leukocyte ligand for VCAM-1, were shown to bind preferentially to pulmonary vessels expressing high levels of VCAM-1 in sites of LIP. Hence interstitial infiltration was highly correlated with VCAM-1/VLA-4 adhesive interactions as well as focal expansion of B cells co-infected with EBV.

The clinical manifestations of LIP can range from asymptomatic disease with isolated radiographic abnormalities to severe bullous lung disease with pulmonary insufficiency. Children with symptomatic LIP often present during the second or third year of life with the insidious onset of mild cough, fatigue, dyspnea, and tachypnea. These respiratory symptoms are associated with generalized lymphadenopathy, hepatosplenomegaly, parotid gland enlargement (parotitis), and lymphocytosis [40, 41]. The chest physical examination is usually normal. Wheezing, oxygen desaturation with cyanosis, and digital clubbing may also be present in more advanced stages of disease [34]. Chest radiographs show fine, bilateral reticulonodular or alveolar infiltrates that are more prominent in the lower lobes (Figure 31.1), but may have no abnormalities other than hyperinflation. When present, these reticulonodular infiltrates are often difficult to differentiate from other infectious pneumonias due to *Candida* spp., CMV, and *Mycobacterium* spp. Chest computed tomography (CT) confirms the interstitial pattern observed on x-ray and is useful for monitoring the severity and extent of disease (Fig 31.2). Gallium scans may reveal a pattern of diffuse pulmonary uptake indistinguishable from that seen with *Pneumocystis carinii* pneumonia (PCP) [42], but concurrent PCP infection occurs infrequently. Patients with LIP can have significant

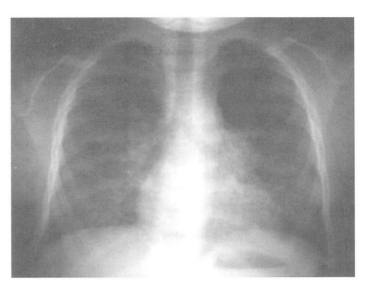

Figure 31.1. Posterior – anterior chest radiograph lymphoid interstitial pneumonitis: Bilateral, diffuse reticulonodular interstitial infiltrates associated with severe LIP.

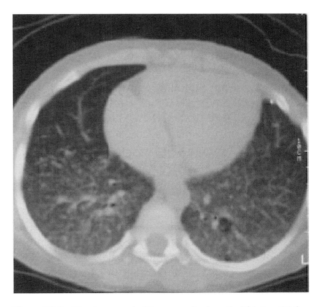

Figure 31.2. Chest computed tomography lymphoid interstitial pneumonitis: Chest CT correlation of radiographic findings in Figure 31.1

pulmonary dysfunction with decreased oxygen saturation at rest or with exercise, a decrease in diffusing capacity, and an increased alveolar-arterial oxygen gradient. Although diagnostic, clinical, radiographic, and laboratory studies may suggest the diagnosis of LIP, only lung biopsy can establish a definitive diagnosis [43]. Biopsy specimens reveal an interstitial infiltrate composed primarily of lymphocytes, with collections of lymphoid aggregates surrounding the airways [44]. However, pulmonary biopsy is now rarely used to confirm the diagnosis, unlike early in the pediatric HIV epidemic. Hence the diagnosis is usually a presumptive one based on clinical criteria supported by radiographic lung findings.

The clinical course of LIP in children is highly variable but generally benign. Historically, HIV-infected children with LIP appeared to have a more indolent course of HIV disease and prolonged survival [13–15]. Lymphoid interstitial pneumonitis can resolve spontaneously, worsen episodically, or worsen slowly and progressively with intercurrent pulmonary infections and bronchiectasis resulting in intermittent pulmonary decompensation or hypoxic respiratory failure [32, 45]. A retrospective study from the National Cancer Institute evaluated the natural history of LIP in 22 HIV-infected children with biopsy-proven LIP for a median period of 4 years (range 0.5–10) [46]. Lymphoid interstitial pneumonitis-related clinical and radiological manifestations as well as abnormal pulmonary function studies resolved or significantly improved over time independent of LIP disease severity or HIV disease status and LIP was not a cause of mortality in the study. Radiographic sequelae included bronchiectasis, emphysema, and bulla formation in a small number of patients.

Broad anecdotal clinical experience indicates that LIP-PLH responds to systemic corticosteroids [47], but no controlled studies have been performed to assess their efficacy in LIP. Bronchodilators and intermittent corticosteroid bursts are currently used for mild to moderately symptomatic LIP (e.g. intermittent cough or wheezing). Treatment with steroids is usually reserved for patients with significant hypoxemia and symptoms of pulmonary insufficiency, including tachypnea, dyspnea on exertion, or exercise intolerance. More severe symptoms may require prolonged corticosteroid therapy. A typical regimen uses 2 mg/kg/day of prednisone administered for 2–4 weeks with subsequent tapering to 1 mg/kg/day titrated to the lowest possible dose that results in control of clinical symptoms and resolution of hypoxemia with normalization of oxygen saturation [48]. Once an adequate response has been documented, steroids should be weaned and discontinued. Most children respond promptly within the first few weeks of treatment, although some with severe, advanced lung disease may be refractory to therapy. Steroids should be discontinued if no response is seen after 4–6 months of therapy [10, 48]. Successful clinical treatment is often associated with an improvement in radiographic abnormalities (Fig 31.3).

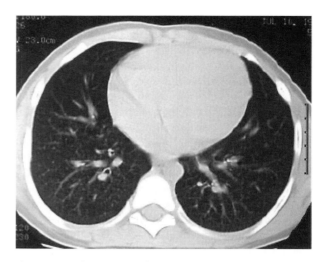

Figure 31.3. Chest computed tomography lymphoid interstitial pneumonitis following treatment with steroids: resolution of LIP interstitial infiltrates in same patient as Figure 31.2 following steroid administration.

31.2.2 Infectious pneumonias

Recurrent invasive bacterial infections

Serious bacterial infections are common in HIV-infected children and are responsible for a substantial degree of the morbidity associated with pediatric HIV disease. Recurrent bacterial pneumonias are a Category C severe manifestation of HIV disease in the CDC classification system [29]. HIV infection is characterized by a state of polyclonal B cell activation, which results in elevated, but functionally ineffective serum immunoglobulins [49, 50]. The bacterial pathogens that cause invasive disease in HIV-infected children are often identical to those seen in immunocompetent pediatric patients, although HIV-infected patients are especially susceptible to infections with the encapsulated bacteria *Streptococcus pneumoniae* and *Haemophilus influenzae* type b [51] (see Chapter 37). While the use of prophylactic vaccines against *H. influenzae* type b has dramatically reduced the incidence of disease caused by this bacterial pathogen, newer conjugated pneumococcal vaccines hold similar promise to decrease the incidence of pneumococcal disease in children of the serotypes present in the vaccine.

Bacterial pneumonia can occur at any time during the course of HIV infection and at any CD4$^+$ lymphocyte count, but the rate of bacterial pneumonia increases with increasing immunosuppression [52]. Pneumococcus remains the most common organism recovered from the blood and causative agent of lobar bacterial pneumonia. A study of *S. pneumoniae* colonization rates revealed that colonization among HIV-infected and indeterminate children was equal to that of controls and was not affected by CDC classification or receipt of oral antibiotic therapy [53]. Importantly, high rates of trimethoprim-sulfamethoxazole (TMP-SMX) antibiotic prophylaxis in HIV-infected children in this study were *not* associated with increased pneumococcal resistance. In contrast, a study of lower respiratory tract infections in HIV-infected children in South Africa documented methicillin and trimethoprim-sulfamethoxazole resistance in 60% of *S. aureus* and 86% of *E. coli* isolates, respectively [54]. Importantly, in this cohort, diagnostic isolates of *Mycobacterium tuberculosis* were as common as *S. pneumoniae*, followed by *H. influenzae* type b, *S. aureus* and *E. coli*. Both the conjugate pneumococcal vaccine (PCV-7) and the pneumococcal polysaccharide vaccine (PPV-23) are routinely recommended for prophylaxis against invasive pneumococcal disease [55]. HIV-infected children often do respond to the immunizations with the production of effective, protective antibodies (see Chapter 3).

Other bacterial pathogens associated with pneumonia include *Streptococcus pyogenes* and *Staphylococcus aureus*, although pneumonia caused by *Pseudomonas aeruginosa* and other Gram-negative organisms appears to be increasing in frequency, particularly in patients with chronic lung disease [48, 52]. Recurrent bacterial pneumonia can result in acute or chronic alterations in pulmonary architecture, including bullous lung disease and bronchiectasis, predisposing patients to lower-airway colonization and recurrent infectious exacerbations (Figure 31.4–31.7). The symptoms of bacterial pneumonia in children are usually non-specific and include high fever, cough, and respiratory distress, with or without mild hypoxemia and/or wheezing. In patients with underlying LIP/PLH, superimposed bacterial pneumonia may significantly worsen the respiratory status. Chest radiographs usually show focal infiltrates or consolidation. Because sputum is extremely difficult to obtain in very young children and non-invasive diagnostic procedures yields an organism in only 30% of cases [48], initial treatment is often empiric. However, if obtainable, an induced sputum should be examined for PCP as well as cultured for routine bacterial, fungal, and mycobacterial pathogens. Broad-spectrum antibiotics such as ticarcillin-clavulanic acid effective against β-lactamase-producing pathogens should be the initial choice. The addition of aminoglycosides should be considered in patients with severe immunocompromise, a history of neutropenia or those infected with resistant Gram-negative bacteria. Bronchoscopic evaluation may be necessary to obtain adequate culture material, especially with severe or rapidly progressive disease.

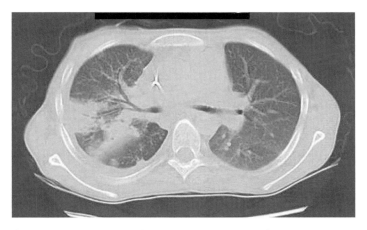

Figure 31.4. Chest computed tomography lobar consolidation and bullous lung disease associated with recurrent bacterial pneumonia due to *Pseudomonas aeruginosa* and *Serratia marcsens*. Day 1: Dense focal lobar consolidation with air bronchogram formation at presentation.

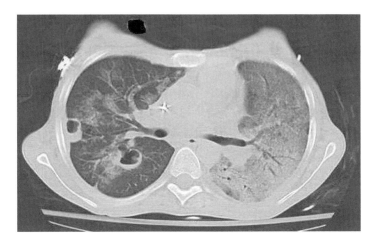

Figure 31.5. Week 1: Progression with extensive infiltrates and cavitary lesions with air fluid levels and cystic bronchiectasis.

Mycobacterial pneumonias

Other pathogens must be considered in the differential diagnosis of any HIV-infected child suspected of having bacterial pneumonia. *Mycobacterium tuberculosis* infection is of particular concern because of its communicability, the emergence of multi-drug resistant organisms and the difficulty in identifying at-risk patients due to their compromised ability to react to PPD-tuberculin skin testing [56]. *Mycobacterium tuberculosis* infection is discussed in more detail in Chapter 38. Despite tremendous advances in the field of antimicrobial therapy, the global burden of tuberculosis (TB) remains enormous, with an estimated global prevalence of 32% or 1.86 billion people [57]. The

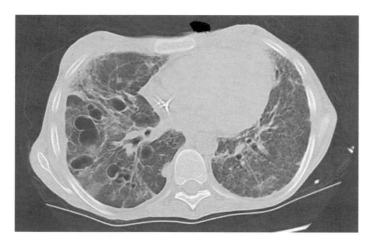

Figure 31.6. Week 2: Persistent infiltrates with multiple cavitary lesions and pleural thickening.

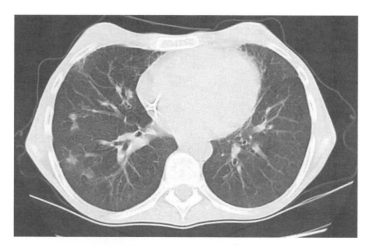

Figure 31.7. Week 6: Almost complete resolution of infiltrates and cavitary lesions status post 6 weeks IV antibiotic treatment.

combined TB and HIV epidemics present a major public health threat as each disease has a negative effect on the other, and mortality in dually infected patients is higher than that associated with either condition alone. Many HIV-infected persons in Africa are also co-infected with TB (32% of TB cases are infected with HIV). Although great variation exists in the co-infection rate among African countries (14–65%), more co-infected individuals reside in India [57, 58]. More importantly, many patients in both resource-rich and resource-poor countries are diagnosed with HIV infection only after presenting with tuberculosis. The primary source of tuberculosis infection in children is almost universally an adult in close contact in the environment,

usually in the household, who has infectious pulmonary TB [10]. Since TB may be the initial manifestation of HIV-associated illness, HIV-infected children with pulmonary illness should be tested for TB, and all children with TB should be tested for HIV.

In general, HIV-infected children with TB tend to have lower $CD4^+$ counts, greater disease severity, more rapid progression, an increased tendency for extrapulmonary or disseminated disease, and a higher mortality rate [59–61]. In areas where TB is endemic, such as India, tuberculosis has been reported in up to 67.5% of pediatric patients with symptomatic HIV infection [9]. Clinical manifestations may vary (see Chapter 38), but fever, cough and lack of weight gain are common. The diagnosis of TB is established based on epidemiologic, clinical, immunologic (the tuberculin skin test) and radiographic criteria, with or without microbiologic confirmation. Because of concerns of drug resistance, efforts should always be made to obtain microbiologic isolates of *M. tuberculosis*. Ideal culture specimens in young children include early morning gastric aspirates, while pulmonary specimens may be more readily obtainable in older children. Tuberculin skin testing should be performed in any child suspected of having TB although pediatric HIV-infected patients are frequently anergic [9, 61]. Although concerns about the development of disseminated disease exists, vaccination with bacilli Calmette–Guerin (BCG) is recommended for asymptomatic HIV-infected children in regions with a high prevalence of tuberculosis. Fortunately, bacteremia due to BCG, *M. tuberculosis*, and *M. bovis* is rare, even among children with recent BCG immunization and symptomatic HIV infection [62]. Children who are suspected of having tuberculosis should be treated promptly and preferably with directly observed therapy. When initiating antituberculosis therapy attention must be given to potential toxicities and drug interactions with antiretroviral drugs.

Infection with nontuberculous mycobacteria, commonly referred to as *Mycobacterium avium* complex (MAC) which includes *M. avium*, *M. intracellulare*, *M. paratuberculosis*, *M. lepremurium*, and *M. scrofulaceum*, results in systemic infection associated with severe immunosuppression and late stage disease. Respiratory symptoms are uncommon in children with systemic MAC infection and isolated pulmonary disease is rare, although the organism may be detected in broncheoalveolar (BAL) fluid [44]. Treatment requires combination therapy with a minimum of 2 or 3 drugs and hence clinical efforts should be directed towards primary prophylaxis against disseminated disease with clarithromycin or azithromycin (Table 31.1). Disease due to MAC is discussed in more detail in Chapter 39.

Table 31.1 Prophylaxis for pulmonary infections in HIV-infected children

Pathogen/indication	First choice	Alternatives
Pneumocystis carinii	TMP-SMX 150/750 mg/m^2/day PO bid 3 days/week on consecutive days	Dapsone (children $\geq$ 1 month of age):
Primary prophylaxis		2 mg/kg (max 100 mg) po qd
All infants aged 1–12 mos, irrespective of HIV status; 1–5 years CD4$^+$ count < 500 μl or 15%; 6–12 years CD4$^+$ count < 200 μl or 15%.	Acceptable alternative dosage schedules: Single dose po 3 days/wk on consecutive days	4 mg/kg (max 200 mg) po q wk Aerosolized pentamidine ($\geq$ 5 years of age): 300 mg q months via Respirgard Nebulizer
Secondary prophylaxis		Atovaquone:
After prior episode PCP	BID dosing qd or 3 days/week on alternate days	Age 1–3 months, >24 months: 30 mg/kg po qd. Age 4–24 months: 45 mg/kg po qd
Mycobacteriumtuberculosis		
Isoniazid sensitive	Isoniazid 10–15 mg/kg (max 300 mg) po qd × 9 months or 20–30 mg/kg (max 900 mg) po 2 days/wk × 9 months	Rifampin 10–20 mg/kg (max 600 mg) po qd × 4–6 months
PPD reaction $\geq$ 5 mm or prior positive result without treatment; or contact with any case of active TB regardless of PPD result		
Isoniazid resistant		
Same as above; high probability of exposure to isoniazid-resistant TB	Rifampin 10–20 mg/kg (max 600 mg) po qd × 4–6 months	Uncertain
Multi-drug (isoniazid/rifampin) resistant		
Same as above; high probability of exposure to multi-drug resistant TB	Choice of drugs requires consultation with public health authorities and susceptibility of isolate from patient	
Mycobacterium avium complex (MAC)		
Primary prophylaxis		
< 1 year CD4$^+$ count < 750 μl; 1–2 years CD4$^+$ count < 500 μl; 2–6 years CD4$^+$ count < 75 μl; $\geq$ 6 years CD4$^+$ count < 50 μl	Clarithromycin 7.5 mg/kg (max 500 mg) po bid or azithromycin 20 mg/kg (max 1200 mg) po q week.	Azithromycin 5 mg/kg (max 250 mg) po qd; children $\geq$ 6 years, rifabutin, 300 mg po qd
Secondary prophylaxis		
After prior disseminated MAC disease	Clarithromycin 7.5 mg/kg (max 500 mg) po BID *plus* ethambutol 15 mg/kg (max 900 mg) po qd; with or without rifabutin 5 mg/kg (max 300 mg) po qd	Azithromycin 5 mg/kg (max 250 mg) po qd *plus* ethambutol 15 mg/kg (max 900 mg) po qd; with or without rifabutin 5 mg/kg (max 300 mg)) po qd
Recurrent invasive bacterial infections	TMP-SMX 150/750 mg/m^2/day po bid qd	Antibiotic chemoprophylaxis with another active agent
> 2 serious infections in 1 year period	IVIG 400 mg/kg IV q 2–4 weeks	

Adapted from USPHS/IDSA Guidelines for the Prevention of Opportunistic Infections, November 2001.

Viral and fungal pneumonias

The same viruses that cause lower respiratory tract infection in immunocompetent children also infect children with HIV infection. They include respiratory syncytial virus (RSV), parainfluenza viruses, influenza A and B, and adenovirus. These viruses may cause a primary pneumonia or worsen pulmonary pathology in the setting of a concurrent opportunistic infection or bacterial pneumonia. Infection is characterized by severe disease, potential systemic involvement and prolonged viral excretion [45]. Culture of nasopharyngeal, sputum, or BAL specimens for respiratory viruses should be performed in children with persistent or significant symptoms of upper or lower respiratory tract infection, particularly during known seasonal peaks of viral disease. All patients should receive inactivated split trivalent influenza vaccine annually before influenza season starts [55]. FluMist, a trivalent, cold-adapted, live-attenuated influenza vaccine, is administered intranasally. It is effective in preventing influenza virus infection and is approved by the US Food and Drug Administration for healthy patients 5–49 years of age. It should not be given to patients with known or suspected immunodeficiency, including HIV infection [63]. Chronic interstitial pneumonitis due to cytomegalovirus (CMV) as a result of acute infection or reactivation, or varicella pneumonitis associated with disseminated infection, are both uncommon in the pediatric population. Even when isolated from pulmonary secretions or tissue specimens, CMV's role as a pathogen remains difficult to assess unless there is direct evidence of CMV inclusions on histopathologic examination. Infections due to herpesviruses, including CMV, are described in more detail in Chapter 41.

Pulmonary mycoses are increasingly encountered in children with HIV infection as a consequence of severe immunodeficiency, although the exact incidence of fungal pneumonia is unknown [64]. Histoplasmosis, cryptococcosis, and coccidioidomycosis may all present with pulmonary involvement and are frequently characterized by progressive pneumonia and disseminated infection. In contrast, some fungal pathogens such as aspergillus, typically present with locally invasive pulmonary and sinus disease (Fig. 31.8) and present extremely challenging management problems [65] (see Chapter 40 for a more extensive discussion of fungal pneumonias).

Diagnostic approach to evaluation of pneumonias

HIV-infected pediatric patients presenting with suspected pneumonia represent a diagnostic challenge. Adequate diagnostic specimens must be rapidly procured and blood cultures should always be obtained. The choice of antimicrobial agent should be based on the sputum Gram stain

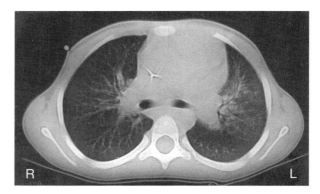

Figure 31.8. Chest computed tomography invasive pulmonary aspergillosis due to *A. fumigatus*: prominent left perihilar interstitial infiltrate with early parenchymal consolidation

and stains for acid-fast bacilli, and the clinical presentation. The treatment of bacterial pneumonia is discussed more extensively in Chapter 37. If the clinician suspects that fungal or viral pathogens may be the etiologic agent for the pneumonia, the evaluation may require broncheoalveolar lavage or an open thorascopic lung biopsy to differentiate simple colonization from invasive disease. This procedure should be considered promptly if disease is severe, progression is rapid, and the response to antibacterial therapy is not good. In patients with recurrent bacterial pneumonias and other recurrent serious bacterial infections, prophylaxis with daily TMP–SMX should be initiated in those who can tolerate it. In a much more costly approach, monthly infusions of intravenous immunoglobulin (IVIG) may be administered at a dose of 400 mg/kg if oral antibiotic prophylaxis fails to reduce the frequency of infections [66]. Shorter dosing intervals can be considered in those individuals determined to have hypogammaglobulinemia.

31.2.3 Chronic cough

Many abnormalities of large and small airways, as well as pulmonary parenchymal disease, can produce chronic cough [67]. Common etiologies in patients without evidence of a specific pulmonary disease include asthma, allergic rhinitis, chronic sinusitis, chronic bronchitis, and gastroesophageal reflux. Cough that occurs at night, after crying spells, intense play, or during exercise is suggestive of asthma [67]. Children with chronic cough who are older than 6 years should have pulmonary function testing, including an assessment of reversibility with bronchodilators, if the history is suggestive of reactive airway disease.

Chronic sinusitis is a source of significant morbidity in HIV disease and aggressive, empiric antibiotic therapy for this condition often results in a dramatic reduction in or complete resolution of cough. CT examination of the sinuses should be performed to determine the extent of disease and response to therapy, particularly in individuals with recurrent episodes.

In younger infants with chronic cough or children with radiographic patterns suggestive of recurrent aspiration pneumonia, significant gastroesophageal reflux (GER) can usually be documented by barium swallow or more definitively by pH probe testing. For patients diagnosed with GER, pharmacologic management should be judicious as many of the drugs used to treat this condition are contraindicated in patients receiving certain antiretroviral agents, particularly protease inhibitors. Rare causes of wheezing on forced exhalation or a seal-like, croupy cough include tracheomalacia or a vascular ring. Young children can also wheeze due to foreign body aspiration.

31.2.4 Asthma/reactive airway disease

Asthma or reactive airway disease (RAD) is a pattern of intermittent recurrent wheezing, dyspnea, dry cough, or chest tightness, precipitated by triggers such as allergens, exercise, or infection [68]. It is often associated with other atopic disorders, such as allergic rhinitis, atopic dermatitis, and food allergy. Patterns of reactivity can be divided into two distinct groups: intermittent and persistent asthma. Many of the basic mechanisms underlying the development of the disease remain unknown. While children commonly wheeze during upper respiratory tract infections, many do not subsequently develop asthma [69]. Elevated total serum IgE levels appear to be linked closely to airway hyper-responsiveness, even in children who have been asymptomatic throughout their lives and have no history of atopic disease [70]. Elevated IgE levels have been reported in individuals with HIV infection, are associated with advanced disease and predictive of worsening immunosuppression [71]. Whether these elevations are associated with an increased incidence of allergic manifestations in HIV-infected persons has not been reported. The incidence of asthma is increasing in the general population, but the incidence in individuals with HIV infection remains unknown.

Asthma can share a similar presentation with other problems commonly seen in HIV patients such as LIP, PCP, chronic bronchitis, and bacterial pneumonia. Wheezing associated with a dry, non-productive cough, without fever may suggest asthma as opposed to a respiratory infection. Infections can exacerbate pre-existing asthma and may be associated with acute wheezing and post-infectious bronchial hyper-responsiveness [52]. Aerosolized pentamidine for PCP prophylaxis is frequently associated with

bronchospasm. Pretreatment with bronchodilators is usually successful in minimizing symptoms; discontinuation of therapy is rarely necessary.

Therapy for wheezing should be tailored to the severity of the episode and frequency of recurrences [72, 73]. Medication delivery devices such as spacers and holding chambers, should be selected according to the child's ability to use them. The goals of asthma therapy are: to minimize chronic symptoms, exacerbations, the use of short-acting inhaled beta$_2$-agonists, and adverse effects from medications; to eliminate limitations on activities of daily living (e.g. missed school), and to maintain normal pulmonary function [73]. Treatment guidelines for mild intermittent and mild, moderate, and severe persistent asthma are outlined in Table 31.2. A stepwise approach is taken to managing asthma, and anti-inflammatory control, with inhaled corticosteroids as the cornerstone of therapy. Pediatric doses of commonly used medications are summarized in Tables 31.3 and 31.4. Infrequent episodic asthma associated only with cough and audible wheezing, may be treated alone with intermittent, short-acting, β$_2$-agonist bronchodilators such as albuterol, using a metered dose inhaler or a nebulizer. Administration of oral β$_2$-agonists (albuterol 0.1 mg/kg/dose given tid–qid) can be considered in younger infants and children for whom aerosol therapy is difficult. Low-dose inhaled corticosteroids are the preferred treatment for mild persistent asthma, although inhaled cromolyn or a leukotriene receptor antagonist such as monteleukast, are clinically acceptable alternatives and may be preferable in patients predisposed to oral thrush. Moderate persistent exacerbations associated with tachypnea, use of accessory muscles or significant dyspnea in addition to wheezing should be treated with low-dose inhaled corticosteroids and long-acting inhaled beta$_2$-agonists or medium-dose inhaled corticosteroids. Alternative treatment can include low-dose inhaled corticosteroids in combination with either a leukotriene receptor antagonist or theophylline. Monitoring of serum drug levels is critical to the safe and successful use of theophylline in asthma management. Severe persistent symptoms require high-dose inhaled corticosteroids, long-acting inhaled beta$_2$-agonists and if needed, oral corticosteroid tablets or syrup long term. Repeated attempts should be made to reduce systemic corticosteroids and maintain control of symptoms with high-dosed inhaled corticosteroids whenever possible.

Every patient with new wheezing, wheezing with a fever, or significant immunocompromise should have a chest x-ray to rule out concurrent pulmonary infection. Further radiographic and diagnostic studies such as chest CT or pulmonary function tests (PFTs) may be warranted if there

Table 31.2 Management of asthma in infants and children

Asthma severity	Symptoms Day / Symptoms Night	Medications required to maintain long-term control	
		5 years of age and younger	Older than 5 years of age
Quick relief All patients		Short-acting inhaled beta$_2$-agonists by nebulizer or face mask and space/holding chamber OR oral beta$_2$-agonist	2–4 puffs short-acting inhaled beta$_2$-agonists as needed for symptoms
Mild Intermittent	≤ 2 days/week / ≤ 2 nights/month	No daily medication needed	No daily medication needed. Severe exacerbations may occur, separated by periods of normal lung function and no symptoms. A course of systemic steroids is recommended.
Mild persistent	> 2/week but < 1 × /day / > 2 night/month	Preferred treatment: Low-dose inhaled corticosteroids (with nebulizer or MDI with holding chamber with or without face mask or DPI) Alternative treatment: Cromolyn (nebulizer preferred or MDI with holding chamber) OR leukotriene receptor antagonist	Preferred treatment: Low-dose inhaled corticosteroids Alternative Treatment: Cromolyn, leukotriene modifier, nedocromil, OR sustained release theophylline to serum concentrations of 5–15 mcg/mL
Moderate persistent	Daily / > 1 night/week	Preferred treatment: Low-dose inhaled corticosteroids and long-acting beta$_2$-agonists OR medium-dose inhaled corticosteroids Alternative treatment: Low-dose inhaled corticosteroids and either leukotriene receptor antagonist or theophylline	Preferred treatment: Low-to-medium dose inhaled corticosteroids and long-acting inhaled beta$_2$-agonists Alternative treatment: Increase inhaled corticosteroids within medium-dosage range OR Low-to medium dose inhaled corticosteroids and either leukotriene modifer or theophylline
Severe persistent	Continual / Frequent	Preferred treatment: High-dose inhaled corticosteroids AND long-acting inhaled beta$_2$-agonists AND if needed, corticosteroid tablets or syrup long term	Preferred treatment: High-dose inhaled corticosteroids AND long-acting inhaled beta$_2$-agonists AND if needed, corticosteroid tablets or syrup long term

Adapted from NAEPP Expert Panel Report July 2002 (NIH Publication No. 02-5075). MDI, metered dose inhaler.

Table 31.3 Pediatric dosages for long-term asthma control medications

Medication	Dosage form	Dose in children ($\leq$ 12 years of age)
Long-acting inhaled beta$_2$-agonists		
Salmeterol	MDI 121 mcg/puff	1–2 puffs q 12 h
Formoterol	DPI 50 mcg/blister	1 blister q 12 h
	DPI 12 mcg/single-use capsule	1 capsule q 12 h
Combined medication		
Flucatisone/Salmeterol	DPI 100, 250, or 500 mcg/50mcg	1 inhalation BID; dose depends on severity of asthma
Cromolyn and nedocromil		
Cromolyn	MDI 1 mg/puff	1–2 puffs TID – QID
Nedocromil	Nebulizer 20 mg/ampule	1 ampule TID – QID
	MDI 1.75 mg/puff	1–2 puffs BID – QID
Leukotriene modifiers		
Monteleukast	4 or 5 mg chewable tablet	4 mg qhs (2–5 years)
	10 mg tablet	5 mg qhs (6–14 years)
	10 or 20 mg tablet	10 mg qhs (> 14 years)
Zafirlukast		20 mg daily (7–11 years)
		(10 mg tablet bid)
Methylxanthines		
Theophylline* *Serum monitoring is critical; target concentration of 5–15 mcg/mL @ steady state	Liquids, sustained-release tablets, and capsules	Starting dose 10 mg/kg/day; usual max: < 1 year: 0.2 (age in weeks) + 5 = mg/kg/day $\geq$ 1 year: 16 mg/kg/day
Systemic corticosteroids		
Methylprednisolone	2, 4, 8,16, 32 mg tablets 5 mg tablets,	Applies to all three corticosteroids: 0.25–2 mg/kg daily in a single dose in a.m. or qod as needed for control.
Prednisolone	5 mg/5 cc, 15 mg/5 cc	
	1, 2.5, 5, 10, 20, 50 mg tablets;	Short-course "burst": 1–2 mg/kg/day,
Prednisone	5 mg/5 cc	maximum 60 mg/day for 3–10 days

Adapted from NAEPP Expert Panel Report July 2002 (NIH Publication No. 02-5075).

is any evidence of anatomic abnormalities, interstitial lung disease, or a clinical history of chronic pulmonary symptoms. For children with mild, infrequent episodic wheezing, intermittent inhaled β_2-agonists may be used to relieve symptoms as daily medication is not indicated. While exacerbation of oral thrush is a well-known and undesirable side-effect of inhaled corticosteroids, no increased incidence of infection or significant adverse effects have been observed in HIV-infected adults receiving them when clinically indicated [52]. Oral rinsing following inhalation and the use of spacers and holding chamber devices, further minimizes the risk of developing oral thrush. Serial monitoring of response to therapy should be done using peak flow meters and pulmonary function testing. The approach

to management of wheezing and reactive airway disease is the same for all children regardless of HIV infection status. However, because wheezing may often be precipitated or exacerbated by the inflammation associated with acute and chronic infection, underlying pulmonary infections should be treated promptly and aggressively in HIV-infected children.

31.3 Other pulmonary problems

31.3.1 Bronchiectasis

Bronchiectasis is a permanent abnormal dilatation of the bronchi and most commonly results from a previous

Table 31.4 Comparative daily pediatric dosages for inhaled corticosteroids

Drug	Low daily dose	Medium daily dose	High daily dose
Beclomethasone CFC			
42 or 84 mcg/puff	84–336 mcg	336–672 mcg	> 672 mcg
Beclomethasone HFA			
40 or 80 mcg/puff	80–160 mcg	400–800 mcg	> 800 mcg
Budesonide DPI			
200 mcg/inhalation	200–400 mcg	400–800 mcg	> 800 mcg
Inhalation suspension for nebulization (child dose)	0.5 mg	1.0 mg	2.0 mg
Flunisolide			
250 mcg/puff	500–750 mcg	1000–1250 mcg	> 1250 mcg
Flucatisone			
MDI: 44, 110, or 220 mcg/puff	88–176 mcg	176–440 mcg	> 440 mcg
DPI: 50, 100, or 200 mcg/inhalation	100–200 mcg	200–400 mcg	> 400 mcg
Triamcinolone acetonide			
100 mcg/puff	400–800 mcg	800–1200 mcg	> 1200 mcg

Adapted from NAEPP Expert Panel Report July 2002 (NIH Publication No. 02-5075).

infectious process that damages the pulmonary mucosa and the bronchial wall, irreversibly altering its shape and function. These alterations in pulmonary architecture predispose to recurrent infection. In HIV disease this bronchial damage can develop as a consequence of viral, bacterial, mycobacterial, fungal, or protozoal pneumonia, or as a consequence of less severe but more protracted bacterial infections that are localized to the bronchus itself, as in the case of chronic bronchitis. These infections compromise local host defenses, thus promoting additional bronchial wall damage and initiating a vicious cycle of infection and further disruption of normal pulmonary architecture [74–77]. In their retrospective study of 164 children with AIDS and respiratory problems, Sheikh and colleagues observed bronchiectasis in 16% of patients. The median age at the time of diagnosis of bronchiectasis was 7.5 years and there was a significant association of bronchiectasis with LIP, recurrent and unresolved pneumonia, and CD4+ T cell counts less than 100 cells/μL [77]. Although chest radiographs often reveal evidence of bronchial wall thickening, the hallmark bronchial dilatation characteristic of bronchiectasis requires confirmation by high-resolution, thin-section CT examination. Elevated levels of BAL neutrophils and decreased diffusion capacity have been associated with bronchial dilatation [76], suggesting that increased pulmonary neutrophils may

be associated with airway damage and lung destruction. Once a diagnosis of bronchiectasis is established, patients should receive aggressive chest pulmonary toilet, prompt antimicrobial therapy for exacerbations, and anti-inflammatory therapy, if indicated, for LIP or recurrent asthma. Patients with bronchiectasis should undergo routine monitoring every 6 months with high-resolution chest CTs and PFTs. Those with bronchiectasis due to recurrent bacterial pneumonias should receive monthly IVIG prophylaxis as previously described to minimize the recurrence of serious bacterial infections and further anatomic distortion.

31.3.2 Spontaneous pneumothorax

Spontaneous pneumothorax (PTX) is a well-recognized complication of AIDS and may occur with *Pneumocystis carinii* infection and pulmonary cryptococcosis [78, 79]. Although the cause of spontaneous PTXs remains unclear, cigarette smoking, aerosolized pentamidine treatment, and the presence of pneumatocoeles have been associated with an increased risk of pneumothorax in adults [78]. Persistent or recurrent PTXs are common in the adult population and mortality is high, especially in individuals with bilateral PTXs or unresolving bronchopleural fistulae [80]. The incidence of PTX in HIV-infected children is unknown. The single report of spontaneous PTX in pediatric HIV disease [81] described the cases of three children with AIDS, one with LIP (without evidence of concurrent PCP) and two with PCP. Although none of the children had any other risk factors for developing a PTX, all had radiographic evidence of subpleural cystic lesions and bilateral pleural adhesions. Regrettably none of the patients responded to conservative medical management with chest tube thoracostomy and chemical pleurodesis. Two patients required pleurectomy. This diagnosis should always be suspected and immediately confirmed in patients with cystic or bullous lung disease associated with LIP or bronchiectasis who experience an acute respiratory decompensation.

31.3.3 Lymphoproliferative thymic cysts

Multilocular thymic cysts (MTCs) are believed to result from an unusual response of the normal thymus gland to infection, inflammation, or neoplasm [82]. Congenital thymic cysts have also been described, but they are typically located in the neck rather than the mediastinum, are small, unilocular, and thin-walled, and lack inflammation. In contrast, multilocular thymic cysts are usually found in the mediastinum, are multilocular by definition and demonstrate significant inflammation and fibrosis on histopathologic examination [82]. Characteristically, MTCs are associated with Sjogren's disease and neoplasms that are accompanied by a heavy inflammatory infiltrate, such as Hodgkin's disease and germinoma. Typically, HIV infection is associated with thymic gland atrophy, although thymic enlargement has been reported in patients with lymphoproliferative syndrome. MTCs appear to be a rare condition in pediatric HIV disease since only two cases have been reported in the literature [83, 84]. It should be considered in the differential diagnosis in HIV-infected children who present with an anterior mediastinal mass. With the advent of HAART this condition is becoming increasingly uncommon.

31.3.4 Pulmonary symptoms associated with Cardiac disease

Underlying cardiac disease must always be considered in the differential diagnosis of patients with respiratory symptoms. The frequency of chronic cardiac disease as an underlying cause of death increases with age in HIV-infected children with prolonged survival [5]. Cardiomyopathy may occur as a primary manifestation of HIV disease or poten-

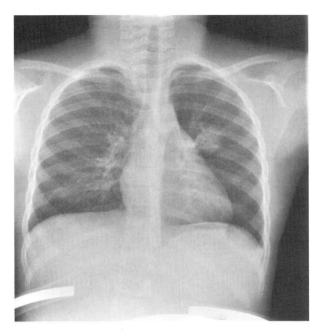

Figure 31.9 and **31.10** Chest X-ray pulmonary mucosa-associated lymphoid tissue (MALT): left upper lobe anterior pulmonary mass projected over the left hilum.

tially be associated with extensive exposure to zidovudine, an antiretroviral agent with known myotoxicity. Pulmonary findings suggestive of cardiomyopathy include recurrent episodes of tachypnea, dyspnea, and bilateral crepitant rales on auscultation that may also be accompanied by wheezing. Chest radiographs typically show bilateral increased interstitial markings and may demonstrate small pleural or lingular effusions. The diagnosis is confirmed by echocardiography and patients usually respond promptly to the initiation of myocardial inotropic support, after-load reduction, and discontinuation of zidovudine, if indicated.

31.3.5 Malignancy

Pulmonary malignancies may present as hilar adenopathy, isolated parenchymal nodules, mediastinal masses or, less commonly, diffuse interstitial disease, and are often incidental findings on routine chest radiographs. These malignancies may occur in the presence of other chronic HIV-associated pulmonary disease and often include non-Hodgkin's lymphomas, tumors of smooth muscle origin, or mucosa-associated lymphoid tissue (MALT) lesions (Figures 31.9–31.12) [85]. While pulmonary Kaposi's sarcoma

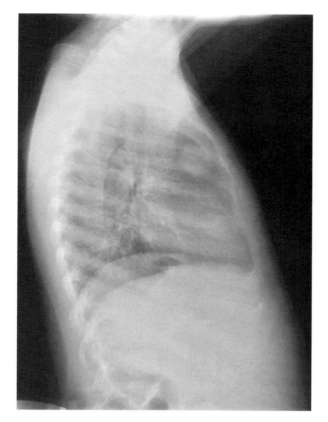

Figure 31.10. Corresponding later chest x-ray or Fig. 31.9.

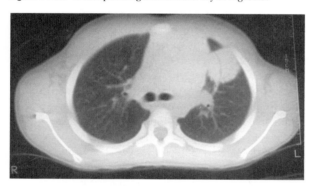

Figure 31.11. Chest computed tomography pulmonary mucosa-associated lymphoid tissue (MALT): Left upper lobe mass adjacent to the mediastinum with a bronchus traversing the lesion.

Figure 31.12. Histopathology of pulmonary MALT (mucosa-associated lymphoid tissue). Panel A. Low power view, hematoxylin and eosin stain. B: bronchiole. Panel B. High power, hematoxylin and eosin stain. GC: germinal center. Panel C. Immunohistochemical staining for the B cell marker. Leu-22. Histologic findings suggestive of a low-grade lymphoma of MALT: extensive infiltration by a dense lymphoid infiltrate (Panel A) composed of germinal centers (Panel B) with marked plasmacytosis and irregular lymphoid cells characteristic of monocytoid B-lymphocytes. Co-expression of Leu-22 by most of the B cells (Panel C).

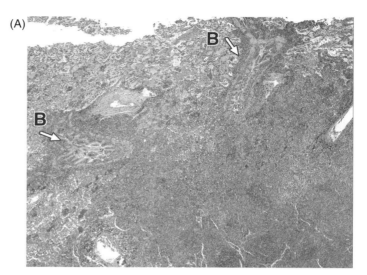

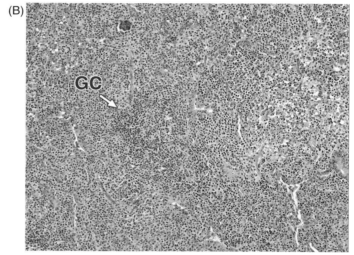

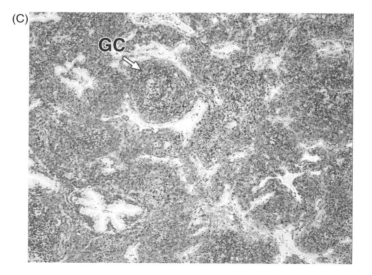

is a well-described phenomenon in adults, it is extremely rare in children [30]. Lung biopsy is always required to definitively establish a diagnosis. See Chapter 36 for an extensive discussion of malignancies associated with pediatric HIV disease.

31.4 Approach to evaluation and management of pulmonary disease

Clinicians evaluating HIV-infected children with respiratory symptoms must first determine whether those symptoms result from a common bacterial infection or an opportunistic infection. A chest x-ray should always be obtained in patients with any pulmonary complaints even if infection is not suspected. An assessment of the acuity, type, and severity of symptoms should guide the practitioner's approach to management (Table 31.5). Children with mild to moderate or chronic symptoms who are clinically stable can often be treated empirically, assessed for response to therapy, and if unimproved, undergo more conclusive diagnostic studies. The suspected clinical condition should also determine the tests performed (Table 31.6). Clinicians should not hesitate to employ additional, more intensive studies to establish a definitive diagnosis, particularly in severely immunosuppressed patients. These studies include induced sputum examination, bronchoscopy with broncheoalveolar lavage (BAL), pulmonary function testing, arterial blood gas analysis or pulse oximetry monitoring, and open lung biopsy.

Pulmonary function tests (PFTs) provide a rapid, albeit non-specific, non-invasive method to evaluate HIV-infected children with cough or dyspnea. Children must be cooperative and generally at least 6 years of age, to generate a valid and accurate study. Pulmonary function tests can be used to confirm the presence of pulmonary disease in symptomatic patients with normal chest radiographs or to detect evidence of diffuse disease in patients with localized infiltrates. In HIV-infected persons without defined lung disease, measurements of forced vital capacity (FVC), forced expiratory volume in 1 second (FEV_1), and FEV_1/FVC are usually normal [11]. The diffusing capacity (DL_{CO}) is a highly sensitive but non-specific test for detecting parenchymal lung disease in HIV-infected patients. The DL_{CO} may be reduced in patients without clinically apparent pulmonary disease, especially in those with advanced immunosuppression [11]. Abnormalities in DL_{CO} may precede the development of resting hypoxemia or infiltrates on chest radiographs [86].

Resting hypoxemia is frequently found in children with interstitial lung disease (ILD), and PFTs typically demonstrate a pattern of restrictive lung disease characterized by a reduced FVC and FEV_1, and a normal FEV_1/FVC [25].

Careful measurements of the respiratory rate are useful in evaluating children with ILD. Resting or sleeping respiratory rates can provide objective documentation of tachypnea that may reflect underlying hypoxemia. Arterial blood gas analysis, especially after exercise, can be used to measure the severity of impairment in gas exchange. Pulse oximetry has the advantage of measuring oxygen saturation without arterial puncture, making it a more attractive diagnostic approach in children, but it is less sensitive for detecting gas exchange abnormalities than blood gas analysis [86]. Assessment of oxygen saturation by either technique should be obtained in any child who presents with significant tachypnea, wheezing, exercise intolerance, or digital clubbing.

Although bronchoscopy may present technical challenges in pediatric patients, analysis of BAL fluid may offer a moderately invasive opportunity to establish a clinical diagnosis and allow refinement of antimicrobial therapy. Patients with unrevealing induced sputum results who are unresponsive to empiric antimicrobial therapy or who have rapidly progressive disease are primary candidates for BAL. Fluid should be sent for Gram, acid-fast, and silver stains; routine bacterial, fungal, and viral cultures; cytology; and enzyme-linked immunosorbent assays or fluorescent antibody studies for *Bordetella pertussis*, *Chlamydia*, and *Legionella*. If BAL analysis is inconclusive, open lung biopsy is the procedure of choice to obtain tissue for definitive histologic diagnosis in children, although thorascopic or CT-guided needle biopsy can be considered for older children and adolescents. Adequate tissue sampling of the lung parenchyma with the most extensive involvement is necessary to ensure that all the appropriate diagnostic studies can be performed. The biopsy specimen should be subdivided into a minimum of four portions for the following diagnostic studies: a portion for bacterial, fungal, AFB and viral cultures, viral probes, smears, or touch preparations with Gram stain and special stains; a frozen portion for immunofluorescence studies; a small portion for electron microscopy; and a large portion for light microscopy examination [34]. Although associated with notable surgical morbidity, when patients are selected appropriately, lung biopsy may have a significant impact on therapy and clinical outcome in HIV-infected children with pulmonary infiltrates [87].

Table 31.5 Approach to the pediatric patient with pulmonary disease

Respiratory symptoms
    Determine if acute or chronic
    Determine severity: mild, moderate, severe
    Identify symptoms: cough, chest tightness, wheezing, tachypnea, dyspnea, sputum
       production, digital clubbing, fever
    Identify physical examination findings: consolidation, crepitant rales, rhonchi, wheezing,
       pleural friction rubs, tachycardia, murmurs, gallops
    Identify precipitants and exacerbators of respiratory symptoms

Relevant clinical history
    CDC Classification (Clinical and Immunologic Category)
    CD4$^+$ T lymphocyte count and HIV-1 RNA level
    Current antiretroviral treatment and prophylaxis for opportunistic infections
    Prior episodes of recurrent serious bacterial or opportunistic infections
    Exposure history

Fever absent		Fever present	
Suspect non-infectious complications		Suspect infectious complications	
↓		↓	
Chest radiograph		Chest radiograph	
Normal or hyperinflated	*Focal or Diffuse Infiltrates, parenchymal nodules*	*Normal*	*Focal or diffuse infiltrates*
Allergic rhinitis	LIP / PLH	Acute/chronic bronchitis	Bacterial, fungal, viral,
Acute/chronic sinusitis	Atypical	Acute/chronic sinusitis	mycobacterial pneumonia.
Foreign body	mycobacterial disease	Viral URI	Atypical pneumonia
Asthma/RAD	Cardiac disease	OIs: PCP, TB, fungal infection	Consider common vs opportunistic pathogens
Bronchiectasis	Bronchiectasis	↓	
Gastroesophageal reflux	Bronchiolitis obliterans	↓	↓
Vocal cord dysfunction	Malignancy	↓	↓
Vascular ring	↓	↓	↓
Tracheomalacia	↓	↓	↓
Diagnostic studies		Diagnostic studies	
CT sinuses	Induced sputum	Expectorated sputum, n/p wash	Blood culture
PFTs	Chest CT	Pathogen identified: treat	Induced sputum
CT chest	PFTs	No pathogen identified: treat empirically	ABG or pulse oximetry
ABG or pulse oximetry	ABG or pulse oximetry	If no improvement consider:	Pathogen identified: treat
Barium swallow	Echocardiogram	induced sputum → BAL	No pathogen identified:
	Consider open lung biopsy		BAL → open lung biopsy

Table 31.6 Diagnostic evaluation of HIV-associated pulmonary problems

Condition	Incidence	Diagnostic and radiographic studies
LIP-PLH	Common	Chest radiograph, high resolution chest CT Pulmonary function studies in older children Assessment of arterial oxygen saturation at rest and with exercise Consider BAL to rule out infectious pathogens Open lung biopsy for definitive diagnosis
Recurrent pneumonias	Common	Chest radiograph Blood cultures Induced sputum or BAL with panmicrobial culture to assess for infectious pathogens; early am gastric aspirates to rule out *Mycobacterium tuberculosis*. *In severe recurrent disease:* High resolution chest CT to assess for bronchiectasis Pulmonary function studies to assess for restrictive lung disease and alterations in diffusion capacity and oxygen saturation
Chronic cough	Common	Assess and treat for acute/chronic bronchitis, allergic rhinitis Consider CT of sinuses to asses for acute/chronic sinusitis Pulmonary function studies to assess for reversible, subacute bronchospasm Barium swallow or pH probe to rule out gastroesophageal reflux
Asthma/wheezing	Common	Chest radiograph to rule out acute infiltrates, foreign bodies, anatomic abnormalities Pulmonary function studies with assessment of response to bronchodilators. Peak flow meters should be used for ongoing monitoring in patients with chronic symptoms Induced sputum or BAL if indicated by radiographic studies to rule out infectious pathogens Consider comprehensive allergy assessment including skin testing in patients with significant clinical or family history of atopic disease
Bronchiectasis	Uncommon	High resolution chest CT Aggressive microbial screening with induced sputum or BAL with exacerbations of recurrent pneumonia to rule out unusual opportunistic pathogens
Spontaneous pneumothorax	Uncommon	Chest radiograph Induced sputum or BAL to rule out infectious pathogens, especially PCP
Lymphoproliferative thymic cysts	Uncommon	High resolution chest CT: assess for intrathoracic adenopathy and other parenchymal lung lesions
Malignancy	Uncommon	Etiologies to consider: non-Hodgkin's lymphoma, leiomyoma, leiomyosarcoma, mucosa-associated lymphoid tumor (MALT) *Tissue histopathology is definitive:* CT guided needle biopsy Open lung biopsy

LIP-PLH, lymphoid interstitial pneumonitis-pulmonary lymphoid hyperplasia; CT, computed tomography; BAL, broncheoalveolar lavage; PCP, *Pneumocystis cariniii* pneumonia.

31.5 Summary

Despite advances in treatment, respiratory symptoms continue to be a very common manifestation of disease in HIV-infected children. Practitioners must determine whether these symptoms are due to an opportunistic infection or to a chronic process such as asthma, chronic bronchitis, recurrent pneumonia, bronchiectasis, or LIP. New patterns of disease will continue to emerge. Clinicians must be prepared to meet this challenge by keeping abreast of the constantly changing spectrum of pulmonary HIV disease.

REFERENCES

1. United States Public Health Service (USPHS). Guidelines for the use of antiretroviral agents in pediatric HIV infection. http://www.aidsinfo.nih.gov/ living document, December 14, 2001.

2. Paella, F. J., Delaney, K. M., Moorman, A. C. *et al.* Declining morbidity and mortality among patients with advanced human immunodeficiency virus infection. *New Engl. J. Med.* **338** (1998), 853–60.

3. Johann-Liang, R., Cervia, J. S. & Noel, G. J. Characteristics of human immunodeficiency virus-infected children at the time of death: an experience in the 1990s. *Pediatr. Infect. Dis. J.* **16** (1997), 1145–50.

4. Frederick, T., Alvarez, J. J., Shin, Y. S. *et al.* Trends in CD4 counts and AIDS-defining conditions (ADCs) in infants and children in Los Angeles County (LAC) before and after HAART. In *9th Conference on Retroviruses and Opportunistic Infectious* February 4–8 **8** (2001), 247 [Abstract no. 675].

5. Langston, C., Cooper, E. R., Goldfarb, J. *et al.* Human immunodeficiency virus-related mortality in infants and children: data from the pediatric pulmonary and cardiovascular complications of vertically transmitted HIV (P(2)C(2)) Study. *Pediatrics* **107** : **2** (2001), 328–38.

6. Bamji, M., Thea, D. M., Weedon, J. *et al.* Prospective study of human immunodeficiency virus 1-related disease among 512 infants born to infected women in New York City. *Pediatr. Infect. Dis. J.* **15** (1996), 891–8.

7. Centers for Disease Control and Prevention. AIDS-indicator conditions reported in 1996, by age group, United States. HIV/AIDS *Surveillance Report* **9** : **2** (1997), 18.

8. Merchant, R. H., Oswal, J. S., Bhagwat, R. V. & Karkare, J. Clinical profile of HIV infection. *Indian Pediatr.* **38** (2001), 239–46.

9. Dhurat, R., Mamta, M., Sharma, R. & Shak, N. K. Clinical spectrum of HIV infection. *Indian Pediatr.* **37** (2000), 831–6.

10. Mato, S. P. & Van Dyke, R. B. Pulmonary infections in children with HIV infection. *Semin. Respir. Infect.* **17** : **1** (2002), 33–46.

11. Rosen, M. J. Overview of pulmonary complications. *Clin. Chest Med.* **17** : **4** (1996), 621–31.

12. Englund, J. A., Baker, C. J., Raksino, C. *et al.* Clinical and laboratory characteristics of a large cohort of symptomatic, human immunodeficiency virus-infected infants and children. *Pediatr. Infect. Dis. J.* **15** (1996), 1025–36.

13. Scott, G. B., Hutto, C., Makuch, R. W. *et al.* Survival in children with perinatally acquired human immunodeficiency type 1 infection. *New Engl. J. Med.* **321** (1989), 1791–6.

14. Morris, C. R., Araba-Owoyele, L. Spector, S. A. & Maldonado, Y. Disease patterns and survival after acquired immunodeficiency syndrome diagnosis in human immunodeficiency virus-infected children. *Pediatr. Infect. Dis. J.* **15** (1996), 321–8.

15. Spira, R., Lepage, P., Msellati, P. *et al.* Natural history of human immunodeficiency virus type 1 infection in children: a five year prospective study in Rwanda. *Pediatrics* **104** (1999), 1–9.

16. Agostini, C., Zambello, R., Trentin, L. & Semenzato, G. HIV and pulmonary immune responses. *Immunol. Today* **17** : **8** (1996), 359–64.

17. Cohen, D., Fitzpatrick, E., Hartsfield, C., Avdiushko, M. & Gillespie, M. Abnormal lung cytokine synthesis by immunodeficient T cells in murine AIDS-associated interstitial pneumonitis. *Ann. N. Y. Acad. Sci.* **796** : **47** (1996), 47–58.

18. Clarke, J. R., Robinson, D. S., Coker, R. J., Miller, R. F. & Mitchell, D. M. AIDS and the lung: update 1995. 4. Role of the human immunodeficiency virus within the lung. *Thorax* **50** : **5** (1995), 567–76.

19. Teruya-Feldstein J., Kingma, D. W., Weiss, A. *et al.* Chemokine gene expression and clonal analysis of B cells in tissues involved by lymphoid interstitial pneumonitis from HIV-infected pediatric patients. *Mod. Pathol.* **14** : **10** (2001), 929–36.

20. Agostini, C. & Semenzato, G. Immunologic effects of HIV in the lung. *Clin. Chest Med.* **17** : **4** (1996), 633–45.

21. Sei, S., Kleiner, D. E., Kopp, J. B., Chandra, R., Klotman, P. E. & Yarchoan, R. Quantitative analysis of viral burden in tissues from adults and children with symptomatic human immunodeficiency virus type 1 infection assessed by polymerase chain reaction. *J. Infect. Dis.* **170** (1994), 325–33.

22. Wallace, J. M., Rao, A. V., Glassroth, J. *et al.* Respiratory illness in persons with human immunodeficiency virus infection. *Am. Rev. Respir. Dis.* **148** (1993), 1523–9.

23. Carrington, C. B. & Liebow, A. A. Lymphocytic interstitial pneumonia. *Am. J. Pathol.* **48** (1966), 36–?.

24. Halprin, G. M., Ramirez, J. & Pratt, P. C. Lymphoid interstitial pneumonia. *Chest* **62** (1972), 418–23.

25. Fan, L. L. & Langston, C. Chronic interstitial lung disease in children. *Pediatr. Pulmonol.* **16** (1993), 184–96.

26. Scott, G. B., Buck, B. E., Letterman, J. G. *et al.* Acquired immunodeficiency syndrome in infants. *New Engl. J. Med.* **310** (1984), 76–81.

27. Rubinstein, A., Morecki, R., Silverman, B. *et al.* Pulmonary disease in children with acquired immune deficiency syndrome and AIDS-related complex. *J. Pediatr.* **108** (1986), 498–503.

28. Schneider, R. F. Lymphocytic interstitial pneumonitis and nonspecific interstitial pneumonitis. *Clin. Chest Med.* **17** : **4** (1996), 763–6.

29. Centers for Disease Control and Prevention. 1994 Revised classification system for human immunodeficiency virus infection in children less than 13 years of age. *MMWR* **43** : **RR-12** (1994), 1–10.

30. Solal-Celigny, P., Couderc, L. J., Herman, D. *et al.* Lymphoid interstitial pneumonitis in acquired immunodeficiency syndrome-related complex. *Am. Rev. Respir. Dis.* **131** : **6** (1985), 956–60.

31. Ziza, J.-M., Brun-Vezinet, F., Venet, A. *et al.* Lymphadenopathy-associated virus isolated from bronchoalveolar lavage fluid in AIDS-related complex with lymphoid interstitial pneumonitis. *New Engl. J. Med.* **313** : **3** (1985), 183.

32. Travis, W. D., Fox, C. H., Devaney, K. O. *et al.* Lymphoid pneumonitis in 50 adult patients infected with the human immunodeficiency virus: lymphocytic interstitial pneumonitis versus nonspecific interstitial pneumonitis. *Hum. Pathol.* **23** : **5** (1992), 529–41.

33. Kazi, S., Cohen, P. R., Williams, F., Schempp, R. & Reveille, J. D. The diffuse infiltrative lymphocytosis syndrome. Clinical and immunogenetic features in 35 patients [see comments]. *AIDS* **10** : **4** (1996), 385–91.

34. Bokulic, R. E. & Hilman, B. C. Interstitial lung disease in children. *Pediatr. Clin. N. Am.* **41** : **3** (1994), 543–67.

35. Vellutini, C., Horschowski, N., Philippon, V., Gambarelli, D., Nave, K. A. & Filippi, P. Development of lymphoid hyperplasia in transgenic mice expressing the HIV tat gene. *AIDS Res. Hum. Retroviruses* **11** : **1** (1995), 21–9.

36. Agostini, C., Sancetta, R., Cerutti, A. & Semenzato, G. Alveolar macrophages as a cell source of cytokine hyperproduction in HIV-related interstitial lung disease. *J. Leukoc. Biol.* **58** : **5** (1995), 495–500.

37. Andiman, W. A., Eastman, R., Martin, K. *et al.* Opportunistic lymphoproliferations associated with Epstein-Barr viral DNA in infants and children with AIDS. *Lancet* **II**: (1985), 498–503.

38. Katz, B. Z., Berkman, A. B. & Shapiro, E. D. Serologic evidence of active Epstein-Barr virus infection in Epstein-Barr virus-associated lymphoproliferative disorders of children with acquired immunodeficiency syndrome. *J. Pediatr.* **120** (1992), 228–32.

39. Brodie, S. J., de la Rosa, C., Howe, J. G., Crouch, J., Travis, W. D. & Diem, K. Pediatric AIDS-associated lymphocytic interstitial pneumonia and pulmonary arterio-occlusive disease: role of VCAM-1/VLA-4 adhesion pathway and human herpesviruses. *Am. J. Pathol.* **154** : **5** (1999), 1453–64.

40. Abrams, E. J. Opportunistic infections and other clinical manifestations of HIV disease in children. *Pediatr. Clin. N. Am.* **47** : **1** (2000), 79–108.

41. Abuzaitoun, O. R. & Hanson, I. C. Organ-specific manifestations of HIV disease in children. *Pediatr. Clin. North. Am.* **47** : **1** (2000), 109–25.

42. Shiff, R. G., Kabat, L. & Kamani, N. Gallium scanning in lymphoid interstitial pneumonitis of children with AIDS. *J. Nucl. Med.* **28** : **12** (1987), 1915–19.

43. Pitt, J. Lymphocytic interstitial pneumonia. *Pediatr. Clin. N. Am.* **38** (1991), 89–95.

44. Bye, M. R. HIV in children. *Clin. Chest Med.* **17** (1996), 787–96.

45. Domachowske, J. B. Pediatric human immunodeficiency virus infection. *Clin. Microbiol. Rev.* **9** (1996), 448–68.

46. Gonzalez, C. E., Samakoses, R., Boler, A. M., Hill, S. & Wood, L. V. Lymphoid interstitial pneumonitis in pediatric AIDS. Natural history of the disease. *Ann. N.Y. Acad. Sci.* **918** (2000), 362–6.

47. Rubinstein, A., Berstein, L. J., Charytan, M. *et al.* Corticosteroid treatment for pulmonary lymphoid hyperplasia in children with the acquired immune deficiency syndrome. *Pediatr. Pulmonol.* **4** (1988), 13–17.

48. Laufer, M. & Scott, G. B. Medical management of HIV disease in children. *Pediatr. Clin. N. Am.* **47** : **1** (2000), 127–53.

49. Ramesh, S. & Schwartz, S. A. Therapeutic uses of intravenous immunoglobulin (IVIG) in children. *Pediatr. Rev.* **16** (1995), 403–10.

50. Borkowsky, W., Rigaud, M., Krasinski, K., Moore, T., Lawrence, R. & Pollack, H. Cell-mediated and humoral immune responses in children infected with human immunodeficiency virus during the first four years of life. *J. Pediatr.* **120** (1992), 371–5.

51. Marolda, J., Pace, B., Bonforte, R. J. *et al.* Pulmonary manifestations of HIV infection in children. *Pediatr. Pulmonol.* **10** (1991), 231–5.

52. Huang, L. & Stansell, J. D. AIDS and the lung. *Med. Clin. N. Am.* **80** : **4** (1996), 775–801.

53. Polack, F. P., Flayhart, D. C., Zahurak, M. L., Dick, J. D. & Willoughby, R. E. Colonization by *Streptococcus penumoniae* in human immunodeficiency virus-infected children. *Pediatr. Infect. Dis. J.* **19** : **7** (2000), 608–12.

54. Madhi, S. A., Petersen, K., Madhi, A., Khoosal, M. & Klugman, K. P. Increased disease burden and antibiotic resistance of bacteria causing severe community-acquired lower respiratory tract infections in human immunodeficiency virus type 1-infected children. *Clin. Infect. Dis.* **31** : **1** (2000), 170–6.

55. United States Public Health Service (USPHS). Guidelines for the prevention of opportunistic infections in persons infected with human immunodeficiency virus. http://www.aidsinfo.nih.gov/ 2001;living document, December 14, 2001.

56. Centers for Disease Control and Prevention. Anergy skin testing and preventive therapy for HIV-infected persons: revised recommendations. *MMWR* **46** : **RR-15** (1997), 1–10.

57. Dye, C., Scheele, S., Dolin, P. *et al.* Global burden of tuberculosis. Estimated incidence, prevalence, and mortality by country. *J. Am. Med. Assoc.* **282** (1999), 677–86.

58. Schluger, N. W. & Burzynski, J. Tuberculosis and HIV infection: epidemiology, immunology and treatment. *HIV Clin. Trials* **2** (2001), 356–65.

59. Chan, S. P., Birnbaum, J., Rao, M. & Steiner, P. Clinical manifestation and outcome of tuberculosis in children with acquired immunodeficiency syndrome. *Pediatr. Infect. Dis. J.* **15** : **5** (1996), 443–7.

60. Haller, J. O. & Ginsberg, K. J. Tuberculosis in children with acquired immunodeficiency syndrome. *Pediatr. Radiol.* **27**:2 (1997), 186–8.

61. Thomas, P., Bornschlegel, K., Singh, T. P. *et al.* Tuberculosis in human immunodeficiency virus-infected and human immunodeficiency virus-exposed children in New York City. The New York City Pediatric Spectrum of HIV Disease Consortium. *Pediatr. Infect. Dis. J.* **19**:8 (2000), 700–6.

62. Waddell, R. D., Lishimpi, K., Fordham von Reyn, C. *et al.* Bacteremia due to *Mycobacterium tuberculosis* or M. bovis, Bacille Calmette–Guerin (BCG) among HIV-positive children and adults in Zambia. *AIDS* **15** (2001), 55–60.

63. Piedra, P. A. Safety of the trivalent, cold-adapted influenza vaccine (CAIV-T) in children. *Semin. Pediatr. Infect. Dis.* **13** (2002), 90–6.

64. Shenep, J. L. & Flynn, P. M. Pulmonary fungal infections in immunocompromised children. *Curr. Opin. Pediatr.* **9**:3 (1997), 213–18.

65. Shetty, D., Giri, N., Gonzalez, C. E., Pizzo, P. A. & Walsh, T. J. Invasive aspergillosis in human immunodeficiency virus-infected children. *Pediatr. Infect. Dis. J.* **16**:2 (1997), 216–21.

66. Working Group on Antiretroviral Therapy. Antiretroviral therapy and medical management of HIV-infected infants and children. *Pediatr. Infect. Dis. J.* **12** (1993), 13–22.

67. Callahan, C. Etiology of chronic cough in a population of children referred to a pediatric pulmonologist. *J. Am. Board Fam. Pract.* **9**:5 (1996), 324–7.

68. Warner, J. O. & Naspitz, C. K. Third International Pediatric Consensus statement on the management of childhood asthma. International Pediatric Asthma Consensus Group. *Pediatr. Pulmonol.* **25**:1 (1998), 1–17.

69. Martinez, F. D., Wright, A. L., Taussig, L. M. *et al.* Asthma and wheezing in the first six years of life. *New Engl. J. Med.* **332** (1995), 133–8.

70. Sears, M. R., Burrows, B., Flannery, E. M., Herbison, G. P., Hewitt, C. J. & Holdaway, M. D. Relation between airway responsiveness and serum IgE in children with asthma and in apparently normal children. *New Engl. J. Med.* **325** (1991), 1067–71.

71. Israel-Biet, D., Labrousse, F., Tourani, J. M. Sors, H., Andrieu, J. M. & Even, P. Elevation of IgE in HIV-infected subjects: a marker of poor prognosis. *J. Allergy. Clin. Immunol.* **89** (1992), 68–75.

72. NAEPP Expert Panel Report. National Heart, Lung, and Blood Institute. *Expert Panel Report 2: Guidelines for the Diagnosis and Management of Asthma.* National Institutes of Health NIH Publication 97–4051(1997), pp. 3B–24.

73. NAEPP Expert Panel Report. National Heart, Lung, and Blood Institute. *Expert Panel Report: Guidelines for the Diagnosis and Management of Asthma- Update on Selected Topics 2002.* National Institutes of Health. NIH Publication 02-5075(2002) pp. 3B-24.

74. McGuinness, G., Naidich, D. P., Garay, S., Leitman, B. S. & McCauley, D. I. AIDS Associated bronchiectasis: CT features. *J. Comput. Assist. Tomogr.* **17** (1993), 260–6.

75. Verghese, A., Al-Samman, M., Nabhan, D., Naylor, A. D. & Rivera, M. Bacterial bronchitis and bronchiectasis in human immunodeficiency virus infection. *Arch. Intern. Med.* **154** (1994), 2086–91.

76. King, M. A., Neal, D. E., St. John, R., Tsai, J. & Diaz, P. T. Bronchial dilatation in patients with HIV infection: CT assessment and correlation with pulmonary function tests and findings at broncheoalveolar lavage. *Am. J. Roentgenol.* **168**:6 (1997), 1535–40.

77. Sheikh, S., Madiraju, K., Steiner, P. & Rao, M. Bronchiectasis in pediatric AIDS. *Chest* **112**:5 (1997), 1202–7.

78. Metersky, M. L., Colt, H. G., Olson, L. K. & Shanks, T. G. AIDS-related spontaneous pneumothorax. Risk factors and treatment. *Chest* **108**:4 (1995), 946–51.

79. Torre, D., Martegani, R., Speranza, F., Zeroli, C. & Fiori, G. P. Pulmonary cryptococcosis presenting as pneumothorax in a patient with AIDS. *Clin. Infect. Dis.* **21**:6 (1995), 1524–5.

80. Sepkowitz, K. A., Telzak, E. E., Gold, J. W. M. *et al.* Pneumothorax in AIDS. *Ann. Intern. Med.* **114** (1991), 455–9.

81. Schroeder, S. A., Beneck, D. & Dozor, A. J. Spontaneous pneumothorax in children with AIDS. *Chest* **108**:4 (1995), 1173–6.

82. Suster, S. & Rosai, J. Multilocular thymic cyst: an acquired reactive process: study of 18 cases. *Am. J. Surg. Pathol.* **15** (1991), 388–98.

83. Ramaswamy, G., Saunders, N., Belmonte, A. H. & Tchertkoff, V. Benign lymphoepithelial cysts of the parotid gland in HIV positive patients [Abstract]. *Am. J. Clin. Pathol.* **90** (1988), 497.

84. Shalaby-Rana E, Selby, D., Ivy, P. *et al.* Multilocular thymic cyst in a child with acquired immunodeficiency syndrome. *Pediatr. Infect. Dis. J.* **15** (1996), 83–6.

85. Joshi, V. V., Gagnon, G. A., Chadwick, E. G. *et al.* The spectrum of mucosa-associated lymphoid tissue lesions in pediatric patients infected with HIV: a clinicopathologic study of six cases. *Am. J. Clin. Pathol.* **107**:5 (1997), 592–600.

86. Vander Els, N. J. & Stover, D. E. Approach to the patient with pulmonary disease. *Clin. Chest Med.* **17**:4 (1996), 767–85.

87. Izraeli, S., Mueller, B. U., Ling, A. *et al.* Role of tissue diagnosis in pulmonary involvement in pediatric human immunodeficiency virus infection. *Pediatr. Infect. Dis. J.* **15**:2 (1996), 112–6.

32

Hematologic problems

William C. Owen, M.D. and Eric J. Werner, M.D.

Division of Pediatric Hematology/Oncology, Eastern Virginia Medical School, Children's Hospital of the King's Daughters, Norfolk, VA

Most HIV-infected children and adolescents have abnormalities of their peripheral blood and/or hemostatic systems. These abnormalities may be caused by direct or indirect effects of HIV on hematopoiesis, by secondary infections, by nutritional deficits, by medications, or by aberrations of the immune system. While in many cases these abnormalities are asymptomatic, on occasion they may cause life-threatening consequences. This chapter will review the common hematologic consequences of HIV infection and will emphasize the diagnostic and therapeutic considerations in their management.

32.1 Anemia

Anemia is a common finding in children infected with HIV. Ellaurie *et al.* noted that 94% of HIV-infected children had a hematocrit < 33% [1]. Anemia is present in 37% of children with perinatally acquired HIV at 1 year of age [2]. In Ellaurie's review, the anemia was more pronounced (hematocrit < 25%) in 21 of 23 infants with opportunistic infection [1]. Forsyth *et al.* followed infants with perinatally acquired HIV and noted that anemia in the first year of life was associated with an increased risk of mortality by 3 years of age [2]. Adult studies have shown that anemia continues to predict decreased survival even with highly active antiretroviral therapy (HAART) [3].

Potential etiologies of anemia in children include decreased red blood cell (RBC) production, defective erythroid maturation, blood loss, and increased RBC destruction (hemolysis). In many anemic HIV-infected children, the anemia is multifactorial. The potential etiologies of anemia in HIV-infected children are listed in Table 32.1.

In addition to direct or indirect effects of HIV infection, occasionally such children will coincidently have congenital RBC disorders, such as hemoglobinopathies or intrinsic RBC defects.

Decreased red cell production is common. It often results from suppression of erythrocyte production by the effect of HIV on the bone marrow microenvironment [4]. Cytokines such as tumor necrosis factor and interleukin-1 are elevated in active HIV infection and may have an inhibitory effect on erythropoiesis [5]. Dyserythropoiesis was noted in 20% of the bone marrow aspirates from HIV-infected children [1]. Additionally, anemic patients with HIV have a relatively poor response to erythropoietin [5].

Several types of infections suppress erythropoiesis, including infections due to *Mycobacterium avium* complex (MAC), cytomegalovirus (CMV), and Epstein–Barr virus (EBV). *Mycobacterium avium* complex may be especially associated with severe anemia [6]. Pure red cell aplasia due to acute or persistent parvovirus B19 occurs in the HIV-infected individual [7].

Medications used to treat HIV or its complications may interfere with RBC production. For instance, the dose-limiting toxicity of zidovudine is anemia that is typically macrocytic. Lack of macrocytosis is sometimes used as an indicator of poor adherence to zidovudine. Trimethoprim-sulfamethoxazole (TMP–SMX), ganciclovir, and acyclovir may inhibit erythropoiesis [8]. Infiltration of the bone marrow by malignancy, a relatively uncommon phenomenon in children with HIV, can result in decreased RBC production.

Anemia may be induced by deficiencies in iron, folate, vitamin B12, protein or rarely pyridoxine, copper, or selenium. Iron deficiency can be due to poor nutritional intake,

Table 32.1 Causes of and treatments for anemia in HIV-infected children and adolescents

Cause	Treatment
Decreased erythrocyte production	
Chronic disease/inflammation	Treat underlying cause
Effect of HIV on erythropoiesis	HAART and/or erythropoietin
Infections	
Mycobacterium avium complex (MAC)	Antibiotics
Parvovirus B19	Intravenous immunoglobulin
Cytomegalovirus	Ganciclovir
Epstein–Barr virus	Supportive care
Histoplasmosis	Antifungal therapy
Medications	
Zidovudine	Medication adjustment and/or erythropoietin
Ganciclovir	Medication adjustment and/or erythropoietin
Trimethoprim-sulfamethoxazole	Change medication
Bone marrow infiltration	
Lymphoma	Chemotherapy
Leukemia	Chemotherapy
Nutritional deficiencies	
Iron	Ferrous sulfate supplementation
Folate	Folate supplementation
Vitamin B-12	Cobalamin supplementation
Hemolysis	
Autoimmune hemolytic anemia (rare)	Corticosteroids, other
Congenital erythrocyte disorder	
G-6-PD deficiency	Change medication
	Transfusion for severe anemia
Hemoglobinopathy	Folate supplementation
	Transfusion for severe anemia
Thalassemia (ineffective erythropoiesis)	Folate supplementation
	Transfusion for severe anemia
Medications	
Primaquine	Change medication
Dapsone	Change medication
Sulfonamide	Change medication
HUS/TTP	Plasmapheresis (TTP)
	Supportive care
Hypersplenism	Splenectomy if severe
Blood loss	Treat underlying cause
	Iron supplementation
	Transfusion for severe anemia

occult intestinal blood loss, or repeated phlebotomy. Folate deficiency is usually caused by poor dietary intake. Vitamin B12 deficiency can be caused by ileitis, intrinsic factor deficiency, or poor nutritional intake as may occur with a strict vegan diet [9].

Hemolysis means a shortened red cell lifespan. An elevated reticulocyte count usually indicates increased RBC production as may occur in response to hemolysis or blood loss. Hypersplenism results in increased filtration and premature destruction of normal RBCs. While autoantibodies are frequently detected by the Coombs' test in HIV-infected children, usually they do not result in clinically significant hemolysis [5]. For instance, in Ellaurie's series, a positive Coomb's test was present in 37% but none had evidence of hemolysis [1]. G-6-PD deficiency is common in many populations. Hemolysis can result in persons deficient in G-6-PD in response to infection or multiple medications including sulfonamides and antimalarials [10]. Hemolyticuremic syndrome (HUS) and thrombotic thrombocytopenia purpura (TTP) are uncommon disorders that appear to occur with increased frequency in patients with HIV [10–12]. In these disorders, there is usually a marked hemolytic anemia with schistocytes on the peripheral blood smear.

The diagnostic evaluation of anemia in the HIV-infected patient begins with a thorough history and physical exam, focusing on persistent fever, weight loss, blood loss, medications, diet, and signs or symptoms of hemolysis such as jaundice or darkening of the urine. If available, the newborn hemoglobinopathy screen should be reviewed. The family history should be evaluated for anemia, hemoglobinopathies, recurrent jaundice, splenectomy, or early cholecystectomy that might indicate a congenital cause of anemia.

The laboratory evaluation begins with a complete blood count, reticulocyte count, and review of the peripheral blood smear. The combination of microcytosis and hypochromia should raise the differential diagnosis of iron deficiency, thalassemia, chronic disease or, less commonly, sideroblastic anemia or lead ingestion. The standard laboratory tests for iron deficiency such as the serum iron : transferrin ratio and serum ferritin concentration may be misleading. The serum iron is often low in the anemia of chronic disease leading to a low iron : transferrin ratio in the presence of adequate iron stores, while ferritin is an acute phase reactant and can be falsely normal in inflammatory states. The combination of an elevated ferritin and low total iron-binding capacity is typical of the anemia of chronic inflammation [13]. When in doubt, the clinical response to a trial of ferrous sulfate supplementation, at a dose of 5–6 mg/kg/day of elemental iron, can be both

diagnostic and therapeutic. A hemoglobin electrophoresis will evaluate for the presence of abnormal hemoglobin. To evaluate the possibility of β-thalassemia trait, it is necessary to perform a quantitative hemoglobin A_2 level and the child should be over the age of approximately 1 year for this to be reliable. A lead level determination will rule out lead intoxication, and a G-6-PD assay will rule out G-6-PD deficiency. Red blood cell or serum folate and vitamin B12 levels may be useful in patients with macrocytosis or to look for concomitant iron and folate and/or vitamin B12 deficiency. As noted above, a positive Coombs' test is common, but autoimmune hemolysis is uncommon. The combination of elevated serum indirect bilirubin, decreased serum haptoglobin, and microspherocytes on the peripheral smear support the diagnosis of autoimmune hemolytic anemia, but hereditary spherocytosis may also cause these findings. For the patient with refractory anemia or unexplained fever, urine and buffy coat cultures for CMV, blood cultures for MAC, serology or PCR for parvovirus, CMV, and EBV, and a bone marrow evaluation are indicated to look for malignancy, to evaluate erythropoiesis or to confirm infection [14]. In addition to routine morphological evaluation, the bone marrow should be stained for iron, cultured for bacteria, MAC, viruses, and fungi, and tested for parvovirus by PCR. Bone marrow cytogenic analysis should be considered for evaluation for myelodysplastic disorders.

Effective treatment depends upon a correct diagnosis. Often, effective antiretroviral therapy alone will ameliorate the anemia [8]; however, this therapy may require modification if it contributes to severe anemia as may be seen with zidovudine. Likewise, supportive care drugs that inhibit erythropoiesis may also require modification. Iron deficiency anemia should be corrected with 6 mg/kg/day of elemental iron. Other nutritional deficiencies (B12 and folate) should be corrected with supplements, and opportunistic infections should be treated appropriately. Intravenous immunoglobulin can reverse parvovirus-induced pure red blood cell aplasia [7]. Erythropoietin at 100–150 units/kg given 3 days per week administered subcutaneously often improves the quality of life [15] and allows continuation of medications that can cause anemia, especially for patients with baseline erythropoietin levels less than 500 IU/L [16]. Coyle [5] recommends a dosage escalation by 50 units/kg every 4 weeks (to a maximum of 300 units/kg) until the hematocrit rises by 5–6% or reaches a level of 36%. He further recommends that if the hematocrit increases to > 40%, the erythropoietin should be held until the hematocrit is ≤ 36% and then resumed at a dose that is 50 units/kg lower. Iron sufficiency must be maintained for erythropoietin to be effective.

For patients with life-threatening anemia or for those who continue to have symptomatic anemia despite appropriate interventions, transfusions of packed RBCs can be utilized. Cytomegalovirus-negative or leukocyte-depleted products are desirable to decrease the risk of new CMV infection. If available, irradiated products should be used to decrease the risk of graft-versus-host disease from transfused lymphocytes, although this risk appears to be very small [5].

32.2 Neutropenia

Neutropenia, defined as an absolute neutrophil count (ANC) less than 1500 cells/μL, is common in HIV-infected children. Ellaurie *et al.* found that 41 of 100 HIV-infected children had an ANC < 1500/μL and 5 had an ANC < 500/μL [1]. Neutropenia was present in 65% of children with opportunistic infections as opposed to 34% without opportunistic infections. In addition to a decreased ANC, neutrophil function defects such as decreased bactericidal activity or abnormal chemotaxis have been described [5, 8]. Quantitative and qualitative neutrophil disorders combined with other abnormalities of the immune system predispose these patients to severe and opportunistic infections.

Potential causes of neutropenia in the HIV-infected patient are listed in Table 32.2. Neutropenia can result from impaired myelopoiesis, drug myelotoxicity, or peripheral destruction of the circulating neutrophils. Causes of impaired myelopoiesis include direct suppression of infected marrow progenitor cells by HIV and/or indirect effects caused by release of soluble glycoproteins that inhibit myelopoiesis in HIV-infected marrow [5]. Opportunistic infections such as CMV, EBV, MAC, and parvovirus can directly suppress myelopoiesis. Deficiencies of nutrients such as vitamin B12 and folate as well as malignant infiltration impair myelopoiesis.

Drugs used to treat HIV infection and its complications often cause neutropenia. Zidovudine, ganciclovir, TMP-SMX, and pentamidine, drugs commonly employed in HIV therapeutic regimens, are potential causes of neutropenia as are less commonly used medications such as alpha-interferon and cancer chemotherapeutic agents. Kline *et al.* reported that 20% of children treated with zidovudine (180 mg/m^2, maximum 200 mg every 6 hours) had an ANC < 400/μL [17]. Although anti-granulocyte antibodies are common in children with HIV infection, their presence does not appear to correlate with the degree of neutropenia [18].

The initial diagnostic approach begins with the history, focusing on signs or symptoms of infection, nutritional factors, and the patient's current medications. The patient should be examined for evidence of active infection, adenopathy, and organomegaly. The laboratory evaluations begin with a complete blood count including a review of the peripheral smear. Appropriate cultures and/or serological tests are useful for diagnosis of bacterial (MAC), viral (CMV, EBV, and parvovirus), and fungal etiologies. Bone marrow evaluation should be performed when two or more cell lines are suppressed or when fever of unknown origin is present [14]. Anti-granulocyte antibody tests are generally not helpful [18].

Treatment of the underlying HIV infection itself with antiretroviral therapy will often improve the neutropenia. However, some antiretroviral medications cause neutropenia. Stavudine have been shown to cause less neutropenia than zidovudine [17]. The cytokines GM-CSF and G-CSF both increase circulating neutrophils and improve neutrophil function [5]. In a randomized controlled clinical trial in HIV-infected individuals > 13 years of age, G-CSF was administered in either daily dosing (1–10 μg/kg/day) vs intermittent (300 μg/dose) with the dose adjusted to maintain a neutrophil count of 2–10 × 10^9/L. The mean G-CSF dosage required to maintain this ANC was 1.2 μg/kg/day for the daily treatment and 300 μg twice a week for the intermittent treatment group. G-CSF treatment significantly reduced the incidence of severe neutropenia, severe bacterial infections, and bacterial infection-related hospital days [19]. Other supportive care drugs such as TMP–SMX may need to be altered if they cause significant neutropenia. G-CSF treatment may allow for the continued use of these agents, but the toxicity of long-term use of G-CSF (or GM-CSF) is unknown.

Opportunistic infections should be aggressively treated (selecting drugs which are the least myelosuppressive) nutritional deficiencies should be corrected, and malignant diseases should be appropriately treated. HIV-infected children who present with fever and severe neutropenia (i.e. an absolute neutrophil count < 500/μL) should receive a prompt and thorough evaluation for a source of the fever and immediate broad-spectrum antibiotics.

32.3 Thrombocytopenia

Thrombocytopenia is present in about one-third of children and adolescents infected by HIV [1, 20]. Mueller found 20% of their HIV-infected children had a platelet count < 50 000/μL [8]. In adults, the frequency of

Table 32.2 Causes of and treatment of neutropenia in HIV-infected children and adolescents

Cause	Treatment
Impaired myelopoiesis	
Effect of HIV infection on myelopoiesis	HAART and/or G-CSF
Drug myelotoxicity	Medication change and/or G-CSF
Zidovudine	
Ganciclovir	
Trimethoprim-sulfamethoxazole	
Pentamidine	
Alpha-interferon	
Cancer chemotherapy	
Other	
Infection	
Mycobacterium avium complex (MAC)	Antibiotics
Parvovirus B19	Intravenous immunoglobulin
Cytomegalovirus	Ganciclovir
Epstein–Barr virus	Supportive care
Histoplasmosis	Antifungal therapy
Bone marrow infiltration	
Lymphoma	Chemotherapy
Leukemia	Chemotherapy
Nutritional deficiencies	
Folate	Folate supplementation
Vitamin B-12	Cobalamin supplementation
Peripheral destruction	
Hypersplenism	Splenectomy (if severe)
Acute infection	

thrombocytopenia increases as the CD4 count decreases or the disease reaches an advanced stage [21]. While spontaneous remissions occur, in most instances untreated thrombocytopenia is persistent or progressive [22].

As noted in Table 32.3, thrombocytopenia can result from decreased platelet production, accelerated platelet destruction, platelet sequestration or a combination of these factors. There are indications that both decreased production and accelerated destruction are contributory to HIV-induced thrombocytopenia. Structural abnormalities are seen in the megakaryocytes of HIV-infected individuals [1, 23] and HIV-1 RNA has been identified in the megakaryocytes [23]. There are decreased megakaryocyte precursor cells in the marrows of HIV-infected individuals [24]. Ballem *et al.* [25] found decreased platelet production in untreated HIV-infected individuals. In addition, bone marrow infiltration by malignancy or infection can inhibit platelet production. Other than myelosuppressive cancer chemotherapy, medications infrequently inhibit platelet production.

Platelet survival is shortened in patients with HIV, even those with normal platelet counts [24, 25]. There are elevated levels of immunoglobulin on the surface of the platelet [26]. An antibody that reacts against platelet glycoprotein IIIa is found in serum and at even higher concentrations in immune complexes isolated from HIV-infected individuals [27]. Lastly, the platelet counts in HIV-infected individuals often increase in response to therapies used to treat immune thrombocytopenia [22, 28]. Together, these findings indicate an immune mechanism for the thrombocytopenia is often present.

In addition to immune thrombocytopenia, other factors contributing to shortened platelet lifespan should be considered. Disseminated intravascular coagulation (DIC) may occur in the HIV patient as a complication of granulocyte colony stimulating factor therapy or infection [29].

Table 32.3 Causes of and treatment of thrombocytopenia in HIV-infected children and adolescents

Cause	Treatment
Impaired thrombopoiesis	
Direct effect of HIV on thrombopoiesis	HAART
Drug myelotoxicity	Adjust medication
	Platelet transfusion
Zidovudine	
Ganciclovir	
Cancer chemotherapy	
Other	
Infection	
Mycobacterium avium complex (MAC)	Antibiotics
Cytomegalovirus	Ganciclovir
Epstein–Barr virus	Supportive care
Bone marrow infiltration	
Lymphoma	Chemotherapy
Leukemia	Chemotherapy
Nutritional deficiencies	
Folate	Folate supplementation
Vitamin B-12	Cobalamin supplementation
Peripheral destruction	
Immune thrombocytopenia	Observation, Anti-D, intravenous immunoglobulin, steroids, splenectomy
Disseminated intravascular coagulation	Supportive care
	Platelet transfusion for severe bleeding, plasma infusion
HUS/TTP	Plasmapheresis (TTP)
	Supportive care
Splenic sequestration	Splenectomy if severe

Thrombotic thrombocytopenia purpura also occurs in this population [11, 12]. Splenomegaly may accentuate platelet sequestration.

Mild thrombocytopenia is generally asymptomatic, but when the platelet count falls below approximately 20–50 000/µL, mucosal bleeding (epistaxis, menorrhagia, mouth bleeding) and post-operative hemorrhage may ensue. Rarely, severe thrombocytopenia leads to intracranial hemorrhage [6]. Thrombocytopenia may be especially problematic in patients with hemophilia affected by HIV [30].

The development of easy bruising, petechiae, or unusual bleeding should prompt a diagnostic evaluation. The physical examination should evaluate the size, distribution, and age of petechiae and/or ecchymoses. Massive adenopathy may indicate malignancy or superimposed viral infection such as EBV or CMV. The child with DIC usually has a toxic appearance. Severe headache or neurologic abnormalities raise the possibility of intracranial hemorrhage, cerebral infarction, or TTP.

The laboratory evaluation begins with a complete blood count and careful review of the peripheral blood smear. Concomitant anemia or neutropenia suggest bone marrow infiltrate, failure, or infection. Red cell fragmentation is a feature of DIC or TTP/HUS. A bone marrow aspirate and biopsy should be considered early in the HIV-infected child with thrombocytopenia. In addition to routine histologic evaluation, marrow samples should be cultured for fungi and acid-fast bacilli. A DIC screen (prothrombin time, activated partial thromboplastin time, fibrinogen, and D-dimer or fibrin degradation products) should be performed in the toxic-appearing child. Platelet associated-immunoglobulin is unlikely to be helpful.

Management depends largely upon the patient's clinical status, the etiology and severity of the thrombocytopenia and physician/patient preference. For DIC, treatment of the underlying cause should be instituted immediately. Platelet and/or plasma transfusion is used to treat clinical bleeding. There might also be a role for anti-thrombin concentrates [31]. Thrombotic thrombocytopenia purpura is a rare life-threatening disorder, for which plasma exchange has been shown to improve survival [11, 32]. Other treatments tried but not studied by randomized clinical trial for TTP include corticosteroids, vincristine, intravenous immunoglobulin and splenectomy [33].

Antiretroviral therapy can raise the platelet count [25, 34, 35] and may provide durable responses. Patients with more severe thrombocytopenia, clinical bleeding or already receiving antiretroviral therapy usually need other treatments. Corticosteroids have long been used to treat immune thrombocytopenic purpura (ITP). Initial prednisone doses of 2–4 mg/kg/day have been used [36, 37]. One approach is to administer prednisone at 2 mg/kg/day for 2 weeks then taper or discontinue the medication. Short-term therapy with dexamethasone has been used in HIV-infected adults with immune thrombocytopenia [38]. High dose methylprednisolone (30 mg/kg/day for 3 days, maximum dose 1 gram) has also been reported to be effective in children with ITP [39], although the effectiveness of this approach in HIV-infected patients is unknown. While steroids often improve platelet counts in the HIV-infected patient, the effect is usually transient [40]. Long-term treatment is best avoided due to the toxicity of corticosteroids, especially osteopenia and fungal infection [41].

Intravenous immunoglobulin (IVIG) is widely used for management of immune thrombocytopenia. The mechanism of action likely involves blockade of the splenic Fc receptor. Advantages include a rapid response and relative safety. Responses to IVIG in HIV-infected patients with thrombocytopenia are well documented [40]. A total of 2 g/kg of IVIG is usually administered over 2–5 days. Common adverse effects include fever, headache, and vomiting. A severe headache requires immediate medical attention in the thrombocytopenic individual, as the differential diagnosis includes intracranial hemorrhage. Other problems with IVIG include its high cost, prolonged infusion time and the very small risk of transfusion-transmitted diseases.

Intravenous anti-D has also been effective in increasing platelet counts in HIV-infected children [28]. Anti-D binds to Rh-positive erythrocytes and causes splenic Fc blockade. It is not effective in patients who have the Rh-negative blood type or who have undergone splenectomy. Scaradavou *et al.* [28] reported on a large series of patients treated with anti-D that included 20 HIV-infected patients under 18 years of age. Seventy percent of this subgroup had an increase of $\geq 20\,000/\mu L$ and 45% increased $> 50\,000/\mu L$. Advantages of anti-D over IVIG include a brief intravenous infusion time and relatively few side-effects. Disadvantages include expense, although it is less expensive than IVIG, a theoretical risk of transfusion transmitted disease, and hemolysis. While hemolysis occurs, generally the decrease in hemoglobin is small and well tolerated. Rarely however, significant or even life-threatening hemolysis occurs.

Splenectomy should be considered for patients who do not tolerate or respond to anti-D or IVIG or who require long-term corticosteroid treatment. Ideally, splenectomy should be deferred for as long as possible in young children [42]. While splenectomy does not appear to accelerate the progression of HIV, it is associated with a risk for overwhelming bacterial infection. Prior to splenectomy, patients should be immunized against *Streptococcus pneumoniae*, *Haemophilus influenzae* type b, and *Neisseria meningitidis* [43]. However, it should be recognized that HIV-infected patients, particularly those with significant immunosuppression may not respond optimally to immunization [43]. Partial (subtotal) splenectomy was reported to be successful in a child with HIV-related immune thrombocytopenia [44]. While an occasional patient will have a prolonged response to splenic irradiation [45], in most patients there is a limited increase in the platelet count and a short duration of effect [45, 46].

32.4 Coagulation abnormalities

Both bleeding and thrombotic abnormalities have been described in HIV-infected children and adolescents. A list of hemostatic abnormalities in this population is provided in Table 32.4.

The population affected by hemophilia was one of the first identified as at risk for AIDS. A large proportion of this population become infected by HIV in the 1970s but the use of HIV-screened donor plasma, viral inactivation of plasma-derived anti-hemophilic factor concentrates and the use of recombinant factor concentrates have made these products safe from further transmission of HIV. Most of the HIV-infected hemophilia population is now outside of the pediatric age-range. Acquired bleeding disorders are also seen in HIV-infected patients including those

Table 32.4 Causes of and treatment for coagulation abnormalities in HIV-infected children and adolescents

Cause	Treatment
Bleeding disorders	
Factor VIII deficiency	Factor VIII concentrate
Factor IX deficiency	Factor IX concentrate
Von Willebrand disease	Desmopressin or von Willebrand factor-containing concentrates
Vitamin K deficiency	Vitamin K supplementation
	Fresh frozen plasma for severe bleeding
Liver disease	Vitamin K supplementation
	Fresh frozen plasma for severe bleeding
Prothrombotic disorders	
Lupus anticoagulant	Treatment for thrombosis
Protein S deficiency	Treatment for thrombosis
Heparin cofactor II deficiency	Treatment for thrombosis

due to medications which inhibit platelet function, vitamin K deficiency, or advanced liver disease, as may occur in individuals concomitantly infected with hepatitis B and/or hepatitis C.

Lupus anticoagulants are common in HIV-infected individuals [47]. While the lupus anticoagulant causes a prolonged partial thromboplastin time (PTT), bleeding is not usually a problem. Paradoxically, there is an increased risk of thrombosis. Deficiencies of the circulating anticoagulants protein S and heparin co-factor II are also seen in the HIV-infected population [48–50]. Deficiencies of these proteins are associated with an increased risk of thrombosis. Despite the laboratory evidence for hypercoagulability, the contribution of these factors to thrombosis in HIV-infected children is less clear. A high incidence of stroke in young adults with HIV has been shown [51]. Stroke in pediatric patients has also been described, although infection or other mechanisms may contribute to this complication [52, 53]. Patsalides *et al.* [54] found radiologic abnormalities in 11 of 426 pediatric HIV-infected patients who had undergone neuroimaging (either MRI or CT). Seven patients had a total of 26 cerebral aneurysms and eight patients had a total of 27 infarctions identified. Most of the infarctions were related to the aneurysms. Protein C deficiency was identified in one patient and protein S in two. Only one of these patients was symptomatic. In contrast, Dubrovsky *et al.* [55] reported a series of five patients in their care who had fatal cerebral aneurysms. In a retrospective review of hospitalized HIV-infected adults, deep vein thrombosis was identified in nearly 1% [56]. Central

venous catheters are a known risk factor for thrombosis in children.

Screening coagulation studies (prothrombin time (PT), PTT) will not detect deficiencies of circulating anticoagulants such as anti-thrombin, protein C, protein S, or heparin co-factor II. Therefore, these specific proteins need to be assayed if a deficiency is to be identified. In the patient with the lupus anticoagulant, the PTT is generally prolonged and does not correct when patient plasma is diluted 1:1 dilution with normal plasma. Confirmatory studies such as the dilute Russell viper venom time are available in many specialized laboratories.

For patients with congenital bleeding disorders, the underlying hemostatic abnormality must be considered as multiple new medications are introduced for management of HIV and its complications. There are reports of severe, unusual bleeding in hemophilia patients treated with protease inhibitors [57, 58]. The use of medications that inhibit platelet function, such as aspirin or non-steroidal anti-inflammatory agents, should be avoided in these individuals.

Anticoagulation is not routinely administered to patients with the lupus anticoagulant or deficiencies of circulating anticoagulants unless thrombosis occurs. However, early intervention is recommended for children and adolescents with thrombosis. A useful article on the management of thrombosis in children has been published [59]. For the patient with severe or recurrent thrombosis, the use of long-term anticoagulation should be entertained.

HIV infection and its treatments induce a wide range of hematologic abnormalities. The advent of improved antiretroviral therapy will likely lessen the direct impact of HIV on hematopoiesis. However, additional research is yet needed to determine the impact of these treatments on the blood. Advances in hematologic supportive care options will also improve the quality of life for HIV-infected individuals.

ACKNOWLEDGMENTS

The authors would like to acknowledge the administrative assistance of Jessica Jones, R.N. and Lorraine Nelson and the editorial assistance of Randall Fisher, M.D. and Hal Jenson, M.D.

REFERENCES

1. Ellaurie, M., Burns, E. R. & Rubinstein, A. Hematologic manifestations in pediatric HIV infection: severe anemia as a prognostic factor. *Am. J. Pediatr. Hematol. Oncol.* **12** (1990), 449–53.

2. Forsyth, B. W., Andiman, W. A. & O'Connor, T. Development of a prognosis-based clinical staging system for infants infected with human immunodeficiency virus. *J. Pediatr.* **129** (1996), 648–55.

3. Moore, R. D. Human immunodeficiency virus infection, anemia, and survival. *Clin. Infect. Dis.* **29** (1999), 44–9.

4. Moses, A., Nelson, J. & Bagby, G. C., Jr. The influence of human immunodeficiency virus-1 on hematopoiesis. *Blood* **91** (1998), 1479–95.

5. Coyle, T. E. Hematologic complications of human immunodeficiency virus infection and the acquired immunodeficiency syndrome. *Med. Clin. N. Am.* **81** (1997), 449–70.

6. Ellaurie, M., Burns, E. R., Bernstein, L. J., Shah, K. & Rubinstein, A. Thrombocytopenia and human immunodeficiency virus in children. *Pediatrics* **82** (1988), 905–8.

7. Koduri, P. R., Kumapley, R., Valladares, J. & Teter, C. Chronic pure red cell aplasia caused by parvovirus B19 in AIDS: use of intravenous immunoglobulin – a report of eight patients. *Am. J. Hematol.* **61** (1999), 16–20.

8. Mueller, B. U. Hematological problems and their management in children with HIV infection. In P. A. Pizzo & C. M. Wilfert (eds.), *Pediatric AIDS*. Baltimore: Williams and Wilkins Publishers (1994), pp. 591–601.

9. Rosenblatt, D. S. & Whitehead, V. M. Cobalamin and folate deficiency: acquired and hereditary disorders in children. *Semin. Hematol.* **36** (1999), 19–34.

10. Luzzatto, L. Glucose-6-phosphate dehydrogenase deficiency and hemolytic anemia. In D. G. Nathan & S. H. Orkin (eds.), *Hematologic Disease of Infancy and Childhood*, Vol. 1. Philadelphia: W. B. Saunders Company (1998), pp. 704–26.

11. Thompson, C. E., Damon, L. E., Ries, C. A. & Linker, C. A. Thrombotic microangiopathies in the 1980s: clinical features, response to treatment, and the impact of the human immunodeficiency virus epidemic. *Blood* **80** (1992), 1890–5.

12. Karpatkin, S., Nardi, M. & Green, D. Platelet and coagulation defects associated with HIV-1-infection. *Thromb. Haemost.* **88** (2002), 389–401.

13. Andrews, N. C. & Bridges, K. R. Disorders of iron metabolism and sideroblastic anemia. In D. G. Nathan & H. O. Stuart (eds.), *Hematology of Infancy and Childhood*, Vol. 1. Philadelphia: W. B. Saunders Company (1998), pp. 423–69.

14. Mueller, B. U., Tannenbaum, S. & Pizzo, P. A. Bone marrow aspirates and biopsies in children with human immunodeficiency virus infection. *J. Pediatr. Hematol. Oncol.* **18** (1996), 266–71.

15. Moore, R. D. Anemia and human immunodeficiency virus disease in the era of highly active antiretroviral therapy. *Semin. Hematol.* **37** (2000), 18–23.

16. Fischl, M., Galpin, J. E., Levine, J. D. *et al.* Recombinant human erythropoietin for patients with AIDS treated with zidovudine. *New Engl. J. Med.* **322** (1990), 1488–93.

17. Kline, M. W., Van Dyke, R. B., Lindsey, J. C. *et al.* A randomized comparative trial of stavudine (d4T) versus zidovudine (ZDV, AZT) in children with human immunodeficiency virus infection. AIDS Clinical Trials Group 240 Team. *Pediatrics* **101** (1998), 214–20.

18. Weinberg, G. A., Gigliotti, F., Stroncek, D. F. *et al.* Lack of relation of granulocyte antibodies (antineutrophil antibodies) to neutropenia in children with human immunodeficiency virus infection. *Pediatr. Infect. Dis. J.* **16** (1997), 881–4.

19. Kuritzkes, D. R., Parenti, D., Ward, D. J. *et al.* Filgrastim prevents severe neutropenia and reduces infective morbidity in patients with advanced HIV infection: results of a randomized, multicenter, controlled trial. G-CSF 930101 Study Group. *AIDS* **12** (1998), 65–74.

20. Eyster, M. E., Rabkin, C. S., Hilgartner, M. W. *et al.* Human immunodeficiency virus-related conditions in children and adults with hemophilia: rates, relationship to CD4 counts, and predictive value. *Blood* **81** (1993), 828–34.

21. Sloand, E. M., Klein, H. G., Banks, S. M., Vareldzis, B., Merritt, S. & Pierce, P. Epidemiology of thrombocytopenia in HIV infection. *Eur. J. Haematol.* **48** (1992), 168–72.

22. Glatt, A. E. & Anand, A. Thrombocytopenia in patients infected with human immunodeficiency virus: treatment update. *Clin. Infect. Dis.* **21** (1995), 415–23.

23. Zucker-Franklin, D. & Cao, Y. Z. Megakaryocytes of human immunodeficiency virus-infected individuals express viral RNA. *Proc. Natl. Acad. Sci. U.S.A* **86** (1989), 5595–9.

24. Cole, J. L., Marzec, U. M., Gunthel, C. J. *et al.* Ineffective platelet production in thrombocytopenic human immunodeficiency virus-infected patients. *Blood* **91** (1998), 3239–46.

25. Ballem, P., Belzberg, A., Devine, D. *et al.* Kinetic studies of the mechanism of thrombocytopenia in patients with human immunodeficiency virus infection. *New Engl. J. Med.* **327** (1992), 1779–84.

26. Karpatkin, S. Hemostatic abnormalities in AIDS. In R. W. Colman, J. Hirsh, V. J. Marder & E. W. Salzman (eds.), *Hemostasis and Thrombosis: Basic Principles and Clinical Practice.* Philadelphia: J. B. Lippincott Company (1994), pp. 969–80.

27. Nardi, M. & Karpatkin, S. Antiidiotype antibody against platelet anti-GPIIIa contributes to the regulation of thrombocytopenia in HIV-1-ITP patients. *J. Exp. Med.* **191** (2000), 2093–100.

28. Scaradavou, A., Woo, B., Woloski, B. M. *et al.* Intravenous anti-D treatment of immune thrombocytopenic purpura: experience in 272 patients. *Blood* **89** (1997), 2689–700.

29. Mueller, B. U., Burt, R., Gulick, L., Jacobsen, F., Pizzo, P. A. & Horne, M. Disseminated intravascular coagulation associated with granulocyte colony-stimulating factor therapy in a child with human immunodeficiency virus infection. *J. Pediatr.* **126** (1995), 749–52.

30. Ragni, M. V., Bontempi, F. A., Myers, D. J., Kiss, J. E. & Oral, A. Hemorrhagic sequelae of immune thrombocytopenic purpura in human immunodeficiency virus-infected hemophiliacs. *Blood* **75** (1990), 1267–72.

31. Kreuz, W. D., Schneider, W. & Nowak-Gottl, U. Treatment of consumption coagulopathy with antithrombin concentrate in children with acquired antithrombin deficiency – a feasibility pilot study. *Eur. J. Pediatr.* **158**: Suppl. 3 (1999), S187–91.

32. Prasad, V. K., Kim, I. K., Farrington, K. & Bussel, J. B. TTP following ITP in an HIV-positive boy. *J. Pediatr. Hematol. Oncol.* **18** (1996), 384–6.

33. Parker, R. I. Etiology and treatment of acquired coagulopathies in the critically ill adult and child. *Crit. Care. Clin.* **13** (1997), 591–609.

34. Hymes, K. B., Greene, J. B. & Karpatkin, S. The effect of azidothymidine on HIV-related thrombocytopenia. *New Engl. J. Med.* **318** (1988), 516–17.

35. Arranz Caso, J. A., Sanchez Mingo, C. & Garcia Tena, J. Effect of highly active antiretroviral therapy on thrombocytopenia in patients with HIV infection. *New Engl. J. Med.* **341** (1999), 1239–40.

36. Blanchette, V., Imbach, P., Andrew, M. *et al.* Randomised trial of intravenous immunoglobulin G, intravenous anti-D, and oral prednisone in childhood acute immune thrombocytopenic purpura. *Lancet* **344** (1994), 703–7.

37. Beardsley, D. S. & Nathan, D. G. Platelet abnormalities in infancy and childhood. In D. G. Nathan & S. H. Orkin (eds.), *Hematology of Infancy and Childhood.* Vol. 2. Philadelphia: W.B. Saunders Company (1998), pp. 1585–1630.

38. Ramratnam, B., Parameswaran, J., Elliot, B. *et al.* Short course dexamethasone for thrombocytopenia in AIDS. *Am. J. Med.* **100** (1996), 117–18.

39. van Hoff, J. & Ritchey, A. K. Pulse methylprednisolone therapy for acute childhood idiopathic thrombocytopenic purpura. *J. Pediatr.* **113** (1988), 563–6.

40. Bussel, J. B. & Haimi, J. S. Isolated thrombocytopenia in patients infected with HIV: treatment with intravenous gammaglobulin. *Am. J. Hematol.* **28** (1988), 79–84.

41. Singh, N., Yu, V. L. & Rihs, J. D. Invasive aspergillosis in AIDS. *South Med. J.* **84** (1991), 822–7.

42. Oksenhendler, E., Bierling, P., Chevret, S. *et al.* Splenectomy is safe and effective in human immunodeficiency virus-related immune thrombocytopenia [see comments]. *Blood* **82** (1993), 29–32.

43. Immunization in special clinical circumstances. In L. K. Pickering, G. Peter, C. J. Baker, M. A. Gerber, N. E. MacDonald & W. O. Orenstein (eds.), *2000 Red Book: Report of the Committee on Infectious Diseases.* Elk Grove, IL: *American Academy of Pediatrics* (2000), pp. 66–7.

44. Monpoux, F., Kurzenne, J. Y., Sirvent, N., Cottalorda, J. & Boutte, P. Partial splenectomy in a child with human immunodeficiency virus-related immune thrombocytopenia. *J. Pediatr. Hematol. Oncol.* **21** (1999), 441–3.

45. Blauth, J., Fisher, S., Henry, D. & Nichini, F. The role of splenic irradiation in treating HIV-associated immune thrombocytopenia. *Int. J. Radiat. Oncol. Biol. Phys.* **45** (1999), 457–60.

46. Marroni, M., Sinnone, M. S., Landonio, G. *et al.* Splenic irradiation versus splenectomy for severe, refractory HIV-related thrombocytopenia: effects on platelet counts and immunological status. *AIDS* **14** (2000), 1664–7.

47. Bloom, E. J., Abrams, D. I. & Rodgers, G. Lupus anticoagulant in the acquired immunodeficiency syndrome. *J. Am. Med. Assoc.* **256** (1986), 491–3.

48. Stahl, C. P., Wideman, C. S., Spira, T. J., Haff, E. C., Hixon, G. J. & Evatt, B. L. Protein S deficiency in men with long-term human immunodeficiency virus infection. *Blood* **81** (1993), 1801–7.

49. Sugerman, R. W., Church, J. A., Goldsmith, J. C. & Ens, G. E. Acquired protein S deficiency in children infected with human immunodeficiency virus. *Pediatr. Infect. Dis. J.* **15** (1996), 106–11.

50. Toulon, P., Lamine, M., Ledjev, I. *et al.* Heparin cofactor II deficiency in patients infected with the human immunodeficiency virus. *Thromb. Haemost.* **70** (1993), 730–5.

51. Qureshi, A. I., Janssen, R. S., Karon, J. M. *et al.* Human immunodeficiency virus infection and stroke in young patients. *Arch. Neurol.* **54** (1997), 1150–3.

52. Park, Y. D., Belman, A. L., Kim, T. S. *et al.* Stroke in pediatric acquired immunodeficiency syndrome. *Ann. Neurol.* **28** (1990), 303–11.

53. Philippet, P., Blanche, S., Sebag, G., Rodesch, G., Griscelli, C. & Tardieu, M. Stroke and cerebral infarcts in children infected with human immunodeficiency virus. *Arch. Pediatr. Adolesc. Med.* **148** (1994), 965–70.

54. Patsalides, A. D., Wood, L. V., Atac, G. K., Sandifer, E., Butman, J. A. & Patronas, N. J. Cerebrovascular disease in HIV-infected pediatric patients: neuroimaging findings. *Am. J. Roentgenol.* **179** (2002), 999–1003.

55. Dubrovsky, T., Curless, R., Scott, G. *et al.* Cerebral aneurysmal arteriopathy in childhood AIDS. *Neurology* **51** (1998), 560–5.

56. Saber, A. A., Aboolian, A., LaRaja, R. D., Baron, H. & Hanna, K. HIV/AIDS and the risk of deep vein thrombosis: a study of

45 patients with lower extremity involvement. *Am. Surg.* **67** (2001), 645–7.

57. Wilde, J. T., Lee, C. A., Collins, P., Giangrande, P. L., Winter, M. & Shiach, C. R. Increased bleeding associated with protease inhibitor therapy in HIV-positive patients with bleeding disorders. *Br. J. Haematol.* **107** (1999), 556–9.

58. Racoosin, J. A. & Kessler, C. M. Bleeding episodes in HIV-positive patients taking HIV protease inhibitors: a case series. *Haemophilia* **5** (1999), 266–9.

59. Monagle, P., Michelson, A. D., Bovill, E. & Andrew, M. Antithrombotic therapy in children. *Chest* **119** (2001), 344S–70S.

Gastrointestinal disorders

Harland S. Winter, M.D.[1] and Jack Moye, Jr, M.D.[2]

[1]Division of Pediatric Gastroenterology and Nutrition, Massachusetts General Hospital for Children, Boston, MA
[2]Pediatric, Adolescent, and Maternal AIDS Branch, NICHD, Bethesda, MS

33.1 Introduction

Gastrointestinal (GI) dysfunction, a common occurrence in children with HIV disease, can be related to infectious agents, malnutrition, immunodeficiency, or HIV infection itself, and can result in retardation of growth, increased caloric requirements, and/or diarrhea/malabsorption. The absorption and utilization of nutrients is a primary function of the GI tract, but the immune system of the gut has been shown to be the major site of CD4$^+$ lymphocyte depletion and viral replication [1]. The mucosal immune and enteric nervous systems interact with the epithelium to regulate intestinal function. Lymphocytes and macrophages produce cytokines and vasoactive peptides that can alter brush border epithelial cell enzyme expression, secretion, motility, or mucosal blood flow. These factors ultimately affect nutrient absorption. As immune function deteriorates in the HIV-infected child, intestinal function declines to a degree greater than might be expected due to opportunistic infections alone. The goal of this chapter is to present the GI aspects of HIV disease so that clinicians will begin intervention in the early stages of the disease, thereby minimizing the impact on growth and development.

33.2 The role of the GI tract in pathogenesis of HIV

HIV is acquired via the mucosa of the genital tract in most cases of heterosexual transmission and via the GI tract in most cases of mother-to-child transmission (MTCT). HIV infection of a child can occur through swallowing infected amniotic fluid in utero, or infected blood or cervical secretions during delivery and/or through ingesting infected breast milk in the postnatal period [2]. The mucosal immune system of the GI tract plays an important role in initial HIV infection as well as in the establishment and progression of HIV disease.

33.2.1 The role of the GI tract in transmission

HIV can cross the intestinal epithelium through ulcerations, damaged epithelial cells, M cells, or dendritic cells. M cells are specialized epithelial cells that cover lymphoid aggregates or Peyer's patches in the intestine. Antigens pass through these cells on their way to be processed by macrophages and presented to T cells. The concentrations of virus in the blood and in the genital tract are correlated, and viral load is a major factor in determining the risk of MTCT during birth [3]. In addition, mucosal infections such as *Mycobacterium avium* complex increase the expression of CCR5, the chemokine receptor for macrophage-trophic HIV [4]. Because most transmitted strains of HIV are macrophage trophic, mucosal infections that increase CCR5 expression potentiate acquisition of the macrophage-trophic (R5) HIV. Conversely, a nucleotide deletion in the gene that encodes for CCR5, a mutation found in about 1% of the white population, results in the inability to acquire macrophage trophic HIV [5]. The newborn GI tract is more permeable than the mucosa of the adult and this might contribute as well to the susceptibility of the neonate to acquisition of HIV infection during delivery.

33.2.2 The role of the GI tract in progression of disease

Once present in the GI tract, HIV is transported by M cells to mononuclear cells. Although there are M cells in human tonsil and rectum that in theory could act as a portal for viral entry into the mucosal system, the presence of virus within these cells has not as yet been demonstrated in humans. However, animal studies in the mouse and rabbit provide evidence of the role of M cells in the pathogenesis of HIV [6]. Dendritic cells can be found in the human tonsil, adenoid, and colon; however, the role of these cells in the pathogenesis of HIV in the human small or large colon is unclear. Dendritic cells bind the HIV envelope protein gp20 by utilizing a C-type lectin [7]. These cells express CD4 and are very efficient at binding HIV and presenting it to T cells that subsequently migrate to other lymphoid tissues. Dendritic cell-specific intercellular adhesion molecule (ICAM)-grabbing non-integrin, DC-SIGN is a C-type lectin that plays an important role in the activation of T lymphocytes. The presence of DC-SIGN at mucosal surfaces provides circumstantial evidence of the role of this lectin in potentiating entry of HIV into deeper tissues [8]. Intestinal epithelial cells also can play a role in the movement of HIV across the mucosa. Intestinal epithelial cells do not express the chemokine receptor for lymphotrophic HIV, X4, or for CD4, the primary receptor on lymphocytes. Smith and colleagues demonstrated, in freshly isolated intestinal epithelial cells, that galactosylceramide (GalCer) is an alternate primary receptor for HIV and CCR5 [9]. Thus, intestinal epithelial cells are capable of transferring macrophage-trophic HIV to cells that express the chemokine receptor CCR5 and could play a role in the acquisition of macrophage-trophic strains of HIV. Irrespective of the mechanism by which HIV enters the lamina propria of the mucosa, intestinal lymphocytes that express both CCR5 and CXCR4 are able to support the replication of both macrophage- and lymphocyte-trophic strains of HIV.

The macaque model has been used to study the early phase of intestinal mucosal infection with SIV. Large numbers of activated CD4+ lymphocytes reside in the lamina propria, close to the site of HIV entry, making them prime targets for infection [1]. Infection of macrophages is rare during initial HIV infection. In the days following an acute HIV infection, the viral load is high in the intestinal mucosa, a finding that seems to correlate with villous atrophy and nutrient malabsorption [10]. About 2 weeks later, cell lysis and apoptosis in the lamina propria lymphoid population results in severe depletion of CD4+ mucosal T cells. These alterations in the mucosal immune system precede depression of the peripheral blood CD4+ count [11, 12]. These data support the hypothesis that mucosal lymphocytes are infected initially, and that these infected lymphocytes then disseminate HIV through the circulation to other lymphoid tissues.

During MTCT of HIV, certain features of the newborn GI tract, such as decreased acid production during the first 3 days of life, can increase the numbers of swallowed viral particles that remain available to infect mucosal lymphocytes. Infection of lamina propria lymphocytes eventually results in a depletion of mucosal lymphocytes and an increase in the viral load in the mucosa. The villous injury and resulting nutrient malabsorption that can accompany primary infection via the GI tract can have particular significance for infants. In the infant, malabsorption of specific nutrients, or a decrease in calories that are absorbed, can lead to malnutrition. Protein-calorie malnutrition, independent of the etiology, will cause or, in the case of an HIV-infected individual, potentiate T cell immunodeficiency. As the systemic and mucosal immune systems deteriorate, the individual becomes more susceptible to both enteric and systemic infection. Fever, as well as naturally occurring or opportunistic infections, increase metabolic needs. Enteric infection also increases the severity of malabsorption. Thus, a cycle of malabsorption, malnutrition, and infection is established and can only be broken by controlling viral load and providing sufficient nutrition to support growth.

In a prospective, longitudinal study of growth in children born to HIV-infected mothers in Europe [13], at 10 years of age, uninfected children weighed approximately 7 kg more and were 7.5 cm taller than infected children. HIV-infected children who were asymptomatic grew at similar rates to those HIV-infected children with mild to moderate symptoms. More severely ill children grew more slowly throughout their first 10 years of life. The uninfected, HIV-exposed child has a growth velocity between 96 and 120 months of age of 6.30 cm/year compared with 5.69 cm/year for the symptomatic HIV-infected child. Weight gain also appears to be delayed (4.27 vs 3.06 kg/year). These observations suggest that the presence of HIV infection, even in the mildly symptomatic or asymptomatic child, can affect growth. In a 24-month study of the impact of highly active antiretroviral therapy (HAART) [14], there was a beneficial effect on both weight and height, especially in children who experienced a reduction in viral load to < 500 copies/mL and an increase in CD4+ T cell number. Correlation with mucosal immune function is not available, but one can speculate that the changes that are observed

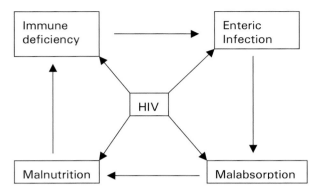

Figure 33.1. The cycle of events leading to clinical deterioration and growth retardation in HIV-infected children.

in the peripheral blood also occur in the mucosa, resulting in restoration of the absorptive surface, enhanced nutrient absorption, and improved growth.

33.3 GI problems of HIV-infected children

During acute infection with HIV, GI symptoms are rare. Older children can experience a "flu-like" illness, but most infants infected through MTCT are asymptomatic. One of the earliest clinical manifestations of HIV infection in children is growth retardation and slow weight gain. These changes in growth can occur as early as 2 months of age and do not appear to be related to concomitant, e.g. opportunistic, infection [15–17]. Older children and adults with HIV disease have decreased lean body mass and relative preservation of fat mass [18]. Alterations in body composition in infants with primary HIV infection have yet to be studied directly, though progressive decrements in body mass index during the first 6 months of life have been observed in HIV-infected infants [2].

With progression of HIV infection, patients can develop enteric infections, increased caloric requirements, and malabsorption. Changes in GI function also can affect nutrient utilization and growth. Decreased acid production in the stomach (achlorhydria), by eliminating the normal gastric acid barrier, predisposes to bacterial overgrowth. Mucosal immune dysfunction can result in decreased mucosal IgA that is targeted against specific pathogens, thereby reducing one of the important mechanisms of protection against enteric pathogens. HIV-infected individuals can produce excessive amounts of antibodies, but the quality or the specificity of the antibody is thought to be poor. Although not yet evaluated in the intestinal lumen of HIV-infected children, one assumes that this process

Table 33.1 Signs and symptoms of GI disease by location of primary lesion

Location of primary lesion	Signs and symptoms
Mouth	Pain with chewing, anorexia, poor weight gain
Esophagus	Dysphagia, odynophagia, retrosternal or subxyphoid pain, anorexia, poor weight gain
Stomach	Nausea, vomiting, early satiety, epigastric pain, hematemesis, pallor, melena
Small intestine	Abdominal pain (usually periumbilical), watery diarrhea, abdominal distention, early satiety, flatulence, poor weight gain, or weight loss
Colon	Abdominal pain (usually lower abdomen), bloody diarrhea, poor weight gain or weight loss
Liver	Fever of unknown origin, jaundice, dark urine, clay-colored stool, pruritis
Pancreas	Abdominal pain (usually during or after meals), anorexia, fever, weight loss, diarrhea

pertains to the mucosal immune system as well as the systemic immune system.

The absorptive capacity of the GI tract is altered in HIV-infected children. Activity of brush border enzymes, particularly lactase, the enzyme required for metabolism of the sugar found in milk, is decreased [19]. Lactose intolerance can present challenges in selecting an appropriate diet for a child because many foods that children like contain milk or milk products. With progression of HIV, systemic immune function declines, and children develop enteric infections that exacerbate malabsorption and malnutrition. Since malnutrition further impairs immune function, particularly T cell function, a cycle of immunodeficiency, enteric infection, malabsorption, and malnutrition results in clinical deterioration and growth retardation. Other brush border enzymes responsible for absorption of proteins and other carbohydrates decrease as HIV continues to drive this cycle (Figure 33.1).

Careful attention to a patient's signs and symptoms should guide the approach to diagnosis and therapy. In the following section, GI tract diseases will be examined by clinical presentation. When possible, a link will be made between symptoms and pathophysiology (Table 33.1).

33.4 Evaluation and management of GI disorders

33.4.1 Anorexia or dysphagia

In the pediatric population, any discomfort with eating can result in anorexia (Table 33.2). Older children can identify pain with chewing or abdominal pain, but younger children and infants can only refuse to eat. In the HIV-infected child, there are many causes of food refusal. The initial manifestation of disease in the mouth is often decreased oral intake and poor weight gain. Although HIV-infected children with parotitis can have decreased caloric intake, impaired salivary secretion of amylase rarely impacts on the digestion of starch. A careful evaluation of the mouth, gums, and teeth should be included in the physical examination. Herpes simplex virus infection, linear gingival erythema, and recurrent aphthous ulcers are commonly found in the oral cavity of HIV-infected children. Culture of the lesion will help identify the pathogen. In addition, children with HIV infection frequently have poor dental hygiene and can have extensive caries, dental abscesses, and gingivitis, causing painful chewing and potential decreases in oral intake (see Chapter 28). Routine dental care is critical for proper management and should be part of the multidisciplinary team approach to caring for HIV-infected children. In children in whom there is no identifiable etiology for anorexia, increased disease activity associated with circulating cytokines such as tumor necrosis factor can decrease appetite. Medications such as megestrol acetate have been prescribed in adults with AIDS wasting and appear to be effective in increasing weight. However, results are not as encouraging in the pediatric population among whom weight is increased, but linear growth is not sustained (see Chapter 16). The side-effect of diabetes mellitus impacts on the use of megestrol in children and it should not be given to any child with lipodystrophy.

Pain with swallowing (odynophagia) should alert the provider to consider an invasive infectious or inflammatory process in the esophageal mucosa (e.g. *Candida* esophagitis). Although esophageal ulceration associated with gastroesophageal acid reflux can cause dysphagia, any symptoms associated with swallowing in the HIV-infected child are likely to be caused by infectious agents such as *Candida* species, cytomegalovirus, or herpes simplex virus (Table 33.3). In the oral cavity, *Candida* infection can be evident as exudative plaques on any mucosal surface, red and atrophic lesions on the palate or tongue, or erythematous fissures at the corners of the mouth, termed angular cheilitis. However, many children with candidiasis of the esophagus may not have evidence for the infection in the mouth. If lesions compatible with thrush are identified, treatment with fluconazole should be effective within 5 days. If dysphagia is not improved during this time, an upper endoscopy is recommended to identify other causes of esophagitis. A barium swallow is usually not sufficiently sensitive to identify esophageal ulcerations. If oral lesions are not identified, upper endoscopy is recommended for the child with chronic dysphagia or odynophagia. Multiple adherent white-yellow plaques can cover the lining of the esophagus and suggest a diagnosis of candidiasis. However, yeast forms on mucosal biopsy or from a mucosal scraping are essential to establish a diagnosis of invasive *Candida* species. *Candida* esophagitis often responds to oral fluconazole (3–6 mg/kg once daily, with a maximum dose of 200 mg). Intravenous amphotericin B should be reserved for those children who fail initial therapy. Improvement in immune function often results in resolution of candidiasis and should not be overlooked as an important component of treatment.

Co-infection with other pathogens is not uncommon. Discrete ulcers with well demarcated borders are suggestive of cytomegalovirus. Intranuclear inclusions with confirmatory immunohistochemical staining support a diagnosis of cytomegalovirus, but culture of mucosal biopsy is necessary for confirmation. Herpes simplex virus esophagitis can be characterized by a diffuse, hemorrhagic appearing esophageal mucosa or by small vesicles with superficial ulcerations. As with other pathogens, mucosal biopsy and culture are confirmatory. Both herpes simplex virus and cytomegalovirus should be treated with ganciclovir, acyclovir, or foscarnet. The decision of which agent to use depends upon the degree of immunodeficiency and the presence of extra-intestinal infections, such as cytomegaloviral retinitis. Rarely in children, *Histoplasma capsulatum* and *Cryptococcus neoformans* can cause painful ulcerations in the oropharynx. Zidovudine or zalcitabine can cause injury to the mouth or esophagus if not cleared rapidly into the stomach. Children should be reminded to always drink a full glass of water when taking medications. Tumors, such as Kaposi's sarcoma of the esophagus and lymphoma, are rare in HIV-infected children in the USA, but should be considered in severely immunocompromised children with intractable progressive weight loss. In some regions of the world, such as sub-Saharan Africa, these malignancies are much more common and should occupy a more prominent consideration in the differential diagnosis of dysphagia and odynophagia.

33.4.2 Nausea and vomiting

Nausea and vomiting are usually caused by gastritis, enteritis, pancreatitis, dysmotility, or medication. By producing

Table 33.2 Recognition and management of GI disorders in HIV-infected children [20]

Signs and symptoms	Differential diagnosis	Evaluation	Management
Dysphagia or anorexia	Disease localized to the mouth and/or esophagus		
	Thrush	Examination, scraping for KOH preparation, culture for *Candida*	Nystatin, clotrimazole, ketoconazole, fluconazole, Amphotericin B with or without flucytosine
	Stomatitis/esophagitis	Culture for cytomegalovirus, herpes simplex virus	Acyclovir, ganciclovir, foscarnet
	Hairy leukoplakia	Exam, biopsy for Epstein-Barr virus, human papilloma virus	May resolve without treatment
	Periodontal disease	Dental evaluation	Dental hygiene, topical chlorhexidine
	Oral ulcers	Check for neutropenia; stop zalcitabine if appropriate	Steroids in some patients
	Medication	Zalcitabine (ddC); stomatitis 2–17%	Often self-limited
		Zidovudine (ZDV); anorexia	Discontinue therapy
		Hydroxyurea; stomatitis 8%	Discontinue therapy
		Ritonavir (RTV); anorexia, dysgeusia 10%	Discontinue therapy
Nausea and vomiting	Diseases localized to the stomach:		
	H. pylori	Serum antibody	Double or triple antibiotic regimen and proton pump inhibitor
		Upper endoscopy and biopsy	
		Urea breath test	
		Rapid urease test on antral biopsy	
		Stool antigen	
	Candidiasis	Upper endoscopy and biopsy	Clotrimazole, ketoconazole, fluconazole, Amphotericin B with or without flucytosine
	Cryptosporidium	Stool analysis using concentration technique prior to staining with modified Kinyoun acid-fast stain or upper endoscopy with biopsy	Paromomycin, azithromycin, nitazoxanide and bovine colostrum (investigational)
	Non-intestinal causes:		Discontinue therapy, substitute as appropriate
	Medication	Review medications: Abacavir (ABC), nausea 45%, vomiting 15%; lamivudine (3TC), zidovudine (ZDV), nausea 4–26%, vomiting 3–8%; stavudine (d4T), 26%; adefovir and ZDV/3TC, mild nausea and vomiting 1–8%; nevirapine (NVP); delavirdine (DLV), nausea 7%; saquinavir (SQC); ritonavir (RTV); indinavir (IDV); amprenavir, vomiting 7–33%; hydroxyurea, nausea 12%, vomiting; trimethoprim-sulfamethoxazole; trimethoprim-dapsone; clindamycin; primaquine; atovaquone; pentamidine isoethionate; sulfadiazine; atovaquone; azithromycin; dapsone; clarithromycin	

Table 33.2 (*cont.*)

Signs and symptoms	Differential diagnosis	Evaluation	Management
	Central nervous system lesion	CT scan of the head	Dependent on cause
Diarrhea	Disease localized primarily to the small intestine:		
	Salmonella	Clinitest or fecal fat, stool cultures, ova and parasite examination, blood culture if fever present	Pathogen-specific therapy
	Shigella		
	Campylobacter		
	Giardia lamblia		
	Cryptosporidium		
	Cytomegalovirus		
	Mycobacterium avium intracellulare		
	Lactose intolerance	Lactose breathe hydrogen test	
	Disease localized to the colon:		
	Cytomegalovirus	Check for blood in the stool, fecal WBC exam, blood culture if fever present Endoscopy, culture or biopsy lesions	Acyclovir, ganciclovir, forcarnet
	C. difficile	*C. difficile* stool toxin assay if indicated	Metronidazole, oral vancomycin, avoid antiperistaltic agents
	Medication	Review medications: didanosine (ddI), 16%; stavudine (d4T), 33%; lamivudine (3TC), mild transient; abacavir (ABC), 25%; adefovir dipivoxil; ZDV-3TC; delavirdine (DLV) 4%; sequinavir; ritonavir (RTV); indinavir (IDV); nelfinavir (NLF) 2–19%; amprenavir; Lopinavir/ritonavir, 10–20%; hydroxyurea	Discontinue therapy if symptoms are severe or persistent
Hepatomegaly, jaundice or elevated aminotransferases	Nutritional	Abdominal ultrasound	Enteral nutrition
	Obstruction of the common bile duct: malignancy, infection	Abdominal ultrasound	Depends on cause and clinical status
	Medication	Review medications: zidovudine (ZDV), steatosis; didanosine (ddI), 6–20%; stavudine (d4T), 65%; abacavir (ABC), 2–5% have hypersensitivity reaction with elevated AST/ALT; adefovir dipivoxil and ZDV3TC, 4%; nevirapine (NVP), 1%; delavirdine (DLV), <5%; ritonavir (RTV), 10–15%; indinavir (IDV), 10%; ABT 378 (lopinavir-ritonavir), 8%; hydroxyurea, 2%	Discontinue medication
Abdominal pain	Enteric pathogen	Stool analysis	Treatment dependent upon stool analysis

(*cont.*)

Table 33.2 (*cont.*)

Signs and symptoms	Differential diagnosis	Evaluation	Management
	Medication	Review medications: stavudine (d4T), 23%; lamivudine (3TC); abacavir (ABC), 15%; saquinavir (SQC); ritonavir (RTV), 20–40%; indinavir (IDV), 4–15%;	For Abacavir, abdominal pain may decrease after weeks of therapy
	Lactose intolerance	Lactose breath test	Lactose free diet
	Pancreatitis: idiopathic	Abdominal ultrasound	Bowel rest
	Cryptosporidium	Serum lipase and amylase	Nutrition support with or without total parenteral nutrition as needed
	Cytomegalovirus	Endoscopic retrograde cholangiopancreatography with culture and/or biopsy	
	Medication	Review medications: didanosine (ddI), 4–8%; zalcitabine (ddC), 0.5–9%; nelfinavir (NLF); stavudine (d4T); clindamycin-primaquine; atovaquone; azithromycin; clarithromycin; pentamidine	Discontinue implicated medication, substitute therapy as appropriate
GI bleeding	Hematemesis	Upper endoscopy	Depends on cause
	Hematochezia	Sigmoidoscopy	Depends on cause

Reference [20].

acid, the stomach serves as an important barrier for the prevention of bacteria colonizing the upper GI tract. To prevent peptic injury to the esophagus from gastroesophageal reflux, clinicians can initiate acid suppression treatment with H_2 blockers or proton pump inhibitors. Prolonged and sustained hypochlorhydria, as achieved with high dose H_2 antagonists or proton pump inhibitors, can result in *Candida* overgrowth in the stomach. Other agents, such as antacids, are not as effective at neutralizing acid and rarely result in severe hypochlorhydria. *Helicobacter pylori*, a common gastric pathogen associated with chronic gastritis and duodenal ulcer, can also cause hypochlorhydria, but has been reported infrequently in the HIV-infected child [21]. Other pathogens such as cytomegalovirus, herpes simplex virus, *Candida*, or the intestinal parasite *Cryptosporidium* can present with nausea and vomiting caused by inflammation in the stomach. Upper endoscopy and mucosal biopsy is often helpful in identifying specific causes and guiding treatment. A diagnosis of *H. pylori* infection can be established by non-invasive methods such as stool antigen or urea breath test. Serologic tests are not reliable in the pediatric population and this is most likely

even more relevant for the HIV-infected child. Many of the medications used to treat children with HIV disease cause nausea and vomiting (Table 33.2). Abacavir (ABC), lamivudine (3TC), zidovudine (ZDV), and stavudine (d4T) are most commonly associated with nausea and vomiting. Although not well characterized in the pediatric population, one suspects that many of these medications injure the mucosa, resulting in gastritis and possible ulceration. When tolerated, giving medications with food can prevent some of these symptoms.

33.4.3 Diarrhea and GI bleeding

Diarrhea is a very common clinical manifestation of HIV disease, especially as the immune system deteriorates and viral load increases. For this reason, diarrhea has been seen throughout the pandemic as a clinical indicator of deteriorating immune function and disease progression. During this phase of the disease, the number of prescribed medications increases. Many cause diarrhea. In the early phases of HIV infection, some patients can experience an acute, self-limited diarrheal illness. With progression of

Table 33.3 Infectious agents causing esophageal injury in HIV-infected children

Bacterial agents
  Mycobacterium avium complex
  Mycobacterium tuberculosis
Viral agents
  Cytomegalovirus
  HIV
  Epstein–Barr virus
  Herpes simplex virus
Fungal agents
  Candida albicans
  Torulopsis glabrata
  Histoplasma capsulatum
Protozoal agents
  Cryptosporidium
  Pneumocystis carinii
  Leishmania species

HIV disease and concomitant immune dysfunction, AIDS enteropathy characterized by malabsorption can develop. The mechanism of this enteropathy is not well understood. There appears to be injury to the epithelium without identification of a specific pathogen. Perhaps the mucosal immune system plays a role in the maintenance of epithelial function and deterioration of immune function results in epithelial dysfunction and malabsorption. In the late stages of the illness, parasitic, viral, bacterial, and fungal infections contribute to diarrhea and malnutrition.

The differential diagnosis of diarrhea in the pediatric population includes infectious agents, allergic conditions (such as milk or soy intolerance in infants), lactose intolerance, inflammatory bowel disorders, antibiotic-associated colitis, and malabsorption syndromes. Intestinal pathogens can be difficult to identify unless they can be found in the stool [22]. Enteric pathogens such as *Mycobacterium avium* complex (MAC) and *Cryptosporidium* may not be evident in the stool in early stages of the infection but can cause profuse diarrhea. Other intestinal pathogens, such as S*almonella, Shigella, Campylobacter, Clostridium difficile,* and *Giardia lamblia*, are easier to identify by examinations of the stool or culture and may not cause the profound diarrhea seen in other enteric pathogens. Herpes simplex virus and cytomegalovirus can cause focal ulcerations that bleed. Patients infected with these pathogens can present with melena, hemetemesis or hematochezia as well as with bloody diarrhea. Endoscopic evaluation, biopsy, and culture of ulcers often establish the diagnosis. Both herpes simplex virus and cytomegalovirus can be cul-

tured from stool of patients without mucosal ulcerations or injury. The most common enteric pathogens found in the pediatric population are listed in Table 33.2. Microsporidia, *Entamoeba histolytica, Isospora bella*, and malignancies such as Kaposi's sarcoma are quite rare in children and are not frequent causes of diarrhea.

In children without an identifiable enteric pathogen, testing for lactose intolerance with a non-invasive test such as the lactose breath hydrogen test can provide a clue to the cause of the symptom. HIV-infected children develop lactose intolerance earlier than expected based upon genetic predisposition. By age 5 years, many will be lactose intolerant, but many may not exhibit classical symptoms [23]. However, there does not appear to be a direct relationship between lactose intolerance, malabsorption, and delayed weight gain or growth. This observation leaves the clinician to determine if removing lactose-containing foods from the diet will result in improvement of diarrheal symptoms or eliminate an important source of calories that will eventually result in reduced caloric intake and weight loss.

The evaluation of diarrhea includes a thorough history and physical examination. Careful assessment of weight and growth provide important clues about malabsorption. Bulky, malodorous stools are found in children with pancreatic insufficiency; whereas, malabsorption from injury to the small intestine usually causes watery diarrhea. Bloody diarrhea is seen in colitis. The presence of fecal leukocytes supports a diagnosis of colitis; whereas carbohydrate in the stool as demonstrated by a positive Clinitest assay for reducing substances or fecal fat detected by Sudan stain of stool supports a disorder associated with small intestinal injury. Radiographic studies have little role in the initial evaluation of diarrhea. Culture of the stool for enteric pathogens yields the best chance to identify treatable causes. For many enteric pathogens, identification may only be possible by endoscopic evaluation that permits sampling of duodenal fluid and/or mucosal tissue. Visual and biopsy findings from endoscopy can change medical management in over two-thirds of children [24].

Melena and hematemesis are usually caused by lesions in the stomach, esophagus, mouth, or nasopharynx. Neutropenic ulcers can be troublesome to manage, but rarely result in significant blood loss. Although rare in the pediatric population, tumors of the GI tract can present with GI bleeding. Kaposi's sarcoma is the most common malignancy associated with HIV disease, followed by lymphoma. The GI tract is involved about one third of the time [25]. Blood loss can occur also with lymphoma, and the cauliflower-like masses also can cause intestinal obstruction. Smooth muscle tumors such as leiomyoma

Table 33.4 Selected therapies for common enterocolonic pathogens in children

Pathogen	Treatment
Salmonella	ampicillin, amoxicillin, trimethoprim-sulfamethoxazole, cefotaxime, ceftriaxone
Shigella	ampicillin, trimethoprim-sulfamethoxazole, cefixime, ceftriaxone, cefotaxime, ciprofloxacin, ofloxacin
Campylobacter	erythromycin, ciprofloxacin
Giardia lamblia	metronidazole, tinidazole, furazolidone, paromomycin
Cryptosporidium	paromomycin, azithromycin, nitazoxanide (investigational), hyperimmune bovine colostrum (investigational)
Cytomegalovirus	Ganciclovir, foscarnet
Mycobacterium avium intracellulare	clarithromycin or azithromycin plus ethambutol; additionally rifabutin, rifampin, clofazimine, ciprofloxacin, or amikacin

and leiomyosarcoma are rare in children, but have been described in association with GI blood loss [26].

Treatment depends on the specific cause of the diarrhea (Table 33.4). For example, several drugs are effective against giardiasis, including metronidazole (15 mg/kg/day in three doses for 5 days) which is effective in over 80% of children. Quinacrine, 2 mg/kg tid for 5 days (maximum dose 300 mg/day) and paromomycin (Humatin), 25–35 mg/kg/day in three doses for 7 days also have been used to treat *Giardia lamblia* infections.

The anti-protozoal agent, nitazoxanide [27] has been approved by the FDA for treatment of diarrhea caused by *Cryptosporidium parvum* and *Giardia lamblia* in children ages 1–11 years old. This medication is available in a liquid formulation, and is well absorbed from the GI tract. Peak serum concentrations are achieved within 1–4 hours. The active metabolite, tizoxanide, is then glucuronidated prior to excretion in the urine (30%) and stool (60%). The mechanism of action of this drug is not known, but inhibition of the pyruvate : ferredoxin oxidoreductase enzyme-dependent electron transfer reactions are thought to be important. Nitazoxanide appears to be effective against

other enteric pathogens such as *Isospora belli, Entamoeba histolytica, Balantidium coli*, and helminthes (*Ascaris lumbridoides, Enterobius vermicularis, Ancylostoma duodenale, Trichuris trichiura, Taenia saginate, Hymenolepsis nana, Strongyloides stercoralis*, and *Fasciola hepatica*). Yellow sclerae rarely occurs, but is related to deposition of the medication and resolves upon completing treatment. Other side-effects such as headache, abdominal pain, diarrhea, and vomiting do not occur more frequently than placebo. The efficacy of nitazoxanide seems to differ in HIV-infected and HIV-uninfected children. In a randomized controlled trial of children less than 3 years of age with cryptosporidiosis, 100 mg nitazoxanide twice daily for 3 days resulted in improvement in 56% of the HIV-uninfected children compared to 23% of HIV-uninfected children who received placebo. However, in the HIV-infected children in the same study, there was no difference in the response rate in the groups treated with nitazoxanide or placebo. For treating giardiasis, nitazoxanide was as effective as metronidazole. The recommended dose for treating giardiasis for children 12–47 months old is 100 mg (5 mL) q12 hours for 3 days. For children 4–11 years old, the dose is 200 mg (10 mL) q12 hours for 3 days. Currently nitazoxanide is not approved for use in adults [27].

33.4.4 Hepatomegaly and jaundice

Although hepatomegaly and mildly elevated liver function tests are common findings in HIV-infected children, chronic and progressive liver disease is unusual. Steatosis, most commonly associated with nutritional deficiencies, is one of the most common causes for an enlarged liver and elevated transaminases. Other conditions in the differential diagnosis include hepatitis B, hepatitis C, MAC infection, Epstein–Barr viral hepatitis, cytomegalovirus, and drug toxicity. Of the medications an HIV-infected child is likely to take, several are associated with elevated transaminases (e.g. rifabutin, isoniazid, fluconazole, itraconazole, ketoconazole, rifampin, trimethoprim–sulfamethoxazole, lamivudine, stavudine, zalcitabine, nevirapine, and ritonavir). Although hepatitis B can occur in HIV-infected children, the infection does not usually cause hepatocellular injury. The injury to the hepatitis B infected hepatocyte is caused by activated lymphocytes. Because of the immunodeficiency associated with HIV infection, immune-mediated injury from hepatitis B is ameliorated. This is not the case with hepatitis C. Infants born to mothers who are co-infected with HIV and hepatitis C are at a significantly increased risk for developing hepatitis C [28]. This infection is a slow, progressive disease and problems with hepatocellular carcinoma may not be evident until adulthood. Nevertheless, all children who are infected with hepatitis C or B should be followed regularly and based upon transaminases and their clinical course treated with interferon or lamivudine.

Jaundice in the HIV-infected child should raise the possibility of common bile duct obstruction or cholestatic hepatitis. Gallstones, fibrosis, or inflammation of the biliary tract can result in symptoms of obstruction. Initial evaluation should include an abdominal ultrasound. *Cryptosporidium* can migrate into the bile duct resulting in inflammation of the epithelium and acalculous cholecystitis. Fever and right upper quadrant abdominal pain, and positive Murphy's sign should increase suspicion for this diagnosis. Cytomegalovirus can cause similar symptoms and an endoscopic retrograde cholangiopancreatography (ERCP) or biopsy of the papilla can help distinguish between these diagnostic possibilities.

Jaundice in the HIV-infected child should cause concern about an obstruction of the common bile duct or severe hepatitis. Drug-induced hepatic injury should be considered in patients with progressive liver disease. In adults, hepatitis and rarely fulminant hepatic failure with lactic acidosis have been associated with receipt of nucleoside analog reverse transcriptase inhibitors. Elevated transaminases should prompt evaluation for known causes of hepatitis, but often no cause is identified. In this setting, malnutrition or HIV itself can be causing the abnormality. If transaminases remain persistently elevated for 6 months, a liver biopsy can be beneficial in finding an etiology. Because HIV can modify the immune response, unusual opportunistic infections may be found when evaluating hepatic tissue.

33.4.5 Abdominal pain

Children with HIV disease can experience crampy abdominal pain in association with increased luminal secretion and enhanced peristalsis from enteric pathogens. In this setting, bowel sounds are increased in frequency, but are normal in pitch. Abdominal pain in conjunction with decreased frequency of bowel sounds or increased pitch (tingles or rushes) should alert the clinician to the possibility of more serious causes. Appendicitis and bowel obstruction (intussusception) can occur in the HIV-infected child, but have not been reported to occur at increased frequency. *Mycobacterium avium* complex often infects the mesenteric lymph nodes before the bacteria can be identified in the mucosa. When the lymph nodes become enlarged they can cause abdominal pain; initiation of diarrhea may begin months later. The mechanism is not known, but transient intussusception led by these enlarged lymphoid aggregates

can play a role. The diagnosis is difficult to establish but may be suspected by identifying enlarged mesenteric nodes on an abdominal CT scan.

Abdominal pain caused by pancreatitis can be the harbinger of clinical deterioration in an HIV-infected child. The diagnosis is established by detecting an elevated amylase and/or lipase. Since many children with HIV may have elevated salivary amylase, total serum amylase is not a reliable indicator of clinical pancreatitis in these children. Fractionation of amylase or measurement of lipase should be determined if pancreatitis is suspected. A plain radiograph of the abdomen may demonstrate a widened duodenal loop suggesting edema of the head of the pancreatitis. Abdominal ultrasound is better at assessing pancreatic parenchyma and size of intrapancreatic ducts. Cytomegalovirus and, less commonly, *Cryptosporidium* can invade the biliary epithelium, resulting in inflammation and eventual obstruction of the pancreatic duct. In addition, antiretroviral drugs, especially didanosine, and medications used to treat opportunistic infections, such as pentamidine and isoniazid, have been associated with pancreatitis. Diagnosis of the infectious pathogens is dependent upon brushings or lavage of the pancreatic duct or biopsy of the papilla.

Treatment of pancreatitis is often palliative. Discontinuing medications that have been implicated in causing pancreatitis can be of some benefit, but monitoring amylase and lipase in children at risk may permit earlier intervention. Because food or using the GI tract for nutritional support exacerbates pancreatic disease, children with pancreatitis may become malnourished rapidly unless total parenteral nutrition is started early in the course of the illness. Even when an etiologic agent such as cytomegalovirus is identified, treatment with an antiviral agent is rarely effective, and management remains primarily supportive. In one series of HIV-infected children, pancreatitis was associated with a high rate of mortality within months of diagnosis [29].

33.5 Conclusions

Gastrointestinal disorders affect the lives of HIV-infected children by causing abdominal pain and discomfort, impairment of nutrient utilization and growth, decreasing caloric intake, and equally important, by depriving them of the simple pleasures surrounding family meal times. The goals of intervention are to recognize the subtle signs and symptoms of GI disease, and to use the multi-disciplinary expertise of nutritionists, nurses, social workers, dietitians, physicians, mental health workers, and pharmacists to formulate a plan that meets the needs of the child as well as the expectations of the family.

REFERENCES

1. Veazey, R. S., DeMaria, M., Chalifous, L. V. *et al.* Gastrointestinal tract as a major site of CD4$^+$ T-cell depletion and viral replication in SIV infection. *Science* **280** (1998), 427–31.

2. Newell, M.-L. Mechanisms and timing of mother-to-child transmission of HIV. *AIDS* **12** (1998), 831–7.

3. Fideli, U. S., Allen, S. A., Musonda, R. *et al.* Virologic and immunologic determinants of heterosexual transmission of human immunodeficiency virus type 1 (HIV) in Africa. *AIDS Res. Hum. Retrovirus.* **17** (2001), 901–10.

4. Wahl, S. M., Greenwell-Wild, T., Peng, G. *et al. Mycobacterium avium* complex augments macrophage HIV production and increases CCR-5 expression. *Proc. Natl. Acad. Sci. U.S.A.* **5** (1998), 12574–9.

5. Samson, M., Libert, F., Doranz, B. J. *et al.* Resistance to HIV infection in Caucasian individuals bearing mutant alleles of the CCR-5 chemokine receptor gene. *Nature* **382** (1996), 722–5.

6. Amerongen, H. M., Weltzin, R., Farnet, C. M. *et al.* Transepithelial transport of HIV by intestinal M cells: a mechanism for transmission of AIDS. *J. AIDS* **4** (1991), 760–5.

7. Geijtenbeek, T. B. H., Kwon, D. S., Torensma, R. *et al.* DC-SIGN, a dendritic cell-specific HIV-binding protein that enhances trans-infection of T cells. *Cell* **100** (2000), 587–97.

8. Soilleux, E. J. DC-SIGN (dendritic cell-specific ICAM-grabbing non-integrin) and DC-SIGN-related (DC-SIGNR): friend or foe? *Clin. Sci.* **104** (2003), 437–46.

9. Meng, G., Wei, X., Wu, X. *et al.* Primary intestinal epithelial cells transfer CCR5 R5 HIV to CCR5+ cells. *Nat. Med.* **8** (2002), 150–6.

10. Kewenig, S., Schneider, T., Hohloch, K. *et al.* Rapid mucosal CD4(+) T-cell depletion and enteropathy in simian immunodeficiency virus-infected rhesus macaques. *Gastroenterology* **116** (1999), 1115–23.

11. Schneider, T., Jahn, H. U., Schmidt, W. *et al.* Loss of CD4 T lymphocytes in patients infected with immunodeficiency virus type 1 is more pronounced in the duodenal mucosa than in the peripheral blood. *Gut.* **37** (1995), 524–9.

12. Clayton, F., Snow, G., Reka, S. *et al.* Selective depletion of rectal lamina propria rather than lymphoid aggregate CD4 lymphocytes in HIV infection. *Clin. Exp. Immunol.* **107** (1997), 288–92.

13. The European Collaborative Study. Height, weight, and growth in children born to mothers with HIV infection in Europe. *Pediatrics* **111** (2003), e52–60.

14. Verweel, G., van Rossum, A. M., Hartwig, N. G., Wolfs, T. F., Scherpbier, H. J. & de Groot, R. Treatment with highly active antiretroviral therapy in human immunodeficiency virus type 1-infected children is associated with a sustained effect on growth. *Pediatrics* **109** (2002), e25.

15. Moye, J., Rich, K. C., Kalish, L. A. *et al.* Women and Infants Transmission Study Group. Natural history of somatic growth in infants born to women infected by human immunodeficiency virus. *J. Pediatr.* **128** (1996), 58–69.

16. McKinney, R. E., Robertson, J. W. R. & Duke Pediatric AIDS Clinical Trials Unit. Effect of human immunodeficiency virus infection on the growth of young children. *J. Pediatr.* **123** (1993), 579–82.

17. Saavedra, J. M., Henderson, R. A., Perman, J. A., Hutton, N., Livingston, R. A. & Yolken, R. H. Longitudinal assessment of growth in children born to mothers with human immunodeficiency virus. *Arch. Pediatr. Adolesc. Med.* **149** (1995), 497–502.

18. Miller, T. L., Evans, S. J., Orav, E. J., McIntosh, K. & Winter, H. S. Growth and body composition in children infected with the human immunodeficiency virus-1. *Am. J. Clin. Nutr.* **57** (1993), 588–92.

19. Miller, T. L., Orav, E. J., Martin, S. R., McIntosh, K. & Winter, H. S. Malnutrition and carbohydrate malabsorption in children with vertically transmitted human immunodeficiency virus 1 infection. *Gastroenterology* **100** (1991), 1296–302.

20. Smith, P. D. & Janoff, E. N. Gastrointestinal infections in HIV-1 disease. M. J. Blaser, P. D. Smith, J. I. Ravdin, H. B. Greenberg & R. L. Guerrant (eds.), In *Infections of the Gastrointestinal Tract*, edn, **2** : **415**. Philadelphia: Lippincott Williams & Wilkins.

21. Marano, B. J. Jr, Smith, F. & Bonanno, C. A. *Helicobacter pylori* prevalence in acquired immunodeficiency syndrome. *Am. J. Gastroenter.* **88** (1993), 687.

22. Chang, T., Pelton, S. I. & Winter, H. S. Enteric infections in HIV-infected children. In M. J. Blaser, P. D. Smith, J. I. Ravdin, H. B. Greenberg & R. L. Guerrant (eds.), *Infections of the Gastrointestinal Tract.* New York: Raven Press (1995), pp. 499–510.

23. Yolken, R. H., Hart, W., Oung, I., Schiff, C., Greenson, J. & Perman, J. A. Gastrointestinal dysfunction and disaccharide intolerance in children infected with human immunodeficiency virus. *J. Pediatr.* **118** (1991), 359–63.

24. Miller, T. L., McQuinn, L. B. & Orav, E. J. Endoscopy of the upper gastrointestinal tract as a diagnostic tool for children with human immunodeficiency virus infection. *J. Pediatr.* **130** (1997), 766–73.

25. Danzig, J. B. *et al.* Gastrointestinal malignancy in patients with AIDS. *Am. J. Gastroenterol.* **86** (1991), 715.

26. Chadwick, E. G. *et al.* Tumors of smooth-muscle origin in HIV-infected children. *J. Am. Med. Assoc.* **263** (1990), 3182.

27. Nitazoxanide (Alinia) – A New Anti-Protozoal Agent. *Med. Letter* **45** (2003), 29–30.

28. Mazza, C., Ravaggi, A., Rodella, A. *et al.* for the Study Group of Vertical Transmission: Prospective study of mother to infant transmission of hepatitis C virus (HCV) infection. *J. Med. Virol.* **54** (1998), 12–19.

29. Miller, T. L., Winter, H. S., Luginbuhl, L. M., Orav, E. J. & McIntosh, K. Pancreatitis in pediatric human immunodeficiency virus infection. *J. Pediatr.* **120** (1992), 223–7.

Renal disease

Somsak Tanawattanacharoen, M.D. and Jeffrey B. Kopp, M.D.

Metabolic Diseases Branch, NIDDK, NIH, Bethesda, MD

34.1 Introduction

HIV infection is associated with a wide range of renal and metabolic disturbances [1, 2]. Electrolyte and acid-base disorders are fairly common, particularly in hospitalized patients. These include hyponatremia, hyperkalemia, and metabolic acidosis. Acute renal failure may occur, most typically as a consequence of drug therapy. Other common syndromes include hematuria, pyuria, and proteinuria; it is important for the physician who cares for patients with HIV disease to have a plan of evaluation for each of these clinical syndromes. Glomerular disease is less common and most typically manifests as focal segmental glomerulosclerosis in African–Americans and proliferative glomerulonephritis in patients of other ethnic backgrounds.

34.2 Fluid and electrolyte disorders: water, sodium, and potassium

Hyponatremia is the most common electrolyte disorder in HIV-infected patients. In a longitudinal study of pediatric HIV patients, the incidence of hyponatremia was about 25% and the major cause was the syndrome of inappropriate secretion of antidiuretic hormone (SIADH) [3]. Volume depletion due to gastrointestinal losses and poor fluid intake is another common cause, and is doubtless the most common cause of hyponatremia in the developing world. Other causes include adrenal insufficiency and drugs, including diuretics. Evaluation of hyponatremic patients involves clinical assessment of intravascular volume status and measurement of random urine sodium and creatinine concentrations. In the setting of hyponatremia and sodium depletion (extracellular volume depletion, as manifested by orthostatic hypotension), urine sodium <10 mEq/L indicates extra-renal saline loss (e.g. diarrhea) and urine sodium >10 mEq/L suggests renal saline losses (e.g. diuretics or renal salt wasting). If a patient has SIADH, the patient will typically have hyponatremia, a normal extracellular volume status, and a urine sodium >20 mEq/L. In HIV-infected patients, SIADH may be due to brain or lung infection, hypothyroidism, hypocortisolism, or medication. Management includes free-water restriction and, in refractory cases, doxycycline therapy (avoid in children < 8 years old due to impairment of tooth development).

Hyperkalemia in the setting of HIV infection can be caused by adrenal insufficiency, hyporeninemic hypoaldosteronism, or acute renal failure [4]. Hyperkalemia may also be due to medication, particularly trimethoprim [5] and pentamidine [6]. These drugs have structural similarities to potassium-sparing diuretics such as triamterene and block apical sodium channels within the collecting duct. This blockade of cellular sodium entry into the tubular cell results in reduced tubular secretion of potassium, which is linked to sodium uptake.

34.3 Acid-base disorders

Hyperchloremic, normal anion-gap, metabolic acidosis secondary to chronic diarrhea or medication is frequently seen in HIV-infected children. Some patients have associated persistent hyperkalemia suggestive of renal tubular acidosis type IV [7]. Type A lactic acidosis (associated with hypotension) is commonly due to sepsis and type B lactic acidosis (associated with normal blood pressure) has been described in association with nucleoside reverse transcriptase inhibitor therapy (NRTIs) [8]. The diagnostic approach to a reduced serum bicarbonate includes the following: exclude hyperventilation with appropriate renal compensation; calculate serum anion gap; if there is an elevated anion gap, measure suspected anions (e.g. lactate); if anion gap is normal, then evaluate for causes of hyperchloremic metabolic acidosis (including urine pH). Therapy is indicated for acute metabolic acidosis guided by arterial blood gas pH (treat with intravenous serum bicarbonate) and for chronic metabolic acidosis with serum bicarbonate <18–20 mEq/L (treat with citrate solutions). The pathogenesis of metabolic disorders associated with antiretroviral therapy is described in Chapter 20.

34.4 Acute renal failure

Acute renal failure (ARF), defined as the acute retention of nitrogenous wastes with or without oliguria, may occur in HIV-infected children, although less commonly than in adults [7–9] (Table 34.1). The major etiologies of ARF are summarized in Table 34.1. Evaluation of these patients involves the following: clinical assessment of intravascular volume status; microscopic examination of the urine including staining for eosinophils; and measurement of random urine sodium and creatinine prior to the administration of diuretics, from which is calculated the fractional excretion of filtered sodium (FE Na = [U Na × P Cr]/[P Na × U Cr] × 100), where U Na is urine sodium, P Cr is plasma creatinine, P Na is plasma sodium, and U Cr is urine creatinine.

Pre-renal ARF is associated with reduced urine output, urine sodium concentration <20 mEq/L, and FE Na <1%. Intrinsic renal causes of ARF include acute tubular necrosis (urinalysis showing muddy brown casts, urine sodium >40 mEq/L, and FE Na > 2%), interstitial nephritis (urinalysis showing leukocytes, sometimes including eosinophils, and sometimes dysmorphic erythrocytes or cellular casts), and rapidly progressive glomerulonephritis (urinalysis showing dysmorphic erythrocytes and frequently red blood cell casts). Postrenal ARF in a child is most commonly due to ureteral obstruction and therefore is best assessed by obtaining renal ultrasound examination in patients at particular risk of stones, or retroperitoneal or pelvic masses.

Referral to a nephrologist should be considered when the etiology of ARF is in doubt and for management of renal causes of ARF. Urology consultation is warranted for postrenal causes of ARF. Patients with developing ARF should

Table 34.1 Acute renal failure in patients with HIV infection

Classification	Etiology
Pre-renal	Intravascular volume depletion (vomiting, diarrhea, glucocorticoid deficiency)
	Capillary leak (sepsis, hypoalbuminemia, therapy with interleukin-2, interferon-α, or interferon-γ)
	Hypotension (sepsis, HIV cardiomyopathy)
	Decreased renal blood flow (non-steroidal anti-inflammatory drugs)
Renal	Acute tubular necrosis (ischemia, sepsis, antimicrobials, radiographic contrast, rhabdomyolysis)
	Interstitial nephritis (penicillins, ciprofloxacin, non-steroidal anti-inflammatory drugs, adenovirus, cytomegalovirus, polyomavirus, microsporidia, *Mycobacteria*)
	Rapidly progressive glomerulonephritis (immune complex glomerulonephritis, thrombotic thrombocytopenic purpura)
Post-renal	Tubular obstruction (sulfadiazine, acyclovir, tumor lysis)
	Extrinsic ureteral and pelvic obstruction (e.g. lymphoma or massive lymphadenopathy)
	Intrinsic reteral obstruction (e.g. stone, fungus ball due to Candida, blood clot, sloughed papilla, indinavir crystals)

have close attention to saline balance, in order to avoid hypotension (which can exacerbate renal injury) and fluid overload. Indications for dialysis include hyperkalemia, metabolic acidosis, volume overload, and severe azotemia.

34.5 Drug-induced renal complications

HIV infection requires the use of multiple medications for prolonged periods and the risk of toxicity, including renal

Table 34.2 Renal complications of drugs commonly used in HIV patients

Antibacterial and antiprotozoal agents	
Aminoglycosides	Acute renal failure, magnesium wasting
Penicillins	Allergic interstitial nephritis
Ciprofloxacin	Allergic interstitial nephritis
Pentamidine	Rhabdomyolysis, azotemia, acute renal failure
Rifampin	Acute renal failure, Fanconi syndrome, renal tubular acidosis, nephrogenic diabetes insipidus, interstitial nephritis, glomerulonephritis
Sulfa drugs	Azotemia without change in GFR, sulfadiazine crystal-induced obstructive nephropathy, allergic interstitial nephritis
Antifungal agents	
Amphotericin	Azotemia, acute renal failure, potassium and magnesium wasting, distal renal tubular acidosis, nephrocalcinosis
Antiviral agents	
Acyclovir	Acyclovir crystal-induced obstructive nephropathy
Dideoxyinosine	Hypokalemia, hyperuricemia, Fanconi syndrome
Indinavir	Nephrolithiasis, flank pain, dysuria, asymptomatic crystalluria, interstitial nephritis, acute renal failure, possibly hypertension
Foscarnet	Acute renal failure, nephrogenic diabetes insipidus
Zidovudine	Rhabdomyolysis
Several reverse transcriptase inhibitors	Lactic acidosis
Anti-inflammatory agents	
Non-steroid anti-inflammatory drugs	Reduced sodium excretion, interstitial nephritis, nephrotic syndrome

toxicity, is high. Renal complications of drugs used commonly in HIV-infected patients are listed in Table 34.2.

34.6 Hematuria

Hematuria may reflect bleeding from kidney, ureter, bladder, or urethra (Table 34.3). Urinary dipsticks will show a positive test for blood in the presence of intact red blood cells (RBCs), hemoglobin, and myoglobin. Ingestion of ascorbate will inhibit this test and therefore mask the assessment of hematuria by dipstick, but will not affect the microscopic examination of urine. When occult blood is present in the urine without RBCs, one must consider the possibility of hemoglobinuria or myoglobinuria. When RBCs are present, a careful microscopic inspection using a phase contrast microscope may reveal dysmorphic changes, such as irregular margins and, particularly, surface blebs, which are helpful clues to the presence of glomerular or tubular injury, as distinguished from bleed-

ing originating from lower in the urinary tract. Causes of the latter include stones or crystalluria (e.g. due to indinavir therapy), urothelial malignancy (which has an increased prevalence in HIV-infected adults [10]), and infection.

Microscopic examination of the urine should be performed in all patients with suspected renal disease, looking for dysmorphic RBCs (evidence of glomerular or tubular disease), RBC casts (evidence of glomerulonephritis or occasionally interstitial nephritis), white blood cell casts (evidence of glomerulonephritis, interstitial nephritis, or pyelonephritis), and broad and waxy casts (evidence of chronic renal disease).

34.7 Pyuria: infection and interstitial nephritis

Pyuria may be due to infection, drug-induced interstitial nephritis, or glomerulonephritis (Table 34.4). Pyuria is typically defined as more than 2–4 leukocytes per high power field, although the precise range of normal depends on the degree of urinary concentration used

Table 34.3 Causes of hematuria in HIV-infected patients

Renal causes	Postrenal causes	Other
Dysmorphic erythrocytes on urinalysis	Nondysmorphic erythrocytes on urinalysis	Erthyrocytes absent from urinalysis
Glomerular diseases: glomerulonephritis, nephrotic syndrome (see Table 34.5)	Kidney stone, crystal aggregates	Hemoglobinuria
Interstitial nephritis (see Table 34.5)	Cancer of kidney or bladder	Myoglobinuria
	Infection in kidney, ureter, bladder, prostate, urethra	

Adapted with permission from [2].

Table 34.4 Causes of pyuria in HIV-infected patients

Bacterial infection	Viral infection	Protozoan infection	Other
Gram-negative bacteria: pyelonephritis, cystitis, prostatitis	Cytomegalovirus: interstitial nephritis	Microsporidian Encephalitozoon species: interstitial nephritis	Drug-induced interstitial nephritis
Neisseria gonorrhoeae, Chlamydia species: urethritis	Adenovirus: interstitial nephritis, ureteritis		Stones and crystalluria, including drug (indinavir, acyclovir)
Mycobacterium species: pyelonephritis	Polyomavirus, especially BK virus: interstitial nephritis, ureteritis		Urothelial cancer

Adapted with permission from [2].

to prepare the sample. Allergic interstitial nephritis may be suspected when the patient exhibits eosinophilia, or when eosinophils are present in the urine, although their absence does not exclude the diagnosis. There appears to be no increased risk of bacterial urinary tract infection among HIV-infected children [11]. Other infectious agents which may present with pyuria include the following: *Mycobacterium tuberculosis, Mycobacterium avium* complex, microsporidians of the genus *Encephalitozoon,* cytomegalovirus (CMV), adenovirus, and BK virus (a polyomavirus) [12–14]. Adenoviral infection may also present with gross hematuria and ureteric obstruction due to cellular injury and clot. Diagnosis of infection with mycobacterial species, cytomegalovirus, and adenovirus is made by culture. Polyomavirus, typically BK virus, but possibly JC virus or SV40 virus, may be suspected when dysmorphic tubular epithelial cells are present on cytologic examination and this finding is confirmed by immunostaining or PCR.

Crystalluria is seen with a number of medications, including particularly sulfa-related compounds, acyclovir, and indinavir. Only with indinavir does crystalluria lead to frequent complications. Indinavir crystals are highly distinctive, taking two forms: irregular, rectangular plates and starburst or rosette forms. Crystalluria is due to the fraction of indinavir that is excreted unchanged in the urine (approximately 20%) and the low solubility of indinavir in aqueous solutions. Crystal-related complications include dysuria, renal obstruction due to sludging, and nephrolithiasis. Two large studies suggested that loin pain (due to sludging or stone) occurs at a frequency of 6.7–8.3 episodes per 100 patient years of indinavir therapy [15, 16]. When multiple urinalyses are performed, indinavir crystalluria is seen in up to 67% of patients, suggesting that the presence of crystals alone is not a useful predictor of the likelihood of developing complications [17]. Indinavir therapy is also associated with interstitial nephritis, with normal or elevated blood urea a nitrogen (BUN) and creatinine, and with pyuria; characteristic crystals are present in urine and within renal parenchyma and the urine frequently has multinucleated giant cells (histiocytes) [18, 19]. All patients receiving indinavir should have periodic urinalysis and measurement of serum creatinine, probably every 3 months. Management of suspected interstitial nephritis involves cessation of indinavir therapy, which is associated with prompt resolution of pyuria. In patients in whom indinavir is continued, there is a risk for irreversible renal function decline and renal atrophy.

34.8 Proteinuria

HIV-associated proteinuria is quite common in children. Thus, of 556 HIV-infected children evaluated over a 12-year period, nearly 13% were found to have persistent urine dipstick findings of 1+ or greater, in the absence of fever or urinary tract infection [20]. All patients with urinary protein on dipstick of 2+ or greater should undergo measurement of 24-hour urine protein and creatinine excretion, or if that is not feasible, should have a random urine protein/creatinine ratio determined [21].

Normal urinary protein is mostly composed of Tamm–Horsfall protein, a product of the distal tubule ($\sim$50%) and low molecular weight serum proteins ($\sim$50%). Normal protein excretion is < 0.3 g/day/m^2 for full-term babies, < 0.25 g/day/m^2 for infants and children <10 years, and < 0.2 g/day/ m^2 for children >10 years [22]. Collection of a 24-hour urine can be difficult in children, and as an alternative one can use the protein/creatinine ratio measured on a random urine sample. The urine protein/creatinine ratio is a dimensionless number, obtained by dividing the urine protein in mg/dl by the urine creatinine in mg/dl. Normal values of protein/creatinine ratio are < 0.5 in children < 2 years and < 0.2 in children > 2 years [22]. Children with nephrotic-range proteinuria, defined as > 3.5 g/day/1.73 m^2, will generally have a random urine protein/creatinine ratio >3.

The degree of pathologic proteinuria provides some clues as to likely source (Table 34.5). Tubular disease

is typically associated with levels of proteinuria of 0.5–2 g/day/1.73 m^2. Urinary protein electrophoresis, which identifies and quantitates the major classes of urinary proteins, is also helpful in distinguishing tubular proteinuria (typically with < 20% albumin) from glomerular proteinuria (typically with $\sim$50% albumin). Glomerular disease syndromes include nephritis (hypertension, edema, hematuria, and protein excretion typically 0.5–3 g/day/1.73 m^2) and nephrotic syndrome (edema, hypoalbuminemia, hypercholesterolemia, and protein excretion >3.5 g/day/1.73 m^2). In patients with tubular proteinuria, it is particularly important to review carefully the use of medications, including prescription medicine, over-the-counter medicines, and complementary and alternative medicines.

The management of tubular proteinuria begins with identifying possible infections or offending medications; those with proteinuria >1 g/day/1.73 m^2 should be referred to a nephrologist. Patients with glomerular proteinuria should be referred to a nephrologist, and consideration should be given to the advisability of renal biopsy. Proteinuria >1 g/day/1.73 m^2 probably merits introduction of angiotensin antagonist therapy (angiotensin converting enzyme [ACE] inhibitors and angiotensin receptor blockers [ARB]) to slow the progression of renal injury, although the data to support such a recommendation derives largely from studies of adults.

34.9 HIV-associated glomerular diseases

Patients with HIV-associated glomerular disease may present with proteinuria or hematuria on routine urinalysis, or with gross hematuria, edema, hypertension, or elevated BUN and creatinine. Since many patients are asymptomatic, routine urinalysis should probably be performed regularly, perhaps semi-annually. The incidence of glomerular disease in children with HIV-1 infection is unknown.

Focal segmental glomerulosclerosis (FSGS) is the most typical glomerular lesion associated with HIV infection and has been termed HIV-associated nephropathy (for recent reviews see [1, 23]. It is a pathologic syndrome characterized by increased accumulation of glomerular extracellular matrix protein that initially affects some portions (hence segmental) of some glomeruli (hence focal). African–Americans have an increased incidence of FSGS and this is particularly true of HIV-associated FSGS, suggesting a genetic basis. The prevalence of FSGS is estimated at 2–10% in longitudinal studies of patient populations which are predominantly African–American [24–26]. Children with HIV-associated FSGS typically

Table 34.5 Causes of proteinuria in patients with HIV infection

	Comment
Glomerular proteinuria	Urine albumin > 50% urine protein and urine protein typically > 2 g/d/1.73 m^2
Focal segmental glomeruloclerosis	Especially in Black patients
Mesangial hypercellularity	Patients of all racial backgrounds
Immune complex glomerulonephritis	Especially in White and Asian patients
IgA nephropathy	Especially in White and Asian patients
Thrombotic microangiopathy	Uncommon
Amyloid nephropathy	Rare
Membranous nephropathy	Rare
Fibrillary/immunotactoid glomerulonephritis	Rare
Histoplasmosis	Rare
Membranoproliferative glomerulonephritis	Generally associated with hepatitis C
Diabetes	Common due to the high prevalence of diabetes in developed countries
Interstitial nephritis	Urine albumin <30% of urine protein and urine protein typically <2 g/d/1.73 m^2
Drugs (see Table 34.2)	
Mycobacteria, both typical and atypical	Common (at autopsy)
Cryptococcus species	Rare
Polyomavirus (BK, JC, and possibly SV40)	Moderately common
Adenovirus	Rare
Cytomegalovirus	
Microsporidia (*Encephalitozoon* species)	Rare

Adapted with permission from [2].

present with heavy proteinuria, and some may have renal insufficiency at presentation. In patients with vertically acquired HIV infection, the modal time for the appearance of proteinuria is between ages 3 and 5 years [24, 25]. Children with HIV-associated FSGS, like adults, have in past years tended to progress to end stage renal disease (ESRD) fairly rapidly, frequently within a year of the appearance of renal disease [25]. With the advent of highly active antiretroviral therapy (HAART), it appears that the course of progressive renal dysfunction has become more indolent. In some patients the introduction of HAART has been associated with marked improvement in renal function and renal histopathology [27, 28] Therapy includes control of hypertension and the use of angiotensin-converting enzyme inhibitors and/or angiotensin blockers. These medications have three favorable effects on chronic kidney disease: they reduce blood pressure, proteinuria, and fibrosis. These recommendations derive from studies of adults with HIV-1 [29, 30] and adults with a range of other kidney diseases

[31]. No similar studies of children with HIV-1 have been reported.

The pathogenesis of HIV-associated FSGS has been the subject of considerable investigation. It appears that several mechanisms contribute. First, podocytes and renal tubular epithelial cells are susceptible to infection by HIV-1, with in situ hybridization studies suggesting low-level viral replication [28]. The consequences of this infection are not clear but at least in the case of renal tubular epithelial cells may include apoptosis [32]. Second, mice transgenic for subgenomic HIV-1 constructs develop FSGS, suggesting that replicating virus is not required and that viral proteins are toxic to renal parenchymal cells, particularly podocytes and renal tubular epithelial cells [33, 34]. This observation is consistent with the observation that other lentiviruses, including simian immunodeficiency virus and feline immunodeficiency virus, also cause FSGS in their host species. Third, there may be a pathogenetic role for the release of cytokines or viral proteins from infected lymphocytes or macrophages, located within the kidney itself or within lymphoid tissue (with products being delivered to kidney via the circulation). Fourth, the approximately 18-fold increased risk for FSGS among Black patients with HIV-1 compared with White patients with HIV-1 suggests that genetic factors contribute to risk, although the genetic loci remain to be identified [35].

A second glomerular lesion, mesangial hypercellularity, has been seen about half as commonly as FSGS in children with HIV-1 infection (and less commonly in adults), and occurs in all racial groups [24–26]. Like patients with FSGS, patients with mesangial hypercellularity typically present with proteinuria or frank nephrotic syndrome. Pediatric patients with mesangial hypercellularity tend to be somewhat older than pediatric patients with HIV-associated FSGS. Mesangial hypercellularity is a diagnosis that represents a subset of minimal change nephrotic syndrome and this disorder is seen chiefly in children (and not in adults), either with or without HIV infection. These patients have slightly increased numbers of mesangial cells and either lack immunoglobulin deposits within the glomerulus or have modest amounts of IgM and/or complement [36]. Patients with mesangial hypercellularity generally appear to have an excellent prognosis, although those with heavy proteinuria may deserve a trial of prednisone.

A third category of HIV-associated glomerular disease is mesangial proliferative glomerulonephritis, which occurs with a frequency comparable with mesangial hypercellularity [24–26, 37–39]. In pediatric patients, HIV-associated glomerulonephritis has included otherwise uncategorized mesangial glomerulonephritis, IgA glomerulonephritis [38, 39] and crescentic glomerulonephritis [40]. Patients with HIV-associated proliferative glomerulonephritis generally have an excellent prognosis over the medium-term, although this may not be true for the more aggressive lesions. No study has followed these patients for more than a few years, and the long-term prognosis is unknown. The pathogenesis of mesangial proliferation in the setting of HIV-1 infection is not well understood. In at least some patients, immune complexes within the mesangium have been shown to include HIV-1 antigens [41]. Mesangial hypercellularity and proliferative glomerulonephritis are the most common glomerular diseases in White and Asian patients with HIV-1 infection, in contrast to more common occurrence of FSGS among patients of African ancestry [42, 43].

Finally, a range of other lesions occur in the setting of HIV infection, including minimal change glomerulopathy (nil disease) and lupus nephritis [40]. Atypical hemolytic-uremic syndrome/thrombotic thrombocytopenic purpura (HUS/TTP) may be seen, and has a poor prognosis [44, 45].

34.10 Evaluation of glomerular disease

In patients with glomerular proteinuria and in those with suspected glomerular hematuria, it is important to exclude other causes of glomerular disease. A serologic evaluation should include C4, CH50, and a streptococcal antigen panel. In selected patients, where particular diseases are diagnostic considerations, it may also be advisable to order one or more of the following: ANA (to evaluate the possibility of lupus, although false positive tests are common in HIV-infected patients), serologic test for syphilis, antibodies to hepatitis B and hepatitis C, anti-neutrophil cytoplasmic antibody (to evaluate the possibility of vasculitis), and anti-glomerular basement membrane antibody (to evaluate the possibility of Goodpasture's syndrome). Ultrasound may be performed to assess the renal parenchyma, since enlarged and echogenic kidneys are typical of, but not diagnostic for, FSGS [46]. Referral to a nephrologist should be considered under the following circumstances: unexplained renal insufficiency, proteinuria in excess of 1 g/day/1.73 m^2 (or a random urine protein/creatinine ratio >1), or unexplained hematuria. Ultimately, renal biopsy may be required to establish the diagnosis and prognosis.

34.11 Treatment for glomerular disease

Therapy for chronic glomerular disease associated with HIV infection includes maximizing antiretroviral therapy (on the assumption that pathology may be related to continued high level viral replication), aggressive measures to control hypertension, and the use of angiotensin antagonist therapy in patients with proteinuria or declining renal function. Edema may be managed symptomatically with sodium restriction and diuretics. Close consultation with a pediatric nephrologist is recommended.

These treatment recommendations are tentative, since no randomized trials have been reported in adults or children. Prednisone therapy for 2 months improved serum creatinine and proteinuria in an uncontrolled study of HIV-infected adults [47, 48]. ACE inhibitors have been shown to improve proteinuria and retard progression of renal insufficiency in various renal diseases and may do so in HIV-associated renal disease, although randomized controlled trials are not available [30, 49]. To date there have been no studies of prednisone or angiotensin antagonist therapy in children. If angiotensin antagonist therapy is instituted, it is important to be alert for hypotension associated with the first dose of the angiotensin antagonist, particularly when diuretics are used concurrently, and for hyperkalemia. Patients with thrombotic microangiopathy, including hemolytic uremic syndrome and TTP, are treated with plasmapheresis and/or fresh frozen plasma infusion.

34.12 Summary

HIV infection is associated with a surprisingly diverse range of renal disease, including renal disease directly associated with HIV infection, complications due to infections associated with HIV disease, and complications of therapy. With new and more effective antiretroviral therapies and longer patient survival, the nature and distribution of HIV-associated renal syndromes will likely continue to evolve. Careful attention to the diagnosis and management of pediatric HIV-associated renal disease may minimize the impact of acute and chronic renal disease on the growth and development of these children.

REFERENCES

1. Kimmel, P. L., Barisoni, L., & Kopp, J. B. Pathogenesis and treatment of HIV-associated renal diseases: lessons from clinical and animal studies, molecular pathologic correlations, and genetic investigations. *Ann. Int. Med.* **139** (2003), 214–26.

2. Kopp, J. B. Renal dysfunction in HIV-1-infected patients. *Curr. Infect. Dis. Rep.* **4**:5 (2002), 449–60.

3. Tolaymat, A., Al-Moushly, F., Sleasman, J., Paryani, S. & Neiberger, R. Hyponatremia in pediatric patients with HIV-1 infection. *South. Med. J.* **88** (1995), 1039–42.

4. Glassock, R. J., Cohen, A. H., Danovitch, G. & Parsa, K. P. Human immunodeficiency virus infection and the kidney. *Ann. Intern. Med.* **112** (1990), 35–49.

5. Choi, M. J., Fernandez, P. C., Patnaik, A. *et al.* Brief report: trimethoprim-induced hyperkalemia in a patient with AIDS. *New Engl. J. Med.* **328** (1993), 703–6.

6. Kleyman, T. R., Roberts, C. & Ling, B. N. A mechanism for pentamidine-induced hyperkalemia: inhibition of distal nephron sodium transport. *Ann. Intern. Med.* **122** (1995), 103–6.

7. Zilleruelo, G. & Strauss, J. HIV nephropathy in children. *Pediatr. Clin. N. Am.* **42** (1995), 1469–85.

8. Smith, K. Y. Selected metabolic and morphologic complications associated with highly active antiretroviral therapy. *J. Infect. Dis.* **185**: Suppl. 2 (2002), S123–7.

9. Pardo, V., Strauss, J., Abitbol, C. & Zilleruelo, G. Renal disease in children with HIV infection. In P. L. Kimmel, J. S. Berns & J. H. Stein (eds.), *Contemporary Issues in Nephrology.* New York: Churchill Livingstone (1995), pp. 135–53.

10. Baynham, S., Katner, H. & Cleveland, K. Increased prevalence of renal cell carcinoma in patients with HIV infection. *AIDS Patient Care STDs* **11** (1997), 161–5.

11. O'Regan, S., Russo, P., Lapointe, N. & Rousseau, E. AIDS and the urinary tract. *J. AIDS* **3** (1990), 244.

12. Aarons, E. J., Woodrow, D., Hollister, W. S., Canning, E. U., Francis, N. & Gazzard, B. G. Reversible renal failure caused by a microsporidian infection. *AIDS* **8** (1994), 1119–21.

13. Shintaku, M., Nasu, K. & Ito, M. Necrotizing tubulo-interstitial nephritis induced by adenovirus in an AIDS patient. *Histopathology* **23** (1993), 588–90.

14. Ito, M., Hirabayashi, M., Uno, Y., Nakayam, A. & Asai, J. Necrotizing tubulointerstitial nephritis associated with adenovirus infection. *Hum. Pathol.* **22** (1991), 1225–31.

15. Herman, J. S., Ives, N. J., Nelson, M., Gazzard, B. G. & Easterbrook, P. J. Incidence and risk factors for the development of indinavir-associated renal complications. *J. Antimicrob. Chemother.* **48**:3 (2001), 355–60.

16. Dieleman, J. P., Sturkenboom, M. C., Jambroes, M. *et al.* Risk factors for urological symptoms in a cohort of users of the HIV protease inhibitor indinavir sulfate: the ATHENA cohort. *Arch. Intern. Med.* **162**:13 (2002), 1493–501.

17. Gagnon, R. F., Tecimer, S. N., Watters, A. K. & Tsoukas, C. M. Prospective study of urinalysis abnormalities in HIV-positive individuals treated with indinavir. *Am. J. Kidney. Dis.* **36**:3 (2000), 507–15.

18. Kopp, J. B., Falloon, J., Filie, A. *et al.* Indinavir-associated interstitial nephritis and urothelial inflammation: clinical and cytologic findings. *Clin. Infect. Dis.* **34**:8 (2002), 1122–8.

19. van Rossum, A. M., Dieleman, J. P., Fraaij, P. L. *et al.* Persistent sterile leukocyturia is associated with impaired renal function in human immunodeficiency virus type 1-infected children treated with indinavir. *Pediatrics* **110**:2 (2002), e19.

20. Strauss, J., Zilleruelo, G., Abitbol, C. *et al.* HIV nephropathy (HIVN) in children: importance of early identification (Abstract). *J. Am. Soc. Nephrol.* **4** (1993), 288.

21. Ginsberg, J., Chang, B., Matarese, R. & Garella, S. Use of single voided urine samples to estimate quantitative proteinuria. *New Engl. J. Med.* **309** (1983), 1543–6.

22. Makker, S. Proteinuria. In K. K. Kher, & S. P. Makker, (eds.), *Clinical Pediatric Nephrology.* New York: McGraw-Hill (1992), pp. 117–36.

23. Herman, E. S. & Klotman, P. E. HIV-associated nephropathy: epidemiology, pathogenesis, and treatment. *Semin. Nephrol.* **23** (2003), 200–8.

24. Ingulli, E., Tejani, A., Fikrig, S., Nicastri, A., Chen, C. & Pomrantz, A. Nephrotic syndrome associated with acquired immunodeficiency syndrome in children. *J. Pediatrics* **119** (1991), 710–16.

25. Strauss, R., Abitbol, C., Zilleruelo, G. *et al.* Renal disease in children with the acquired immunodeficiency syndrome. *New Engl. J. Med.* **321** (1989), 625–30.

26. Rajpoot, D., Kaupke, M., Vaziri, N., Rao, T., Pomrantz, A. & Fikrig, S. Childhood AIDS nephropathy: a 10-year experience. *J. Natl. Med. Assoc.* **88** (1997), 493–8.

27. Wali, R. K., Drachenberg, C. I., Papadimitriou, J. C., Keay, S. & Ramos, E. HIV-1-associated nephropathy and response to

highly-active antiretroviral therapy. *Lancet* **352**: **9130** (1998), 783–4.

28. Winston, J. A., Bruggeman, L. A., Ross, M. D. *et al.* Nephropathy and establishment of a renal reservoir of HIV type 1 during primary infection. *New Engl. J. Med.* **344**: **26** (2001), 1979–84.

29. Burns, G. D., Matute, R., Onyema, D., Davis, I. & Toth, I. Response to inhibition of angiotensin-converting enzyme in human immunodeficiency virus-associated nephropathy: a case report. *Am. J. Kidney. Dis.* **23** (1994), 441–3.

30. Kimmel, P. L., Mishkin, G. J. & Umana, W. O. Captopril and renal survival in patients with human immunodeficiency virus nephropathy. *Am. J. Kidney. Dis.* **28** (1996), 202–8.

31. Nakao, N., Yoshimura, A., Morita, H., Takada, M., Kayano, T. & Ideura, T. Combination treatment of angiotensin-II receptor blocker and angiotensin-converting-enzyme inhibitor in nondiabetic renal disease (COOPERATE): a randomised controlled trial. *Lancet* **361**: **9352** (2003), 117–24.

32. Conaldi, P. G., Biancone, L., Bottelli, A. *et al.* HIV-1 kills renal tubular epithelial cells in vitro by triggering an apoptotic pathway involving caspase activation and Fas upregulation. *J. Clin. Invest.* **102**: **12** (1998), 2041–9.

33. Kopp, J. B., Klotman, M. E., Adler, S. H. *et al.* Progressive glomerulosclerosis and enhanced renal accumulation of basement membrane components in mice transgenic for HIV-1 genes. *Proc. Natl. Acad. Sci. U.S.A.* **89** (1992), 1577–81.

34. Kajiyama, W., Klotman, P. E., Dickie, P. & Kopp, J. B. HIV-1 genes are expressed in glomerular and tubular epithelial cells in HIV-transgenic mouse kidney. *AIDS Res. Hum. Retrovirus.* **11**: Suppl. 1 (1995), S153.

35. Kopp, J. B. & Winkler, C. A. HIV-associated nephropathy in African Americans. *J. Am. Soc. Nephrol.* **63** (2003), S43–9.

36. Southwest Pediatric Nephrology Study Group. Childhood nephrotic syndrome associated with diffuse mesangial hypercellularity. *Kidney Int.* **23** (1983), 87–94.

37. Connor, E., Gupta, S., Joshi, V. *et al.* Acquired immunodeficiency syndrome-associated renal disease in children. *J. Pediatr.* **113** (1988), 39–44.

38. Trachtman, H., Gauthier, B., Vinograd, A. & Valderrama, E. IgA nephropathy in a child with human immunodeficiency virus type 1 infection. *Pediatr. Nephrol.* **5** (1991), 724–6.

39. Schoeneman, M. J., Ghali, V., Lieberman, K. & Reisman, L. IgA nephritis in a child with human immunodeficiency virus: a unique form of human immunodeficiency virus-associated nephropathy? *Pediatr. Nephrol.* **6** (1992), 46–9.

40. Landor, M., Bernstein, L. & Rubinstein, A. A steroid-responsive nephropathy in a child with human immunodeficiency virus infection. *Am. J. Dis. Child.* **147** (1993), 261–2.

41. Kimmel, P. L., Phillips, T. M., Ferreira-Centeno, A., Farkas-Szallasi, T., Abraham, A. A. & Garrett, C. T. Idiotypic IgA nephropathy in patients with human immunodeficiency virus infection. *New Engl. J. Med.* **327** (1992), 702–6.

42. Nochy, D., Gloz, D., Dosquet, P. *et al.* Renal disease associated with HIV infection: a multicentric study of 60 patients from Paris hospitals. *Nephrol. Dial. Transplant.* **8** (1993), 11–19.

43. Praditpornsilpa, K., Napathorn, S., Yenrudi, S., Wankrairot, P., Tungsaga, K. & Sitprija, V. Renal pathology and HIV infection in Thailand. *Am. J. Kidney Dis.* **33**: **2** (1999), 282–6.

44. Jorda, M., Rodriques, M. M. & Reik, R. A. Thrombotic thrombocytopenic purpura as the cause of death in an HIV-positive child. *Pediatr. Pathol.* **14** (1994), 919–25.

45. Turner, M. E., Kher, K., Rakusan, T. *et al.* Atypical hemolytic uremic syndrome in human immunodeficiency virus-1-infected children. *Pediatr. Nephrol.* **11** (1997), 161–3.

46. Zinn, H. L. & Haller, J. O. Renal manifestations of AIDS in children. *Pediatr. Radiol.* **29**: **7** (1999), 558–61.

47. Eustace, J. A., Nuermberger, E., Choi, M., Scheel, P. J., Jr., Moore, R. & Briggs, W. A. Cohort study of the treatment of severe HIV-associated nephropathy with corticosteroids. *Kidney Int.* **58**: **3** (2000), 1253–60.

48. Smith, M. C., Austen, J. L., Carey, J. T. *et al.* Prednisone improves renal function and proteinuria in human immunodeficiency virus-associated nephropathy. *Am. J. Med.* **101** (1996), 41–8.

49. Burns, G. C., Paul, S. K., Toth, I. R. & Sivak, S. L. Effect of angiotensin-converting enzyme inhibition in HIV-associated nephropathy. *J. Am. Soc. Nephrol.* **8** (1997), 1140–6.

35

Endocrine disorders

Daina Dreimane, M.D. and Mitchell E. Geffner, M.D.

Childrens Hospital Los Angeles, Los Angeles, CA

Although growth failure is common among HIV-infected children, especially those with more advanced disease, primary endocrinopathies are relatively uncommon. Also, despite the prevalence of encephalopathy among HIV-infected children, hypothalamic-pituitary function is rarely affected. Highly active antiretroviral therapy (HAART) with protease inhibitors (PIs) can cause specific derangements of body composition and metabolism. When true endocrine dysfunction occurs in HIV-infected children, it usually results either from infection or malignancy affecting specific glandular function or from the effects of pharmacological agents on hormone synthesis or action.

35.1 Growth failure (failure-to-thrive) and pubertal delay

Growth failure [1–3] occurs in 20–80% of symptomatic HIV-infected children regardless of route of acquisition. In perinatally infected children, failure-to-thrive (FTT) presents as early as 6 months of age. As the infection becomes more advanced, growth failure may progress to a distinct wasting syndrome (analogous to that which occurs in adults).

35.1.1 Proposed mechanisms of growth failure

Mechanisms include the non-specific effects of chronic disease, decreased intake (anorexia, esophagitis, and abdominal pain), and enteropathy (diarrhea, malabsorption, and gut infection)[2]. In addition, affected children manifest hypermetabolism (increased resting expenditure)/

catabolism. Their caloric intake, even if normal or increased for age, may not meet their energy needs. Hormonal aberrations also have been implicated, including deficiencies of growth hormone (GH), sex steroids (during adolescence), and thyroid hormones (see below).

35.1.2 Growth hormone/insulin-like growth factor-I (IGF-I) axis

Growth hormone deficiency diagnosed by pharmacological provocation or under physiological conditions, i.e. sleep, has been reported, but appears to occur less often than might be predicted based on the prevalence of AIDS encephalopathy in children [2]. Levels of the GH-dependent surrogates, IGF-I and insulin-like growth factor binding protein-3 (IGFBP-3), even without GH deficiency, are typically low secondary to undernutrition, and there is enhanced IGFBP-3 proteolysis as well in HIV-infected children. GH/IGF-I resistance has been documented in vitro using hormonally responsive erythroid progenitor cells isolated from short, well-nourished, non-acutely ill children with HIV infection [4].

35.1.3 Sex steroid deficiency

Delayed sexual maturation is associated with perinatal HIV infection. Puberty is delayed by up to 2 years in girls, and 1 year in boys [5]. The mechanism of delay remains unknown, but is most likely related to the HIV virus per se. Unfavorable environmental factors may contribute, but are not the cause of delay, since delayed puberty is frequently observed in HIV-infected boys with hemophilia [6].

35.1.4 Non-hormonal causes of growth failure

Growth failure also can result from the effects of opportunistic infections and tumors [7, 8]. Pituitary infections caused by *Toxoplasma gondii*, cytomegalovirus (CMV), and *Pneumocystis carinii* have been reported in adults; Kaposi's sarcoma also has been found in the hypothalamus and pituitary at autopsy. Cytomegalovirus, *Mycobacterium avium complex* (MAC), *Cryptococcus neoformans,* and *Pneumocystis carinii* (even without pulmonary involvement), as well as Kaposi's sarcoma, have been found in thyroid glands of adults at autopsy. Lastly, CMV (most common), MAC, *Toxoplasma gondii, Mycobacterium tuberculosis,* and Kaposi's sarcoma may invade the testes of adult males. Additionally, drug effects could alter the hormonal systems necessary for normal growth. For example, rifampin, used to treat tuberculosis, induces hepatic microsomal enzymes and thereby increases thyroid hormone clearance. This may be clinically relevant in subjects on levo-thyroxine replacement or in those with diminished thyroid or pituitary reserve. Ketoconazole, used at high doses to treat fungal disease, inhibits testicular steroidogenesis and can prevent the onset or slow the progression of puberty. Megestrol acetate, an appetite stimulant, can lower testosterone levels by central feedback inhibition on luteinizing hormone (LH).

35.1.5 Diagnostic approach

The pediatrician should first assess for undernutrition by performing a calorie count and by ordering appropriate biochemical measurements of nutritional adequacy. If these evaluations are normal, a bone age x-ray should be ordered which, if significantly delayed, suggests an endocrinological cause for growth delay. This would include a possible diagnosis of hypothyroidism (see below). If, however, thyroid function is normal, the endocrinologist may wish to perform provocative GH testing to detect disturbances of the GH-IGF-I axis. Lastly, if there is a suspicion of sex steroid deficiency on clinical grounds (lack of pubertal changes in girls over 13 years old and in boys over 14 years old), the endocrinologist may order random or stimulated gonadotropin (LH and follicle-stimulating hormone [FSH] by immunochemiluminescent assay [ICMA]) levels which may help to distinguish primary from central forms of hypogonadism.

35.1.6 Treatment

The pediatrician should correct any nutritional inadequacy, including use of parenteral nutrition and appetite-stimulating drugs, e.g. progestational agents, such as megestrol acetate [9]. Administration of HAART including PIs improves linear growth and weight gain [10]. Of note, these approaches all tend to stimulate weight gain out of proportion to lean body mass. Alternatively, with the guidance of a pediatric endocrinologist, specific hormonal therapies may be considered. These include anabolic agents, e.g. oxandrolone or human GH (approved for use in adults with wasting). The use of these latter agents is associated with preferential gains in lean body mass. Growth hormone deficiency is corrected by treatment with human GH at standard doses (0.15–0.3 mg/kg/week). However, the GH regimen approved for treatment of HIV-related wasting in adults is up to 6 mg/day for 3 months [11]. These high doses are presumably required to overcome underlying GH/IGF-I resistance. There is no evidence that GH stimulates HIV activity in vivo. Limited studies of GH use in HIV-infected patients have been performed to date [12]. A multicenter research protocol employing GH administration in infected children is currently underway in the US to assess effects on growth and immune function. For documented hypothyroidism, thyroid hormone replacement is initiated (see below). Sex steroid deficiency involves replacement of estrogen and progesterone in girls and of testosterone in boys, and should be initiated by the pediatric endocrinologist.

35.2 Hypothyroidism

Clinically significant derangements of thyroid function in HIV-infected children are infrequent. Much more common is biochemical evidence of the sick euthyroid syndrome in the setting of overwhelming illness. Symptoms of hypothyroidism include linear growth failure, relative preservation of weight, constipation, cold intolerance, fatigue, and hair loss [13–15].

35.2.1 Proposed mechanisms

In most but not all studies, overt primary thyroid failure is rare. However, anti-thyroid autoantibodies may be present in up to 34% of perinatally infected children [16]. Thyroid dysfunction is observed early in the course of perinatally acquired infection. It is pronounced in children with high viral load early in the course of HIV disease and severe immunosuppression, and precedes worsening of disease [17]. Subtle central hypothyroidism in children has been reported to be manifested as a failure to observe the expected rise in nocturnal thyroid-stimulating hormone (TSH) on serial sampling. The sick euthyroid syndrome also has been described in children with advanced disease as have, for unknown reasons, elevated thyroxine-binding globulin levels.

35.2.2 Diagnostic approach

If clinical signs and symptoms suggest the presence of hypothyroidism, the pediatrician should have serum levels of ultrasensitive TSH and free thyroxine (T_4) measured. If these thyroid test results suggest an abnormality, but are not absolutely diagnostic, consultation with a pediatric endocrinologist for additional thyroid assessments, e.g. thyrotropin-releasing hormone (TRH) testing and nocturnal TSH sampling, may be required.

35.2.3 Treatment

For documented hypothyroidism, levo-thyroxine (50–100 $\mu g/m^2/day$) is prescribed. This can be done by the pediatrician under the direction of an endocrinologist.

35.3 Body composition, energy expenditure, and metabolic abnormalities related to protease inhibitor therapy

Recently, an association has been noted between PI therapy in HIV-infected adults and a metabolic syndrome, consisting of peripheral fat wasting and truncal obesity (lipodystrophy), hypertriglyceridemia, and insulin resistance or diabetes mellitus. Children have similar changes in body fat distribution [18]. Total cholesterol levels and low-density lipoprotein (LDL) cholesterol levels are increased in children treated with PIs, with lesser elevations of triglycerides and apolipoprotein B [19]. Insulin resistance in children is less pronounced than in adults. A similar syndrome may occur in HIV-infected adults who have not received PI therapy.

35.3.1 Proposed mechanisms

The exact cause of these metabolic abnormalities is unknown. It has been suggested that PIs bind to two proteins that regulate lipid metabolism, that, in turn, cause abnormal lipoproteins, insulin resistance, and characteristic body composition [20].

35.3.2 Diagnostic approach

Fasting plasma lipids should be monitored if PIs are used. Diagnosis of glucose intolerance is discussed below. An elevated fasting c-peptide level may be a useful screening test for the presence of insulin resistance. These tests should be ordered by the pediatrician every 3–6 months and, if abnormal, should prompt referral to a pediatric endocrinologist.

35.3.3 Treatment

No uniform treatment recommendations are available. In severe cases in adults, which are more often linked to use of ritonavir than to other PIs, switching to a different PI or to an antiretroviral regimen that does not employ PIs may result in improvement in the metabolic derangements. Whether such an association occurs and whether a similar therapeutic approach is efficacious in children is unclear. Further studies are needed to assess long-term risk for developing cardiovascular disease as a result of the lipodystrophy syndrome in light of improved survival of HIV-infected children who are treated with PIs. See Chapter 20 for further information regarding the metabolic complications of antiretroviral therapy.

35.4 Adrenocortical insufficiency

Signs and symptoms of HIV infection mimic those of adrenal insufficiency [21, 22], e.g. nausea, vomiting, anorexia, weight loss, fever, diarrhea, fatigue, and orthostatic hypotension, yet the hypothalamic-pituitary-adrenal (HPA) axis and mineralocorticoid production are normal in ~90% of infected adults. The adrenals are the most common endocrine glands affected by opportunistic infections and malignancy based on autopsy studies (49–92%). Elevated serum cortisol levels are frequently found in adults and children and may reflect stress, cytokine activation, or, in some cases, cortisol resistance [23]. The fat redistribution syndrome associated with protease inhibitor therapy has similarities with Cushing's syndrome; however, plasma cortisol and urinary free cortisol excretion are not increased in affected individuals [24].

35.4.1 Proposed mechanisms

Opportunistic infections that may infiltrate the adrenal cortices, include CMV (most frequent, i.e. found in as many as 50% of adult adrenals), MAC, and *Cryptococcus*. Since glandular destruction in these settings rarely exceeds 50% of total adrenal tissue, clinically significant adrenocortical insufficiency is not likely. Tumors, e.g. Kaposi's sarcoma, also can invade or there may be autoimmune destruction of the adrenal cortices. Cortical lipid depletion, a non-specific finding associated with many severe wasting diseases, also has been reported. Drugs also can alter adrenocortical function. For example, ketoconazole inhibits adrenocortical steroidogenesis; megesterol acetate lowers serum cortisol levels and decreases responsiveness to provocative testing; and rifampin increases cortisol metabolism. Theoretically, central adrenocortical insufficiency secondary to hypothalamic and/or pituitary destruction could occur. Lastly, cortisol resistance with actual hypercortisolemia in the setting of clinical adrenocortical insufficiency has been described in a subset of adults.

35.4.2 Diagnostic approach

If there are multiple clinical findings suggestive of glucocorticoid insufficiency, the pediatrician should screen the integrity of the HPA axis by measuring an 8:00 am cortisol level. A serum cortisol level over 18 μg/dL at any time is evidence of normal glucocorticoid function. If, however, the cortisol result is low or low-normal, further testing under the direction of a pediatric endocrinologist is required. Insulin-induced hypoglycemia or adrenocorticotropin (ACTH) stimulation is used for testing of HPA axis. Corticotropin-releasing hormone (CRH) may be used if the above tests are inconclusive, to detect mild or partial central adrenal insufficiency. To assess the adequacy of mineralocorticoid function (affected only in primary adrenal insufficiency), the pediatrician should measure serum electrolytes. If hyponatremia and reciprocal hyperkalemia are found, the pediatric endocrinologist should continue the investigation, including measurement of peripheral renin activity (PRA) and aldosterone before the electrolytes are corrected. It also should be noted that hyponatremia without hyperkalemia may occur with isolated glucocorticoid deficiency (as occurs with ACTH deficiency).

35.4.3 Treatment

If clinical adrenocortical insufficiency (either primary or central) is suspected, the pediatrician should consult immediately with an endocrinologist and give intravenous stress doses of hydrocortisone (50–100 μg/m^2/day as a bolus followed by a similar dose given as an infusion over the next few days) as soon as HPA-axis testing is completed. If adrenal insufficiency is primary, mineralocorticoid replacement with fludrocortisone (0.05–0.1 mg/day orally) also must be given. There is no pure *parenteral* mineralocorticoid available, but high-dose hydrocortisone provides significant mineralocorticoid effect. For central adrenocortical insufficiency, mineralocorticoid replacement is unnecessary. Lastly, volume support through fluids and pharmacological agents should be given as needed.

After a few days, maintenance glucocorticoid replacement is provided as oral hydrocortisone (15 mg/m^2/day in three doses with one-half given in the morning and one-quarter given both in the mid-afternoon and at bedtime) and, for cases of primary adrenal insufficiency, maintenance mineralocorticoid continued as oral fludrocortisone (at a dose of between 0.05–0.1 mg once-daily depending on body size). Principles of stress-dosing of hydrocortisone are taught, including provision of an injectable formulation for home use, and Medic-Alert registration is strongly encouraged.

35.5 Abnormal glucose metabolism

Clinically significant hyperglycemia, despite abnormal pancreatic histology in ~50% of adults at autopsy, is unusual [7, 8]. Severe hyperglycemia is experienced by less than 2% of HIV-infected adults; half of those have pre-existing conditions [25]. It is, however, becoming more common with the use of PI therapy. In contrast, heightened sensitivity to the metabolic actions of insulin has been described in adults (in contrast to sepsis, in which there is insulin resistance).

35.5.1 Proposed mechanisms

Hypoglycemia may result from use of drugs such as pentamidine isothionate, which chronically stimulates unregulated release of insulin in 14–33% of adults, or from trimethoprim–sulfamethoxazole, the latter component of which stimulates insulin secretion. Hyperglycemia may result from: opportunistic infections, including infections with CMV (most common), *Cryptococcus, Candida,* and *Toxoplasma gondii*; tumors, including Kaposi's sarcoma and lymphoma; possible direct HIV invasion of the pancreas; and drugs, including pentamidine (which, in some patients, if used chronically, may induce pancreatitis and destroy β-cells). High-dose glucocorticoids, megestrol acetate, and PI-related lipodystrophy cause insulin resistance, which, if severe, can lead to hyperglycemia [26].

35.5.2 Diagnostic approach

The pediatrician should check the patient for hypoglycemia by obtaining *pre*-prandial blood glucose measurements by bedside meter and for hyperglycemia by obtaining either *post*-prandial blood glucose measurements by meter or by checking for urinary glucose. Additionally, quarterly glycosylated hemoglobin (hemoglobin A$_{1c}$) measurements may be ordered.

35.5.3 Treatment

If a derangement in glucose metabolism is drug-induced, the pediatrician should first discontinue the offending agent, if possible. To treat non-acute hypoglycemia, appropriate dietary measures should be attempted, perhaps with the assistance of a pediatric dietitian. If diabetes is found, a pediatric endocrinologist should be consulted promptly. If diabetes is associated with ketoacidosis, insulin will be required, whereas, if diabetes is due to insulin resistance, oral hypoglycemic therapy, such as metformin, may be attempted. The treatment strategy employed in HIV-infected children with hyperglycemia would be similar.

35.6 Abnormal calcium metabolism

Both hypo- and hypercalcemia have been described in association with HIV infection [21, 22]. However, parathyroid gland involvement in infected adults is rare and, even when CMV and MAC have been found at autopsy, there has usually been no evidence of premortem hypocalcemia.

35.6.1 Proposed mechanisms

Hypocalcemia may result from: critical illness; drugs, including foscarnet treatment of CMV retinitis (by complexing ionized calcium), pentamidine, aminoglycosides and amphotericin B (secondary to magnesium depletion), and ketoconazole (by inhibiting renal 1α-hydroxylase activity); and reduced parathyroid hormone (PTH) responsiveness to hypocalcemia in infected adults. Hypercalcemia has been described with: HIV-related lymphoma and other hematological malignancies as a result of production of $1,25(OH)_2$ vitamin D, PTH-related peptide, or cytokines; and with granulomatous disease, e.g. MAC, as a result of disordered extra-renal synthesis of $1,25(OH)_2$ vitamin D.

35.6.2 Diagnostic approach

If there are symptoms and signs of hypocalcemia (paresthesias, sensorial changes, arrhythmias, seizures, or positive Chvostek's or Trousseau's signs) or hypercalcemia (bone pain, abdominal pains, and sensorial changes), the pediatrician should check a serum *ionized* calcium (along with phosphorus and magnesium). If the ionized calcium is abnormal, a simultaneous PTH level should be measured.

35.6.3 Treatment

To correct hypocalcemia, the pediatrician, with the assistance of an endocrinologist, should attempt to eliminate any causative factor, if possible, and to normalize the serum calcium with parenteral and oral calcium and, if associated with decreased production or action of PTH, active vitamin D (calcitriol). For hypercalcemia, the pediatrician, again with the assistance of an endocrinologist, should eliminate any causative factor if possible, and reduce the serum calcium through hydration and staged administration of calcium-lowering agents, such as furosemide, prednisone, bisphosphonates, and calcitonin.

35.7 Conclusion

Although endocrinological problems are relatively uncommon among HIV-infected children, if the clinical presentation suggests the presence of a hormonal abnormality, the first-line tests outlined above should enable the pediatrician to begin the appropriate evaluation in a cost-effective manner. For assistance with interpretation of initial laboratory data, initiation of second-line hormonal testing (e.g. stimulation tests), or introduction of specific hormonal therapies, consultation with a pediatric endocrinologist becomes mandatory.

REFERENCES

1. Geffner, M. E., Van Dop, C., Kovacs, A. A. *et al.* Intrauterine and postnatal growth in children born to women infected with HIV. *Pediatr. AIDS HIV Infect.* **5** (1994), 162–8.

2. Frost, R. A., Lang, C. H. & Gelato, M. C. Growth hormone/insulin-like growth factor axis in human immunodeficiency virus-associated disease. *Endocrinologist* **7** (1997), 23–31.

3. Miller, T. L., Easley, K. A., Zhang, W. *et al.* Maternal and infant factors associated with failure to thrive in children with vertically transmitted human immunodeficiency virus-1 infection: the prospective P2C2 human immunodeficiency virus multicenter study. *Pediatrics* **108** (2001), 1287–96.

4. Geffner, M. E., Yeh, D. Y., Landaw, E. M., Scott, M. L., Stiehm, E. R., Bryson, Y. J. & Israele, V. *In vitro* insulin-like growth factor-I, growth hormone, and insulin resistance occurs in symptomatic human immunodeficiency virus-1-infected children. *Pediatr. Res.* **34** (1993), 66–72.

5. De Martino, M., Tovo, P., Galli, L. *et al.* Puberty in perinatal HIV-1 infection: a multicentre study of 212 children. *AIDS* **15** (2001), 1527–34.

6. Mahoney, E., Donfield, S. M., Howard, C., Kaufman, F., Gertner, J. M. and the Hemophilia Growth and Development Study. HIV-associated immune dysfunction and delayed pubertal development in a cohort of young hemophiliacs. *J. AIDS* **21** (1999), 333–7.

7. Balter-Seri, J. & Ashkenazi, S. The effects of infectious diseases on the endocrine system. *J. Pediatr. Endocrinol. Metab.* **10** (1997), 245–56.

8. Grinspoon, S. Neuroendocrine manifestations of AIDS. *Endocrinologist* **7** (1997), 32–8.

9. Clarick, R. H., Hanekom, W. A., Yogev, R. & Chadwick, G. E. Megestrol acetate treatment of growth failure in children infected with human immunodeficiency virus. *Pediatrics* **99** (1997), 354–7.

10. Dreimane, D., Nielsen, K., Deveikis, A., Bryson, Y. J. & Geffner, M. E. Effect of protease inhibitors combined with standard antiretroviral therapy on linear growth and weight gain in human immunodeficiency virus type-1 infected children. *J. Pediatr. Infect. Dis.* **20** (2001), 315–16.

11. Schambelan, M., Mulligan, K., Grunfeld, C., Daar, E. S., LaMarca, A. & Kotler, D. P. Recombinant human growth hormone in patients with HIV-associated wasting. *Ann. Intern. Med.* **125** (1996), 873–82.

12. Hirschfeld, S. Use of human recombinant growth hormone and human recombinant insulin-like growth factor-I in patients with human immunodeficiency virus infection. *Hormon. Res.* **46** (1996), 215–21.

13. Laue, L., Pizzo, P. A., Butler, K. & Cutler, Jr G. B. Growth and neuroendocrine dysfunction in children with acquired immunodeficiency syndrome. *J. Pediatr.* **117** (1990), 541–5.

14. Hirschfeld, S., Laue, L., Cutler, Jr G. B. & Pizzo, P. A. Thyroid abnormalities in children infected with human immunodeficiency virus. *J. Pediatr.* **128** (1996), 70–4.

15. Heufelder, A. E. & Hofbauer, L. C. Human immunodeficiency virus infection and the thyroid gland. *Eur. J. Endocrinol.* **134** (1996), 669–74.

16. Fundaro, C., Olivieri, A., Rendeli, C. *et al.* Occurrence of antithyroid autoantibodies in children vertically infected with HIV-1. *J. Pediatr. Endocrinol. Metab.* **11** (1998), 745–50.

17. Chiarelli, F., Galli, L., Verrotti, A., di Ricco, L., Vierucci, A. & de Martino, M. Thyroid function in children with perinatal human immunodeficiency virus type 1 infection. *Thyroid* **10** (2000), 499–505.

18. Arpadi, S. M., Cuff, P. A., Horlick, M., Wang, J. & Kotler, D. P. Lipodystrophy in HIV-infected children is associated with high viral load and low CD4+-lymphocyte count and CD4+-lymphocyte percentage at baseline and use of protease inhibitors and stavudine. *J. AIDS* **27** (2001), 30–4.

19. Melvin, A. J., Lennon, S., Mohan, K. M. & Purnell, J. Q. Metabolic abnormalities in HIV type-1-infected children treated and not treated with protease inhibitors. *AIDS Res. Hum. Retrovirus.* **17** (2001), 1117–23.

20. Carr, A., Samaras, K., Chisholm, D. J. & Cooper, D. A. Pathogenesis of HIV-1-protease inhibitor-associated peripheral lipodystrophy, hyperlipidemia, and insulin resistance. *Lancet* **531** (1998), 1881–3.

21. Danoff, A. Endocrinologic complications of HIV infection. *Med. Clin. N. Am.* **80** (1996), 1453–69.

22. Sellmeyer, D. E. & Grunfeld, C. Endocrine and metabolic disturbances in human immunodeficiency virus infection and acquired immune deficiency syndrome. *Endocr. Rev.* **17** (1996), 518–32.

23. Oberfield, S. E., Kairam, R., Bakshi, S. *et al.* Steroid response to adrenocorticotropin stimulation in children with human immunodeficiency virus infection. *J. Clin. Endocrinol. Metab.* **70** (1990), 578–81.

24. Yanovski, J. A., Miller, K. D., Kino, T., Friedman, T. C., Chrousos, G. P. & Falloon, J. Endocrine and metabolic evaluation of human immunodeficiency virus-infected patients with evidence of protease inhibitor-associated lipodystrophy. *J. Clin. Endocrinol. Metab.* **84** (1999), 1925–31.

25. Kilby, J. M. & Tabereaux, P. B. Severe hyperglycemia in an HIV clinic: pre-existing versus drug-associated diabetes mellitus. *J. AIDS Hum. Retrovirol.* **17** (1998), 46–50.

26. Dube, M. P., Johnson, D. L., Currier, J. S. & Leedom, J. M. Protease inhibitor-associated hyperglycaemia. *Lancet* **2** (1997), 713–14.

Neoplastic disease in pediatric HIV infection

Richard F. Little, M.D.

HIV and AIDS Malignancy Branch, National Cancer Institute, NIH, Bethesda, MD

36.1 Introduction

One of the striking features of HIV infection is the increased incidence of malignancies. Approximately 40% of adults infected with HIV develop cancer during the course of HIV infection [1, 2]. The risk of neoplastic disease is also increased in children, but due to the low incidence of cancer in the general pediatric population, it is seen relatively infrequently in the USA and Europe. In certain parts of Africa, malignancy complications are more frequently seen in pediatric populations [3]. Three malignancies constitute AIDS-defining diagnoses in HIV-infected patients: Kaposi's sarcoma (KS), non-Hodgkin's lymphoma (NHL), and cervical cancer. Indeed, in the early 1980s, KS in young men with a history of sexual contact with other men (MSM) was one of the features which initially alerted the Centers for Disease Control and Prevention to the emerging epidemic. In the USA, KS remains rare except among HIV-infected MSM and their sex partners, up to 35% of whom may develop KS at some point in their disease. In contrast, KS is the most common cancer in certain parts of Africa [3]. Non-Hodgkin's lymphoma is greatly increased among those with HIV infection, but unlike KS, the risk of developing HIV-related NHL is equivalent among all groups at risk for acquiring HIV infection. Among HIV-infected patients up to age 19 years, NHL is increased by a factor of 360 compared with that expected in the general population [4]. Pediatric HIV-related NHL is still relatively rare, because of the very low incidence of NHL in pediatric patients. In the developing world, NHL, especially Burkitt's lymphoma, is seen more commonly in the

pediatric population compared with Western countries [3]. Cervical cancer is an important disease because it may be prevented, and in HIV-infected adolescent girls and women, it can be highly aggressive. Other neoplasms encountered in the HIV-infected pediatric population include leiomyoma, leiomyosarcoma, Hodgkin's disease, and lymphomas of mucosa-associated lymphoid tissue (MALT). These conditions are not considered AIDS-defining diagnoses, although they are clearly increased in frequency compared with the background population. Although the overall risk of neoplastic disease is elevated by a factor of 130, only 2–5% of children with HIV infection in rich countries are diagnosed with malignancy [5]. Yet, the occurrence of cancer in the HIV-infected patient creates a series of difficult psychosocial and medical challenges to patients, their families, and the entire medical team. Patients with neoplastic disease and HIV infection should ideally receive their care from specialists experienced in AIDS-related malignancy, but this may not be feasible in many cases. Close co-operation between oncologists and infectious disease specialists is essential in managing these patients.

36.2 Epidemiology of AIDS-related cancers

36.2.1 Kaposi's sarcoma

Kaposi's sarcoma, which is found rarely in pediatric AIDS, has a distinct epidemiologic pattern in the USA: it primarily affects MSM, and their female sexual partners [2]. The epidemiology of KS in the USA suggested that an infectious agent is likely to be a co-factor for KS, and the recently discovered human herpes-virus 8 (HHV-8), also known as the Kaposi's sarcoma-associated herpes virus (KSHV) has been shown to be a necessary component of KS etiology [6–9]. Prior to HAART, approximately 50% of patients infected with both HIV and KSHV/HHV-8 will develop KS within 10 years [10]. HAART appears to forestall development of KS for a period in patients who have good immunologic and virologic results of therapy [11]. There is evidence to support sexual transmission and perhaps mother-to-child transmission of KSHV/HHV-8 [12]. Although KSHV/HHV-8 may be common, clinical KS is exceedingly rare among North American children under the age of 13 years. When KS is encountered in pediatric practice it is most likely to be in an adolescent with hemophilia. In Africa however, HIV-associated KS occurs frequently, affecting women and men who have acquired HIV via heterosexual contact, and children [13]. This differing epidemiology probably reflects the much higher prevalence of KSHV/HHV-8 infection in Africa, where KS is the most common malignancy among men [14]. The seroprevalence of KSHV/HHV-8 varies substantially in different regions and in different populations. For example, KSHV/HHV-8 seroprevalence is less than 1% in the blood donor population of the USA [8], but 16% of MSM who are not HIV infected are KSHV-infected [15], and in one small study nearly 30% of healthy children without HIV infection in southwest Texas were found to be KSHV positive [16]. Antibodies for KSHV/HHV-8 can be found in approximately 50% of some African blood donor populations [17]. Evidence suggests that the highest risk of KS in the African pediatric population are children under the age of 5 years, and that males are approximately five times more likely than females to be affected [18].

36.2.2 HIV-related non-Hodgkin's lymphoma

In the USA, the overall incidence of NHL as an initial AIDS-defining diagnosis in the pediatric population is 1.7% [19]. However, this figure may be an underestimate of the true incidence since HIV-related NHL is not required to be reported if there is a prior AIDS diagnosis (e.g. if the patient already has AIDS by virtue of CD4$^+$ cell count less than 200 cells/mL). Some autopsy series have found the presence of NHL in up to 20% of HIV-infected individuals who had not been diagnosed with NHL antemortem [20]. The Italian Registry reported that 8% of children surviving less than 5 years and 2% of children surviving more than 5 years following perinatal HIV infection developed NHL [21]. Of NHL cases, approximately 15%–18% will be primary central nervous system lymphoma (PCNS) in populations without access to HAART [22]. Burkitt's lymphoma was a relatively

common cancer in African children before the beginning of the HIV epidemic, and HIV infection increases the risk of the Burkitt's. African children with Burkitt's lymphoma are significantly more likely to have HIV infection than children without lymphoma [23].

36.2.3 Cervical cancer

Cervical cancer has been an AIDS-defining condition in adults since 1993, and is an increasingly important contributor to morbidity and mortality for HIV-infected women, making it imperative to screen the sexually active adolescent population for this disease. The prevalence of cervical dysplasia (15%) in HIV-infected women may be up to twice that in women who are not HIV-infected (7%) [24]. Cervical intraepithelial neoplasia (CIN) has been associated with human papillomaviruses (HPV), especially types 16 and 18 [25]. Human papillomavirus HPV can be found in a high percentage of sexually active adolescents and young women [26]. The effect of the AIDS epidemic on the incidence of cervical cancer in Africa are not clear, but appears to be relatively small [27]. More information on HPV infection and cervical cancer can be found in Chapters 14 and 15.

36.2.4 Non-AIDS-defining malignancies in HIV-infected patients

Other non-AIDS-defining malignant and premalignant lesions are found in the pediatric HIV population. Leiomyosarcoma and leiomyomas appear at rates greater than in the general population [28] and, interestingly, appear to be Epstein–Barr virus (EBV)-associated in this setting [29]. Hodgkin's disease, leukemias, and other cancers common in childhood are seen in the HIV-infected pediatric patient, also at levels notably above those seen in the HIV-uninfected patient population.

36.2.5 Incidence: HAART and future prospects

It is unclear how HAART will affect the incidence of HIV-related malignancies in the long term. Since the advent of HAART, there has been a profound decrease in the incidence of KS among populations where these drugs are widely available [30]. There has also been a decrease in the incidence of HIV-related NHL since the advent of HAART [31]. The highest incidence of NHL is among individuals with the greatest degree of immune depletion, and the incidence is lower among individuals with better preserved immune function. HAART-induced immune reconstitution has resulted in fewer severely immunosuppressed individuals, thus substantially decreasing the proportion of the HIV-infected population at greatest risk of NHL. Within CD4 strata, there has been no change in NHL incidence since the advent of HAART.

Many factors may influence the incidence of neoplastic disease among patients treated with HAART, including the degree of resultant immune reconstitution. If HAART prolongs the lifespan of HIV-infected individuals, with only partial immune reconstitution, an even higher incidence of HIV-related malignancies may ultimately occur. Also, as currently available antiretroviral therapy begins to fail for larger numbers of patients and they develop renewed HIV disease progression, an increased incidence of malignant conditions may follow.

36.3 Clinical manifestations, diagnosis, and management of HIV-associated malignancies

36.3.1 Kaposi's sarcoma

Kaposi's sarcoma is a highly vascular tumor resulting in violaceous skin nodules, which can present anywhere on the skin or in the viscera (see Figs. 36.1–36.3, color plates). Disease can be minimal, with indolent waxing and waning of lesions, or it can be aggressive and characterized by explosive growth leading to death. The lesions can be flat or nodular, and can vary in size from a few millimeters in diameter to extensive lesions that completely circumscribe a limb. In affected African children, involvement of the lymph nodes, face and oral cavity, and inguinal-genital region is common [13]. Kaposi's sarcoma-associated edema can result in severe morbidity. Kaposi's sarcoma also affects internal organs, most commonly the gastrointestinal tract and lungs. Rarely, KS can affect the internal organs without cutaneous involvement. Chest radiographs are useful in assessing the patient for the presence of pulmonary KS, but in the absence of clinical signs or symptoms of organ involvement, aggressive searches for other involved internal sites require invasive measures, such as endoscopy, and would be unlikely to change management. Computed tomography scanning is not generally helpful in assessing the presence of gastrointestinal KS.

Staging for KS is based on the tumor extent (T), severity of immunosuppression (I), and history of other systemic HIV-associated illness (S) [32]. Patients are classified as good (subscript 0) or poor risk (subscript 1) based on each of these factors (see Table 36.1). Patients with poor risk on any of the TIS factors have decreased survival compared with those with no poor risk features.

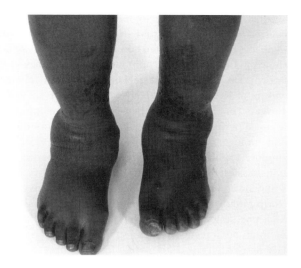

Figure 36.1. Kaposi's sarcoma involving the skin with associated edema.

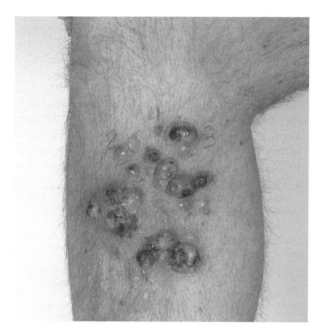

Figure 36.2. Ulcerating nodular lesions in AIDS- Kaposi's sarcoma

A pathologist experienced in KS should evaluate biopsy specimens and confirm the diagnosis prior to initiation of therapy. The pathologic diagnosis is a difficult one. Kaposi's sarcoma can be confused with prominent vascularity in lymph nodes or a variety of granulomatous conditions. Minimal KS may not require treatment unless the psychological impact causes the patient problems; this aspect of the disease can be profound and must not be

Table 36.1 Summary of ACTG Staging Classification for Kaposi's sarcoma

	Good risk	Poor risk
Tumor	T_0: KS confined to the skin and/or lymph nodes, and/or minimal (non-nodular) oral KS	T_1: ulcerated KS, KS-associated edema, nodular oral KS, or KS involvement of any non-nodal visceral organ
Immune status	I_0: CD4$^+$ lymphocyte count of 150/mL or higher	I_1: CD4$^+$ lymphocyte count less than 150/mL
Systemic illness	S_0: Karnofsky performance status $\geq$ 70; no fever, diarrhea, AIDS-defining opportunistic infections, oropharyngeal candidiasis, or unexplained weight loss	S_1: Karnofsky performance status < 70; presence of fever, diarrhea, AIDS-defining opportunistic infections, oropharyngeal candidiasis, or unexplained weight loss

Adapted from the Aids Clinical Trial Group Staging Classification for KS [32].

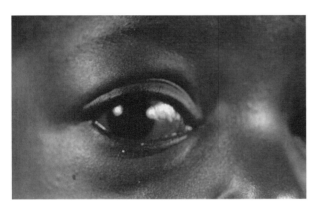

Figure 36.3. Child from Uganda with lymphadenopathic form of Kaposi's sarcoma with conjunctival involvement. (Photo courtesy of Dr. Sam Mbulaiteye, Viral Epidemiology Branch, National Cancer Institute, NIH).

underestimated. The psychosocial aspects of KS can be disabling because KS serves as a constant reminder of the underlying HIV infection and the visible lesions stigmatize patients, resulting in social withdrawal and reduction in the quality of life.

The first step in the treatment of AIDS-associated KS is to optimize antiretroviral therapy [33]. For cases that are not causing substantial physical or psychological morbidity, specific anti-KS therapy can be delayed for a period to assess the efficacy of antiretroviral therapy alone. Antiretroviral naïve patients who begin HAART and have good HIV suppression and CD4$^+$ lymphocyte recovery are more likely to have KS regression than those who do not. Additional specific therapy for KS is needed in such cases, or for those

in whom morbidity is too severe to wait for the potential effects of HAART, which may in some cases require several months to show an effect.

Kaposi's sarcoma can be treated with local modality treatment (intralesional chemotherapy, cryotherapy, radiation therapy), with systemic interferon-α or with systemic cytotoxic chemotherapy. Local modality therapy can be effective if there are few lesions, but often the cosmetic result is not satisfactory. Cryotherapy permanently destroys melanocytes, leaving cosmetically disturbing white spots following cryotherapy, most obvious in dark-skinned individuals. Radiation therapy can be effective when there is severe edema and pain, as the tumor is quite radioresponsive, but the cosmetic outcome is often not acceptable to patients. Post radiotherapy telangiectasias and darkened skin of toughened texture can be bothersome. Interferon-α can be effective in KS, with responses most likely to be seen in patients with CD4$^+$ lymphocyte counts over 200/mL in patients receiving nucleoside analogue monotherapy [34]. Trials using interferon in patients receiving HAART have not been reported, and it is not known if the responses are improved in this setting. Many patients do not tolerate the flu-like symptoms associated with interferon-α.

A number of systemic chemotherapy regimens have utility against KS, but these can produce significant drug-related toxicity (Table 36.2). Moreover, no current regimens can cure KS; chemotherapy requires continuing indefinite cycles, although with HAART, progression free survival may be prolonged after stopping chemotherapy [35]. Without adequate treatment of the underlying HIV disease, the KS will usually begin to grow again after chemotherapy is stopped. Recently, monotherapy with

Table 36.2 Selected chemotherapy regimens for Kaposi's sarcoma, and response rates

Chemotherapy	Dose and schedule	Response	Common toxicity
Liposomal Doxorubicin (Doxil®)	20 mg/m^2 every 2 to 3 weeks	45% [74]	Myelosuppression Palmar plantar erythrodysesthesia
Liposomal Daunorubicin (DaunoXome®)	40 mg/m^2 every 2 weeks	28% [37]	Myelosuppression
Paclitaxel (Taxol®)	135 mg/m^2 every 3 weeks; 100 mg/m^2 every 2 weeks; 50 mg/m^2 weekly	59–71% (refs [38, 75])	Myelosuppression, neurotoxicity, alopecia;
ABV (doxorubicin, bleomycin, vinca alkaloids	ABV every 2–4 weeks: Doxorubicin, 10–40 mg/m^2; Bleomycin 15 U; Vincristine 1 mg (OR vinblastine, 6 mg/m^2)	24–88% (higher response rates but increased toxicity at higher doxorubicin doses) [37, 76]	Myelosuppression, alopecia, mucositis, neurotoxicity
Vincristine/vinblastine	Vincristine, 1 mg, alternating with vinblastine, 2–4 mg every week	45% [39]	Myelosuppression; neurotoxicity

liposomal doxorubicin (Doxil®) or liposomal daunorubicin (DaunoXome®) has been shown to be as efficacious as the combination of doxorubicin, bleomycin, and vincristine (or vinblastine) (ABV) with less toxicity [36, 37]. Paclitaxel was recently approved as monotherapy, with response rates of up to 71% [38], which is higher than the response rates reported for the liposomal anthracyclines. A randomized trial is currently being conducted by the AIDS Malignancy Consortium to determine the relative efficacy and toxicity of liposomal doxorubicin versus paclitaxel in KS. Currently, the FDA has approved liposomal daunorubicin as first line KS therapy, and liposomal doxorubicin and paclitaxel as second line therapy for KS in adults. Many AIDS oncologists frequently use paclitaxel as first line for particularly severe disease. These studies have been conducted in adult patients, and therapy for children with KS is not defined.

Where HAART and the costly liposomal anthracyclines are unavailable, monotherapy with vincristine or vinblastine is sometimes used for palliative care. Also, a schedule of alternating vincristine and vinblastine is useful for palliative care and is well tolerated (Table 36.2) [39, 40].

Because KS is a highly vascular tumor, it serves as an ideal model in which to test antiangiogenesis agents. Several trials with such agents are in development, and preliminary reports suggest that thalidomide may have activity in KS [41]. Such agents may be of limited value as long-term therapy in the pediatric population, as inhibition of new blood vessel formation could lead to significant adverse effects on the developing child. However, it may be reasonable to consider this type of approach in the older adolescent population.

36.3.2 Non-Hodgkin's lymphoma

Since NHL is a rare childhood disease, all children who develop NHL should be tested for HIV infection. Among vertically infected children, the mean age at NHL diagnosis is 35 months, with a range of 6–62 months [42]. Compared to the general population, patients with HIV-related NHL more often present with: "B" symptoms characterized by fever, drenching night sweats, and greater than 10% loss of baseline body weight unexplained by other causes; subtle behavioral or personality changes, or cranial nerve palsies, seizures, or hemiparesis, possibly indicative of leptomeningeal or intraparenchymal brain disease; and extranodal disease. Central nervous system disease occurs in 15%–20% of cases. Physical examination may reveal jaundice, abdominal distention, or abdominal organomegally. In adults, most cases (60–80%) will present with advanced stage (III or IV) disease. The NCI experience suggests that children may present with less extensive disease. Cytopenias can reflect either HIV-associated bone marrow dysfunction, HIV-related immune thrombocytopenia purpura (ITP), or involvement by lymphoma (occurring in approximately 20% of cases).

Staging for HIV-related NHL should include history and physical examination; CT scans of the chest, abdomen and pelvis; head MRI with gadolinium or CT with contrast if MRI is not available; bilateral bone marrow biopsy; and lumbar puncture for cytological examination of the cerebrospinal fluid. Laboratory evaluation should include complete blood count with differential, T-cell subsets, electrolytes, renal and hepatic function, and LDH.

The World Health Organization lymphoma classification recognizes three main histologic subtypes of AIDS-related lymphoma (ARL): Burkitt's lymphoma, diffuse large B-cell lymphoma (DLBCL), and primary effusion lymphoma (PEL) [43]. These tumors behave aggressively in the setting of HIV infection. Lymphoblastic T-cell lymphomas are not considered AIDS-related NHLs, though they can certainly occur in patients with HIV infection. It has been reported that the Burkitt's and centroblastic DLBCL type occurs most frequently in the pediatric AIDS population and at an earlier point in the natural history of HIV infection while the CD4$^+$ cell count remains relatively preserved, whereas immunoblastic DLBCL more often occur in older age groups, later during infection when CD4$^+$ lymphocytes are depleted [44]. Burkitt's lymphoma peaks in incidence in AIDS patients in the first two decades of life (as in non-AIDS patients) and may represent the AIDS defining diagnosis in children, whereas DLBCL increases in incidence with age [4]. Central nervous system lymphomas do not appear to be age-related. Anaplastic large cell lymphomas represent a higher proportion of cases than expected, and the CDC consistently reports a greater proportion of pediatric AIDS-defining lymphoma cases as being large cell. It is not clear what the predominant histologic type is in this population.

In Uganda, the increase in ARL incidence is due primarily to an increase in Burkitt's lymphoma among children [27]. There has been a recent three-fold increase in this tumor due to the expanding AIDS epidemic in Africa, as more children are infected with HIV.

Prognostic features in the pediatric population are not as well-defined as for their adult counterparts. For adults, prognostic features predictive of poor outcome are CD4$^+$ lymphocyte count less than 200 cells/mL, prior AIDS-related opportunistic illness, age greater than 40 years, advanced stage disease, elevated LDH, and poor performance status. Adult patients with less than 200 CD4$^+$ lymphocyte cells/mL have a median survival of less than

4 months from diagnosis, and those with higher CD4$^+$ lymphocyte counts have a median survival of 11 months. These survival estimates are based on the pre-HAART experience. It appears that since with HAART, the median overall survival has improved to approximately 2 years in patients with ARL [31]. To what extent these prognostic factors can be extrapolated to the pediatric HIV-related patient population is unknown.

There are no published results from clinical trials for the treatment of HIV-related lymphomas in the pediatric population, and optimal therapy has not been determined, though data from ongoing trials should be available in the future. Whenever possible, these patients should be referred for participation in a clinical trial. Treatment of HIV-related lymphoma should not be based solely on the experience with NHL in the general pediatric population. HIV-associated Burkitt's lymphoma occurring in a patient with a normal CD4$^+$ lymphocyte count and no history of opportunistic infections should probably be treated in the same way as the cancer in a patient without HIV infection. However, markedly immunosuppressed patients are much less likely to tolerate the high dose induction regimens shown to be effective in curing NHL, including Burkitt's lymphoma, in patients not infected with HIV. Moreover, it has not been shown in adults with ARL that dose-intensive regimens are necessary for Burkitt's lymphoma. In HIV infection, the risk of prolonged neutropenia from myelosuppressive therapy may increase the risk of fatal infectious complications and there does not appear to be added survival benefit from intensive regimens in these patients [45, 46]. A number of combination chemotherapy regimens that have been explored, generally used in a much less intensive fashion than for non-HIV-infected patients, include various combinations of drugs, such as doxorubicin, cyclophosphamide, vincristine, methotrexate, and prednisone (Tables 36.3 and 36.4).

The recent clinical research in adult ARL has focused primarily on combining antiretroviral therapy with combination chemotherapy. Trial results have shown that this is a feasible approach. Additionally, the epidemiologic data have shown an increased survival since the era of HAART [31]. A subset analysis of adult patients with prior long-term successful HAART therapy receiving combination chemotherapy for ARL showed a higher response rate compared with patients failing HAART [47]. Based on these and other results demonstrating combined HAART and chemotherapy such as CHOP (cyclophosphamide, doxorubicin, vincristine, and prednisone) to be feasible [48], a conventional wisdom has emerged that combined HAART and chemotherapy are required to optimize the treatment outcome. However, patients with good clinical benefit on

Table 36.3 Low and standard dose m-BACOD for AIDS-releated lymphoma [45]

Drug	Standard-Dose	Low-Dose
Methotrexate (IV)	200 mg/m^2, day 15	200 mg/m^2, day 15
Bleomycin (IV)	4 U/m^2, day 1	4 U/m^2, day 1
Doxorubicin (IV)	45 mg/m^2, day 1	25 mg/m^2, day 1
Cyclophosphamide (IV)	600 mg/m^2, day 1	300 mg/m^2, day 1
Vincristine (IV)	1.4 mg/m^2, day 1	1.4 mg/m^2, day 1
Dexamethasone (oral)	6 mg/m^2, day 1–5	3 mg/m^2, day 1–5
GM-CSF (SC)	5 μg/kg days 4–13	5 μg/kg days 4–13, as needed

Meningeal lymphoma prophylaxis in all patients: Cytarabine 50 mg, IT, days 1, 8, 15, and 22 of cycle 1 only

Table 36.4 Low and Standard dose CHOP in AIDS-releated lymphoma [48]

Drug	Standard Dose	Low Dose
Cyclophosphamide (IV)	750 mg/m^2, day 1	375 mg/m^2, day 1
Doxorubicin (IV)	50 mg/m^2, day 1	25 mg/m^2, day 1
Vincristine (IV)	1.4 mg/m^2 (2 mg maximum dose)	1.4 mg/m^2 (2 mg maximum dose)
Prednisone (oral)	100 mg, days 1–5	100 mg, days 1–5
G-CSF (SC)	300–480 μg/day days 4–13 if needed	

HAART given to all patients (stavudine, lamivudine, indinavir)

long-term HAART appear to be more likely to develop non-immunoblastic tumors that may be more chemosensitive. Thus, HAART changes the immune environment in which the tumor evolves, but there are no data showing that HAART changes the actual response to chemotherapy once the tumor has formed. Decisions on combining HAART or not should be individualized.

Even though there is no consensus on the optimal treatment of DLBCL in pediatrics (regardless of HIV infection status), many such patients can be successfully treated. Long-term survival appears to be primarily related to the ability to control the underlying HIV infection once the lymphoma is in remission. Future results from ongoing clinical trials will help to determine the optimal therapy for HIV-related NHL.

36.3.3 Primary central nervous system lymphoma

The outcome for primary central nervous system lymphoma (PCNSL) is particularly poor. Median survival among adults with PCNSL receiving radiation therapy alone is significantly less for AIDS-related PCNSL (2.6 months) compared to non-AIDS-related PCNSL (16.6

months) [49]. The major differential in diagnosis is CNS *Toxoplasma gondii* infection (but other possibilities include fungal infections and tuberculosis) and this can be resolved by stereotactic brain biopsy, shown to be generally safe in HIV-infected patients with CNS lesions. However, not infrequently, brain biopsies are omitted in AIDS patients because of a concern that the potential morbidity associated with the procedure may not be justified by any apparent improvement in outcome ensuing from a histologically-confirmed diagnosis of PCNSL. Therefore, definitive therapy is often delayed because of diagnostic uncertainty. A frequently employed approach is to treat the patient for toxoplasmosis for 2–3 weeks; if there is no response, or rapid progression, a presumed diagnosis of PCNSL is made and the patient is treated presumptively for PCNSL with radiation therapy and/or chemotherapy. This is one of the few settings in oncology where antineoplastic treatment is commenced without tissue diagnosis. Recent advances in diagnosing PCNSL are based on the finding that 100% of PCNSL contain Epstein–Barr virus (EBV). Investigators have shown that combining thallium-201 single photon emission computed tomography (SPECT) imaging with qualitative EBV PCR on the cerebrospinal fluid can accurately identify lymphoma [50]. If both tests are positive, the positive predictive value for lymphoma is 100%. Conversely, if both tests are negative, the negative predictive value for lymphoma is 100%. Thus, definitive therapy for lymphoma can be instituted earlier. Similarly, lymphoma can be excluded from the differential diagnosis with negative tests. If there are discordant findings, then biopsy remains necessary.

36.3.4 Cervical cancer

Clinical, epidemiologic, and molecular evidence support the relationship between HPV infection, cervical intraepithelial neoplasia, and squamous cell cervical carcinomas [24, 51]. A high percentage of cervical cancers have genomically integrated HPV DNA [51]. Human papillomavirus types 16, 18, 31, and 33 are associated with malignant transformation and high-grade CIN. Among women who are not HIV infected, a slow progression from CIN to invasive carcinoma occurs over a period in excess of 15 years, suggesting an important role for the host immune response to HPV infection. Patients with HIV and other immunodeficiencies who are infected with HPV develop CIN more frequently and at an earlier age than the general population with HPV infection [25]. Puberty and first pregnancy are periods when the cervical squamocolumnar metaplastic process occurs at a more rapid rate, and the highest risk of neoplasia coincides with periods of greatest metaplastic activity. Sexually active adolescents who are HIV infected should therefore be considered at risk for developing HPV-related atypical squamous metaplasia that can progress to CIN. Semiannual cervical cytological examination (Papanicolaou smears) with aggressive follow up for abnormal cytology has been recommended for HIV-infected women, and it is reasonable to include sexually active HIV-infected adolescents in this group.

Currently there is a paucity of data on the treatment of HIV-associated CIN and cervical cancer. Moreover, there is little information on how to prevent CIN from developing or progressing to squamous carcinoma. There is some interest in utilizing antiviral agents effective against HPV or differentiating agents such as isotretenoin in attempts to help eradicate HPV and prevent development of CIN or invasive cervical carcinoma. However, current standard treatment is conization of the cervix or hysterectomy. Frank carcinoma of the cervix is treated according to stage. Cervical cancer in HIV-infected women often behaves aggressively, requiring radical hysterectomy and pelvic lymphadenectomy or radiation therapy. In general, the clinical outcomes are relatively poor, so preventive care should be emphasized.

36.3.5 Other cancers (not AIDS-defining)

Leiomyosarcoma and leiomyomas

In addition to Kaposi's sarcoma, other soft tissue sarcomas occur with increased frequency among HIV-infected individuals. Whereas KS occurs primarily in adults and indicates a diagnosis of AIDS, leiomyomas and leiomyosarcoma occur with a higher frequency in HIV-infected children [28], but have not, as yet, been considered to be AIDS-defining illnesses. Leiomyoma is a benign smooth muscle tumor occurring most frequently in the uterus and gastrointestinal tract, but can also occur in the skin and subcutaneous tissues, probably arising from the smooth muscle of small blood vessels in these tissues. Leiomyosarcomas are malignant neoplasms that arise from smooth muscle anywhere in the body. They can arise in the viscera or blood vessels of internal organs such as the lungs and spleen. Leiomyosarcomas commonly arise in the retroperitineum and are highly aggressive in this case. The histological distinction between leiomyoma and leiomyosarcoma is difficult.

Clinical presentation is often characterized by fever, radiographic evidence of pulmonary infection unresponsive to antibiotics, bloody diarrhea, abdominal pain, or obstruction, depending on the site of disease. Hepatic and meningeal metastases have been reported [52, 53].

Epstein–Barr virus DNA has been found in large amounts within the cells of these tumors in HIV-infected patients, and rarely in patients not HIV infected who are undergoing immunosuppressive therapy following transplantation [54, 55].

Therapy consists of complete excision when possible. The role of adjuvant radiation and chemotherapy in children is not defined, but some cases have been treated with infusion doxorubicin, interferon-alpha, and/or radiotherapy, although with very limited response [56]. The prognosis is generally poor, and the malignancy tends to recur.

Lymphoproliferative lesions of mucosa-associated lymphoid tissue

Extranodal marginal zone B-cell lymphomas (low grade B-cell lymphoma of MALT type) have been reported in the HIV-infected pediatric population, and probably occur with increased frequency compared with the general pediatric population [57, 58]. Lymphomas of MALT type have been identified in many extranodal sites, including the gastrointestinal tract (as well as Waldeyer's ring and salivary glands), respiratory tract, thyroid, lung, breast, and skin. Pathologic features include reactive lymphoid follicles with prominent marginal zones containing cells that resemble, but can be distinguished from, the small centrocyte of the germinal center [59]. There is infiltration by malignant plasma cells and immunoblasts into the benign germinal centers of these lesions. These lymphomas are generally considered to be low-grade lymphomas (not intermediate- or high-grade lymphomas seen in AIDS-related NHL), and while they do constitute true cancer, they are not classified as AIDS-related lymphoma, and thus do not confer an AIDS diagnosis in the affected patient. Lymphomas of MALT type seen in HIV-infected patients appear to be associated with EBV, but perhaps less frequently with *Helicobacter pylori* compared with cases seen in HIV-uninfected patients [58, 60]. They can be removed surgically, but some cases associated with *H. pylori* have been observed to regress following treatment with appropriate antibiotics in patients not HIV infected [61].

Other non-malignant lymphoproliferative lesions occur in HIV-infected children. For example, early myoepithelial sialadenitis (MESA) represents a benign reactive lymphoproliferative lesion, which can occasionally progress to MALT [62, 63]. Polyclonal, polymorphic B-cell lymphoproliferative disorder (PBLD) involving the lungs, liver, kidneys, lymph nodes, and spleen may represent an intermediate between benign and malignant lymphoproliferation [64]. The progression from benign polyclonal to malignant clonal lymphoproliferation may involve accumulated genetic changes (e.g. those associated with EBV infection) which persist due to insufficient immune surveillance occurring with progressive HIV-induced immune dysfunction.

Lymphoproliferative disorders have been treated with varying degrees of success utilizing a variety of approaches including interferon-α, radiation, corticosteroids, cytotoxic chemotherapy, or HAART [58, 65]. It is not clear how often non-malignant lymphoproliferative lesions progress to malignancy, and a period of observation may be useful in determining individual therapy in these cases.

Other malignancies

Other cancers may be seen in HIV-infected pediatric patients, at frequencies above the general population. These include leukemias (most of B-cell origin), Hodgkin's disease, Ewing's sarcoma, malignant germ cell tumors, seminomas, and brain tumors. The curative potential in such cases depends not only on the tumor and stage, but also on the status of the underlying HIV disease.

36.3.6 Antiretroviral therapy and antineoplastic therapy

While it is generally assumed that the administration of antiretroviral therapy should be continued during antineoplastic chemotherapy for HIV-related malignancies, there is little information to guide such management. Ideally, one would wish to completely suppress HIV replication, without interruption, throughout the course of life-long HIV therapy. This may not be a realistic therapeutic goal for all HIV-infected patients, and in the setting of neoplastic disease, this goal may be even more difficult to achieve.

For a potentially curable malignancy requiring combination antineoplastic drugs, timely courses of adequately dose-intensive chemotherapy will optimize the chance of tumor eradication. The impact on survival of concurrently administered HAART regimens given with curative-intent antineoplastic therapy is not known. In deciding upon a therapeutic plan, consideration should be given to the potentially beneficial versus harmful effects of combining the two treatments. HIV suppression may prevent progressive HIV-induced immunosuppression during chemotherapy. However, attention should be given to overlapping toxicities anticipated with combining the various agents. Such toxicities can prompt chemotherapy dose reductions or cycle delays, possibly reducing the chances of tumor eradication. For example, one might predict an increase in neurotoxicity when using vincristine and stavudine simultaneously, or an increase in myelotoxicity when using zidovudine and cyclophosphamide, doxorubicin, or methotrexate together. Unclear and sometimes unpredictable pharmacokinetic interactions can lead to altered drug clearance and changes in toxicity profiles and therapeutic effects as a result of combining certain drug classes. An example of such interactions is the simultaneous use of cyclophosphamide and protease inhibitors, where plasma cyclophosphamide levels may be increased. This may result in exaggerated myelotoxicity, leading to prolonged neutropenia which may be more immediately life-threatening than uncontrolled HIV viremia for the finite period it takes to deliver the courses of antineoplastic chemotherapy. There are few examples in the literature to help guide clinicians. Didanosine resulted in lower than expected etoposide levels when the agents were used simultaneously, which could theoretically reduce the cure rate of the underlying cancer [66]. An increase in mucositis was observed when combination chemotherapy for NHL was combined with HAART (didanosine and/or stavudine with saquinavir) [67]. Zidovudine has been reported to increase the myelotoxic effects of chemotherapy, even in the presence of myeloid growth factors [68]. Other authors have utilized antiretroviral drugs with attenuated dose chemotherapy to avoid toxicity without improvement in overall survival [69]. In adults, low vs standard-dose m-BACOD (methotrexate, bleomycin, doxorubicin, cyclophosphamide, vincristine, and dexamethasone) appears to result in similar overall survival in AIDS-associated NHL, but there may be a higher proportion of patients with active lymphoma at the time of death among patients receiving low-dose m-BACOD [45]. Even though the low-dose group experienced fewer hospitalizations from febrile neutropenic episodes, there were no differences in the occurrence of opportunistic infections between the two treatment groups. It may be possible that the subset of patients with less advanced immunosuppression may benefit from more dose-intensive chemotherapy, and strategies to minimize precipitating factors that increase the likelihood of dose reductions may be useful.

Another important concern is the effect of chemotherapy-associated toxicity on the patient's ability to maintain antiretroviral therapy compliance. Chemotherapy-related mucositis, or nausea and vomiting may cause the patient to miss multiple doses of HAART, increasing the risk of drug-resistant virus emerging, thereby creating constraints on future options for effective HIV control. Attention to appropriate prophylaxis for opportunistic infections during the courses of antineoplastic therapy may reduce the risk of opportunistic complications, making it possible to deliver antineoplastic therapy without concomitant antiretroviral therapy. Profound lymphocyte depletion occurs with lymphocytotoxic chemotherapy in patients not HIV-infected, and antiretroviral therapy is unlikely to prevent this effect [70]. Following chemotherapy, immune recovery to baseline requires in excess of 1 year in HIV-infected adults responding to HAART, and this is similar to the CD4$^+$ lymphocyte dynamics in adults not HIV-infected [71]. CD4$^+$ lymphocyte recovery occurs much more quickly in children who are not HIV infected following chemotherapy, but data are unavailable for HIV-infected children [72].

There are inadequate clinical data to formulate recommendations as to the role of antiretroviral therapy during treatment for lymphoma at present. Physicians should be alert to the potential toxicities and drug interactions of antiretroviral and antineoplastic drugs, and should consult reference guides such as the Drug Information Manual published by the American Hospital Formulary Service for guidance in individual cases [73].

In the management of oncologic cases where palliation, not cure, is the therapeutic goal, the anti-HIV therapy and the antineoplastic therapy should be managed in a way to optimize control of both processes for as long as possible. For example, patients with KS can benefit from well-managed care for years, even though the KS is not cured. Therefore, it is important that HAART be integrated into the treatment plan without interruption if possible. Currently available monotherapeutic, antineoplastic options for KS make this easier to accomplish. As cautioned above, however, appropriate reference to drug information literature should be a part of the therapeutic planning for such cases.

36.4 Summary

The pediatric patient with HIV disease and neoplastic complications represents a particular challenge. There is relatively little clinical literature to provide guidance in the management of such cases. Historically, patients with HIV-related malignancies have had a poor prognosis. It remains to be seen whether the recent improvements in anti-HIV therapy and refinements in antineoplastic therapy will translate into substantial therapeutic benefits for pediatric patients with AIDS and cancer.

REFERENCES

1. Biggar, R. J. & Rabkin, C. S. The epidemiology of AIDS–related neoplasms. *Hematol. Oncol. Clin. N. Am.* **10**:**5** (1996), 997–1010.
2. Levine, A. M. AIDS-related malignancies: the emerging epidemic. *J. Natl. Cancer Inst.* **85**:**17** (1993), 1382–97.
3. Banda, L. T., Parkin, D. M., Dzamalala, C. P. & Liomba, N. G. Cancer incidence in Blantyre, Malawi 1994–1998. *Trop. Med. Int. Health* **6**:**4** (2001), 296–304.
4. Beral, V., Peterman, T., Berkelman, R. & Jaffe, H. AIDS-associated non-Hodgkin lymphoma. *Lancet* **337** (1991), 805–9.
5. Mueller, B. U. & Pizzo, P. A. Malignancies in pediatric AIDS. *Curr. Opin. Pediatr.* **8**:**1** (1996), 45–9.
6. Chang, Y., Cesarman, E., Pessin, M. *et al.* Identification of Herpesvirus-like DNA sequences in AIDS-associated Kaposi's sarcoma. *Science* **266** (1994), 1865–9.
7. Moore, P. S. & Chang, Y. Detection of herpesvirus-like DNA sequences in Kaposi's sarcoma in patients with and without HIV infection. *New Engl. J. Med.* **332**:**18** (1995), 1181–5.
8. Gao, S. J., Kingsley, L., Li, M. *et al.* KSHV antibodies among Americans, Italians and Ugandans with and without Kaposi's sarcoma. *Nat. Med.* **2**:**8** (1996), 925–8.
9. Kedes, D. H., Operskalski, E., Busch, M., Kohn, R., Flood, J. & Ganem, D. The seroepidemiology of human herpesvirus 8 (Kaposi's sarcoma-associated herpesvirus): distribution of infection in KS risk groups and evidence for sexual transmission. *Nat. Med.* **2**:**8** (1996), 918–24.
10. Martin, J. N., Ganem, D. E., Osmond, D. H., Page-Shafer, K. A., Macrae, D. & Kedes, D. H. Sexual transmission and the natural history of human herpesvirus 8 infection. *New Engl. J. Med.* **338**:**14** (1998), 948–54.
11. Bower, M., Portsmouth, S., Mandalia, S., Nelson, M. & Gazzard, B. HIV-1 related Kaposi's sarcoma (KS) in the highly active antiretroviral therapy (HAART) era. Non-nucleoside reverse transcriptase inhibitors (NNRTIs) are as effective at preventing

KS as protease inhibitors (PI's). In *Sixth International Conference on Malignancies in AIDS and Other Immunodeficiencies: Basic, Epidemiologic and Clinical Research*, Bethesda, April 22–24, 2002.

12. Whitby, D., Smith, N., Ariyoshi, K. *et al.* Serologic evidence for different routes of transmission of HHV-8 in different populations. In *Second National AIDS Malignancy Conference*, Bethesda, April 6–8, 1998.

13. Ziegler, J. L. & Katongole-Mbidde E. Kaposi's sarcoma in childhood: an analysis of 100 cases from Uganda and relationship to HIV infection. *Int. J. Cancer* **65** : 2 (1996), 200–3.

14. Bassett, M. T., Chokunonga, E., Mauchaza, B., Levy, L., Ferlay, J. & Parkin, D. M. Cancer in the African population of Harare, Zimbabwe, 1990–1992. *Int. J. Cancer* **63** : 1 (1995), 29–36.

15. Casper, C., Wald, A., Pauk, J., Tabet S. R., Corey, L. & Celum, C. L. Correlates of prevalent and incident Kaposi's sarcoma-associated herpesvirus infection in men who have sex with men. *J. Infect. Dis.* **185** : 7 (2002), 990–3.

16. Baillargeon, J., Leach, C. T., Deng, J. H., Gao, S. J. & Jenson, H. B. High prevalence of human herpesvirus 8 (HHV-8) infection in south Texas children. *J. Med. Virol.* **67** : 4 (2002), 542–8.

17. Enbom, M., Urassa, W., Massambu, C., Thorstensson, R., Mhalu, F. & Linde, A. Detection of human herpesvirus 8 DNA in serum from blood donors with HHV-8 antibodies indicates possible bloodborne virus transmission. *J. Med. Virol.* **68** : 2 (2002), 264–7.

18. Amir, H., Kaaya, E. E., Manji, K. P., Kwesigabo, G. & Biberfeld, P. Kaposi's sarcoma before and during a human immunodeficiency virus epidemic in Tanzanian children. *Pediatr. Infect. Dis. J.* **20** : 5 (2001), 518–21.

19. *MMWR: US HIV and AIDS cases reported through December 1994. HIV/AIDS Surveillance Report*, Vol. 6. Atlanta: Centers for Disease Control and Prevention (1995), pp. 1–39.

20. Wilkes, M. S., Fortin, A. H., Felix, J. C., Godwin, T. A. & Thompson, W. G. Value of necropsy in acquired immunodeficiency syndrome. *Lancet* **2** (1988), 85–8.

21. Arico, M., Caselli, D., D'Argenio, P. *et al.* Malignancies in children with human immunodeficiency virus type 1 infection. The Italian Multicenter Study on Human Immunodeficiency Virus Infection in Children. *Cancer* **68** : 11 (1991), 2473–7.

22. Irwin, D. & Kaplan, L. Clinical aspects of HIV-related lymphoma. *Curr. Opin. Oncol.* **5** : 5 (1993), 852–60.

23. Newton, R., Ziegler, J., Beral, V. *et al.* A case-control study of human immunodeficiency virus infection and cancer in adults and children residing in Kampala, Uganda. *Int. J. Cancer* **92** : 5 (2001), 622–7.

24. Motti, P. G., Dallabetta, G. A., Daniel, R. W. *et al.* Cervical abnormalities, human papillomavirus, and human immunodeficiency virus infections in women in Malawi. *J. Infect. Dis.* **173** : 3 (1996), 714–17.

25. Northfelt, D. W. Cervical and anal neoplasia and HPV infection in persons with HIV infection. *Oncology (Huntingt)* **8** : 1 (1994), 33–7; Discussion 38–40.

26. Carter, J. J., Koutsky, L. A., Wipf, G. C. *et al.* The natural history of human papillomavirus type 16 capsid antibodies among a cohort of university women. *J. Infect. Dis.* **174** : 5 (1996), 927–36.

27. Parkin, D. M., Wabinga, H., Nambooze, S. & Wabwire-Mangen, F. AIDS-related cancers in Africa: maturation of the epidemic in Uganda. *AIDS* **13** : 18 (1999), 2563–70.

28. Chadwick, E. G., Connor, E. J., Hanson, I. C. *et al.* Tumors of smooth-muscle origin in HIV-infected children. *J. Am. Med. Assoc.* **263** : 23 (1990), 3182–4.

29. Jenson, H. B., Leach, C. T., McClain, K. L. *et al.* Benign and malignant smooth muscle tumors containing Epstein–Barr virus in children with AIDS. *Leuk. Lymphoma* **27** : 3–4 (1997), 303–14.

30. Jacobson, L. P., Yamashita, T. E., Detels, R. *et al.* Impact of potent antiretroviral therapy on the incidence of Kaposi's sarcoma and non-Hodgkin's lymphomas among HIV-1-infected individuals. Multicenter AIDS Cohort Study. *J. Acquir. Immune Defic. Syndr.* **21** : Suppl. 1 (1999), S34–41.

31. Besson, C., Goubar, A., Gabarre, J. *et al.* Changes in AIDS-related lymphoma since the era of highly active antiretroviral therapy. *Blood* **98** : 8 (2001), 2339–44.

32. Krown, S. E., Testa, M. A. & Huang, J. AIDS-related Kaposi's sarcoma: prospective validation of the AIDS Clinical Trials Group staging classification. AIDS Clinical Trials Group Oncology Committee. *J. Clin. Oncol.* **15** : 9 (1997), 3085–92.

33. Yarchoan, R. & Little, R. F. Immunosuppression-related malignancies. In V. T. De Vita Jr., S. Hellman & S. A. Rosenberg (eds.), *Cancer, Principles and Practice of Oncology*, 6th Edition. Philadelphia: Lippincott Williams and Wilkins (2001), pp. 2575–97.

34. Krown, S. E. Interferon and other biologic agents for the treatment of Kaposi's sarcoma. *Hematol. Oncol. Clin. N. Am.* **5** : 2 (1991), 311–22.

35. Dupont, C., Vasseur, E., Beauchet, A. *et al.* Long-term efficacy on Kaposi's sarcoma of highly active antiretroviral therapy in a cohort of HIV-positive patients. CISIH 92. Centre d'information et de soins de l'immunodeficience humaine. *AIDS* **14** : 8 (2000), 987–93.

36. Northfelt, D. W., Dezube, B. J., Thommes, J. A. *et al.* Efficacy of pegylated-liposomal doxorubicin in the treatment of AIDS-related Kaposi's sarcoma after failure of standard chemotherapy. *J. Clin. Oncol.* **15** : 2 (1997), 653–9.

37. Gill, P. S., Wernz, J., Scadden, D. T. *et al.* Randomized phase III trial of liposomal daunorubicin versus doxorubicin, bleomycin, and vincristine in AIDS-related Kaposi's sarcoma. *J. Clin. Oncol.* **14** : 8 (1996), 2353–64.

38. Welles, L., Saville, M. W., Lietzau, J. *et al.* Phase II trial with dose titration of paclitaxel for the therapy of human immunodeficiency virus-associated Kaposi's sarcoma. *J. Clin. Oncol.* **16** : 3 (1998), 1112–21.

39. Kaplan, L., Abrams, D. & Volberding, P. Treatment of Kaposi's sarcoma in acquired immunodeficiency syndrome with an alternating vincristine-vinblastine regimen. *Cancer Treat. Rep.* **70** : 9 (1986), 1121–2.

40. Stein, M. E., Spencer, D., Ruff, P., Lakier, R., MacPhail, P. & Bezwoda, W. R. Endemic African Kaposi's sarcoma: clinical

and therapeutic implications. 10-year experience in the Johannesburg Hospital (1980–1990). *Oncology* **51**:1 (1994), 63–9.

41. Little, R., Welles, L., Wyvill, K. *et al.* Preliminary results of a phase II study of oral thalidomide in patients with AIDS-related Kaposi's sarcoma (KS). In *Second National AIDS Malignancy Conference*, Bethesda, April 6–8, 1998.

42. Mueller, B. U., Shad, A. T., Magrath, I. T. & Horowitz, M. E. Malignancies in children with HIV infection. In P. A. Pizzo & C. M. Wilfert (eds.), *Pediatric AIDS: The Challenge of HIV Infection in Infants, Children, and Adolescents*. Baltimore: Williams & Wilkins (1994), pp. 603–22.

43. Jaffe, E. S., Harris, N. L., Stein, H. & Vardiman, J. W. *World Health Organization Classification of Tumors: Pathology and Genetics: Tumors of Haematopoietic and Lymphoid Tissues*. Lyon: IARC Press (2001), p. 351.

44. Gaidano, G., Pastore, C., Lanza, C., Mazza, U. & Saglio, G. Molecular pathology of AIDS-related lymphomas. Biologic aspects and clinicopathologic heterogeneity. *Ann. Hematol.* **69**:6 (1994), 281–90.

45. Kaplan, L. D., Straus, D. J., Testa, M. A. *et al.* Low-dose compared with standard-dose m-BACOD chemotherapy for non-Hodgkin's lymphoma associated with human immunodeficiency virus infection. National Institute of Allergy and Infectious Diseases AIDS Clinical Trials Group. *New Engl. J. Med.* **336**:23 (1997), 1641–8.

46. Walsh, C., Wernz, J. C., Levine, A. *et al.* Phase I trial of m-BACOD and granulocyte macrophage colony stimulating factor in HIV-associated non-Hodgkin's lymphoma. *J. AIDS* **6**:3 (1993), 265–71.

47. Antinori, A., Cingolani, A., Alba, L. *et al.* Better response to chemotherapy and prolonged survival in AIDS-related lymphomas responding to highly active antiretroviral therapy. *AIDS* **15**:12 (2001), 1483–91.

48. Ratner, L., Lee, J., Tang, S. *et al.* Chemotherapy for human immunodeficiency virus-associated non-Hodgkin's lymphoma in combination with highly active antiretroviral therapy. *J. Clin. Oncol.* **19**:8 (2001), 2171–8.

49. Forsyth, P. A., Yahalom, J. & DeAngelis, L. M. Combined-modality therapy in the treatment of primary central nervous system lymphoma in AIDS. *Neurology* **44**:8 (1994), 1473–9.

50. Antinori, A., De Rossi G, Ammassari, A. *et al.* Value of combined approach with thallium-201 single-photon emission computed tomography and Epstein-Barr virus DNA polymerase chain reaction in CSF for the diagnosis of AIDS-related primary CNS lymphoma. *J. Clin. Oncol.* **17**:2 (1999), 554–60.

51. Klein, R. S., Ho, G. Y., Vermund, S. H., Fleming, I. & Burk, R. D. Risk factors for squamous intraepithelial lesions on Pap smear in women at risk for human immunodeficiency virus infection. *J. Infect. Dis.* **170**:6 (1994), 1404–9.

52. Holloway, H., Walsh, C. B., Thomas, R. & Fielding, J. Primary hepatic leiomyosarcoma. *J. Clin. Gastroenterol* **23**:2 (1996), 131–3.

53. Morgello, S., Kotsianti, A., Gumprecht, J. P. & Moore, F. Epstein–Barr virus-associated dural leiomyosarcoma in a man infected with human immunodeficiency virus. Case report. *J. Neurosurg.* **86**:5 (1997), 883–7.

54. McClain, K. L., Leach, C. T., Jenson, H. B. *et al.* Association of Epstein–Barr virus with leiomyosarcomas in children with AIDS. *New Engl. J. Med.* **332**:1 (1995), 12–18.

55. Kingma, D. W., Shad, A., Tsokos, M. *et al.* Epstein–Barr virus (EBV)-associated smooth-muscle tumor arising in a post-transplant patient treated successfully for two PT-EBV-associated large-cell lymphomas. Case report. *Am. J. Surg. Pathol.* **20**:12 (1996), 1511–19.

56. McClain, K. L., Joshi, V. V. & Murphy, S. B. Cancers in children with HIV infection. *Hematol. Oncol. Clin. N. Am.* **10**:5 (1996), 1189–201.

57. Teruya-Feldstein, J., Temeck, B. K., Sloas, M. M. *et al.* Pulmonary malignant lymphoma of mucosa-associated lymphoid tissue (MALT) arising in a pediatric HIV-positive patient. *Am. J. Surg. Pathol.* **19**:3 (1995), 357–63.

58. Joshi, V. V., Gagnon, G. A., Chadwick, E. G. *et al.* The spectrum of mucosa-associated lymphoid tissue lesions in pediatric patients infected with HIV: A clinicopathologic study of six cases. *Am. J. Clin. Pathol.* **107**:5 (1997), 592–600.

59. Aisenberg, A. C. Coherent view of non-Hodgkin's lymphoma. *J. Clin. Oncol.* **13**:10 (1995), 2656–75.

60. Eidt, S., Schrappe, M. & Fischer, R. Analysis of antral biopsy specimens for evidence of acquired mucosa-associated lymphoid tissue in HIV1-seropositive and HIV-1-negative patients. *Scand. J. Gastroenterol.* **30**:7 (1995), 635–9.

61. Montalban, C., Manzanal, A., Boixeda, D. *et al.* Helicobacter pylori eradication for the treatment of low-grade gastric MALT lymphoma: follow-up together with sequential molecular studies. *Ann. Oncol.* **8**: Suppl. 2 (1997), 37–9.

62. Isaacson, P. G. Gastrointestinal lymphoma. *Hum. Pathol.* **25**:10 (1994), 1020–9.

63. Harris, N. L. Extranodal lymphoid infiltrates and mucosa-associated lymphoid tissue (MALT). A unifying concept. *Am. J. Surg. Pathol.* **15**:9 (1991), 879–84.

64. Joshi, V. V., Kauffman, S., Oleske, J. M. *et al.* Polyclonal polymorphic B-cell lymphoproliferative disorder with prominent pulmonary involvement in children with acquired immune deficiency syndrome. *Cancer* **59**:8 (1987), 1455–62.

65. Craven, D. E., Duncan, R. A., Stram, J. R. *et al.* Response of lymphoepithelial parotid cysts to antiretroviral treatment in HIV-infected adults. *Ann. Intern. Med.* **128**:6 (1998), 455–9.

66. Sparano, J., Wiernik, P., Hu, X., Sarta, C. & Schwartz, E. Pilot trial of infusional cyclophosphamide, doxorubicin, and etoposide plus didanosine and filgrastim in patients with human immunodeficiency virus-associated non-Hodgkin's lymphoma. *J. Clin. Oncol.* **14**:11 (1996), 3026–35.

67. Sparano, J., Wiernik, P., Hu, X., Sarta, C., Henry, D. & Ratech, H. Pilot trial of saquinavir and nucleoside analogues plus infusional cyclophosphamide, doxorubicin, and etoposide in patients with HIV-associated non-Hodgkin's lymphoma. In

Second National AIDS Malignancy Conference, Bethesda, MD, April 6–8, 1998.

68. Gabarre, J., Lepage, E., Thyss, A. *et al.* Chemotherapy combined with zidovudine and GM-CSF in human immunodeficiency virus-related non-Hodgkin's lymphoma. *Ann. Oncol.* **6**:**10** (1995), 1025–32.

69. Levine, A. M., Wernz, J. C., Kaplan, L. *et al.* Low-dose chemotherapy with central nervous system prophylaxis and zidovudine maintenance in AIDS-related lymphoma. A prospective multi-institutional trial. *J. Am. Med. Assoc.* **266**:**1** (1991), 84–8.

70. Mackall, C. L., Fleisher, T. A., Brown, M. R. *et al.* Lymphocyte depletion during treatment with intensive chemotherapy for cancer. *Blood* **84**:**7** (1994), 2221–8.

71. Little, R., Pearson, D., Gutierrez, M., Steinberg, S., Yarchoan, R. & Wilson, W. Dose-adjusted EPOCH chemotherapy (CT) with suspension of antiretroviral therapy (ART) for HIV-associated non-Hodgkin's lymphoma (HIV-NHL). In *Fourth International AIDS Malignancy Conference*, Bethesda, MD, May 16–18, 2000.

72. Mackall, C. L., Fleisher, T. A., Brown, M. R. *et al.* Age, thymopoiesis, and CD4+ T-lymphocyte regeneration after intensive chemotherapy. *New Engl. J. Med.* **332**:**3** (1995), 143–9.

73. McEvoy, G. K. American Hospital Formulary Service. In: K. Litvak, H. Olin & J. Welsh (eds.), *AHFS 96 Drug Information, 1996 edn.* Bethesda, MD: American Society of Health-System Pharmacists, Inc. (1996), p. 2813.

PART V

Infectious problems in pediatric HIV disease

Serious infections caused by typical bacteria

Shirley Jankelevich, M.D.

Medical Officer, Pediatric Medicine Branch, National Institute of Allergy and Infectious Diseases, NIH, Bethesda, MD

37.1 Introduction

HIV-infected children are at risk for the same minor and serious bacterial infections that affect immunocompetent children, although they occur more frequently and may be more severe in HIV-infected children. Because of this increased risk, the US Centers for Disease Control and Prevention (CDC) added a new category of invasive bacterial infections to the list of pediatric AIDS-defining illnesses in 1987 [1].

Bacterial infections in HIV-infected children often present in a manner similar to HIV-uninfected children and respond to the same antibiotics, although disseminated infection or frequent recurrences are often seen in HIV-infected children. The differential diagnosis may be large because some of these infections can present in a manner similar to opportunistic and endemic infections, including those due to viruses, unusual bacteria, fungi, and parasites. In addition, bacteria that are unusual in the immunocompetent host may cause significant disease in immunosuppressed HIV-infected children (Tables 37.1 and 37.2).

Multiple immunologic abnormalities in HIV-infected children prevent these children from mounting a robust immune response to a broad range of bacterial pathogens (See Chapter 3). These abnormalities include defects in the cell-mediated (T cell) and the humoral (B cell) arms of the immune system, decreases in neutrophil number, multiple defects in neutrophil function, impairment in macrophage and monocyte function [2], functional asplenia [3] and defects in three components of complement [3] (Table 37.1). Other factors that increase susceptibility to infection in HIV-infected children include frequent use of broad-spectrum antibiotics, frequent hospitaliza-

tions, use of indwelling intravascular catheters, and disruption of the integrity of skin and mucous membranes by invasive procedures or other pathogenic organisms [4]. Additional factors in resource-poor countries include malnutrition, micronutrient deficiencies, and lack of adequate medical care. The results of these abnormalities and deficiencies are increased susceptibility to infection with encapsulated bacteria beyond the age of 2 years [5], increased nasopharyngeal colonization rates for *Streptococcus pneumoniae* [6] and, presumably, *Haemophilus influenzae*, recurrent infections with the same bacterial species, increased susceptibility to infections with bacteria unusual in immunocompetent hosts, and increased morbidity and mortality. Certain vaccines against bacterial agents or their toxins administered to HIV-infected children often produce antibody titers that are lower and less persistent than those seen in HIV-uninfected children. These include *H. influenzae* type b (Hib) polysaccharide conjugate vaccine [7], pneumococcal polysaccharide vaccine, a 5-valent pneumococcal conjugate vaccine [8] and pertussis vaccine [9], as well as diphtheria and tetanus toxoids [10].

The antimicrobial regimens used in the treatment of many bacterial infections in HIV-infected children are often the same as for HIV-uninfected children. Suggested empiric regimens are listed in Table 37.3. The duration of therapy is often greater and should be based, in part, on the clinical course of the child. Lack of response to a regimen of appropriate duration and targeted to the pathogen(s) isolated should prompt a re-evaluation of the child since co-infection with several different pathogens, including mycobacteria, fungus, viruses, and parasites can occur.

Table 37.1 Selected immunologic defects and correlation of susceptibility to specific types of bacterial infections

Immunologic defect	Type of bacteria
Cell-mediated immunity (T cell)	*Salmonella* spp. *Listeria monocytogenes* *Nocardia* spp. *Treponema pallidum*
Humoral immunity (B cell)	*Streptococcus pneumoniae* *Haemophilus influenzae* *Moraxella catarrhalis* *Campylobacter* spp. *Shigella* spp. *Pseudomonas* spp.
Neutrophil abnormalities (defects in neutrophil function and number)	*Staphylococcus aureus* *Klebsiella pneumoniae* *Escherichia coli* and other *Enterbacteriaceae* *Pseudomonas aeruginosa*

The Integrated Management of Childhood Illness (IMCI) strategy developed by the World Health Organization (WHO) is currently being used as a guideline for the care and treatment of many bacterial diseases affecting children less than 5 years of age in some resource-poor countries but are often not specific for HIV-infected children in resource-poor countries. This chapter recommends diagnostic procedures and antibiotic treatment based on current practices in healthcare institutions in resource-rich countries. These recommendations and antibiotics chosen should be used in accordance with the capabilities and limitations of the healthcare institutions providing treatment for these children and with the type and prevalence of antibiotic resistance in each geographic region.

While this chapter generally addresses infections due to bacterial infections, it is important for the practitioner to have a low threshold for consulting experts in the care of immunosuppressed patients and for expanding the differential diagnosis, the diagnostic work-up and therapeutic coverage to include other less likely potential pathogens. All HIV-infected children with constitutional symptoms and suspected severe bacterial infection should have blood cultures drawn in addition to other appropriate diagnostic tests. As is the case with children not infected with HIV, practitioners caring for HIV-infected infants and children should have a low threshold for considering bacterial meningitis in the appropriate clinical setting.

37.2 Epidemiology of serious infections in HIV-infected children

Serious bacterial infections (SBIs) occur much more frequently in HIV-infected children than in non-infected children. The rate of SBIs in an HIV-infected population of 3331 children between ages 0.1–20.9 years old enrolled in Pediatric AIDS Clinical Trials Group (PACTG) studies was 15.1/100 person-years [11]. The median age, CD4$^+$ lymphocyte count and percentage of CD4$^+$ lymphocytes for these children was 3.8 years old, 420 cells/μL and 17%, respectively. Children in this study who developed PCP had a median age, CD4$^+$ lymphocyte and CD4% of 3.9, 42 cells/μL and 6%, respectively, indicating that SBI may occur at a much higher CD4$^+$ lymphocyte count and percentage than that at which PCP occurs [11, 12].

The two most common SBIs in HIV-infected children in the USA and their event rates per 100 person-years were pneumonia (11.1) and bacteremia (3.3) and were most frequently caused by *Streptococcus pneumoniae* [11]. These rates are much higher than those seen in the general population. In HIV-uninfected children, the rate of pneumonia was 3–4 events per 100 person-years and, in a population-based study in children less that 5 years old, the rate of bacteremia due to *Streptococcus pneumoniae* was 0.007 events per 100 person-years. In HIV-infected children, the event rate for urinary tract infections (UTI) was 1.6 per 100 person-years while the clinical syndromes of osteomyelitis, meningitis, abscess, and septic arthritis had event rates per 100 person-years of < 0.2. Other SBIs in HIV-infected children include cellulitis, sinusitis, adenitis, and mastoiditis [5]. The rate of SBI in HIV-infected children decreases with age. In the Pediatric Spectrum of Disease (PSD) study, SBI occurred most frequently in children less than 1 year old (21.5 episodes per 100 person-years) while in those of ages 1 and 2 years, the rates decreased to 14.3 and 11.2 episodes per 100 person-years, respectively [5]. By age 10 years, the estimated rate decreased to 3.3 episodes per 100 person-years.

The high rates of SBI in HIV-infected children have led researchers to examine agents for prophylaxis of bacterial infections. One randomized clinical trial of intravenous immunoglobulin (IVIG) given in doses of 400 mg per kilogram of body weight every 28 days to HIV-infected children demonstrated a significant decrease in serious and minor bacterial infections only in children with CD4$^+$ lymphocyte counts greater than 200 cells/μL but not in children whose CD4$^+$ lymphocyte counts were less than 200 cells/μL [13] during the median follow-up period of 17 months. In a second randomized clinical trial of IVIG given to children with advanced HIV disease who were treated with

Table 37.2 Infections observed in HIV-infected persons due to less common and newly emerging pathogens

Type of bacteria	Sites of infection	Diagnosis	Comments
Nocardia spp.	Lungs; hematogenous spread to multiple organs, including liver, brain and kidney	Requires 2–4 weeks for growth in culture; special microbiologic stains available	Patients with low CD4 count, absence of either TMP–SMX prophylaxis for PCP and IVIG are predisposed to infection
Rhodococcus equi	Pneumonia +/− with cavitary lesions, pleural effusion or empyema; bacteremia	Easily be isolated from respiratory specimens or blood	Usually subacute lung infection
Bartonella henselae	Cat-scratch disease; bacillary angiomatosis, peliosis hepatis, persistent or relapsing bacteremia with fever; endocarditis	Special culture and staining procedures; PCR for *Bartonella*-specific DNA	Cat is mammalian reservoir; cat flea is arthropod vector
Bartonella quintana	Trench fever; bacteremia in some homeless persons; bacillary angiomatosis	Special culture and staining procedures; PCR for *Bartonella*-specific DNA	Arthropod vector is body louse

TMP–SMX, trimethoprim–sulfamethoxasole; PCP, *Pneumocystis carinii* pneumonitis; IVIG, intravenous immunoglobulin; PCR, polymerase chain reaction.

zidovudine, IVIG decreased the risk of SBI in children compared with placebo [12]. However, an analysis of children stratified by concurrent administration of trimethoprim-sulfamethoxazole (TMP–SMX) three times per week for *Pneumocystis carinii* pneumonia (PCP) showed that IVIG provided no additional benefit in reducing risk of SBI in children already receiving TMP–SMX. The increased use of (TMP–SMX) for SBI and PCP prophylaxis, however, will result in increased colonization with bacteria resistant to TMP–SMX, resulting in decreased effectiveness of TMP–SMX as an agent for SBI prophylaxis.

HIV-infected children in South Africa also have a significantly higher rate of SBIs than HIV-uninfected children. However, because of differences in diagnostic criteria and methodologies, direct comparisons between rates of infections in the USA and in South Africa are often difficult to make. Acute lower respiratory tract infections (ALRI), diarrhea and bacteremia accounted for the majority of infections in 108 hospitalized HIV-infected children in Cape Town, South Africa, whose median age was 61 months (1.5–214 months) [14]. Also seen, but with less frequency, were skin infections, meningitis, and urinary tract infections (UTIs). In this study, none of these children received pneumococcal or *H. influenzae* vaccines, IVIG, or antiretroviral therapy. These children had 136 episodes; 85% of infections occurred in children less than 2 years old and 40% had two or more clinical syndromes. The most frequent syndromes were ALRI (44%), diarrhea (29%), septicemia (17%),

and skin infections (5%). All other syndromes, including meningitis and UTI accounted for less than 2% of SBIs. Bacterial cultures were positive in 24%, 18%, and 45% of children with ALRI, diarrhea and septicemia, respectively. *S. pneumoniae*, *Campylobacter* spp., and Gram-negative bacilli accounted for the majority of the isolates in patients with ALRI, diarrhea and septicemia, respectively. Of note, 33% of these episodes occurred in patients receiving TMP–SMX 3 times a week.

37.3 Antibiotic resistance in bacterial pathogens

Resistance of numerous bacterial pathogens to many antibacterial agents continues to increase globally. Frequencies, patterns and distributions of resistant bacteria vary significantly with geographic regions and may often reflect inappropriate usage patterns of antibiotics. Factors that increase antibiotic resistance include total antibiotic consumption as well as under use through lack of access, inadequate dosing, poor adherence, or the use of drugs that have been stored inadequately or manufactured poorly [15]. Thus, certain areas in many developing countries may have increases in certain antimicrobial resistance patterns not seen in industrialized countries. These increases in bacterial resistance create barriers to the treatment of severe and recurrent infections in HIV-infected children and adults, especially in resource-poor countries, because

Table 37.3 Clinical syndromes, bacterial and non-bacterial pathogens and empiric treatment

Clinical syndrome	[1]Commonly isolated bacteria/ less commonly isolated bacteria	[2]Non-bacterial pathogens	[3,4]Empiric treatment targeted at most commonly isolated bacterial pathogens
Meningitis/ Meningo- encephalitis syndrome	*Streptococcus pneumoniae* *Haemophilus influenzae type* b *Neisseria meningitidis* *Salmonella* spp. *Listeria monocytogenes* Group B streptococcus *Treponema* pallidum Other aerobic bacteria and anaerobic bacteria	Viruses Enterovirus HSV VZV CMV Measles EBV JC virus *Mycobacteria* *Mycobacterium tuberculosis* *Mycobacterium avium* complex Parasites *Acanthamoeba* spp. *Naegleria fowleri* *Malaria falciparum* *Toxoplasma gondii* *Trypanosoma cruzi* Fungi *Cryptococcus neoformans* *Coccidioides immitis*	For children >1 month old: (1) Vancomycin plus cefotaxime or ceftriaxone if: strains with intermediate-level or high-level resistance to both penicillins and cephalosporins are present in the geographic area cefotaxime or ceftriaxone alone if no intermediate-level or high-level resistance to both penicillins and cephalosporins are present in the geographic area or (2) Vancomycin and ceftazidime if: CSF shunt present
Pneumonia	*Streptococcus pneumoniae* *Haemophilus influenza type* B *Staphylococcus aureus* Viridans streptococci *Streptococcus pyogenes* *Listeria monocytogenes* *Haemophilus influenzae* *Pseudomonas* spp. *Bordetella pertussis* *Salmonella* spp. *Escherichia* coli *Klebsiella pneumoniae* *Moraxella catarrhalis* *Nocardia* spp. Other aerobic bacteria and anaerobic bacteria	Viruses CMV RSV Influenza A and B Parainfluenza Adenovirus Atypical bacteria *Mycoplasma pneumoniae* *Chlamydia pneumoniae* *Legionella* spp. *Mycobacteria* *Mycobacterium tuberculosis* *Mycobacterium avium* complex, other atypical mycobacterial spp. Fungi *Pneumocystis carinii* *Aspergillus* spp. *Cryptococcus neoformans* *Histoplasma capsulatum* *Coccidioides immitis* Parasites *Strongyloides stercoralis* Malaria	(1) Cefuroxime or cefotaxime or ceftriaxone (2) Ceftazidime if neutropenia Start TMP-SMX for patients at risk for PCP until PCP ruled out if patient is: less than 12 months old regardless of CD4$^+$ count 1–5 years old with <500 CD4$^+$ cells/μL >5 years old with <200 CD4 cells/μL

Table 37.3 (*cont.*)

Clinical syndrome	[1]Commonly isolated bacteria/ less commonly isolated bacteria	[2]Non-bacterial pathogens	[3,4]Empiric treatment targeted at most commonly isolated bacterial pathogens
Suspected Bacteremia/ sepsis syndrome (no CVC present)	*Streptococcus pneumoniae* *Staphylococcus aureus* *Haemophilus influenzae* type b non-typhoidal *Salmonella* spp. *Campylobacter jejuni* viridans streptococci *Streptococcus pyogenes* *Escherichia coli* *Listeria monocytogenes* *Enterococcus* spp *Neisseria meningitidis* *Klebsiella pneumoniae* *Enterobacter* spp *Proteus mirabilis* *Citrobacter freundii* *Rhodococcus equii* *Actinomyces isrealii* Other aerobic bacteria and anaerobic bacteria In patient with CD4 count <50 cells/μL or ANC < 500 cells/μL, consider: *Pseudomonas* spp.	Viruses HSV VZV CMV Influenza A and B Adenovirus Enterovirus *Mycobacteria* *Mycobacterium tuberculosis* *Mycobacterium avium* complex, other atypical mycobacterial spp. Fungi *Candida* spp. Parasites Malaria	1) Ceftriaxone (cefotaxime) if: CD4 count > 200 cells/μL and an ANC > 500, +/− presence of CVC 2) Ceftazidime or other antipseudomonal drug if: CD4 count < 50 cells/μL and ANC < 500 cells/μL Add Vancomycin to above if: (1) CVC plus high prevalence of oxacillin-R *S. aureus* or (2) the child is toxic appearing and the geographic region has substantial numbers of penicillin-resistant and cephalosporin-resistant pneumococci
Bacteremia (CVC present)	*Staphylococcus aureus* *Staphylococcus epidermidis* *Pseudomonas* spp. Acinetobacter spp. Other Gram-negative rods *Bacillus cereus* *Enterococcus* spp. Other aerobic and anaerobic bacteria	Fungi *Candida* spp.	(1) Vancomycin plus (a) Ceftriaxone (cefotaxime) if: CD4 count > 200 cells/μL and an ANC > 500, +/− presence of CVC or (b) Ceftazidime or other antipseudomonal drug if: CD4 count < 50 cells/μL or ANC < 500 cells/μL

(*cont.*)

Table 37.3 (*cont.*)

Clinical syndrome	[1]Commonly isolated bacteria/ less commonly isolated bacteria	[2]Non-bacterial pathogens	[3,4]Empiric treatment targeted at most commonly isolated bacterial pathogens
Urinary tract infections	*Escherichia coli* *Klebsiella* spp. *Enterobacter* spp *Enterococcus* spp. *Pseudomonas* spp *Proteus* spp. *Morganella* spp. Other aerobic and anaerobic bacteria	*Viruses* Adenovirus CMV Polyoma virus *Mycobacteria* *Mycobacterium tuberculosis*	Ampicillin and gentamicin or Cefotaxime (ceftriaxone)
Cellulitis	*Staphylococcus aureus* group A streptococcus *Haemophilus influenzae type b* group B streptococcus *Pseudomonas aeruginosa* Other aerobic and anaerobic bacteria		(1) First generation cephalosporin or an antistaphylococcal penicillin if: infection on extremity and patient is well appearing (2) Ceftriaxone (cefotaxime) if: facial cellulitis or patient is ill-appearing or cellulitic area has a purplish hue: (3) Add: Ceftazidime (or other antipseudomonal drugs) to above regimen if: Severely immunocompromised or gravely ill patients
Central catheter-related soft tissue infections	*Staphylococcus aureus* *Staphylococcus epidermidis* Other aerobic bacteria		Regimen should include vancomycin Catheter removal is necessary for bacterial eradication in cases of catheter tunnel infections
Ecthyma gangrenosum	*Pseudomonas aeruginosa*	Fungi *Aspergillus* spp.	Two antipseudomonal antibiotics
Lymphadenitis	*Staphylococcus aureus* group A streptococci Viridans streptococci *Enterobacter* spp. *Staphylococcus epidermidis* Other aerobic and anaerobic bacteria *Bartonella henselae*	*Mycobacteria* MAC and other atypical mycobacteria *Mycobacterium tuberculosis*	Nafcillin (oxacillin)

Table 37.3 (*cont.*)

Clinical syndrome	[1]Commonly isolated bacteria less commonly isolated bacteria	[2]Non-bacterial pathogens	[3,4]Empiric treatment targeted at most commonly isolated bacterial pathogens
Perirectal abscesses	*Bacteroides* spp. *Prevotella melaninogenica* *Peptostreptococcus* spp. *Escherichia coli* *Klebsiella pneumoniae* *Staphylococcus aureus.* *Enterococcus* spp. *Acinetobacter* spp. Other aerobic and anaerobic bacteria		Clindamycin or metronidazole plus an aminoglycoside, ceftriaxone (cefotaxime)
Septic arthritis	*Streptococcus pneumoniae* *Staphylococcus aureus* Viridans streptococci *Streptococcus pyogenes* *Haemophilus Influenzae type b* *Salmonella* spp. *Klebsiella* spp Other aerobic and anaerobic bacteria		Nafcillin (oxacillin) or ceftriaxone (cefotaxime)
Osteomyelitis	*S. aureus* *Streptococcus pyogenes* Non-typhoidal *Salmonella* spp. *Haemophilus influenzae* type b *Moraxella catarrhalis* Other aerobic and anaerobic bacteria	*Mycobacteria* *Mycobacterium tuberculosis* MAC, other atypical mycobacteria BCG *Fungi* *Candida* spp.	Nafcillin (oxacillin) or ceftriaxone (cefotaxime)
Syphilis – congenital or acquired			Aqueous crystalline penicillin G

Note:

1. Bacterial species predominance and resistance patterns may vary with geographic locations.

2. The differential diagnosis for infectious and non-infectious causes of these syndromes is broad; unusual and endemic infections must be considered in the diagnosis.

3. Empiric treatment recommended is targeted at the most commonly isolated bacteria. See text for treatment for specific organisms. All antibiotics should be IV.

4. Following isolation of an organism or if an unusual pathogen is suspected, antibiotic therapy should be modified appropriately. HSV, herpes simplex virus; VZV, varicella-zoster virus; CMV, cytomegalovirus; EBV, Epstein–Barr virus; JC, JC virus, a virus named after the initials of the person in which it was first found; CSF, cerebrospinal fluid; RSV, respiratory syncytial virus; TMP–SMX, trimethoprim-sulfamethoxazole; PCP, *Pneumonocystis* carinii pneumonia; MAC, *Mycobacterium avium* complex; ANC, absolute neutrophil count.

complex regimens with expensive antibiotics are often needed to provide coverage for these resistance pathogens. Resistance to TMP–SMX is of particular concern because it is the least expensive and most useful prophylactic antimicrobial agent for PCP and bacterial infections. For example, TMP–SMX resistance in clinically important bacteria has been increasing in Malawi and is thought to be linked to the use of sulfadoxine-pyrimethamine to treat patients with chloroquine-resistant malaria [16]. The widespread use of TMP–SMX and increasing bacterial resistance may lead to decreased effectiveness of TMP–SMX prophylaxis for the prevention of SBI globally.

37.3.1 Antibiotic resistance in *Streptococcus pneumoniae*

Streptococcus pneumoniae is responsible for the majority of SBI in HIV-infected children globally, but treatment is becoming more problematic because of continually increasing resistance to many available antibiotics. Antibiotic resistance of *S. pneumoniae* to penicillin is characterized as intermediate resistance, with MICs of 0.1–1 μg/mL, and high resistance, with MICs of ≥ 2 μg/mL. High doses of penicillin and related, β-lactam antibiotics provide antibiotic levels that are sufficient to overcome intermediate resistance of *S. pneumoniae* in serum and in all tissue except for that in the central nervous system. While non-meningeal infections with intermediately resistant *S. pneumonia* can be treated with higher doses on penicillins, such a strategy can not be used for any types of invasive infections with highly resistant *S. pneumoniae*. In the USA, 24% of *S. pneumoniae* isolates from cases of invasive pneumococcal disease in 1998 were found to be resistant to penicillin [17]; 14% of these isolates had an MIC of ≥ 2 μg/mL. Resistance was also found to cefotaxime, meropenem, and erythromycin and 14% of the isolates had resistance to at least three different antibiotic classes. Furthermore, 29% of these were resistant to TMP–SMX. Of the nine pneumococcal serotypes (19A, 9V, 6A, 23F, 6B, 19F, 14, 18C, and 4) that were isolated frequently from children less than 5 years old with invasive disease, more than 33% of each of seven of these serotypes (19A, 9V, 6A, 23F, 6B, 19F, 14) were resistant to penicillin. Further complicating treatment of these strains is that penicillin-resistant strains often have some degree of cross-resistance to cephalosporins, and carbapenems. A new property termed vancomycin tolerance, the ability of *S. pneumoniae* to escape lysis and killing by vancomycin, has recently been found in 3% of 116 clinical isolates of pneumococci in the USA [18]. Such resistance may result in treatment failure, particularly in cases of meningitis in which bactericidal activity is critical for eradication. The incidence of *S. pneumoniae* resistant to ceftriaxone, cefotaxime, and cefuroxime are also increasing.

Mortality due to infection with penicillin-resistant pneumococci may be increased in some HIV-infected persons. In the USA [19], the mortality rate of HIV-infected adults in San Francisco co-infected with high-level penicillin resistant pneumococci (≥ 2 μg/mL) was 7.8 times higher than that of the same population infected with susceptible (≤ 0.06 μg/mL) or intermediately resistant pneumococcus

(0.1–1 μg/mL). In HIV-uninfected children, non-CNS invasive infections due to *S. pneumoniae* with intermediate penicillin resistance were not associated with a higher mortality rate than infections due to susceptible *S. pneumoniae*, although there was a significant increase in length of hospitalization and longer time to defervescence [20].

Pneumococcal resistance to TMP–SMX is also increasing (reviewed in [21, 22]. A recent survey comparing resistance data from 1997–98 with the period of 1998–99 in 96 institutions revealed that resistance of *S. pneumoniae* to TMP–SMX increased from 13.8% to 27.3%. Furthermore, the selection pressure caused by prolonged use of TMP–SMX for the prophylaxis of PCP is apparently causing the evolution of resistance in other bacteria. TMP–SMX resistance in *E. coli* isolated from HIV-infected adults at San Francisco General Hospital has increased from 24% in 1988 to 74% in 1995 [22].

The resistance pattern of *S. pneumoniae* in the general population in South Africa is somewhat different from that in the USA Antibiotic resistance was found to differ in public and private healthcare settings as demonstrated by the increased resistance of *S. pneumoniae* to macrolides in the private sector where antibiotics are more available [23]. While approximately 45% of *S. pneumoniae* isolates from children in South Africa had penicillin-resistance, high-level resistance was infrequently seen [23]. In India, resistance to penicillin, TMP–SMX and chloramphenicol were found in 1.3%, 56%, and 17%, respectively, of pneumococcal isolates [24]. Of concern is the increase in macrolide resistance from 1% to 21% in *S. pneumoniae* isolates 2 months following a mass azithromycin prophylaxis campaign to eradicate trachoma in an aboriginal village in Australia [25]. Thus, the campaign to eradicate trachoma with the use of azithromycin may have led to an increase in macrolide-resistant *S. pneumoniae*, making erythromycin treatment for *S. pneumoniae* ineffective.

37.3.2 Antibiotic resistance in pathogens associated with diarrhea

Resistance of the three major bacterial pathogens associated with diarrhea, *Shigella* spp., non-typhoidal *Salmonella* spp. and *Campylobacter* spp., to numerous antibiotics have been increasing globally [26]. Resistance to ampicillin, TMP–SMX, tetracycline, and quinolones as well as some β-lactam antibiotics have been detected worldwide in *Shigella* spp., although the antibiotic susceptibility patterns vary by geographical regions. Antibiotic resistance in non-typhoidal *Salmonella* spp. to ampicillin, chloramphenicol, streptomycin, sulfamethoxazole, and tetracycline is also being observed worldwide. Some isolates are simultaneously resistant to five different antibiotics, although many remain susceptible to cefotaxime and ceftriaxone. *Campylobacter* spp. has also been developing resistance to tetracycline, ampicillin, and quinolones in various geographic regions and multidrug resistance has also been reported [27]. For example, in Kenya, 90% of primary isolates of these three bacterial species tested had resistance to ≥1 antibiotics, 74% had resistance to ≥3 antibiotics, while all *Shigella dysenteriae* type 1 tested were resistant to ≥ 6 antibiotics [28]. In South Africa, *Shigella* spp., *Campylobacter* spp., non-typhoidal *Salmonella* spp., and V. *cholerae* isolates with high levels of antibiotic resistance to multiple antibiotics were found [19]. Thus, treatment of these infections requires current knowledge of the antibiotic resistance patterns for the geographic area.

37.3.3 Antibiotic resistance in *H. influenzae*

Beta-lactam resistance of *H. influenzae* in the USA has remained stable at approximately 33% [29]. In India, antibiotic-resistant *H. influenzae* type b continues to be responsible for invasive infections in children with 46–60% of isolates resistant to chloramphenicol, ampicillin, TMP–SMX, or erythromycin and 32% resistant to three or more antibiotics [30]. Fortunately, resistance to third-generation cephalosporins was not detected. South Africa has a relatively low incidence of β-lactamase producing *H. influenzae* (∼10%) [31].

37.3.4 Antibiotic resistance in nosocomial pathogens

The increase in bacterial resistance is also seen in nosocomial pathogens [29]. In 1997, vancomycin-resistant enterococci had increased to 15% and many Gram-negative nosocomial pathogens, including *Klebsiella pneumoniae*, *E. coli*, *Proteus mirabilis*, and *Citrobacter* spp., were found to be resistant to many cephalosporins, including third – and some fourth – generation cephalosporins. *Pseudomonas aeruginosa* and *Acinetobacter* spp. are often multi-drug resistant. Many isolates of *Pseudomonas* are resistant to multiple antibiotics, including β-lactam antibiotics and aminoglycosides, with some isolates now resistant to several quinolones and imipenem-cilastatin [32]. Antibacterial resistance among *Pseudomonas* species may develop in patients while receiving appropriate antipseudomonal antibiotics. Methicillin-resistant *Staphylococcus aureus* (MRSA) is significantly increased in frequency in South Africa relative to that found in the USA (50% vs 23%). Of note is that MRSA was found to be more common in HIV-infected children than in HIV-uninfected children [31].

37.4 Bacteria most commonly associated with serious infections in HIV-infected children

37.4.1 *Streptococcus pneumoniae*

Streptococcus pneumoniae is the most common bacterium causing SBIs, including bacteremia, pneumonia, and meningitis in HIV-infected adults and children. The risk of pneumococcal invasive disease is higher in HIV-infected children than in adults [33]. Invasive pneumococcal disease may occur in HIV-infected children despite active immunization with the pneumococcal polysaccharide vaccine or passive immunization and chemoprophylaxis [3]. In HIV-infected children in the USA, *S. pneumoniae* is the most common pathogen causing invasive bacterial infections (reviewed in [33]). An incidence rate of 6.1 SBIs due to *S. pneumoniae* per 100 person-years for children through age 7 years [34] was seen and was similar to that seen in children with sickle cell disease through age 6 years. However, this rate was 100 to 300-fold the rates seen in the USA and several other industrialized countries in immunocompetent, HIV-uninfected children. Mortality due to invasive pneumococcal disease is high and may be associated with isolates that are resistant to penicillin.

37.4.2 Non-typhoidal *Salmonella* spp.

A low CD4$^+$ lymphocyte count and an advanced stage of HIV disease increases the risk of *Salmonella* infection [33]. The incidence of salmonellosis in HIV-infected persons in the USA appears to be decreasing, possibly due to the use of PCP prophylaxis with TMP–SMX. *Salmonella* infections may be particularly severe in HIV-infected persons, with a very high incidence of disseminated infection, resulting in bacteremia, pneumonia, osteomyelitis, and meningitis, and relapses despite antibiotic treatment [35, 36]. Treatment must be extended for 4–6 weeks to prevent relapse [37]. Initial treatment of *Salmonella* infection should consist of either cefotaxime or ceftriaxone because of widespread multi-drug resistance. Antibiotics can then be tailored to the antibiotic susceptibility of the isolate.

37.4.3 *Campylobacter* spp.

Campylobacter spp., especially *jejuni*, is one of several bacteria causing gastroenteritis that may disseminate and cause widespread serious infection, including bacteremia, in HIV-infected patients. If *Campylobacter jejuni* is suspected, both blood and stool cultures should be obtained. No studies have established the optimal treatment of *Campylobacter* bacteremia. Intravenous therapy for bacteremia with ampicillin/clavulanate, cefotaxime, imipenem/cilastatin, meropenem, or gentamicin, based on the results of susceptibility testing, should provide appropriate coverage.

37.4.4 *Pseudomonas* spp. (predominantly *aeruginosa*)

HIV-infected persons have an increased frequency of *Pseudomonas* infections due to the underlying immunodeficiency and invasive procedures, such as placement of a central venous catheter (CVC) [38, 39]. Infections caused by *Pseudomonas* spp. include bacteremia, pneumonia, urinary tract infections, otitis media and externa, skin and soft tissue infections, sinusitis, and epiglottitis. Bacteremia due to *Pseudomonas* carries a high mortality [32]. Treatment of *Pseudomonas* infection with two antipseudomonal drugs that are active against the isolate may substantially decrease mortality from *Pseudomonas* bacteremia in patients with AIDS [40].

37.4.5 *Staphylococcus aureus*

Staphylococcus aureus is a common cause of bacterial skin infections in HIV-infected patients [41], but is also associated with catheter-related infections, bacteremia, pneumonia, and sinusitis. While *S. pneumoniae* was the most frequent bacterial pathogen in HIV-infected children without a CVC, *S. aureus* was the predominant pathogen in those children with these catheters [38]. Most strains of hospital-acquired *S. aureus* are resistant to penicillin. While the mainstay of treatment of penicillin-resistant *S. aureus* strains has been methicillin, nafcillin, or oxacillin, resistant strains have been appearing in hospitals at an alarming rate. Vancomycin often remains the only active antibiotic against these strains, although vancomycin tolerance has been observed. First or second generation cephalosporins may be used cautiously for patients with penicillin allergy if the *S. aureus* isolate is methicillin-susceptible. Vancomycin may be necessary for the 5–10% of these patients who are also allergic to cephalosporins.

37.4.6 *Staphylococcus epidermidis*

Staphylococcus epidermidis is often associated with CVC-related infections but occasionally may cause more invasive infections. Because most strains of *S. epidermidis* are resistant to penicillin and methicillin/oxacillin, vancomycin remains the treatment of choice.

37.4.7 *Haemophilus influenzae*

Haemophilus influenzae type b is responsible for severe invasive infection in children, including meningitis, bacteremia, pneumonia, epiglottis, septic arthritis, cellulitis, and empyema. The incidence has decreased in countries with wide use of the *H. influenzae* type b conjugate vaccine although HIV-infected children are still at risk for these infections despite vaccination. Resistance to ampicillin requires the initial use of cefotaxime, ceftriaxone, or ampicillin in combination with chloramphenicol for invasive infections until the resistance pattern of the isolate is known. Duration of therapy is for 7–10 days or longer in complicated cases. Chemoprophylaxis with rifampin should be considered for the index case and household contacts [37].

37.5 Clinical syndromes and treatment

37.5.1 Bacteremia

The incidence of bacteremia is increased among patients with low CD4$^+$ lymphocyte counts [38]. It is not uncommon for patients to have more than one episode of bacteremia or to have polymicrobial bacteremia. The bacterial species most often associated with bacteremia in HIV-infected children are shown in Table 37.3. Bacteremia often occurs secondary to infection of the lung, gastrointestinal tract, vascular catheters and skin and soft tissue (reviewed in [4]). Infections at other sites, such as ear, sinuses, and urinary tract may also lead to bacteremia. Often, no source of bacteremia can be identified, especially in cases of *S. pneumoniae* bacteremia. Complications include septic shock and disseminated intravascular coagulation and mortality is high in HIV-infected children.

Blood cultures should be obtained before treatment whenever possible, and a source for the bacteremia should be sought and specifically treated. In a patient with a CVC, blood cultures from the CVC and peripheral vein should be obtained. If the CVC is removed, the catheter tip should be sent to the microbiology laboratory for culture. Empiric treatment of suspected bacteremia is shown in Table 37.3.

Streptococcus pneumoniae
Streptococcus pneumoniae is the most frequently isolated bacteria from bacteremic HIV-infected children. Bacteremia frequently occurs during pneumococcal pneumonia. For non-meningeal infections, the antibiotics that may be used include penicillin G, cefotaxime/ceftriaxone, vancomycin, chloramphenicol, clindamycin,

Gram-positive cocci and Gram-negative bacilli can also cause these infections (Table 37.3). Exit site infections do not necessarily require surgical removal of the catheter and may often be treated with antibiotic therapy alone. Initial treatment for exit site infections with vancomycin will provide coverage for *S. aureus* and *S. epidermidis*. If *S. aureus* and *S. epidermidis* are isolated and are shown to be susceptible to oxacillin, vancomycin should be stopped and oxacillin or nafcillin therapy instituted. Antibiotics should be tailored to bacteria isolated from the exit site. Seven to 14 days of antibiotic treatment is often necessary for bacterial eradication. Catheter removal, however, is necessary for bacterial eradication in cases of catheter tunnel infections. Initial antibiotic therapy should include vancomycin and then be directed toward the bacteria isolated from the infected site and catheter. Since the infection is deep-seated, antibiotic treatment often must be continued for at least 7 days following catheter removal.

Skin lesions secondary to *Pseudomonas aeruginosa* infection

Skin lesions caused by *P. aeruginosa* infection are more common in the late stages of HIV infection than in children who are uninfected or in the early stages of HIV infection. The skin lesions may present as ecthyma gangrenosum, erythematous macular or macular-papular lesions, or violaceous nodules [54], and *P. aeruginosa* can be cultured from these lesions. Ecthyma gangrenosum is a painless, round, indurated, ulcerated lesion containing a central black eschar. It usually occurs during *P. aeruginosa* bacteremia, but may occur following infection of hair follicles. The erythematous and macular, maculo-papular, or nodular lesions occur following disseminated *P. aeruginosa* infection [54]. Blood cultures should be obtained and a work-up for widely disseminated infection should be considered as appropriate. Treatment with two antipseudomonal antibiotics for 10–14 days should be instituted.

Lymphadenitis

Adenitis may be caused by typical bacterial pathogens, such as *S. aureus* and group A streptococci, but may also include bacteria such as *S. viridans*, *Enterobacter* spp. and *S. epidermidis* [51]. The etiologic agent of cat-scratch disease, *Bartonella henselae*, should also be considered in the diagnosis. Initial treatment should be directed against *S. aureus* and group A streptococcus. An aspirate or biopsy of an infected lymph node may be necessary, especially for those not responsive to antibiotics that are active against *S. aureus* and group A streptococci, in order to rule out cat-scratch disease, mycobacterial infection, or malignancy.

Perirectal abscess

Perirectal abscesses are seen more frequently in immunosuppressed patients, especially those with neutropenia [55]. The most frequently isolated bacteria include *Bacteroides* spp., *P. melaninogenicus*, *Peptostreptococcus* spp., *E. coli*, *K. pneumoniae*, and *S. aureus*. In addition, *Enterococcus* spp. and *Acinetobacter* spp. have been reported in HIV-infected children [51]. Rectal exam is usually sufficient to detect a perianal abscess, although computed tomographic (CT) imaging may be needed in systemically ill children who are thought to have deep abscesses. Infected material obtained at the time of perianal abscess drainage should have a microbiologic evaluation. A combination of clindamycin or metronidazole plus an aminoglycoside, ceftriaxone, or cefotaxime will be active against most of the bacteria associated with these infections. In the nonneutropenic child, consideration should be given to surgical drainage or aspiration of the abscess even if local fluctuance is not palpable [55, 56]. Material obtained from drainage or aspiration of the abscesses should be sent for Gram stain and aerobic and anaerobic culture. Antibiotics should be tailored to the bacterial isolates obtained from the infected material. In an HIV-infected child with severe neutropenia, drainage is often not attempted because of the lack of pus formation. In these cases, IV antibiotics are given for 2–3 weeks, and surgical drainage or aspiration performed if there is disease progression with abscess formation [55, 56].

37.5.6 Septic arthritis

Septic arthritis is thought to occur following bleeding into a joint with secondary seeding of bacteria from another site [57], and may account for the larger number of cases of septic arthritis that have been reported in patients with hemophilia and HIV infection, especially those with low CD4[+] lymphocyte counts [57]. Although fever, increased leukocyte counts and elevated erythrocyte sedimentation rates are often present, the classic signs of joint swelling, pain, redness, and warmth are usually modified. Joint aspiration with appropriate chemistries, hematologic and microbiologic studies should be performed. The predominant bacteria isolated from infected joints are *S. pneumoniae*, *S. aureus*, viridans streptococci, *S. pyogenes*, *H. influenzae*, *Salmonella* spp., *Klebsiella* spp. (Table 37.3) [13]. Treatment consists of intravenous antibiotics targeted against the isolated bacteria for 3 weeks. Arthrotomy, arthroscopic lavage, or repeated aspiration is needed as adjunctive therapy to decrease joint cartilage destruction by proteolytic enzymes that accumulate in the infected joint.

37.5.7 Osteomyelitis

Although osteomyelitis occurs in HIV-infected children [13, 38], it is seen less frequently than other serious bacterial infections in HIV-infected patients. A variety of organisms have been reported in HIV-infected patients and include *S. aureus*, *S. pyogenes*, non-typhoidal *Salmonella* spp., *H. influenzae*, and *Moraxella catarrhalis* (Table 37.3). Occasionally, mixed infection may be seen. Diagnosis involves appropriate radiographic studies and culture of blood and material obtained from infected bone by needle aspirate or biopsy. Treatment requires prolonged IV therapy with antibiotics that achieve high bone penetration and are directed against the identified or presumed causative bacteria. There are no published studies of optimum treatment of osteomyelitis other than that due to *Salmonella* spp. in HIV-infected children. Thus, the length of therapy should be guided by the bacteria isolated, the mode of acquisition of the infection (e.g. hematogenous, direct inoculation by injury), whether drainage is performed, and by the patient's clinical course. If *Salmonella* spp. have been isolated, therapy may be required for 4–6 weeks [37]. In some instances, blood and/or bone cultures may not identify an organism. In such cases, patients are treated with empirically chosen antibiotics in consultation with an infectious diseases specialist. Home IV therapy may be an option for children who require prolonged IV therapy.

37.5.8 Congenital syphilis

The diagnosis and treatment of syphilis in mothers with HIV infection and their infants is often challenging because the serologic responses to syphilis and the clinical course are often different from that seen in non-immunosuppressed patients [58]. The altered serologic responses may result in a delay in diagnosis [58]. Treatment failures in HIV-infected patients with single dose intramuscular penicillin in early primary syphilis and with erythromycin in secondary syphilis may occur. Rapid progression of disease to neurosyphilis and uveitis is also seen.

Evaluation of newborn infants for congenital syphilis [37] should be performed in all neonates whose mother has a positive non-treponemal test (VDRL and RPR tests) or a history of syphilis and (1) no or inadequate treatment, (2) lack of serologic response or information regarding serologic response following therapy, and (3) syphilis during pregnancy and lack of serologic response following treatment with penicillin or treatment with a non-penicillin antibiotic or treatment instituted within the month before delivery. Infants born to HIV-infected mothers should also be evaluated for syphilis if mothers or infants have lesions suggestive of syphilis, even without a positive non-treponemal test.

Evaluation of the infant for congenital syphilis includes appropriate physical examination and standard blood tests including complete blood count (CBC), liver function tests, a non-treponemal serologic test in the neonatal serum [37]; CSF cell count, protein concentration, and VDRL on CSF, and long-bone radiographs. Neonatal serum for IgM against treponemal antigens may also be determined by the CDC [37]. The interpretation of serologic tests in infants co-infected with *T. pallidum* and HIV may be difficult since they may have delayed, elevated, or absent treponemal (FTA-ABS) and non-treponemal serologic tests [58]. All syphilis serologic tests should be performed on the neonate's serum rather than cord blood since non-treponemal screening on cord blood may be yield false-negative results. All positive non-treponemal tests should always be confirmed with a treponemal test [58].

Evaluation of neonates for neurosyphilis may be difficult for several reasons. Neonatal CSF may show a positive VDRL test because of transfer of maternal VDRL antibodies into the neonate's CSF. The normally broad range of normal CSF cell counts and protein concentrations found in neonates is complicated by the findings that HIV-infected adults and infants both sometimes exhibit increased cell counts and protein concentrations even in the absence of neurosyphilis.

The most effective treatment of the infant with proven or probable congenital syphilis or infants who have required a work-up for congenital syphilis but in whom the diagnosis can not be excluded is either aqueous crystalline penicillin G, 100 000 to 150 000 U/kg day given q12h for the first 7 days of life and then q8h thereafter for 10 days or procaine penicillin G 50 000 U/kg per dose intramuscularly a day in a single dose for 10 days [37]. Aqueous crystalline penicillin is preferred because of its high penetration into the CSF. It is essential that these infants have good follow-up because of the potential failure of even the most effective antibiotic therapy in eradicating syphilis in HIV-infected patients.

37.6 Summary

HIV-infected children are at increased risk for a wide variety of typical bacterial pathogens. Increasing resistance of these bacteria worldwide to commonly used agents as well as other more expensive antibiotics present greater challenges to the treatment of these children, especially in resource-poor nations. Repeated infections often occur, especially in those children who are more severely immunosuppressed. Many of the typical bacterial infections have common presentations but may require prolonged antibiotic treatment. Prompt recognition and treatment of these infections often results in a successful outcome.

REFERENCES

1. Center for Disease Control and Prevention. *Revised Classification System for Human Immunodeficiency Virus Infection in Children Less Than 13 Years of Age.* Vol. **43** (1994), RR-12.

2. Chaisson, R. E. Infections due to encapsulated bacteria, Salmonella, Shigella, and Campylobacter. *Infect. Dis. Clin. N. Am.* **2**:2 (1988), 475–84.

3. Krasinski, K. Bacterial infections. In P. A. Pizzo (ed.), *Pediatric AIDS.* Baltimore: Williams & Wilkins (1994), pp. 241–53.

4. Kovacs, A., Leaf, H. L. & Simberkoff, M. S. Bacterial infections. *Med. Clin. N. Am.* **81**:2 (1997), 319–43.

5. Pizzo, P. A. & Wilfert, C. M. (eds.), *Pediatric AIDS: the Challenge of HIV Infection in Infants, Children and Adolscents* (3rd edn). Baltimore: Williams & Wilkins (1998).

6. Cruciani, M., Luzzati, R., Fioredda, F. *et al.* Mucosal colonization by pyogenic bacteria among children with HIV infection. *AIDS* **7**:11 (1993), 1533–4.

7. Gibb, D., Spoulou, V., Giacomelli, A. *et al.* Antibody responses to *Haemophilus influenzae* type b and *Streptococcus pneumoniae* vaccines in children with human immunodeficiency virus infection. *Pediatr. Infect. Dis. J.* **14**:2 (1995), 129–35.

8. King, J. C., Jr., Vink, P. E., Farley, J. J., Smilie, M., Parks, M. & Lichenstein, R. Safety and immunogenicity of three doses of a five-valent pneumococcal conjugate vaccine in children younger than two years with and without human immunodeficiency virus infection. *Pediatrics* **99**:4 (1997), 575–80.

9. de Martino, M., Podda, A., Galli, L. *et al.* Acellular pertussis vaccine in children with perinatal human immunodeficiency virus-type 1 infection. *Vaccine* **15**:11 (1997), 1235–8.

10. Barbi, M., Biffi, M. R., Binda, S. *et al.* Immunization in children with HIV seropositivity at birth: antibody response to polio vaccine and tetanus toxoid. *AIDS* **6**:12 (1992), 1465–9.

11. Dankner, W. M., Lindsey, J. C. & Levin, M. J. Correlates of opportunistic infections in children infected with the human immunodeficiency virus managed before highly active antiretroviral therapy. The Pediatric AIDS Clinical Trials Group. *Pediatr. Infect. Dis. J.* **20**:1 (2001), 40–8.

12. Spector, S. A., Gelber, R. D., McGrath, N. *et al.* Intravenous immune globulin for the prevention of serious bacterial infections in children receiving zidovudine for advanced human immunodeficiency virus infection. *New Engl. J. Med.* **331** (1994), 1181–7.

13. National Institute of Child Health and Human Development Intravenous Immunoglobulin Study Group. Intravenous immune globulin for the prevention of bacterial infections in children with symptomatic human immunodeficiency virus infection. *New Engl. J. Med.* **325** (1991), 73–80.

14. Westwood, A. T., Eley, B. S., Gilbert, R. D. & Hanslo, D. Bacterial infection in children with HIV: a prospective study from Cape Town, South Africa. *Ann. Trop. Paediatr.* **20**:3 (2000), 193–8.

15. World Heath Organization. *WHO Global Strategy for Containment of Antimicrobial Resistance.* In WHO/CDS/CRS/DRS/2001.2; 2001.

16. Feikin, D. R., Dowell, S. F., Nwanyanwu, O. C. *et al.* Increased carriage of trimethoprim/sulfamethoxazole-resistant *Streptococcus pneumoniae* in Malawian children after treatment for malaria with sulfadoxine/pyrimethamine. *J. Infect. Dis.* **181**:4 (2000), 1501–5.

17. Whitney, C. G., Farley, M. M., Hadler, J. *et al.* Increasing prevalence of multidrug-resistant *Streptococcus pneumoniae* in the United States. *New Engl. J. Med.* **343**:26 (2000), 1917–24.

18. Henriques Normark, B., Novak, R., Ortqvist, A., Kallenius, G., Tuomanen, E. & Normark, S. Clinical isolates of *Streptococcus pneumoniae* that exhibit tolerance of vancomycin. *Clin. Infect. Dis.* **32**:4 (2001), 552–8.

19. Nuorti, J. P., Butler, J. C., Gelling, L., Kool, J. L., Reingold, A. L. & Vugia, D. J. Epidemiologic relation between HIV and invasive pneumococcal disease in San Francisco County, California. *Ann. Intern. Med.* **132**:3 (2000), 182–90.

20. Rowland, K. E. & Turnidge, J. D. The impact of penicillin resistance on the outcome of invasive *Streptococcus pneumoniae* infection in children. *Austr. N. Z. J. Med.* **30** (2000), 441–9.

21. Huovinen, P. Resistance to trimethoprim-sulfamethoxazole. *Clin. Infect. Dis.* **32**:11 (2001), 1608–14.

22. Martin, J. N., Rose, D. A., Hadley, W. K., Perdreau-Remington, F., Lam, P. K. & Gerberding, J. L. Emergence of trimethoprim-sulfamethoxazole resistance in the AIDS era. *J. Infect. Dis.* **180**:6 (1999), 1809–18.

23. Klugman, K. P. Emerging infectious diseases – South Africa. *Emerg. Infect. Dis.* **4**:4 (1998), 517–520.

24. Kurien, T. L. Invasive Bacterial Infection Surveillance Group, International Clinical Epidemiology Network. Prospective multicenter hospital survellance of *Streptococcus pneumoniae* disease in India. *Lancet* **353** (1999), 1216–21.

25. Leach, A. J., Shelby-James, T. M., Mayo, M. *et al.* A prospective study of the impact of community-based azithromycin treatment of trachoma on carriage and resistance of *Streptococcus pneumoniae. Clin. Infect. Dis.* **24** (1997), 356–62.

26. Sack, R. B., Rahman, M., Yunus, M. & Khan, E. H. Antimicrobial resistance in organisms causing diarrheal disease. *Clin. Infect. Dis.* **24**: Suppl. 1 (1997), S102–5.

27. Tee, W., Mijch, A., Wright, E. & Yung, A. Emergence of multidrug resistance in *Campylobacter jejuni* isolates from three patients infected with human immunodeficiency virus. *Clin. Infect. Dis.* **21** (1995), 634–8.

28. Shapiro, R. L., Kumar, L., Phillips-Howard, P. *et al.* Antimicrobial-resistant bacterial diarrhea in rural western Kenya. *J. Infect. Dis.* **183** : **11** (2001), 1701–4.

29. Jones, R. N. Resistance patterns among nosocomial pathogens. *Chest* **2** (2001), 397S–404S.

30. Steinhoff, M. Invasive *Haemophilus influenzae* disease in India: a preliminary report of prospective multihospital surveillance. IBIS (Invasive Bacterial Infections Surveillance) Group. *Pediatr. Infect. Dis. J.* **17** : Suppl. 9 (1998), 172–5.

31. Madhi, S. A., Petersen, K., Madhi, A., Khoosal, M. & Klugman, K. P. Increased disease burden and antibiotic resistance of bacteria causing severe community-acquired lower respiratory tract infections in human immunodeficiency virus type 1-infected children. *Clin. Infect. Dis.* **31** : **1** (2000), 170–6.

32. Tacconelli, E., Tumbarello, M., Ventura, G., Lucia, M. B., Caponera, S. & Cauda, R. Drug resistant *Pseudomonas aeruginosa* bacteremia in HIV-infected patients. *J. Chemother.* **7** : Suppl. 4 (1995), 180–3.

33. Ruiz-Contreras, J., Ramos, J. T., Hernandez-Sampelayo, T. *et al.* Sepsis in children with human immunodeficiency virus infection. The Madrid HIV Pediatric Infection Collaborative Study Group. *Pediatr. Infect. Dis. J.* **14** : **6** (1995), 522–6.

34. Moa, C., Harper, M., McIntosh, K. *et al.* Invasive pneumococcal infections in Human Immunodeficiency Virus–infected children. *J. Infect. Dis.* **173** (1995), 870–6.

35. Rubinstein, A. Pediatric AIDS. *Curr. Probl. Pediatr.* **16** : **7** (1986), 361–409.

36. Jacobs, J. L., Gold, J. W., Murray, H. W., Roberts, R. B. & Armstrong, D. Salmonella infections in patients with the acquired immunodeficiency syndrome. *Ann. Intern. Med.* **102** : **2** (1985), 186–8.

37. Committee on Infectious Diseases. *2000 Red Book: Report of the Committee on Infectious Diseases*, 25th edition. Elk Grove Village, IL: American Academy of Pediatrics (2000).

38. Roilides, E., Marshall, D., Venzon, D., Butler, K., Husson, R. & Pizzo, P. A. Bacterial infections in human immunodeficiency virus type 1-infected children: the impact of central venous catheters and antiretroviral agents. *Pediatr. Infect. Dis. J.* **10** : **11** (1991), 813–19.

39. Roilides, E., Butler, K. M., Husson, R. N., Mueller, B. U., Lewis, L. L. & Pizzo, P. A. Pseudomonas infections in children with human immunodeficiency virus infection. *Pediatr. Infect. Dis. J.* **11** : **7** (1992), 547–53.

40. Mendelson, M. H., Gurtman, A., Szabo, S. *et al.* *Pseudomonas aeruginosa* bacteremia in patients with AIDS. *Clin. Infect. Dis.* **18** : **6** (1994), 886–95.

41. Geusau, A. & Tschacler, E. HIV-related skin disease. *J. Royal Coll. Physicians Lond.* **31** (1997), 374–9.

42. Johann-Liang, R., Cervia, J. S. & Noel, G. J. Characteristics of human immunodeficiency virus-infected children at the time of death: an experience in the 1990s. *Pediatr. Infect. Dis. J.* **16** (1997), 1145–50.

43. Ruiz-Contreras, J., Ramos, J. T., Hernandez-Sampelayo, T., de Jose, M., Clemente, J. & Gurbindo, M. D. Campylobacter sepsis in human immunodeficiency virus-infected children. The Madrid HIV Pediatric Infection Collaborative Study Group. *Pediatr. Infect. Dis. J.* **16** : **2** (1997), 251–3.

44. Cotton, D. J., Gill, V. J., Marshall, D. J., Gress, J., Thaler, M. & Pizzo, P. A. Clinical features and therapeutic interventions in 17 cases of Bacillus bacteremia in an immunosuppressed patient population. *J. Clin. Microbiol.* **25** : **4** (1987), 672–4.

45. Sheikh, S., Madiraju, K., Steiner, P. & Rao, M. Bronchiectasis in pediatric AIDS. *Chest* **112** : **5** (1997), 1202–7.

46. Gallant, J. E. & Ko, A. H. Cavitary pulmonary lesions in patients infected with human immunodeficiency virus. *Clin. Infect. Dis.* **22** : **4** (1996), 671–82.

47. Izraeli, S., Mueller, B. U., Ling, A. *et al.* Role of tissue diagnosis in pulmonary involvement in pediatric human immunodeficiency virus infection. *Pediatr. Infect. Dis. J.* **15** (1996), 112–16.

48. Baron, A. D. & Hollander, H. *Pseudomonas aeruginosa* bronchopulmonary infection in late human immunodeficiency virus disease. *Am. Rev. Respir. Dis.* **148** : **4** (1993), 992–6.

49. Spach, D. H. & Jackson, L. A. Bacterial meningitis. *Neurol. Clin.* **17** : **4** (1999), 711–35.

50. Bernstein, L. J., Krieger, B. Z., Novick, B., Sicklick, M. J. & Rubinstein, A. Bacterial infection in the acquired immunodeficiency syndrome of children. *Pediatr. Infect. Dis.* **4** : **5** (1985), 472–5.

51. Krasinski, K., Borkowsky, W., Bonk, S., Lawrence, R. & Chandwani, S. Bacterial infections in human immunodeficiency virus-infected children. *Pediatr. Infect. Dis. J.* **7** : **5** (1988), 323–8.

52. Brown, P. D., Freeman, A. & Foxman, B. Prevalence and predictors of trimethoprim-sulfamethoxazole resistance among uropathogenic *Escherichia coli* isolates in Michigan. *Clin. Infect. Dis.* **34** : **8** (2002), 1061–6.

53. Smith, K. J., Wagner, K. F., Yeager, J., Skelton, H. G. & Ledsky, R. *Staphylococcus aureus* carriage and HIV-1 disease: association with increased mucocutaneous infections as well as deep soft-tissue infections and sepsis. *Arch. Dermatol.* **130** (1994), 521–2.

54. Flores, G., Stavola, J. J. & Noel, G. J. Bacteremia due to *Pseudomonas aeruginosa* in children with AIDS. *Clin. Infect. Dis.* **16** : **5** (1993), 706–8.

55. Arditi, M. & Yogev, R. Perirectal abscess in infants and children: report of 52 cases and review of literature. *Pediatr. Infect. Dis. J.* **9** (1990), 411–15.

56. Shaked, A., Shinar, E. & Fruend, H. Managing the granulocytopenic patient with acute perianal inflammatory disease. *Am. J. Surg.* **152** (1986), 510–12.

57. Gilbert, M. S., Aledort, L. M., Seremetis, S., Needleman, B., Oloumi, G. & Forster, A. Long term evaluation of septic arthritis in hemophilic patients. *Clin. Orthop.* **Jul** : **328** (1996), 54–9.

58. Lambert, J. S., Stephens, I., Christy, C., Abramowicz, J. S. & Woodin, K. A. HIV and syphilis: maternal and fetal considerations. *Pediatr. AIDS HIV Infect. Fetus Adolesc.* **6** (1995), 138–44.

38

Tuberculosis

Rohan Hazra, M.D.

HIV and AIDS Malignancy Branch, National Cancer Institute, NIH, Bethesda, MD

The HIV/AIDS epidemic has led to a resurgence in the rates of tuberculosis in the developed world. In the developing world, co-infection with HIV and tuberculosis is extremely common and a major cause of morbidity and mortality. Tuberculosis in HIV-infected children can be more severe than disease in HIV-uninfected children, and treatment is complicated by drug–drug interactions between antiretrovirals and tuberculosis medications. Nevertheless, effective treatment of tuberculosis in the HIV-infected child is critically important for prolonged survival, even in the absence of antiretroviral therapy.

38.1 Epidemiology

Mycobacterium tuberculosis, the etiologic agent of tuberculosis, is the major species of the *M. tuberculosis* complex, which also includes *M. bovis*, *M. ulcerans*, *M. microti*, a rodent pathogen, and *M. africanum*, a rare cause of tuberculosis in Africa. Humans are the only reservoir for *M. tuberculosis*. In the USA the number of cases of tuberculosis in 2001 reached an all-time low of 15 991 cases [1]. The incidence rate had risen from the mid-1980s until 1992, secondary to the HIV epidemic and decreased attention to public health. Since 1992 there has been a steady decline in the number of cases per year. Pediatric surveillance data, which began in 1953, demonstrates a similar pattern of decline in the incidence until 1988, increase until 1992, and subsequent decline [2].

Internationally, the global burden of disease is staggering. World Health Organization (WHO) data for 1997 estimated almost 8 million new cases that year, 16.2 million existing cases, 1.87 million deaths attributable to tuberculosis, and global prevalence of infection of 32% [3]. The WHO estimates that the worldwide prevalence of tuberculosis and HIV co-infection is 0.18%, with 8% of new cases of tuberculosis occurring in patients who are HIV seropositive. This rate of HIV seropositivity among incident tuberculosis cases is as high as 65% in some African nations. The two countries with the highest number of tuberculosis cases, together accounting for approximately 40% of new cases worldwide, India and China, have a relatively low rate of co-infection with HIV, but the obvious concern is that the HIV epidemics in these countries are in their incipient phases [3]. The global epidemic has serious ramifications for the US tuberculosis elimination program, since recent data indicate that almost half the cases of tuberculosis in the USA are in foreign-born patients.

In an adult, a case of tuberculosis can result from either reactivation of endogenous latent infection or exogenous primary infection or reinfection [4]. A case of tuberculosis in a child should be considered a public health emergency, because it represents recent infection and thus is indicative of ongoing transmission in the community. Since children with tuberculosis are rarely infectious, tuberculosis infection in a child most likely represents transmission from an adult contact [5]. Limited data in the USA demonstrate that 12% of children diagnosed with tuberculosis are HIV-infected [2].

38.2 Pathogenesis

Advances in mycobacterial molecular genetics and the sequencing of the *M. tuberculosis* genome have led and will continue to lead to major progress towards an improved understanding of tuberculosis pathogenesis and the identification of new targets for medications and vaccines [6, 7]. However, the current vaccine against tuberculosis, which is used in most of the world, is of limited effectiveness and was developed about 80 years ago, and no new class of antituberculosis medication has been developed in over 30 years. There is a great need for new ways to prevent, diagnose, and treat tuberculosis.

Tuberculosis is spread from person to person via airborne droplet nuclei. These particles, 1–5 microns in diameter, are produced when patients with pulmonary or laryngeal tuberculosis cough, sneeze, or speak. They can also be released by procedures to induce sputum and during bronchoscopy. Droplet nuclei are small enough to bypass the filtering mechanisms of the upper airway and reach the terminal alveoli, where tuberculosis organisms then replicate. Alveolar macrophages ingest the organisms but are unable to kill them. *Mycobacterium tuberculosis* evades killing by activated macrophages by inhibiting phagosome acidification and phagosome–lysosome fusion [8, 9]. After infection begins in the alveoli, the infection can disseminate rapidly to regional lymph nodes, the bloodstream and to sites throughout the body, before cellular immunity develops.

Bacterial replication can continue at the primary site of infection and at metastatic foci until cellular immunity develops 2–12 weeks after infection when bacteria are contained and walled-off within granulomas. The development of immunity is marked by a positive tuberculin skin test (TST). With the onset of cellular immunity, most adults are able to control their infection. Although necrosis of the initial pulmonary focus can occur with subsequent calcification evident on chest radiograph, in most cases infection controlled by cellular immunity is clinically and radiographically inapparent. Patients such as these are considered to have latent tuberculosis infection, and approximately 5–10% of them will develop active disease during their lifetime in the absence of therapy.

The macrophage has long been thought to be the primary site of *M. tuberculosis* replication and the vector responsible for the dissemination of infection throughout the body. However, a recent study argues against this view and instead suggests that infection of pneumocytes is necessary for *M. tuberculosis* dissemination [10]. In this study, *M. tuberculosis* mutants were created in which the gene encoding heparin-binding hemagglutinin adhesin (*hbhA*), a surface protein that mediates adherence and entry into epithelial cells, was deleted. These deletional mutants grew normally in liquid culture and macrophage culture, but were unable to infect pneumocytes. Mice administered with an intratracheal challenge of such tuberculosis mutants had markedly decreased extrapulmonary bacillary loads.

Latent tuberculosis infection is poorly understood. Organisms can remain in this state, walled-off within granulomas, for decades without causing disease or invoking an immune response capable of eradicating the organism but can then re-emerge when cellular immunity decreases, secondary to HIV infection, steroid treatment, or old age. Under certain in vitro conditions, such as oxygen withdrawal, the organism's glyoxylate shunt enzymes are activated. When isocitrate lyase, part of the glyoxylate shunt pathway, is experimentally deleted, the resulting tuberculosis mutants grow normally in mice during initial infection but die off during the period of chronic infection [11]. The relevance of this finding to latency is uncertain, but it does raise the hope that an improved understanding of latent infection is possible and that drugs may be developed that can target latent infection.

Children less than 4 years of age are more likely to develop active disease after tuberculosis infection and are more likely to have a negative tuberculin skin test (TST) at the time of diagnosis than older children and adults [2]. The age distribution for pediatric tuberculosis has two peaks, at less than 4 years of age and in late adolescence [12, 13]. Children between 5 and 15 years of age are relatively resistant to the development of active disease but not to infection. In the USA, over one-third of children with tuberculosis are foreign-born or born to recent immigrants. Data from the UK are similar [14]. Most children with tuberculosis in the USA live in households in which other members have risk factors for tuberculosis, including recent immigration, history of tuberculosis treatment, TST positivity, occupations in healthcare, incarceration, HIV infection, intravenous drug use, alcoholism, homelessness, and diabetes [13].

Numerous factors have been identified that increase the risk for tuberculosis, including host genetic polymorphisms in genes such as HLA loci, vitamin D receptors, and the gene for the natural resistance-associated macrophage protein [15, 16], but by far the leading risk factor for the development of active disease is co-infection with HIV. HIV-infected patients are at much increased risk for the development of active disease. The annual risk of developing tuberculosis in a TST-positive, HIV-infected adult can be as high as 8–12% [17], and the risk for progressive disease after newly acquired infection is up to 50% [18]. To contain tuberculosis macrophages must become activated, which requires the secretion of lymphokines by CD4$^+$ T lymphocytes exposed to mycobacterial antigens in association with major histocompatibility class II. As CD4$^+$ counts decrease as a result of HIV infection, the risk for active tuberculosis increases [19]. HIV patients with high or normal CD4$^+$ counts are also at increased risk of active tuberculosis. HIV infection can alter the production of interferon gamma (IFN-γ), a key component of immunity to mycobacterial disease. When lymphocytes from HIV-infected patients are exposed to *M. tuberculosis* they produce similar amounts of IL-4 and IL-10 but less IFN-γ than lymphocytes from HIV-negative subjects [20]. These data suggest that HIV infection increases susceptibility to tuberculosis by decreasing the Th1 response. When HIV-infected adults experience immune recovery following highly active antiretroviral therapy (HAART) they enjoy a lower rate of tuberculosis and improved survival when co-infected with *M. tuberculosis*, providing additional evidence that the immune dysregulation that accompanies HIV infection damages the capability to effectively contain the infection [21, 22].

The impact of tuberculosis on HIV infection is also significant. Studies have shown that tuberculosis leads to immune activation, increased viral replication, decreased CD4$^+$ counts, increased risk of opportunistic infections and increased risk of death [23, 24]. Although the immune response to *M. tuberculosis* is important in controlling disease, immune activation is also associated with increased HIV viral load and thus accelerated progression of HIV disease. A recent study demonstrated a 5- to 160-fold increase in plasma viral RNA during the acute phase of untreated tuberculosis [25]. Tuberculosis is thought to have a local effect on HIV replication also, since HIV viral load in bronchoalveolar lavage (BAL) specimens from segments of lung involved with tuberculosis are higher than the viral load in BAL specimens from uninvolved areas of lung [26]. In this study, the BAL viral load was also higher than plasma viral load, with evidence of sequence divergence. Others have shown that this HIV sequence heterogeneity in the lung may lead to increased viral diversity in the plasma of HIV-infected patients with tuberculosis, and thus potentially increase the risk of HIV drug resistance [27].

38.3 Clinical presentations

Clinical manifestations at the time of initial infection vary according to the age of the patient and the immune response. Published data on children with HIV and tuberculosis consist largely of small series and individual case reports [28–32]. In contrast, many studies have examined the clinical presentation of tuberculosis in children without regard to HIV infection [2, 12, 13, 33]. In general, the clinical features of tuberculosis in HIV-infected children are very similar to those in immunocompetent children,

although disease is usually more severe. Pulmonary disease is evident in most cases, but rapidly progressive disseminated disease, including meningitis, can be seen without obvious pulmonary findings. HIV infection and young age both increase the risk for miliary disease and tuberculous meningitis. Therefore, tuberculosis should be considered in the HIV-infected child with meningitis, and disseminated disease should be considered in the HIV-infected child diagnosed with tuberculosis.

Disease in children less than 5 years of age is marked by pneumonitis, hilar and mediastinal adenopathy, bronchial collapse secondary to compression by lymph nodes, and subsequent atelectasis. The primary complex, named the Ghon complex after the person who described it in 1916, consists of a relatively small area of alveolar consolidation, lymphangitis, and regional lymphadenitis. HIV-infected children are more likely to be symptomatic, with fever and cough, and to have atypical findings, such as hilar lymphadenopathy, multilobar infiltrates, and diffuse interstitial disease. In patients in whom hypersensitivity develops, hilar and mediastinal lymphadenopathy greatly increase and often cause compression of bronchi, resulting in a segmental lesion. This lesion can consist of both atelectasis and consolidation. A less frequent result of the enlarging lymphadenopathy is hyperaeration of a segment, lobe, or entire lung. While a pleural effusion often accompanies the primary complex in older children and adults, it is uncommon in children less than 5 years of age. Pulmonary tuberculosis in adolescents can resemble primary disease in young children, but the more common clinical scenario in this population is that of chronic upper lobe disease with cavitation.

Lymphohematogenous spread of *M. tuberculosis* probably occurs in all cases of tuberculosis. In adults the most common result is occult infection, or extrapulmonary disease years later, such as renal tuberculosis. Young children and HIV-infected patients are at increased risk of hematogenous spread resulting in miliary tuberculosis. In the absence of treatment, meningitis usually ensues several weeks after hematogenous spread.

Approximately 25% of pediatric tuberculosis cases are complicated by extrapulmonary disease. HIV-infected children seem to have an even higher rate of extrapulmonary disease, with an increased risk of tuberculous meningitis. By far, the most common extrapulmonary site of disease are lymph nodes. The tonsillar and submandibular nodes are involved most often. The clinical presentation is usually of painless, non-tender lymphadenitis, with minimal systemic symptoms. In the USA, the more common diagnosis of this presentation among immunocompetent children is lymphadenitis caused by non-tuberculous mycobacteria [34]. Other forms of extrapulmonary disease include tuberculosis infection of the bones and joints, and rarely disease of the eye, middle ear, GI tract, and kidney.

38.4 Diagnosis

The cornerstone of diagnostic methods for tuberculosis is the tuberculin skin test. The test, known as the Mantoux, consists of the intradermal injection of 5 tuberculin units of purified protein derivative and measurement of induration 48–72 hours after placement. Multiple puncture tests (e.g. Tine) and other PPD strengths (e.g. 250 tuberculin units) should not be used as they are not accurate [35]. The cut-off size for a positive result for the Mantoux TST depends upon the immune status of the person tested and epidemiologic factors. For HIV-infected children and adults, ≥ 5 mm is considered positive and indicative of infection. Among immunocompetent children with active tuberculosis, approximately 10% will have a negative TST [12]. This rate of negative TST seems to vary depending upon the host immune status and type of disease. In immunocompetent patients, 17% of children with miliary disease have a negative TST vs only 3% of children with pulmonary tuberculosis [2]. There are no data on the overall rate of negative TSTs in HIV-infected children with tuberculosis, though a small series of HIV-infected children with tuberculosis clearly shows that the rate of negative TSTs is much higher than that seen among immunocompetent children with tuberculosis [28–32]. Given the risk of negative TST despite disease, an HIV-infected child with exposure to an infectious contact should receive treatment even if the child's TST is negative [36]. Control antigens to test for anergy are no longer recommended on a routine basis for either children or adults [35].

Despite widespread use for decades and extensive experience, the TST has several serious drawbacks, including false positive responses secondary to exposure to non-tuberculous mycobacteria or prior vaccination with BCG, the necessity for two patient visits, false negative responses secondary to HIV or other immunosuppression, and the variability in the interpretation of the test. A new whole-blood IFN-γ assay, QuantiFERON®-tuberculosis (Cellestis Limited, St. Kilda, Australia) detects cell-mediated immunity to *M. tuberculosis* by quantifying IFN-γ release from lymphocytes that are obtained from the patient and exposed to antigens from *M. tuberculosis*, non-tuberculous mycobacteria, and controls. A study evaluating the IFN-γ assay concluded that it has good overall agreement with the TST, was less affected by prior BCG vaccination, discriminated between exposure to *M. tuberculosis* and non-tuberculous mycobacteria, and lacks the

subjectivity associated with the TST [37]. The US Food and Drug Administration (FDA) approved the test in November 2001 for the diagnosis of tuberculosis in immunocompetent adults, but it is not yet in widespread use. It is not approved for use in children or in HIV-infected patients.

Diagnostic microbiology for tuberculosis consists of microscopic visualization of acid-fast bacilli (AFB) from clinical specimens, the isolation in culture of the organism, and drug susceptibility testing. Because *M. tuberculosis* replicates very slowly, with a generation time of 15–20 hours, visible growth on solid media emerges only after 3–6 weeks. Fortunately, more rapid liquid culture detection methods have been developed. The yield for detecting AFB and culturing *M. tuberculosis* from pediatric samples is low, because the bacillary load in children is lower than that in adults, and because specimen collection, such as sputum collection, is more difficult in children than in adults. In most studies of children with tuberculosis, the positive yield from culture is < 50%, with an even lower yield from AFB smear [2, 38]. The yield from culture appears higher in HIV-infected children and in both HIV-infected and HIV-uninfected infants [28–33]. Explanations for this higher yield include higher bacillary loads in these patients secondary to immunocompromise, or more aggressive sampling acquisition secondary to their being sicker and thus more likely to be hospitalized. Obtaining early morning gastric aspirates for AFB stain and culture is the method of choice when attempting to diagnose tuberculosis in young children who are often unable to produce sputum. A standardized protocol for obtaining the gastric aspirates can improve the yield from these specimens to 50%, and the yield is maximized with the culture of three samples obtained separately [39].

Because of the difficulty in diagnosing tuberculosis in children, clinical and historical factors must sometimes be used, such as history of close contact with an adolescent or adult with tuberculosis, and clinical and radiographic findings compatible with tuberculosis [38]. Fortunately, the adult contact can usually be identified, and the drug susceptibility of the contact's isolate can be used to guide the child's treatment [40].

Two nucleic acid amplification tests can identify *M. tuberculosis* from clinical specimens within 24 hours [19]. The Amplified *Mycobacterium tuberculosis* Direct test (MTD, Gen-Probe, San Diego, CA) is approved by the FDA for detection of *M. tuberculosis* ribosomal RNA from both AFB positive and negative respiratory specimens. The AMPLICOR® *Mycobacterium tuberculosis* Test (Roche Molecular Systems, Branchburg, NJ) is approved for detection of *M. tuberculosis* ribosomal DNA from AFB positive respiratory specimens. The United States Centers for Disease Control and Prevention (CDC) has published an algorithm for the use of the two tests [41]. These tests have shown limited ability to detect *M. tuberculosis* in gastric aspirates, and thus are of limited value in children [12, 42].

38.5 Treatment

38.5.1 Latent tuberculosis infection

No studies of latent tuberculosis therapy in HIV-infected children have been reported, so recommendations about this population are derived from the guidelines for HIV-uninfected children and HIV-infected adults. See Table 38.1 for recommended pediatric doses. Isoniazid (INH) given to HIV-uninfected adults for the treatment of latent tuberculosis for 9–12 months decreases the risk of active disease by approximately 80%; results in children are similar [35]. For children who are HIV-infected and TST positive, the recommended regimen is INH daily or twice-a-week for 9 months, with monitoring of liver function tests [35]. Factors to consider when choosing the frequency of dosing include expected adherence to the regimen and the need for directly observed therapy. Some experts recommend at least 12 months for children who are HIV-infected [36]. Data in adults show no added protection for therapy given for more than 12 months [43]. Isoniazid is also recommended for HIV-infected children with recent contact with an adult with tuberculosis, even if the child's TST is negative.

In HIV-infected adults a 2-month regimen of daily rifampin and pyrazinamide (PZA) is as effective as 12 months of INH for latent tuberculosis treatment, but this regimen is more toxic and has been associated with cases of severe and fatal hepatitis [44–46]. It has not been studied in children, and therefore, is not recommended for the pediatric population. However, studies of this shortened regimen have been proposed, targeting HIV-infected children in areas of high tuberculosis prevalence [35]. In the UK, a 3-month regimen of rifampin and INH or a 6-month regimen of INH alone are the recommended regimens for latent tuberculosis in both adults and children [47, 48]. If INH resistance is known or expected in the contact, the recommendation is treatment with rifampin for 6 months. As detailed below, the use of rifampin with certain non-nucleoside reverse transcriptase inhibitors (NNRTIs) and protease inhibitors (PIs) is contraindicated.

38.6 Tuberculosis disease

For an HIV-infected child not receiving treatment with NNRTIs or PIs, recommended therapy for active tuberculosis is an initial 2-month, 4-drug regimen, consisting of INH, rifampin, PZA, and a fourth drug, either ethambutol or streptomycin, followed by INH and rifampin for an additional 4 months [43]. In the USA, ethambutol is preferred, even for children too young to have visual acuity and red-green color perception evaluated, because these toxicities are exceedingly rare in children at the recommended dose. Nevertheless, renal function, ophthalmoscopy and, if possible visual acuity, should be determined prior to initiation of therapy with ethambutol and monitored regularly during therapy with ethambutol. If renal function is abnormal dose modification is essential. Use of streptomycin is hampered by the need for injection, which can be especially problematic in children with low body mass, and the potential for ototoxicity and nephrotoxicity. If the isolate from the adult contact is known to be drug-susceptible the ethambutol can be excluded. Therapy should include ongoing assessment of response, and be administered as directly observed therapy (DOT) if possible. It is important to recognize that DOT alone in the absence of vigilance on the part of the family and healthcare team does not ensure adherence [38]. Daily administration of the drugs for the first 2 weeks to 2 months followed by daily, two (as long as CD4$^+$ count is not low – see below) or three times per week therapy to complete 6 months is acceptable. Some experts recommend a longer course of treatment, up to 9 months total [36]. The less frequent dosing regimens (i.e. two or three times per week) should be used under direct observation if non-adherence with treatment is likely.

Treatment for active tuberculosis in an HIV-infected child receiving treatment with NNRTIs or PIs is more complicated. Overall, as outlined below, the options include the use of rifampin in some circumstances, the use of rifabutin with altered doses, or discontinuing HAART while treating tuberculosis.

The use of rifampin with the PIs and NNRTIs was initially contraindicated, because rifampin is a potent inducer of the hepatic cytochrome CYP450 enzyme system and thus drastically decreases the levels of the drugs metabolized by that system, such as the PIs and NNRTIs [43]. Additional data led to the revision of these guidelines in March 2000, which suggested that rifampin can be administered in patients receiving the following [49]:

• efavirenz and 2 NRTIs
• ritonavir and one or more NRTIs
• ritonavir-boosted saquinavir therapy.

It is important to note that these revised guidelines are based upon limited data in adults, and thus their applicability to children is questionable. Given that data on HIV-infected children treated with ritonavir-boosted saquinavir are limited, and the fact that drug–drug interactions are amplified with the addition of rifampin, the use of rifampin in HIV-infected children also receiving efavirenz, ritonavir,

Table 38.1 Commonly used drugs for the prevention and treatment of tuberculosis in children [43]

Drug	Dosage forms (United States)	Doses in mg/kg (maximum dose)[a]	Adverse reactions	Drug Interactions[a]
Isoniazid (INH)	50 mg/5 ml susp. 100 mg tablet 300 mg tablet	Daily: 10–20 (300 mg) Two times/week: 20–40 (900 mg) Three times/week: 20–40 (900 mg)	Rash, hepatic enzyme elevation, peripheral neuropathy	Increases levels of phenytoin and disulfiram
Rifampin	150 mg capsule 300 mg capsule Suspension can be formulated from capsule contents	Daily: 10–20 (600 mg) Two times/week: 10–20 (600 mg) Three times/week: 10–20 (600 mg)	Rash, hepatitis, fever, orange-colored body fluids	Major effects on PIs and NNRTIs. Refer to [42] for dose adjustments
Rifabutin	150 mg capsule	Daily: 10–20 (300 mg) Two times/week: 10–20 (300 mg)	Leukopenia, gastrointestinal upset, anterior uveitis, arthralgias, rash, hepatic enzyme elevation, skin discoloration, orange-colored body fluids	Major effects with PIs and NNRTIs. Refer to [42] for dose adjustments
Pyrazinamide	500 mg tablet	Daily: 15–30 (2.0 g) Two times/week: 50–70 (3.5 g) Three times/week: 50–70 (2.5 g) 15 mg/kg/dose qd, max. 2.5 g qd (treatment only)	Gastrointestinal upset, hepatitis, rash, arthralgias, hyperuricemia	Might make glucose control more difficult in patients with diabetes
Ethambutol	100 mg tablet 400 mg tablet	Daily: 15–25 (1600 mg) Two times/week: 50 (4000 mg) Three times/week: 25–30 (2000 mg)	Optic neuritis, decreased red-green color vision, rash,	No known important interactions
Streptomycin	1 g vial (IM or IV only)	Daily: 20–40 (1 g) Two times/week: 25–30 (1.5 g) Three times/week: 25–30 (1.5 g)	Ototoxicity, nephrotoxicity	

[a] Life-threatening drug interactions may occur with these and other drugs that affect hepatic metabolism – review all potential interactions before adding these or other drugs to a patient's regimen.
PI, protease inhibitors; NNRTIs, non-nucleoside analogue reverse transcriptase inhibitors.

or ritonavir-boosted saquinavir therapy should only be undertaken with great caution, and potentially with the aid of therapeutic drug monitoring of antiretrovirals and rifampin.

A related rifamycin, rifabutin, is a much less potent inducer of the CYP450 system and thus can be used with some CYP450-metabolized drugs with dose adjustments. Rifapentine, a new, long-acting rifamycin, is not recommended as a substitute for rifampin because its safety and effectiveness have not been established for the treatment of patients with HIV-related tuberculosis [43]. Depending upon the degree of inhibition or activation of the

CYP450 system, the dose of the PI may need to be increased in the presence of rifabutin and the dose of rifabutin may need to be decreased. Specific guidelines about the replacement of rifampin with rifabutin have been published [43, 49]. Again, they are based upon data from HIV-infected adults, so their applicability to HIV-infected children is not clear. In summary, they include the following points:

- Dose of rifabutin should be halved in the presence of amprenavir, nelfinavir, or indinavir.
- Dose of rifabutin should be halved and administered 2–3 times per week in the presence of ritonavir (including situations in which ritonavir is used as a pharmacokinetic enhancer of another PI, such as combination lopinavir/ritonavir (Kaletra).
- Dose of indinavir co-administered with rifabutin should be increased by 25%.
- Dose of nelfinavir co-administered with rifabutin should probably be increased by 33%.
- Dose of rifabutin co-administered with efavirenz should be increased by 50–100%.
- It is unknown whether dose of rifabutin should be decreased in the presence of nevirapine or saquinavir.
- Rifabutin should not be administered with delavirdine (because of the marked decrease in delavirdine concentrations when administered with rifabutin).

The use of intermittent therapy with rifabutin after the initial 2–8 weeks of daily therapy was initially recommended without benefit of data from clinical trials [49]. As a result, the CDC initiated a single-arm trial of twice-weekly rifabutin-based treatment for tuberculosis in HIV-infected adults [50]. The overall treatment failure rate in this study was low (4.1%), reinforcing the expected efficacy of this regimen. However, the Data Safety and Monitoring Board for this study suspended enrollment in March 2002 because of five cases of acquired rifamycin resistance. All five patients had CD4$^+$ counts < 60, and four out of five received twice-weekly therapy during the first 2 months of treatment. Similar development of acquired rifamycin resistance in adults with advanced HIV has been seen with intermittent rifampin and rifapentine therapy [51–53]. The mechanisms for this increased risk for acquired rifamycin resistance are unclear, but possibilities include non-adherence to tuberculosis therapy, prior use of rifabutin for prophylaxis against *Mycobacterium avium* complex, persistence of actively replicating organisms in severely immunocompromised hosts, selective malabsorption, and inadequate tissue penetration [43, 51, 54].

While the guidelines endorse use of rifampin or rifabutin-based regimens for the treatment of tuberculosis with co-administration of HAART, some have argued that the effect of the rifamycins on PI drug levels is too unpredictable, and the subsequent risk of HIV resistance too great, and therefore recommend the deferral of HAART until rifampin-based tuberculosis treatment is completed [55]. Another alternative is to use a rifamycin-sparing regimen of INH, streptomycin, pyrazinamide (PZA), and ethambutol for 8 weeks, followed by intermittent INH, streptomycin, and PZA for an additional 7 months [43]. As new antiretroviral agents and additional pharmacokinetic data become available, recommendations for the use of these agents during the treatment of tuberculosis are likely to be revised.

Tuberculosis resistant to standard antibiotics has become a major problem in many areas. WHO data, from surveys in 64 countries in 1997, estimate that the prevalence of resistance to at least one drug ranges from 1.7% of cases in Uruguay and 12% of cases in the USA, to 36.9% of cases in Estonia [56, 57]. Estimates of rates of multi-drug resistance (MDR), defined as resistance to at least INH and rifampin, ranged from 0% in Cuba, Uruguay, Venezuela, Finland, France, Northern Ireland, Switzerland, and New Caledonia, 1.2% in the USA, to 14% of cases in Estonia. The prevalence of MDR tuberculosis is also high (> 4 %) in the Chinese provinces of Henan and Zhejiang, Latvia, Dominican Republic, Russia, Iran, Ivory Coast, and Argentina. One shortfall of these data is that in some countries with high burdens of disease, such as China, India, and Russia, only one or a few administrative units were surveyed. In addition, resistance surveys have not been done in many countries with predicted high rates of MDR tuberculosis, such as Afghanistan, Armenia, Cambodia, Egypt, Pakistan, Sudan, and Yemen.

Patients with HIV infection and tuberculosis are at increased risk of having rifampin resistance, as discussed above, but they are also at increased risk of having INH resistance and MDR. The presence of drug resistance is associated with higher rates of treatment failure and relapse. HIV-infected patients with MDR tuberculosis have a higher death rate than HIV-uninfected patients with MDR tuberculosis [58]. The recommendation for the treatment of rifampin-resistant tuberculosis is INH, streptomycin, pyrazinamide, and ethambutol for 2 months, followed by an additional 7 months of INH, streptomycin, and PZA. The recommendation for the treatment of INH-resistant tuberculosis is a rifamycin, pyrazinamide, and ethambutol for 6–9 months [43].

A thorough review of the treatment of MDR tuberculosis is beyond the scope of this chapter, but two review articles by the same author offer an excellent overview with recommendations [58, 59]. In most of the world where in vitro susceptibility tests are not readily available, resistance is assumed if response to treatment is poor.

In this setting where susceptibility results are not available, the WHO recommends empiric therapy with an initial phase of an aminoglycoside, ethionamide, pyrazinamide, and ofloxacin, and a continuation phase consisting of ethionamide and ofloxacin to complete at least 24 months of therapy. Of course, this approach is problematic, since lack of response can be due to poor adherence to therapy and not to drug resistance, and use of empirically chosen therapy without susceptibility results carries the risk of exposure to toxic medications without benefit.

In the setting where susceptibility results are available, treatment can be individualized. General recommendations are that referral should be made, if possible, to an expert in HIV and tuberculosis treatment; a multiple-drug regimen consisting of medications that have not been administered to the patient before and that show activity against the patient's strain in vitro, such as an aminoglycoside and quinolone, should be considered; and treatment should continue until 24 months after conversion to negative culture and always be administered as directly observed therapy (DOT). Patients who fail second- or third-line regimens may benefit from surgical resection of involved lung.

38.7 Directly observed therapy

The WHO's goals for global tuberculosis control by 2005 are to detect 70% of all AFB smear positive cases and treat 85% of them successfully [60]. The strategy utilizes directly observed therapy, known as DOT, or DOTS, with the "S" referring to short course therapy. The five elements of DOTS are (1) government commitment, (2) diagnosis by sputum smear microscopy, (3) standardized short-course therapy, (4) adequate and reliable drug supply, and (5) reporting and recording system that allows for data collection and treatment evaluation. The strategy has met with success, for example, in India, where many of the DOTS principles were developed though only recently implemented [1]. In other areas, such as parts of Russia, DOTS has been less effective [61]. The reasons for lack of success are varied and complex, but include logistical issues that lead to treatment interruptions, lack of qualified staff, shortage of laboratory equipment, decentralization of health services, and war [60, 61]. Another important reason for lack of success with DOTS that the WHO has highlighted is the lack of collaboration between tuberculosis and HIV programs [60]. WHO also states that in countries that have consistently high tuberculosis treatment success rates, DOTS need not be used for all patients as long as adequate reporting and recording of cases is in place.

38.8 Prevention and control of tuberculosis

38.8.1 Bacillus of Calmette and Guerin (BCG)

Bacillus of Calmette and Guerin (BCG) is a live, attenuated vaccine for controlling tuberculosis. It was derived from *M. bovis* by Calmette and Guerin at the Pasteur Institute in 1921, and has been administered to more people in the world than any other vaccine (see also Chapter 10). The recommendations regarding the use of the vaccine differ around the world, based upon local rates of tuberculosis incidence and prevalence, divergent results of studies conducted in different areas of the world, local practice and custom. Differences about the particular strain that is used, the recommended age at vaccination, and the need for booster doses of vaccine also exist.

A meta-analysis of 18 studies showed a protective effect of 75–86% for the prevention of meningeal and miliary tuberculosis, but did not calculate a protective effect against pulmonary disease because of the great heterogeneity of results [62]. The authors of this meta-analysis, Rodrigues *et al.*, abstracted data from ten randomized controlled trials and eight case-control studies published since 1950. The studies originated from many parts of the world, including the USA, the UK, India, Brazil, Puerto Rico, Colombia, Cameroon, and Indonesia. The protective efficacy of BCG against pulmonary tuberculosis varies greatly (0–80%), but another meta-analysis of 26 studies concluded that the average efficacy is 50% [63]. This meta-analysis abstracted data from 14 prospective trials and 12 case-control studies, and included a majority of the studies analyzed by Rodrigues *et al.* Data on BCG vaccination of HIV-infected children are limited, but in one study of Haitian children, the complication rates after a higher than normal dose of BCG vaccination were 9.6% in infants born to HIV-negative women, 13.3% in HIV-uninfected infants born to HIV-infected women, and 30.8% in HIV-infected infants [64]. In this study, and in others cited by the authors, the reactions were usually mild. The authors' review of BCG complications in HIV-infected children revealed only four reported cases of disseminated BCG infection among 431 HIV-infected or exposed children who received BCG.

The USA and the Netherlands are the only countries to have never adopted a program of universal vaccination with BCG. In the USA, where the overall risk of tuberculosis is low, the variable effectiveness of BCG, including minimal protection in a major United States Public Health Service trial in the southern USA [65], and the difficulties in interpretation of the TST in a BCG-vaccinated person led to an alternative to BCG as a strategy to control tuberculosis. The aim of this strategy is to minimize the risk of

change to a domed opaque phenotype occurs during in vitro culture; primary isolates may also be of this phenotype and rough colony types are also sometimes observed. Some of the less commonly identified mycobacteria grow poorly in culture or require specially supplemented growth media so that it may be difficult to document the presence of infection despite obtaining multiple cultures. The use of broth culture methods with radiometric or other methods of growth detection give positive results more quickly than traditional agar plate-based methods. These have come into widespread use, and have been adapted to determine susceptibility to some of the more commonly used antimycobacterial agents.

Nucleic acid probes are available to provide rapid identification of members of the *M. avium* complex (*M. avium*, *M. intracellulare*, and other uncommon closely related species) and members of the *M. tuberculosis* complex (*M. tuberculosis*, *M. bovis*, and *M. africanum*). Other mycobacterial species must be identified using traditional methods, which may require several additional weeks. Because of the need for special expertise, media and equipment, many clinical microbiology laboratories do not perform mycobacterial cultures, and send out samples to reference laboratories. Susceptibility testing of non-tuberculous mycobacteria is not standardized, and is recommended only for determining susceptibility to clarithromycin (which also defines susceptibility to azithromycin) [8].

39.3 Pathogenesis

Relatively little is known about the pathogenesis of DMAC infection in children or adults with AIDS. A severe deficit in cell-mediated immunity and exposure to the organisms are the only known conditions necessary for the development of DMAC infection. Disseminated *M. avium* complex infection is rare in adults with more than 100 CD4$^+$ lymphocytes/mL and typically occurs in those who have < 50 CD4$^+$ lymphocytes/mL. In children, DMAC infection also occurs primarily in those with severe immune deficiency. Data from a large cohort of HIV-infected children treated with antiretroviral therapy in the pre-HAART era indicate that DMAC infection can occur in children < 6 years of age at higher levels of CD4$^+$ lymphocytes than in older children or adults [9]. In this study, although the median CD4$^+$ lymphocyte count at which DMAC infection occurred was ≤ 50 for each age group, 45% of DMAC infection in 1 to 2-year-old and 30% of DMAC infection in 2 to 6-year-old children occurred in those with > 50 CD4$^+$ lymphocytes/mL. In contrast, among those greater than 6 years of age, 89% of infections occurred in children with < 50 CD4$^+$ lymphocytes/mL. This age dependence of the relation between CD4$^+$ lymphocyte count and degree of immunosuppression has led to the development of guidelines that incorporate age-specific CD4$^+$ lymphocyte counts at which prophylactic therapy should be introduced to prevent DMAC infection [10].

The mode of acquisition of *M. avium* infection is not clearly established. Gastrointestinal and respiratory colonization are thought to be primary portals of entry that can then lead to disseminated infection. Person to person transmission has not been documented and is not believed to be a significant mode of infection. The presence of colonization may be predictive of subsequent disseminated infection, although in one prospective study, the occurrence of disseminated infection occurred commonly in the absence of documented prior colonization [11]. When DMAC infection occurs, mycobacteria are found in blood, bone marrow, lymph nodes (especially abdominal lymph nodes), bone, and solid organs including liver and spleen.

In DMAC infection the mycobacteria are typically found within macrophages. In the absence of effective cell-mediated immunity the infected macrophages are unable to kill the organisms, resulting in large numbers of intracellular bacilli that may be seen on acid-fast staining of pathologic specimens. Granulomas are typically absent or poorly formed, reflecting the absence of effective cell-mediated immunity required to control DMAC infection. In the absence of treatment, ongoing bacterial replication results in persistent bacteremia and an extremely large systemic organism burden, making subsequent treatment more difficult.

39.4 Clinical presentation and diagnosis

Clinical and laboratory findings in children and adults with DMAC are non-specific. The most common symptoms associated with DMAC infection include weight loss or failure to gain weight (65–100%), persistent diarrhea (15–89%), abdominal pain (27–90%), persistent or recurrent fever (80–100%), sweats (22–32%), and fatigue (23%) [12–15]. Laboratory abnormalities may include anemia, leukopenia, and thrombocytopenia. Serum chemistries are generally not markedly abnormal, although some patients may have elevations of alkaline phosphatase, serum transaminases, or lactate dehydrogenase. Although these clinical and laboratory findings are common in children with AIDS and DMAC infection, they are also relatively common in children with advanced immune suppression who do not have documented DMAC infection.

In some patients, an "immune reconstitution syndrome" has occurred within weeks to months of starting HAART accompanied by significant increases in CD4$^+$ lymphocyte counts. This syndrome, with new onset of constitutional symptoms, especially fever or abdominal pain, often occurs in association with focal lymphadenopathy [16, 17]. Other sites of focal infection, including bone, have been described as sites of symptomatic inflammation in patients with this syndrome. This syndrome has occurred both in persons with previously documented DMAC infection and in those in whom the infection was not known to be present. In these patients, immune reconstitution in response to HAART appears to have generated a more vigorous cell-mediated immune response to mycobacterial infection that was previously asymptomatic, with the resulting signs and symptoms of infection. Markers of enhanced cell-mediated immune responses to *M. avium* have been documented in vitro following the initiation of HAART in HIV-infected individuals with DMAC infection [18]. Pathologically, in contrast to the poorly formed granulomas of DMAC infection in those with severe immune suppression, well-formed granulomas are seen [17].

Disseminated *M. avium* complex infection is diagnosed by blood culture or culture of a normally sterile site, e.g. lymph node or bone marrow. Bone marrow culture has been shown to contain higher numbers of organisms than blood, but is not commonly performed [19]. Blood or bone marrow samples can be inoculated into any of several commercially available mycobacterial liquid growth media, and typically take 2 to several weeks to grow. Once established, mycobacteremia is persistent, so that multiple cultures within a short period of time are generally not necessary. Early in the course of DMAC infection, however, organ involvement with symptoms may occur prior to persistent bacteremia, so that multiple blood cultures over time in a persistently symptomatic patient with advanced immunosuppression may yield a positive result when initial cultures are negative [15].

In settings where tuberculosis is not common, histology from bone marrow, lymph node, or other sites demonstrating macrophages containing acid-fast bacilli strongly suggests the diagnosis of DMAC in a patient with typical signs and symptoms. Culture is essential, however, to distinguish non-tuberculous mycobacteria from *M. tuberculosis* and, when *M. tuberculosis* is not present, to determine which species of non-tuberculous mycobacterium is the cause of infection.

In a patient with advanced immune suppression based on age-specific CD4$^+$ lymphocyte counts who has clinical findings or laboratory abnormalities consistent with DMAC infection, a blood culture for *M. avium* infection should be obtained. As noted previously, all of the clinical findings associated with DMAC infection are non-specific, so that other causes of the symptoms should also be sought. Because of the potential benefit of treatment, physicians should have a low threshold for obtaining mycobacterial blood cultures in any HIV-infected child with symptoms consistent with DMAC infection. If symptoms persist in the absence of an alternative diagnosis, repeated blood cultures over time are warranted.

Cultures from stool or respiratory specimens do not indicate disseminated infection per se. Positive cultures from these non-sterile sites may be an initial sign of disseminated infection, however, and should prompt evaluation for DMAC infection [12]. Where disseminated infection is not demonstrated, a substantial proportion of patients with positive MAC cultures from non-sterile sites will subsequently develop DMAC infection within months (31% within 32 weeks in one study). [20]. Positive respiratory cultures for MAC organisms in a patient with pulmonary infiltrates indicates the presence of MAC lung disease that requires treatment, although MAC pulmonary disease is uncommon in adults and children with AIDS [21]. As noted above, pulmonary MAC infection may be localized to the lung or associated with disseminated infection.

Because of the potential toxicity of the treatment regimens and the possibility of alternative causes of symptoms, empiric therapy of DMAC infection based on persistent symptoms despite negative cultures or diagnostic histopathology is rarely warranted. In the setting of a child with severe immune suppression, persistent symptoms and repeated negative mycobacterial blood cultures, diagnostic imaging may be of value. Chest and abdominal lymphadenopathy is a common finding in children with advanced HIV infection and may represent evidence of DMAC infection in the absence of positive blood cultures. One study documented significantly enlarged lymph nodes on abdominal (mesenteric or retroperitoneal lymph nodes) or chest (hilar or posterior mediastinal lymph nodes) in 100% of 16 HIV-infected children with documented DMAC infection; findings in a control group of HIV-infected children without DMAC infection were not presented, however [22]. A study evaluating abdominal lymphadenopathy in HIV-infected children identified enlarged lymph nodes in 8 (28%) of 30 children. Of these three (38% of those with enlarged nodes) were found to have DMAC infection [23]. Taken together, these data suggest that the DMAC infection is a common cause of abdominal or chest lymphadenopathy, but that other etiologies may also cause this finding, as has been shown in adults [24]. In settings where tuberculosis is prevalent, this infection is the most common cause of lymph node enlargement in HIV-infected children [25]. In assessing a child at risk for DMAC infection with abdominal or chest lymphadenopathy but with negative mycobacterial blood cultures, efforts should be made to obtain tissue for histopathology and culture to document the presence of DMAC or of an alternative cause of the lymphadenopathy and associated symptoms.

39.5 Prevention

The most effective strategy for the prevention of DMAC infection in children with HIV infection is to preserve the child's immune system through early diagnosis and effective antiretroviral treatment. Despite the overall decline in the incidence of DMAC infection associated with HAART, DMAC remains among the most common opportunistic infections in HIV-infected individuals [1]. In adults receiving HAART, the risk of infection remains strongly correlated with low CD4+ lymphocyte counts; the risk of DMAC infection in persons whose counts have recovered above threshold values for the initiation of prophylaxis is comparable with the risk among persons whose counts never fell to this level [26]. Viral load appears to be an independent, though less strong, risk factor for several opportunistic infections including DMAC in persons receiving HAART [27].

The most recent US Public Health Service/Infectious Disease Society of America guidelines for the prevention of opportunistic infections in HIV-infected individuals were published in November 2001 [10]. These guidelines specifically address initiation of primary prophylaxis and discontinuation of primary and secondary prophylaxis for DMAC infection in adults and adolescents. The major additions to these guidelines relevant to DMAC prophylaxis in these populations include (1) the increased strength of clinical data supporting discontinuation of primary prophylaxis in patients whose CD4+ lymphocytes have increased to >100 cells/μL for $\geq$ 3 months in response to HAART, and (2) new recommendations to consider discontinuation of secondary prophylaxis in patients who have completed $\geq$ 12 months of macrolide-based therapy for DMAC, are asymptomatic and whose CD4+ lymphocytes have increased to >100 cells/μL for $\geq$ 6 months in response to HAART. While the recommendations for discontinuation of primary prophylaxis are supported by extensive data in adults [28–30], the data supporting the recommendations for the discontinuation of secondary prophylaxis (maintenance therapy) are more limited [31–33].

These guidelines include previously developed age-specific CD4+ lymphocyte thresholds for the initiation of DMAC prophylaxis in children < 13 years old. The applicability of the guidelines regarding discontinuation of

prophylaxis to children is uncertain, however, because of limited data. Discontinuation of primary prophylaxis in children <13 years of age has not been studied, although many experts would do so in a child with sustained levels of CD4+ lymphocytes in response to HAART that are well above the age-specific criterion for initiation of prophylaxis. It is recommended that secondary prophylaxis in children with a history of DMAC infection be continued for life. Specific prophylactic strategies for DMAC infection are described in Chapter 11. It is essential to exclude the presence of DMAC infection before initiating prophylaxis by obtaining a blood culture for mycobacteria.

39.6 Treatment

Treatment has been shown to decrease symptoms and prolong survival in persons with AIDS and DMAC infection [34–36]. In one study survival increased three-fold between 1991 and 1997 with improved survival associated with clarithromycin therapy as well as combination antiretroviral therapy [37]. As is the case for preventive therapy, the treatment of established DMAC infection in HIV-infected children is based on inference from adult data, limited published pediatric information and experience of clinicians who treat HIV-infected children.

While treatment has been shown to be clinically beneficial and to decrease mycobacteremia, effective therapy of DMAC infection is often limited by toxicities and drug interactions. In addition, when DMAC infection occurs in a patient who has had prophylaxis with azithromycin or clarithromycin, a substantial minority of the breakthrough MAC strains will be resistant to these agents. In early studies, resistance occurred in 29–58% of breakthrough isolates from adults receiving clarithromycin prophylaxis, and in 11% of isolates from those receiving azithromycin prophylaxis [38–40]. Additional analysis has shown that breakthrough with resistant strains is more likely when prophylaxis is initiated in patients with more profound immune suppression [41], so that early initiation of prophylaxis is likely to be beneficial in preventing the emergence of resistance during prophylactic therapy. When macrolide resistance occurs, effective treatment is much more difficult because these agents are the cornerstone of effective therapy against DMAC.

When DMAC infection is documented by a positive culture of blood or other sterile site, multi-drug therapy should be initiated (Table 39.1). The addition of ethambutol to macrolide-based treatment regimens decreases the rate of relapse so that initial therapy should include clarithromycin or azithromycin plus ethambutol [42].

Table 39.1 Commonly used drugs for the prevention and treatment of DMAC infection in children with HIV infection

Drug	Dosage forms	Doses[a]	Major toxicities	Drug interactions[b]
Clarithromycin	125 mg/5 ml susp. 250 mg/5 ml susp. 250 mg tablet 500 mg tablet	7.5–12.5 mg/kg/dose bid, max. 500 mg bid (treatment or prophylaxis – use lower dose for prophylaxis)	Nausea, diarrhea, abdominal pain Uncommon: headache, leukopenia, elevation of transaminases, altered taste	Decreases hepatic metabolism of many drugs. Protease inhibitors may increase clarithromycin concentration; efavirenz may reduce clarithromycin concentration. Minor effect on hepatic metabolism
Azithromycin	100 mg/5 ml susp. 200 mg/5 ml susp. 250 mg capsule 600 mg tablet 1000 mg packet for single dose susp.	5–10 mg/kg/dose qd, max. 500 mg qd (treatment or prophylaxis – use lower dose for prophylaxis) *or* 20–25 mg/kg/dose q week, max 1200 mg q week (prophylaxis only)	Nausea, diarrhea, abdominal pain, possible ototoxicity Uncommon: headache, leukopenia, elevation of transaminases	
Rifabutin[c,d]	150 mg capsule	5–6 mg/kg/dose qd, max. 300 mg qd (treatment or prophylaxis)	Leukopenia, gastrointestinal upset, anterior uveitis, arthralgias, rash, elevation of transaminases, skin discoloration, secretion discoloration	Increases hepatic metabolism of many drugs. Drugs that slow hepatic metabolism may increase rifabutin concentration and toxicity – may require dose adjustment or discontinuation. Should not be used with saquinavir or delavirdine; major dose adjustment required for other protease inhibitors and NNRTIs
Ethambutol[c]	100 mg tablet 400 mg tablet	15 mg/kg/dose qd, max. 2.5 g qd (treatment only)	Optic neuritis (rare at 15 mg/kg – monitor visual acuity and red-green color vision monthly); headache, peripheral neuropathy, rash, hyperuricemia	No known important interactions. Drug is cleared by renal excretion; check baseline renal function and do not use in patients with significant renal impairment

[a] Limited data from clinical trials are available to support the doses of these agents for the prevention and treatment of DMAC infection in children. Doses provided in this table are those that have been used by persons expert in the care of HIV-infected children. Azithromycin or clarithromycin are first choice agents for prophylaxis; established infection is treated with clarithromycin (first choice) or azithromycin (alternative) plus ethambutol, with or without rifabutin (see text).

[b] Life threatening drug interactions may occur with these and other drugs that affect hepatic metabolism – review all potential interactions before adding these or other drugs to a patient's regimen. See [10] for specific dose adjustments and contraindications for these drugs.

[c] Not approved for children under 13 years of age.

[d] Rifabutin, alone or in combination with weekly azithromycin, is a second-line agent for the prevention of DMAC infection in children who cannot receive clarithromycin or azithromycin.

Most experts initiate therapy with clarithromycin if possible, because of its greater potency in vitro and one study demonstrating bacteriologic superiority of clarithromycin plus ethamubtol vs azithromycin plus ethambutol, although a separate study did not identify significant differences between these regimens [43, 44].

Ethambutol is not available as a liquid preparation and is not approved for use in children because of concern for optic nerve toxicity that may be difficult to monitor or recognize. Despite these issues, it is essential that DMAC infection in children be treated with combination therapy including ethambutol. This agent has been used in children without a high incidence of toxicity, so long as renal function is normal. Monotherapy with a macrolide alone in this setting provides transient benefit and results in the rapid emergence of macrolide-resistant strains, severely limiting subsequent effective therapy [35]. Renal function, ophthalmoscopy, and if possible visual acuity, should be determined prior to initiation of therapy. If renal function is abnormal, dose modification and regular monitoring of renal function is essential. Monitoring of vision, including visual acuity, peripheral vision, and color discrimination should be performed regularly in patients receiving ethambutol. Rifabutin may be included as a third drug, although the added benefit of this drug to the two-drug regimen is less clear and its use may be limited by drug interactions and toxicity [45]. Though not available in a liquid preparation, a rifabutin suspension can be formulated from the contents of the capsules.

Nearly all isolates from patients not receiving clarithromycin or azithromycin as prophylaxis are susceptible to these agents, and a majority from those who have received prophylaxis are susceptible. Susceptibility testing of isolates from patients who have not been receiving macrolide prophylaxis prior to the diagnosis of DMAC infection is generally not necessary. For patients who develop DMAC infection despite prophylactic therapy, testing of the initial isolate for susceptibility to clarithromycin should be performed. Susceptibility testing should also be performed on isolates from patients who fail to respond to therapy, or who have recurrent symptoms and new positive cultures following an initial response to macrolide-based therapy for DMAC [8]. Susceptibility to clarithromycin predicts susceptibility to azithromycin, so that separate testing for azithromycin susceptbility is not recommended.

Among other available drugs with antimycobacterial activity, correlation between in vitro susceptibility and clinical response has not been clearly demonstrated. Clofazamine is active in vitro against most MAC strains from AIDS patients. This agent does not appear to impact mycobacterial clearance in patients receiving macrolide-containing regimens, however, and use of clofazamine has been associated with increased mortality in clinical trials of DMAC therapy in adults, so its use is not recommended [46]. Streptomycin and amikacin are active against some strains and may be useful as second-line agents, but are available only for intramuscular or intravenous administration. Quinolones including ciprofloxacin and ofloxacin may also have a role as second-line agents against strains that are susceptible. Linezolid, a relatively new antimicrobial agent, is active against some MAC strains in vitro, though its utility as a therapeutic agent against DMAC has not been studied.

Treatment options for a patient who has relapsed while receiving a macrolide-based treatment regimen, or who cannot tolerate clarithromycin or azithromycin, are severely limited. No regimen that does not contain clarithromycin or azithromycin has been shown to be of clinical benefit, although microbiologic response has been seen in small numbers of patients treated with multiple drugs, both in the pre-macrolide era and in patients with acquired resistance macrolide [47–49]. Combinations of rifabutin, ethambutol, clofazamine, amikacin, and a quinolone may be tried, but the risk of toxicities must be weighed against the low likelihood of substantial clinical benefit. Because of the likely persistence of macrolide-susceptible organisms even after resistant isolates have emerged, it is reasonable to continue macrolide therapy when initiating new therapy with combinations of second-line agents in the treatment of macrolide-resistant DMAC infection. Whether there is a role for linezolid in this setting is not known.

The major limitations to therapy for DMAC infection are toxicities and drug interactions. The major toxicities of the drugs commonly used for treatment and prophylaxis are shown in Table 39.1. The important drug interactions for each of these drugs result from their effect on the hepatic metabolism of other agents, including many of the protease inhibitors and non-nucleoside reverse transcriptase inhibitors (NNRTIs) [10, 50, 51], and are shown in Table 39.1 and discussed further in Chapter 19. Clarithromycin, though not azithromycin, decreases the clearance of many drugs that are eliminated by hepatic metabolism. Rifabutin induces the metabolism of many of these same drugs. Conversely, concentrations of clarithromycin and rifabutin may be altered significantly in patients receiving other drugs that affect hepatic metabolism. For example, major dose reductions of rifabutin or use of an alternative are required in patients receiving many of the currently available protease inhibitors and NNRTIs, in order to avoid toxicity. Specific contraindications and dose adjustment recommendations resulting from drug interactions of clarithromycin and rifabutin with specific antiretroviral agents are addressed in the US Public Health Service/Infectious Disease Society of America guidelines [10].

Management of immune reconstitution syndrome associated with focal MAC infection is not well established. Antiretroviral therapy should be maintained and anti-DMAC therapy should be initiated. Although these therapies alone may be sufficient, corticosteroids have been used in some patients and may be beneficial when the symptoms or pathologic consequences associated with the focal inflammatory response are severe [16, 52]. In this setting, the use of corticosteroids requires careful consideration of potential risks and benefits. The potential value of other immune modulators remains to be determined.

39.7 Other mycobacteria

Several other non-tuberculous mycobacterial species have been found to cause infection in AIDS patients including *M. kansasii, M. gordonae, M. genavense, M. hemophilum, M. xenopi*, and the rapid growers *M. chelonae, M. abscessus*, and *M. fortuitum*. Most of these infections are disseminated and have clinical manifestations that are similar to those of DMAC infection. *Mycobacterium kansasii* is a relatively common cause of disseminated and pulmonary infection in adults with AIDS in certain populations [53, 54]. The appropriate treatment for these infections depends on the species causing the infection; in some cases no effective regimen has been defined. Therapy of these infections should be designed in consultation with an expert in the treatment of mycobacterial infections.

REFERENCES

1. Palella, F. J., Jr., Delaney, K. M., Moorman, A. C. *et al.* Declining morbidity and mortality among patients with advanced human immunodeficiency virus infection. HIV Outpatient Study Investigators. *New Engl. J. Med.* **338** : **13** (1998), 853–60.

2. von Reyn, C. F., Waddell, R. D., Eaton, T. *et al.* Isolation of *Mycobacterium avium* complex from water in the United States, Finland, Zaire, and Kenya. *J. Clin. Microbiol.* **31** : **12** (1993), 3227–30.

3. von Reyn, C., Maslow, J., Barber, T., Falkinham J., III & Arbeit, R. Persistent colonisation of potable water as a source of *Mycobacterium avium* infection in AIDS. *Lancet* **343** (1994), 1137–41.

4. Pettipher, C. A., Karstaedt, A. S. & Hopley, M. Prevalence and clinical manifestations of disseminated *Mycobacterium avium* complex infection in South Africans with acquired immuno-deficiency syndrome. *Clin. Infect. Dis.* **33** : **12** (2001), 2068–71.

5. Inderlied, C., Kemper, C. & Bermudez, L. The *Mycobacterium avium* complex. *Clin. Microbiol. Rev.* **6** (1993), 266–310.

6. Guthertz, L., Damsker, B., Bottone, E., Ford, E., Midura, T. & Janda, J. *Mycobacterium avium* and *Mycobacterium intracellulare* infections in patients with and without AIDS. *J. Infect. Dis.* **160** (1989), 1037–41.

7. Hazra, R., Lee, S. H., Maslow, J. N. & Husson, R. N. Related strains of *Mycobacterium avium* cause disease in children with AIDS and in children with lymphadenitis. *J. Infect. Dis.* **181** : **4** (2000), 1298–303.

8. Woods, G. L. Susceptibility testing for mycobacteria. *Clin. Infect. Dis.* **31** : **5** (2000), 1209–15.

9. Dankner, W. M., Lindsey, J. C. & Levin, M. J. Correlates of opportunistic infections in children infected with the human immunodeficiency virus managed before highly active antiretroviral therapy. *Pediatr. Infect. Dis. J.* **20** : **1** (2001), 40–8.

10. USPHS/IDSA Prevention of Opportunistic Infections Working Group. *2001 USPHS/IDSA Guidelines for the Prevention of Opportunistic Infections in Persons Infected with Human Immunodeficiency Virus* (2001), pp. 1–65.

11. Chin, D. P., Hopewell, P. C., Yajko, D. M. *et al.* *Mycobacterium avium* complex in the respiratory or gastrointestinal tract and the risk of *M. avium* complex bacteremia in patients with human immunodeficiency virus infection. *J. Infect. Dis.* **169** : **2** (1994), 289–95.

12. Hoyt, L., Oleske, J., Holland, B. & Connor, E. Nontuberculous mycobacteria in children with acquired immunodeficiency syndrome. *Pediatr. Infect. Dis. J.* **11** (1992), 354–60.

13. Lewis, L., Butler, K., Husson, R. *et al.* Defining the population of human immunodeficiency virus-infected children at risk for *Mycobacterium avium-intracellulare*. *J. Pediatr.* **121** (1992), 677–83.

14. Gleason-Morgan D., Church, J. A. & Ross, L. A. A comparative study of transfusion-acquired human immunodeficiency virus-infected children with and without disseminated *Mycobacterium avium* complex. *Pediatr. Infect. Dis. J.* **13** : **6** (1994), 484–8.

15. Gordin, F., Cohn, D., Sullam, P., Schoenfelder, J., Wynne, P. & Horsburgh, C. J. Early manifestations of disseminated *Mycobacterium avium* complex disease: A prospective evaluation. *J. Infect. Dis.* **176** (1997), 126–32.

16. Race, E. M., Adelson-Mitty, J., Kriegel, G. R. *et al.* Focal mycobacterial lymphadenitis following initiation of protease-inhibitor therapy in patients with advanced HIV-1 disease. *Lancet* **351** : **9098** (1998), 252–5.

17. Cinti, S. K., Kaul, D. R., Sax, P. E., Crane, L. R. & Kazanjian, P. H. Recurrence of *Mycobacterium avium* infection in patients receiving highly active antiretroviral therapy and antimy-cobacterial agents. *Clin. Infect. Dis.* **30** : **3** (2000), 511–14.

18. Havlir, D. V., Schrier, R. D., Torriani, F. J., Chervenak, K., Hwang, J. Y. & Boom, W. H. Effect of potent antiretroviral therapy on immune responses to *Mycobacterium avium* in human immunodeficiency virus-infected subjects. *J. Infect. Dis.* **182** : **6** (2000), 1658–63.

19. Hafner, R., Inderlied, C. B., Peterson, D. M. *et al.* Correlation of quantitative bone marrow and blood cultures in AIDS patients with disseminated *Mycobacterium avium* complex infection. *J. Infect. Dis.* **180** : **2** (1999), 438–47.

20. Bogner, J. R., Rusch-Gerdes, S., Mertenskotter, T. *et al.* Patterns of *Mycobacterium avium* culture and PCR positivity in immunodeficient HIV-infected patients: progression from localized to systematic disease, German Aids Study Group (GASG/IDKF). *Scand. J. Infect. Dis.* **29** : **6** (1997), 579–84.

21. Kalayjian, R. C., Toossi, Z., Tomashefski, J. F., Jr. *et al.* Pulmonary disease due to infection by *Mycobacterium avium* complex in patients with AIDS. *Clin. Infect. Dis.* **20** : **5** (1995), 1186–94.

22. Pursner, M., Haller, J. O. & Berdon, W. E. Imaging features of *Mycobacterium avium-intracellulare* complex (MAC) in children with AIDS. *Pediatr. Radiol.* **30** : **6** (2000), 426–9.

23. Chung, C. J., Sivit, C. J., Rakusan, T. A. & Ellaurie, M. Abdominal lymphadenopathy in children with AIDS. *Pediatr. AIDS HIV Infect.* **5** : **5** (1994), 305–8.

24. Saikia, U. N., Dey, P., Jindal, B. & Saikia, B. Fine needle aspiration cytology in lymphadenopathy of HIV-positive cases. *Acta Cytol.* **45** : **4** (2001), 589–92.

25. Jeena, P. M., Coovadia, H. M., Hadley, L. G., Wiersma, R., Grant, H. & Chrystal, V. Lymph node biopsies in HIV-infected and non-infected children with persistent lung disease. *Int. J. Tuberc. Lung Dis.* **4** : **2** (2000), 139–46.

26. Kaplan, J. E., Hanson, D., Dworkin, M. S. *et al.* Epidemiology of human immunodeficiency virus-associated opportunistic infections in the United States in the era of highly active antiretroviral therapy. *Clin. Infect. Dis.* 30 : Suppl. 1 (2000) S5–14.

27. Kaplan, J. E., Hanson, D. L., Jones, J. L. & Dworkin, M. S. Viral load as an independent risk factor for opportunistic infections in HIV-infected adults and adolescents. *AIDS* **15** : **14** (2001), 1831–6.

28. Currier, J. S., Williams, P. L., Koletar, S. L. *et al.* Discontinuation of *Mycobacterium avium* complex prophylaxis in patients with antiretroviral therapy-induced increases in CD4+ cell count. A randomized, double-blind, placebo-controlled trial. AIDS Clinical Trials Group 362 Study Team. *Ann. Intern. Med.* **133** : **7** (2000), 493–503.

29. Dworkin, M. S., Hanson, D. L., Kaplan, J. E., Jones, J. L. & Ward, J. W. Risk for preventable opportunistic infections in persons with AIDS after antiretroviral therapy increases CD4+ T lymphocyte counts above prophylaxis thresholds. *J. Infect. Dis.* **182** : **2** (2000), 611–15.

30. El-Sadr, W. M., Burman, W. J., Grant, L. B. *et al.* Discontinuation of prophylaxis for *Mycobacterium avium* complex disease in HIV-infected patients who have a response to antiretroviral therapy. Terry Beirn Community Programs for Clinical Research on AIDS. *New Engl. J. Med.* **342** : **15** (2000), 1085–92.

31. Aberg, J. A., Yajko, D. M. & Jacobson, M. A. Eradication of AIDS-related disseminated *Mycobacterium avium* complex infection after 12 months of antimycobacterial therapy combined with highly active antiretroviral therapy. *J. Infect. Dis.* **178** : **5** (1998), 1446–9.

32. Soriano, V., Dona, C., Rodriguez-Rosado, R., Barreiro, P. & Gonzalez-Lahoz, J. Discontinuation of secondary prophylaxis for opportunistic infections in HIV-infected patients receiving highly active antiretroviral therapy. *AIDS* **14** : **4** (2000), 383–6.

33. Zeller, V., Truffot, C., Agher, R. *et al.* Discontinuation of secondary prophylaxis against disseminated *Mycobacterium avium* complex infection and toxoplasmic encephalitis. *Clin. Infect. Dis.* **34** : **5** (2002), 662–7.

34. Horsburgh, Jr. C., Havlik, J., Ellis, D. *et al.* Survival of patients with acquired immune deficiency syndrome and disseminated *Mycobacterium avium* complex infection with and without antimycobacterial chemotherapy. *Am. Rev. Respir. Dis.* **144** (1991), 557–9.

35. Husson, R., Ross, L. A., Sandelli, S. *et al.* Orally administered clarithromycin for the treatment of systemic *Mycobacterium avium* complex infection in children with acquired immunodeficiency syndrome. *J. Pediatr.* **124** (1994), 807–14.

36. Shafran, S. D., Singer, J., Zarowny, D. P. *et al.* A comparison of two regimens for the treatment of *Mycobacterium avium* complex bacteremia in AIDS: rifabutin, ethambutol, and clarithromycin versus rifampin, ethambutol, clofazamine and ciprofloxacin. *New Engl. J. Med.* **335** (1996), 377–83.

37. Horsburgh, C. R. Jr, Gettings, J., Alexander, L. N. & Lennox, J. L. Disseminated *Mycobacterium avium* complex disease among patients infected with human immunodeficiency virus, 1985–2000. *Clin. Infect. Dis.* **33** : **11** (2001), 1938–43.

38. Havlir, D., Dube, M., Sattler, F. *et al.* Prophylaxis against disseminated *Mycobacterium avium* complex with weekly azithromycin, daily rifabutin, or both. *New Engl. J. Med.* **335** (1996), 392–8.

39. Pierce, M., Crampton, S., Henry, D. *et al.* A randomized trial of clarithromycin as prophylaxis against disseminated *Mycobacterium avium* complex infection in patients with advanced acquired immunodeficiency syndrome. *New Engl. J. Med.* **335** (1996), 384–91.

40. Benson, C. A., Williams, P. L., Cohn, D. L. *et al.* Clarithromycin or rifabutin alone or in combination for primary prophylaxis of *Mycobacterium avium* complex disease in patients with AIDS: A randomized, double-blind, placebo-controlled trial. The AIDS Clinical Trials Group 196/Terry Beirn Community Programs for Clinical Research on AIDS 009 Protocol Team. *J. Infect. Dis.* **181** : **4** (2000), 1289–97.

41. Craft, J. C., Notario, G. F., Grosset, J. H. & Heifets, L. B. Clarithromycin resistance and susceptibility patterns of *Mycobacterium avium* strains isolated during prophylaxis for disseminated infection in patients with AIDS. *Clin. Infect. Dis.* **27** : **4** (1998), 807–12.

42. Dube, M., Sattler, F., Torriani, F. *et al.* A randomized evaluation of ethambutol for prevention of relapse and drug resistance during treatment of *Mycobacterium avium* complex bacteremia with clarithromycin-based combination therapy. *J. Infect. Dis.* **176** (1997), 1225–32.

43. Ward, T. T., Rimland, D., Kauffman, C., Huycke, M., Evans, T. G. & Heifets, L. Randomized, open-label trial of azithromycin plus ethambutol vs. clarithromycin plus ethambutol as therapy for

Mycobacterium avium complex bacteremia in patients with human immunodeficiency virus infection. Veterans Affairs HIV Research Consortium. *Clin. Infect. Dis.* **27** : **5** (1998), 1278–85.

44. Dunne, M., Fessel, J., Kumar, P. *et al.* A randomized, double-blind trial comparing azithromycin and clarithromycin in the treatment of disseminated *Mycobacterium avium* infection in patients with human immunodeficiency virus. *Clin. Infect. Dis.* **31** : **5** (2000), 1245–52.

45. Gordin, F. M., Sullam, P. M., Shafran, S. D. *et al.* A randomized, placebo-controlled study of rifabutin added to a regimen of clarithromycin and ethambutol for treatment of disseminated infection with *Mycobacterium avium* complex. *Clin. Infect. Dis.* **28** : **5** (1999), 1080–5.

46. Chaisson, R. E., Keiser, P., Pierce, M. *et al.* Clarithromycin and ethambutol with or without clofazimine for the treatment of bacteremic *Mycobacterium avium* complex disease in patients with HIV infection. *AIDS* **11** : **3** (1997), 311–7.

47. Hoy, J., Mijch, A., Sandland, M., Grayson, L., Lucas, R. & Dwyer, B. Quadruple-drug therapy for *Mycobacterium avium-intracellulare* bacteremia in AIDS patients. *J. Infect. Dis.* **161** (1990), 801–5.

48. Kemper, C., Meng, T.-C., Nussbaum, J. *et al.* Treatment of

Mycobacterium avium complex bacteremia in AIDS with a four-drug regimen. *Ann. Int. Med.* **116** (1992), 466–72.

49. Dube, M. P., Torriani, F. J. See, D. *et al.* Successful short-term suppression of clarithromycin-resistant *Mycobacterium avium* complex bacteremia in AIDS. California Collaborative Treatment Group. *Clin. Infect. Dis.* **28** : **1** (1999), 136–8.

50. Piscitelli, S., Flexner, C., Minor, J., Polis, M. & Masur, H. Drug interactions in patients infected with human immunodeficiency virus. *Clin. Infect. Dis.* **23** (1996), 685–91.

51. Tseng, A. & Foisy, M. Management of drug interactions in patients with HIV. *Ann. Pharmacother.* **31** (1997), 1040–58.

52. DeSimone, J. A., Pomerantz, R. J. & Babinchak, T. J. Inflammatory reactions in HIV-1-infected persons after initiation of highly active antiretroviral therapy. *Ann. Intern. Med.* **133** : **6** (2000), 447–54.

53. Witzig, R. S., Fazal, B. A., Mera, R. M. *et al.* Clinical manifestations and implications of coinfection with *Mycobacterium kansasii* and human immunodeficiency virus type 1. *Clin. Infect. Dis.* **21** : **1** (1995), 77–85.

54. Corbett, E. L., Blumberg, L., Churchyard, G. J. *et al.* Nontuberculous mycobacteria: defining disease in a prospective cohort of South African miners. *Am. J. Respir. Crit. Care Med.* **160** : **1** (1999), 15–21.

Fungal infections

Corina E. Gonzalez, M.D.

Division of Pediatric Hematology/Oncology, Georgetown University Hospital, Washington, DC

40.1 Introduction

HIV-infected patients, like others with impaired T-cell function, are at increased risk for developing fungal infections [1]. Other HIV-associated conditions, such as depletion of gut-associated lymphoid tissue, decreased gastric acidity, viral esophagitis, depressed mucosal immunity, and possibly altered epithelial attachment sites also may increase the susceptibility of these patients to mycoses [2–3].

Fungal infections represent an important cause of morbidity and mortality in HIV-infected children. Most children with low CD4$^+$ lymphocyte counts develop mucosal candidiasis that increases in severity with worsening immunosuppression [2–4]. Invasive fungal infections due to pathogens such as *Cryptococcus neoformans*, *Coccidioides immitis*, *Histoplasma capsulatum*, *Penicillium marneffei* and others occur less frequently in pediatric than in adult patients with the acquired immunodeficiency syndrome (AIDS), but carry similar high morbidity and mortality. The basis for such differences in susceptibility between pediatric and adult AIDS populations is probably related to lower exposure to the sources of these fungal pathogens at younger ages. More recently, invasive pulmonary aspergillosis has emerged as an HIV-associated complication.

Fungal infections may present with atypical clinical manifestations, making their recognition a true challenge (Table 40.1). Thus, when fungal cultures or serologic or antigenic markers are negative, biopsies of affected sites are often important in making a diagnosis [5].

In the past decade, the therapeutic options for invasive fungal infections have broadened with the introduction of the triazole compounds fluconazole and itraconazole, the lipid formulations of amphotericin B, the allilamine terbinafine, and the echinocandin caspofungin [6–11]. These antifungal drugs have different pharmacological properties and clinically important drug interactions that must be considered when managing patients receiving multiple medications, such as those with HIV infection (Tables 40.2 and 40.3) [7, 11–16]. Despite these advances, however, there are still a limited number of effective and safe antifungal agents for treatment of fungal infections (Table 40.4). This chapter reviews the clinical manifestations and current therapy for fungal infections in HIV-infected children.

40.2 Cutaneous infections

40.2.1 Cutaneous candidiasis

Cutaneous candidiasis may develop as diaper dermatitis or as a more generalized eruption [17]. Candida diaper dermatitis is characterized by erythema bordered by scales, with satellite papules and pustules. In HIV-infected infants, this condition tends to be recurrent and require protracted therapy. Treatment includes attentive local care with frequent diaper changes and good hygiene as well as antifungal therapy. Initial treatment often consists of topical nystatin. Clotrimazole or miconazole cream may be used for further treatment. Simultaneous administration of oral antifungal agents, such as nystatin, may further reduce colonization. Treatment may require 1–3 weeks. Persistence of dermatitis during nystatin treatment may indicate dermatophytosis [17–20].

Table 40.1 Diagnosis and physical findings of selected mycoses complicating pediatrc HIV infection

Fungal infection	Physical findings	Diagnostic methods
Oral candidiasis	Mucosal erythema, white-beige plaques	KOH preparation, culture
Esophageal candidiasis	Dysphagia, odynophagia, retrosternal pain	Barium swallow: evidences of plaques and ulceration "moth eaten" appearance. These findings are suggestive but not diagnostic Endoscopy: mucosal erythema, white-beige plaques. Culture and biopsy of the lesions
Disseminated candidiasis	Fever, endophthalmitis, and cutaneous lesions	Blood cultures, biopsy of skin lesions
Cryptococcosis	Fever, headaches, pulmonary infiltrates, Alteration of mental status, and septic shock	Cryptococcal antigen titers in serum and CSF Sputum and BAL direct examination and culture Blood and CSF culture
Histoplasmosis	Fever, pulmonary infiltrates, hepato-splenomegaly, lymphadenopathy, cutaneous lesions, and septic shock	Antigen detection in serum and urine Sputum, BAL, and bone marrow direct examination and culture. Blood culture. Bone marrow, skin or pulmonary biopsy
Coccidioidomycosis	Fever, headaches, pulmonary infiltrates, confusion, and cutaneous lesions	Sputum and BAL direct examination and culture Skin or pulmonary biopsy
Aspergillosis	Fever, pulmonary infiltrates	Sputum and BAL direct examination and culture Pulmonary biopsy
Penicillinosis	Fever, pulmonary infiltrates, hepatosplenomegaly, lymphadenopathy and cutaneous lesions	Skin biopsy direct examination and culture. Blood culture. Lymph node biopsy Sputum and BAL direct examination and culture

KOH, potassium hydroxide; BAL, bronchoalveolar lavage; CSF, cerebrospinal fluid.

40.2.2 Dermatophyte infections

Dermatophytosis is caused by *Microsporum* spp., *Trichophyton* spp., and *Epidermophyton floccosum*. Common dermatophyte infections are tinea capitis, tinea corporis, and tinea fascialis. Tinea capitis is highly infectious. It may present with a variety of lesions, including gray patch scaling, conditions mimicking seborrheic dermatitis, black dot alopecia, folliculitis, pustules, and kerion [17, 21]. Tinea facialis and corporis appear as scaling macular eruptions on the facial area, hairline, or body. Potassium iodide (KOH) direct examination, calcofluor examination, and culture can be used to verify the diagnosis. The treatment of choice for tinea capitis remains griseofulvin, administered twice daily with a fatty meal, ideally accompanied by 2.5% selenium sulfide, 4% povidone iodine, or ketoconazole shampoos [18–20, 22]. Any of the shampoos will lessen the risk of transmission of dermatophyte infection and may be used to decrease the incidence of infection in households [23].

Treatment duration is guided clinically and by negative hair cultures. Relapses are managed with systemic azoles or terbinafine. Treatment of tinea facialis or corporis includes topical azoles or terbinafine [18–20].

40.2.3 Other superficial fungal infections

Tinea versicolor, due to *Malassezia furfur*, presents with hyper- or hypopigmented macules on the shoulders, neck, and upper chest. Infectious folliculitis is another manifestation of *M. furfur* infection of the skin. Both conditions can be treated with topical azoles, but recurrence is common. Alternatively, a short course of an oral azole for 2 weeks may result in substantial resolution of the infection [17, 18]. Onychomycosis may be managed with grisefulvin or oral azoles, but long duration therapy is required. Terbinafine has recently been introduced as an effective therapeutic alternative for onychomycosis [17–20].

Table 40.2 Systemic antifungal agents used for treatment of fungal infections

Antifungal Polyenes

Mechanism of action: polyenes bind to membrane ergosterol and appear to form pores which increase membrane permeability and leakage of cell molecules. An additional mechanism of action may include oxidative damage of the fungal cell.

Spectrum of activity: *Candida* spp., *Cryptococcus neoformans, Torulopsis glabrata, Blastomyces dermatitides, Histoplasma capsulatum, Coccidioides immitis, Paracoccidioides brasilensis, Aspergillus* ssp., *Penicillium marneffei,* and the agents of zygomycosis.

	Administration	Pharmacokinetic profile	Toxicity
Deoxycholate Amphotericin B (AMB) (Fungizone) 100 mg vial	AMB is a colloidal suspension that must be prepared in electrolyte-free D5W at 0.1 mg/mL to avoid precipitation. There is no need to protect the suspension from the light. The duration of the IV infusion can range from 1 to 6 hours depending on patient tolerance to acute adverse reactions. Manufacturer recommends a test dose of 1 mg, but its value predicting the occurrence of side-effects is unknown	Oral bioavailability is negligible. At recommended dosages, peak concentrations of AMB are higher than the MICs reported for most fungi. AMB appears to accumulate extensively in tissues. Little drug penetrates into CSF, vitreous humor, or amniotic fluid. Elimination and metabolism of the drug is not well understood. Because of its tissue binding, release is very slow with a terminal phase half life of about 15 days. Requires dose adjustment with renal insufficiency	Infusion-related adverse reactions are common (~70–90%) and include fever and rigors, which may also be accompanied by headaches, nausea, vomiting, hyperpnea, hypo or hypertension, and arrhythmias. Phlebitis is associated with the peripheral administration of AMB. A reduction in the infusion rate and premedication with acetaminophen or hydrocortisone may decrease the incidence of these side-effects. Rigors respond to meperidine. Toxicity of major concern is nephrotoxicity (~80%) which may manifest as a tubulopathy by kaliuresis, hypokalemia, hypomagnesemia, or RTA type II, or as a decrease in GFR with rising BUN and serum creatinine. Normal saline loading pre or post infusion may restore GFR to normal. Avoid use of concomitant nephrotoxic drugs (e.g. aminoglycosides), if possible. Less common adverse reactions include anemia, thrombocytopenia and anaphylaxis
Amphotericin B lipid complex (ABLC) (Abelcet) 100 mg vial	ABLC must be administered at a rate of 2.5 mg/kg/hour usually over 1–2 hours. If the infusion time exceeds 2 hours, mix the suspension by shaking the infusion bag. Do not dilute with saline solutions or mix with electrolytes or other drugs. Do not use in-line filters	Compared to AMB, it has a larger volume of distribution, rapid blood clearance and higher tissue concentrations particularly in the RES	Fever and rigors ~20%; increased creatinine ~15%; anemia 4%
Amphotericin B colloidal dispersion (ABCD) (Amphocil) 100 mg vial	ABCD must be diluted in D5W and infused at 1 mg/kg/hour. Do not use in-line filter	Compared with AMB, it has a larger volume of distribution, and higher tissue concentrations particularly in the RES	Fever and rigors ~50%; increased creatinine ~20%
Amphotericin B liposome (Ambisome) 50 mg vial	Ambisome must be diluted with D5W and infused over a period of 1–2 hours.	Compared with AMB, it achieves higher peak plasma concentrations this may translate into better penetration into tissue sites, such as CSF	Fever and rigors 8–20%; nausea ~10%; vomiting ~5%; increased creatinine ~20%
Nystatin (Mycotastin) 30 gm cream 500,000U tabs	Topical and oral	Very minimal gastrointestinal absorption	Virtually no side-effects. Bitter taste

The lipid formulations of AMB enable AMB to be administered in higher doses (2 to 10 mg/kg/day) with less nephrotoxicity and acute side-effects. Lipid formulations of AMB are appropriate alternatives to conventional AMB and may represent an advance in antifungal therapy. They are as efficacious and have a more favorable safety profile than AMB. While some would restrict the use of these lipid formulations as a secondary alternative to AMB because of their high costs and lack of data showing superior efficacy, consideration for their use as initial therapy should be given on a case-by-case basis. Their use is warranted on patients with renal impairment, with unacceptable toxicity associated with AMB, or in patients with fungal infections refractory to AMB.

Table 40.2 (*cont.*)

Antifungal Azoles

Mechanism of Action: inhibit the cytochrome P 450-dependent enzyme involved in the conversion of lanosterol to ergosterol, a major component of the fungal cell wall. Azoles may also inhibit the cytochrome c oxidative and peroxidative enzymes, with the resultant increase in intracellular peroxide generation, which may contribute to the degeneration of subcellular structures.

Spectrum of activity: Dermatophytes, *Blastomyces dermatitides, Histoplasma capsulatum, Coccidioides immitis, Paracoccidioides brasilensis, Penicillium marneffei*, and *Sporotrix schenckii*. One notable exception is the lack of activity of miconazole against *B. dermatitides*. In addition, all azoles are active against *Candida albicans* but somewhat less active against many of the non-*albicans* spp of *Candida*. Ketoconazole, fluconazole and itraconazole are active against *Cryptococcus neoformans*. Itraconazole and voriconazle are the only azoles with substantial activity against *Aspergillus* ssp.

	Administration	Pharmacokinetic Profile	Toxicity
Ketoconazole (Nizoral) 200 mg tablets 2% topical cream 1% shampoo	Topical and oral. Absorption can be improved when the drug is administered with a high lipid content meal or orange juice.	Oral bioavailability of ketoconazole is variable among individuals. In normal subjects can be as high as 75%. Reduced gastric acidity due to achlorhydria, AIDS, antacids, or the ingestion of a high carbohydrate meal decrease its absorption. It is widely distributed in the body but penetrates poorly into the CSF. Ketoconazole is extensively metabolized in the liver with a terminal half life of 7–9 hrs.	GI: nausea and vomiting are the most frequent dose dependent side effects, 10–40%. Less frequent are abdominal pain, and anorexia. Skin: pruritus and rash, 2–4%. Liver: asymptomatic elevations of transaminases, 2–10%, hepatitis. Endocrine system: adrenal insufficiency (rare), decreased libido, impotence, gynecomastia, menstrual irregularities. Other: disulfiram-like reactions, fever, chills, photophobia (rare). Safety during pregnancy has not been established.
Fluconazole (Diflucan) 50, 100, and 200 mg tablets, 350 and 1400 mg oral suspension, and 2 mg/mL intravenous formulation	Oral and intravenous. Intravenous infusion is well tolerated. It is recommended that fluconazole be dosed twice daily in children with severe fungal infections. A 72 hr dosing interval seems appropriate for premature infants.	Fluconazole is rapidly and completely absorbed from the gastrointestinal tract. It is widely distributed in the body. In contrast to other systemic azoles, has low protein binding and penetrates well into virtually all tissue sites, including into the CSF. Steady state plasma concentrations are achieved after several days, but can be rapidly attained by doubling the dose on the first day of therapy. It is eliminated primarily by renal excretion. Dose modification is recommended in individuals with renal impairment. Terminal half-life is 27–37 hrs in adults, 14–17 hrs in children, and 55–88 hrs in premature infants	GI: nausea and vomiting 5%. Skin: rash, possible exfoliative (Stevens–Johnson syndrome), alopecia in scalp or pubic area. Liver: asymptomatic elevations of plasma transaminases 1–7%, hepatitis (rare). other: headache, seizures Few cases of craniofacial and skeletal abnormalities following prolonged in-utero exposure to fluconazole have been reported.
Itraconazole (Sporanox) 100 mg capsules 10 mg/ml Oral solution with cyclodextrin	Oral and intravenous. Absorption of capsules can be improved when the drug is administered with a high lipid content meal or orange juice. The drug is poorly absorbed in patients with hypo or achlor-hydria. By comparison, the oral solution of the drug does not need to be administered with food and its absorption is not affected by the level of gastric acidity.	Oral bioavailability of itraconazole is variable among individuals. In normal subjects can be as high as 70%. Reduced gastric acidity decreases its absorption. It is widely distributed in the body but penetrates poorly into the CSF or vitreous humor. However, tissue concentrations, including nervous tissue, are 2 to 5 times higher than those of plasma. Steady state plasma concentrations are achieved after 14 days, thus a loading dose during the first 3 days of therapy is recommended for treatment of serious infections. Itraconazole is extensively metabolized in the liver with a terminal half-life of 30 hrs. Itraconazole in cyclodextrin solution has improved bioavailability of the drug by as much as 30%, when administered to healthy volunteers. Children <than 12 yrs with neoplastic disease may require higher doses on a mg/kg basis (>5 mg/kg/d) than adults for equivalent therapeutic benefits. Because the pharmacokinetics of the drug are related nonlinearly to dose, monitoring serum levels is recommended when treating severe fungal infections, plasma concentrations of at least 250–500 ng/mL are desirable.	GI: nausea and vomiting 5%, abdominal pain diarrhea Skin: pruritus, rash. Liver: asymptomatic elevations of plasma transaminases (1–5%), hepatitis (rare). other: headache, dizziness, hypokalemia, hypertension, edema, impotence (rare). Safety during pregnancy has not been established.

(*cont.*)

Table 40.2 (*cont.*)

	Administration	Pharmacokinetic Profile	Toxicity
Voriconazole (V-fend) 50 and 100 mg tablets 200 mg vial for intravenous use	Oral and intravenous Tablets should be taken at least 1 hour before or 1 hour following a meal	Oral bioavailability of voriconazole is estimated to be 96%. Voriconazole is widely distributed in the body and penetrates well into tissues. Steady state plasma concentrations are achieved within one day following the loading dose on first day of therapy. It is eliminated via hepatic metabolism by the cytochrome P450 enzymes with less than 2% of the dose eliminated unchanged in the urine. The CYP2C19 is significantly involved in its metabolism. This enzyme exhibits genetic polymorphism. For example, 15–20% of Asians may be expected to be poor metabolizers and may require dose reduction. The pharmacokinetics of voriconazole are non-linear due to saturation of its metabolism. Dose modification is recommended in individuals with mild to moderate hepatic cirrhosis; after the standard loading dose patients should receive 50% of the maintenance dose. No dose adjustments are necessary for patients with renal impairment.	Visual disturbances: approximately 30% of patients have experienced altered/enhanced visual perception, blurred vision, color vision change, and/or photophobia. These disturbances are generally mild and rarely resulted in discontinuation of the drug. Skin: rash 6%, photosensitivity usually associated with long-term treatment GI: anorexia, nausea, vomiting, dry mouth Liver: asymptomatic elevations of plasma transaminases (1–2%), hepatitis (rare). Other (<1%): fever, chills, headaches, and chest pain most likely associated with IV therapy. Tachycardia, hyper/hypotension, vasodilation, hallucinations, dizziness. Safety during pregnancy has not been established.
Miconazole (*Monistat IV*) ampoule 200 mg Only indicated for the treatment of invasive infections due to *Pseudallescheria boydil.*	Intravenous route of administration. The drug should be diluted in D5W or 0.9% NS and infused over a period of 60–120 minutes per ampoule.	Miconazole is widely distributed to body tissues. It also penetrates well into infected joints and vitreous humor, but only relatively low concentrations are reached in the CSF. The drug is extensively metabolized in the liver with a terminal half life of 20–25 hrs.	GI: nausea and vomiting ~15%. Skin: pruritus 30%, rash 10%. Hematologic: anemia 45%, leucopenia thrombocytosis or thrombocytopenia Other: phlebitis, fever, psychosis, hyperlipidemia, hyponatremia. Rapid infusion of the drug has been associated with translent tachycardia, cardiac arrhytmias, anaphylaxis and cardiac and respiratory arrest. Initial dose requires careful observation.

40.3 Mucosal infections

40.3.1 Oropharyngeal candidiasis

Oropharyngeal candidiasis is the most common opportunistic infection in HIV-infected children. Almost all children with HIV infection will develop this condition during their disease [24]. The clinical manifestations of oral candidiasis are variable, including punctate or diffuse mucosal erythema, angular cheilitis, and the more classical white-beige plaques on the oropharyngeal mucosa. These lesions may become confluent, involving extensive regions of the oral mucosa. The plaques can be removed with difficulty to reveal a granular base that bleeds easily [4, 24]. Oropharyngeal candidiasis can be so severe that it impairs alimentation. The diagnosis is based on clinical signs and symptoms and ultimately confirmed by the response to antifungal treatment. Definite diagnosis requires direct microscopic examination of scrapings of the lesions and culture confirmation.

Topical antifungal treatment is usually effective in controlling most cases of oropharyngeal candidiasis and is recommended as the initial therapeutic intervention. Nystatin has limited activity in moderate to advanced forms of oropharyngeal candidiasis in immunocompromised hosts [25]. Clotrimazole, administered 4–5 times per day, appears to be more active than nystatin, but clotrimazole troches must be retained in the mouth until completely dissolved, which may be difficult in younger children. Children with oropharyngeal candidiasis refractory to topical therapy are candidates for systemic therapy using oral fluconazole. Fluconazole, a triazole agent, is usually effective for treatment of oropharyngeal and esophageal candidiasis [25–27]. However, there have been an increasing number of

Table 40.3 Drug interactions involving azole antifungal drugs

Effect and drug involved	Clinically important interaction	Potentially important interaction[a]
Decrease plasma concentration of the azole		
Decrease absorption		
Antacids	Ketoconazole, itraconazole[a]	
H2-receptor antagonist drugs	Ketoconazole, itraconazole[a]	
Sucralfate		Ketoconazole
Increase metabolism		
Isoniazid	Ketoconazole	
Phenytoin	Ketoconazole, itraconazole[a]	
Rifampin, Rifabutin	Ketoconazole, itraconazole[a], Voriconazole[i]	Fluconazole
Carbamazepine	Voriconazole[i]	
Long-acting barbiturates	Voriconazole[i]	
Increase plasma concentrations of the azole		
Ritonavir		Ketoconazole, itraconazole, Miconazole
Increase plasma concentration of the coadministered drug		
Cyclosporine and tacrolimus	Ketoconazole, Fluconazole, itraconazole, Voriconazole	
Methylprednisolone		Itraconazole
Digoxin		Itraconazole
Nifedipine, amlodipine, felodipine	Itraconazole	Voriconazole
Lovastatin, and simvastatin[h]		
Phenytoin	Ketoconazole, Fluconazole, Voriconazole	Itraconazole
Sulfonilurea drugs, especially Tolbutamide		Ketoconazole, Itraconazole, Fluconazole, Voriconazole
Terfenadine, aztemizole, pimozide Cisapride, and Quinidine[b]	Ketoconazole, Itraconazole, Voriconazole	
Midazolam, triazolam, and alprazolam[c]	Ketoconazole, Itraconazole, Fluconazole	Voriconazole
Rifabutin	Itraconazole, Voriconazole	
Sildenafil citrate	Itraconazole, Fluconazole	
Buspirone	Itraconazole	
Busulfan	Itraconazole	
Oxibutinin	Itraconazole	
Theophilline		Itraconazole, Fluconazole, Voriconazole
Warfarin		Ketoconazole, Itraconazole, Voriconazole
Zidovudine		Fluconazole
Saquinavir[d]	Fluconazole	
Indinavir[e]		Ketoconazole, Itraconazole, Voriconazole
Vinca alkaloids		Voriconazole
Decrease plasma concentration of the coadministered drug		
Theophylline	Ketoconazole	
Didanosine[f]	Ketoconazole, Itraconazole	

[a] This information is based on results of controlled studies or limited observations in patients. Monitoring of plasma concentrations and an adjustment in the dose may be indicated.

[b] Elevated plasma levels of their metabolites may prolong QT intervals on EKG and cause cardiac arrhytmias. Therefore, administration of these drugs with ketoconazole, itraconazole, and voriconazole is contraindicated.

[c] Elevated plasma levels of both drugs may prolong hypnotic and sedative effects.

[d] No dose adjustment of saquinavir is required.

[e] A dose reduction of indinavir should be considered when coadministered with ketoconazole.

[f] Give at least two hours between administration of didanosine and azoles.

[g] Elevated plasma levels of these drugs have been associated with rhabdomyolysis. Therefore, their administration with itraconazole is contraindicated.

[h] Voriconazole is contraindicated for use when co-administered with these drugs.

Table 40.4 Drugs of choice for selected fungal infections

Infection	Drug of choice	Dosage	Alternative therapy
Aspergillosis	Amphotericin B or Lipid formulations[a], Voriconazole 6 mg/kg BID on day 1 IV/PO and 4 mg/kg BID IV/PO thereafter	1–1.5 mg/kg/day, IV 5–8 mg/kg/day, IV	Itraconazole[b,c,d] 5–12 mg/kg/day, PO/IV Caspofungin 70 mg/m^2 on day 1 and 50 mg/m^2/day IV thereafter
Blastomycosis	Amphotericin B	0.5–1 mg/kg/day, IV	Itraconazole[b,c] 5–12 mg/kg/day, PO/IV Ketoconazole 5–10 mg/kg/day, PO
Candidiasis			

Oropharyngeal	Nystatin or
	  Clotrimazole
	  (trouches)
	Fluconazole
		200–600.000 U q6h, PO
		10 mg 5 times a day, PO
		
		3–12 mg/kg/day, PO
			Itraconazole[b,c] 5–12 mg/kg/day, PO
			Amphotericin B 100 mg qid, PO
			Amphotericin B 0.5–1 mg/kg/day, IV
			Ketoconazole 5–10 mg/kg/day, PO

Esophageal	Fluconazole Amphotericin B	3–12 mg/kg/day, PO/IV 0.5–1 mg/kg/day, IV	Itraconazole[b,c] 5–12 mg/kg/day PO/IV Ketoconazole 5–10 mg/kg/day, PO
Chronic suppression[e]	Fluconazole[f]	3–12 mg/kg/day, PO	Itraconazole[b,c] 5–12 mg/kg/day, PO Ketoconazole 5–10 mg/kg/day, PO
Vaginal	Topical azole formulation Fluconazole	 150 mg/d, PO	
Disseminated	Amphotericin B ± Fluocytosine[g,h]	0.5–1 mg/kg/day, IV 1–1.5 mg/kg/day for *C. tropicalis* and *C. parapsillosis* 100–150 mg/kg/day ÷ q6h, PO	Fluconazole[i] 8–12 mg/kg/day, IV
Coccidioidomycosis	Amphotericin B	0.5–1mg/kg/day, IV[k]	Fluconazole 8–12 mg/kg/dPO/IV[i] Itraconazole[b,c] 5–12 mg/kg/day, PO/IV
Chronic suppression[e]	Fluconazole[a]	8–12 mg/kg/day PO	Amphotericin B 0.5–1 mg/kg/weekly, IV Itraconazole[b,c] 5–12 mg/kg/day, PO
Cryptococcosis	Amphotericin B + Fluocytosine[h]	0.7–1 mg/kg/day, IV[b] 100–150 mg/kg/d ÷ q6h, PO	Fluconazole 12 mg/kg/day, PO/IV[a]
Chronic suppression[e]	Fluconazole[j]	12 mg/kg/day, PO/IV	Amphotericin B 0.5–1 mg/kg weekly, IV Itraconazole[b,c] 5–12 mg/kg/day, PO
Histoplasmosis	Amphotericin B or Lipid formulations[a]	0.5–1 mg/kg/day, IV 3–5 mg/kg/day, IV	Itraconazole[b,c] 5–12 mg/kg/day, PO/IV Ketoconazole 5–10 mg/kg/day, PO
Chronic suppression[e]	Itraconazole[b,c]	5–12 mg/kg/day, PO	Amphotericin B 0.5–0.8mg/kg/weekly, IV
Paracoccidioidomycosis	Amphotericin B	0.5 mg/kg/day, IV	Itraconazole[b,c] 5–12 mg/kg qd or bid, PO Ketoconazole 5–10 mg/kg qd or bid, PO or a sulfonamide[l]
Chronic suppression[e]	Fluconazole[j]	12 mg/kg/day, PO/IV	Amphotericin B 0.5–1 mg/kg weekly, IV Itraconazole[b,c] 5–12 mg/kg/day, PO

(*cont.*)

Table 40.4 (*cont.*)

Infection	Drug of choice	Dosage	Alternative therapy
Penicillinosis Chronic suppression[e]	Amphotericin B Itraconazole[b,c]	0.5–1 mg/kg/day, IV 5–12 mg/kg/day	Itraconazole[b,c] 12 mg/kg/day, IV/PO
Phaeohyphomycosis	Amphotericin B ± Fluocytosine[h]	1–1.5 mg/kg/day, IV 100–150 mg/kg/day, PO	Itraconazole[b,c] 12 mg/kg/day, IV/PO
Pseudoallescheriasis	Itraconazole	5–12 mg/kg/day, IV/PO	Ketoconazole 5–10 mg/kg/day, PO
Sporotrichosis Cutaneous Systemic	Itraconazole[b,c] Amphotericin B	5–12 mg/kg/d, IV/PO 0.5–1 mg/kg/d, IV	Potassium iodide 1–5 ml tid, PO Itraconazole[b,c] 12 mg/kg/d, IV/PO
Trichosporonosis Systemic	Amphotericin B + Fluconazole + Flucytosine	1–1.5 mg/kg/d, IV 8–12 mg/kg/d, IV 100–150 mg/kg/d ÷ q6h, PO	
Zygomycosis	Amphotericin B Lipid formulation	1–1.5 mg/kg/d, IV 5–10 mg/kg/d, IV	No dependable alternative

[a] Ambisome, Amphotericin B colloidal dispersion, and Amphotericin B lipid complex.

[b] Dosage adjustment required if absorption impaired by reduced gastric acidity.

[c] For life-threatening infections, requires a loading dose; 4 mg/kg TID for 3 days is sufficient.

[d] For aspergillosis, itraconazole is appropriate after completion of a course of amphotericin B, in stable patients.

[e] There are no data on which to base specific recommendations in children, but lifelong suppressive therapy is appropriate.

[f] Recommended only if subsequent episodes are frequent or severe.

[g] Flucytosine may be useful in combination with amphotericin B when there is a deep-seated infection, particularly in the central nervous system.

[h] To minimize bone marrow suppression, peak plasma concentrations should be maintained between 40–60 μg/mL. Monitoring serum levels is required.

[i] Only in uncomplicated candidemia.

[j] For life-threatening or severe infections in children, higher doses are recommended, 10–12 mg/kg in two divided doses. Loading dose is twice the target dose on first day of therapy.

[k] Recent findings indicate that fluconazole is effective against coccidioidal meningitis in adults. Thus, a trial of fluconazole appears warranted before starting intrathecal amphotericin B. Intraventricular, intralumbar, or intracisternal injection has been recommended in addition to IV amphotericin B for coccidioidal meningitis, the initial dosage of 0.1 mg three times a day per week is increased gradually to a maximum of 0.5 mg, with hydrocortisone (10–15 mg) added as required to relieve headache.

[l] Sulfadiazine 4–6 g/day, or a long term sulfonamide such as sulfamethoxypyridazine 1–2 g/day.

reports of *Candida* infections refractory to fluconazole [4, 28–30]. These cases usually occur in children with severely depressed cell-mediated immunity and involve *Candida* strains that also demonstrate in vivo and in vitro resistance to fluconazole [31]. Such patients may respond well to short and intermittent courses of amphotericin B. Cyclodextrin itraconazole, an itraconazole formulation with improved bioavailability, has also been used with success in children

and adults with fluconazole-refractory oropharyngeal candidiasis [32].

40.3.2 Esophageal candidiasis

Esophageal candidiasis can occur with or without oropharyngeal candidiasis, or other infections of the esophagus such as herpes simplex, cytomegalovirus, and bacterial

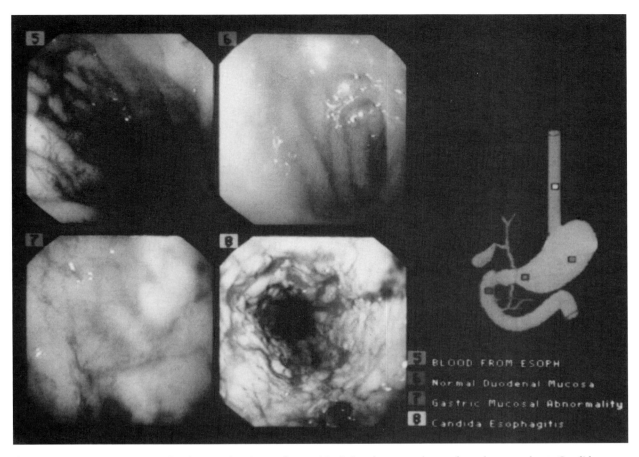

Figure 40.1. Upper gastrointestinal endoscopy showing confluent white-beige plaques on the esophageal mucosa due to *Candida albicans*.

infections. Symptoms can include substernal pain, dysphagia, and odynophagia [33–35]. Some patients may be asymptomatic. Esophagoscopy with mucosal biopsy is the most definitive method for establishing a diagnosis (Figure 40.1). However, this practice may not be feasible or safe in many children, and an empirical approach based on clinical presentation and a positive barium swallow with the typical moth-eaten appearance (Figure 40.2) is often warranted. Children with HIV infection may initially receive therapy, depending upon severity of symptoms and level of immunosuppression, with oral or intravenous triazoles or amphotericin B. Nystatin is ineffective.

40.3.3 Vulvovaginal candidiasis

Vulvovaginal candidiasis is a common infection in HIV-infected adolescents [36, 37]. Recurrent episodes of vulvo-

vaginal candidiasis often precede the oropharyngeal infection. Symptoms include vulvar pruritus, burning, or pain, thick and curdy vaginal discharge, and external dysuria. Rapid microscopic examination of a fresh wet mount is the recommended method for confirmation of vaginal candidiasis [36]. Treatment includes topical azoles or short courses of oral fluconazole.

40.3.4 Other mucosal fungal infections

Laryngeal candidiasis or *Candida* epiglottitis typically occurs in the setting of oropharyngeal candidiasis. Patients may develop hoarseness, laryngeal stridor and respiratory compromise [38–40]. Treatment includes amphotericin B or intravenous fluconazole.

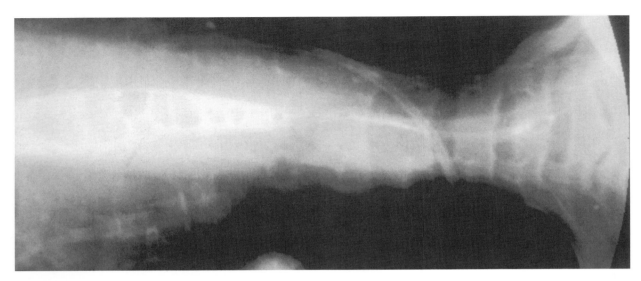

Figure 40.2. Esophagogram of a patient with esophageal candidiasis; typical moth-eaten appearance.

40.4 Invasive fungal infections due to opportunistic fungi

40.4.1 Disseminated candidiasis

Disseminated candidiasis is unusual in HIV-infected children [41, 42]. It may arise from the gastrointestinal tract, particularly when herpes simplex or cytomegalovirus infections disrupt mucosal barriers, but more typically it occurs in association with indwelling central venous catheters [41–43]. It may develop as isolated candidemia or as a disseminated disease with deep organ involvement. Common complications include endophthalmitis, renal candidiasis, arthritis, and osteomyelitis. About half of all reported cases of fungemia in HIV-infected children have been due to non-*albicans Candida* species [42]. Successful management of candidemia or disseminated candidiasis depends on early detection by blood cultures, removal of the central venous catheter, and rapid institution of amphotericin B for an average duration of 2–3 weeks. Since non-*albicans* species of *Candida* are frequently involved, fluconazole is not recommended as a first line therapy.

40.4.2 Cryptococcosis

The predominant portal of entry of *Cryptococcus* is the respiratory tract. However, in the majority of cases, pulmonary involvement remains clinically silent while the organism seeds the central nervous system and causes meningoencephalitis. Mortality has been associated with fulmin-

ant cryptococcemia and disseminated disease. Clinical manifestations include fever of unknown origin, chronic meningitis, pulmonary infection, and septic shock [44, 45]. Meningitis is probably the most common manifestation of cryptococcosis in children. Fever, headache, and altered mental status are frequent symptoms. These can be indolent evolving over weeks. Such subtle manifestations, as well as the benefit of early treatment on outcome, clearly justify a low threshold for initiating appropriate diagnostic investigations in symptomatic HIV-infected children. Diagnosis is established by lumbar puncture, direct examination of cerebrospinal fluid (CSF) with India ink stain, and culture. Latex agglutination cryptococcal polysaccharide antigen titers in serum and CSF correlate with the tissue burden of *C. neoformans* are an important tool in the diagnosis and evaluation of the therapeutic response [46].

The choice of antifungal drugs and duration of treatment are not well defined in children. Data from the adult population indicate that induction therapy with the combination of amphotericin B plus flucytosine results in earlier CSF clearance and fewer relapses than amphotericin B alone [47]. Lipid formulations of amphotericin B also have been found to be very effective for induction therapy of cryptococcosis [48–50]. Induction therapy can be limited to the period of clinical response (2–6 weeks). Fluconazole plus flucytosine is a potent oral antifungal regimen in adults, however, little is known about this combination in children [51, 52]. HIV-infected children with cryptococcosis must be treated indefinitely. Fluconazole is typically used for

patients with AIDS. *Antimicrob. Agents Chemother.* **46** (2002), 248–50.

66. Wheat, L. J., Hafner, R., Wulfsohn, M. *et al.* Prevention of relapse of histoplasmosis with itraconazole in patients with the acquired immunodeficiency syndrome. *Ann. Intern. Med.* **118** (1993), 610–16.

67. MacDonald, N., Steinhoff, M. C. & Powell, K. R. Review of coccidiodomycosis in immunocompromised children. *Am. J. Dis. Child.* **135** (1981), 553–6.

68. Stevens, D. A. Coccidiodomycosis. *New Engl. J. Med.* **332** (1995), 1077–82.

69. Galgiani, J. N., Catanzaro, A., Cloud, G. A. *et al.* Fluconazole therapy for coccidioidal meningitis. The NIAID-Mycoses Study Group. *Ann. Intern. Med.* **119** (1993), 28–35.

70. Shehab, Z. M., Britton, H. & Dunn, J. H. Imidazole therapy in coccidioidal meningitis in children. *Pediatr. Infect. Dis. J.* **7** (1988), 440–4.

71. Chariyalertsak, S., Sirisanthana, T., Saengwonloey, O. & Nelson, K. E. (2001). Clinical presentation of patients with acquired immunodeficiency syndrome in Thailand, 1994–1998: regional variation and temporal trends. *Clin. Infect. Dis.* **32** (2001), 955–62.

72. Sirisanthana, V. & Sirisanthana, T. *Penicillium marneffei* infection in children infected with human immunodeficiency virus. *Pediatr. Infect. Dis. J.* **12** (1993), 1021–5.

73. Sirisanthana, V. & Sirisanthana, T. Disseminated *Penicillium marneffei* infection in human immunodeficiency virus infected children. *Pediatr. Infect. Dis. J.* **14** (1995), 935–40.

74. Sirisanthana, T., Supparatpinyo, K., Perriens, J. & Nelson, K. E. Amphotericin B and itraconazole for the treatment of disseminated *Penicillium marneffei* infection in human immunodeficiency virus-infected patients. *Clin. Infect. Dis.* **26** (1998), 1107–10.

75. Supparatpinyo, K., Nelson, K. E., Merz, W. G., Breslin, B. J., Cooper, C. R. Jr, Kamwan, C. & Sirisanthana, T. Response to antifungal therapy by human immunodeficiency virus-infected patients with disseminated *Penicillium marneffei* infections and *in vitro* susceptibilities of isolates from clinical specimens. *Antimicrob. Agents Chemother.* **37** (1993), 2407–11.

76. Supparatpinyo, K., Perriens, J., Nelson, K. & Sirisanthana, T. A controlled trial of itraconazole to prevent relapse of *Penicillium marneffei* infection in patients with the human immunodeficiency virus. *New Engl. J. Med.* **339** (1998), 1739–43.

Herpesvirus infections

Richard M. Rutstein, M.D.[1] and Stuart E. Starr, M.D.[2]

[1]Division of General Pediatrics, Children's Hospital of Philadelphia, Philadelphia, PA
[2]Division of Allergy, Immunologic and Infectious Diseases, Children's Hospital of Philadelphia, Philadelphia, PA

41.1 Introduction

The eight known herpesviruses share a common structure consisting of double-stranded DNA, surrounded by a protein capsid and then a lipid and glycoprotein envelope. Herpesviruses infect humans worldwide, but prevalence varies among populations.

For most herpesviruses, primary infection usually occurs during childhood or early adult years. Beyond the neonatal period, infection rarely results in serious illness in the immunocompetent host. Herpesvirus infections are usually controlled by elements of the cellular immune system (see Chapters 1 and 3); patients significantly compromised by HIV infection can develop serious, sometimes life-threatening herpesvirus infections. In the normal host, after primary infection, herpesviruses establish life-long, latent infection, in which virus is sequestered in a non-replicative state, with the potential for recurrent or chronic disease after reactivation. The sites of latent infection for herpes simplex virus (HSV) and varicella-zoster virus (VZV) are believed to be sensory ganglia. For cytomegalovirus (CMV), Epstein–Barr virus (EBV) and human herpesvirus 6 (HHV-6), lymphocytes represent the reservoir of latent infection. With EBV, the target cell appears to be B lymphocytes, for HHV-6, T lymphocytes. The site of latency for CMV appears to be bone marrow-derived monocytes and monocyte precursors. A complex interplay exists between herpesviruses and HIV [1]. In some in vitro systems, infection with CMV, or HSV may increase susceptibility of cells to infection with HIV. In cells chronically infected with HIV, CMV or HSV infections appear capable of upregulating expression of HIV, with enhanced viral replication.

Co-infection of cells with HIV and CMV enhances CMV replication compared with cells infected with CMV alone.

In immunocompromised hosts, including HIV-infected children with immunologic impairment, primary infections with some herpesviruses may be more severe than such infections in healthy children. Reactivation infections occur more frequently in HIV-infected children and may be more severe.

In this chapter we will discuss those herpesvirus which cause significant morbidity in HIV-infected individuals: CMV, HSV, VZV, and EBV (Table 41.1). We also touch briefly on Human Herpesvirus-6 (HHV-6), as well as Human Herpesvirus-8 (HHV-8 or Kaposi's sarcoma-associated herpesvirus, KSHV) and its relation to Kaposi's sarcoma (KS). More information about HHV-8 and KS can be found in Chapter 36.

41.2 Cytomegalovirus

41.2.1 Epidemiology

Cytomegalovirus is transmitted by exposure to blood, urine, saliva, tears, breast milk, stool, and genital secretions of infected individuals. Cytomegalovirus can be transmitted in utero, perinatally, or postnatally. In children, infection usually occurs secondary to exposure to infected saliva or urine. In young adulthood, the rate of CMV seropositivity rises secondary to sexual activity.

In developed countries, 10–15% of children are infected by early adolescence, with increased rates seen among those in lower socioeconomic groups. In developing countries, where the majority of infants are breast fed, CMV

Table 41.1 Clinical syndromes caused by herpesviruses in HIV-infected Children

Cytomegalovirus	Herpes simplex virus	Varicella-zoster virus
Retinitis	Gingivostomatitis	Chicken pox (varicella)
Pneumonitis	Labial/genital	Herpes zoster
Colitis	Esophageal ulcers	Persistent skin infection
Esophageal ulcers	Encephalitis	Encephalitis
Hepatitis		
Pancreatitis		
Encephalitis		
Polyradiculopathy		

is frequently acquired in infancy. Prevalence increases to nearly 50% in women of child-bearing age. Seropositivity increases with advancing age, and virtually all individuals seroconvert eventually.

Congenital CMV infection is the most common intrauterine infection in the USA affecting 1–2% of all live-born infants. Symptomatic infection occurs in 5–10% of those infected, and is associated with a high incidence of mental retardation, sensorineural hearing loss, chorioretinitis, and neurologic defects [2]. Transmission from mother to fetus occurs as a consequence of both primary and recurrent maternal infection, though infants are much more likely to be symptomatic if infected during primary maternal infection.

Perinatal CMV infection occurs in 25–50% of neonates exposed to CMV in the birth canal. In one US based study, in a population of younger mothers, 89% were CMV seropositive, and 11% of mothers had CMV detected in cervical fluid in the third trimester [3]. Infection also occurs in 40–60% of infants who are breast fed for more than 1 month by mothers with infectious CMV in their breast milk; the risk is highest for women with recent, or primary infection [2]. Beyond the neonatal period, CMV infection is typically asymptomatic. Young adults, and occasionally children, can develop an EBV-negative mononucleosis syndrome.

The rate of CMV seropositivity is much greater among adults with life styles associated with high risk for HIV infection than in the general population. In healthy gay adults, rates of CMV seropositivity are in the range of 85–90%; while in gay men with AIDS, the rate approaches 100%. Among hemophiliacs, rates vary from 26–64%, equivalent to those found in age-matched controls. Several researchers have noted increased seropositivity and an increased incidence

of active CMV infection in women with HIV infection, possibly as a result of interaction between the two viruses. In addition, HIV-infected infants have an increased incidence of congenital/perinatal CMV infection when compared with HIV-exposed, but uninfected infants, and to infants born to HIV-negative women.

41.2.2 Possible influence of CMV infection on rate of progression of HIV infection

Several studies suggest that in HIV-infected adults, co-infection with CMV results in a more rapid progression of HIV infection and shortened survival. This has been related to the immunosuppressive effects of CMV, independent of HIV infection, as well as the potential up-regulation of HIV replication by CMV.

Likewise, several pediatric studies also have noted a trend towards more rapidly progressive disease in co-infected infants. In a prospective study of HIV-exposed neonates, dually infected children were more likely to experience rapid progression to an AIDS-defining condition and to develop progressive encephalopathy. Dually infected children also had higher CD8$^+$ cell counts and lower CD4$^+$ lymphocyte counts. Another study reported more rapid progression to AIDS and death in HIV-infected children with detectable levels of CMV DNA in serum [4, 5].

Other studies in children or adults did not find a link between dual infection and rapid progression of HIV disease. One of the difficulties in interpreting these studies involves the issue of association versus causation. It is apparent that severely immunocompromised HIV-infected infants (and adults) are more likely to have viremia and/or to excrete CMV; it is not clear that CMV infection leads to more rapid disease progression. In addition, studies have linked rapid progression of HIV in infants to the severity of illness in their mothers. It may be that the mothers more likely to have infants with rapidly progressive HIV disease (based on their own stage of illness) are also more likely to transmit CMV to their newborns.

41.2.3 Clinical manifestations

End organ disease from CMV is the most frequent manifestation of viral opportunistic infection in HIV-infected persons. Up to 10% of deaths in adults with AIDS are related to CMV infection, and evidence of CMV disease is found at autopsy in 50–75% of HIV-infected adults. While pneumonitis is the most common CMV disease in bone marrow transplant recipients, retinal and gastrointestinal manifestations of CMV are more common in adults with HIV infection [6].

Clinical syndromes related to CMV infection include retinitis, colitis, esophagitis, gastritis, encephalitis, polyradiculitis, hepatitis, and adrenalitis. In adults, retinitis is the most common manifestation of CMV disease (50–80% of cases) followed by colitis and pneumonitis. Clinical manifestations of CMV disease generally do not occur until the CD4$^+$ lymphocyte count falls below 100/mL. The risk of developing retinitis over 24 months is 20% and 40%, for adults with CD4$^+$ counts of < 100/mL and < 50/mL, respectively. The median CD4$^+$ count at time of diagnosis of retinopathy is below 50 cells/μL.

In children, CMV is responsible for 8–10% of AIDS-defining illnesses, with retinitis accounting for only one-quarter of the total cases, with the other 75% consisting of CMV end organ disease of the liver, colon, lung, or brain. The overall lifetime incidence of CMV-related disease in perinatally acquired HIV infection prior to the advent of HAART had been reported to be 30–60%. Through 2001, CMV-end organ disease was reported in 10% of children with AIDS. In one large cohort study, the prevalence of retinitis was 4%, lower than the 15–40% prevalence rate of retinitis in adults with AIDS. One quarter of children with a history of at least one CMV positive blood or urine culture had evidence of CMV disease at autopsy [7–9].

The incidence of CMV infection and excretion increases with HIV-related disease progression. Symptomatic HIV-infected children have a higher rate of CMV viruria than asymptomatic HIV-infected children and HIV-exposed children (46% vs 14%). Once shedding of CMV is detected, HIV-infected infants generally continue to excrete virus in the urine. Overall, one third of HIV-infected children are CMV-shedders (up to 60% in children with AIDS), compared with 15–20% of HIV-exposed, but uninfected children, and <15% of unexposed infants. In one longitudinal study, 45% of children with evidence of CMV infection before 6 months of age developed symptomatic CMV infection. A higher percentage of HIV-infected infants had congenital CMV infection (defined as a positive urine CMV conventional culture or shell vial viral culture assay at <3 weeks of age) than HIV-exposed infants (21% vs 3.4%). In addition, CD4$^+$ counts were lower in co-infected infants and there was a trend towards decreased survival [5, 7–9].

Specific organ systems

Retinitis
Cytomegalovirus retinitis occurs in at least 10–20% of adult AIDS patients, and autopsy studies indicate that up to 30% had evidence of CMV retinal infections. The disease typically begins unilaterally, but progression to bilateral disease is common. Affected adults most commonly complain of painless loss of vision, visual field cuts, or floaters. In children, however, the disease is frequently asymptomatic, and discovered on routine ophthalmologic examination. At times, fever and irritability may be the only signs of CMV retinitis in infancy. Practitioners caring for HIV-infected children should therefore have a low threshold for investigating the possibility of CMV disease, particularly CMV retinitis (see also Chapter 27).

Ophthalmologic examination of the CMV-diseased retina reveals large yellowish-white, granular areas with perivascular exudates and hemorrhage. Histological findings include coagulation necrosis and microvascular abnormalities. Cytomegalovirus retinitis must be differentiated from HIV-related retinopathy. In the latter condition, cotton wool spots, representing areas of ischemic atrophy, appear on the retina. These lesions are common in HIV, usually asymptomatic and frequently regress over time in patients receiving antiretroviral therapy.

Compared with adults, retinal disease due to CMV is less common in HIV-infected children. Many investigators recommend regular eye exams for severely immunocompromised infants known to be CMV-infected.

Gastrointestinal manifestations
HIV-infected patients can develop CMV disease at any site in the gastrointestinal (GI) tract. The incidence of CMV GI disease in adults with AIDS ranged from 4–52% in different cohorts, with a mean incidence of 30% [10]. Cytomegalovirus disease of the GI tract is the most common condition leading to emergency or elective abdominal surgery in HIV-infected adults. Patients presenting with sudden severe abdominal pain must be evaluated for CMV-related gastrointestinal perforation and/or hemorrhage.

Examination of biopsy and autopsy specimens has shown that many gastrointestinal tract cell types can be infected with CMV, most commonly vascular endothelial cells, but also fibroblasts, smooth muscle cells, and glandular epithelium. Mucosal infection leads to inflammation with tissue necrosis, vascular endothelial involvement, and subsequent ischemic mucosal injury. Ulcerations, erosions, and mucosal hemorrhage are the primary macroscopic findings.

The most common GI manifestation, CMV colitis, occurs in at least 5–10% of adults with AIDS. Presenting symptoms are non-specific and include diarrhea, abdominal pain, weight loss, hematochezia, anorexia, and fever. Other possible causes of colitis in an HIV-infected patient include common bacterial pathogens (*Mycobacterium avium* complex (MAC), *Giardia lamblia*, *Cryptosporidium parvum*, *Clostridium difficile*) and primary HIV colitis. Massive acute bleeding from CMV colitis, as well as perforation, has been reported in several HIV-infected infants. Toxic megacolon may occur as a complication of CMV colitis. In the small intestine, CMV may mimic Crohn's disease, causing mucosal erosions and ulcers. There are also several reports of pseudomembranous colitis secondary to CMV infection.

In HIV-infected patients, oral and esophageal ulcers and esophagitis are most commonly due to fungal or HSV infections, but CMV also can cause disease in these locations. Symptoms are non-specific, and may include substernal pain, dysphagia, odynophagia, and decreased appetite, with or without fever. Up to 50% of patients also have thrush at the time of diagnosis [11]. Esophageal strictures have been described as a consequence of CMV-related esophageal ulcers.

Hepatic involvement with CMV is common, but generally mild. Histologic evidence of CMV hepatitis is seen in 25–33% of patients with end organ CMV disease. Although liver enzymes and alkaline phosphatase may be elevated, bilirubin levels are usually normal.

A more serious syndrome, ascending cholangiopathy, also has been associated with CMV infection in HIV-infected adults. In one series, 25% of patients with ductal abnormalities had microscopic evidence of CMV infection. The disease presents with fever, abdominal pain localized to the right upper quadrant, and elevated serum alkaline phosphatase levels.

Infrequently, CMV infects gastric tissue, resulting in epigastric pain, nausea, and vomiting. The infection can progress to overt gastric ulcers, with or without bleeding, as well as gastric outlet obstruction and/or perforation. Rarely, CMV has been implicated as the etiology of pancreatitis in HIV-infected adults and children.

Pulmonary disease

Although CMV is the most common cause of pneumonia in bone marrow transplants, it is an infrequent pulmonary pathogen in HIV-infected individuals. Even when CMV is isolated from lung secretions or lung tissue, its role in causing lung disease may be difficult to assess. In adults and children with pneumonia, in whom both *Pneumocystis carinii* and CMV were recovered from lung fluid, clinical recovery was independent of CMV culture results when treatment was directed against *P. carinii*. This indicates that most patients had *P. carinii* pneumonia and infection with CMV, but not disease. In general, the diagnosis of CMV pneumonia should be considered if other pathogens are ruled out, or if patients fail to respond to therapy directed against other pathogens [12, 13].

Cytomegalovirus pneumonia is generally an interstitial process, with gradual onset of shortness of breath and a dry, non-productive cough. Usually, auscultatory findings are minimal. Cytomegalovirus pneumonia is more common in adults with other end organ CMV disease, and severe immunosuppression (CD4$^+$ < 25/mL). Median survival after diagnosis is less than 30 days [14].

Central nervous system

A syndrome of CMV-related subacute encephalopathy, indistinguishable from HIV-related encephalopathy, has been reported in HIV-infected adults and children. In addition, a small number of adults have been described with ventriculitis thought to be secondary to CMV infection. Several autopsy series have reported evidence of central nervous system (CNS) CMV infection in 10–40% of AIDS patients [15].

The relative role of CMV infection in the development of dementia or progressive encephalopathy in HIV-infected patients is hard to discern. Both HIV- and CMV-related encephalopathy are characterized by diffuse increased white matter signal density on magnetic resonance imaging (MRI) studies, and CMV culture of the CSF often remains negative, even in proven cases of CMV in encephalopathy.

Though rarely reported in children, CMV has been implicated in axonal polyradiculopathy in adults. This disease presents much like Guillain–Barré syndrome, with painful, ascending muscle weakness, loss of deep tendon reflexes, and loss of bladder/bowel control.

41.2.4 Diagnosis

It can be difficult to distinguish between CMV infection and CMV disease. Patients with HIV infection, in particular, may be infected with CMV, but their serious end organ disease may be caused by other etiologies. In general, detection of anti-CMV antibodies, or culturing CMV from the blood or other body fluids confirms CMV infection, but not necessarily end organ disease secondary CMV.

In a child over 12 months of age, detection of anti-CMV antibody indicates prior infection with the virus, but not necessarily disease. Antibody detection prior to 12 months of age may be secondary to maternally derived anti-CMV antibodies. At any age, a positive CMV urine culture or detection of CMV antigen in shell vial cultures is indicative of CMV infection. As HIV-infected children may excrete virus for prolonged periods, a positive urine culture does not define the time of primary infection, except in instances where the urine culture had previously been negative.

Isolation of virus in cultured cells remains the gold standard for establishing the presence of CMV infection. Classic culture methods require 1–3 weeks for isolation of CMV; with the advent of centrifugation-assisted shell vial culture amplification techniques, CMV may be detected within

24 hours of inoculation of cultures. However, CMV can be isolated in only one-third of patients with documented CMV colitis, and from oropharyngeal secretions of only one-third of patients with esophageal lesions histopathologically proven due to CMV [10]. Several diagnostic methods, including detection of pp65 antigenemia, qualitative and quantitative PCR, and DNA hybridization have been studied for their ability to identify patients most at risk for CMV disease. In general, all of these methods detect CMV infection 3–6 months prior to the development of clinically recognized disease.

The detection of CMV antigenemia involves the staining of neutrophils with monoclonal antibody directed against the CMV matrix protein pp65. Typically, cells are counted by flow cytometry and results are reported as the number of stain-positive cells per 50 000 or 200 000 counted cells.

Plasma PCR DNA is more sensitive for detecting CMV than urine or blood cultures. Quantitative PCR may be the most sensitive test for identifying patients at high risk for CMV disease, including CMV retinitis, i.e. patients with plasma DNA PCR levels above 100–1000 copies/μL. In one study of adults receiving HAART, CD4$^+$ counts < 75 cells/μL, positive plasma CMV DNA and pp65 antigenemia >100 positive cells/200 000 cells, all were predictive of risk of CMV disease over a 24-month follow-up period [16, 17]. Several prospective studies have confirmed that the detection of CMV DNA by PCR and/or antigenemia accurately predicts the risk of development of CMV end organ disease. In addition, patients on anti-CMV therapy who convert from positive to negative CMV PCR DNA status have an improved outcome. Effective therapy also leads to a decrease in the level of pp65 antigenemia [18, 19].

The appearance of the retina is usually sufficient for a presumptive diagnosis of CMV retinitis. For other end organ CMV disease, diagnosis is based on isolation of CMV and/or demonstration of characteristic histopathologic findings (the pathognomonic "owl's eye" intranuclear and smaller intracytoplasmic inclusion bodies) in biopsy specimens.

In patients with CMV-related colitis, sigmoidoscopy reveals diffuse areas of erythema, submucosal hemorrhage, and diffuse mucosal ulcerations, which may be indistinguishable from ulcerative colitis. The most frequent finding in patients with esophagitis is a large, solitary distal ulcer. Histopathologic changes in the GI tract include vasculitis, neutrophil infiltration, and non-specific inflammation. The presence of CMV inclusions and/or positive cultures for CMV helps to confirm the diagnosis.

The diagnosis of CMV-related pneumonia is based on the exclusion of other pathogens, and isolation of CMV from lung tissue or bronchial fluid, with histologic evidence of CMV disease (cells with intranuclear inclusions). Treatment should be limited to those with histopathologic changes at lung biopsy, or if too ill for biopsy, those with worsening pulmonary disease in the absence of other pathogens.

In CMV CNS disease, examination of the CSF reveals pleocytosis in approximately 50% of cases, frequently with a polymorphonuclear predominance; the protein concentration is elevated in 75%, and hypoglycorrhachia occurs in 30%. Up to 20% of patients may have completely normal CSF findings. Detection of CMV DNA in CSF by PCR has been found to be highly sensitive and specific for adults with autopsy-proven CMV encephalopathy, ventriculitis, or polyradiculopathy [20].

41.2.5 Treatment

Three drugs are available to treat CMV disease: ganciclovir, cidofovir, and foscarnet. Ganciclovir and cidofovir, as nucleoside and nucleotide analogues respectively have mechanisms of action that closely resemble the nucleoside and nucleotide analogue antiretroviral reverse transcriptase inhibitors. Treatment for CMV disease and other herpesvirus infections is outlined in Table 41.2.

The drug generally used as first-line therapy for CMV end organ disease is intravenous ganciclovir, since the other two agents have significant toxicities. (Oral valganciclovir, a ganciclovir pro-drug, may have an increasing role in therapy, see below.) Ganciclovir is a guanosine nucleoside analogue that is converted in vivo to ganciclovir triphosphate, the intracellularly active form of the drug. Ganciclovir is phosphorylated first to the monophosphate by a product of the CMV gene (or open reading frame, ORF) UL97. Since the phosphorylase is only expressed in CMV-infected cells, phosphoryation of ganciclovir by UL97 helps to selectively target the effects of ganciclovir to infected cells. After the initial phosphorylation step, the monophosphate is then phosphorylated to the active triphosphate form of the drug by cellular enzymes. Ganciclovir triphosphate competitively inhibits the native deoxyguanosine triphosphate from interacting with the viral DNA polymerase, which inhibits viral DNA replication. Futhermore, after the viral DNA polymerase cleaves ganciclovir triphosphate to ganciclovir monophosphate as it adds the ganciclovir monophosphate to the growing viral DNA chain, no further nucleotides can be added because ganciclovir lacks a free 3' OH group, causing termination of the growing viral DNA chain.

Two mechanisms cause resistance to ganciclovir, mutations in the UL97 phosphorylase and mutations in the CMV DNA polymerase. Laboratory and clinical CMV isolates

Table 41.2 Treatment of herpesvirus infection in HIV-infected children

Virus	Syndrome	Drug	Dose/route	Common side-effects
CMV	Retinitis-induction	Ganciclovir	IV: 5 mg/kg, BID for 14 days	Myelosuppression
	Alternative drugs:	Foscarnet	IV: 90 mg/kg,BID or 60 mg/kg, TID for 14 days	Nephrotoxicity
		Cidofovir	IV: 5 mg/kg qwk for 2 doses, pretreat with probenicid and saline loading	Nephrotoxicity
	Maintenance	Ganciclovir	IV: 5 mg/kg/day	
	Alternative drugs:	Ganciclovir	PO: 1g TID	
		Foscarnet	IV: 90–120 mg/kg/day	
		Cidofovir	5 mg/kg q2wks, pretreat with probenicid and saline loading	
		Valganciclovir	Adult: 900 mg bid	Neutropenia
	Gastrointestinal/ Pulmonary	same as for retinitis induction		
HSV 1, 2	Primary oral/genital	Acyclovir	IV: 750 mg/m^2/day in 3 doses PO: 1200 mg/m^2 per day, in 3 doses	Phlebitis, nephrotoxicity, nausea, vomiting
	Alternative drugs:	Famciclovir	Adults: 125–500 mg BID	rash
		Valacyclovir	Adults: 0.5–1 g BID	Gastrointestinal upset
	For acyclovir resistance	Foscarnet		
	Recurrent	Acyclovir	same as above	
	encephalitis	Acyclovir	IV: 1500 mg/m^2/day or 30 mg/kg/day in 3 divided doses	
Varicella-zoster virus	Varicella	Acyclovir	IV-1500 mg/m^2/day in 3 doses PO-80 mg/kg/day in 4 divided doses	Phlebitis, nephrotoxicity nausea,vomiting, rash
		Famciclovir	Adults: 500 mg TID	
		Valacyclovir	Adults: 1 g TID	
	Zoster	Same as for varicella		
	Acyclovir resistant virus	Foscarnet		

with certain point mutations in the UL97 gene are unable to phosphorylate ganciclovir and demonstrate low-level resistance. Mutations in the CMV DNA polymerase gene (UL54) confer high-level resistance to ganciclovir. High-level resistance to ganciclovir is generally associated with mutations in both UL97 and UL54. In patients with newly diagnosed CMV retinitis, less than 2–5% will have evidence of resistance-related mutations prior to therapy. On therapy, 10–25% of patients develop resistance-related mutations [21, 22].

The starting dose of ganciclovir is 5 mg/kg twice a day for 2 weeks, followed by 5 mg/kg/day, 5–7 days per week. The major side-effect is myelosuppression. Dosage reduction or use of filgrastim (G-CSF) frequently is necessary owing to anemia, thrombocytopenia, or neutropenia.

Cidofovir is a nucleotide analogue of cytosine. Thus, it is already monophosphorylated and does not require phosphorylation by the CMV UL97 gene product. Similarly to ganciclovir, cidofovir is further phosphorylated to the triphosphate by cellular phosphorylases. The phosphorylated cidofovir competitively inhibits binding of the native cytosine to the viral DNA polymerase, and incorporation of cidofovir into the growing viral DNA chain causes chain termination because it does not have a free 3′ OH group. Since cidofovir does not require phosphorylation by the UL97 viral phosphorylase, CMVs resistant to ganciclovir due to mutations in UL97 retain sensitivity to cidofovir. However, mutants in the viral DNA polymerase can confer resistance against both ganciclovir and cidofovir. If a virus demonstrates high-level resistance to ganciclovir it will likely be resistant to cidofovir.

Cidofovir has a significant and potentially difficult to manage set of toxicities, including potentially severe proximal tubular injuries resulting in proteinuria, glycosuria, and bicarbonate and phosphate wasting. A substantial incidence of neutropenia has also been observed. Renal function should be carefully monitored in patients treated with cidofovir. Cidofovir is dosed at 5 mg/kg intravenously every week for 2 weeks as induction therapy, and then every other week for maintenance therapy. Cidofovir must be given with oral probenecid and saline loading.

Foscarnet is another drug used to treat CMV infections. Unlike ganciclovir or cidofovir, foscarnet is not a nucleic acid analogue. Instead, foscarnet is a pyrophosphate analogue, one of the structurally simplest approved drugs. Foscarnet inhibits viral DNA polymerase. Since it is not a nucleic acid analogue, foscarnet does not require phosphorylation to an active form. Therefore, ganciclovir-resistant strains of CMV due to mutations in the UL97 phosphorylase gene are sensitive to foscarnet. There are mutations in the viral DNA polymerase that can confer resistance to foscarnet. Some of these may be distinct from those DNA polymerase mutations conferring resistance to ganciclovir and cidofovir. Some viruses resistant to all three approved CMV antivirals, ganciclovir, cidofovir, and foscarnet, have been described. Foscarnet also appears to have some degree of antiviral activity against HIV itself.

Foscarnet, however, can produce significant, severe toxicities. The main toxicity of foscarnet is decreased renal function. Renal toxicity can lead to serious electrolyte and calcium imbalances, with secondary seizures. The renal toxicity of foscarnet may be increased when other nephrotoxic agents are also given, particularly amphotericin B, pentamidine, and aminoglycosides. Electrolytes should be carefully monitored in patients receiving foscarnet. Renal side-effects may be minimized by infusing foscarnet over 1 hour, with saline fluid loading.

Approximately 80–90% of CMV retinitis cases respond initially to treatment, but relapse invariably occurs if therapy is discontinued. Relapses are delayed if maintenance therapy is given with ganciclovir or foscarnet. Dual therapy with ganciclovir and foscarnet has been used successfully for some cases of rapidly progressive CMV disease or disease that was not responsive to monotherapy.

The difficulty of continuing daily intravenous therapy, and the ongoing potential for drug toxicity, has made the development of alternative maintenance therapies for CMV disease a high priority. Strategies tested to date for prevention of recurrent retinitis include: oral ganciclovir, intravitreal administration of medication (as with implants impregnated with either ganciclovir or or cidofovir, see Chapter 27), or cidofovir, an agent with a longer half life [23–26]. There have been two main problems with local therapy: risk of ophthalmologic side-effects, such as retinal detachment, and development of extraocular CMV disease. One study comparing treatment options for maintenance therapy for CMV retinitis found a breakthrough rate of new CMV disease at 6 months of 44.3% for patients treated with a ganciclovir implant, 24.3% for patients treated with the implant plus oral ganciclovir, and 19.6% in the intravenous ganciclovir treatment group [24]. Local treatment of CMV retinitis has no effect on other, systemic CMV disease. Interestingly, patients who were treated with protease inhibitor-containing HAART regimens had a low rate of new CMV disease, irregardless of treatment group.

Studies are under way employing valganciclovir (VGC) in CMV-related disease. Valganciclovir is an orally administered pro-drug of ganciclovir. A dose of 900 mg orally provides serum levels comparable with those found with a 5 mg/kg intravenous dose of ganciclovir. In a randomized trial in HIV-infected adults with newly diagnosed CMV retinitis, oral VGC was as effective as intravenous ganciclovir in treating the first episode and delaying progression of illness.

There may be a role for using VGC in a pre-emptive manner, in patients with low CD4$^+$ counts despite HAART, and evidence of CMV infection, prior to the development of end organ disease. Studies in adults are under way.

The necessity of maintenance therapy for CMV-related hepatitis, pneumonia, or colitis has not been firmly established. In several small series, therapy with ganciclovir or foscarnet resulted in symptomatic improvement, but maintenance therapy did not seem to prevent relapse or development of CMV disease in other end organs [27].

Newer agents under development for the treatment of CMV-related disease include intravitreous fomivirsen, for CMV retinitis. Fomivirsen has been shown to have considerable activity, when injected every 2–4 weeks (after an induction period) for patients with eye disease that progressed, or relapsed, while on other anti-CMV therapies [28]. Other potential agents, not yet in advanced clinical trials, include maribavir (a protein kinase inhibitor), and inhibitors of the terminase complex that cleaves viral produced DNA, such as tomeglovir and GW-275175X [29].

Limited options are available for treatment of HIV-infected children with CMV end organ disease (see also Chapter 27 for information about ophthalmic disease). Use of intravitreal ganciclovir and intravenous cidofovir is still investigational in children. Intravenously administered ganciclovir or foscarnet is available for such children. Frenkel *et al.* reported on the use of an oral ganciclovir liquid formulation in HIV-infected children [30]. In this pharmacokinetic study, a dose of 30 mg/kg every 8 hours resulted in serum levels similar to those found in adults treated with 1 g every 8 hours. The relative bioavailability of the liquid formulation was essentially equivalent to that of capsules and was well tolerated. The main, and expected side-effect was neutropenia. The volume of the suspension required (at 25 mg/ml, daily dosing for a 30 kg child would be 36 ml every 0.8 hours) or the high pill burden (four 250 capsules every 8 hours) represents a major impediment to adherence to long-term therapy [30].

41.2.6 Cytomegalovirus infection in patients treated with highly active antiretroviral therapy

Since the advent of combination therapy employing three or more drugs, termed highly active antiretroviral therapy (HAART), the incidence of opportunistic infections among HIV-infected adults has dropped markedly. Overall, the incidence of end-organ disease secondary to CMV infection among HIV-infected persons has declined from 15–20/100 patient-years to 1–5/100 patient-years [31, 32]. Clearing of CMV viremia has been reported following immunologic improvement associated with HAART [33].

The immune reconstitution that follows successful HAART has been associated with certain distinct inflammatory syndromes, including syndromes related to pre-existing CMV disease, such as an inflammatory vitritis related to quiescent or subclinical CMV retinitis. This vitreal inflammatory response may be severe, and may respond to intraocular steroid therapy [34].

Effective HAART may produce such substantial immune reconstitution that certain patients with existing CMV disease may be able to discontinue maintenance ganciclovir therapy without experiencing recurrence of CMV disease. Such patients should have been treated with HAART for at least 6 months, with an increase of CD4+ count to levels above 100–150 cells/μL, and have negative CMV blood markers prior to the anticipated discontinuation of anti-

CMV therapy [35]. Children may have the potential to experience a more substantial immune reconstitution than adults. However, no clinical trials have established whether maintenance therapy for CMV disease may be discontinued for pediatric patients. Even as the overall incidence of CMV disease in HIV-infected adults is decreasing, active surveillance for CMV end organ involvement must continue, as CMV disease in patients on HAART is now occurring at CD4+ levels once thought protective against CMV disease.

41.3 Herpes simplex virus

41.3.1 Epidemiology

As with other herpesviruses, HSV-1 and 2 affect all populations. HSV-1 is transmitted primarily by contact with infected oral secretions, and HSV-2 primarily through infected genital secretions. Primary HSV-1 infection usually is asymptomatic. Lesions, when present, are usually located in the oropharynx. Primary infection in young adults has been associated with pharyngitis and, less commonly, a mononucleosis-like syndrome. In resource-rich countries, children of lower socioeconomic class acquire HSV-1 earlier than children of higher classes. Only 30–40% of individuals from middle and upper socioeconomic classes are seropositive by the second decade of life, compared with 75–90% of individuals from lower socioeconomic classes [36]. HSV-2 is generally acquired through contact with genital lesions, and as such the seroprevalence is low until late adolescence and early adulthood, increasing with the onset of sexual activity. Overall, 20–30% of adults in the USA have serologic evidence of HSV-2 infection [37, 38].

After primary infection with HSV, the virus remains latent within sensory ganglia. With immunosuppression or acquired immunodeficiency, reactivation of latent virus occurs more frequently than in immunocompetent hosts. Reactivation typically involves mucocutaneous areas near the original site of entry, the lips or face for HSV-1, and the genital areas for HSV-2. In severely immunocompromised patients, recurrent infection may spread beyond the original involved area. Sites distant to the originally involved area also may be affected secondary to an associated viremia [37].

Co-infection with HSV-1 and -2 has not been associated with an effect on HIV disease progression among adults. Co-infected adults tend to have more episodes of HSV reactivation, as defined by days of viral shedding; many such episodes are asymptomatic.

41.3.2 Clinical manifestations

Orolabial herpes

Primary infection with HSV usually occurs in the perioral, ocular, or genital areas, but any skin site may be involved. Lesions can be extensive, and may mimic herpes zoster if present in a dermatomal distribution, although pain usually is less severe than with herpes zoster.

Primary oral infections or recurrences may be accompanied by high fever, extensive mucosal ulceration, drooling, and anorexia. In immunocompetent hosts, the disease lasts 10–14 days. The most common symptom of reactivation is herpes labialis, estimated to occur in 25–50% of infected individuals, frequently in association with a febrile illness, local trauma, or sun exposure. Painful vesicles appear at the vermillion border, progress to ulcers and then crust over 2–4 days.

Reactivation of HSV occurs more frequently, and tends to be more severe in immunosuppressed hosts. Both adults and children with HIV infection may develop chronic, severe, or recurrent orolabial herpes. In some such patients, chronic ulcerative lesions and virus shedding persists for weeks. From 5–10% of children with AIDS and primary gingivostomatitis subsequently develop frequent recurrences associated with severe ulcerative lesions and symptoms usually encountered only with primary infection.

Esophagitis

Up to 25% of autopsy-proven esophagitis in HIV-infected adults is secondary to HSV, with 25–50% having evidence of HSV infection elsewhere. Though rarely reported in normal children, esophageal disease due to HSV infection is relatively common in immunocompromised children. Symptoms include retrosternal pain and odynophagia. Herpetic lesions usually are not seen in the oral cavity. Definitive diagnosis requires endoscopy with biopsy and viral culture. In HIV-infected children presenting with symptoms consistent with esophagitis, endoscopic examination is recommended for those with a low probability of candidal esophagitis, the most frequent cause of esophagitis in this population. This would include those without thrush at the time of initial presentation, and those not responding to initial anti-candidal therapy.

Nervous system

HSV causes infrequent, but life-threatening encephalitis in immunocompetent hosts. Though HSV-1 is the primary etiologic agent, encephalitis may also occur secondary to HSV-2, particularly in the newborn, and in immunocompromised patients. The temporal lobe is the principal site of the necrotizing hemorrhagic encephalitis caused by HSV. In HIV-infected adults, herpes encephalitis may not present with such a classic localization, owing to the presence of other pathogens in the brain. For example, many patients with HSV-1 encephalitis also have evidence of ongoing CNS infection with CMV.

The usual symptoms are those associated with acute encephalitis, namely headache, fever, behavior changes and seizures. Electroencephalogram (EEG), MRI and computerized axial tomography (CAT) scans reveal changes consistent with HSV encephalitis by day 4 in many cases. Magnetic resonance imaging is now the imaging procedure of choice, and shows localized edema in the temporal and orbital surface of the frontal lobes, and deeper areas. The EEG, early in the disease, may only show non-specific slowing. Later in the course, epileptiform discharges may be found in the temporal areas. Cerebrospinal fluid findings (pleocytosis of 10–200 cells/μL, normal CSF glucose and increased protein) are non-specific and mimic those found with encephalitis due to other viruses.

Genital disease

Primary genital herpes rarely occurs in immunocompetent infants, unless a caregiver inadvertently inoculates the genital area via contaminated hands, or an infant has been abused sexually. In adolescents, symptoms of primary genital herpes are similar to those in adults and include fever, pain, itching, dysuria, discharge, and regional adenopathy. Vesicular lesions or ulcers may be noted in the perineal/vaginal/anal area. Lesions tend to last 2–3 weeks before complete healing.

In HIV-infected patients, the frequency and severity of recurrences of genital herpes increase as immunodeficiency worsens. Chronic deep necrotic ulcers secondary to HSV infection have been described in some severely immunodeficient, HIV-infected adults.

Disseminated disease

HSV-1, and rarely, HSV-2 can cause disseminated disease, with involvement of the liver, adrenals, lungs, kidney, spleen and brain, in severely immunocompromized hosts. In addition to a widespread vesicular eruption, patients may develop a hemorrhagic shock syndrome, with hemorrhage, evidence of intravascular coagulation, seizures, renal failure, and death, despite antiviral therapy.

41.3.3 Diagnosis

The diagnosis of HSV infection may be suspected clinically based on the typical appearance of vesicles and ulcers. Isolation of the virus remains the definitive diagnostic test. HSV grows rapidly, and is usually detected in tissue culture cells within 1–3 days. New methodologies (shell vial culture, enzyme-linked culture system) may decrease further the time to detection. Definitive diagnosis of esophageal disease requires endoscopy with biopsy and culture.

Cells collected from scrapings of skin lesions, conjunctiva, or mucosa lesions can be examined for HSV antigens by direct immunofluorescence. This method allows for quick identification of the virus, and can distinguish between VZV and HSV. Histologic examination reveals intranuclear inclusions and multi-nucleated giant cells.

In the evaluation of possible HSV encephalitis, detection of HSV DNA in CSF by PCR has replaced brain biopsy as the diagnostic test of choice. Infectious virus is rarely present in the CSF, but HSV DNA usually is detected by PCR. In one large adult study, HSV PCR on CSF had 100% sensitivity and 99.6% specificity for HSV encephalitis confirmed at autopsy [39]. The test has a 95% sensitivity and specificity. False negative results may occur early, or late, in the course of the illness. As early institution of treatment is critical, immunocompromised patients presenting with acute neurologic symptoms consistent with possible HSV encephalitis should be considered for empiric acyclovir therapy pending full evaluation.

41.3.4 Treatment

The drug of choice for HSV infections is acyclovir. Acyclovir is an acyclic purine nucleoside analogue. It is phosphorylated by viral kinase, and then further phosphorylated by the host cell kinases into active drug, which inhibits viral DNA polymerase. It acts by competing with native guanosine triphosphate for the viral DNA polymerase, by chain termination of the replicating viral genomic DNA, and by inactivating the viral DNA polymerase. Acyclovir has an excellent therapeutic index, partly based on a very high affinity for the viral thymidine kinase that mediates the first step in acyclovir's activation pathway. Concentrations of the drug are as much as 100-fold higher in cells infected with HSV, compared with uninfected cells. In addition, normal cells lack the thymidine kinase enzyme. Acyclovir penetrates well into all tissues, including the brain and CSF.

Symptomatic HIV-infected children with primary gingivostomatitis should be treated with intravenous acyclovir at a dose of 750 mg/m^2/day, in three divided doses, or oral acyclovir at a dose of 1200 mg/m^2/day in three divided doses. For disseminated disease or encephalitis, a higher parenteral dose, 1500 mg/m^2/day or 30 mg/kg/day in three divided doses is recommended.

Severe oral recurrences should be treated with oral acyclovir. Daily suppressive therapy is recommended for children with more than 3–6 recurrences per year. Acyclovir-resistant HSV infection has been reported, generally in patients who have received multiple courses of therapy or who are receiving chronic suppressive therapy. The most common basis for resistance is a mutation leading to diminished or absent viral thymidine kinase activity. In addition, several acyclovir-resistant isolates have been noted to have altered DNA polymerase.

For patients with acyclovir-resistant HSV infections, foscarnet is a reasonable alternative, since it inhibits most acyclovir-resistant strains in vitro. Foscarnet generally is given at a dose of 40 mg/kg every 8 hours [40, 41], although foscarnet can be toxic (see above). For chronic skin lesions unresponsive to intravenous or oral acyclovir anecdotal reports have noted success with topical creams compounded from foscarnet or cidofovir.

Valacyclovir and famciclovir are oral prodrugs that have activity against HSV and better bioavailability than acyclovir. Both are effective in reducing the duration of symptoms and viral shredding in adults with recurrent genital herpes. Neither of these newer agents has been well studied in children. In addition, neither drug is active against acyclovir-resistant HSV.

41.4 Varicella-zoster virus

41.4.1 Epidemiology

Primary infection with VZV causes chickenpox, one of the most contagious infections of humans.

Following primary infection, VZV establishes latent infection in sensory ganglia of peripheral and cranial nerves. This state of latency may persist for life, or VZV may reactivate to cause herpes zoster, also known as shingles. Herpes zoster is a disease primarily of the elderly, but the incidence of herpes zoster also is increased in younger, immunocompromised individuals, including patients with acquired immunodeficiency owing to chemotherapy or immunosuppression.

Transmission of VZV is thought to occur by the respiratory route through inhalation of droplets containing viral particles. Potential source(s) of such droplets include vesicular or ulcerating skin lesions and the respiratory tract of infected individuals. Humans are the only known source of VZV. Infected individuals can transmit infection from 1–2 days before rash appears until all lesions are crusted. Individuals with chickenpox are more likely to transmit infection than individuals with herpes zoster. Transmission occurs more frequently after household exposures than exposures in school, suggesting that close contact with an infected individual increases the risk of acquiring infection.

Most individuals acquire chickenpox during childhood. Currently, the highest incidence of chickenpox in the USA is in 5 to 10-year-old children. Chickenpox also occurs in susceptible adolescents and young adults. The incubation period is usually 14–16 days, with a range of 10–21 days. After administration of Varicella-zoster immune globulin (VZIG) the incubation period may be as long as 28 days.

While precise epidemiologic data are not available, HIV-infected children are probably as likely to be exposed to VZV infection and to develop chickenpox as non-infected children. HIV-infected children are more likely to develop recurrent VZV infection, as described below.

41.4.2 Clinical manifestations

Varicella

In healthy children, chickenpox is usually an annoying, but benign illness. A variety of complications, including skin infections, pneumonia, and encephalitis, occur in a small percentage of such children. Less common, life-threatening complications include bacterial sepsis, toxic-shock syndrome and Reye's syndrome.

Manifestations of chickenpox in HIV-infected children appear to be less severe than initially thought. Jura *et al.* reported that chickenpox was severe, prolonged, and frequently complicated in HIV-infected children observed between 1985 and 1989 [42]. Most of these children had evidence of lung or liver involvement, and one, at autopsy, had evidence of widespread dissemination to lung, liver, brain, and pancreas. More recently, almost all cases of chickenpox in HIV-infected children have been uncomplicated [43, 44]. In a recent prospective study, only one of 30 cases of chickenpox was considered severe [44]. In this study, two-thirds of the children received either intravenous or oral acyclovir, which may have prevented complications from developing in some of them. Also, children who developed chickenpox in recent years were usually on antiretroviral therapy and probably had better immune function than children who acquired chickenpox prior to the advent of effective antiretrovirals.

41.4.3 Herpes zoster

In HIV-infected adults, the incidence of zoster has been estimated at 2.5–4 cases/100 patient years. Recently, reports have noted an increased incidence of zoster within the first 6 months of initiating HAART. Two reports noted an incidence of 6.2 and 19 cases/100 patient years, respec-

tively, among adults recently started on HAART. These studies indicate that zoster may represent one of the many "immunoreconstitution syndromes" now recognized in adults following the initiation of HAART [45, 46]. It is apparent that zoster is also much more common among HIV-infected children than among non-infected children. The incidence of zoster in immunocompetent children less than 10 years of age is reported as less than 1/1000. In contrast, various reports have noted a 10–70% risk of zoster in HIV-infected children followed longitudinally [47, 48].

In one prospective study of VZV infections in HIV-infected children, 8 of 30 children who acquired chickenpox after 1 year of age developed herpes zoster [47]. The mean interval between varicella and zoster in these children was 1.9 years. Zoster occurred more frequently in HIV-infected children who had low $CD4^+$ cell counts at the onset of varicella. In fact, in this small study, 70% of HIV-infected children with <15% $CD4^+$ cells at the onset of varicella developed herpes zoster.

In HIV-infected children, recurrent VZV infection may present as a disseminated rash typical of chickenpox, rather than as herpes zoster [47]. Compared with herpes zoster, in which a few lesions may appear outside the involved dermatome(s), the disseminated rash of recurrent VZV infection is much more generalized. In contrast to healthy children, HIV-infected children may have multiple episodes of recurrent disease. HIV-infected children who have low $CD4^+$ cell counts are more likely to develop multiple recurrences than those with higher counts.

Persistent VZV infection

Following primary or recurrent VZV infections, HIV-infected children may develop persistent skin lesions. In one series, persistent infection, defined as continued appearance of new varicella or zoster lesions for more than one month, occurred in 14% of HIV-infected children who developed VZV infections [48]. Lesions persisted in these children for 2–24 months, despite treatment of most of these children with oral or intravenous acyclovir. In occasional children, the persistent lesions have led to the diagnosis of HIV infection. HIV-infected children who develop persistent VZV infection generally have low $CD4^+$ cell counts. Some may become infected with acyclovir-resistant strains of VZV [48]. Resistance to acyclovir is more likely to appear in children receiving chronic therapy with acyclovir or multiple courses of acyclovir for persistent or recurrent infection.

VZV-related retinal disease

A rare, but devastating complication of VZV infections in HIV-infected adults is acute retinal necrosis (ARN).

Patients generally present with ocular pain and decreased acuity. Up to 85% of cases result in blindness. Diagnosis is made by ophthalmologic exam. Findings are described in Chapter 27.

In severely immunocompromised patients, VZV can cause encephalitis, as well as myelitis or meningitis. In a retrospective review of adult patients with VZV-related neurologic disease (all with positive CSF PCR for VZV), a zoster rash was noted at the time of diagnosis in 71% of patients while 12% had ARN. Almost 60% had fever at the time of presentation. The median CD4+ count at presentation was 11 cells/μL. Cerebrospinal fluid findings included mild pleocytosis (mean WBC 126/mL) and elevated protein. A small number of patients (9%) had no history of zoster, nor rash or eye findings at the time of presentation [49].

Effect of highly active antiretroviral therapy

Initial observations on VZV infections in HIV-infected children were made prior to the availability of HAART. Now that antiretroviral regimens are available that can reduce plasma viral loads of HIV-infected children, with concomitant rises in CD4+ cell counts, the incidence and severity of VZV infections needs to be reassessed. In addition, it remains to be seen if the increased incidence of zoster seen in adults commencing HAART also occurs in HIV-infected children.

Diagnosis

A clinical diagnosis of VZV infection often can be made on the basis of physical findings. Skin lesions in HIV-infected children with VZV infection usually are indistinguishable from those of healthy children. Hyperkeratotic, slow-healing lesions, not seen in healthy children, may appear with persistent infection in HIV-infected children. The differential diagnosis of VZV infection includes insect bites, other viruses associated with vesicular rashes (including HSV and certain enteroviruses) and contact dermatitis. Primary or recurrent HSV infection can present with vesicular lesions in a dermatomal distribution.

Several methods are available for laboratory diagnosis of VZV infection. Detection of multi-nucleated giant cells with intranuclear inclusions in Tzanck smears of scrapings from vesicular lesions would be consistent with the diagnosis of VZV infection, but other viruses, including HSV, can produce similar changes. Immunofluorescent staining of scrapings from lesions can provide a more specific diagnosis. Cells scraped from the bases of lesions and allowed to adhere to glass slides are incubated with fluorescein-conjugated antibodies that react with antigens of VZV or HSV. After incubation with such antibodies, cells containing VZV or HSV antigens can be visualized by fluorescence microscopy. Using this method, VZV and HSV infections can be diagnosed rapidly and with great accuracy,

Varicella zoster virus also can be isolated from vesicular fluid or from swabs of ulcers. Prompt delivery of specimens to a clinical virology laboratory increases the yield of virus culture. Specimens that cannot be delivered to a laboratory within a few hours should be kept frozen at –70 °C. Polymerase chain reaction methods also can be used to detect VZV DNA in vesicular lesions, however, such tests are available only in a small number of research laboratories; PCR techniques are highly sensitive for detecting VZV DNA, however, false positive results may be obtained owing to contamination within a laboratory.

Serologic assays also may be useful for diagnosis of VZV infection, particularly if viral isolation and PCR assays are not available or yield negative results. Acute and convalescent sera, with the latter collected 2–3 weeks after onset of illness, should be tested simultaneously. Detection of a 4-fold or higher rise in antibody titer in the fluorescent antibody membrane antigen (FAMA) test, or seroconversion (initial negative titer with subsequent positive titer) would be strong evidence of a recent VZV infection. Fluorescent antibody membrane antigen assays are technically demanding and generally are not available in clinical laboratories. Commercially available enzyme-linked immunoabsorbent and latex agglutination assays are useful for detecting seroconversion, but are less reliable for detecting rises in antibody titer.

Acute retinal necrosis generally is diagnosed by its classic appearance on ophthalmologic examination. Neurologic complications of VZV infection are diagnosed based on symptoms and a clinical exam consistent with VZV, and a positive CSF VZV PCR assay.

Treatment

Acyclovir is the drug of choice for VZV infections in HIV-infected children. Since the severity of infection cannot be predicted with certainty at the onset of disease, all HIV-infected children with primary varicella should be treated with acyclovir. In most cases, the intravenous route of administration is preferred, based on the cellular concentration of drug required to inhibit VZV, since only about 5% of oral acyclovir is absorbed. The recommended dose of intravenous acyclovir for VZV infections is 1500 mg/m^2/day in three divided doses. Oral administration may be considered for HIV-infected children who have normal or only slightly decreased CD4+ cell counts. An oral dose of 80 mg/kg/day should be used, since administration of acyclovir at this dose was associated with modest clinical benefit in previously healthy children with chickenpox.

Lower doses of acyclovir are unlikely to be efficacious, and higher doses have not been studied.

Acyclovir also is the drug of choice for herpes zoster in HIV-infected children. In most cases, acyclovir can be given orally, since herpes zoster is less likely than chickenpox to disseminate and to cause life-threatening disease in this patient population. Patients with very low $CD4^+$ cell counts, trigeminal or ocular involvement or extensive herpes zoster elsewhere should be treated, at least initially, with intravenous acyclovir. Two newer antivirals, famciclovir (prodrug of penciclovir) and valacylovir (pro-drug of acyclovir) are well absorbed when given orally, and both have been shown to be effective for treating herpes zoster in adults. The results of a preliminary pharmacokinetic study on the use of the tablet formulation of valacyclovir in immunocompromised children (ages 5–12 years) revealed acceptable bioavailability and minimal toxicity. The authors estimate a valacyclovir dose of 30 mg/kg three times a day to achieve serum concentrations of acyclovir equivalent to that found with three times a day of intravenous acyclovir, at a dose of 250 mg/m^2 [50].

After acyclovir is started, new lesions may continue to appear for up to 72 hours. Crusting of all lesions may take considerably longer, usually 5–7 days. Patients who continue to develop new lesions, or whose lesions fail to heal, despite therapy with acyclovir, could be infected with strains of VZV that are resistant to acyclovir. As with HSV isolates resistant to acyclovir, most VZV resistance to acyclovir appears to be based on the development of mutations leading to absent, or greatly decreased, activity of viral thymidine kinase [51]. Occasional isolates have been noted to be resistant based on changes in the viral DNA polymerase. Isolates of VZV from such patients should be tested for susceptibility to acyclovir in specialized laboratories. Isolates that are resistant to acyclovir also will be resistant to famciclovir and valacylovir.

Patients who fail to respond clinically to acyclovir, including those from whom acyclovir-resistant strains of VZV are isolated, may be switched to foscarnet which has activity against most acyclovir-resistant strains of VZV. Foscarnet can cause severe nephrotoxicity and therefore should be used only if acyclovir resistance is documented or strongly suspected based on clinical findings. Foscarnet-resistant VZV is uncommon, but has been reported.

Prophylaxis

Varicella-zoster immune globulin should be given to susceptible HIV-infected children within 72 hours after a significant exposure to VZV infection. To hasten administration of VZIG after such exposures, HIV-infected children should be prescreened for antibodies to VZV on a yearly basis. Post-exposure acyclovir may be considered as well, based on a study in non-infected children, which indicated efficacy in decreasing incidence of clinical disease following household exposure.

Varicella vaccine was recently licensed for use in normal children. Although it is a live virus vaccine, it perhaps has some utility in HIV-infected children. A recently concluded trial of varicella vaccine in asymptomatic HIV-infected children with normal $CD4^+$ counts has led to the recommendation that such children should routinely receive the vaccine [52]. In this study, 41 HIV-infected children received two doses of varicella vaccine. Following the second dose of vaccine, 60% had detectable anti-varicella serum antibodies, and 83% a positive lymphoproliferative response to varicella antigen. Systemic side-effects were minimal. There was no statisically significant change in viral load. Consequently, all asymptomatic, or mildly symptomatic HIV-infected children, with normal or near normal $CD4^+$ counts, should receive two doses of varicella vaccine, at least 3 months apart (see also Chapter 10).

A current study is targeting symptomatic HIV-infected children with lower $CD4^+$ counts to assess safety and efficacy of the vaccine in this population. In addition, another ongoing study is evaluating the feasibility of boosting varicella immunity, by active immunization, to decrease the risk of zoster in HIV-infected children who have already experienced primary varicella.

A cautionary note must be made of the report of a 16-month-old, who developed disseminated varicella, with a chronic skin rash, and CNS symptoms after receiving the varicella vaccine prior to diagnosis of HIV infection. The initial $CD4^+$ count at the time of presentation was only 8 cells/μL. This case clearly illustrates the potential risk in immunizing HIV-infected children with severe immunocompromise [53].

Epstein–Barr virus

As with other members of the family Herpesviridae, EBV infection is worldwide in distribution. Transmission occurs through close interpersonal contact. In many parts of the world almost all school-age children have evidence of EBV infection. In developed countries, improved sanitary conditions and decreased crowding are associated with delayed acquisition of EBV, so that in these countries transmission often occurs during adolescence.

Primary infection in infants or young children may be unapparent or may result in a short febrile illness. In older children and adults, EBV infection may result in the infectious mononucleosis syndrome, with fever, pharyngitis, adenopathy, and hepatic or splenic enlargement.

Epstein–Barr virus is a potent stimulator of B cells and has been associated with lymphoproliferative syndromes in immunosuppressed hosts. It is therefore not surprising that EBV has been linked to HIV-related lymphoproliferative syndromes. The most common EBV-related syndromes in HIV-infected children are lymphocytic interstitial pneumonitis (LIP, see Chapter 31) and non-Hodgkin's lymphoma (discussed in Chapter 36).

Human Herpesvirus 6

Human Herpesvirus 6 is a member of the Roseolovirus genus of herpesviruses. It is the causative agent for most cases of roseola, a febrile illness of early childhood associated with a distinctive rash and, occasionally, febrile seizures. Many cases of primary infections are asymptomatic. Primary infection generally occurs before the age of 2. During latency, cellular reservoirs include CD4$^+$ lymphocytes and, possibly, epithelial cells of the salivary glands.

The CD4$^+$ lymphocyte is the primary target of HHV-6. In cell cultures HHV-6 can infect HIV-infected CD4$^+$ lymphocytes. In vitro experiments indicate that HHV-6 can upregulate HIV expression in co-infected cells, possibly through transactivation of the HIV promotor [54]. Preliminary data suggest that HHV-6 infection may play a role in progression of HIV infection in children [55].

Human Herpesvirus 8

Human Herpesvirus 8 (also known as Kaposi's sarcoma-associated herpesvirus, KSHV) is a recently identified member of Herpesviridae with similarities in DNA sequences to EBV, and a more distant related herpesvirus, saimiri, which primarily infects monkeys. Clear epidemiologic and clinical links exist between HHV-8 and Kaposi's sarcoma, and between the virus and other neoplastic diseases, such as body cavity-based lymphomas (primary effusion lymphomas), and multicentric Castleman's disease. HHV-8 and related disorders are discussed more extensively in Chapter 36).

41.5 Summary

Herpesviruses can produce troublesome, and sometimes lethal, opportunistic infections in immunocompromised patients, particularly those with advanced HIV disease. With the introduction of HAART and resulting improved immunologic reconstitution, herpesvirus infections may become less bothersome in HIV-infected children. Nevertheless, it is likely that some HIV-infected children will continue to acquire symptomatic herpesvirus infections.

Therefore, development of more effective, less toxic antivirals as well as vaccines against members of this family of viruses, remains an important goal.

REFERENCES

1. Heng, M. C., Heng, S. Y. & Allen, S. G. Co-infection and synergy of human immunodeficiency virus-1 and herpes simplex virus-1. *Lancet* **343** (1994), 255–8.
2. Alford, C. A., Stagno, S., Pass, R. F. *et al.* Congenital and Perinatal Cytomegalovirus Infections. *Rev. Infect. Dis.* **12** (1990), S745–53.
3. Stagno, S., Reynold, D., Tsiantos, A. *et al.* Cervical cytomegalovirus excretion in pregnant and nonpregnant women: suppression in early gestation. *J. Infect. Dis.* **131** (1975), 522–7.
4. Nigro, G., Krzysztofiak, A., Gattinara, G. C. *et al.* Rapid progression of HIV disease in children with cytomegalovirus DNAemia. *AIDS* **10** (1996), 1127–33.
5. Doyle, M., Atkins, J. T. & Rivera-Matos, I. R. Congenital cytomegalovirus infection in infants infected with human immunodeficiency virus type. *Pediatr. Infect. Dis. J.* **15** (1996), 1102–6.
6. Ives, D. V. Cytomegalovirus disease in AIDS. *AIDS* **11** (1997), 1791–7.
7. Frenkel, L. D., Gaur, S., Tsolia, M. *et al.* Cytomegalovirus infection in children with AIDS. *Rev. Infect. Dis.* **12** (1990), S820–1.
8. Kitchen, B. J., Engler, H. D., Gill, V. J. *et al.* Cytomegalovirus infection in children with human immunodeficiency virus infection. *Pediatr. Infect. Dis. J.* **16** (1997), 358–63.
9. Chandwani, S., Kaul, A., Bebenroth, D. *et al.* Cytomegalovirus infection in human immunodeficiency virus type 1-infected children. *Pediatr. Infect. Dis. J.* **15** (1996), 310–14.
10. Goodgame, R. W. Gastrointestinal cytomegalovirus disease. *Ann. Intern. Med.* **119** (1993), 924–35.
11. Wilcox, C. M., Diehl, D. L., Cello, J. M. *et al.* Cytomegalovirus esophagitis in patients with AIDS: a clinical, endoscopic, and pathologic correlation. *Ann. Intern. Med.* **113** (1990), 589–93.
12. Bozzette, S. A., Arcia, J., Bartok, A. E. *et al.* Impact of *Pneumocystis carinii* and cytomegalovirus on the course and outcome of atypical pneumonia in advanced human immunodeficiency virus disease. *J. Infect. Dis.* **165** (1992), 93–8.
13. Jacobson, M. A., Mills, J., Rush, J. *et al.* Morbidity and mortality of patients with AIDS and first episode *Pneumocystis carinii* pneumonia unaffected by concomitant pulmonary cytomegalovirus infection. *Am. Rev. Respir. Dis.* **144** (1991), 6–9.
14. Salomon, N., Gomez, T., Perlman, D. C., Laya, L., Eber, C. & Mildvan, D. Clinical features and outcome of HIV-related cytomegalovirus pneumonia. *AIDS* **11** (1997), 319–24.
15. Roullet, E. Opportunistic infections of the central nervous system during HIV-1 infection (emphasis on cytomegalovirus disease). *J. Neurol.* **246** (1999), 237–43.

16. Dodt, K. K., Jacobsen, P. H. & Hofmann, B. Development of cytomegalovirus (CMV) disease may be predicted in HIV-infected patients by CMV polymerase chain reaction and the antigenemia test. *AIDS* **11** (1997), F21–8.

17. Salmon-Ceron, D., Mazeron, M.-C., Chaput, S. *et al.* Plasma cytomegalovirus DNA, pp65 antigenemia and a low CD4 count remain risk factors for cytomegalovirus disease in patients receiving highly active antiretroviral therapy. *AIDS* **14** (2000), 1041–9.

18. De Jung, M. D., Galasso, G. J., Gazzard, B. *et al.* Summary of the II International Symposium on cytomegalovirus. *Antiv. Res.* **39** (1998), 141–62.

19. Spector, S. A., Hsia, K., Crager, M. *et al.* Cytomegalovirus (CMV) DNA load is an independent predictor of CMV disease and survival in advanced AIDS. *J. Virol.* **73** (1999), 7027–30.

20. Cinque, P., Vago, L., Brytting, M. *et al.* Cytomegalovirus infection of the central nervous system in patients with AIDS: diagnosis by DNA amplification from cerebrospinal fluid. *J. Infect. Dis.* **166** (1992), 1408–11.

21. Liu, W., Shum, C., Martin, D. F. *et al.* Prevalence of antiviral drug resistance in untreated patients with cytomegalovirus retinitis. *J. Infect. Dis.* **182** (2000), 1234–8.

22. Jabs, D. A., Martin, B. K., Forman, M. S. *et al.* Longitudinal observations on mutations conferring ganciclovir resistance in patients with acquired immunodeficiency syndrome and cytomegalovirus retinitis: the cytomegalovirus and viral resistance study group report number 8. *Am. J. Ophthalmol.* **132** (2001), 700–10.

23. Martin, D., Kuppermann, B. D., Wolitz, R. A., Palestine, A. G., Li, H. & Robinson, C. A. Oral ganciclovir for patients with cytomegalovirus retinitis treated with a ganciclovir implant. *New Engl. J. Med.* **340** (1999), 1063–70.

24. The Studies of Ocular Complications of AIDS Research Group, in Collaboration With The AIDS Clinical Trials Group. The ganciclovir implant plus oral ganciclovir versus parenteral cidofovir for the treatment of cytomegalovirus retinitis in patients with acquired immunodeficiency syndrome: The ganciclovir cidofovir cytomegalovirus retinitis trial. *Am. J. Opthalmol.* **131** (2001), 457–67.

25. Drew, W. L., Ives, D., Lalezari, J. P. *et al.* Oral ganciclovir as maintenance for cytomegolovirus retinitis in patients with AIDS. *New Engl. J. Med.* **333** (1995), 615–20.

26. Spector, S. A., McKinley, G. F., Lalezari, J. P. *et al.* Oral ganciclovir for the prevention of cytomegalovirus disease in persons with AIDS. *New Engl. J. Med.* **334** (1996), 1491–7.

27. Blanshard, C., Benhamou, Y., Dohin, E. *et al.* Treatment of AIDS-associated gastrointestinal cytomegalovirus infection with foscarnet and ganciclovir: a randomized comparison. *J. Infect. Dis.* **172** (1995), 622–8.

28. The Vitravene study group. Randomized dose-comparison studies of intravitreous fomiversen for treatment of cytomegalovirus retinitis that has reactivated or is persistently active despite other therapies in patients with AIDS. *Am. J. Ophthalmol.* **133** (2002), 475–83.

29. Emery, V. C. & Hassan-Walker, A. F. Focus on new drugs in development against human cytomegalovirus. *Drugs* **62** (2002), 1853–8.

30. Frenkel, L. M., Capparelli, E. V., Danker, W. M. *et al.* Oral ganciclovir in children: pharmacokinetics, safety, tolerance, and antiviral effects. *J. Infect. Dis.* **182** (2000), 1616–24.

31. Pallela, F. J., Delaney, K. M., Moorman, A. C. *et al.* Declining morbidity and mortality among patients with advanced human immunodeficiency virus infection. *New Engl. J. Med.* **338** (1998), 853–60.

32. Casado, J. L., Arrizabalage, J., Montes, M. *et al.* Incidence and risk factors for developing cytomegalovirus retinitis in HIV-infected patients receiving protease inhibitor therapy. *AIDS* **13** (1999), 1497–501.

33. O'Sullivan, C. E., Drew, W. L., McMullen, D. J. *et al.* Decrease of cytomegalovirus replication in human immunodeficiency virus infected-patients after treatment with highly active antiretroviral therapy. *J. Infect. Dis.* **180** (1999), 847–9.

34. Karavellas, M. P., Lowder, C. Y., Macdonal, J. C., Avila, C. P. Jr & Freeman, W. R. Immune recovery vitritis associated with inactive cytomegalovirus retinitis. *Arch. Ophthalmol.* **116** (1998), 169–75.

35. Salmon-Ceron, D. Cytomegalovirus infection: the point in 2001. *HIV Med.* **2** (2001), 255–9.

36. Arvin, A. M. & Whitley, R. J. Herpes Simplex Virus Infections. In J. S. Remington & J. O. Klein (eds.), *Infectious Diseases of the Fetus and Newborn Infant*, 5th edn. Philadelphia, PA: WB Saunders Company (2001), pp. 425–46.

37. Cavert, W. Viral infections in human immunodeficiency virus disease. *Med. Clin. N. Am.* **81** (1997), 411–27.

38. Scott, L. L. Perinatal herpes: current status and obstetric management strategies. *Pediatr. Infect. Dis. J.* **14** (1995), 827–32.

39. Cinque, P., Vago, L., Marenz, I. R. *et al.* Herpes simplex virus infections of the central nervous system in human Immunodeficiency virus-infected patients: clinical management by polymerase chain reaction assay of cerebrospinal fluid. *Clin. Infect. Dis.* **27** (1998), 303–9.

40. Gately, A., Gander, R. M., Johnson, P. C. *et al.* Herpes simplex virus type 2 meningoencephalitis resistant to acyclovir in a patient with AIDS. *J. Infect. Dis.* **161** (1990), 711–5.

41. Hardy, W. D. Foscarnet treatment of acyclovir-resistant herpes simplex virus infection in patients with acquired immunodeficiency syndrome: preliminary results of a controlled, randomized, regimen-comparative trial. *Am. J. Med.* **92** (1992), 30S–5S.

42. Jura, E., Chadwick, E. G., Josephs, S. H. *et al.* Varicella-zoster virus infections in children infected with human immunodeficiency virus. *Pediatr. Infect. Dis. J.* **8** (1989), 586–90.

43. Kelley, R., Mancao, M., Lee, F., Sawyer, M., Nahmias, A. & Nesheim, S. Varicella in children with perinatally acquired human immunodeficiency virus infection. *J. Pediatr.* **124** (1994), 271–3.

44. Gershon, A. A., Mervish, N., LaRussa, P. *et al.* Varicella-zoster virus infection in children with underlying human immunodeficiency virus infection. *J. Infect. Dis.* **176** (1997), 1496–500.

45. Aldeen, T., Hay, P., Davidson, F. & Lau, R. Herpes zoster infection in HIV-seropositive patients associated with highly active antiretroviral therapy. *AIDS* **12** (1998), 1719–20.

46. Martinez, E., Gatell, J., Moran, Y. *et al.* High incidence of Herpes zoster in patients with AIDS soon after therapy with protease inhibitors. *Clin. Infect. Dis.* **27** (1998), 1510–13.

47. Von Seidlein, L., Gillette, S. G., Bryson, Y. *et al.* Frequent recurrence and persistence of varicella-zoster virus infections in children infected with human immunodeficiency virus type 1. *J. Pediatr.* **128** (1996), 52–7.

48. Pahwa, S., Biron, K., Lim, W. *et al.* Continuous varicella-zoster infection associated with acyclovir resistance in a child with AIDS. *J. Am. Med. Assoc.* **260** (1988), 2879–82.

49. Blanchardiere, A. D. L., Rozenberg, F., Caumes, E. *et al.* Neurologic complications of Varicella-zoster virus infection in adults with human immunodeficiency virus infection. *Scand. J. Infect. Dis.* **32** (2000), 263–9.

50. Nadal, D., Leverger, G., Sokal, E. M. *et al.* An investigation of the steady-state pharmacokinetics of oral valacyclovir in immunocompromised children. *J. Infect. Dis.* **186** Suppl. 1 (2002), S123–30.

51. Roberts, G. B., Fyfe, J. A., Gaillard, R. K. & Short, S. A. Mutant varicella-zoster virus thymidine kinase: correlation of clinical resistance and enzyme impairment. *J. Virol.* **65** (1991), 6407–13.

52. Levin, M. J., Gershon, A. A., Weinberg, A. *et al.* Immunization of HIV-infected children with varicella vaccine. *J. Pediatr.* **139** (2001), 305–10.

53. Kramer, J. M., LaRussa, P., Tsai, W. C. *et al.* Disseminated vaccine strain varicella as the acquired immunodeficiency syndrome-defining illness in a previously undiagnosed child. *Pediatrics* (2001), **108** e39.

54. Horvat, R. T., Wood, C., Josephs, S. F. & Balachandran, N. Transactivation of the human immunodeficiency virus promoter by human herpesvirus 6 (HHV-6) strains GS and Z-29 in primary human T lymphocytes and identification of transactivating HHV-6(GS) gene fragments. *J. Virol.* **65** (1991), 2895–902.

55. Kositanont, U., Wasi, C., Wanprapar, N. *et al.* Primary infection of Human Herpesvirus 6 in children with vertical infection of human immunodeficiency virus type 1. *J. Infect. Dis.* **180** (1999), 50–5.

42

Pneumocystis carinii pneumonia

Leslie K. Serchuck, M.D.

Pediatric, Adolescent and Maternal AIDS Branch, NICHD/NIH, Rockville, MD

Pneumocystis carinii pneumonia (PCP) is the most common AIDS-defining condition and most life-threatening opportunistic infection in children infected with HIV in developed countries. The incidence of PCP has decreased dramatically with the introduction of highly active antiretroviral therapy (HAART) and with routine use of prophylaxis regimens.

42.1 Biology and taxonomy

In 1909 and 1910, Chagas and Carini first described *Pneumocystis carinii*, incorrectly, as the sexual state of *Trypanosoma cruzi* [1, 2]. The organism was identified as a unique microbe in 1912 in Parisian sewer rats and named after Carini. It was recognized as a human pathogen in 1952 by the Czech parasitologist, Jirovec [3] who causally related the organism to plasma cell pneumonia in 3 to 6-month-old preterm and malnourished infants living in European orphanages after World War II. From that time until the 1980s, PCP was uncommon, occurring primarily in patients who were immunocompromised because of cancer therapy or congenital immune deficiencies [4].

Pneumocystis is a unicellular eukaryotic organism with a nuclear membrane and intracellular organelles. It exists in three morphologic forms: sporozoites, trophozoites, and cysts. Trophozoites (2–5 μm) adhere to alveolar epithelium where they multiply and mature into cysts (5–8 μm). These cysts are round or crescent-shaped thick-walled structures that contain up to 8 sporozoites (1–2 μm) which when released mature to become trophozoites. The cyst and trophozoite forms are found in lung and pleural fluid.

Pneumocystis organisms were initially thought to be a single strain that infected a broad range of hosts. It is now known through molecular and immunologic studies that there are in fact multiple strains of *Pneumocystis* that are restricted to infecting a single host species [2]. Mouse-derived *Pneumocystis* will not infect rats or humans, while a human-derived *Pneumocystis* will not infect mice or rats. The organism first known as *P. carinii* is found exclusively in rats. Consequently, in keeping with the International Code of Botanical Nomenclature, the correct biological and taxonomical name to refer to the human *Pneumocystis* organism is *P. jiroveci* (PJ) (formerly *P. carinii* special family *hominis*) rather than *P. carinii* [5]. For convenience, the organism causing the human disease will be referred to in this chapter as *Pneumocystis* and the pulmonary infection will be referred to as PCP. Molecular typing of isolates using the internally transcribed spacer region of the ribosomal RNA has shown that there are approximately 50 unique isolates of human *Pneumocystis* [6]. Co-infection with multiple isolates has been reported in up to 30% of PCP cases [7]. Some recurrent episodes demonstrated type variation suggesting that the recurrence may be the result of re-infection with a new type rather than reactivation of the initial PCP type [8].

The taxonomic classification of *Pneumocystis* has been the subject of considerable debate. The organism was once thought to be protozoan based on its morphological appearance, ultrastructure, failure to grow on fungal culture media, and susceptibility to antiprotozoal agents, such as pentamidine and trimethaprim/sulfamethoxazole (TMP–SMX). However ample evidence, including sequence analysis of ribosomal RNA genes, sequence analysis of the *Pneumocystis* enzymes dihydrofolate reductase and thymidylate synthetase, and finally the discovery in 1992 of the presence of a translation elongation factor 3 gene found exclusively in fungi, have shown that *Pneumocystis* is phylogenetically closer to fungi than protozoa [9, 10]. Additionally, antifungal compounds that inhibit β-glucan synthesis, such as echinocandins and papulocandins, reduce *Pneumocystis* cysts and trophozoites (whose cell wall contain β-glucan) in immunosuppressed rats [11]. However, *Pneumocystis* has some features that are atypical for fungi. It is resistant to standard antifungal agents (e.g. amphotericin and azoles) since it lacks ergosterol, the sterol characteristic of fungal cell membranes. Unlike most fungi that contain hundreds of copies of ribosomal RNA genes, *Pneumocystis* contains only a limited number [12].

42.2 Epidemiology

Serum antibodies to *Pneumocystis* can be found in greater than 80% of all children by age 2–4 years, suggesting that primary asymptomatic infection occurs commonly in immunocompetent hosts [13, 14]. Although there is no well-defined clinical syndrome associated with *Pneumocystis* infection in immunocompetent hosts, *Pneumocystis* DNA has been found in children with focal pneumonitis and with upper and lower respiratory tract infections. Since the 1980s patients most at risk for PCP remain those with advanced HIV disease with impaired cell-mediated immunity. HIV-infected infants are also at increased risk of developing PCP, but at much higher $CD4^+$ cell counts than older children or adults. In addition, the $CD4^+$ count can fall precipitously in HIV-infected infants. All HIV-exposed infants should receive prophylaxis for PCP from the age of 6 weeks. Prophylaxis may subsequently be discontinued for infants found to be uninfected (see Chapter 9).

Pneumocystis carinii pneumonia is the most common AIDS-defining illness in children in developed countries. As of December 2000 it had been reported in 33% of 8908 pediatric AIDS cases in the USA, with the greatest percentage of those cases occurring in children < 1 year old, peaking between the ages of 3–6 months [15]. An analysis of 3300 HIV-infected children participating in Pediatric AIDS Clinical Trials Group studies from 1988–98 reported a PCP event rate of 1.3 per 100 person years [16]. With the advent of routine PCP prophylaxis for HIV exposed/infected infants in developed countries, PCP occurs mainly in infants born to HIV-infected women who are unaware of their serostatus.

Autopsy and clinical studies suggest that the incidence of PCP in HIV-infected African children hospitalized with severe pneumonia (defined by WHO criteria as presence of tachypnea or lower chest retractions) [17] ranges from 10–48% dependent on diagnostic technique [18–20]. The reported incidence was less when a negative result obtained using induced sputum was not followed by another attempt at diagnosis using specimens obtained by bronchoscopy with alveolar lavage, a technique with superior sensitivity. The peak age of occurrence, 2–6 months, is similar to that observed in developed countries. Reports from South Africa and the UK suggest that co-infection with cytomegalovirus occurs commonly in HIV-infected children with pneumonia and that survival is significantly worse in these infants [21, 22]. Concomitant treatment with anti-CMV therapy in addition to PCP treatment should be strongly considered, particularly for those patients on corticosteroids. In Bangkok, Thailand PCP caused at least one-third of all severe pneumonias, while presumptive PCP was the most common AIDS-defining condition in Thai children during from 1988–1995 [23]. In Barbados, more than 37% of children presented with PCP as their initial clinical presentation of HIV infection. It was the primary cause of death in 65% of the AIDS-related deaths in these children [24]. It is a significant cause of death in HIV-infected children in many populations. In some African studies, mortality due to PCP occurs in greater than 60% of pediatric patients, even when patients are treated with cotrimoxazole and prednisone. In the USA and UK, mortality in patients with PCP ranges from 38–62% [25–28]. The mortality rate in untreated cases approaches 100%.

42.3 Pathogenesis

$CD4^+$ lymphocytes are necessary for an effective host response to *Pneumocystis*. $CD8^+$ cells appear to play a minor role in controlling *Pneumocystis* infection. Patients with impaired cell-mediated immunity (i.e. infants, patients with HIV, severe malnutrition, or patients exposed to cytotoxic agents or corticosteroids) are at highest risk of developing PCP. The reservoir for human infection is unknown, but may include environmental sources including soil and water as well as other humans [1, 29]. It is hypothesized that persons most likely become infected by inhalation of the organism. Since most immunocompetent persons have antibodies to *Pneumocystis*, it has been traditionally believed that illness in immunocompromised hosts represents reactivation of latent infection in the setting of immunosuppression. However, there have been clusters of cases reported among immunosuppressed patients, and molecular epidemiologic studies in healthcare workers suggest that new infection can also occur [32, 33]. Molecular typing of BAL samples in some HIV-infected patients with separate episodes of PCP greater than 6 months apart, showed different sequence types detected in the second and subsequent episodes compared with the first, suggesting infection with a different *Pneumocystis* strain [8, 34]. It has also been clearly demonstrated in rats and mice that infection can be transmitted from animal to animal via the airborne route. Whether this occurs in humans is still not known [30, 31].

Pneumocystis carinii pneumonia impairs lung function by causing alveolar erosion after the trophozoite's surface glycoprotein binds to the surface of the type I pneumocyte through extracellular proteins [35]. This attachment does not involve fusion between the cell wall and alveolar epithelium or tissue invasion but rather degeneration and subsequent erosion of the type I pneumocyte leading to disruption of the epithelium and the underlying basement membrane [36]. Cellular infiltration, interstitial fibrosis and increased inflammation characterize the ensuing alveolar damage. As infection progresses, alveolar septal hypertrophy occurs, with an accumulation of interstitial edema and mononuclear cell infiltration [36]. Increased alveolar-capillary permeability leads to early impairment of gas exchange and ultimately decreased compliance, total lung capacity, and vital capacity [37]. The host inflammatory response may further impair lung function. Light microscopy of lung tissue may show prominent eosinophilic, foamy intra-alveolar exudates with a mild interstitial pneumonitis, along with proliferation of type II pneumocytes.

42.4 Clinical features of disease due to *Pneumocystis*

42.4.1 Pulmonary disease

The onset of illness is usually abrupt in children with AIDS, though it may be insidious, developing over a period of weeks. The classic presentation includes high-grade fever (> 40 °C), tachypnea, dyspnea, and non-productive cough. Rarely, children may present without fever [38] or with increasing lethargy and weight loss. One case report described chest pain as the only presenting clinical symptom in a young child [39]. Physical examination frequently reveals an acutely ill child with nasal flaring, inter-, sub-, or supracostal retractions, bibasilar rales and evidence of respiratory distress. Hypoxia is a prominent feature of PCP and may be less responsive to oxygen than in the case of bacterial pneumonia [26]. The hypoxia may be worse than would be expected on the basis of the physical exam and chest x-ray. Cyanosis may be present or rapidly develop.

42.4.2 Extrapulmonary pneumocystosis

Extrapulmonary pneumocystosis (EP) may be the initial presentation of *Pneumocystis* infection. Between 0.06–2.5% of *Pneumocystis* disease cases are EP [40]. Autopsy findings indicate that dissemination of the infection most likely occurs by direct spread or by hematogenous or lymphatic routes [41]. The use of aerosolized pentamidine for PCP prophylaxis was thought to be associated with an increase in incidence of EP, since it is not systemically absorbed. However, cases of EP have been reported in patients receiving systemic prophylaxis with dapsone and pyrimethamine.

Extrapulmonary pneumocystosis has been reported to occur in the ear; eye; thyroid; spleen; and gastrointestinal (GI) tract, including peritoneum, stomach, duodenum, small intestine, transverse colon, liver, and pancreas. It has less frequently been reported to occur in the adrenal glands; bone marrow; heart; kidney and ureter; lymph nodes; meninges and cerebral cortex; and muscle. HIV-infected patients with EP often do not have clinically significant pulmonary involvement, and present with symptoms resulting from infection at an extrapulmonary site, such as hearing loss, abdominal pain, and ascites [40, 42]. Extrapulmonary pneumocystosis may occur at single extrapulmonary sites or at numerous, non-contiguous sites simultaneously and should be considered in the differential of unexplained hearing loss, visual field loss, thyroiditis, new onset ascites, or clinical signs consistent with colitis.

42.5 Laboratory features of *Pneumocystis carinii* pneumonia

Hypoxemia is the most consistent feature with alveolar-arterial oxygen gradient often greater than 30 mm Hg, and arterial oxygen tension (PaO_2) between 34–73 mm Hg. Arterial CO_2 tension (PaO_2) may remain stable, although pH increases with increasing severity of disease, as the ventilation rate increases with worsening hypoxia, leading to respiratory alkalosis. Lactate dehydrogenase is often increased greater than 500 U/L, but most likely represents lung damage and is not specific for PCP [43]. Serum total protein and albumin concentrations are frequently depressed.

42.6 Radiographic features of *Pneumocystis carinii* pneumonia

Chest radiographs most commonly show hyperinflation or bilateral diffuse parenchymal infiltrates with a "ground glass" or reticulogranular appearance, but may be normal or show very mild parenchymal abnormalities (Figure 42.1). A diffuse reticular pattern with alveolar densities and air bronchograms may be present [44] (Figure 42.2). Patients receiving aerosolized pentamidine prophylaxis may present with upper lobe disease. HIV-infected patients with PCP often have multiple pulmonary cysts and cavities resulting from lung destruction and necrosis due to the organism. Pneumothoraces from rupture of a cavity or cyst been reported as a presenting feature [45]. Localized nodular densities in the periphery, lobar infiltrates, pulmonary air cysts, and pleural effusions may occur in severe disease (Figures 42.3 and 42.4). Cavitary granulomas with central calcifications may also occur. High-resolution computerized tomography (HRCT) has an increased sensitivity and specificity over chest radiography for respiratory complications in immunocompromised adults (see Figure 42.5). When a respiratory infection such as PCP is suspected clinically, HRCT may reveal abnormalities despite a normal radiograph; it is also useful to guide biopsy (transbronchial or open) to the site of affected lung, when tissue sampling is required to make the diagnosis. The HRCT appearance of PCP includes ground-glass attenuation, consolidation, nodules, thickening of interlobular septa, and thin-walled cysts [46]. Hilar lymphadenopathy may also be present. Radionuclide gallium scans frequently show increased uptake of gallium by the lungs but are not specific for PCP [47].

42.7 Diagnosis of *Pneumocystis carinii* pneumonia

The differential diagnosis of patients with clinical presentations suggestive of PCP includes bacterial, viral, and fungal pneumonias, including Epstein–Barr virus infection; cytomegalovirus pneumonitis; *Mycobacterium avium* complex pulmonary infection; and lymphoid interstitial pneumonitis (pulmonary lymphoid hyperplasia). Lymphoid interstitial pneumonitis (LIP), like PCP, also presents with multiple, small widespread nodules, although the clinical course of LIP is generally much more indolent.

Neither clinical presentation, laboratory tests, nor radiography is pathognomonic for PCP. Since it is not possible to culture *Pneumocystis* in vitro, the diagnosis of infection in both pulmonary and extrapulmonary sites relies on a variety of direct staining, histologic, and molecular diagnostic techniques. The definitive diagnosis can only be made by histopathologic demonstration of organisms in nasopharyngeal aspirates, induced sputum tissue, bronchoalveolar lavage fluid, or tissues. Spontaneously expectorated

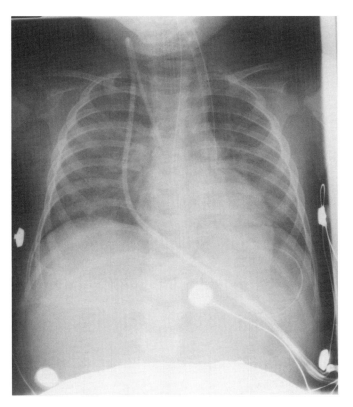

Figure 42.1. Chest x-ray of a child with *Pneumocystis carinii* pneumonia demonstrating diffuse "ground glass" infiltrates.

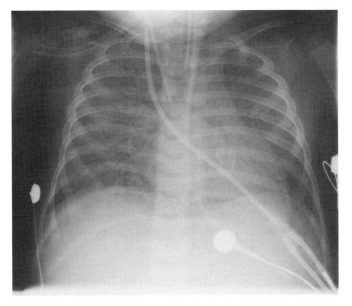

Figure 42.2. Chest x-ray of a patient with *Pneumocystis carinii* Pneumonia showing a diffuse reticular pattern with alveolar densities and air bronchograms.

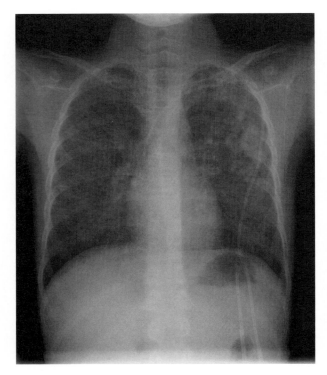

Figure 42.3. Chest x-ray (PA view) of a child with *Pneumocystis carinii* pneumonia showing localized nodular disease.

sputum has very low sensitivity and is not useful for diagnosis of PCP in children.

42.7.1 Diagnostic procedures

Several diagnostic procedures can be used to obtain specimens for the diagnosis of PCP. These procedures vary in their yields of diagnostic specimens and in the skill required to effectively perform them. The choice of diagnostic procedures will vary from case to case, depending on the clinical features of the case, and from institution to institution depending upon the available expertise.

Nasopharyngeal aspirate
Nasopharyngeal aspirate (NPA) is performed using a modified feeding catheter attached to a 5 ml syringe containing 3–5 ml of normal saline. The catheter is passed through either nostril into the nasopharynx, saline flushed, and immediately aspirated [19]. *Pneumocystis* is identified using a direct monoclonal antibody immunofluorescent stain. Immunofluorescence assay (IFA) has high sensitivity when applied to deep lung secretions, but may be able to identify *Pneumocystis* organisms from NPA only in cases of overwhelming infection [18].

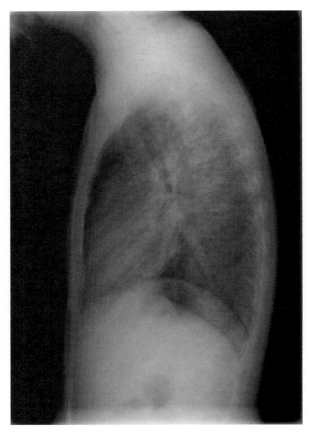

Figure 42.4. The lateral Chest X-ray corresponding to Figure 42.3.

Induced sputum analysis
Induced sputum analysis (ISA) is an easy, non-invasive test wherein a patient produces sputum after inhalation of nebulized 3% hypertonic saline. The sensitivity ranges from 25–90%. Best results depend on good specimen collection and preparation, and on analysis by experienced personnel [49]. However, the negative predictive value is only 48%. Therefore, bronchoalveolar lavage (BAL) should follow a negative ISA. Complications of ISA include nausea, vomiting, and bronchospasm.

Fiberoptic bronchoscopy with bronchoalveolar lavage
Bronchoalveolar lavage is the diagnostic procedure of choice in hospitals where the prevalence of PCP is low, ISA is difficult to obtain or negative, or hospital personnel are inexperienced in performing ISA. Sensitivity of BAL (which requires at least 15–25 ml of lavage fluid) ranges from 55–97% and is not affected by previous aerosolized pentamidine prophylaxis [49, 50]. Importantly, BAL remains positive for at least 72 hours after PCP treatment has been instituted. PCP treatment should not be delayed while awaiting the results of the procedure [51]. Complications of

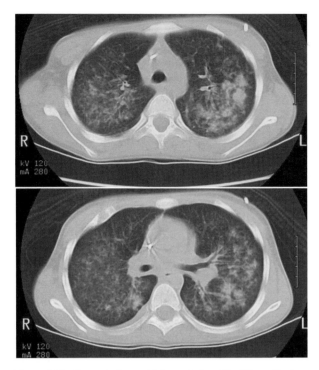

Figure 42.5. Two cuts from a high resolution CT of the patient with PCP in Figures 42.3 and 42.4.

BAL include hemoptysis, pneumothorax, transient hypoxemia, transient increase in pulmonary infiltrates at the lavage site, and post-bronchoscopy fever.

Fiberoptic bronchoscopy with transbronchial biopsy

Transbronchial biopsy has been used as the initial diagnostic procedure of choice in patients with diffuse lung disease [52]. However, because of the increased risk of pneumothorax, this procedure is not recommended routinely unless the BAL is negative or non-diagnostic in a patient with a clinical picture consistent with PCP. The sensitivity of TBB ranges from 87–95% and cysts may be commonly identified up to 10 days after treatment has begun (up to 4–6 weeks in some patients) [53]. Complications of TBB include pneumothorax and hemorrhage. This procedure may be contraindicated in patients with severe thrombocytopenia or other bleeding disorders.

Non-bronchoscopic bronchoalveolar lavage

This technique has been used with infants and children in whom bronchoscopy is technically difficult. Although a larger specimen can be obtained using this procedure than through ISA, the procedure carries a significant risk of aspiration because the catheter is placed blindly.

Open lung biopsy

This diagnostic procedure is the most sensitive for PCP (> 95%), but is seldom used today, as it requires thoracotomy and subsequent chest tube drainage. The histopathology of specimens obtained by this method is often characteristic, showing diffuse alveolar damage with alveoli filled with eosinophilic, acellular, proteinaceous material that contains cysts and trophozoites yet few inflammatory cells. Unlike typical foamy, alveolar exudates, the pulmonary alveolar proteinosis seen in PCP is finely granular, with occasional clumps and cholesterol clefts [54]. Interstitial fibrosis is commonly seen. Complications include pneumothorax, pneumomediastinum, and hemorrhage.

42.7.2 Diagnostic methods

Histological diagnostic methods – stains

Pneumocystis carinii cysts are 5–7 μm and require special stains for identification. They appear as helmet, crescent, or banana shapes with darkly stained foci resulting from thickening of the capsule. There are three different stains used in the diagnosis of *Pneumocystis* organisms in clinical specimens. These include: Gomori-Methenamine-Silver Stain, which stains the cyst wall brown or black; Toluidine Blue Stain, which stains the cyst wall blue or lavender and also stains fungal elements; and Giemsa and/or Wright's Stain, which stains *Pneumocystis* trophozoites and intracystic sporozoites pale blue with a punctate red nucleus. This stain does not stain the cyst wall. Many laboratories are currently diagnosing *Pneumocystis* with monoclonal immunofluorescent antibodies, which stain the cyst wall of *Pneumocystis*.

Molecular diagnostic methods – polymerase chain reaction

It is possible to amplify *P. jiroveci* DNA sequences by polymerase chain reaction (PCR) directly from blood or serum samples as well as from nasopharyngeal aspirates and BAL specimens [55]. The highest sensitivity is found using either a multi-copy gene target (such as mitochondrial ribosomal RNA) or a nested PCR procedure. There have been reports of individuals with positive PCR but negative confirmatory stain [13]. While most patients had clinical disease, some did not, suggesting either asymptomatic colonization or carriage. Polymerase chain reaction remains predominantly a research tool.

42.8 Treatment

Children with known or suspected HIV infection who present with a clinical picture consistent with PCP, and

CD4$^+$ lymphocyte counts or age that place them at risk for PCP infection, should be treated presumptively, without delay, and without waiting for confirmation by diagnostic examinations (Table 42.1). As noted above, BAL can remain positive for up to 72 hours of treatment, while evidence of cysts can be found in transbronchial biopsy specimens up to 10 days after treatment has begun. Intravenous trimethoprim-sulfamethoxazole should be the first-line agent used (unless patient is known to be allergic) regardless of the patient's prior prophylactic regimen. The recommended duration of treatment is a minimum of 21 days in patients with HIV infection. Prophylaxis to prevent recurrence should be instituted for all children once treatment for confirmed PCP has been completed.

Prior to beginning adjunctive corticosteroid treatment, it is prudent to determine if cytomegalovirus co-infection is present. *Pneumocystis carinii* pneumonia has been reported to occur in pulmonary infections with cytomegalovirus (CMV) pneumonitis, *Candida albicans*, *Mycobacterium avium* complex (MAC), *Mycobacterium tuberculosis*, *Aspergillus fumigatus*, and *Streptococcus pneumoniae*. If a patient with known or suspected PCP does not improve within 4–7 days following initiation of appropriate treatment, other etiologies should be pursued. If additional diagnoses are not confirmed, treatment failure should be considered and a change in PCP therapy may be warranted.

Treatment failure is defined as a clinical deterioration, with worsening respiratory status and arterial blood gases. Without corticosteroids, early and reversible deterioration can be expected within the first several days of PCP treatment due to the inflammatory response caused by antibiotic-induced lysis of organisms in the lung. Organisms may persist in specimens even when treatment is effective and do not indicate treatment failure [56].

42.8.1 Supportive measures

Oxygen should be given to maintain PaO$_2$ > 70 mm Hg. Assisted ventilation should be initiated when PaO$_2 \leq 60$ mm Hg with $\geq 50\%$ FiO$_2$. Continuous positive airway pressure (CPAP) by face mask improves oxygenation in cases with tachypnea and desaturation refractory to standard masks, thereby mitigating the need for mechanical ventilation in some cases.

42.8.2 Pharmacologic therapy for *Pneumocystis* infections

Trimethoprim–sulfamethoxazole

Trimethoprim–sulfamethoxazole (TMP–SMX) is preferred for initial treatment of PCP because of its excellent tissue penetration and oral bioavailability, rapid in vivo activity, and wide availability [57, 58]. Trimethoprim inhibits dihydrofolate reductase, while SMX inhibits dihydropteroate synthase, blocking sequential steps in the folic acid biosynthetic pathway of *Pneumocystis* leading to inhibition of tetrahydrofolic acid synthesis.

Dosage and administration

Trimethoprim–sulfamethoxazole should be used only in children older than 4–6 weeks of age because sulfonamides may cause displacement of bilirubin bound to albumin, possibly leading to jaundice and kernicterus. At disease onset, the patient should be given the combination, dosed at 15–20 mg/kg/day of the TMP component (75–100 mg/kg of the SMX component) intravenously in four divided doses with each dose infused over 1 hour. Oral treatment (20 mg/kg/day of TMP component in 3 or 4 divided doses) to complete a 21-day course may be considered once pneumonitis has resolved or in those with mild to moderate disease, without malabsorption or diarrhea.

Adverse reactions

Intolerance to TMP–SMX is common. HIV-infected adults appear to have a much greater incidence of adverse reactions than patients not infected with HIV. Approximately 15% of children will experience toxicity with TMP–SMX, such as rash (including Stevens–Johnson syndrome), neutropenia, thrombocytopenia, or megaloblastic or aplastic anemia. Hepatitis and renal disorders such as interstitial nephritis have been reported.

Precautions

Manufacturers recommend using TMP–SMX with caution in patients with impaired renal or hepatic function, severe allergy, bronchial asthma or glucose-6-phosphate dehydrogenase (G-6-PD)-deficiency, where hemolysis may occur. Patients with renal impairment with creatinine clearance (CrCl) of 15–30 ml/min should decrease the TMP–SMX dose by 50%. It should not be used in patients with CrCl < 15 ml/min.

Pentamidine isothionate

Pentamidine isothionate (PI) is the drug of choice in patients unable to tolerate TMP–SMX or who have not shown improvement after 5–7 days of TMP–SMX therapy. The mechanism of action of PI against *Pneumocystis* is unknown. It is postulated that PI interferes with oxidative phosphorylation or nucleic acid synthesis [57]. Combination therapy with TMP–SMX and PI does not appear to be more beneficial than PI alone and is potentially more toxic [59]. In patients with clinical improvement after 7–10 days

Table 42.1 Treatment of *Pneumocystis* Infection

Drug	Dosage	Mode of action	Adverse effects	Comments
Trimethoprim-sulfamethoxazole (TMP–SMX)	15–20 mg/kg/day as TMP IV divided q6h. May complete treatment PO if clinically recovered, 20 mg/kg/day as TMP PO divided every 6–8 hours, Duration: 21 days	Blocks sequential steps in folic acid metabolism	Rash-erythematous maculopapular, Stevens Johnson syndrome; neutropenia; thrombocytopenia; megaloblastic or aplastic anemia; increased liver function tests	Use only in children > 4–6 weeks. May consider change to oral therapy to complete 21 days in mild-moderate disease
Pentamidine isothionate	4 mg/kg/day IV/ IM q day (infuse IV over 60–90 min.) Duration: 21 days	Mechanism unknown May interfere with nucleic acid synthesis	Hypotension; pancreatitis; renal failure; insulin-dependent diabetes; fever; neutropenia; hypo/hyperglycemia; torsades de pointe (prolonged QT interval)	For patients who do not tolerate TMP–SMX or are not responding after 5–7 days. Do not give with didanosine. Rx may be complicated by toxicities in 80% patients
Clindamycin / Primaquine	Clindaymycin: 10 mg/kg IV or PO every 6 hrs Primaquine 0.3 mg/kg as base PO every 24 hours Duration: 21 days	Mechanism unknown	Skin rashes; nausea, neutropenia, hemolytic anemia (in G6PD), diarrhea (*C. difficile*)	Effective in mild-moderate PCP in adults Contraindicated in G6PD deficiency
Atovaquone	Adult dose: 750 mg bid Duration 21 days	Mechanism unknown May interupt pyrimidine synthesis	Diarrhea; nausea skin rashs (after first week) transaminitis	Effective in mild to moderate PCP May be used in patients with G6PD Bioavailability significantly increased by administration with fatty food. Administer with meals
Trimetrexate / Leucovorin	Trimetrexate: 45 mg/m² IV every 24 hours for 21days Leucovorin: 20 mg/m² IV every 6 hours for 24 d (72 hours after Trimetrexate discontinuation)	1500× more potent than TMP for dihydrofolate reductase	Reversible neutropenia; skin rashes; stomatitis, transaminitis; anemia; thrombocytopenia	Most effective as salvage therapy in patients who fail TMP–SMX Must use with Leucovorin which protects host cells from disruption of dihydrofolate reductase pathway
Dapsone/ Trimethoprim	Dapsone: 2 mg/kg PO every 24 hours (maximum 100 mg) Trimethoprim: 5 mg/kg PO every 8 hours Duration: 21 days	Inhibitor of dihydropteroate synthase	Methemoglobinemia; hemolytic anemia; neutropenia; thrombocytopenia	Effective in mild-moderate PCP in adults Contraindicated in G6PD deficiency

of intravenous PI, an oral regimen (i.e. atovaquone) to complete a 21-day course may be considered.

Dosage and administration

Pentamidine isothionate should be administered at a dose of 4 mg/kg/day given intravenously or intramuscularly (IV given over 60–90 minutes to reduce incidence of hypotension).

Adverse reactions

The most common adverse drug reaction is renal toxicity, which characteristically occurs in the second week of treatment, and can be averted by adequate hydration and careful monitoring of renal function and electrolytes. Severe hypotension, prolonged QT interval (torsades de pointe) and cardiac arrhythmias may occur. Hypoglycemia (usually occurs after 5–7 days of therapy) or hyperglycemia, hypercalcemia, hyperkalemia, pancreatitis, and insulin-dependent diabetes mellitus have also been reported. Many patients complain of a metallic and/or bitter taste, which may lead to a decrease in adequate oral intake.

Precautions

Caution should be used when concomitantly using other nephrotoxic agents such as aminoglycosides, amphotericin B, cisplatin, or vancomycin.

Clindamycin/Primaquine

There is evidence in adults to suggest that this combination is effective in the treatment of mild-to-moderate PCP [57]. A large meta-analysis supported the use of this combination as the most beneficial alternative for patients not responding to TMP–SMX or pentamidine [60]. The mechanism of action against *Pneumocystis* is unknown. Primaquine is contraindicated in patients with G-6-PD deficiency as it may cause hemolytic anemia.

Dosage and administration

Data on dosing in children are unavailable. Drug doses are extrapolated from approved pediatric dosing for other indications. Children should receive clindamycin 10 mg/kg (to a maximum of 600 mg) intravenously every 6 hours for 21 days. Primaquine should be administered as 0.3 mg/kg (30 mg base) orally once daily for 21 days. This is equivalent to the adult dose of primaquine when used for malaria.

Adverse reactions

Adverse reactions observed with this combination include skin rashes, neutropenia, anemia, nausea, and diarrhea, which may include *Clostridium difficile*-associated colitis.

Atovaquone

Atovaquone is recommended for mild to moderately severe PCP in patients who are intolerant of TMP–SMX. It is beneficial for patients with G-6-PD-deficiency unable to tolerate dapsone-containing regimens and in patients with pre-existing bone marrow suppression. Atovaquone is a hydroxynapthoquinone that interferes with electron transport at the cytochrome bc_1 complex, indirectly inhibiting nucleic acid and ATP biosynthesis [61]. It is an antimalarial agent that interrupts pyrimidine synthesis in plasmodium, but its precise mechanism of action against *Pneumocystis* is unknown. Bioavailability of atovaquone is greatly increased by administration with fatty foods.

Dosage and administration

Infants and children, ages 3–24 months require 45 mg/kg/day suspension [62] while children 2–12 years old should receive 30–40 mg/kg/day suspension orally given in two divided doses with fatty foods. Food increases the bioavailability of atovaquone by 1.4-fold that achieved in the fasting state. For 13–16 year olds, the recommended dose is 750 mg (5 mL) suspension administered orally with meals twice daily for 21 days (total daily dose 1500 mg).

Adverse reactions

Most adverse reactions with this agent appear after the first week of therapy. Skin rashes, nausea, and diarrhea have been reported. Patients may have elevated liver enzyme concentrations.

Precautions

Fluconazole and prednisone increase the concentration of atovaquone whereas acyclovir, opiates, cephalosporins, rifampin, and benzodiazepines decrease its plasma concentration.

Trimetrexate glucuronate/Leucovorin

Trimetrexate is effective as initial and salvage therapy in severe PCP in adults who are intolerant or refractory to treatment with TMP–SMX. Trimetrexate is a lipid-soluble analogue of methotrexate. Data in adults suggest that this agent is better tolerated than TMP–SMX for primary therapy of PCP but was associated with a lower response rate and a higher incidence of relapse than TMP–SMX therapy [63]. There are limited pediatric data [64]. Trimetrexate is 1500 times more potent an inhibitor of dihydrofolate reductase (DHFR) than TMP. Because of its toxic effect on mammalian cells it must be used in conjunction with leucovorin, a reduced folate. Trimetrexate inhibits the growth of *Pneumocystis* trophozoites.

Dosage and administration

Based on limited pediatric data available for this agent, trimetrexate should be administered at 45 mg/m^2 per day intravenously for 21 days with concomitant leucovorin 20 mg/m^2 intravenously every 6 hours for 24 days or for 72 hours after the last dose of trimetrexate.

Adverse reactions

Reversible neutropenia is the primary adverse event with this agent. Skin rashes, stomatitis, transaminitis, anemia, and thrombocytopenia may occur, as well as an elevation of serum transaminases. Most events are reversible even with continued drug administration at reduced dose.

Dapsone/Trimethoprim

This combination has been shown to be effective in the treatment of mild-to-moderate PCP in adults [57]. Data regarding its toxicity and efficacy in children with PCP is lacking. It is contraindicated in patients with G6PD deficiency due to the risk of hemolytic anemia.

Dosage and administration

Based on limited pediatric data available for this agent, dapsone should be administered 2 mg/kg by mouth once daily (maximum 100 mg) for 21 days. Trimethoprim is administered 5 mg/kg by mouth thrice daily for 21 days.

Adverse reactions

Adverse reactions observed with this combination include methemoglobinemia, transaminitis, anemia, neutropenia, and thrombocytopenia.

42.9 Adjunctive therapies

42.9.1 Corticosteroids

The respiratory status of patients often deteriorates after initiation of PCP therapy. This may be due to an inflammatory response to the dying organisms [65]. Numerous adult studies have shown that corticosteroid therapy, if initiated within 72 hours of beginning anti-pneumocystis therapy, improves clinical outcomes and decreases mortality, respiratory failure, and deterioration of oxygenation [66, 67]. Several small pediatric studies have shown a reduction in acute respiratory failure, a decrease in ventilatory support requirements, and a significant decrease in mortality with early use of adjunctive corticosteroids [68–70].

Adjunctive use of corticosteroids may not be helpful when the patient is infected with both *Pneumocystis* and cytomegalovirus. There are data from South Africa and the UK reporting decreased survival time in patients co-infected with cytomegalovirus infection and PCP. Importantly, adjunctive corticosteroids did not impart a survival advantage in these co-infected patients and some data suggest that corticosteroids may adversely affect the course of the CMV disease [22, 71]. The dosage in children varies among studies. Alternatives include: (1) Prednisone: Days 1–5 = 40 mg twice daily; Days 6–10 = 40 mg daily; Days 11–21 = 20 mg daily. (2) Prednisone (or methylprednisolone sodium): Days 1–5 = 1 mg/kg twice daily; Days 6–10 = 0.5 mg/kg per dose twice daily; Days 11–18 = 0.5 mg/kg once a day. (3) Methylprednisolone sodium intravenously: Days 1–7 = 1 mg/kg every 6 hours; Days 8–9 = 1 mg/kg twice a day; Days 10–11 = 0.5 mg/kg twice a day; Days 12–16 = 1 mg/kg once a day.

42.9.2 Surfactant

A few case reports have suggested that patients with PCP have decreased amounts of pulmonary surfactant. Surfactant therapy has been associated with improved pulmonary function in case reports of infants with confirmed PCP, with ARDS, and respiratory failure requiring assisted ventilation [72, 73]. Surfactant therapy may offer a possible treatment strategy in desperately ill infants. Surfactant should be used in consultation with a pediatric infectious disease specialist.

42.10 Resistance

Drug resistance in *Pneumocystis* is difficult to confirm by conventional means since the organism cannot be grown in culture and in vitro drug sensitivities cannot be performed. Several investigators have looked for drug resistance mutations in the dihydropteroate synthase (DHPS) gene [74–76]. Studies show that individuals receiving PCP prophylaxis had significantly more mutations than those not receiving prophylaxis. However, the presence of these mutations does not appear to affect either response to treatment or survival [76, 77]. Despite detection of these mutations, there is currently no compelling evidence to change the approach to the treatment or prevention of PCP [1]. Trimethoprim–sulfamethoxazole at full treatment doses remains the first line treatment of choice in patients who develop PCP while receiving TMP–SMX prophylaxis.

42.11 Summary

Pneumocystis carinii pneumonia remains a significant cause of morbidity and mortality in immunocompromised children throughout the world. Although the incidence of PCP is decreasing in developed countries with improved identification of HIV-infected pregnant women and their infants, the use of HAART, and primary PCP prophylaxis, the disease still occurs and continues to be prevalent in developing countries in children with severe pneumonia. Transmission may occur through reactivation of latent infection, through environmental sources via the airborne route, or potentially from human to human. The treatment of choice for established PCP is high dose trimethoprim–sulfamethoxazole, with corticosteroids in moderate to severe disease. Alternatives to TMP–SMX for the patient who cannot tolerate it or who did not respond to the drug include intravenous pentamidine, atovaquone, clindamycin with primaquine, trimetrexate glucuronate with leucovorin, or dapsone with trimethoprim.

REFERENCES

1. Kovacs, J. A., Gill, V. J., Meshnick, S. & Masur, H. New insights into transmission, diagnosis, and drug treatment of *Pneumocystis carinii* pneumonia. *J. Am. Med. Assoc.* **286**:**19** (2001), 2450–60.

2. Stringer, J. R. *Pneumocystis carinii*: what is it, exactly? *Clin. Microbiol. Rev.* **9**:**4** (1996), 489–98.

3. Frenkel, J. K. *Pneumocystis* pneumonia, an immunodeficiency-dependent disease (IDD): a critical historical overview. *J. Eukaryot. Microbiol.* **46**:**5** (1999), 89S-92S.

4. Hughes, W. T., Feldman, S., Aur, R. J., Verzosa, M. S., Hustu, H. O. & Simone, J. V. Intensity of immunosuppressive therapy and the incidence of *Pneumocystis carinii* pneumonitis. *Cancer* **36**:**6** (1975), 2004–9.

5. Stringer, J. R., Beard, C. B., Miller, R. F. & Wakefield, A. E. A new name (*Pneumocystis jiroveci*) for pneumocystis from humans. *Emerg. Infect. Dis.* **8**:**9** (2002), 891–6.

6. Lee, C. H., Helweg-Larsen, J., Tang, X. *et al.* Update on *Pneumocystis carinii* f. sp. *hominis* typing based on nucleotide sequence variations in internal transcribed spacer regions of rRNA genes. *J. Clin. Microbiol.* **36**:**3** (1998), 734–41.

7. Nahimana, A., Blanc, D. S., Francioli, P., Bille, J. & Hauser, P. M. Typing of *Pneumocystis carinii* f. sp. *hominis* by PCR-SSCP to indicate a high frequency of co-infections. *J. Med. Microbiol.* **49**:**8** (2000), 753–8.

8. Keely, S. P., Stringer, J. R., Baughman, R. P., Linke, M. J., Walzer, P. D. & Smulian, A. G. Genetic variation among *Pneumocystis carinii hominis* isolates in recurrent pneumocystosis. *J. Infect. Dis.* **172**:**2** (1995), 595–8.

9. Edman, J. C., Kovacs, J. A., Masur, H., Santi, D. V., Elwood, H. J. & Sogin, M. L. Ribosomal RNA sequence shows *Pneumocystis carinii* to be a member of the fungi. *Nature* **334**:**6182** (1988), 519–22.

10. Stringer, J. R. & Walzer, P. D. Molecular biology and epidemiology of *Pneumocystis carinii* infection in AIDS. *AIDS* **10**:**6** (1996), 561–71.

11. Schmatz, D. M., Romancheck, M. A., Pittarelli, L. A. *et al.* Treatment of *Pneumocystis carinii* pneumonia with 1,3-beta-glucan synthesis inhibitors. *Proc. Natl. Acad. Sci. U. S. A.* **87**:**15** (1990), 5950–4.

12. Giuntoli, D., Stringer, S. L. & Stringer, J. R. Extraordinarily low number of ribosomal RNA genes in *P. carinii*. *J. Eukaryot. Microbiol.* **41**:**5** (1994), 88S.

13. Vargas, S. L., Hughes, W. T., Santolaya, M. E. *et al.* Search for primary infection by *Pneumocystis carinii* in a cohort of normal, healthy infants. *Clin. Infect. Dis.* **32**:**6** (2001), 855–61.

14. Sheldon, W. Subclinical *pneumocystis* pneumonitis. *Am. J. Dis. Child.* **97** (1959), 287–97.

15. Centers for Disease Control and Prevention. *HIV/AIDS Surveillance Report* **13**:**2** (2001), Atlanta.

16. Dankner, W. M., Lindsey, J. C. & Levin, M. J. Correlates of opportunistic infections in children infected with the human immunodeficiency virus managed before highly active antiretroviral therapy. *Pediatr. Infect. Dis. J.* **20**:**1** (2001), 40–8.

17. Mulholland, E. K., Simoes, E. A., Costales, M. O., McGrath, E. J., Manalac, E. M. & Gove, S. Standardized diagnosis of pneumonia in developing countries. *Pediatr. Infect. Dis. J.* **11**:**2** (1992), 77–81.

18. Zar, H. J., Dechaboon, A., Hanslo, D., Apolles, P., Magnus, K. G. & Hussey, G. *Pneumocystis carinii* pneumonia in South African children infected with human immunodeficiency virus. *Pediatr. Infect. Dis. J.* **19**:**7** (2000), 603–7.

19. Ruffini, D. D. & Madhi, S. A. The high burden of *Pneumocystis carinii* pneumonia in African HIV-1-infected children hospitalized for severe pneumonia. *AIDS* **16**:**1** (2002), 105–12.

20. Lucas, S. B., Peacock, C. S., Hounnou, A. *et al.* Disease in children infected with HIV in Abidjan, Cote d'Ivoire. *Br. Med. J.* **312**:**7027** (1996), 335–8.

21. Jeena, P. M., Coovadia, H. M. & Chrystal, V. *Pneumocystis carinii* and cytomegalovirus infections in severely ill, HIV-infected African infants. *Ann. Trop. Paediatr.* **16**:**4** (1996), 361–8.

22. Williams, A. J., Duong, T., McNally, L. M. *et al. Pneumocystis carinii* pneumonia and cytomegalovirus infection in children with vertically acquired HIV infection. *AIDS* **15**:**3** (2001), 335–9.

23. Chokephaibulkit, K., Wanachiwanawin, D., Chearskul, S. *et al. Pneumocystis carinii* severe pneumonia among human immunodeficiency virus-infected children in Thailand: the effect of a primary prophylaxis strategy. *Pediatr. Infect. Dis. J.* **18**:**2** (1999), 147–52.

24. Kumar, A. & St John, M. A. HIV infection among children in Barbados. *West Indian Med. J.* **49**:**1** (2000), 43–6.

25. Eppes, S. C., Turner, B. J. & Markson, L. E. *Pneumocystis carinii* pneumonia in children with perinatally acquired HIV infection. *J. Am. Med. Assoc.* **271**:**2** (1994), 102; discussion 103.

26. Graham, S. M., Mtitimila, E. I., Kamanga, H. S., Walsh, A. L., Hart, C. A. & Molyneux, M. E. Clinical presentation and outcome of *Pneumocystis carinii* pneumonia in Malawian children. *Lancet* **355**:**9201** (2000), 369–73.

27. Simonds, R. J., Oxtoby, M. J., Caldwell, M. B., Gwinn, M. L. & Rogers, M. F. *Pneumocystis carinii* pneumonia among US children with perinatally acquired HIV infection. *J. Am. Med. Assoc.* **270** : **4** (1993), 470–3.

28. Sheikh, S., Bakshi, S. S. & Pahwa, S. G. Outcome and survival in HIV-infected infants with *Pneumocystis carinii* pneumonia and respiratory failure. *Pediatr. AIDS HIV Infect.* **7** : **3** (1996), 155–63.

29. Morris, A., Beard, C. B. & Huang, L. Update on the epidemiology and transmission of *Pneumocystis carinii*. *Microbes Infect.* **4** : **1** (2002), 95–103.

30. Hughes, W. T., Bartley, D. L. & Smith, B. M. A natural source of infection due to *pneumocystis carinii*. *J. Infect. Dis.* **147** : **3** (1983), 595.

31. Dumoulin, A., Mazars, E., Seguy, N. *et al.* Transmission of *Pneumocystis carinii* disease from immunocompetent contacts of infected hosts to susceptible hosts. *Eur. J. Clin. Microbiol. Infect. Dis.* **19** : **9** (2000), 671–8.

32. Beck, J. M. *Pneumocystis carinii* and geographic clustering: evidence for transmission of infection. *Am. J. Respir. Crit. Care Med.* **162** : **5** (2000), 1605–6.

33. Helweg-Larsen, J., Tsolaki, A. G., Miller, R. F., Lundgren, B. & Wakefield, A. E. Clusters of *Pneumocystis carinii* pneumonia: analysis of person-to-person transmission by genotyping. *Quart. J. Med.* **91** : **12** (1998), 813–20.

34. Tsolaki, A. G., Miller, R. F., Underwood, A. P., Banerji, S. & Wakefield, A. E. Genetic diversity at the internal transcribed spacer regions of the rRNA operon among isolates of *Pneumocystis carinii* from AIDS patients with recurrent pneumonia. *J. Infect. Dis.* **174** : **1** (1996), 141–56.

35. Henshaw, N. G., Carson, J. L. & Collier, A. M. Ultrastructural observations of *Pneumocystis carinii* attachment to rat lung. *J. Infect. Dis.* **151** : **1** (1985), 181–6.

36. Benfield, T. L., Prento, P., Junge, J., Vestbo, J. & Lundgren, J. D. Alveolar damage in AIDS-related *Pneumocystis carinii* pneumonia. *Chest* **111** : **5** (1997), 1193–9.

37. Coleman, D. L., Dodek, P. M., Golden, J. A. *et al.* Correlation between serial pulmonary function tests and fiberoptic bronchoscopy in patients with *Pneumocystis carinii* pneumonia and the acquired immune deficiency syndrome. *Am. Rev. Respir. Dis.* **129** : **3** (1984), 491–3.

38. Hughes, W. T. *Pneumocystis carinii* pneumonia: new approaches to diagnosis, treatment and prevention. *Pediatr. Infect. Dis. J.* **10** : **5** (1991), 391–9.

39. Mueller, B. U., Butler, K. M., Husson, R. N. & Pizzo, P. A. *Pneumocystis carinii* pneumonia despite prophylaxis in children with human immunodeficiency virus infection. *J. Pediatr.* **119** : **6** (1991), 992–4.

40. Ng, V. L., Yajko, D. M. & Hadley, W. K. Extrapulmonary pneumocystosis. *Clin. Microbiol. Rev.* **10** : **3** (1997), 401–18.

41. Raviglione, M. C. Extrapulmonary pneumocystosis: the first 50 cases. *Rev. Infect. Dis.* **12** : **6** (1990), 1127–38.

42. Hagmann, S., Merali, S., Sitnitskaya, Y., Fefferman, N. & Pollack, H. *Pneumocystis carinii* infection presenting as an intra-abdominal cystic mass in a child with acquired immunodeficiency syndrome. *Clin. Infect. Dis.* **33** : **8** (2001), 1424–6.

43. Boldt, M. J. & Bai, T. R. Utility of lactate dehydrogenase vs radiographic severity in the differential diagnosis of *Pneumocystis carinii* pneumonia. *Chest* **111** : **5** (1997), 1187–92.

44. Sivit, C. J., Miller, C. R., Rakusan, T. A., Ellaurie, M. & Kushner, D. C. Spectrum of chest radiographic abnormalities in children with AIDS and *Pneumocystis carinii* pneumonia. *Pediatr. Radiol.* **25** : **5** (1995), 389–92.

45. Solomon, K. S., Levin, T. L., Berdon, W. E., Romney, B., Ruzal-Shapiro, C. & Bye, M. R. Pneumothorax as the presenting sign of *Pneumocystis carinii* infection in an HIV-positive child with prior lymphocytic interstitial pneumonitis. *Pediatr. Radiol.* **26** : **8** (1996), 559–62.

46. Ambrosino, M. M., Roche, K. J., Genieser, N. B., Kaul, A. & Lawrence, R. M. Application of thin-section low-dose chest CT (TSCT) in the management of pediatric AIDS. *Pediatr. Radiol.* **25** : **5** (1995), 393–400.

47. Coleman, D. L., Hattner, R. S., Luce, J. M., Dodek, P. M., Golden, J. A. & Murray, J. F. Correlation between gallium lung scans and fiberoptic bronchoscopy in patients with suspected *Pneumocystis carinii* pneumonia and the acquired immune deficiency syndrome. *Am. Rev. Respir. Dis.* **130** : **6** (1984), 1166–9.

48. Kroe, D. M., Kirsch, C. M. & Jensen, W. A. Diagnostic strategies for *Pneumocystis carinii* pneumonia. *Semin. Respir. Infect.* **12** : **2** (1997), 70–8.

49. Levine, S. J., Masur, H., Gill, V. J. *et al.* Effect of aerosolized pentamidine prophylaxis on the diagnosis of *Pneumocystis carinii* pneumonia by induced sputum examination in patients infected with the human immunodeficiency virus. *Am. Rev. Respir. Dis.* **144** : **4** (1991), 760–4.

50. de Blic, J., McKelvie, P., Le Bourgeois, M., Blanche, S., Benoist, M. R. & Scheinmann, P. Value of bronchoalveolar lavage in the management of severe acute pneumonia and interstitial pneumonitis in the immunocompromised child. *Thorax* **42** : **10** (1987), 759–65.

51. Mitchell, D. M., Emerson, C. J., Collins, J. V. & Stableforth, D. E. Transbronchial lung biopsy with the fibreoptic bronchoscope: analysis of results in 433 patients. *Br. J. Dis. Chest* **75** : **3** (1981), 258–62.

52. Shelhamer, J. H., Ognibene, F. P., Macher, A. M. *et al.* Persistence of *Pneumocystis carinii* in lung tissue of acquired immunodeficiency syndrome patients treated for *pneumocystis* pneumonia. *Am. Rev. Respir. Dis.* **130** : **6** (1984), 1161–5.

53. Tran Van Nhieu, J., Vojtek, A. M., Bernaudin, J. F., Escudier, E. & Fleury-Feith, J. Pulmonary alveolar proteinosis associated with *Pneumocystis carinii*. Ultrastructural identification in bronchoalveolar lavage in AIDS and immunocompromised non-AIDS patients. *Chest* **98** : **4** (1990), 801–5.

54. Weig, M., Klinker, H., Bogner, B. H., Meier, A. & Gross, U. Usefulness of PCR for diagnosis of *Pneumocystis carinii* pneumonia in different patient groups. *J. Clin. Microbiol.* **35** : **6** (1997), 1445–9.

55. Roger, P. M., Vandenbos, F., Pugliese, P. *et al.* Persistence of *Pneumocystis carinii* after effective treatment of *P. carinii*

pneumonia is not related to relapse or survival among patients infected with human immunodeficiency virus. *Clin. Infect. Dis.* **26** : **2** (1998), 509–10.

56. Warren, E., George, S., You, J. & Kazanjian, P. Advances in the treatment and prophylaxis of *Pneumocystis carinii* pneumonia. *Pharmacotherapy* **17** : **5** (1997), 900–16.

57. Hughes, W. T. Current issues in the epidemiology, transmission, and reactivation of *Pneumocystis carinii. Semin. Respir. Infect.* **13** : **4** (1998), 283–8.

58. Walzer, P. D. *Pneumocystis carinii.* In G. D. R. Mandell & J. Benett (eds.), *Principles and Practices of Infectious Diseases.* New York: Churchill Livingstone (1990), pp. 2103–10.

59. Smego, R. A., Jr., Nagar, S., Maloba, B. & Popara, M. A meta-analysis of salvage therapy for *Pneumocystis carinii* pneumonia. *Arch. Intern. Med.* **161** : **12** (2001), 1529–33.

60. Deresinski, S. C. Treatment of *Pneumocystis carinii* pneumonia in adults with AIDS. *Semin. Respir. Infect.* **12** : **2** (1997), 79–97.

61. Hughes, W., Dorenbaum, A., Yogev, R. *et al.* Phase I safety and pharmacokinetics study of micronized atovaquone in human immunodeficiency virus-infected infants and children. *Antimicrob. Agents Chemother.* **42** : **6** (1998), 1315–18.

62. Sattler, F. R., Frame, P., Davis, R. *et al.* Trimetrexate with leucovorin versus trimethoprim-sulfamethoxazole for moderate to severe episodes of *Pneumocystis carinii* pneumonia in patients with AIDS: a prospective, controlled multicenter investigation of the AIDS Clinical Trials Group Protocol 029/031. *J. Infect. Dis.* **170** : **1** (1994), 165–72.

63. Smit, M. J., De Groot, R., Van Dongen, J. J., Van der Voort, E., Neijens, H. J. & Whitfield, L. R. Trimetrexate efficacy and pharmacokinetics during treatment of refractory *Pneumocystis carinii* pneumonia in an infant with severe combined immunodeficiency disease. *Pediatr. Infect. Dis. J.* **9** : **3** (1990), 212–14; discussion 215.

64. Masur, H. Prevention and treatment of *pneumocystis* pneumonia. *New Engl. J. Med.* **327** : **26** (1992), 1853–60.

65. Sistek, C. J., Wordell, C. J. & Hauptman, S. P. Adjuvant corticosteroid therapy for *Pneumocystis carinii* pneumonia in AIDS patients. *Ann. Pharmacother.* **26** : **9** (1992), 1127–33.

66. NIH Panel. Consensus statement on the use of corticosteroids as adjunctive therapy for *pneumocystis* pneumonia in the acquired immunodeficiency syndrome. The National Institutes of Health-University of California Expert Panel for Corticosteroids as Adjunctive Therapy for *Pneumocystis* Pneumonia. *New Engl. J. Med.* **323** : **21** (1990), 1500–4.

67. Bye, M. R., Cairns-Bazarian, A. M. & Ewig, J. M. Markedly reduced mortality associated with corticosteroid therapy of *Pneumocystis carinii* pneumonia in children with acquired immunodeficiency syndrome. *Arch. Pediatr. Adolesc. Med.* **148** : **6** (1994), 638–41.

68. McLaughlin, G. E., Virdee, S. S., Schleien, C. L., Holzman, B. H. & Scott, G. B. Effect of corticosteroids on survival of children with acquired immunodeficiency syndrome and *Pneumocystis carinii*-related respiratory failure. *J. Pediatr.* **126** : **5** (1995), 821–4.

69. Sleasman, J. W., Hemenway, C, Klein, A. S. & Barrett, D. J. Corticosteroids improve survival of children with AIDS and *Pneumocystis carinii* pneumonia. *Am. J. Dis. Child.* **147** : **1** (1993), 30–4.

70. Jensen, A. M., Lundgren, J. D., Benfield, T., Nielsen, T. L. & Vestbo, J. Does cytomegalovirus predict a poor prognosis in *Pneumocystis carinii* pneumonia treated with corticosteroids? A note for caution. *Chest* **108** : **2** (1995), 411–14.

71. Creery, W. D., Hashmi, A., Hutchison, J. S. & Singh, R. N. Surfactant therapy improves pulmonary function in infants with *Pneumocystis carinii* pneumonia and acquired immunodeficiency syndrome. *Pediatr. Pulmonol.* **24** : **5** (1997), 370–3.

72. Marriage, S. C., Underhill, H. & Nadel, S. Use of natural surfactant in an HIV-infected infant with *Pneumocystis carinii* pneumonia. *Intensive Care Med.* **22** : **6** (1996), 611–12.

73. Helweg-Larsen, J., Benfield, T. L., Eugen-Olsen, J., Lundgren, J. D. & Lundgren, B. Effects of mutations in *Pneumocystis carinii* dihydropteroate synthase gene on outcome of AIDS-associated *P. carinii* pneumonia. *Lancet* **354** : **9187** (1999), 1347–51.

74. Ma, L., Borio, L., Masur, H. & Kovacs, J. A. *Pneumocystis carinii* dihydropteroate synthase but not dihydrofolate reductase gene mutations correlate with prior trimethoprim-sulfamethoxazole or dapsone use. *J. Infect. Dis.* **180** : **6** (1999), 1969–78.

75. Huang, L., Beard, C. B., Creasman, J. *et al.* Sulfa or sulfone prophylaxis and geographic region predict mutations in the *Pneumocystis carinii* dihydropteroate synthase gene. *J. Infect. Dis.* **182** : **4** (2000), 1192–8.

76. Kazanjian, P., Armstrong, W., Hossler, P. A. *et al. Pneumocystis carinii* mutations are associated with duration of sulfa or sulfone prophylaxis exposure in AIDS patients. *J. Infect. Dis.* **182** : **2** (2000), 551–7.

PART VI

Medical, social, and legal issues

43

Clinical trials for HIV-infected children

James G. McNamara, M.D.

Pediatric Medicine Branch, Division of AIDS, NIAID, NIH, Bethesda, MD

The past two decades of fighting the HIV/AIDS epidemic has led to an explosion of therapies developed to limit viral replication or to combat the complications of HIV infection. More antiviral agents are licensed and available to treat HIV than any other viral infection. In the USA, 20 drugs are currently approved in adults for use in HIV infection and 12 have pediatric label information. These approvals are the result of hundreds of clinical studies performed in adults and children through collaborations of clinical investigators, industry, and government partners to support drug development. All too frequently, clinicians find that drugs approved for use in adults or some pediatric populations have insufficient dosing information for their younger patients. Pediatricians know that children are not just small adults. Typically dose recommendations for children are not obtained by simply scaling an adult dose by weight. Additionally, potential risks may well be different in a child that is growing and developing. As a result we have a critical need to conduct clinical studies in children to ensure that they too have the potential to benefit from drug discoveries that are of benefit to older patient populations. It is well recognized though, that children, since they are not able to consent for research themselves, are a population that warrant special protections. Thus, clinical trials in pediatric populations are conducted with due caution for the child's safety while being balanced with moving forward as quickly as possible to open new treatment options.

The cornerstone of all clinical research is that it is conducted in an ethically sound fashion. Principles for the ethical conduct of clinical studies have been articulated in pivotal reports frequently as a result of a need to enhance the protection of research subjects after research scandals, some of which have involved children [1–3]. Unfortunately, communities that have disproportionately born the brunt of research violations in the past frequently may have a continuing distrust of research studies today. Guidelines for assessing the ethical status of research studies provide a tool to help clinicians and investigators evaluate such studies [4]. It is necessary to assess at each step if appropriate protections are in place for children in order to conduct safe, ethically sound research studies.

Participation in a clinical trial presents benefits and risks for the patient. A clinical study often provides access to cutting-edge interventions or investigational therapies and to care by expert clinicians. Pediatric Phase I studies typically follow adult studies that have shown preliminary safety and some drug activity suggesting that patients may benefit from participation in a Phase I study with access to highly investigational drug therapies as well as from Phase II/III studies that typically compare standard and investigational treatments. Each type of study has its own complement of benefits and risks. As for all therapies, the clinician and patient also must weigh the anticipated benefit against other treatment options. For the patient who has been treated with many antiretroviral agents and who has evidence of disease progression and limited standard treatment options, participation in a clinical study offers new treatment possibilities and hope. The decision process may be quite different for the treatment-naïve patient where study participation is one of several alternatives. For the patient considering a comparative Phase II/III study, participation brings less treatment risk since the study is predicated on the assumption that the new treatment arm is as good or better than a standard of care comparative arm. Additional benefits to be considered include the expert healthcare that is available to the study participant and

Table 43.1 Phases of drug development

Phase of investigation	Description	Typical sample size (number of subjects)
I	Safety and dose-seeking	4–12/dose level
II	Expanded safety and preliminary activity data	Several dozen
III	Efficacy trials	Several hundred or more
IV	Post-licensure studies	Thousands

research-related health evaluations that are usually at no charge to the patient, including state-of-the-art virology assessments. However, the decision to enroll in a clinical trial should be based on an evaluation of the merits of the proposed study intervention, and not possible ancillary benefits. Excessive ancillary benefits could be seen as unfair inducements to partake in a study.

Clinical trial participation is not for all patients. A clinical trial requires a special relationship between patients and clinicians; enrolling in a clinical trial is, in essence, a contract between study subjects and clinical investigators. Study participants agree to comply with scheduled visits, to take the study drugs as prescribed, and report any untoward effects that may occur. Investigators agree to consider the safety of the child of paramount importance and conduct the overall study in as safe and scientifically rigorous a way as possible. A bond of trust is needed from both sides of the relationship if the study is to be successfully completed as safely as possible. Similarly, physicians need to be comfortable with separating the role of investigator from that of clinician in discussing clinical study options with their patients. In practice, clinicians are usually in the position of making therapeutic recommendations to their patients. However, clinicians in a research environment need to deliver a balanced voice on the therapeutic potential of a research study versus alternative options. An investigator's enthusiasm for the study should never mislead a potential study participant to overestimate the therapeutic impact or potential benefit of enrolling in a study. It is particularly important that optimism for a study not be attributable to potential conflicts of interest. While it is expected that physicians engaged in research should be compensated for their efforts and costs incurred, many have voiced concerns that physicians should be aware that perceived or real conflicts of interest erode confidence in the integrity of the ethical conduct of studies. Excessive financial compensation or a substantial financial holding in the development of a drug represent two examples of situations in which physicians could be criticized as being conflicted in representing the interests of the subject versus their own financial interests [5].

In addition to investigational new therapies, clinical trials often use approved drugs in new ways – such as different doses, dose schedules, or in novel combinations that merit investigational study. At times these may come in conflict with labeled information or published guidelines. However, guidelines are state-of-the-art treatment summaries while clinical studies are designed to develop new knowledge and support the advancement of new treatment strategies.

43.1 What are clinical trials?

Clinical trials are investigations that aim to address one or more specific research questions that are conducted with a principal concern for the safety of study participants. The research questions must be clearly defined and the outcome measures used to assess the study must be carefully chosen. Studies are designed to enroll the minimum number of participants required to answer a research question, so as to place as few as possible research subjects at risk. On the other hand, studies must strive to enroll the number of patients needed to answer the research question since, if an insufficient number of children are enrolled to answer it, the children are exposed to unnecessary risks. Sample size needs are monitored during trials and enrollment targets are modified if new information indicates that changes would be appropriate. Changes in study design frequently occur, particularly in the earlier phases, and should not raise undue concern.

Traditionally, drugs are developed and studied in phases (Table 43.1). "Phase I" studies in humans are frequently referred to as "proof-of-principle" studies. These studies are quite small and have precise but limited questions. There is no single way to perform Phase I studies, but generally they aim to obtain essential safety, tolerability, and pharmacokinetic information. Patients in Phase I studies are followed intensively with particular attention to safety.

Later, larger studies build on the initial safety data obtained in a Phase I study and produce much more comprehensive safety information. Small trials search for common toxicities and are unlikely to detect rare, but perhaps quite serious toxicities, which may only be seen in large clinical trials or even post-licensure marketing studies. Pediatric Phase I studies usually follow after preliminary Phase I studies in adults, permitting the design of studies for children based on adult experiences, and focus more directly on particular pharmacokinetic and safety issues. After an appropriate dose is selected, Phase II studies are conducted to examine potential toxicities more extensively and to provide the information needed to progress to larger studies. Phase III studies are large clinical trials performed to assess the efficacy of a product or strategy. Drugs that reach this stage of development have passed earlier safety hurdles and frequently have double-blind study designs (i.e. neither the patient nor the investigator know if the patient is receiving the study drug or the comparative therapy). Generally such studies aim to determine whether a new therapy is better than an existing one.

Pediatric HIV studies today are frequently much more complex than standard drug development plans. For example, it is rare today to find a traditional dose escalation study for an antiretroviral drug. Concerns about the rapid development of drug resistance due to suboptimal drug levels need to be balanced with the Phase I safety and tolerability concerns of any investigational antiviral drug. In early adult studies of new agents it is not unusual to find that preliminary pharmacokinetic studies have been conducted in adult volunteers that are not HIV-infected in order to identify drug dosing that achieves target levels the investigators believe will have antiviral activity based on in vitro studies. In initial studies in HIV-infected volunteers it is not uncommon to see an approach in which relatively brief single-drug dose-escalation studies are combined with subsequent combinations of antiretroviral drugs. This strategy is also employed because antiretroviral agents almost certainly will be employed in combinations and it may be useful to obtain safety and tolerability data for new drugs in the context of likely drug combinations. Brief exposure to monotherapy is justifiable only with drugs known to more slowly induce resistance or demonstrate little cross-resistance with other agents, in order to obtain valuable information on the toxicity profile of the drug given alone. However, when new drugs are studied in combination without much monotherapy experience, particularly in patients who may have disease that affects many organ systems, it may be difficult to accurately attribute any observed toxicities. It is also not unusual to find that Phase I and II studies are merged together if safety and pharmacokinetic data in adults adequately support a more aggressive approach to drug development in children. Another variation is the blending of Phase II and III studies. Phase III studies have traditionally focused on clinical endpoints. However, the development of HIV RNA as a reliable marker of disease activity, and one that is clinically used to guide therapeutic choices, has resulted in shorter duration adult and pediatric studies that have fewer study participants, but are still capable of detecting significant antiviral effects. While this approach is entirely reasonable and is supported by a significant amount of clinical data, investigators and clinicians should be aware that such studies are evaluating surrogate endpoints and not the clinical endpoints of greatest concern to the patients and their clinicians, i.e. disease progression and death. Thus, studies that plan to enroll the number of patients needed to determine Phase II safety information also may have sufficient statistical power to assess "virologic efficacy" [6].

Bringing new drugs and innovative therapies to the clinical arena safely and rapidly entails many significant challenges. Different types of studies present different risks and demand different kinds of monitoring. The earliest studies have the greatest potential risks and require intensive safety and pharmacologic monitoring. Studies of drugs or combinations of drugs with a previous safety record require less intensive monitoring since the perceived risk is lower. Some families may not be able to make the commitment of time, effort, and energy needed to safely and effectively participate in an intensive study. Clinical staff need to assess the suitability of a study for a family and child and discuss with that family their needs, the nature of the study, and its participation requirements. Not all children and families are equally suited for all studies. In considering a patient for a study intended for children who are treatment experienced but have elevated HIV viral loads, the clinician and family need to assess why the child is failing the current regimen. If compliance with the current regimen is poor, the issues that have led to poor compliance need to be addressed prior to initiating any new regimens.

43.2 How are clinical trials conducted?

Clinical trial protocols are written by individuals with different areas of expertise and responsibility. The principal investigator and/or study chair have overall responsibility for protocol design and management, and are responsible for answering queries about eligibility issues, administrative concerns, and toxicity management. Protocols frequently have an investigator as a vice-chair who addresses these matters when the chair is not available. Other protocol team members frequently include: a pharmacologist; statisticians and data managers; other investigators who may have specific expertise in such disciplines as virology, immunology, mathematical modeling, molecular virology, evolutionary biology, neuropsychology or nursing; a pharmacist; pharmaceutical company representatives; and a specialist adept at bringing this diverse group together and translating ideas and concepts into a protocol document.

Protocols define a specific study population through precise inclusion and exclusion criteria for several important reasons. Studies generally aim to enroll as homogenous a study population as possible. If a study team decides to assess a drug's effect on a particular clinical parameter, it must set an enrollment limit for the measurement of that parameter. For example, a study to assess the ability of a therapy to decrease viral RNA frequently will require a minimum level of RNA as entry criteria. A subject without any detectable RNA could not provide any data concerning the ability of the therapy to decrease viral RNA. Similar restrictive entry criteria may also apply to the clinical features of a disease. Studies designed for infants first identified as HIV-infected are very different from those designed for children with advanced stages of disease. For their protection, subjects are frequently required to have only mildly abnormal clinical laboratory measures so potential toxicities are more easily identified.

Once it is determined that a family and child are interested in, and the child is potentially eligible for, a clinical trial, informed consent for study participation must be obtained. The consent process is a critical aspect in the conduct of a protocol. In the USA, it is generally considered that children under 18 years of age are not capable of providing informed consent for enrollment into a clinical trial. Instead, parent(s) or legal guardian(s), depending on the kind of study, give permission for their child to participate in a study. At an age when children can begin to understand and partake of the consent process, which is established locally by the Institutional Review Board (IRB), children are asked to assent to participation in studies. In language appropriate for the study population, the consent process covers a number of important elements, such as why the study is being conducted, essential information about the conduct of the study (length of study, number of participants, etc.), the potential risks and benefits, alternatives to participation, as well as the organization sponsoring the study, sources of financial support for the study (especially if the study involves the support or collaboration of a for-profit company), and contact information for study personnel. The consent form should inform the patient about special procedures they may be asked to undergo that may entail increased risks, such as invasive procedures or exposure to diagnostic radiographic procedures not otherwise indicated for clinical care. The consent form also should indicate whether any unusual tests will be performed with specimens collected from the patient (e.g. if patient genetic information will be obtained, if the investigators plan to store specimens for possible future studies, or if the investigators may try to create cell lines using material from the patient). Concerns about study misconceptions remaining after the consent process underscore the importance and attention to the informed consent that is needed [7]. Enrollment then proceeds and typically involves notifying a study data center that in turn notifies the research pharmacist at the site who disburses the study drug(s).

Once a child is enrolled, it is critical that the IRB approved protocol be followed; the family and investigator must follow the protocol unless direct safety concerns for the patient demand otherwise. Regardless of whether a study is conducted at one or many sites, a plan for monitoring the conduct of the study is essential. For Phase I studies, a core group of protocol team members usually review safety data on a frequent, sometimes weekly, basis. Phase II studies also are monitored by the study team and frequently by external reviewers as well. Phase III studies require the use of a Data Safety and Monitoring Board (DSMB), a completely external panel of experts. The DSMB reviews safety issues at scheduled intervals or after the accumulation of a specified number of endpoints. The DSMB assesses if the protocol is progressing in a sound scientific and ethical manner. Participants and investigators must be confident that the safety of the overall study is being monitored and that, if changes are needed to address safety concerns, they will be undertaken. The DSMB may make recommendations to halt the trial if it determines that the study objective has been reached, or if the patients in one arm are doing better than those in another arm. Other safeguards for the study subjects are in place as well. For studies involving investigational agents, serious adverse events that are experienced during the study are also reported to the local IRB as well as to the US Food and Drug Administration (FDA). Typically those reports describe the event that was experienced, whether the investigator thought it was related to the investigational agent or not, as well as whether changes in the protocol are needed in the view of the investigator and study sponsor. The IRB and FDA have the authority to request more information or changes to the protocol. Safety reports on adverse experiences that go to the FDA from the sponsor are distributed to all sites participating in multi-centered trials for review and submission to the local IRB. As a result, investigators are kept informed of serious events that may occur at other study sites. Studies aimed at obtaining information that will be submitted to regulatory agencies in the USA (the FDA) or outside the USA generally are required to adhere to a set of clinical trial conduct standards termed "good clinical practices," or GCP. A uniform set of standards acceptable to the regulatory agencies in the USA, European Union, and Japan have been developed by the International Committee on Harmonisation so that studies conducted anywhere according to these standards can be used to seek regulatory approval from many different national regulatory agencies [8]. Very similar GCP guidelines have been developed by the World Health Organization for use in clinical trials [9]. Even in the absence of regulatory approval requirements, utilizing GCP guidelines to conduct clinical trials should be strongly encouraged. Doing so provides a reassuring standard for the ethical and scientific conduct of studies that have the safety of trial participants as a primary concern.

When patients get ill or develop toxicities that could be related to study drugs, they may not always be able to reach the study staff immediately. Patients also can become ill and not recognize a potential link to the study drug and first appear for evaluation in a private office, clinic, or emergency room. It is critically important that the clinician evaluating the patient be aware of the patient's status as a clinical trial participant. It also is critically important for the patient to realize that he/she should not independently change the drugs prescribed under the study, and that the study investigators should be consulted when the use of any other drug(s) is contemplated. Once the clinician has identified the patient as a trial participant and completed the necessary preliminary evaluations, study staff should be contacted for management advice. Protocols usually outline management plans for commonly observed toxicities as well as identify the toxicities that are particularly worrisome. Notifying study personnel is critical so that the study team is alerted to potentially serious toxicities that could affect the management of other trial participants. If study-related toxicities are suspected, the treating clinician may request unblinding of the patient's treatment assignment. As unblinding may compromise the essential elements of the study, this request is not taken lightly and is evaluated on a case-by-case basis. The treating physician is unblinded only if knowledge about the treatment assignment is critical to the patient's welfare. If a participant is evaluated in a clinic other than the study site, staff will frequently request copies of the evaluation that was done, after appropriate permission is obtained, to provide adequate study documentation of the care that was delivered for a potential adverse event.

A study is not completed at the last study visit; clinicians need to address several issues in anticipation of the last visit. Most pressing is the issue of drug availability following the trial's completion. During protocol development, investigators should consider the continued provision of the study drug if it benefits the participant – but this may not be simple, especially for Phase I studies. While a drug may appear promising, problems ranging from toxicities to drug formulation and production may make it impossible to promise that the drug will be available to the individual at the end of the study. Phase I studies may identify problems critical in the drug development process that can seriously affect the availability of the drug. At a minimum, study sponsors should be able to commit that, if drug development progresses, as anticipated, future availability of the product would be assured, especially for patients who appear to be benefiting significantly from the study drug. This is much less of an issue for Phase II or III studies which have presumably cleared many development hurdles. For a drug or formulation that is not approved by the FDA, provisions to continue to receive the drug usually come from the pharmaceutical company. Frequently this is as a simplified protocol that continues to monitor safety parameters. Additionally, investigators need to inform study participants what treatment assignment they had (for a blinded study), what the final study findings were, and how their participation contributed to the findings.

43.3 Who runs clinical trials?

Many different organizations conduct HIV/AIDS-related clinical trials. All have the same goal – the development of drugs or biologics to treat HIV infection and its complications. Today there is considerable overlap in the studies that are conducted by industry and non-industry sponsors. However, industry-sponsored trials are primarily focused on a path that leads to drug licensure, while academic and government-sponsored studies seek to complement this role by placing an additional emphasis on pathogenesis. Particularly for pediatric trials, where a strong ethical imperative for therapeutic intent exists, trials with an emphasis on pathogenesis often necessarily also involve the testing of new drugs in ways that also will produce data useful for licensure. All organizations that sponsor clinical studies abide by the same regulatory, ethical and study conduct guidelines. In the USA, the mandate for regulatory oversight of investigational drug studies resides with the FDA. All sponsors of studies involving these agents must submit an IND application to the FDA for review prior to initiating a clinical study. The FDA holds the organization that submits the IND responsible for the safe and proper conduct of the study. A pharmaceutical company, a governmental or non-governmental organization, or an

Table 43.2 Further information regarding pediatric and perinatal HIV/AIDS-related clinical trials

Organization	Internet address (http://) and/or telephone number
Clinical trial information	
AIDS Clinical Trials Information Service (AIDSInfo)	www.aidsinfo.nih.gov 1-800-TRIALS-A (1-800-HIV-0440)
Pediatric AIDS Clinical Trials Group (PACTG)	pactg.s-3.com
HIV and AIDS Malignancy Branch (formally Pediatric Branch), National Cancer Institute, NIH	www-dcs.nci.nih.gov/aidstrials/301-435-4627
HIV Prevention Trials Network (HPTN)	www.hptn.org
Paediatric European Network for the Treatment of AIDS (PENTA)	www.ctu.mrc.ac.uk/penta
CDC Division of HIV/AIDS Prevention	www.cdc.gov/hiv/dhap.htm
Clinical Trials.gov (database for clinical trials)	clinicaltrials.gov
HIV InSite (AIDS information site and trial database)	hivinsite.ucsf.edu
Center Watch (clinical trials listing service)	www.centerwatch.com
Additional clinical trial resources	
The Elizabeth Glaser Pediatric AIDS Foundation	www.pedaids.org
National Pediatric and Family HIV Resource Center	www.pedhivaids.org
Project Inform	www.projinf.org
AIDS Education Global Information System (AEGIS)	www.aegis.com
USA Food and Drug Administration (FDA)	www.fda.gov
European Agency for the Evaluation of Medicinal Products (EMEA)	www.emea.eu.int
UNAIDS	www.unaids.org
National Institutes of Health	www.nih.gov
Office of Human Research Protections (OHRP)	www.hhs.gov/ohrp

individual investigator can submit an IND to conduct a study. The European Agency for the Evaluation of Medicinal Products (EMEA) is analogous to the FDA and has authority for the review, approval, and oversight of drug interventions for European Union member nations. In resource-poor nations, regulatory approval for initiating clinical trials as well the registration of drugs for use in that country typically resides within the Ministry of Health for that country.

Table 43.2 outlines some of the organizations that sponsor pediatric clinical trials for treatment of HIV infection and its complications. The Pediatric AIDS Clinical Trials Group (PACTG) conducts by far the largest number of trials in the world involving the largest number of study participants. The group is co-funded by the National Institute of Allergy and Infectious Diseases (NIAID) and the National Institute of Child Health and Human Development (NICHD). The PACTG consists of over 50 clinical sites located throughout the USA, as well as sites in four other countries; laboratories for specialized virology, immunol-

ogy, and pharmacology assessments; a data management and statistical center; as well as an operations office to manage this large clinical trial network. The PACTG has a broad scientific agenda that includes the treatment of HIV and its complications, as well as studies to reduce maternal-infant transmission of HIV. Studies range from those involving HIV-infected pregnant women and infants to adolescents and young adults through age 21 years. Investigations include drug treatments and immune-based therapies for HIV infection, as well as therapies for opportunistic infections and other illnesses associated with HIV disease.

The HIV and AIDS Malignancy Branch (formerly the Pediatric Branch) of the National Cancer Institute (HAMB-NCI) also plays an important role in supporting the evaluation of new therapies for children with HIV infection through its program on the NIH campus in Bethesda, MD. This program focuses much of its work on Phase I and I/II trials and on pathogenesis studies which complement the work done by the PACTG. Studies done by the PACTG and the HAMB-NCI program, in collaboration with the pharmaceutical industry, have contributed information that has led to many drug label indications for children. Studies sponsored directly by pharmaceutical companies, usually at the Phase I level but occasionally at the Phase II/III level, also have led to the availability of many new drug treatments for children. Adult HIV/AIDS clinical trial groups allow the participation of children over 13 years old in many of their studies. Adolescents participating in these trials, as well as in pediatric studies, play an important role in contributing to the scientific evaluation of treatment opportunities in this population. Recently, the Adolescent Medicine Trials Network (ATN) was formed with sponsorship from NICHD. The ATN is giving greater focus and resources to the examination of adolescent HIV/AIDS research concerns through the conduct of collaborative clinical trials. The Paediatric European Network for the Treatment of AIDS (PENTA) is an important resource for trial opportunities within Europe as well as with their collaborators in Canada and Brazil. PENTA has also contributed important pediatric antiretroviral drug label and safety information for the EMEA.

Clinical trial research opportunities are increasing in regions beyond North America and Europe. In studies seeking to reduce mother-to-child transmission of HIV, the French Agence Nationale de Recherches sur le SIDA (ANRS), US Centers for Disease Control and Prevention (CDC) and NIH (through the HIV Prevention Trials Network [HPTN] and other investigator-initiated studies) have all sponsored pivotal clinical trials in resource-poor nations and have ongoing clinical research projects. Pediatric HIV treatment research projects in resource-poor settings are just beginning. As an example, the PACTG has established collaborative trial sites with investigators in Thailand, South Africa, Brazil, and the Bahamas.

43.4 How do I find out about what clinical trials are available for my patients?

The most direct way of finding out information about clinical trials, in addition to discussing studies with clinicians who are involved with protocols locally, is to contact AIDSInfo. This service is funded by the US Department of Health and Human Services and provides information on clinical trials sponsored by industry as well as by government agencies. AIDSInfo can be contacted by phone where information is provided in either English or Spanish (1-800-448-0440) or for the hearing impaired (1-888-480-3739 [TTY]). AIDSInfo also has a very useful internet site (Table 43.2), where access to several large

databases is available to the user 24 hours a day. The AIDSInfo Home Page has a Clinical Trials link where you are able to review studies by clinical categories or use a search engine to identify studies of interest. A brief synopsis of the studies is available including the drugs under investigation, subject eligibility criteria and study contacts. More detailed information on licensed and experimental antiretroviral drugs as well as drugs to treat the complications of HIV can be obtained from the Drugs link to on the AIDSInfo website. The AIDS Education Global Information System (AEGIS) and HIV InSite home pages both have information on many industry and government sponsored pediatric clinical trials. The PACTG and the HAMB-NCI have their own web sites and contact phone numbers (Table 43.2).

43.5 Conclusion

Clinical trials in children are the critical path for the development of appropriate drug dosing and safety information in diverse pediatric populations. Passing down this path is an exciting but challenging process of families working collaboratively with investigators to provide more and better therapeutic options. Clinical trials, particularly in the arena of HIV, are part of a dynamic process of monitoring and defining advances in our knowledge of HIV and its complications. Studies conducted through clinical trials have, in a few short years, dramatically changed the outlook for HIV-infected children [10]. However, many challenges remain as we strive to develop new, more potent drugs with less frequent dosing and improved toxicities profiles. Ultimately, our goal is to continue the rapid and safe development of new therapies that will enhance the health of our patients.

REFERENCES

1. The Nuremberg Code. *J. Am. Med. Assoc.* **276** (1996), 1691.
2. Protection of human subjects: Belmont Report – ethical principles and guidelines for the protection of human subjects of research. *Fed. Regist.* **44** (1979), 23192–7.
3. World Medical Association Declaration of Helsinski. Ethical principles for medical research involving human subjects. *J. Am. Med. Assoc.* **284** (2000), 3043–5.
4. Emanuel, E. J., Wendler, D. & Grady, C. What makes clinical research ethical? *J. Am. Med. Assoc.* **283** (2000), 2701–11.
5. Joffe, S., Cook, E. F., Cleary, P. D., Clark, J. W. & Weeks, J. C. Quality of informed consent in cancer clinical trials: a cross-sectional survey. *Lancet* **358** (2001), 1772–7.

6. Gilbert, P. B., DeGruttola, V., Hammer, S. M. & Kuritzkes, D. R. Virologic and regimen termination surrogate end points in AIDS clinical trials. *J. Am. Med. Assoc.* **285** (2001), 777–84.

7. Morin, K., Rakatansky, H., Riddick, Jr. F. A. *et al.* Managing conflicts of interest in the conduct of clinical trials. *J. Am. Med. Assoc.* **287** (2002), 78–84.

8. International Conference on Harmonisation; Good Clinical Practice; Consolidated Guideline; availability – FDA. Notice. *Fed. Regist.* **62** (1997), 25691–709.

9. World Health Organization. Guidelines for good clinical practice (GCP) for trials on pharmaceutical products. WHO Technical Report Series, No. 850, 1995, Annex 3 access at   www.who.int/medicines/library/par/ggcp/GCPGuide-Pharmatrials.pdf.

10. Gortmaker, S. L., Hughes, M., Cervia, J. *et al.* Effect of combination therapy including protease inhibitors on mortality among children and adolescents infected with HIV-1. *New Engl. J. Med.* **345** (2001), 1522–8.

Medical issues related to the care for HIV-infected children in the home, day care, school, and community

Stephen J. Chanock, M.D.

Pediatric Oncology Branch, National Cancer Institute, NIH, Bethesda, MD

44.1 Introduction

Children with HIV infection spend very little time in hospital; they live, learn, grow, and play in different settings in the community. Despite significant advances in the understanding of HIV transmission infection, a number of misconceptions continue, spawning misunderstandings that can harm children with HIV infection. In some circumstances, these misunderstandings have led to fear and the ostracism of children with HIV infection in situations which present no discernible risk to others. A major challenge for those caring for children with HIV infection is to promote an acceptance of HIV-infected children in the community. Healthcare providers bear an important responsibility to adequately educate children, their caretakers and the community at large on the risk of transmission of both HIV and other infections. Recommended practices for reducing the risk for transmission should be implemented in a balanced manner and should neither minimize nor exaggerate the relative risk for transmission. Every effort should be made to promote understanding, confidentiality, and compassion for children with HIV infection [1, 2].

44.1.1 Transmission of HIV

Risk for transmission of HIV is directly related to exposure to contaminated body fluids [1]. Since HIV preferentially replicates in cells expressing CD4+ and its co-receptors, transmission is highly associated with exposure to infected cells bearing the CD4 antigen (e.g. T-lymphocytes and monocytes) [3, 4]. HIV has been isolated from many body fluids (see Table 44.1), but HIV transmission is most commonly associated with exposure to body fluids, such as blood or semen, which are especially rich in lymphocytes and monocytes [1].

Transmission of HIV requires that a sufficient quantity of virus be introduced to infect host cells [4]. Over the past two decades, four major modes of transmission for HIV infection have been established: (1) between sex partners; (2) from an HIV-infected mother to her child during pregnancy, delivery, or breastfeeding; (3) by direct inoculation of infected blood or blood-containing tissues including transfusion, transplantation, re-use of contaminated needles, or penetrating injuries with contaminated needles; (4) splattering or spraying of mucous membranes or non-intact skin with infected blood [3, 6, 7]. The risk of HIV transmission by one of these four modes depends upon a number of factors listed in Table 44.2 [6]. Inhalation of aerosols, bites from bloodsucking insects, or ingestion of food prepared or served by an infected person have not been associated with transmission of HIV.

44.1.2 The risk for HIV transmission to and from children

The active nature of children and their tendency to liberally spread body fluids have led to the investigation of HIV transmission by casual contact [1, 2]. The data do not support casual contact as a risk factor for transmission. Unless a body fluid is contaminated with blood (usually visibly apparent), the risk for transmission following casual contact is non-existent. For example, HIV is rarely isolated from saliva and tears; transmission has not been observed to be a consequence of exposure to either body secretion [1]. In a handful of reported cases of HIV transmission outside the hospital environment, transmission is via the same modes

Table 44.1 Body fluids from which HIV has been isolated (in general order of frequency of recovery)*

Blood
Semen
Vaginal and cervical secretions
Amniotic fluid
Breast milk
Saliva
Tears
Throat swabs
Cerebrospinal fluid
Synovial, pleural, peritoneal, and pericardial fluid

*HIV has not been routinely isolated from stool or vomitus; however, these fluids theoretically may contain HIV if contaminated with blood.

Table 44.2 Factors upon which risk for transmission of HIV is dependent

Volume of exposed blood or contaminated body fluid
Titer of HIV in source person (related to the stage of
     infection)
Antiretroviral therapy
Route of exposure (in order of less efficient
     transmission)
     Intravenous
     Mucosal (broken ≫ intact)
     Percutaneous (non-intact ≫ intact skin)
Strain of HIV
Underlying health of exposed individual

Table 44.3 Appropriate precautions outside the hospital environment*

Education
     Prevention of exposure
     Recognition of exposure
     Knowledge that HIV is only transmitted via intimate
          contact (intimate sexual contact or inoculation of
          contaminated material)
     Proper clean-up procedure/use of standard
          precautions
     Appreciation of importance of good handwashing
          technique between contacts
     Need to remain calm
     Access to medical advice (if needed)
Materials
     Gloves and gowns for anticipated exposure to any
          body fluid
     Masks and goggles only if splattering or spraying of
          material is likely
     Bleach (for 1:10 or 1:100 dilution in water)
     Disposable vessel for cleaning fluid
     Disposal bags or container

*Standard precautions [10] were designed for hospital-based conditions but should be applied to any location where exposure to body fluids is anticipated.

documented for occupational exposure. Moreover, accidental spilling or splattering of contaminated body secretions is an inefficient method of transmission, which is in sharp contradistinction to the more efficient modes, intimate sexual contact (including exchange of infected secretions) or infusion of a contaminated transfusion product. The reported cases of HIV transmission in a household setting have occurred in circumstances that mirror occupational exposure, namely exposure to a high concentration of infected material via a recognized portal of entry (i.e. bloodstream, mucous membrane, or non-intact skin) [1, 3, 6].

HIV does not survive on environmental surfaces for an extended period of time. Acquisition of HIV results from direct, or intimate exposure to virus, which in turn infects susceptible host cells [4]. The HIV virion is labile and highly susceptible to disinfectants. Consequently, the risk for transmission from environmental surfaces is

non-existent. Still, in the event of a spill, the recommended solution for cleaning a spill is diluted bleach (at 1:10 to 1:100 concentration) [8, 9, 10]. Appropriate materials, including gloves, materials to soak up the spill and adequate disposal containers (Table 44.3) should be available in all settings where children play, learn, or rest [1, 11].

Because children frequently place objects (including hands) in their mouths, transmission via oral secretions has been extensively investigated. In horizontal household exposure studies, transmission via casual contact is exceptionally rare, if it occurs at all [1, 7]. Biting is common among children, but rarely results in direct blood contact. Transmission following a bite is unlikely unless blood is inoculated percutaneously. In prospective studies of individuals bitten by HIV-infected patients, no seroconversions have been reported. In a handful of reported cases, individuals have seroconverted following a severe human bite, notable for exposure to blood-contaminated secretions. Furthermore, the data do not support the likelihood that HIV can be transmitted by kissing, particularly between children and loved ones. In the two cases of possible transmission following passionate or deep kissing, at least one of the partners was noted to have bleeding gums and blood-stained saliva, which probably account for transmission [1]. These cases

Table 44.4 Activities in household contact that have not resulted in transmission of HIV infection

Sharing the same bed
Bathing together
Kissing on lips
Sharing comb
Sharing toilet
Sharing eating utensil
Giving injection
Sharing toothbrush*

* Sharing of toothbrush or razor is not recommended.

emphasize the unlikely possibility of transmission following exposure to contaminated bloody secretions.

The risk of HIV transmission from contact among children in households, schools, day-care centers, and other out-of-home child-care settings is extremely small. A handful of case reports of HIV transmission in the home environment have been reported [1, 2]. In several cases, sequence analysis of viral isolates has pinpointed the source to the home exposure. In each case, exposure to blood or blood-tinged material appears to be the mode of transmission, particularly through non-intact skin or mucous membranes. Nearly 20 studies have been published addressing HIV infection among adult and child household members of infected persons. Including more than 1300 household contacts, new cases of HIV have only occurred in individuals with other major, risk factors for acquisition of infection [1]. Many of these studies have specifically demonstrated the absence of transmission associated with household activities that might involve contact with blood or other potentially infected body fluids, such as sharing razors or toothbrushes (see Table 44.4) [7].

Reported cases of HIV transmission have been associated with the provision of home healthcare. The primary mode has been a needlestick injury or splattering of contaminated material onto non-intact skin or mucosal membranes [3, 6, 12]. In prospective studies of healthcare workers who have sustained a needlestick injury, the estimated risk of HIV transmission following a single percutaneous exposure to HIV-infected blood is about 0.3% [6, 13, 14]. Factors that appear to influence the risk for transmission of HIV include a deep penetrating injury, visible blood on the contaminated device, a high viral titer load in the source individual, recent placement of the catheter in a blood vessel or death of the source patient within 60 days post exposure [5, 12, 14, 15]. HIV transmission following exposure of non-intact skin or mucous membranes to HIV-infected blood has rarely been reported. The estimated risk for this mode of transmission is less than 0.1% [1, 13].

Table 44.5 Techniques of standard precautions that should be practiced outside of hospital

Handwashing	Before and after contact with body fluids. Always after removing gloves
Gloves	Worn if contact with body fluid is anticipated
Masks/eye wear	If splattering of body fluid is likely
Non-sterile gown	Protect skin/clothing from splashes Dispose of properly for cleaning
Patient equipment	Handle carefully to avoid splattering
Linen	Change and dispose of without exposure to others
Surface cleaning	Thorough cleaning of exposed surface
	Removal of fluid
	Disinfect with bleach solution (see Table 44.3)

These rare cases have resulted from extensive exposure to concentrated HIV-contaminated body fluids, splashed into an open wound or mucous membrane.

44.1.3 Precautions and HIV transmission

Originally, guidelines for universal precautions were intended to develop a set of recommendations for minimizing the risk for transmission of *all* blood-borne pathogens [1, 8]. Recommended as a standard of care in all medical facilities in the USA, the guidelines are known as "standard precautions" [10]. They streamline the approach to prevent percutaneous, mucous membrane, and skin exposures to blood-borne pathogens, including HIV. These guidelines are certainly applicable outside of the hospital and should be practiced in schools, camps, athletic, home, and institutional care facilities. Standard precaution guidelines should always be observed, regardless of the presumed infection status of a patient; knowledge of an individual's disease status is not necessary to implement appropriate precautions in or out of the hospital setting. Particular care should be taken when handling blood or blood-tinged solutions from anyone. There are several other blood-borne infectious agents, including hepatitis B and C, which are transmitted more efficiently than HIV [5].

The principles of standard precautions include directives for safe practices in all settings and when indicated, appropriate barrier precautions when contact with blood or body fluids is anticipated (Tables 44.3 and 44.5) [8, 10]. Gloves should be used for handling blood, body fluids, excretions, secretions, mucous membranes, and non-intact skin in all

Table 44.6 HIV infection in the home: What to say and do

Assurance that transmission of HIV results from inoculation of contaminated blood only

　Home transmission only results from accidental inoculation

　Need to have intimate contact with infected material

Casual or physical contact has never been associated with transmission

　Sharing and casual contact are to be encouraged

Use barrier protection for anticipated contact with blood or blood-tinged material

Avoid exposure to blood or blood-contaminated materials

　Prevent access to medical supplies and drugs

Immediately report blood spillage

Clean up spills with appropriate materials

　Keep children away during clean-up

Protect confidentiality of family unit

---

settings. To prevent skin and mucous membrane exposures gowns and gloves should be worn when contact with blood or potentially infected materials is anticipated. Masks, protective eyewear, face shields and gowns should be reserved for circumstances in which there is a chance of splattering infected material to the face or body. Generally, this is applicable in the hospital setting. It cannot be overemphasized that hands should be washed immediately after contact with blood or body fluids, including after removal of gloves. It is worth emphasizing several points that are of particular importance for the care of children in and out of the hospital environment. For the care of children, gloves are not recommended for routine diaper changes and cleaning of nasal secretions [2]. Gloves do not need to be worn when feeding a child, including breast milk. However, some experts have argued that standard precautions be used as a precautionary measure when preparing or offering breast milk, if the HIV status of the mother or breast milk donor is unknown.

With children, the cornerstone of preventing transmission by needlestick or exposure to contaminated sharp items is avoidance. Children should not have access to sharp items. Tamper-proof waste disposals must be kept out of reach of children [16]. Because many children receive home-based care, for instance in conjunction with venous-catheter devices, home care providers should receive proper education in precautions to all occupants. Furthermore, only non-recapping equipment should be used out of hospital. Under no circumstances should needles, syringes, or other such equipment be used for more than one person without sterilization. Blood or potentially infected body fluids spilled on environmental surfaces should be promptly removed and disposed of properly. The contaminated surfaces must be cleaned with a bleach solution (diluted 1:10 to 1:100, depending on the amount of organic material present) after the liquid material has been absorbed and disposed of properly [8, 10].

Appropriate infection control practices should be rigorously followed in other healthcare settings such as clinics, offices, or homes. Common play areas on pediatric wards, in clinics, and in offices need to be supervised by staff trained to handle situations, such as bleeding episodes, that may pose a risk of disease transmission. Toys should be cleaned and disinfected before being used by another child if they are contaminated by blood. Otherwise, there should be no restriction on availability of toys.

44.1.4 General principles for approaching the child with HIV infection outside the hospital

In order to promote a program that is sensitive to the emotional and social as well as medical needs of the HIV-infected child, a co-ordinated approach must be developed that protects both the patient and others (Table 44.6). First and foremost, confidentiality must be protected at all times. Knowledge of HIV status should be restricted to only those who are responsible for medical decisions. Otherwise, there is no indication for public revelation of HIV infection, unless the child and providers believe it suitable.

Mandatory HIV testing is not indicated for attendance at schools, nor for participation in athletics and day care. It has been advocated that HIV testing be conducted in children at risk (e.g. born to infected mothers or those at high risk who refuse testing) prior to adoption or placement in foster care, primarily to provide suitable medical direction for antiretroviral and supportive care of the child.

The principles of infection control practiced within the hospital environment are applicable outside the hospital. Education of lay people (e.g. coaches, day care providers, foster parents, and teachers) who may supervise HIV-infected children is essential. Blood exposures from fights, unintentional injuries, nosebleeds, shed teeth, menstruation, and other causes can occur in many different venues. All institutions which care for and educate children should educate staff about safe practices, establish current policies for protecting confidentiality, provide suitable cleaning materials, and use appropriate infection control practices, including standard precautions, for all children (Tables 44.3 and 44.5).

Because of the advances in antiretroviral therapy, many children are living longer and attending activities outside of the home environment. Many choose to disclose their HIV status. Consequently, educational programs should be available in all settings, and in addition, support systems are needed to counsel and advise infected children. At the same time, public educational programs should be instituted to provide the general public with the knowledge of facts pertinent to effective infection control practices. Since it is estimated that perhaps as many as 20% of infected adults acquired HIV in adolescence, appropriate infection control practices should be reviewed in all settings where children play, learn, or rest [2, 17].

Although HIV-infected children pose only a trivial risk to their uninfected peers, they may acquire from their healthy peers secondary infections which can be life-threatening in the setting of significant immunosuppression [18]. It is important to maintain an active awareness of infectious diseases in the community. Restriction from activity will most likely be determined by concern for acquisition of a serious, secondary infection [19, 20]. Table 44.7 reviews the recommended precautions for contagious diseases that may be particularly dangerous to children with HIV infection.

44.1.5 Specific issues pertaining to children outside the hospital environment

Schools

In the past, children with HIV infection have been discriminated against in schools and on occasion, barred from attendance. These instances have galvanized public attention but more importantly propagated the unfounded notion that HIV is likely to be transmitted in schools. HIV transmission has never been documented to have taken place in school. An educational program for both the staff and student body can help create an accepting environment for children with HIV infection. Many HIV-infected children have chosen to disclose their HIV infection. They attend school with the full support of their teachers and peers and have an extremely positive experience (see Chapter 46).

Children with HIV infection can participate in all school activities to the extent that their health permits [21, 22]. Coordinating a child's medical and educational needs requires ongoing communication among the family, healthcare providers, and school health staff. Like other children with special health needs, children with HIV infection benefit from educational programs that provide needed medical services, such as management of emergencies and administration of medications. All educational institutions should have a policy regarding students and staff who have HIV infection.

In the school, confidentiality is a particularly important issue; privacy rights must be protected at all times [23–25]. A child's HIV status should be disclosed only with the informed consent of the parents or other legal guardians and, when age-appropriate, assent of the child. There is no justification for routine testing of children prior to admission to school. School personnel aware of the child's HIV infection should be limited to the school medical advisor, school nurse, and teacher. The administration of HIV-related medications in school may compromise confidentiality; an infected child should be encouraged to self-administer most medications.

Athletic activities

Since children naturally engage in physical play and often gravitate towards athletic competition, supervision of playgrounds, playing fields, and athletic programs is a major responsibility. Suitable first-aid training and kits should be available wherever children engage in active, physical activities (Tables 44.3 and 44.5) [10, 26]. Participation in contact sports carries a minimal risk of exposure to blood because forceful contact with hard surfaces, equipment, or other players may result in laceration or abrasion. Theoretically, close contact between participants could lead to direct exposure to another person's blood. However, the risk of HIV transmission during sporting activities is extremely low.

HIV testing of athletes should not be a prerequisite for participation in sports. Athletes with HIV infection should be permitted to participate in competitive sports at all levels, as long their condition permits. Notable exceptions to be addressed on a case-by-case basis include the likelihood of blood contact (e.g. intramural touch football vs varsity tackle football), the athlete's propensity to bleed (e.g. thrombocytopenia), and the presence of skin lesions that cannot be covered during active sport. The American Academy of Pediatrics recommends that an HIV-infected athlete considering a sport such as football or wrestling be encouraged to consider an alternative sport after discussing the risk factors for transmission of HIV [2, 26]. Finally, the respect and authority held by many coaches may provide them the opportunity to educate athletes and others about the risk of HIV transmission through unprotected sex and through the sharing of needles or syringes for injection of anabolic steroids or other drugs.

Day care centers

Transmission of HIV in a child-care setting is theoretically possible, but very unlikely, especially if appropriate

Table 44.7 Appropriate precautions for common childhood infections[a]

Organism	Special precautions in			Comments
	Hospital[b]	School	Day Care	
Candida	None	No	No	Ubiquitous
Cytomegalovirus	None	No	No	Ubiquitous
Coccidioidomycosis	None	No	No	No person-to-person transmission
Cryptococcus	None	No	No	No person-to-person transmission
Cryptosporidia	Contact	No	Yes	Child with diarrhea should be excluded from day care
Epstein–Barr virus	None	No	No	Ubiquitous
Haemophilus influenza type[b]	Droplet	No	No	Prophylaxis of contacts[c]
Hepatitis B	None	No	Yes	Avoid biting and blood contact[c]
Histoplasmosis	None	No	No	No person-to-person transmission
Herpes simplex	Contact	No	Yes	Exclude child with mouth sores and drooling
Influenza	Droplet	No	No	Common in winter
Isospora hominis	Contact	No	yes	Pathogenicity negligible in immunocompetent children
Mycobacterium avium intracellulare	None	No	No	No person-to-person transmission
Measles	Airborne	Yes	Yes	Exclude child until resolved[c]
Pertussis	Droplet	Yes[d]	Yes[d]	Exclude child until treated[c]
Pneumococcus	None	No	No	Ubiquitous in normal children
Pneumocystis carinii	None	No	No	Ubiquitous
Respiratory syncytial virus	Contact	No	No	Common in winter/spring
Rotavirus	Contact	No	Yes	Child with diarrhea should be excluded from day care
Salmonella	Contact	No	Yes	Infected child should be excluded until 3 stools negative
Staphylococcus	Contact	Yes[d]	Yes[d]	Exclude child until resolved
Streptococcus	Contact	Yes[d]	Yes[d]	High rate of carriage among children
Syphilis	Contact	No	No	Should have been treated in infancy
Toxoplasma	None	No	No	No person to person transmission
Tuberculosis	Airborne	Yes	Yes	Until treated[e]
Varicella-zoster	Airborne + Contact	Yes	Yes	Exclude child until lesions scabbed

[a] Adapted from [1]

[b] Based upon standard precautions recommendations [10].

[c] Immunization recommended for all children.

[d] Precautions can be discontinued once the patient has been on therapy for at least 24 hours.

[e] Consultation with physician recommended, particularly in area with high prevalence of resistant strains of tuberculosis.

precautions are taken. The lack of data supporting transmission of HIV through casual contact following household exposure is pertinent to the child-care setting. The CDC, AAP, and the American Public Health Association have recommended that children with HIV infection be allowed to attend child care in nearly all cases [16, 27, 28]. Exceptional circumstances that argue against attendance at day care include a strong propensity for aggressive biting, the likelihood of having uncontrollable bleeding episodes, the presence of oozing skin lesions that cannot be covered (e.g. on the face), or a degree of immunosuppression which would place the patient at risk in the day-care setting [1]. The latter is probably most pertinent and requires an awareness of secondary infections in the community that may imperil the child with severe immunosuppression. It is recommended that the child's physician participate in the decision to enroll a child in day care.

In some communities, day care centers designed to meet the special medical, developmental, and other needs of children with HIV infection have been successfully established. The success of these programs is not a reason to mandate that all children with HIV should attend a specialized program. In fact, most experts agree that infected children benefit greatly from participation in normal activities with other children.

Adoption

Adoption of the child with HIV entails responsibility for medical care. Prospective adoptive or foster parents of HIV-infected children and children at risk for whom the diagnosis has not been excluded should be aware of the diagnosis, treatment plan, and prognosis of the child [1, 23]. They should be instructed in appropriate infection control measures designed to minimize the risk for transmission [29]. Children born to infected mothers should be tested with permission of the biologic mother. On occasion, this may not be possible. Most states can request HIV testing through the legal system. Because nearly all HIV-infected children who are to be adopted or placed in foster care have acquired infection perinatally, great care should be taken to protect the confidentiality of the biologic mother's HIV status.

Summer camp and other recreational activities

Recently, a number of camping opportunities have become available to children with HIV infection [30]. Some are restricted to children with HIV infection while others integrate children into a general camp setting. On occasion, family camps have been offered to provide a nurturing environment for children and families together. Proper training in the management of blood and potentially infectious fluid spills is required of all staff. Generally, medical and nursing support should be available to handle both standard emergencies and serious intercurrent illnesses. Suitability for attendance should be based upon the condition of the child. In the camp environment, children should not be restricted in their activities on the basis of their HIV status. However, secondary conditions, such as diarrhea or cryptosporidiosis may preclude specific activities, such as swimming in an enclosed public pool. It is notable, that lake swimming also presents a risk for acquisition of a waterborne pathogen.

44.1.6 Management of exposure to HIV

Despite efforts to avoid direct exposures to HIV-infected blood and other body fluids by educational and preventive measures, children are still at risk for accidental exposure to HIV outside the hospital environment [1, 14, 31]. Exposure following a bite or splashing of contaminated material is also possible, but the efficiency of transmission is greatly reduced relative to percutaneous needlestick injuries [1]. In the rare instance in which a child is exposed to HIV-infected body fluids, immediate consultation of medical care is critical for assessment and intervention [31]. Post-exposure prophylaxis for HIV is described in Chapter 24. Other post-exposure prophylaxis measures may be indicated if there is a concomitant exposure to other infectious agents (e.g. hepatitis B). Because blood and body fluid exposures also may occur in the home or outside the hospital environment, the availability of access to information regarding post-exposure management should be established for persons outside of medical centers.

Recommended management of an accidental exposure to HIV includes reporting exposures promptly, evaluating the nature of the exposure, counseling the exposed person regarding management, and testing the source person (with consent) for hepatitis B surface antigen and HIV antibody. During the follow-up period, the exposed person should seek medical evaluation for any acute illness and refrain from blood, semen, and organ donation. Updated information on HIV post-exposure prophylaxis is available from the Internet at CDC's home page (http://www.cdc.gov) and the National AIDS Clearinghouse (800-458-5231). Policy statements from the American Academy of Pediatrics can be found on their web site (http://www.aap.org).

44.2 Precautions for other infections

Children with HIV are more susceptible to severe or life-threatening complications of opportunistic and common pediatric infections. Opportunistic infections can generally not be prevented by limiting person-to-person exposure, since they are usually present in the environment, carried by the at-risk host, and are associated with immunosuppression rather than with exposure [18, 19]. Generally, opportunistic infections are not transmitted to other children as opposed to common pediatric infections (such as varicella or measles) which can be transmitted to other children, including those without HIV infection.

The greater danger is to the child with HIV whose immune function is significantly depressed because of the greater risk for more severe or chronic complications of the secondary infection. Prophylaxis for opportunistic infections is discussed in Chapter 11.

A major challenge to providers of care, education, and recreation for children with HIV is preventing acquisition of preventable infections. Because the consequences of routine, viral infections, such as varicella or measles, can be so severe in HIV children, providers must be vigilant and knowledgeable of ongoing outbreaks in the community. Restricting a child from participation in school, day care or athletics should only be recommended if an outbreak or documented cases have been reported and the likelihood is high that exposure may take place.

Strategies to prevent acquisition of a secondary infection include immunization (both passive and active), protecting a child from exposure (which may be unrealistic), and prophylaxis with antimicrobial agents [19]. While the latter is effective in decreasing the risk for infection, it is not fully protective and in fact, intensifies the pressure to develop infection with resistant organisms.

Standard precautions should be followed for all patients, regardless of their presumed infection status [10]. Recommendations for isolation have been streamlined into three categories, based upon the mode of transmission; droplet, contact, and airborne [10]. Recommendations have been generated for specific clinical syndromes highly suspicious for infection but requiring temporary implementation of precautions until a definitive diagnosis is confirmed. Standard precautions have only been recommended for hospital-based practice, but their application is appropriate for the care of children with HIV outside the hospital. Recommendations concerning attendance in school or day care should be based upon these precautions and can easily be applied to other settings, such as family gatherings, athletic events, summer camps, or recreational programs [11, 21, 22, 29].

44.3 Conclusion

On the basis of the published literature and extensive clinical experience with HIV infection, it is appropriate to conclude that the presence of HIV infection, per se, should not restrict children from participating in athletics, day care, and school unless an exceptional circumstance intervenes. Accordingly, children with HIV infection should be able to enjoy the same access to healthcare, privacy, education, and social interactions as other children. Management of children with HIV infection outside of the hospital environment should be routine as long as the proper guidelines for infection control practices and confidentiality are followed. Educated and caring healthcare professionals need to help the community better understand HIV infection and the needs of infected children. The activities of children with HIV should be restricted only due to either a debilitating complication or the risk of a secondary infection that may be more severe in the compromised host. Because of the evolving nature of the HIV epidemic, updated recommendations will most likely continue to be issued by organizations including the American Academy of Pediatrics and the Centers for Disease Control and Prevention.

REFERENCES

1. Chanock, S. J., Donowitz, L., & Simonds, R. J. Medical issues related to provision of care for the HIV-infected child in the hospital, home, day care, school and community. In P. A. Pizzo, & C. Wilfert (eds.), *Pediatric AIDS: the Challenge of HIV Infection in Infants, Children and Adolescents*, 3rd edn. Philadelphia, PA: Lippincott, Williams & Wilkins (1998), pp. 645–62.

2. American Academy of Pediatrics Committee on Pediatric AIDS and Committee on Infectious Diseases. Issues related to human immunodeficiency virus transmission in schools, child care, medical settings, the home and community. *Pediatrics* **104** (1999), 318–24.

3. Curran, J. W., Jaffe, H. W., Hardy, A. M. *et al.* Epidemiology of HIV infection and AIDS in the United States. *Science* **239** (1988), 610–16.

4. Pantaleo, G. & Fauci, A. S. Immunopathogenesis of HIV infection. *Ann. Rev. Microbiol.* **50** (1996), 825–54.

5. American Academy of Pediatrics. Human immunodeficiency virus infection. In G. Peter (ed.), *2000 Red Book: Report of the Committee on Infectious Diseases*, 25th edn. Elk Grove, Il: American Academy of Pediatrics (2000), pp. 325–50.

6. Tokars, J. I., Marcus, R., Culver, D. H. *et al.* Surveillance of HIV infection and zidovudine use among health care workers after occupational exposure to HIV infected blood. *Ann. Intern. Med.* **118** (1993), 913–19.

7. Simonds, R. J. & Chanock, S. J. Medical issues related to caring for HIV-infected children in and out of the home. *J. Pediatr. Infect. Dis.* **12** : 845–52 (1993)

8. Centers for Disease Control. Recommendations for prevention of HIV transmission in health-care settings. *MMWR* **36**: Suppl. 2S (1987), 1–18S.

9. Occupational Safety and Health Administration. Occupational exposure to bloodborne pathogens. *Fed. Regist.* **56** (1991), 64175–82.

10. Hospital Infection Control Practices Advisory Committee. Guidelines for isolation precautions in hospitals. *Infect. Control Hosp. Epidem.* **17** (1996), 53–80.

11. Hale, C. M. & Polder, J. A. *The ABCs of Safe and Healthy Child Care: A Handbook for Child Care Providers*. Atlanta, GA: DHHS/USPHS/CDCP (1997).

12. Tokars, J. I., Bell, D. M., Culver, D. H. *et al.* Percutaneous injuries during surgical procedures. *J. Am. Med. Assoc.* **267** (1992), 2899–904.

13. Ippolito, G., Puro, V. & De Carli, G. The risk of occupational human immunodeficiency virus infection in health care workers: Italian multicenter study: Italian study group on occupational risk of HIV infection. *Arch. Intern. Med.* **153** (1993), 1451–8.

14. Cardo, D. M., Culver, D. H., Ciesielski, C. A. *et al.* A case-control study of HIV seroconversion in health care workers after percutaneous exposure. *New Engl. J. Med.* **337** (1997), 1485–90.

15. Henderson, D. K. Post-exposure treatment of HIV – taking some risk for safety's sake. *New Engl. J. Med.* **337** (1997), 1542–3.

16. Simmons, B., Trusler, M., Roccaforte, J., Smoth, P. & Scott, R. Infection control for home health. *Infect. Control Hosp. Epidemiol.* **11** (1990), 362–70.

17. American Academy of Pediatrics Committee on Pediatric AIDS and Committee on Adolescence. Adolescents and human immunodeficiency virus infection: the role of the pediatrician in prevention and intervention. *Pediatrics* **107** (2001), 188–90.

18. Mueller, B. M. & Pizzo, P. A. Pediatric AIDS and childhood cancer. In P. Pizzo, & D. Poplack, (eds.), *Principles and Practice of Pediatric Oncology*, 3rd edn. Philadelphia, PA: Lippincott-Raven (1997), pp. 1005–25.

19. Centers for Disease Control and Prevention. 1997 USPHS/IDSA guidelines for the prevention of opportunistic infections in persons infected with human immunodeficiency virus. *MMWR.* **46**: **RR-12** (1997), 1–46.

20. Centers for Disease Control. Guidelines for preventing the transmission of tuberculosis in health-care settings, with special focus on HIV-related issues. *MMWR.* **39**: **RR-17** (1990), 1–29.

21. American Academy of Pediatrics Task Force on Pediatric AIDS. Education of children with human immunodeficiency virus infection. *Pediatrics* **88** (1991), 645–8.

22. Centers for Disease Control. Education and foster care of children infected with human T-lymphotrophic virus type III/lymphadenopathy-associated virus. *MMWR* **34** (1985), 517–21.

23. Fraser, K. *Someone at School has AIDS*. Alexandria, VA: National Association of State Boards of Education. (1989), pp. 1–35.

24. Grier, E. C. & Hodges, H. E. HIV/AIDS: a challenge in the classroom. *Public Health Nurs.* **15** (1998), 257–62.

25. Santelli, J. S., Birn, A. E. & Linde, J. School placement for human immunodeficiency virus-infected children: the Baltimore city experience. *Pediatrics* **89** (1992), 843–8.

26. American Academy of Pediatrics, Committee on Sports Medicine and Fitness. Human immunodeficiency virus [acquired immunodeficiency syndrome (AIDS) virus] in the athletic setting. *Pediatrics* **88** (1991), 640–1.

27. American Public Health Association, American Academy of Pediatrics. *Caring for our Children*. (1989), pp. 231–6.

28. American Academy of Pediatrics Committee on Infectious Diseases. Health guidelines for the attendance in day-care and foster care settings of children infected with human immunodeficiency virus. *Pediatrics* **79** (1987), 466–71.

29. American Academy of Pediatrics Task Force on Pediatric AIDS. Guidelines for human immunodeficiency virus (HIV)-infected children and their foster families. *Pediatrics* **89** (1992), 681–3.

30. Pearson, H. A., Johnson, S., Simpson, B. J. *et al.* A Residential Summer Camp for children with vertically transmitted HIV/AIDS: A six-year experience at the Hole in the wall gang camp. *Pediatrics* **100** (1997), 709–13.

31. Merchant, R. C. & Kershavarz, R. Human immunodeficiency virus postexposure prophylaxis for adolescents and children. *Pediatrics* **108**: E38 (2001), 1–13.

Contact with social service agencies

Sandra Y. Lewis,[1] Psy.D. and Heidi J. Haiken, L.C.S.W., M.P.H.[2]

[1] Montclair State University and National Pediatric and Family HIV Resource Center, UMDNJ – New Jersey Medical School, Newark, NJ
[2] Francois-Xavier Bagnoud Center, UMDNJ – New Jersey Medical School, Newark, NJ

45.1 Introduction

Though a cure for HIV disease remains elusive, medical advances have demonstrated that the virus can be reduced to undetectable levels and disease progression can be significantly slowed. The use of antiretroviral prophylaxis and cesarian section reduces the rate of perinatal transmission of HIV infection, thus increasing the likelihood that a child born to a mother with HIV infection will not be infected. Medical advances, nutritional support, psychosocial support, co-ordination of key services, and attention to quality of life issues have contributed to improved treatment and prevention outcomes for HIV-exposed and HIV-infected children. Children with HIV infection are living well into their teen years and even their 20s. Parents living with HIV who have access to HIV care are able to be primary caregivers for their children for a longer period of time. Although this chapter is primarily oriented to the experience of patients living in the USA, some of the information, particularly the information concerning broader psychological and social concerns should be helpful to patients in other parts of the world.

45.2 Psychosocial concerns

Amidst the notable successes in HIV care, there continue to be a number of important psychosocial issues. Among the most critical issues facing children and families living with HIV are the psychosocial developmental needs of children with HIV infection. Children growing into teenagers with HIV face profoundly challenging adolescent psychosocial developmental issues. With the changing characteristics of the HIV epidemic, the developmental difficulties faced by children and families have changed, producing new challenges in parenting and planning for the future. In the past, parents did not expect their child to live into adolescence. As children grow older, issues such as disclosure, development of intimacy, career and school choices and the usual tasks of adolescence may offer overwhelming challenges for parents and frequently require support from health and mental health professionals.

Other crucial psychosocial issues are the special concerns of uninfected children living in a family with other HIV-infected members. In recent years, investigators have begun to describe the needs of affected children [1–3]. This research has noted that HIV-uninfected children of HIV-infected mothers evidenced greater psychosocial adjustment difficulties when compared with their peers whose mothers are HIV-uninfected [1]. This is sometimes a forgotten group of children because families may be focused on the children who are HIV-positive. It is important that such children have access to services such as healthcare, mental healthcare, recreation, and other services that help to normalize their lives. In many cases, services are available through the HIV care programs used by infected family members.

Permanency planning for children can be an urgent issue for families. The decrease in perinatal HIV transmission makes it more likely that children will be uninfected while their parents will be HIV-infected. While parents are living longer, healthier lives, there is a real risk that their children will be orphaned due to HIV disease. Levine [4] estimated that by the year 2000, more than 200 000 children would have lost their mothers to HIV infection in the USA. Planning for AIDS orphans is a worldwide concern. Within the

USA, parents have a number of options for permanency planning and can get assistance through HIV care facilities (See also Chapter 48). In sub-Saharan Africa, organizations such as the Association François Xavier Bagnoud and The International Partnership Against AIDS are leading efforts to ensure orphans of the AIDS epidemic are able to grow up in nurturing environments.

Like other chronic illnesses, HIV infection can disrupt the child's ability to engage in normal daily activities such as school, cause serious psychological and emotional problems, and may lead to premature death [5, 6]. Distinctive psychosocial issues set pediatric and family HIV apart from other chronic illnesses: stigma; family secrecy about diagnosis; lack of social support; isolation; interactions between HIV and other family problems such as drug abuse and poverty; the multi-generational nature of HIV among women and children; and the multiple losses due to HIV experienced by members of families affected by the disease. All of these can increase the psychosocial burden and emotional distress experienced by many families living with HIV/AIDS [7, 8]. Sherwen and Storm [9] examined the studies that describe the psychosocial challenges of families of children with HIV infection. Stress and isolation were identified as recurring themes, contributing to the psychological vulnerability of families. Families living with HIV are often simultaneously coping with poverty, limited access to health and educational resources, homelessness, and other social problems that can require that they interface with numerous social service agencies in addition to medical providers.

45.3 Assessing family needs

Families living with HIV infection can have widely varying compositions, ranging from the nuclear family consisting of parents and children, to grandparents caring for their ill adult children and their grandchildren, to foster families. Determining which family members constitute the key caregivers is essential for the optimal provision of healthcare and psychosocial services. In many states, foster parents receive specialized training and financial supplements for caring for HIV-infected children. Biological family members who assume this same responsibility are often not eligible for monetary support [10]. In some states, providers and legislators are realizing that this lack of support for biological family members hinders keeping families together. They are beginning programs such as the Kinship Navigator Program in New Jersey, which provides additional support for family members. More information about this program can be accessed at their website:

http://www.state.nj.us/humanservices/DHS%20Publications/kinshipbro1.html.

While foster parents may provide the day-to-day care and assume responsibility for making sure a child's medical needs are met, the biological parent and/or the state retains the legal guardianship of the child. Thus, foster parents are often unable to legally consent for certain medical interventions, including enrollment in clinical trials, or simple surgical procedures. Foster parents may also face difficulty in decisions about disclosure and in assuming responsibility for making funeral arrangements when children die. The limits of foster parents' legal rights to make medical and other decisions may vary from state to state and must be evaluated with each family.

Families with HIV-infected members face many challenges. They often live under significant stress and may be fragile. However, they also have strengths that have helped them manage previous difficult situations. Past coping strategies provide clues for developing effective plans for families.

Social issues, such as poverty and homelessness, faced by families necessitate that providers assess whether basic needs such as food and shelter are being satisfied. For example, when a family comes for medical services, the medical provider may focus on providing the child with the newest state of the art medications and treatments. However, unless the family's basic needs are met, it will be difficult to assist them in implementing the best medical care for their child. In addition, when a family comes for a medical visit, their expectations regarding the visit must be assessed. With time constraints, and with desires to provide the best possible care to children, a question to ask the parent or guardian is: What are the concerns for today? This should include both medical and social concerns. In a setting where a multi-disciplinary team approach is utilized, the services of a social worker or psychologist can be enlisted to address those concerns on site. If not, it is worthwhile to keep available a list of community resources that provide support with basic needs such as housing and food. Ryan White Comprehensive AIDS Resources Emergency (CARE) Act funding is available in many communities. It supports a variety of services for persons infected and affected by HIV.

Other, more basic, concerns may arise. For example, the possibility that a child may be in danger because the basic needs for food and shelter are not being met or because the child is at risk of being physically abused. Providers who care for children with HIV infection should compile lists of organizations that can provide resources and treatment facilities where troubled parents can seek help. Local community or county social service departments will often have this information. When referring a family to a social service agency, it is helpful to assess their previous history with the organization. If their experiences have been negative, it may be necessary to broker this relationship in order to obtain the needed services for the child and family.

45.4 Managed care and other insurance coverage

In the USA, the complicated system of medical insurance and reimbursement present a specific set of challenges to those who would deliver excellent care to the HIV-infected child. Managed care is a system where a primary healthcare provider (PCP) functions as the gatekeeper of medical services needed by the client. The PCP will make referrals to specialists that he or she determines as needed. Health Maintenance Organizations (HMOs) are one type of managed care program. In this type of plan, all of the healthcare providers who see the patient must be enrolled in the HMO or there will not be financial coverage for the services. There are certain special circumstances where the HMO may allow the patient to be covered by the HMO for care provided by a clinician not employed by the HMO, called "to go out of network," if the needed service is not available in network. These situations are negotiated with the PCP and HMO. Some states use HMOs to deliver services under their Medicaid programs. Preferred Providers Organizations (PPOs) and Point of Service (POS) plans also use PCPs and have various rules about referrals to specialists who are considered "in-network" and those out of network. With these plans, there may be no cost or the patient may have to make a co-payment at the time of the visit to see the PCP or to the specialist if the specialist is in-network. The PCP bills the HMO, PPO, or POS insurance company for the remainder of the fees beyond the co-payment if the healthcare provider is in-network. Written referrals are usually needed for specialists, although some plans do not require referrals for certain specialists, for example gynecologists. There are also traditional health insurance plans, also known as "fee for service" plans, in which each physician who sees the client charges the patient for the service. In these plans either the patient pays the healthcare provider and is then reimbursed by the insurance company, or the physician bills the insurance company directly. Each plan varies, and if families have a choice of insurance plans, they should carefully examine the benefits offered by each plan and consult with the insurance companies or their benefits specialist to determine which plan is best suited for them. If a patient has a wish to see a particular specialist, it is imperative that they ensure that the specialist will be covered by the healthcare plan. Families should carefully monitor the benefits offered by insurance plans and the healthcare providers and hospitals that are considered in-network, since these can change frequently and with little warning. Families can sometimes face unpleasant surprises when they discover that the insurance arrangements have changed for a healthcare provider that they have seen for a long time. It is important to also verify where lab work and other tests can be done.

45.5 Organizational considerations in the psychosocial care of pediatric HIV infection

HIV infection can exert extreme stresses on many families. Providers should make themselves aware of these stresses and often must provide concrete recommendations for patients in order to provide optimal care. Medical specialists and generalists, social workers and case managers who provide care for HIV-infected children must be aware of some of the key features of the medical insurance system. Careful planning can help. Recommendations that providers caring for patients with HIV may want to consider include:

1. Maintaining an automated list of your clients, their health insurance plan, their primary care provider (PCP), and the number of referrals that have already been made to specialists since insurance companies often limit such referrals.
2. Determination of the relationship between each client and their PCP and the establishment of a working relationship with their PCP. The insurance company may need to be consulted to determine: Which provider sees the client and for what specific conditions? Can the specialist provide primary care? When should the child see the PCP? Other key points to consider include: Whether the family has a clear idea of when to see whom. Whether the specialist and the PCP agree about the services required and the treatment plan. Whether the HMO directly provides any additional services (e.g. education, home visits) or other help that could support your efforts (e.g. transportation)?
3. Assess whether the family can obtain their own referrals? If not, determine who from your office is responsible for calling the PCP when a referral is needed, if the insurance company requires that referrals be made through the PCP.
4. Evaluate why families are not able to obtain their own referrals. Assist with skill training as needed.
5. Have readily accessible the phone numbers to the most commonly used insurance companies, their complaint

lines, and, if needed, information for families being cared for by Medicaid HMOs. (Certain jurisdictions require that patients receiving care through Medicaid be enrolled in a Medicaid HMO, but certain patients with complicated diseases may sometimes be exempted from this requirement.)

Using insurance benefits, public and private, can create significant barriers for HIV-infected children and their families. Some families continue to fear discrimination when they utilize their insurance coverage. Very often, this desire not to use insurance is related to the secrecy around the diagnosis. However, it also could be due to accounts in the press or personal experiences of people who had difficulty accessing care or who have experienced negative consequences from seeking care for HIV infection. Before a patient applies for insurance benefits the provider should consider whether the benefit is likely to be granted and what patients and providers can do to ensure that the patient receives all the benefits that should be available. For example, it is important to know if your state has exceptions for pre-existing conditions. Some state laws prohibit denial of coverage for pre-existing conditions. While laws may not calm families' fears, they may help to ensure families get appropriate medical coverage.

Communication between the medical provider and the insurer is essential. Success in dealing with managed care requires education and negotiation skills. The representative of the insurance company may not understand HIV disease. For example, the representative may question HIV wasting and why tube feedings are being done on a child who can eat. In this example, it may be helpful to enlist the aid of a nutritionist who can explain why the tube feedings are essential. To maximize the likelihood that an insurance claim will be honored the provider must maintain clear, detailed records. Some insurance companies may require growth charts if they are asked to pay for special nutritional services. However, meticulous records may not be sufficient. The individual providing the initial review at the insurance company may be ignorant of HIV disease, insufficiently trained, and inexperienced, so providing a complete explanation with the pertinent records may enhance the likelihood that a claim will be honored.

45.6 Social security and Medicaid

In the USA, Social Security and Medicaid Programs are also available for clients. The regulations for social security change based upon the current federal and state legislation and funding levels. Supplemental Security Income (SSI) is available for children with AIDS if they meet certain requirements [11]. The Social Security Administration publishes this information online in the *Online Social Security Handbook: Your Guide to Basic Social Security Programs*. It can be accessed at: http://www.ssa.gov/OP_Home/handbook/ssa-hbk.htm. Specific requirements for children can be accessed at: http://www.ssa.gov/OP_Home/handbook/handbook.05/handbook-0516.html. The requirements include "marked and severe functional limitations," length of disability and "inability to have gainful activity due to a physical or mental impairment." There is also a financial criterion for SSI eligibility. The calculations that determine financial eligibility are complicated, and it may be helpful to consult with someone with extensive experience in obtaining SSI for children with HIV disease. In most states, children eligible for SSI are eligible for Medicaid. States can contribute to or match federal entitlements, so that the eligibility and funding levels can vary significantly from state to state. (Further information can also be found in Chapter 48.)

In certain circumstances, presumptive SSI is available to eligible clients with HIV infection. This means that they are given SSI for 6 months based on minimal documentation substantiating a diagnosis of AIDS or HIV infection with low $CD4^+$ count, and/or certain opportunistic infections, and other medical or functional criteria. The reviewers use criteria that may change with new classification systems and new healthcare guidelines. During these 6 months, a more complete medical evaluation is done to determine if the client is eligible for SSI benefits. To expedite this process, it may be helpful to have the presumptive SSI applications in your office. It is also helpful to provide the client with the following to take to the Social Security office:

Medical and laboratory records

The name and phone number of the person in your office who handles SSI medical request forms.

The name and address of the medical practitioner who is responsible for completing the form.

The family should take the following with them:

Their own and their child's social security card

Recent pay or entitlement stubs

Outstanding medical bills

Utility receipts

Rent receipts

Bank account information

Reports from other medical practitioners or physical/occupational therapists.

These items are needed in order to determine the level of physical and cognitive functioning of the child as well as their financial eligibility for the program. There are times when the whole family's income is counted and times when the child's income is counted as the determining factor.

This depends upon the relationship the child has with the guardian. For instance, a child who is living with a relative who has not adopted the child or with a family in which the guardianship relationship is not formalized may be eligible as an individual without using family income. This may also occur with some non-kinship adoptions through the child welfare agency.

Social Security officials recommend that you inform clients of the basic eligibility requirements before they apply. For example, you may have a client who wants to have their child apply for SSI. However, the child is asymptomatic and functions appropriately, physically and cognitively, for their age. They should be informed that they do not meet the criteria and advised against applying for SSI until their child meets the eligibility criteria. The Social Security Administration has guides available for clients on Social Security and HIV infection.

Due to the recent changes in SSI eligibility, some children are losing their benefits. They may lose their Medicaid if they do not meet the financial criteria for other state-controlled Medicaid Programs. Some adolescents are being re-evaluated when they become 18 years old. These re-evaluations can have quick and disastrous effects for children who are on medications. Insurance coverage may be denied in such situations and resources may need to be found without delay to prevent a lapse in their medication regimen. Programs such as the AIDS Drug Distribution Program (ADDP) can often provide resources for HIV-related medications. Another alternative is to seek medications through the indigent assistance programs of the pharmaceutical companies. While it is important that effective antiretroviral therapies be maintained even when insurance coverage changes, clinicians should carefully and thoughtfully explain the options for insurance coverage and funding for the drugs, so that patients and their families understand that alternatives are available and do not experience needless anxiety.

45.7 Medicaid model waivers

Model waivers are federally funded and state-administered funds available for medical services. The most common waiver for children with AIDS is the AIDS Community Care Alternatives waiver, commonly known as ACCAP. In order to apply for this waiver, the child must be HIV infected and under the age of 13 years, or have the disability diagnosis of AIDS if they are 13 years and older. They must also be in need of home care services. The concept behind the waivers is to keep people out of institutions and in the community. With ACCAP, patients can receive home-care ser-

vices, including services from a home health aide, a licensed practical nurse (LPN) or registered nurse (RN), inpatient and outpatient medical services, and other services traditionally provided by Medicaid, which may vary from state to state. ACCAP does have a financial cap on the services provided to a child. ACCAP is also available for adults. Some states have other waiver programs for children. There are no financial criteria to be eligible for ACCAP. It is best to consult with your local or state Medicaid office about other available waivers.

Families on waiver programs may have private insurance and Medicaid. Questions about billing and services covered arise. When Medicaid is involved, the insurance company is billed first. Providers must build relationships with case managers from the insurance companies. It may take extensive negotiation to get services from the two entities, Medicaid and a private insurer, as each may expect the other to pay. It is important for families to bring in their insurance booklets describing services covered for the social worker to review. Experienced social workers can sometimes identify approaches that will provide for reimbursement that are not immediately apparent to the patient and family.

Federal funding is available for certain patient services. This ranges from program staff to client medications, transportation, home care, and hospice care. Currently, most of funding specifically for children infected with AIDS is through the Ryan White CARE Act Title I, Title II, Title IIIb, Title IV, and Special Projects of National Significance (SPNS). Questions and requests for technical assistance regarding this funding can be directed to the AIDS Policy Center and the National Pediatric and Family HIV Resource Center (numbers and website addresses to follow).

45.8 Alternative sources for resources

As listed in Table 45.1 there are other sources of private funding. Sometimes, these sources will consider paying for short-term nursing or medications needed upon discharge. Hospital foundations are also an option for patient funding. Often there are private organizations and foundations available to local hospitals and clinics. This table is not exhaustive but includes some key resources, services, and grants provided.

45.9 Discharge planning

The frequency of hospitalization among HIV-infected children makes discharge planning a key element of medical

Table 45.1 Alternate sources of resources

Organization	Services/grants offered
The Elizabeth Glaser Pediatric AIDS Foundation	Emergency funding for services to HIV infected children and families Educational grants for student interns and research Application usually due in the Fall Grants up to $10 000.00 Projects in Africa aimed at reduction of perinatal HIV transmission
Association Francois Xavier Bagnoud	Orphan projects Human rights HIV/AIDS prevention and treatment programs Training for providers
Children Affected by AIDS	Emergency direct service grants Direct service grants Education grants Administration grants
M.A.C. Cosmetics	Donations to pediatric HIV/AIDS programs through their Kids Helping Kids Program Profits from Viva Glam lipsticks support AIDS organizations
Children's Hope Foundation	Serves the New York City, New Jersey, and nearby area emergency funding (applications due in the Fall) Hospital equipment and child-care necessities (available year-round) Recreational events

Helpful Web Sites

Africare – http://www.africare.org

The Elizabeth Glaser Pediatric AIDS Foundation – http://www.pedaids.org

Medicaid – http://www.hcfa.gov/

Social Security – http://www.ssa.gov

FXB Center – www.fxbcenter.org

AFXB – www.afxb.org

FXB International Training Program – www.fxbtrain.org

Kids Connect (For Kids who are HIV infected and their families) – www.kidsconnect.org

Children Affected by AIDS Foundation – http://www.caaf4kids.org/International Partnership Against HIV/ AIDS in Africa (IPAA) – http://www.unaids.org/aricapartneship/whatis.html

National Pediatric and Family HIV Resource Center – www.pedhivaids.org

Various information – www.hivpositive.com; www.thebody.com; www.hivatis.org; www.hivfiles.org

Helpful Phone Numbers

The Elizabeth Glaser Pediatric AIDS Foundation 310-314-1459

Children Affected by AIDS 310-258-0850

Children's Hope Foundation 212-233-5133

M.A.C. Cosmetics 800-611-1613 x2518

Social Security Administration 1-800-772-1213

National Pediatric and Family HIV Resource Center 1-800-362-0071

François-Xavier Bagnoud Center, Newark NJ 1-973-972-0400

services. Most private insurance companies and government programs only permit patients to be hospitalized under very specific circumstances and sometimes, for prescribed periods of time. Often, upon discharge, professionals find it difficult to offer the care that they believe a patient needs because of the constraints imposed by insurance companies and government programs. It is at this point that the family is often exposed to additional providers, such as home-care agencies. Social work involvement in discharge planning at the beginning of an admission can reduce the length of stay [12]. Social workers can assist the medical team in defining and addressing the physical, social, and emotional needs of the family during a hospital stay, and can help make plans so the plan for the patient's care continues effectively after discharge. HIV-infected children often have complicated, multi-system medical problems and a challenging social setting. Additional resources, which are optimally suited for the needs of each family and which the social worker can work to have in place, can make a significant difference for the patient and the family and can comprise an essential part of an effective therapeutic plan. Such additional resources may include a visiting nurse, health aides, and the provision of needed medical equipment and training. Children with HIV infection sometimes become heavily dependent on complicated medical technology. The staff may question the caregiver's abilities in providing highly technical services at home, such as total parenteral nutrition (TPN), tube feedings, and respiratory therapy equipment. Certain criteria must be met for some of these technologies, for example access to utilities, refrigeration, and a stable caregiver. Many caregivers who may initially appear not to be capable of delivering highly technical care frequently can if effective instruction is provided. If the parent wants to provide highly technical care at home, they can be taught and should be able to demonstrate competency prior to discharge. Repeated teaching sessions begun well in advance of discharge are frequently effective. These sessions are not only to teach the family members, but also to allow them the opportunities to gain confidence in the procedure by demonstrating their proficiency to hospital staff. An overnight stay, during which the parents are responsible for most of the child's care, is also helpful. Such a stay gives the family caregiver the opportunity to assess their abilities. Caregivers should have a back-up person for any highly technical care at home. This is sometimes difficult due to isolation or issues of secrecy. It works best when there are two people who are very knowledgeable about the treatments. Older children, cognitively above the age of 10 years, are often involved in their own care. However, they ought not be the sole providers of this care. This is particularly the case for antiretroviral therapy, because poor adherence can promote the development of resistance. Some families who are unable to cope with the situation may expect this of their child but it is not in the best interests of the child.

Upon discharge the parent should receive specific instructions and contact information should trouble develop. Such information should include instructions about filling prescriptions, the follow-up appointment, and contingency plans if the problem that resulted in the hospitalization recurs. The contact at the hospital or clinic should be available and the parent should receive instructions outlining additional back-up contacts.

45.10 Interacting with multiple agencies

Patients and their families are often uncertain what information and documentation they will be expected to provide to insurance companies and government agencies. It is helpful to provide clients with guidance regarding the information that agencies will be asking of them. Another reliable adult should keep copies of these papers. Clinics and social service agencies may also choose to keep copies of some items (with the client's permission and released with permission by the client), because this information will often be requested, for example when applying for the indigent programs of pharmaceutical companies. For those clients who are homeless, it is very helpful for them to know that their personal records are being kept safe and confidential. Following is a guideline of what may be helpful for the client to keep in a folder.

- Social Security cards
- Income tax returns
- Proof of address (this can be two items mailed to the patient).
- Birth certificates
- Legal guardianship papers
- Standby guardianship papers
- Insurance/Medicaid cards
- Rent and utility receipts.

Clients can also be educated about interviewing with various agencies. Some clients do not receive services because they are not able to ask for services in the way that the agency expects them to ask. Basics of service referrals include:

- Make sure that the services are available prior to referring clients (funding cuts may be sudden).
- Locate a contact person within frequently used agencies.
- Establish a rapport with frequently used agencies.
- Assess whether or not ongoing meetings would be useful with certain agencies to prevent duplication of services.

45.11 Working with child welfare agencies

Boyd-Franklin & Boland [10] highlight the role child welfare agencies can play in the care of HIV-infected children. First, child welfare workers provide a source of support to foster families who may be overwhelmed negotiating the many medical and social services agencies. Their services can range from concrete assistance with transportation to support with community reactions to caring for an HIV-infected child.

Child welfare agencies can be helpful in placing children when parents become unable to provide care due to the parent's deteriorating health, substance abuse, or social issues such as homelessness or inadequate housing. It is important that providers collaborate with parents around the use of child welfare services so that these interventions are not utilized in a punitive way. Even in situations where abuse or neglect is suspected, these concerns must be discussed with the parent and a plan developed in consultation with the parent. It may be that a respite placement or foster placement of a parent and child are viable options for a family.

In order to be effective, child welfare workers require ongoing education regarding the medical and psychosocial aspects of HIV infection. Disease and treatment information change rapidly. Child welfare workers need current information in order to help families make treatment decisions or provide appropriate information to superiors when the agency is legally responsible for the child's care.

45.12 Global issues in accessing care and treatment

A number of agencies and organizations are involved in addressing the global AIDS epidemic. Among these are UNICEF, the Centers for Disease Control and Prevention Global AIDS Program (CDC-GAP), United States Agency for International Development (USAID), UNAIDS, the International Partnership Against AIDS in Africa (IPAA), Association François-Xavier Bagnoud (AFXB), and the Elizabeth Glaser Pediatric AIDS Foundation (EGPAF). Each agency has a variety of global programs. In sub-Saharan Africa, prevention of mother-to-child transmission (PMTCT) represents a major focus in pediatric and family HIV. In many areas, women are able to access HIV preventive care through their antenatal clinics. In these clinics, women can receive voluntary HIV counseling and testing, education about HIV, and safer sex education. Some clinics may also offer voluntary counseling and testing to partners/husbands. (PMTCT is discussed in more detail in Chapter 8.) Ongoing primary HIV care may not be as accessible as prevention services. However, efforts are underway in some countries to extend PMTCT programs so that HIV-positive mothers and infants can receive care. IPAA, CDC-GAP, and EGPAF have been among those agencies with efforts focused on helping pregnant women access preventive care. AFXB and USAID's Food for Peace under the LIFE Initiative (Leadership and Investment in Fighting an Epidemic) for Children Affected by HIV/AIDS have dedicated resources to building capacity and infrastructure. AFXB has a program specifically dedicated to addressing the AIDS orphan crisis. It is important that providers learn about the variety of resources available to families in their area. The websites of these agencies can be accessed for substantial detail on their global efforts and resources they offer.

45.13 Putting it all together

HIV in women and children is a multi-generational family disease distinguished by a number of emotional and social issues. Many families affected by HIV/AIDS face many other severe challenges, such as poverty, homelessness, limited access to healthcare and health information, and discrimination. Coping with HIV often requires the involvement of numerous social service and healthcare systems. The multi-systems model of care provides a much-needed framework for healthcare providers to facilitate this co-ordination, limit duplication of service, and clarify the roles of various providers [10, 13].

Empowerment of families is the guiding principle of the multi-systems approach. Families are coached in understanding how various service systems can meet their needs and how to negotiate those systems. Families become active participants in developing a plan and deciding how to utilize the various services available. When a number of service systems, medical providers, or other professionals are involved with a family, it is crucial that representatives from each of those programs meet on a regular basis to update each other and clarify their roles.

The advantage of the multi-systems approach is a co-ordinated response to the myriad of socio-environmental, emotional, and medical issues faced by families living with HIV. Various needs are addressed and the family builds a strong support network. Both families and providers are empowered when service systems complement each other and all the pieces of the puzzle come together for the family. The information and resources outlined in this chapter are offered as a map to guide professionals and families through the maze of social issues, managed care, funding sources, discharge planning, and other complexities of meeting social service needs.

REFERENCES

1. Forehand, R., Steele, R., Armistead, L., Morse, E., Simon, P. & Clark, L. The Family Health Project: psychosocial adjustment

of children whose mothers are HIV infected. *J. Consult. Clin. Psychol.* **66** : 3 (1998), 513–20.

2. Geballe, S., Greundal, J. & Andiman, W. (eds.), *Forgotten Children of the AIDS Epidemic.* New Haven, CT: Yale University Press (1995).

3. Geballe, S. & Greundal, J. The crisis within the crisis: the growing epidemic of AIDS orphans. In S. Books (ed.), *Invisible Children in the Society and its Schools (Sociocultural, Political, and Historical Studies in Education).* Mahway, NJ: Lawrence Erlbaum Associates (1998), pp. 47–66.

4. Levine, C. Orphans of the HIV epidemic: unmet needs in six US cities. *AIDS* **7** (1995), S57–62.

5. Boland, M., Czarniecki, L. & Haiken, H. Providing care for HIV-infected children. In M. Stuber (ed.), *Children and AIDS.* Washington, DC: American Psychiatric Press (1992), pp. 165–81.

6. Yoos, L. Chronic childhood illness: developmental issues. *Pediatr. Nurs.* **13** (1987), 25–8.

7. Lewis, S., Haiken, H. & Hoyt, L. A psychocial perspective on long-term survivors of pediatric immunodeficiency virus infection. *J. Dev. Behav. Pediatr.* **15** (1994), S12–17.

8. Steiner, G., Boyd-Franklin, N. & Boland, M. Rational and overview of the book. In N. Boyd-Franklin, G. Steiner & M. Boland, (eds.), *Children, Families, and HIV/AIDS: Psychosocial and Therapeutic Issues.* New York: Guilford Press (1995), pp. 3–18.

9. Sherwen, L. & Storm, D. Looking toward the twenty-first century: the role of nursing research in care of children and families affected by HIV. *Nurs. Clin. N. Am.* **31** (1996), 165–78.

10. Boyd-Franklin, N. & Boland, M. A multisystems approach to service delivery for HIV/AIDS families. In N. Boyd-Franklin, G. Steiner & M. Boland (eds.), *Children, Families, and HIV/AIDS: Psychosocial and Therapeutic Issues.* New York: Guilford Press (1995), pp. 199–215.

11. Social Security Administration. Supplemental security income; determining disability for a child under age 18; interim final rules with request for comments. *Fed. Regist. (USA)* **68** (1997), 6407–32.

12. Boone, C., Coulton, C. & Keller, S. The impact of early and comprehensive social services on length of stay. *Soc. Work Health Care* **7** (1981), 1–9.

13. Boyd-Franklin, N. *Black families in Therapy: a Multisystems Approach.* New York: Guilford Press (1989).

46

Disclosure

Lori S. Wiener, Ph.D.

HIV and AIDS Malignancy Branch, National Cancer Institute, NIH, Bethesda, MD

As increasing numbers of children with perinatally acquired human immunodeficiency virus type 1 (HIV) infection are surviving to ages at which they are developmentally ready to learn their diagnosis, the management of disclosure becomes an increasingly crucial component of medical, psychological, and social care [1, 2]. Even though much more is now understood about the transmission of HIV than when AIDS was first reported, most families still keep the diagnosis a closely guarded secret.

The decision to disclose an HIV diagnosis to a child is difficult and emotion-laden. Most parents do eventually disclose the diagnosis to their child, though some families or cultures are not as open about discussing personal subjects with their children as professionals might expect [3, 4].

46.1 Parents' perspectives: reasons cited for the decision not to disclose

A child diagnosed with HIV identifies an entire family at risk of infection [5]. Following a child's positive test result, the whole family is usually tested. In just a matter of days, the family's hopes and expectations for their future together are radically altered. Parents often keep the diagnosis a secret as they worry about a negative reaction by family. They may fear the psychological effect that disclosure might have on non-infected siblings and that (if disclosed to), the infected child may not be able to keep the information confidential [6–8]. Parents often wish to preserve the innocence of childhood and avoid burdening children with the knowledge of their disease for as long as possible

[9], fearing that disclosure might result in severe depression and subsequent declines in physical health. Some parents choose to administer medication without telling the child what the medication is used for. However, as children live longer, the secrecy of the diagnosis becomes more difficult to manage [10]. Families and children may be faced with questions from school personnel about repeated absences, poor school performance, medicines, and hospitalizations. Fears associated with changes in family relationships [11] and guilt surrounding life choices and transmission may further increase a parent's hesitancy to disclose the diagnosis to a child and others [7].

While parents have cited many understandable reasons for deferring or delaying disclosure about the HIV diagnosis, research has shown that greater disclosure, in general, is related to increased social support, social self-competence, and decreased problem behavior [12]. It is also well known that a child's capacity to trust develops from his or her relationships with the parents. Postponement of disclosure and the fabrications that often accompany delayed disclosure can disturb this trust. Children sense when something is out of the ordinary and silence and secrecy can deprive them of the opportunity to explore their emotions or fears and ask relevant questions. When children are not included in this process, they may feel confused, alone, forgotten, or abandoned. When a family decides to disclose a diagnosis, they may require assistance relating the information to their child in a style that takes into account emotional development, and cognitive abilities. It is essential that all interventions related to disclosure are planned from a developmentally based understanding of children's needs.

46.2 The decision to disclose the diagnosis to an HIV-infected child: considerations

Parents' reasons for disclosing the diagnosis are frequently linked to a desire to be honest with their children. Research has shown that parents eventually disclose the diagnosis and cite the reasons for doing so as being opposed to family secrets, not wanting someone outside the family to tell the child before they did, because they felt their child had the right to know what was going on inside his/her own body [4], and due to a desire to establish additional support for their child [11].

Several factors must be taken into consideration prior to a family's decision to disclose a diagnosis of HIV. Disclosing parents should identify a supportive adult who will be available to assist the children in processing and coping with the information. Support groups, extended family members, close family friends, and social workers are very helpful in this role.

A parent's decision to discuss his or her HIV diagnosis may lead to other important disclosures, many of which may be long-kept family secrets, including the true identity of biological parents, other family members with AIDS, and facts concerning disease transmission [4]. Most parents decide that they want to tell their children in the comfort of their own home, without others present, but a social worker's offer to be present is often appreciated, especially if a parent fears becoming too upset to complete the discussion.

Timing of the disclosure is also of great importance. Careful thought should be given to the child's age, emotional development and cognitive abilities, the location of disclosure, the words used, how questions concerning transmission will be answered and plans for the future including the identification of alternative caregivers. Information must be supplied in a developmentally appropriate manner. Anticipating the child's responses along with careful planning and back-up supports will increase the chances of a more positive outcome. Once a diagnosis is disclosed, it remains disclosed forever. Parents should be made aware of all sources of support that are available to the child and the family. Information about local AIDS organizations and community agencies providing emotional and financial support may be helpful. Parents and families should be encouraged to seek help from their local communities, such as local clergy or culturally appropriate support networks.

Disclosure of a diagnosis to a child takes place best in a supportive atmosphere of co-operation between healthcare professionals and parents [4]. Accurate, simple, developmentally appropriate, yet complete explanations about the virus and medical procedures should be provided, so that the child does not perceive the required treatments as punishment. The child needs to be reassured that he or she did not cause the illness. Parents should be prepared to answer a barrage of questions ranging from the simple and innocent to the accusing, angry, and emotionally upsetting. Parents may find it helpful to first discuss disclosure with another parent who has already been through the disclosure process successfully. Role playing can help in identifying particularly challenging questions or planning answers to more difficult issues that may arise [7]. Box 46.1 outlines how to help a family throughout the disclosure process. As children asked to keep secrets tend to display more behavioral problems than children not asked to keep secrets [13], the goal of helping parents work through the issue of disclosure in order to create open and honest communication with their child will help optimize future treatment decisions and enhance the response to other challenges the patient will face during adolescence and beyond [5].

46.3 The aftermath of disclosure

Disclosure is a process. It may be days or weeks after the initial disclosure before a child has the courage to ask additional questions [7]. Some parents make the mistake of feeling so relieved about the disclosure that they prematurely view the situation as "out in the open and over," and incorrectly assume that they need never discuss the issue again. Children need to continue sharing their concerns about both the disease itself and its impact on family members. How the child or adolescent initially understands his or her disease initially will be very different from how they come to terms with their diagnosis after a major infection or the loss of a friend or family member to AIDS. Most adolescents focus more on their fear of being rejected by their friends than on their concerns of potentially dying from AIDS [5]. Social workers can help adolescents decide how to disclose their diagnosis to peers and whom to tell, including sexual partners. All healthcare providers must be prepared to answer questions about sex and child-bearing. For both children and adolescents, ongoing contact with social service agencies or on-going counseling can be immensely helpful.

46.4 Adolescent disclosure challenges

A more difficult set of issues arises when parents are reluctant to disclose the diagnosis to their HIV-infected adolescent. Typically, healthcare providers believe honesty to be

Box 46.1. The disclosure process

Step One – Preparation
- Have a meeting with the parent/caregivers involved in the decision-making process. Staff members that the family trusts should be present.
- Address the importance of disclosure and ascertain whether the family has a plan in mind. Respect the intensity of feelings about this issue. Obtain feedback on the child's anticipated response. Explore the child's level of knowledge and his or her emotional stability and maturity.
- If the family is ready to disclose, guide them in various ways of approaching disclosure (Step Two).
- If the family is not ready, encourage them to begin using words that they can build on later, such as immune problems, virus, or infection. Provide books for the family to read with the child on viruses. Strengthen the family through education and support and schedule a follow-up meeting. Let the family know that you will meet with them on a regular basis to help guide them through the disclosure process and to support the child and family after disclosure. Respect the family's timing, but strongly encourage the family not to lie to the child if he or she asks directly about having HIV, unless significant, identifiable safety concerns render the decision to disclose inadvisable. Also remind the family to avoid disclosure during an argument or in anger.

Step Two – Disclosure
- In advance, have the family think through or write out how they want the conversation to go. They need to give careful consideration to what message they want their child to walk away with. Encourage the family to begin with "Do you remember . . .," to include information about the child's life, medications, and/or procedures so that the child is reminded of past events before introducing new facts.
- Have the family choose a place where the child will be most comfortable to talk openly.
- Provide the family with questions the child may ask so they are prepared with answers. Such questions include "How long have you known this?" "Who else has the virus?", "Will I die?"; "Can I ever have children?"; "Who can I tell?"; "Why me?"; and "Who else knows?"
- Encourage having present only the people with whom the child is most comfortable. The healthcare provider may offer to facilitate this meeting, but if at all possible, preparation should be done in advance so that the family can share the information on their own.
- Medical facts should be kept to a minimum (immunology, virology, the effectiveness of therapy) and hope should be reinforced. Silence as well as questions need to be accepted. The child should be told that nothing has changed except a name is now being given to what they have been living with. The child also needs to hear that they didn't do or say anything to cause the disease and that their family will always remain by their side.
- If the diagnosis is to be kept a secret, it is important that the child is given the names of people they can talk to, such as a healthcare provider, another child living with HIV, and/or a family friend. Stating, "You can't tell anyone," makes the child feel ashamed and guilty.
- Provide the child with a journal or diary to record their questions, thoughts, and feelings. If appropriate, provide books about children living with HIV.
- Schedule a follow-up meeting.

Step Three – After Disclosure
- Provide individual and family follow-up 2 weeks after disclosure and again every 2–4 weeks for the first 6 months to assess impact of disclosure, answer questions, and to help foster support between the child and family.
- Ask the child to tell you what they have learned about their virus. This way misconceptions can be clarified. Writing and art may be useful techniques.
- Assess changes in emotional well-being and provide the family with information about symptoms that could indicate the need for more intensive intervention.
- Support parents for having disclosed the diagnosis and, if interested and available, refer them to a parents' support group. Encourage them to think about the emotional needs of the other children in the family in the disclosure process.
- Remind parents that disclosure is not a one time event. Ongoing communication will be needed. Ask parents what other supports they feel would be helpful to them and their child. Provide information about HIV camp programs for HIV infected and affected youth.

the best policy, and most will support and encourage parents to disclose the diagnosis of HIV infection to their children as early as is possible and practical. In cases where parents refuse to do so, numerous ethical issues arise. Doctors may feel that a teenager deserves to know the truth about HIV treatments and medical regimens. A high percentage of HIV-infected adolescents are sexually active, and parents may be unaware of this. HIV-infected adolescents need to know that by engaging in sex, they place their partner(s) at risk of infection and that having sex with someone without informing them of the HIV infection raises enormous moral concerns and can, in some jurisdictions, subject them to potential criminal penalties. They also need to be educated about the use of safe sexual practices, should they choose to have sex.

Social support and open communication about the diagnosis are essential, particularly at an age at which decisions about relationships, sexual activity, drug use, and plans for the future are the focus of adolescent development and individuation [12]. The longer an adolescent goes without learning the truth about the diagnosis, the more mistrustful they become of the healthcare provider, of the medical system, and of their parents. Many hospitals and other healthcare organizations have bioethicists, social work staff, and counselors who can help orient the parents to the legal and ethical consequences of withholding a diagnosis.

46.5 Disclosure to the school

Parents are often concerned about whether they need to inform the child's school personnel of the diagnosis. Healthcare providers can assist the family in researching the school's HIV policy and advise the family. They can also help parents anticipate the responses of school administrators and other parents while building supports for the child. While negative events can occur stemming from peer fear and ignorance, most children have found compassion, sympathy, and support from their teachers. The range of potential reactions to disclosure needs to be discussed openly and honestly with the parent(s), child, teachers, and principal.

46.6 Challenges for the healthcare provider

The majority of parents struggle for years prior to disclosing the diagnosis of HIV infection to their child. They also rely on the healthcare provider for guidance and support. It is the issue of disclosure itself that initially brings most parents to seek mental health services [7]. A comprehensive psychosocial assessment identifying each family's strengths and vulnerabilities is essential in providing support to HIV-infected children and families [5]. Such a tool will allow a healthcare team to best anticipate psychological, social, and concrete needs of the family, as well as assist them in planning appropriate interventions [5]. It is equally important for healthcare providers to be aware of circumstances when disclosure is not advisable. A very young child can not understand the meaning of the diagnosis and should not be expected to comprehend the seriousness of their situation. A parent who is emotionally unstable, experiencing significant anger or guilt about the infection, in a crisis, or unprepared to allow ongoing discussions about the virus to occur should not be encouraged to disclose at that time. Some children are not able to keep information confidential. In such circumstances, where disclosure of the diagnosis could lead to serious financial, social, societal, or even physical threats to the family, disclosure should be delayed until a time when the family's well-being will not be jeopardized or the child is developmentally capable of keeping the information to him or herself.

Many families have inaccurate or dated perceptions about HIV. Providing children and families with accurate, up-to-date information about HIV transmission, new treatments, and the improved prognosis can help provide significant hope and encouragement. Promoting awareness about confidentiality anti-discrimination laws and legislation pertaining to custody, guardianship, the rights of foster parents, and medical decisions are all important aspects of guiding the family throughout the disclosure process and in providing effective care to the HIV-infected child [7].

The issue of disclosure strikes at the heart of all persons infected and affected by HIV-1. Specific issues related to disclosure are most challenging in resource-poor countries where the burden of HIV-1 infection is greatest. In such countries, such as in sub-Saharan Africa, the stigma associated with HIV infection is so great, that women cite refusing to disclose the diagnosis to anyone due to fear of discrimination, and domestic violence or divorce [14, 15]. All families, regardless of location, could benefit from intensive and culturally sensitive counseling and supportive intervention programs around prevention of mother-to-child HIV-1 transmission, disclosure, and treatment options and availability.

REFERENCES

1. Abrams, E. J. & Nicholas, S. W. Pediatric HIV infection. *Pediatr. Ann.* **19** : **8** (1990), 482–3, 485–7.

2. Lipson, M. Disclosure within families. *AIDS Clin. Care* **5** (1993), 43–4.

3. Melvin, D. Don't forget the children: families living with HIV infection. In L. Bennett (ed.), *AIDS as a Gender Issue: Psychosocial Perspectives. Social Aspects of AIDS.* London: Taylor & Francis (1997), pp. 215–34.

4. Wiener, L. S., Battles, H. B., Heilman, N., Sigelman, C. K. & Pizzo, P. A. Factors associated with disclosure of diagnosis to children with HIV/AIDS. *Pediatr. AIDS HIV Infect.* **7**:**5** (1996), 310–24.

5. Wiener, L., Septimus, A. & Grady, C. Psychological support and ethical issues for the child and family. In C. Wilfert (ed.), *Pediatric AIDS: The Challenge of HIV Infection in Infants, Children, and Adolescents*, 3rd edn. Philadelphia: Lippincott, Williams & Wilkins (1998), pp. 703–27.

6. Olsen, R., Huszti, H., Mason, P. & Seibert, J. Pediatric AIDS/HIV infection: an emergency challenge to pediatric psychology. *J. Pediatr. Psychol.* **14** (1989), 1–21.

7. Wiener, L. Helping a parent with HIV tell his or her children. In B. Thompson (ed.), *HIV and Social Work: A Practitioner's Guide.* Binghamton, NY: Haworth Press (1998), pp. 327–38.

8. Wiener, L., Fair, C. & Garcia, A. HIV/AIDS: pediatric. In J. Hopps (ed.), *Encyclopedia of Social Work*, 19th edn. Washington, DC: NASW Press (1995), pp. 1314–24

9. Tasker, M. *How Can I Tell You?* Washington, DC: Association of the Care of Children's Health (1992).

10. Lewis, S. Y., Haiken, H. J. & Hoyt, L. G. Living beyond the odds: a psychosocial perspective on long-term survivors of pediatric human immunodeficiency virus infection. *J. Dev. Behav. Pediatr.* **15**:**3** (1994), S12–17.

11. DeMatteo, D., Wells, L. M., Salter G. R. & King, S. M. The 'family' context of HIV: a need for comprehensive health and social policies. *AIDS Care* **14**:**2** (2002), 261–78.

12. Battles, H. B. & Wiener, L. S. From adolescence through young adulthood: psychosocial adjustment associated with long-term survival of HIV. *J. Adolesc. Health* **30**:**3** (2002), 161–8.

13. Kirshenbaum, S. B. & Nevid, J. S. The specificity of maternal disclosure of HIV/AIDS in relation to children's adjustment. *AIDS Educ. Prev.* **14**:**1** (2002), 1–16.

14. Kilewo, C., Massawe, A., Lyamuya, E. *et al.* HIV counseling and testing of pregnant women in sub-Saharan Africa: experiences from a study on prevention of mother-to-child HIV-1 transmission in Dar es Salaam, Tanzania. *J. AIDS* **28**:**5** (2001), 458–62.

15. Ladner, J., Leroy, V., Msellati, P. *et al.* A cohort study of factors associated with failure to return for HIV post-test counselling in pregnant women: Kigali, Rwanda, 1992–1993. AIDS **10**:**1** (1996), 69–75.

47

Psychosocial factors associated with childhood bereavement and grief

Lori S. Wiener, Ph.D.

HIV and AIDS Malignancy Branch, National Cancer Institute, NIH, Bethesda, MD

While recent advances in the treatment of HIV disease have resulted in dramatic reductions in morbidity and mortality in the USA [1], in many countries in the Far East and parts of Africa, the aftermath of high AIDS-related mortality has moved the HIV/AIDS epidemic beyond a health crisis. Disruptions to work patterns caused by absenteeism due to illness and funerals, the lack of physical space in morgues and burial grounds, reach deep into everyday life, and are a constant reminder of the fatal nature of this disease [2]. Populations are trying to exist in a state of daily and ongoing loss.

The number of individuals who have lost friends, parents, children, and other family members remains vast. For each individual infected with the disease, many more are affected by the loss associated with HIV/AIDS, including children, parents, siblings, and caregivers. Individuals vary greatly in ways that they cope with loss and death, depending on their attachment to the deceased, their past experiences of death, and their developmental stage.

Bereavement is one of the most frequent and potent life stressors occurring to individuals infected with or affected by HIV [3]. Bereavement related to HIV differs from grief related to other chronic illnesses mainly in that those affected by the epidemic are typically exposed to multiple losses over a relatively short period of time, decreasing the likelihood that there will be adequate time to process and mourn the loss prior to the next death. One of the most potent barriers to successful mourning is the social stigma related to this disease [4]. In fact, the unique social context in which these losses take place must be considered in order to understand the potential mental health consequences.

The term disenfranchised grief, was defined by Doka [5] as the grief that persons experience when they incur a loss that is not or cannot be openly acknowledged. HIV/AIDS is still a stigmatized disease and as a result, most people keep the diagnosis and losses suffered a secret. When a parent, for example, loses a child to AIDS, people may believe that the child died of something else. Consequently, the family finds themselves further embedded in lies at a time when they most need to openly share their grief. Distancing and unsupportive bereavement-related social interactions have been found to contribute to depression in people who have experienced AIDS-related multiple loss [6]. Hospital personnel, who provide enormous support for the child and family during a child's illness, may no longer be available. This leaves the parent with few opportunities to receive bereavement support. Many communities have limited sources of support for people living with HIV/AIDS. The burden of secrecy and emotional isolation further complicates the bereavement and subsequent healing process.

The grieving process may begin at the time of HIV diagnosis and is referred to as *anticipatory grief* [7]. People with HIV experience a wide range of losses other than the imminence of death [8], including the loss of certainty, hopes for the future, relationships, health, control, sexual desirability and body image, accustomed lifestyle, status, dignity, privacy, and security. Chronic illness, in and of itself, is often experienced as a loss as it is often marked by feelings of varying degrees of sadness related to the fact that as of yet, no cure exists. The legal, financial, stigmatizing, and emotional factors that surround the disease further complicate AIDS-related deaths.

There is no single portrait of a grieving child from an HIV-infected family. Children living in HIV-infected families are of all ages, cultural backgrounds, and races [9]. The majority of these children have already experienced the burdens of poverty, seen the effects of substance abuse and violence, and endured many other types of loss and trauma in their families [10]. Death of a family member is often one more destabilizing factor.

47.1 Loss in childhood

Each year, millions of children throughout the world experience the death of a parent, grandparent or other close relative [11]. Often, adults strive to hide their true feelings about death in an effort to protect their children. This is not an effort to exclude the child, but rather, the result of not knowing how to assist their child with the emotional impact of the death of a loved one.

Each child's experience of grief varies dramatically, based on the developmental stage and the information shared with the child. Children should be made aware of family illnesses; hiding an illness is often more frightening for children than the truth, and may complicate the grieving process. However, AIDS-related grieving presents unique challenges, especially concerning issues surrounding disclosure (see Chapter 46). Many HIV-infected parents remain ambivalent about informing their children and the rest of the family. Many parents do not wish to disclose a diagnosis of HIV in order to protect their child and to allow as normal and as happy a childhood as possible. Parents fear children's reactions to the news and fear the reactions of other family members and the general public. (See Chapter 46 for a discussion of the psychosocial issues of disclosing the diagnosis of HIV infection.) After a parent discloses the news, children will begin to struggle with fears about a parent's or their own death. This is an appropriate time to begin discussions about the fatal nature of the disease in terms that reflect the age, cognitive ability, coping style, and developmental stage of the child. Pennells & Smith [11] review age-related grief reactions, which are summarized in Box 47.1.

47.2 Social and emotional development as a factor

Young children experience the loss of a loved one, but do not understand the permanence of that loss, and continue to seek the presence of the deceased. The experience of death may cause feelings of insecurity and instability. A child may cry, yearn for the deceased, become clingy, and make attempts at reunion with the deceased when playing [12]. Parents or elders mistakenly substantiate this belief/misconception by explaining death in terms of sleeping. For children between the ages of 5–9, death often elicits fear and fantasy behaviors. Feelings of guilt or responsibility for their loved one's death is common. At this age, children manifest an almost morbid curiosity about rituals surrounding death and about the function of dead bodies. For children between the ages of 9–12, the finality and irreversibility of death is understood and they begin to fear their own death. Children grieve in a manner similar to adults at this stage, and may attempt to deny their overwhelming feelings of loss in an effort to "get on with life." Adolescents are capable of grieving as adults do, with appropriate crying, feelings of remorse and loss, anger and depression. They may question their own identity and the meaning of life. Periods of social isolation can occur, as peers are uncertain how to respond to a grieving friend. The death may cause an adolescent to feel painfully different from his/her peers. Role changes can occur as well, as the adolescent assumes increased responsibility around the home. A journal, which allows the adolescent to record memories, feelings, and hopes for the future, is almost always beneficial.

47.3 Grief in children who lose a parent

For any child, the loss of a parent is devastating and has long-lasting effects. When a youngster faces the loss of multiple family members, the impact stretches for years into the future. Parental loss brings with it uncertainty, instability, mistrust, isolation, feelings of abandonment and fear of the future [8]. For many, the stable family environment never existed at all, and there may be serious concerns of who will care for them now.

In the USA, the majority of children infected with HIV are from communities of color [13], live in deteriorating urban centers, and as a result of poverty and/or substance abuse, have limited access to or poor medical resources, and few social supports. Coupled together, these factors lead to a compromising environment for children who are already vulnerable to numerous stresses. Their disease doubly affects children whose families endure both HIV/AIDS as well as the aforementioned stresses and deprivations [4]. Most children who have lost a parent to AIDS have also lost multiple members of their families to drug addiction, violence, incarceration, and suicide. Helping restore these children's ability to invest in emotional relationships without excessive fear of future losses is one of the greatest challenges to working with them [14].

Box 47.1. When children grieve: developmental considerations

0–2 Years
- The child will seek the presence of the deceased person and will experience a loss, but does not have the capabilities to understand the permanence of that loss. They cannot comprehend the word "forever."

2–5 Years
- Experience of death at this age may cause the child's world to feel unsafe and unpredictable.
- Reactions may include tearfulness, temper tantrums, clinginess, bed-wetting, and sleep problems.
- In play, they may make attempts to reunite with the deceased person.
- Child may still believe that death is reversible . . . simple, repeated explanations that the deceased person cannot come back to life are needed.
- If a child is terminally ill, their greatest fears are associated with separation from their loved ones.

5–9 Years
- Children have a wider social network at this point and consequently, children are more sensitive to other people's reactions, remarks from peers, etc.
- Children are learning who they can trust with their feelings.
- They are watching adults' reactions to grief and will sometimes deny their own grief in order to protect an adults' feelings.
- They have a greater awareness of guilt and may feel they were responsible for the death by illogical reasoning (i.e. "Mommy died yesterday because I was naughty the night before").
- This is also the age of fear and fantasy and the child may personalize death as a monster, boogie man, etc.
- Children think more logically about death and begin to focus on rituals surrounding death and about the functions of dead bodies, such as do they need clothes and food.
- If the child is terminally ill, they often question "Why me?," they may feel they have done something wrong to deserve their illness and subsequent death, and frequently have a difficult time accepting that they are truly going to die.

9–12 Years
- Child is aware of the finality of death and that death is common to all living things.
- Child may become fearful of his/her own death, which may cause psychosomatic symptoms to appear.
- The child is grieving more like an adult at this point and may try to deny feeling a sense of loss in order to just try to "get on with life."
- The terminally ill child is responsive to honest discussions (though it is still difficult to accept), to being included in decision-making, and responds to open and honest discussions about what will be happening to their bodies.

Adolescence
- Adolescents are able to grieve more like adults do, with appropriate crying, sadness, confusion, somatic complaints, anger, denial of feelings and/or depression.
- These powerful emotions may lead them to question their identity and the meaning of life.
- Interest in the occult, afterlife, and the rites of different cultures are not uncommon.
- They may feel social pressure to take on more responsibility and find themselves fulfilling the deceased parents' household duties.
- Members of the adolescent's peer group may not know how to handle the bereavement of one of their friends, leading to a sense of isolation for the bereaved adolescent.
- The terminally ill adolescent often has great difficulty with the physical assaults that the illness has on their body, and has a great need to feel in control of medical decisions. Tendencies to withdraw or reach out to others prior to death reflect how they responded to other stresses in their life prior to their illness.

What do bereaved children need?
- Adults who can respond to them with genuine caring, understanding, warmth, and empathy.
- Children should be told about death in a language appropriate for their age and development stage.

- Try to create opportunities for them to acquire knowledge and a vocabulary about death.
- Euphemisms and ambiguous answers are not helpful.
- Children need to be involved in the family's grieving process as much as possible and invited to express their feelings.
- Children need help understanding contradictions in the way people talk about death (i.e. "Mommy is happier in Heaven;" "Your sister is asleep now and will be watching over you").
- Children need reassurance that their world has not disintegrated.
- Children need help to deal with anticipated additional losses (if other family members are also HIV-infected), secondary losses, such as new care providers, house moves, or a parent remarrying.
- It is important to keep the memory of the deceased person alive.
- One cannot replace the loss though it is important to also provide seeds of hope for a future with less emotional pain.

47.4 Grief in children who lose a sibling

The childhood sibling bond has the potential of lasting longer than any other familial relationship [15] and when a sibling dies, the surviving child's sense of abandonment is not unusual. If the surviving child is also HIV-infected, the death of a sibling can be a particularly frightening event, as his/her own mortality must be faced. For an uninfected child, losing a sibling may bring a complex mixture of feelings ranging from relief, to sorrow and guilt. A child may feel relieved that family circumstances may return to normal, followed by severe guilt for feeling this way or for escaping infection. Children who are not infected may have suffered from lack of attention. Professionals must be especially attentive to the previous losses experienced and the sibling's, as well as the family's reaction to the illness and death. One must question whether the sibling's HIV-infected mother has already died, or if the sibling anticipates this loss or others as well, and whether the child knows who will be the caregiver if the parent dies (see Box 47.1). Age-appropriate information should be shared with the child, permanency plans made, and a support system identified swiftly and with compassion [16]. Support groups as well as individual counseling can also be of assistance in alleviating some of the fears and concerns that children may experience. A list of national support groups available for affected children can be found in Box 47.2.

47.5 Recommendations for assisting grieving children

Clinicians need to explain death in simple, easy to understand, and developmentally appropriate language. Ambiguity and euphemisms are not helpful. Children should be encouraged and given permission to take an active part in the grief process. Children must be reassured that their whole world has not been shattered, and they need help to deal with additional anticipated losses and secondary losses such as re-location of family due to moving, new care providers, new school, or a parent re-marrying. It is useful to learn how the child understands and how that understanding evolves. Adults should be prepared to answer any questions openly and directly. Understanding and utilizing the strengths of each child's spiritual beliefs, rituals, and community is essential. It is important that caregivers communicate with the child about any matter of importance in a language that the child understands well and in which the child is comfortable.

It is not uncommon for children to alternate between periods of mourning and periods of refusing to acknowledge the loss and pain [17]. It is natural for a child to avoid discussing a parent's death soon after the event, and denial or disinterest may be manifest in their behavior. When a child exhibits certain signs or symptoms, referrals to a bereavement specialist may be warranted (see Box 47.3). Many behaviors may not appear for one to several years after the death. Box 47.4 provides a guideline of appropriate questions when interviewing bereaved children.

The way the surviving parent or relative responds to the child, the availability of social support, and subsequent life circumstances can influence whether a child develops problems [18]. Increased risk of developing behavioral problems is associated with a lack of continuity in the child's daily life after the death of a parent [19]. Numerous variables will influence this outcome, including how close a child is to either parent and the stability or instability of the child's home environment leading up to and surrounding the circumstances of the death. Maternal loss may have a more profound effect on a child than paternal loss [18]. In children as well as adults, death is not merely the loss of a person, but a dramatic change in a way of life [16].

Box 47.2. National resources

Camp Heartland
1845 N. Farwell Ave.
Milwaukee, WI 53202

Centering Corporation
1531 N. Saddle Creek Rd
Omaha, NE 68104
http://www.centering.org

Center for Grieving Children and Teenagers
819 Massachusetts Ave. Arlington
Massachusetts 02476
http://www.childrensroom.org

Center for Grief Recovery
Southern Human Services
1700 West Irving Park Road
Chicago, IL 60613

Children's Hospice International
901 North Pitt St.
Alexandria, VA 22314

Compassionate Friends
P.O. Box 3693
Oakbrook, IL 60522-3696
http://www.compassionatefriends.org

Dougy Center
3909 SE 52nd
Portland, OR 97206
http://www.dougy.org

Fernside: A Center for Grieving Children
P.O. Box 8944
Cincinnati, OH 45208
http://www.fernside.org

Resources on the Internet

Beareavement and Hospice Support Netline
http://www.hospiceslo.org/links.htm

DyingWell.org
www.dyingwell.org

Growth House
http://www.growthhouse.org

Hospice Foundation of America
http://www.hospicefoundation.org

Journey Program
c/o Children's Hospital
4800 Sand Point Way
Seattle, WA 98103

Kids Grieve Too
451 SW 10th St.
Renton, WA 98055
www. allkidsgrieve.org

The Children's Legacy
P.O. Box 300305
Denver, CO 80203

National Childhood Grief Institute
3300 Edinborough Way, Suite 512
Minneapolis, MN 55435

National Pediatric and Family HIV
Resource Center
University of Medicine & Dentistry of NJ
15 South 9th Street
Newark, NJ 07107
http://www.thebody.com/nphrc/nphrcpage.html

The Good Grief Program
Judge Baker Guidance Center
295 Longwood Avenue
Boston, MA 02115
http://www.bmc.org/pediatrics/special/GoodGrief/
overview.html

Wendt Center for Loss and Healing
730 11th St., NW
Washington, DC 20001

National Association for Home Care
http://www.nahc.org

The Association for Death Education and Counseling
http://www.adec.org

Box 47.3. Indicators that the child may need to be referred for professional help

- Persistent anxiety about their own death
- Changes in appetite or sleep patterns
- Destructive outbursts, self-destructive behavior, acting-out (including attempts to become HIV-infected themselves)
- Threats of hurting oneself or others
- Compulsive care giving
- Euphoria
- Unwillingness to speak about the deceased person (especially if a conflicted relationship existed)
- Expression of only positive or only negative feelings about the deceased person
- Inability or unwillingness to form new relationships
- Daydreaming – resulting in poor academic performance
- Stealing or hoarding household items
- Excessive separation anxiety and/or school phobia
- Withdrawal from peers or previously enjoyable activities
- Sudden unexplained change in behavior, attitude, or mood

Box 47.4. Interview questions of a school-age child or adolescent whose parent or sibling has died

Relationship with deceased
1. Can you tell me a little something about [cite person's name]?
2. What was your relationship like with [cite person's name]?
3. What kind of things did you do together?
4. Can you tell me a little something about [cite person's name] death?
5. Were you there? (If not) what had you heard?
6. Did you realize that [cite person's name] was sick enough to die?
7. Had you known that [cite person's name] had HIV/AIDS?
8. If yes, when had you learned this information?
9. Who told you?
10. What was your response when you first learned this?
11. Were you able to share this with anyone else?
12. Who knew the truth about [cite person's name] illness?
13. Does anyone else in your family have HIV/AIDS?
14. (If the child is not also HIV-infected) Are you concerned that you might have HIV/AIDS?
15. Before [cite person's name] died, were you able to tell him (her) the things you wanted to say?
16. (If no) What happened that you weren't able to say the things you wanted to say?
17. Is there anything that you wanted to do together that you didn't have a chance to do?
18. Do you have anything of [cite person's name] that you hold on to?
19. (If yes). Can you tell me about them?

Adjustment after death
20. I have talked to many other children who had a [cite relative's relationship to the child] die, and some of them are worried that they might have done something to cause the death. Does this worry you?
21. (If yes). Tell me about how this worries you.
22. Since [cite person's name] died, what has life been like for you?
23. What has life been like for your family (go through each significant person individually) since [cite person's name] died?

24. Other children have told me that sometimes when something bad like this happens, other things are also not going well for them either at school or at home. Has anything else not been going well for you?
25. (If yes) tell me about (each one).
26. Have you been through any other bad times like this before?
27. (If yes). Tell me about them – what helped you get through those times?
28. Tell me about your friends. (Trying to get a sense of quality of relationships and how these might have changed since the death).
29. Now can you tell me about how you have been eating?
30. And sleeping? Has your sleeping changed? (If yes) Tell me about how it has changed. (Also get a sense of the kind of dreams he or she is having).
31. Tell me about your teacher(s). Do they know about [cite person's name] death? The nature of [cite person's name] illness?
32. How are you doing with your schoolwork? Homework? Grades?
33. Have you been seeing a doctor for any health problems of your own?
34. (If yes) Tell me about that.
35. Do you think about dying too?
36. (If yes) What do you think about? (If they are suicidal, do an assessment for suicide risk).
37. Is there something else that I haven't asked about?
38. Is there anything else you think I should know about how you are getting along?
39. (If yes). Tell me about that.
40. Do you have any questions that you would like to ask me?
41. (If yes) Go ahead.
42. Thank-you for talking to me. If you have any questions or if you want to talk to me at any time, here is my card.

Source: Adapted from [35]

Children try to maintain the relationship with the parent they have lost. Memorializing the person who died continues throughout an entire life [20]. Assisting the child to remember and maintain a connection to the deceased parent is important, and helps the child to express emotions that are difficult to voice. Memory books and videotapes are effective tools in assisting bereaved individuals to remember their loved ones, validate their life together, and understand past events.

47.6 Adult grief – grief in parents who lose a child to HIV/AIDS

Grief in adults usually consists of the passage through various stages identified by several theorists including Kubler-Ross [21] and Worden [22]. These stages can vary significantly but most grieving adults experience shock, denial, anger, bargaining, depression, and finally, acceptance.

The period immediately prior to the death of a child is often confusing and overwhelming. One of the most important aspects of assisting families at this stage is to allow them to enjoy the remaining time left with their child [23]. Healthcare providers should encourage families to decide where the child's final days will be spent and whether

or not drastic measures to prolong life will be employed. Help may be required to plan and pay for funeral arrangements.

The loss of a child is a devastating and life-altering experience. Parents often feel guilty at what they believe to be "failure" to save their child and the circumstances surrounding their infection. Some HIV-infected parents describe a sense of relief that they lived long enough to care for and comfort their child. Others cannot tolerate living without their child and do not pursue treatment for themselves.

Extensive literature on parental bereavement shows a high incidence of difficulties in parental emotional adjustment. Grieving parents may experience strained marital relationships, difficulties with surviving siblings, and unresolved grief. Survivors often manifest serious medical problems, including hypertension, ulcers, somatic complaints, colitis, and obesity [24, 25]. For parents who are themselves HIV-infected, it is important to differentiate these symptoms from manifestations of HIV disease. Many require psychiatric intervention following the death of a child [24, 26]. Factors associated with better adjustment include family participation in the care of a child, open discussion with the infected child about the illness and the dying process, a strong marital relationship, and ongoing contact with the healthcare team [27]. Feeling as if one was able to care for, comfort (physically, emotionally, and spiritually), and communicate openly with the dying child positively affects the grief process.

47.7 Grief in parents who die before their child(ren)

One of the most difficult aspects of the illness for parents who face the inevitability of dying before their children is the realization that they may not see their children grow to adulthood. Acknowledging that someone else will have to care for his or her children is often described as too painful to bear. Including children in future planning and open discussions about their wishes may assist the parent and the child. This is important for both practical and emotional reasons (see Chapter 48). Children want desperately to hold onto any part of their parent. Helping parents to create and leave concrete legacies for their children, in the form of letters or series of essays, life review books, drawings, audiotapes, portraits, or even videotapes or home movies is often therapeutic for the parent and especially helpful to the surviving child(ren) [28, 29].

47.8 Grandparents

Many grandparents have become the primary caretakers of two generations and they may witness the illness and eventual death of both their children and their grandchildren. A feeling of overload and overwhelming grief is common. Grandparents need a great deal of support, guidance, and education about HIV disease in dealing with the losses they will be forced to encounter. Many express the sentiment that they have already raised their children, and feel resentful that they are now forced to take on the responsibilities of raising a new generation. Through a sensitive response, with individual, community, and group support, financial aid, and the availability of in-home support and respite care, these individuals can carry on their responsibilities while working through the painful consequences of AIDS and multiple deaths [30].

47.9 Caregiver's own grief

Loss and grief may be a frequent and painful experience for the professional caregiver working in the field of HIV/AIDS. Burnout becomes an issue as workers are faced with multiple deaths and little hope of an imminent cure in the chronically ill population. Just as the grief process may begin for the patient and family at the time of diagnosis, the same process may begin for the provider as well [7]. Some clinicians harbor unrealistic expectations concerning their

ability to affect the disease course. This feeling is exacerbated when the patient is a child. Whole families may, in fact, succumb to the disease, leading to "bereavement overload." Unresolved bereavement, also coined "complicated mourning" by Rondo [31], can pose a significant risk for the development of adverse health outcomes ranging from emotional distress (e.g. depression) to somatic disorder (e.g. insomnia), and even death (e.g. by suicide). Following consecutive, and often overlapping losses, healthcare professionals, along with the patients and families who are cared for, are at risk for bereavement overload and complicated mourning [32, 33]. Balancing identification, personal investment, and emotional detachment is not possible for every practitioner. Individuals working with HIV/AIDS may also be overwhelmed by the psychosocial needs of infected children and families. Simultaneously facing the illness and eventual death of a parent and child, while dealing with the needs of other family members can be exceedingly difficult and may, at times, seem to offer little in the way of rewarding experiences [34]. It is essential that staff focus on each family's unique strengths, draw on the resources available within their healthcare team, and recognize their own need for support. While HIV is more of a chronic disease today than an imminently fatal one, healthcare providers must also be attuned to the difficulty some people experience accepting hopeful news about a disease for which they have lost significant people in their lives. Those who have lost loved ones to AIDS need to know that their grief will not be forgotten [35].

47.10 Conclusion

Even though therapy has greatly improved, the losses associated with AIDS will be with us for some time to come. Several interventions can assist families through the grief process. One must remember that bereavement is not a state that ends at a certain point or from which one recovers [20]. Children need to express their emotions and have a clear understanding of what has happened. Keepsakes, rituals, and other methods of preserving legacies are of utmost importance. Keeping in touch with the family after the death, especially on anniversaries, birthdays, and holidays is greatly appreciated. Positive bereavement-related social support and social interactions could help reduce depression in individuals who have suffered multiple losses [6]. Lastly, helping the bereaved to continue on with life and planning for the future is important for the healing process. Although the emotional losses are significant, the rewards of helping a child and family beyond their grief are even greater. Many other additional resources may be helpful for children and families coping with grief. Table 47.1 lists

Table 47.1 Books and Reading Materials for Parents, Children and Professionals

Children's books

Agee, J. *A Death in the Family*. New York: Bantam, 1969. Blackburn, L. B. *The Class in Room 44: When a Classmate Dies*. Omaha, NE: Centering Corporation, 1991.

Bartoli, J., Nonna. New York: Harvey House, Inc., 1975.

Brack, P. & Brack, B. *Moms Don't Get Sick*. Aberdeen, SD Melius Publishing, Inc., 1990.

Braithwaite, A. *When Uncle Bob Died*. London: Dinosaur Publications, 1982.

Bratman, F. *Everything You Need to Know When a Parent Dies*. New York: Rosen Group, 1992.

Buscaglia, L. *The Fall of Freddie the Leaf*. New Jersey: Charles B. Slack Inc., 1982.

De Paola, T. A. *Nana Upstairs and Nana Downstairs*. New York: Penguin, 1973.

Coerr, E. Sadako and the Thousand Paper Cranes. New York: Dell Publishing, 1977.

Crawford, C. P. *Three-Legged Race*. New York: Harper & Row, 1974.

Donahue, M. The Grandpa Tree. Boulder, Co: Robert Rinehart, Publishers, 2000.

Draimin, B. H. *Coping When a Parent Has AIDS*. New York: Rosen Group, 1993.

Fitzgerald, H. *The Grieving Teen: A Guide for Teenagers and Their Friends*, 2000.

Girard, L. W. *Alex, the Kid with AIDS*. Morton Grove, Illinois: Albert Whitman and Co., 1991.

Gootman, M. E. *When a Friend Dies*. Minneapolis: Free Spirit Publishing, 1994.

Greene, C. C. *Beat the Turtle Drum*. New York: Viking, 1976.

Grollman, E. A. *Straight Talk About Death for Teenagers: How to Cope with Losing Someone You Love*, Boston, MA: Beacon Press, 1993.

Hichman, M. *Last Week My Brother Anthony Died*. Nashville, TN: Abingdon, 1983.

Holms, C. D. *Red Balloons, Fly High!* Warminster, PA: mar*co products, inc. 1997.

Johnson J. & Johnson, M. *Where's Jess?* Omaha, NE: Centering Corporation, 1982.

Jordan, M. Losing Uncle Tim. Morton Grove, Illinois: Albert Whitman and Co., 1989.

Krementz, J. *How It Feels When A Parent Dies*. New York: Knopf, 1981.

Lee, V. *The Magic Moth*. New York: Seabury Press, 1972.

Linn, E. *Children Are Not Paper Dolls: A Visit with Bereaved Children*. Incline Village, NV: Publishers Mark, 1982.

McNamara, J. W. *My Mom is Dying: A Child's Diary*. Minneapolis: Augsburg Fortress, 1994.

Mellonie, B. & Ingpen, R. *Lifetimes: The Beautiful Way to Explain Death to Children*. New York: Bantam, 1983.

Merrifield, M. *Come Sit by Me*. Toronto, Canada: Woman's Press, 1990.

Miles, M. *Annie and the Old One*. Boston: Little Brown, 1971.

Peterkin, A. *What About Me? When Brothers and Sisters Get Sick*. New York: Magination Press, 1992.

Powell, E. S. *Geranium Morning*. Minneapolis: Carolrhoda Books, 1990.

Richter, E. *Losing Someone You Love*. New York: Putnam, 1986.

Rofes, E. *The Kids' Book About Death and Dying*. Boston: Little, Brown, 1985.

Sanders, P. *Let's Talk About Death and Dying*. London: Aladdin Books, 1990.

Shriver, M. *What's Heaven?* Golden Books Publishing Co, 1999.

Sims, A. M. *Am I Still a Sister?* Slidell, Louisiana: Big A & Company / Starline Printing, Inc., 1986.

Starkman, N. *Z's Gift*. Seattle: Comprehensive Health Education Foundation, 1988.

Stiles, N. I'll miss you Mr. Hooper. New York: Random House, 1984.

Varley, S. *The Badger's Parting Gifts*. Mulberry Books, 1992.

Vigna, J. *Saying Goodbye to Daddy*. Morton Grove, Illinois: Albert Whitman and Co., 1991.

Viorst, J. *The Tenth Good Thing About Barney*. New York: Atheneum, 1971.

White, E. B. *Charlotte's Web*. New York: Harper and Row, 1952.

Wiener, L.; Best, A. & Pizzo, P. *Be A Friend: Children Who Live With HIV Speak*. Morton Grove, Illinois: Albert Whitman and Co., 1994.

Williams, M. *The Velveteen Rabbit*. Garden City, NY: Doubleday, 1971.

Zim, H.; Bleeker, S. *Life and Death*. New York: Morrow, 1970.

(cont.)

Table 47.1 (*cont.*)

Books for siblings

Alexander, S. Nadia the Willful. New York: Pantheon Books, 1983.

Adler, C. Ghost Brother. New York: Clarion Books, 1990.

Cleaver, V. Belle Pruitt. New York: J. B. Lippincott Co., 1988.

Books for parents

Fitzgerald H. *The Grieving Child*: A Parent's Guide. New York: Simon & Schuster, 1992.

Grollman, E. *Talking About Death*. Boston: Beacon Press, 1976.

Kander, J. *So Will I Comfort You*. Cape Town: Lux Verbi, 1990.

Kushner, H *When Bad Things Happen To Good People*, 1994.

LeShan, E. *Learning to Say Goodbye*. New York: Macmillan, 1976.

McCracken, A. and Semel, A. A Broken Heart Still Beats: When Your Child Dies. Center City, MN; Hazeiden Publishing and Educational Services, 1988.

Rosof, B. The Worst Loss. New York: Henry Holt Publishing, 1995.

Schaefer, D.; Lyons, C. *How Do We Tell the Children? Helping Children Understand and Cope When Someone Dies* (revised edition). New York: Newmarket, 1988.

Schiff, H. *The Bereaved Parent*. UK: Souvenir Press, 1979.

Tasker, M. *How Can I Tell You? Secrecy and Disclosure with Children When a Family Member Has AIDS*. Bethesda, MD: Association for the Care of Children's Health, 1992.

Wolfelt, A. Healing Your Grieving Heart: 100 Practical Ideas. Colorado: Companion Press, 2000.

Videotapes

A Child's View of Grief. Center for Loss and Life Transition. CO: Fort Collins, 1991.

A Family in Grief: The Ameche Story. Champagne, IL: Research Press, 1989.

How Children Grieve. Portland, OR: The Dougy Center.

Living with Loss: Children and HIV (Part 4 of the *Hugs InVited* series). Washington, DC: Child Welfare League of America, 1991

What do I Tell My Children? Wayland, MA: Aquarius Productions, 1990.

When Grief Comes to School. Bloomington, IN: Blooming Educational Enterprises, 1991.

With Loving Arms. Washington, DC: Child Welfare League of America, 1989.

Resources for health care providers

Baxter, G. & Stuart, W. *Death And The Adolescent: A Resource Handbook For Bereavement Support Groups In Schools*. Toronto: University Of Toronto Press, 1999.

Crowley, R. & Mills, J. *Cartoon Magic: How to Help Children Discover Their Rainbows Within*. New York: Magination Press, 1989.

Dougy Center Staff. *35 Ways to Help a Grieving Child*. Dougy Center, 1999.

Geballe, S.; Gruendel, J. & Andiman, W. *Forgotten Children of the AIDS Epidemic*. New Haven: Yale University Press, 1995.

Haasal, B. & Marnocha, J. *Bereavement Support Group Program for Children: Leader's Manual*. Muncie, Indiana: Accelerated Development, Inc, 1990.

Lagorio, J. *Life Cycle Education Manual*. Solana Beach, CA: Empowerment in Action, 1991.

O'Toole, D. *Growing through Grief*. Burnsville, NC: Mt. Rainbow Publications, 1989.

Worden, J. W. *Grief Counseling and Grief Therapy: A Handbook for the Mental Health Practitioner*. Springer, 1982.

Zunin, L. & Zunin, H. S. The Art of Condolence. New York: Harper Collins Collins, 1991.

books for children (non-fiction and fiction) and books and other resources for adults.

REFERENCES

1. Deeks, S. G., Smith, M., Holodniy, M. & Kahn, J. O. HIV-1 protease inhibitors. A review for clinicians. *J. Am. Med. Assoc.* **277**:**2** (1997), 145–53.

2. Macintyre, K., Brown, L. & Sosler, S. "It's not what you know, but who you knew": examining the relationship between behavior change and AIDS mortality in Africa. *AIDS Educ. Prev.* **13**:**2** (2001), 160–74.

3. Goodkin, K., Blaney, N. T., Tuttle, R. *et al.* Bereavement and HIV Infection. *Int. Rev. Psychiatry* **8** (1996), 201–16.

4. Dane, B. Children, HIV infection, and AIDS. In C. A. Corr & D. M. Corr (eds.), *Handbook of Childhood Death and Bereavement.* New York: Springer Publishing Company (1996), pp. 51–70.

5. Doka, K. Disenfranchised Grief. In K. L. Doka (ed.), *Disenfranchised Grief: Recognizing Hidden Sorrow.* Lexington, MA: Lexington Books (1989), pp. 3–11.

6. Ingram, K., Jones, D. & Smith, N. Adjustment among people who have experienced AIDS-related multiple loss: the role of unsupportive social interactions, social support, and coping. *Omega* **43**:**4** (2001), 287–309.

7. Elia, N. Grief and loss in AIDS work. In M. Winiarski (ed.), *HIV Mental Health Care for the 21st Century.* New York: New York University Press (1997), pp. 67–81.

8. Scherr, L. & Green, J. Dying, bereavement and loss. In J. Green & A. McCreaner (eds.), *Counseling in HIV Infection and AIDS,* 2nd edn. Oxford: Blackwell Science (1996), pp. 179–94.

9. The Working Committee on HIV C, and Families. *Families in Crisis.* New York: Federation of Protestant Welfare Agencies (1997).

10. Fitzgerald H. *The Grieving Child: A Parent's Guide.* New York: Simon & Schuster (1992).

11. Pennells, S. & Smith, S. *The Forgotten Mourners.* Bristol, PA: Jessica Kingsley Publishers (1995).

12. O'Donnell, M. *HIV/AIDS: Loss, Grief, Challenge, and Hope.* Washington, DC: Taylor & Francis (1996).

13. Prevention CfDCa. *HIV/AIDS Surveillance Report.* **7**:**1** (2001).

14. McKelvy, C. Counseling children who have a parent with AIDS or who have lost a parent to AIDS. In M. Shernoff (ed.), *The Second Decade of AIDS: A Mental Health Practice Handbook.* New York: The Hatheleigh Company Limited (1995), pp. 137–59.

15. Stahlman, S. Children and the death of a sibling. In D. Corr (ed.), *Handbook of Childhood Death and Bereavement.* New York: Springer Publishing Company (1996), pp. 149–64.

16. Fanos, J. & Wiener, L. Tomorrow's survivors: siblings of human immunodeficiency virus-infected children. *J. Dev. Behav. Pediatr.* **15**:**3** (1994), S43–8.

17. Siegel, K. & Freund, B. Parental loss and latency age children. In C. Levine (ed.), *AIDS and the New Orphans.* Westport, CT: Auburn House (1994), pp. 43–58.

18. Silverman, P. R. & Worden, J. W. Children's reactions in the early months after the death of a parent. *Am. J. Orthopsychiatry* **62**:**1** (1992), 93–104.

19. Reese, M. Growing up: the impact of loss and change. In D. Belle (ed.), *Lives in Stress: Women and Depression.* Beverly Hills, CA: Sage (1982). pp. 65–88.

20. Silverman, P., Nickman, S. & Worden, J. Detachment revisited: the child's reconstruction of a dead parent. In K. Doka (ed.), *Children Morning Mourning Children.* Washington, DC: Hospice Foundation of America (1995), pp. 131–48.

21. Kubler-Ross, E. *On Death and Dying.* New York: Macmillan Publishing Co. (1969).

22. Worden, J. W. *Grief Counseling and Grief Therapy: A Handbook for the Mental Health Practitioner.* New York: Springer (1982).

23. Wiener, L., Fair, C. & Pizzo, P. Care for the child with HIV infection and AIDS. In A. Armstrong-Dailey & S. Goltzer (eds.), *Hospice Care for Children.* New York: Oxford University Press (2001), pp. 113–36.

24. Kaplan, D. M., Grobstein, R. & Smith, A. Predicting the impact of severe illness in families. *Health Soc. Work* **1**:**3** (1976), 71–82.

25. Tietz, W., McSherry, L. & Britt, B. Family sequelae after a child's death due to cancer. *Am. J. Psychother.* **31**:**3** (1977), 417–25.

26. Binger, C. M., Ablin, A. R., Feuerstein, R. C., Kushner, J. H., Zoger, S. & Mikkelsen, C. Childhood leukemia. Emotional impact on patient and family. *New Engl. J. Med.* **280**:**8** (1969), 414–8.

27. Fry, P. S. Grandparents' reactions to the death of a grandchild: an exploratory factor analytic study. In B. de Vries (ed.), *Kinship Bereavement in Later Life.* New York: Baywood Publishing Company (1997), pp. 119–40.

28. Wiener, L. Helping a parent with HIV tell his or her children. In B. Thompson (ed.), *HIV and Social Work: A Practitioner's Guide.* Binghamton, NY: Haworth Press (1998), pp. 327–38.

29. Taylor-Brown S. & Wiener, L. Making videotapes of HIV-infected women for their children. *Families Soc.* **74**:**8** (1993), 468–80.

30. Wiener, L., Septimus, A. & Grady, C. Psychological support and ethical issues for the child and family. In C. Wilfert (ed.), *Pediatric AIDS: The Challenge of HIV Infection in Infants, Children, and Adolescents,* 3rd edn. Philadelphia: Lippincott, Williams & Wilkins (1998), pp. 703–27.

31. Rondo, T. The increasing prevalence of complicated mourning: the onslaught is just beginning. *Omega* **26** (1992), 43–59.

32. Kastenbaum, R. *Death and Bereavement.* Springfield, IL: Charles C. Thomas (1969).

33. Mallinson, R. K. The lived experience of AIDS-related multiple losses by HIV-negative gay men. *J. Assoc. Nurses AIDS Care* **10**:**5** (1999), 22–31.

34. Lewert, G. Children and AIDS. In H. Land (ed.), *AIDS: A Complete Guide to Psychosocial Intervention.* Milwaukee: Family Service America, Inc. (1992), pp. 153–68.

35. Demmer, C. Dealing with AIDS-related loss and grief in a time of treatment advances. *Am. J. Hosp. Palliat. Care* **18**:**1** (2001), 35–41.

Legal issues for HIV-infected children

Carolyn McAllaster

Clinical Professor of Law, Duke University School of Law, Box 90360, Durham, NC

48.1 Introduction

HIV-infected children face a host of issues, many of which involve the legal system. These children often need to have future plans made for their care, or they may want to apply for government benefits or to participate in clinical trials. This chapter is designed to describe some common legal issues confronting the HIV-infected child in the USA. Each country will have different legal approaches to the subjects discussed in this chapter. The USA legal response to the needs of HIV-infected children is illustrative of how one legal system has dealt with the issues discussed here.

48.1.1 Permanent custody planning for children

Introduction

Since the vast majority of HIV-infected children have a mother who is also infected, it is important that plans be made for a time when the mother either becomes unable to care for her child or dies. Permanency planning is the process by which plans are made for the long-term legal custody or adoption of children at risk of losing their custodial parent or guardian. Such plans are particularly important when the HIV-infected parent is a single parent.

The ideal custody plan includes the identification of a stable future guardian who: (a) already has a bond with the child; (b) has the physical, emotional, and financial ability to care for the child; (c) has a long-term commitment to the child; and (d) understands and is willing to meet the special needs of an HIV-infected child.

Obstacles to making permanent plans

HIV-infected parents face considerable obstacles to seeking the legal help necessary to make permanent plans for their children. Parents may deny the need for permanency planning, particularly during the asymptomatic phase of their illness. They may fear breaches of confidentiality relating to their HIV status. Clients may be intimidated at the prospect of dealing with an unknown lawyer or have trust issues surrounding the process. Many clients face transportation problems, financial constraints or more immediate priorities that can interfere with their ability to make legally binding plans for their children. Healthcare professionals, case managers and social workers can help by working collaboratively with attorneys to assist parents as they work through many of these issues.

Assessing the rights and responsibilities of non-custodial biological parents

When making long-term plans for an HIV-infected child, it is important to assess first the rights and responsibilities of the non-custodial parent. In some cases, the absent parent is a reasonable candidate for future custody of the child. If that is the case, plans should be made for a smooth transition of future custody to that parent should the custodial parent die or no longer be able to care for the child, by actively involving the non-custodial parent in the planning for a future change of custody. It may also be that the absent parent will consent to the custodial parent's plan to appoint a non-parent caregiver.

If it appears, however, that the absent parent is not an appropriate future caregiver for the child and might interfere with the implementation of an optimal plan, the custodial parent may want to consider terminating the absent parent's rights. The decision to terminate parental rights should not be made lightly. As a result of a court order terminating a parent's rights, the legal parent–child relationship is ended. Termination of parental rights involves not only a termination of the parent's right to seek custody or visitation, it also involves a termination of the parent's obligations, including child support, and terminates the child's right to collect benefits on his or her parent's record. For example, once a parent's rights are terminated, the child can no longer collect Social Security benefits to which he or she might be entitled as a result of an absent parent's death or disability. Before a decision to terminate is made, it is important to assess the effect on potential benefits for the child.

Assessing present and future benefits to which the child may be entitled

When developing a long-term custody plan for an HIV-infected child, it is important to evaluate the sources of financial support that may be available to the child both currently and once the plan is implemented. Depending on the family's financial situation and the child's health, the parent or HIV-infected child may be entitled to certain benefits, such as TANF (Temporary Assistance for Needy Families), SSI (Supplemental Security Income), SSDI (Social Security Disability Income), Medicaid, Food Stamps, Veteran's Administration Benefits, or state welfare benefits. When considering the permanent plan for the child, one must determine whether the benefits follow the child or are dependent on the status of the caretaker. For example, if the long-term plan involves the appointment of a non-relative as guardian for the child, that person would not be eligible for benefits which are limited to biological or adoptive parents or blood relatives of the child.

Powers of attorney for decisions relating to HIV-infected children

Many states allow custodial parents to sign a power of attorney authorizing another adult to make certain decisions regarding their minor child. For example, a typical power of attorney will authorize the adult to make healthcare decisions for the child. An HIV-infected parent who cannot be consistently available to make decisions for a child should consider signing such a power of attorney as a short-term measure. This may ensure that healthcare, schooling, and other decisions regarding the child are made in a timely manner. By signing a power of attorney, the parent is not relinquishing his/her rights to make decisions for the child. He/she is agreeing to share that power with another adult.

Guardianship arrangements

Guardianship laws vary from state to state. In many states, a guardian may be appointed while the parent is still alive.

Although the procedures vary, they most certainly will require either consent or legal notification of any absent biological parent. Once appointed, the guardian can immediately make legal decisions on behalf of the child and the parent has the peace of mind of knowing that his/her choice of guardian is firmly established. Appointment of a guardian also has its disadvantages. The primary disadvantage is that the parent must relinquish custody and control over the child in order to have a guardian appointed. This is often a difficult and wrenching decision.

A parent may also opt to designate a guardian in his or her will. The designation takes effect only after the parent's death. If there is no surviving parent, the parent's nomination of a guardian in the will generally will be given deference. A guardianship designation in a will is not binding on the court, however, and only becomes effective if there is not a surviving parent. Furthermore, this method allows the parent to retain custody of the child, but does not effectively plan for the possibility that the parent, while still alive, will become unable to care for his or her child.

Several states [1] have now legislated solutions to the problem of requiring a parent to relinquish custody in order to make stable future plans for a child. These solutions allow HIV-infected parents to maintain custody of their children while at the same time solidifying a plan for the children's guardianship in the event the parent dies or becomes incapacitated. There are two types of alternative guardianships that have now been recognized in a minority of states – joint guardianships or standby guardianships. These laws allow a parent with a progressively chronic or terminal illness to have a guardian appointed while the parent is still alive and competent. Typically the statutes do not require the parent to give up custody or legal decision-making authority, but allow the standby guardian to act legally for the child if the parent becomes mentally or physically incapacitated or dies. The statutes often also allow the parent to consent to sharing decision-making authority with the standby guardian. The standby or joint guardianship option gives the parent the flexibility of having someone who can step in to care for and make decisions for the child when the parent is unable to do so. During periods of good health, the parent can resume her parental role. The child may be able to stay with the parent throughout the parent's illness while at the same time having the stability and security of knowing he or she will be cared for in the future.

None of the guardianship options discussed here result in a final termination of a biological or adoptive parent's rights. Rights to seek custody, visitation, or child support remain, as does the child's right to inherit and collect benefits on the non-custodial parent's record.

Adoption

A parent may choose to relinquish her child for adoption. This difficult decision might be made because of the combined effect of a parent's declining health and the lack of an identifiable caretaker for the child. Once a child is adopted, the parental rights of the biological parents are terminated and the adoptive parent assumes all the rights and responsibilities of a biological parent. State adoption laws vary, but may or may not provide for contact between the child and the biological parent after the adoption is final. The child may also become ineligible for public assistance and/or Medicaid after being adopted.

The Federal Adoption Assistance and Child Welfare Act of 1980 does make additional subsidies available to "special needs" children, including those children who meet financial eligibility requirements and who are HIV-infected [2]. Adoption assistance payments can be crucial in enabling prospective adoptive parents to afford adoption of an HIV-infected child.

Foster Care

Many HIV-infected children end up in the foster care system, either because their parent voluntarily places them in foster care or because of involuntary intervention by a child welfare agency based on a finding of abuse or neglect or in situations where a parent is unable to meet the needs of his or her child. In the case of a voluntary placement, the parent may be seeking a temporary respite from the child's care and may be able to regain custody after showing the ability to resume care of the child. In the case of an involuntary removal of the child from the home, the burden on the parent to regain custody will be higher and will be dictated in most situations by the terms of a court order.

In some cases, relatives of the child may be eligible to become licensed foster parents. This is known as kinship foster care and enables the child to remain within his or her extended family. Federal law requires that states consider giving preference to an adult relative over a non-related caregiver for children needing foster care [3]. If licensed, an adult relative would receive the same foster care payments a non-relative foster parent would.

48.1.2 Supplemental Security Income (SSI) for disabled children

Definition of disability

Low-income HIV-infected children may be eligible for SSI benefits. Supplemental Security Income is a federally financed and administered needs-based program that provides a monthly income benefit to disabled children, among others. Under welfare reform passed by Congress in August of 1996 [4], a child under age 18 would be considered disabled if he or she has a medically determinable mental or physical impairment which results in marked and severe functional limitations and which can be expected to result in death or which has lasted or can be expected to last for a continuous period of not less than 12 months.

The Social Security Administration publishes a list of HIV-related impairments, which include specific criteria about the level of severity that will be required for a child to be considered disabled [5]. An HIV-infected child applying for SSI benefits must either have one of the listed conditions or have a condition which is medically or functionally equivalent in severity to a listed condition. In order for a child's impairment to be medically equivalent to a listed condition, the child's *medical* findings must be of equal medical equivalence to the listed condition. In order for a child's impairment to be *functionally* equivalent to a listed condition, the impairment must cause the same disabling limitations in a child's day-to-day functioning as those of the listed condition.

In evaluating the functional limitations of HIV-infected children, several factors are considered, including ". . . symptoms, such as fatigue or pain; characteristics of the illness, such as the frequency and duration of manifestations or periods of exacerbation and remission in the disease course; and the functional impact of treatment for the disease, including the side effects of medication" [6].

Information needed to apply for SSI

Parents or guardians of disabled children can apply for SSI benefits by calling or visiting their local Social Security Office. In order to expedite the process, they should have the following information and documentation when they apply: the child's birth certificate and Social Security number, and records documenting the parent and child's income and assets. In order to document the severity of the child's disability, it also will be important to provide names, addresses and phone numbers of the child's doctors and hospitals where she/he has received treatment, and the same information for teachers, child care providers, counselors, social workers, and other professionals who have worked with the child. The parent can also expedite the process by providing copies of the child's medical records to Social Security. Parents who are considering filing an SSI claim on behalf of their child should keep a daily journal documenting specifically how the child's disability limits the child's day-to-day activities.

Presumptive disability

For children who are severely disabled, there are special provisions in the law which allow them to collect SSI benefits for up to 6 months while the formal disability decision is being made. If the child is later determined not to be disabled, the benefits do not have to be paid back.

Appeal process

If the initial SSI application is denied, the parent or guardian will receive a Notice of Denial of Benefits in the mail. The parent then has 60 days to appeal the initial decision. The Notice will explain how to file an appeal. The appeal process has four steps: [1] Reconsideration by a disability examiner; [2] A hearing before an Administrative Law Judge; [3] Social Security Appeals Council Review; and [4] Appeal to Federal Court. A substantial number of initial Social Security Determinations that are appealed are reversed at the hearing level, so for children with serious disabilities it is important to pursue the appeal process at least through the hearing level. If denied at the initial application step, it is generally advisable for the parents to seek legal representation from an attorney who specializes in handling SSI cases.

48.1.3 Consent to medical treatment for minor children

In general

It is generally required that a child's legal guardian consent to medical treatment for a child under age 18. There are exceptions to this general rule.

Emancipation

Many states recognize the emancipation of children under age 18 by statute or case law. Emancipation is typically recognized in situations where a minor has married, entered the armed services, or is living apart from parents and is financially independent [7]. Emancipation confers upon the child some or all of the rights and responsibilities of adulthood, depending on the state law where the minor child lives.

Laws allowing minors to consent to certain medical procedures

Many states also have laws which specifically allow minors to consent to their own medical treatment in certain enumerated situations, typically pregnancy, sexually transmitted diseases, birth control, and substance abuse [8].

Medical neglect: parental refusal to seek treatment

All states have a mechanism for overriding the requirement of parental consent for medical treatment where the child's life may be threatened or the parent's refusal to consent to medical treatment rises to the level of child abuse or neglect [9]. The child's parent or legal guardian ordinarily has the authority to make medical decisions on behalf of his or her child. In order to override that authority, the healthcare provider or social worker must seek a court order. In situations where the child's life may be threatened, the court can directly authorize the needed treatment. Where the refusal to seek medical treatment is not immediately life threatening, but does constitute neglect, welfare agencies may seek legal custody from the court in order to be able to give consent to the needed treatment.

Consent for participation in clinical trials

In order for an HIV-infected non-foster child to participate in a clinical trial, it is necessary to obtain the consent of the custodial parent or legal guardian [10]. Clinical trials investigators must, in most circumstances, also obtain the assent of the children who enroll as subjects and who are capable of assenting [11]. In cases of children in foster care, the legal custodian is usually, but not always, the child welfare agency. Many states, however, do not allow children in the foster care system to participate as research subjects [12]. "Most child protection agencies . . . have only the authority to consent to 'standard' medical treatment for foster children" [13]. When clinicians believe that there is a compelling need for a patient to receive investigational therapy, but the child welfare agency cannot consent to enrollment in a clinical trial, an attorney should be consulted. The laws and regulations concerning such situations vary considerably from state to state.

48.2 Conclusion

It is hoped that this chapter has provided a useful guide to those working with HIV-infected children regarding the basic US law that applies in the areas of custody planning, disability benefits, and consent to medical treatment for children. This chapter is designed to provide information illustrative of how one legal system has addressed the issues discussed here. The chapter should not be considered a substitute for legal advice from an attorney. For representation in individual cases or more detailed information, readers are urged to refer to the appendix in this textbook entitled "Selected Legal Resources for HIV-infected Children." This Appendix lists on a state-by-state basis several organizations that provide direct legal services or referrals to HIV-infected individuals.

REFERENCES

1. Ark. Code Ann. § 28-65-221 (LexisNexis Supp. 2001); Cal. Prob. Code § 2105 (West Supp. 2002); Colo. Rev. Stat. Ann. § 15-14-202 (2) (Bradford Publishing 2001); Conn. Gen. Stat. §§ 45a-624 to 625 (West Supp. 2002); Fla. Stat. § 744.304 (West Supp. 2002); Ill. Comp. Stat. Ann ch. 755 § 5/11–5.3 (West Supp. 2002); Mass. Gen. Laws Ann. ch, 201 §§ 2A-2H (LexisNexis Supp. 2002); Md. Code Ann., Est. & Trusts §§ 13–901 to 908 (Lexis 2001); Minn. Stat. Ann. §§ 257B.01- 257B.10 (West Supp. 2002); Neb. Rev. Stat. § 30-2608 (Lexis 2001); N.J. Rev. Stat. §§ 3B:12–67 to 78 (West Supp. 2001): N.Y. Surr. Ct. Proc. Act §§ 1726 (West 2001–2002); N. C.Gen. Stat. §§ 35A-1370 to 1382 (West 2000); Pa. Con. Stat. Ann. ch. 23 §§ 5601–5616 (West 2001); Va. Code Ann. §§ 16.1-349 to 355 (Michie 1999); W. Va. Code §§ 44A-5-1 (LexisNexis Supp. 2001); Wis. Stat. Ann. § 48.978 (West Supp. 2001).

2. 42 U.S.C.A. § 670 *et seq.*

3. 42 U.S.C.A. § 671(a)(19).

4. Personal Responsibility and Work Opportunity Reconciliation Act of 1996, Pub.L.No. 104–193 (1996).

5. 20 C.F.R. pt. 404, subpt. P, App. 1, Part B, § 114.08 (2002).

6. 20 C.F.R. pt. 404, subpt. P, App. 1, Part B, § 114 D.8 (2002).

7. See, for example, N.M. Stat. Ann. §§ 32A-21-1 to -21-7 (Michie 1999); Cal. Fam. Code § 7001 *et seq.* (West 1994).

8. See, for example, N.C.G.S. § 90-21.5 (West 2000).

9. Mnookin, R. H. & Weisberg, D. K. *Child, Family and State*, 3rd edn. Little, Brown and Company (1995), pp. 558–61.

10. For research not involving greater than minimal risk, or for research involving greater than minimal risk but presenting the prospect of direct benefit to the individual subjects, the permission of only one parent is necessary. For research involving greater than minimal risk and no prospect of direct benefit to the subject, but likely to yield generalizable knowledge about the subject's disorder or condition, or for research not otherwise approvable which presents an opportunity to understand, prevent, or alleviate a serious problem affecting the health or welfare of children, the permission of both parents is required, "unless one parent is deceased, unknown, incompetent, or not reasonably available, or when only one parent has legal responsibility for the care and custody of the child." 45 C.F.R. § 46.408(b).

11. Assent is defined as "a child's affirmative agreement to participate in research. Mere failure to object should not, absent affirmative agreement, be construed as assent." 45 C.F.R. § 46.402(b). "In determining whether children are capable of assenting, the IRB shall take into account the ages, maturity and psychological state of the children involved." 45 C.F.R. § 46.408(a).

12. *See* Martin & Sacks, Do HIV-Infected Children in Foster Care Have Access to Clinical Trials of New Treatments?, 5 *AIDS Pub. Policy J.* **3** (1990).

13. McNutt, The Under-Enrollment of HIV-Infected Foster Children in Clinical Trials and Protocols and the need for Corrective State Action, 20 *Am. J. Law Med.* **231** (1994).

Appendices

Formulary: Antiretroviral agents

Paul Jarosinski, Pharm.D.

Pharmacy Department, National Institutes of Health, Bethesda, MD

Formulary – Antiretroviral Agents

Generic name (synonyms)/forms	FDA approved dose	Other doses	Comments
Nucleoside Reverse Transcriptase Inhibitors			
Zidovudine (Retrovir®, AZT, ZDV)/100 & 300 mg tabs, 10 mg/ml oral solution, 10 mg/ml for iv infusion.	Neonates: 2 mg/kg po q6h or 1.5 mg/kg iv q6h 6 wk-12 years: 160 mg/m^2 (max 200 mg) po q8h >12 yo: 600 mg/day in 2 or 3 doses	Premature neonates: 2 mg/kg po or 1.5 mg/kg iv Q12H until 2 weeks of age then 2 mg/kg po q8h*	Can be taken without regard to food, only HIV antiretroviral available for iv infusion after dilution, not recommended for use with stavudine.
Zalcitabine (Hivid®, ddC)/ 0.375 and 0.750 mg tablets	No approved dose for < 13 yo Adult: 0.75 mg q8h	0.01 mg/kg q8h*	Cmax decreased 40% and AUC 14% when given with food – significance unknown. Best given on an empty stomach. Not recommended for use with lamivudine and didanosine.
Didanosine (Videx®, ddI)/ 25, 50,100, 150 chew tabs, 100/167/250 powder packets, 10 mg/ml oral solution, and 125/200/250/400 mg enteric coated tabs	Children ≥ 6 mo: 120 mg/m^2 bid Adult ≥ 60 kg: 200 mg (tablets)/250 mg (buffered powder) bid, 400 (EC) qd <60kg 125 mg (tablets)/167 mg (buffered powder) bid, 250 mg (EC) qd	Neonates < 90 days: 50 mg/ m2 q12h* Ped dose: 90–150 mg/m^2 q12h*	10 mg/ml buffered solution is stable for 30 days refrigerated, dose on empty stomach, two tablets required for sufficient antacid, children < 3 may require additional antacid with oral solution, EC daily tablet available for adults with compliance problems on bid (less optimal). Beware of interaction related to antacid content. Not recommended for use with zalcitabine.

(cont.)

Generic name (synonyms)/forms	FDA approved dose	Other doses	Comments
Lamivudine (Epivir®, /Epivir-HBV, 3TC)/100, 150, and 300 mg tablet and 5 and 10 mg/ml solutions.	Children 3 mo – 16 yo: 4 mg/kg bid – max 150 mg bid Adult: 150 mg bid or 300 mg qd	Neonate (<30 days): 2 mg/kg bid*	Oral liquid is stable at room temperature, can be given without regard to food, not recommended for use with zalcitabine. 5 mg/ml solution and 100 mg tablet are marketed for HBV, but can be used for pediatric HIV treatment.
Stavudine (Zerit®, Zerit XR, d4T)/15, 20, 30, 40 mg caps, 1 mg/ml solution, and 37.5, 50, 75, and 100 mg XR caps	Children < 30 kg: 1 mg/kg q12h Adults 30 kg-<60 kg: 30 mg q12h Adults ≥60 kg: 40 mg q12h or 100 mg XR qd for ≥ 60 kg or 75 mg qd for < 60 kg (use of XR tablets has not been studied in children)	Neonatal dose under study in PACTG 332	Oral solution is stable for 30 days refrigerated, can be given without regard to food, XR (extended release) caps may be mixed with 2 tablespoons of yogurt or applesauce as long as beads are not chewed or crushed, not recommended for use with zidovudine.
Abacavir (Ziagen®,1592U89)/300 mg tab and 20 mg/ml oral solution	Children 3 mo –16 yo: 8 mg/kg bid – max 300 mg bid Adults: 300 mg bid	Infants (1 – 3 mo): 8 mg/kg bid is under study.	Oral solution is stable at room temperature, can be given without regard to food.
Emtricitabine (Emtriva®, FTC) 200 mg capsules	Adults 18 and over: 200 mg daily		Chemically related to lamivudine. May be taken with or without food.

Non-nucleoside Reverse Transcriptase Inhibitors

Generic name (synonyms)/forms	FDA approved dose	Other doses	Comments
Nevirapine (Viramune®, NVP)/200 mg tablets and 10 mg/ml suspension	Children 2 mo or older: 4 mg/kg once daily × 14 days then 7 mg/kg bid (2 mo-<8 yo) or 4 mg/kg bid (>8 yo) – max 200 mg bid† Adults: 200 qd × 14 days then bid	Neonatal dose (PACTG 356): under study** 120 mg/m2 qd × 14 days then 120–200 mg/m² bid, max 200 mg/dose*	Oral suspension is stable at room temperature, lead-in dose lessens occurrence of rash, new lead-in period required for any 7-day interruption in therapy, can be given without regard to food, induces 3A4 liver enzymes.
Delavirdine (Rescriptor®, DLV)/100 and 200 mg tablets	Not approved for children Adults: 400 mg tid		100 mg tablet only can be dispersed in water, can be given without regard to food, separate from didanosine and any antacid by one hour, inhibits liver enzymes 3A4 and 2C9.
Efavirenz (Sustiva®, Stocrin®, DMP266)/50, 100, and 200 mg capsules, 600 mg tablet, 30 mg/ml liquid in some countries	For children 3 yo and above 10-<15 kg 200 mg daily 15-<20 kg 250 mg daily 20-<25 kg 300 mg daily 25-<32.5 kg 350 mg daily 32.5 kg-<40 kg 400 mg daily ≥40 kg 600 mg	No information on dosing to younger children	Should be taken on an empty stomach preferably at bedtime to minimize side effects, induces liver enzymes 3A4, 2C9, and 2C19. For patients that cannot swallow the smallest capsule (50 mg), there are reports of opening the capsule for administration in food or liquids, with grape jelly mentioned as effective in disguising the peppery taste.*

Formulary – Antiretroviral Agents (*cont.*)

Generic name (synonyms)/forms	FDA approved dose	Other doses	Comments
Nucleotide Reverse Transcriptase Inhibitors			
Tenofovir (Viread®, PMPA prodrug)/ 300 mg tablets	Not approved for children Adult: 300 mg once daily	Children 4–18 yo: 175 mg/m^2 daily being studied at the NCI	No liquid formulation, tablets cannot be crushed or dissolved, should be taken with a meal.
Protease Inhibitors			
Ritonavir (Norvir®, RTV)/100 mg caps and 80 mg/ml oral solution	For children 2 yo and above: 400 mg/m^2 bid starting at 250 mg/m^2 and increasing by 50 mg/m^2 q2-3d to full dose, Max dose = adult dose = 600 mg bid	Neonates: Under study in PACTG 354	Oral solution (43% ethanol) is stable at room temperature, refrigerate capsules unless used w/in 30 days, take with food, unpleasant taste of solution may be minimized by chocolate, peanut butter, etc., potent inhibitor of 3A4 liver enzymes as well as 2D6 (check drug interactions).
Indinavir (Crixivan®, IDV)/100, 200, 333, and 400 mg caps	Not approved for children Adults: 800 mg q8h	Neonates: Not used due to hyperbilirubinemia. Older children: 350–450 mg/m2 q8h+	No liquid formulation, should be taken on an empty stomach not with an antacid or at the same time as didanosine, drink plenty of fluids – at least 1.5 liters for adult doses, inhibitor of 3A4 liver enzymes
Nelfinavir (Viracept®, NFV)/250 and 625 mg tablets and oral powder	Children 2–13 yo: 20–30 mg/m^2 tid using the chart in the package insert. Children ≥ 23 kg get adult dose of 750 mg q12h. Alternate adult dose: 1250 mg bid	Neonates: 40 mg/kg q12h under study in PACTG 353	Oral powder may be mixed with water, milk, formula, and dietary supplements, administer with food, tablets may be dissolved in water or crushed, inhibitor of 3A4 liver enzymes.
Amprenavir (Agenerase®, APV, VX-478, 141W94)/ 50 and 150 mg caps and 15 mg/ml solution	Children 4–12 yo or 13–16 yo and < 50 kg: 22.5 mg/kg bid or 17 mg/kg tid as solution, max 2800 mg/day as OR 20 mg/kg bid or 15 mg/kg tid as capsules, max 2400 mg/day.	Neonates: Not recommended in children ≤ 3 yo.	Oral solution is stable at room temperature, solution dose does not equal capsule dose, may be taken with or without food, avoid taking with high fat meal, do not take vitamin E supplements, inhibitor of 3A4 liver enzymes.
Lopinavir/RitonavirKaletra®/ caps of 133/33 mg and 80/20 mg/ml oral solution.	Children ≥ 50 kg and adults: 1400 mg bid as solution or 1200 mg bid as capsules		Oral solution contains 42% ethanol, capsules and solution should be refrigerated or used within 2 months if stored at room temperature, take with food, potent inhibitor of 3A4 liver enzymes as well as 2D6 (check drug interactions).
	Children 6 mo–12 yo (LPV/RTV)[§] 7-<15 kg: 12/3 mg/kg bid 15–40 kg: 10/2.5 mg/kg bid, max 400/100 mg bid >40 kg and adult: 400/100 mg bid	Children 6 mo–12 yo: 230/57.5 mg/m^2 bid (max 400/100 bid)*	

(*cont.*)

Formulary – Antiretroviral Agents (*cont.*)

Generic name (synonyms)/forms	FDA approved dose	Other doses	Comments
Saquinavir (SQV, Invirase® 200 mg hard gel caps, Fortovase® 200 mg soft gel caps)	Not approved for children under < 16 yo. Adult doses Invirase®: 600 mg tid Fortovase®: 1200 mg tid	Pediatric dose under study: 50 mg/kg q8h as single protease therapy or 33 mg/kg q8h with nelfinavir	Invirase® and Fortovase® may not be used interchangeably. Invirase® should be stored at room temperature and Fortovase® should be refrigerated or stored at room temperature and used within 3 months, should be taken with a meal, inhibitor of 3A4 enzymes.
Atazanavir (Reyataz®) 200 mg caps	Adult dose: 400 mg qd	There are insufficient data for a pediatric dosage recommendation	Take with food. Antacids (including didanosine tablets and powder) allowed ≥ 2 hours after atazanavir or ≥ 1 hour before. Notify MD if white portion of eyes or skin yellows. Many drug interactions.
Fusion Inhibitors Enfuvirtide (Fuzeon®, T-20)/ lyophilized powder reconstituted to 90 mg/ml	6–16 yo: 2 mg/kg sc bid (max dose 90 mg) Adults: 90 mg bid		Injections should be into upper arm, anterior thigh, or abdomen. 86% of patients have their first injection site reaction in first week of therapy. Injections should be not given in a site where there is a remaining reaction from a previous dose. Do not administer into moles, scars, navel, or bruises.

Dosing to prevent mother to child transmission of HIV is discussed in Chapter 8.

FDA = United States Food and Drug Administration; PACTG = Pediatric AIDS Clinical Trial Group; yo = years old; mo = month; N/V = nausea/vomiting; Cmax = Peak blood concentration; AUC = Area under the curve (reflective of total absorption); EC = Enteric Coated tablet for once daily dosing; sc = subcutaneous.

* Guidelines for the Use of Antiretroviral Agents in Pediatric HIV Infection, 12/14/01 edition.

[†] The FDA approved dose was based on pharmacokinetic modeling to achieve similar plasma concentrations as dosing of 150 mg/m^2. Nevirapine clearance is highest during the first 2 years of life and decreases gradually until reaching adult clearance around 12 years of age. The current FDA regimen results in an abrupt 43% decrease in dose on the eighth birthday that is not consistent with the gradual change in clearance. The majority of pediatric clinical studies were done with the 120 mg/m^2 dosing regimen.

**PACTG 356 dosing for neonates through 2 months of age: 5 mg/kg or 120 mg/m^2 qd $\times$ 14 days then 120 mg/m^2 q12h for 14 days, then 200 mg/m^2 q12h.

+ Two studies (NCI/PACTG) have now confirmed a significant incidence of renal toxicity at a 500 mg/m^2 pediatric dose. The optimal indinavir dose for children is somewhere between the 350 mg/m^2 dose in the NCI study and 450 mg/m^2 (10% below the 500 mg/m^2 dose).

[§]The FDA doses are extrapolated from the pediatric trials that were dosed on body surface area at LPV 230/ RTV 57.5 mg/m^2 bid.

Formulary: Drugs for opportunistic infections associated with HIV

Paul Jarosinski, Pharm.D.

Pharmacy Department, National Institutes of Health, Bethesda, MD

Formulary – Drugs for Opportunistic Infections Associated with HIV

Generic name (Synonyms)/Dosage Form	FDA approved dose	Other doses	Comments
Acyclovir (Zovirax®) 200 mg caps, 400 and 800 mg tabs, 40 mg/ml suspension	HSV 1, 2: 250 mg/m^2 iv q8h or (adults) 200 mg q4h × 5 daily for 10 days. VZV: 500 mg/m^2 iv q8h or 20 mg/kg po qid (max is adult dose of 800 mg qid) × 5 days HZ: 500 mg/m^2 iv q8h and, in adults, 800 mg q4h × 5 daily for 7–10 days	Oral HSV in children: 400 mg/m2 po tid. Oral HZ in children: 20 mg/kg po qid (max dose 800 mg qid)	Crystallization of drug in renal tubules can lead to renal failure if hydration is not adequate especially with high iv doses for zoster.
Atovaquone (Mepron®) 250 mg tabs and 150 mg/ml suspension	PCP treatment: (13 yo-adult) 750 mg bid with meals for 21 days. PCP prophylaxis: (13–16 yo) 1500 mg qd with a meal.	PCP treatment and PCP/Toxo prophylaxis: (3–24 months) 45 mg/kg/day and (1–3 mo or 2–12 yo) 30 mg/kg/day once daily	Must be taken with meals to maximize absorption, suspension must be shaken, drug interactions possible due to high protein binding (>99%) and metabolism. Effective for mild/moderate PCP in adults. May be taken by G6PD deficient patients.

(cont.)

(Synonyms)/Dosage Form	FDA approved dose	Other doses	Comments
Azithromycin (Zithromax®) 250 mg cap, 600 mg tab, 20 mg and 40 mg/ml susp, 1 g single dose packet	MAC prophylaxis (adults):1200 mg po q week	MAC prophylaxis (Children) 20 mg/kg (max 1200 mg) po q week or 5–10 mg/kg/dose (max 500 mg) qd (lower dose for prophylaxis/higher for treatment)	Capsules should be taken on an empty stomach while the suspension and tablets can be taken without regard to food. Shake suspension before used. Can be refrigerated, but not required. Less drug interactions than clarithromycin.
Cidofovir (Vistide®) 75 mg/ml for iv infusion in 375 mg vials	CMV: 5 mg/kg iv q week × 2, then 5 mg/kg iv q2 week. Probenecid 2 g po required 3 hours before each dose and 1 g 2 and 8 hours after each cidofovir dose.		Cidofovir should be given over 1 hour. Saline hydration required. Giving food before probenecid may reduce nausea.
Clarithromycin (Biaxin®) 250 and 500 mg tabs, 125 and 250 mg/ml susp, and 500 mg XL tabs	MAC prophylaxis (Children) 7.5 mg/kg (max 500 mg) bid, (adults) 500 mg bid	MAC Treatment (Children) up to 12.5 mg/kg (max 500 mg) bid	May be given without regard to food. Shake suspension before use and do not refrigerate. Some drug interactions. XL (sustained release) form is not indicated for MAC therapy.
Clindamycin (Cleocin®) 75, 150, and 300 mg caps and 150 mg/ml injection in 2, 4, or 6 ml sizes		PCP treatment: 10 mg/kg iv (max 600 mg) q6h with primaquine 0.3 mg/kg (as base) po qd. × 21 days	Effective to mild-moderate PCP in adults. Contraindicated in G6PD deficiency. Drug must be diluted and given iv over 30 minutes or more.
Dapsone 25 and 100 mg tabs		PCP treatment: 2 mg/kg po daily (max 100 mg with 5 mg/kg trimethoprim po × 21 d. PCP/toxo prophylaxis (Children > 1 mo): 2 mg/kg qd (max 100 mg) or 4 mg/kg q week (max)	Effective to mild-moderate PCP in adults. Avoid in patients with G6PD deficiency. Do not give with antacids (e.g. didanosine) as this may significantly lower absorption. Toxo prophylaxis regimen must also include pyrimethamine 1 mg/kg qd plus leucovorin 5 mg po q3d
Ethambutol (Myambutol®)100 and 400 mg tablets	For TB with other agents: Children ≥ 13 yo – 15–20 mg/kg (1 gm max) qd or 50 mg/kg (2.5 gm max) 2 × per week. See CDC dosing chart for adults and children ≥ 15 yo or 40 kg	For TB with other agents: Children 5–12 yo – 15–20 mg/kg (1 g max) qd or 50 mg/kg (2.5 g max) 2 × per week. May use in younger children if resistant to other agents	Not recommended by manufacturer for children under 13 due to optic neuritis. Visual testing recommended before and monthly
Famciclovir (Famvir®) 125, 250, and 500 mg tablets	HSV (adults) 125 mg bid × 5 days Suppression of recurrent HSV (adults): 250 mg bid HZ (adults): 500 mg q8h × 7 days	Not tested in children	Start w/in 72 hours of rash onset. May be taken without regard to food

Formulary – Drugs for Opportunistic Infections Associated with HIV (*cont.*)

(Synonyms)/Dosage Form	FDA approved dose	Other doses	Comments
Foscarnet (Foscavir®) 24 mg/ml inj in 250 ml or 500 ml bottles	CMV: 90 mg/kg q12h or 60 mg/kg q8h iv × 14–21 days induction, then 90–120 mg/kg iv qd. Acyclovir resistant HSV: 40 mg/kg iv over 1 hour q 8–12h × 2–3 weeks		IV solution must be diluted to 12 mg/ml or lower. 90 mg/kg dose given over 1.5–2 hours and 60 mg/kg over 1 hour. Maintenance doses given over 2 hours. 90 mg/kg is preferred maintenance dose due to lower toxicity. Hydration is required.
Ganciclovir (Cytovene®, DHPG) 250 and 500 mg caps plus 500 mg vials for reconstitution	CMV: 5 mg/kg iv × 14–21 days induction, then 5 mg/kg iv qd or 6 mg/kg iv qd × 5 days per week or 1000 mg po tid or 500 mg 6 × qd	Some clinicians use 5 mg/kg iv qd for 5 days/week for maintenance	Infusion should be given over one hour with adequate hydration. Capsules should be taken with food, but absorption is still poor. Valganciclovir is preferred agent for oral dosing. Drug can cause birth defects in pregnant women. Causes elevation of didanosine levels and neutropenia with zidovudine.
Isoniazid (INH) 100, 300 mg tabs and 10 mg/ml solution and 100 mg/ml injection	Positive TB skin Test or exposure: 10–15 mg/kg (max 300 mg) qd × 9 mo or 20–30 mg/kg (max 900 mg) twice weekly for 9 months, same dose for treatment in combination with other agents. Adult dose: 5 mg/kg/days (300 max) or 15 mg/kg (900 mg max) once, twice, or thrice weekly		Syrup should be shaken before use. Doses ideally given on an empty stomach.
Oseltamavir (Tamiflu®) 75 mg caps and 12 mg/ml suspension	13 yo and above: 75 mg bid × 5 days Children 1 yo and greater; ≤15 kg – 30 mg twice daily >15 to 23 kg – 45 mg twice daily >23 to 40 kg – 60 mg twice daily >40 kg – 75 mg twice daily		Inactivated influenza vaccine is the first choice for influenza prophylaxis. Treatment should begin within 2 days of onset of symptoms of influenza. The oral suspension should be shaken before use, stored in the refrigerator, and used within 10 days.
Pentamidine Isothionate (Pentam®) 300 mg vial for reconstitution	PCP Treatment: 4 mg/kg iv/im qd × 21 days, may switch to another agent PO to complete 21 days if clinically recovered. PCP prophylaxis (Children > 5 yo): 300 mg via Respirgard II nebulizer q month		Second choice drug for PCP treatment, iv route is preferred for treatment, administer iv over 60–90 minutes to avoid hypotension. Use with caution with other nephrotoxic agents. Do not give with didanosine due to association with pancreatitis.

(*cont.*)

(Synonyms)/Dosage Form	FDA approved dose	Other doses	Comments
Primaquine 26.3 mg tablet		PCP treatment: 0.3 mg/kg (as base) po qd with clindamycin 10 mg/kg iv (max 600 mg) q6h × 21 days	Effective in mild-moderate PCP in adults. Contraindicated in G6PD deficiency. Each 26.3 mg tablet contains 15 mg primaquine base
Pyrazinamide 500 mg scored tablet	For TB with other agents: 15–30 mg/kg (2 g max) qd or 50 mg/kg (2 g max) 2×/week. See CDC dosing chart for adults and children ≥ 15 yo or 40 kg		Can be taken without regard to meals
Rifabutin (Mycobutin®) 150 mg capsule	MAC prophylaxis (adults): 300 mg qd or 150 mg bid	For TB with other agents: 5 mg/kg (300 mg max) qd or 2–3×per week, children 5–6 mg/kg qd or 2×/wk	Patients with nausea may take 150 mg bid with food. May color body fluids brown-orange and permanently discolor soft contact lenses. Several drug interactions
Rifampin (Rifadin®) 150 and 300 mg caps, 600 mg powder for reconstitution.	Positive TB skin test or exposure: 10–20 mg/kg (max 600 mg) po/iv qd × 4–6 mo, same dose for treatment of TB in combination with other agents qd or 2×/week		For prevention in INH resistant strains or intolerance. Given orally on an empty stomach. IV formulation available, but no liquid prep. Pharmacist can prepare 4-week suspension supply. May color body fluids brown-orange and permanently discolor soft contact lenses. Many drug interactions
Streptomycin 1 g vials of 400 mg/ml	For TB with other agents: 20–40 mg/kg (max 1 g) qd or 20 mg/kg (max 1.5 g) 2 × per week, adults < 60 yo and children ≥ 15 yo or 40 kg – 15 mg/kg (1 g max) qd (5–7 days per week) decreased to 2–3 × week after culture conversion.		Only available as IM injection although there are reports of the IM injection being given intravenously, rotate injection sites, adults should not exceed total dose of 120 g
Trimethoprim–Sulfamethoxazole (TMP–SMX, Bactrim®, co-trimoxazole, Septra®, and others)/as TMP 80 and 160 mg tab, 80 mg/ml inj, and 40 mg/ml suspension	PCP treatment: 15–20 mg/kg/day as TMP IV divided q6h × 21 days, may complete treatment PO if clinically recovered. PCP prophylaxis: 75/375 mg/m^2/days (TMP–SMX) po bid 3 consecutive days/wk Toxoplasma prophylaxis: same dose as PCP given qd.	PCP prophylaxis: 75/375 mg/m^2/days bid three times week on alternate days, bid every day, or double dose up to adult max (160/800) qd × 3 days per week.	TMP–SMX not used for PCP therapy in children less that 4–6 weeks due to displacement of bilirubin. Use with caution in those with renal or hepatic dysfunction, severe allergy or asthma, or G6PD deficiency when hemolysis could occur. Hydration is important especially with PCP doses to avoid crystalluria and stone formation.

(*cont.*)

Formulary – Drugs for Opportunistic Infections Associated with HIV (*cont.*)

(Synonyms)/Dosage Form	FDA approved dose	Other doses	Comments
Trimetrexate (Neutrexin®, TMTX) 25 mg vial for reconstitution	PCP treatment (adults): 45 mg/m^2 IV qd × 21 days with leucovorin 20 mg/m^2 IV q6h × 21 days (72 hours after last TMTX)	Pediatric PCP treatment: 45 mg/m^2 IV qd × 21 days with leucovorin 20 mg/m^2 IV q6h × 21 days (72 hours after last TMTX)	Salvage regimen for patients who fail or cannot tolerate TMP–SMX. Drug interactions exist related to CYP 3A4 metabolism
Valganciclovir (Valcyte®) 450 mg tablets	CMV induction (adults): 900 mg bid × 21 days followed by 900 mg qd maintenance	No pediatric recommendations	A 900 mg dose of valganciclovir provides drug levels similar to a 5 mg/kg IV ganciclovir dose. Tablets should be taken with food. Drug can cause birth defects in pregnant women. Causes elevation of didanosine levels and neutropenia with zidovudine
Valacyclovir (Valtrex®) 500 mg and 1 g tablets	HSV (adults): 1 g bid × 10 days. Suppression of recurrent HSV (adults): 500–1000 mg qd HZ (adults): 1 g tid × 7 days	Not tested in children	Start w/in 72 hours of rash onset

National Institute of Health sponsored clinical trials for pediatric HIV disease

James G. McNamara

Pediatric Medicine Branch, Division of AIDS, NIAID, NIH, Rockville, MD

NIAID Pediatric AIDS Clinical Trials Group Units – USA

ALABAMA

Children's Hospital of Alabama
University of Alabama at Birmingham
Department of Pediatrics, Infectious Dis.
1600 Seventh Avenue, S. Suite 752
Birmingham, AL 35233-0011
(205) 939-9590
Fax: (205) 975-6549

CALIFORNIA

University of California at Los Angeles
UCLA School of Medicine
Dept. of Pediatric Infectious Dis., 22-442 MDCC
175217 Le Conte Avenue
Los Angeles, CA 90095-1752
(310) 825-5235
Fax: (310) 206-5529

University of California at San Diego
Dept. of Pediatrics, Division of Infectious Diseases
Clinical Sciences Bldg, Room 430
9500 Gilman Dr., Mail Code 0672
La Jolla, CA 92093-0672
(858) 534-7170
Fax: (858) 534-7411

University of California at San Francisco
UCSF, Moffitt Hospital, M-679
505 Parnassus Avenue, Box 0105
San Francisco, CA 94143-0105
(415) 476-2865
Fax: (415) 476-3466

FLORIDA

University of Miami School of Medicine
Division of Pediatric Infect. Dis. & Immunology
Batchelor Building, Room 296
1580 N.W. 10th Avenue
Miami, FL 33136-1013
(305) 243-6522
Fax: (305) 243-5562

ILLINOIS

Chicago Children's Memorial Hospital
Division of Infectious Diseases
2300 Children's Plaza, Box #20
Chicago, IL 60614-3394
(773) 880-4757
Fax: (773) 880-3208

LOUISIANA

Charity Hospital of New Orleans
Tulane University School of Medicine
Pediatric Infectious Diseases
1430 Tulane Avenue
New Orleans, LA 70112-2699
(504) 588-5422
Fax: (504) 586-3805

MARYLAND

Johns Hopkins University Hospital
Department of International Health

615 North Wolfe Street, Hygiene 5-5515
Baltimore, MD 21205-2103
(410) 955-6964
Fax: (410) 502-6733

MASSACHUSETTS
Children's Hospital of Boston
Infectious Diseases, Enders 6
300 Longwood Avenue
Boston, MA 02115-5724
(617) 355-7621
Fax: (617) 566-4721

University of Massachusetts Medical Center
Dept. of Peds./ Molecular Med.
Biotech II, Suite 318
373 Plantation Street
Worcester, MA 01605-2377
(508) 856-6282
Fax: (508) 856-5500

NEW JERSEY
New Jersey Children's Hospital
UMDNJ-New Jersey Medical School
Division of Pulmonary, Allergy, Immunology & Infectious
    Diseases
185 South Orange Ave., F570A
Newark, NJ 07103-2714
(973) 972-5066
Fax: (973) 972-6443

NEW YORK
Bronx-Lebanon Hospital Center
Pediatric ID Services
Dept. of Peds., Milstein Bldg.-2C
1650 Selwyn Avenue
Bronx, NY 10457
(718) 960-1010
Fax: (718) 960-1011

Columbia Presbyterian Medical Center
Dept. of Pediatrics
630 West 168th Street
New York, NY 10032-3796
(212) 305-9445
Fax: (212) 342-5218

NORTH CAROLINA
Duke University Medical Center
2200 West Main Street, Suite 200B
DUMC Post Office Box 3461

Durham, NC 27710-3461
(919) 684-6335
Fax: (919) 416-9268

PENNSYLVANIA
Children's Hospital of Philadelphia
Div. Allergy, Imm & Inf Diseases
Abramson Research Bldg., Suite 1208
34th Street and Civic Ctr. Blvd.
Philadelphia, PA 19104-4399
(215) 590-3561
Fax: (215) 590-3044

PUERTO RICO
University of Puerto Rico
University Pediatric Hospital
4th Floor South
P.O. Box 365067
San Juan, PR 00936-5067
(787) 759-9595
Fax: (787) 767-4798

TENNESSEE
St. Jude Children's Research Hospital
Dept. of Infectious Diseases
332 North Lauderdale Street
Memphis, TN 38105-2794
(901) 495-3485
Fax: (901) 495-3099

TEXAS
Baylor College of Medicine
Texas Children's Hospital
Allergy/Immunology Service
Abercrombie Bldg., Room A380
6621 Fannin Street, MS 1-3291
Houston, TX 77030
(832) 824-1319
Fax: (832) 825-7131

NAIDS Pediatric AIDS Clinical Trials Group Units – International

SOUTH AFRICA
Red Cross Children's Hospital
University of Cape Town
Dept. of Pediatrics & Child Health
46 Sawkins Road
Rondebosch

Cape Town, South Africa, 7700
+27 21 685 4103
Fax: +27 21 689 5403

Chris Hani Baragwanath Hospital
University of Witwatersrand
Wits Pediatric HIV Research Unit
PO Bertsham, 2013
Johannesburg, South Africa
+27 11 728 3771
Fax: +27 11 728 0460

THAILAND

Siriraj Hospital
Mahidol University
Pediatric Infectious Diseases
Department of Pediatrics, Faculty of
    Medicine
2 Prannok Rd, Bangkoknoi
Bangkok 10700, Thailand
+66 2 418 0545
Fax: 66 2 418 0544

Institute for Research Development
Perinatal HIV Prevention Trial
29/7-8 Samlan Road, Soi 1
Prasing, Muang
Chiang Mai 50200, Thailand
+66 (0) 53 814 270-1
Fax: +66 (0) 53 814 269

NICHD Clinical Trials Network Sites

CALIFORNIA

Los Angeles County/USC Medical Center
Maternal Child Program
Health Science Campus (CHB-HSC)
1640 Marengo Street
Los Angeles, CA 90033
(323) 226-6447 & 226-5068
Fax:(323) 226-8362 & 226-5960

Children's Hospital of Los Angeles
Division of Adolescent Medicine, 4th Floor
5000 Sunset Boulevard
Los Angeles, CA 90027
(323) 669-2390
Fax: (323) 913-3614

COLORADO

University of Colorado Health Science Center
The Children's Hospital
Department of Pediatrics
Infectious Disease Section
4200 East Ninth Avenue
Campus Box C227
Denver, CO 80262
(303) 315-4620
Fax: (303) 315-7909

CONNECTICUT

Yale University School of Medicine
Department of Pediatrics
Division of Infectious Diseases
420 LSOG, P. O. Box 3333
333 Cedar Street
New Haven, CT 06510-8064
(203) 785-4730
Fax: (203) 785-6961

DISTRICT OF COLUMBIA

Howard University Hospital
Department of Pediatrics
2041 Georgia Avenue, NW
Corridor 6N, Room 6E15
Washington, DC 20060
(202) 865-4583
Fax: (202) 865-7335

Children's National Medical Center
Special Immunology Service
111 Michigan Avenue, NW, WW 3.5–105
Washington, DC 20010-2970
(202) 884-2980 & 884-2937
Fax: (202) 884-3051

FLORIDA

South Florida Children's Diagnostic & Treatment
    Center
1401 South Federal Highway
Ft. Lauderdale, FL 33316
(954) 728-1017
Fax: (954) 712-5072

University of Florida Health Science Center
Pediatric Infectious Diseases/Immunology
653-1 West 8th Street
Jacksonville, FL 32209
(904) 244-3051
Fax: (904) 244-5341

University of Florida College of Medicine
Department of Pediatrics
1600 S.W. Archer Road
P.O. Box 100296
Gainsville, FL 32610-0296
(352) 392-2691
Fax: (352) 846-1810

University of South Florida Physicians Group
College of Medicine
Department of Pediatrics
17 Davis Boulevard, Suite 313
Tampa, FL 33606-3475
(813) 259-8800
Fax: (813) 259-8805

ILLINOIS
University of Illinois College of Medicine
Department of Pediatrics, M/C 856
840 S. Wood Street
Chicago, IL 60612
(312) 996-6711
Fax: (312) 413-1526

MICHIGAN
The Children's Hospital of Michigan
Division of Clinical Immunology & Rheumatology
3901 Beaubien Boulevard
Detroit, MI 48201
(313) 993-8794 & (313) 745-4450
Fax: (313) 993-3873

Hutzel Hospital
Wayne State University
School of Medicine
Department of OB/GYN
4707 St. Antoine Boulevard
Detroit, MI 48201
(313) 745-0734
Fax: (313) 993-2685; (313) 993-0689

NEW YORK
Children's Hospital at SUNY Downstate
Department of Pediatrics
450 Clarkson Avenue, Box 49
Brooklyn, NY 11203
(718) 245-4486
Fax: (718) 270-3185

Harlem Hospital Center
Department of Pediatrics
506 Lenox Avenue, Room 16-119
New York, NY 10037
(212) 939-4040
Fax: (212) 939-4048

Lincoln Medical Center
Pediatric Infectious Disease and Immunology
Room 4G183
234 East 149th Street
Bronx, NY 10451
(718) 579-5141
Fax: (718) 579-5381

Jacobi Medical Center
Family Based HIV Services
JACP-5C-15
1400 Pelham Parkway South
Bronx, NY 10461
(718) 918-4903
Fax: (718) 918-4699

Montefiore Medical Center
Adolescent AIDS Program
111 East 210th Street
Bronx, NY 10467
(718) 882-0023
Fax: (718) 882-0432

Mt. Sinai University
Pediatric Infectious Diseases
1 Gustave Levy Place
Annenberg 17-92, Box 1657
New York, NY 10029
(212) 241-6930 & (212) 241-1468

New York University of Medicine
Department of Pediatrics
550 First Avenue, Room 8W51
New York, NY 10016
(212) 263-6426
Fax: (212) 263-7806

SUNY Health Science Center at Stony Brook
Department of Pediatric Infectious Disease
HSC - T09-030
Stony Brook, NY 11794-811
(631) 444-7692
Fax: (631) 444-7248

SUNY Upstate Medical University
Division of Infectious Diseases
750 East Adams Street
Syracuse, NY 13210
(315) 464-6331
Fax: (315) 464-7564

University of Rochester
Strong Memorial Hospital
Department of Pediatrics
601 Elmwood Avenue, Box 690
Rochester, NY 14642
(585) 275-0588 & (585) 275-8760
Fax: (585) 273-1104

OREGON
Oregon Health and Science University
707 SW Gaines Road, CDRC-P
Portland, OR 97239
(503) 494-3197
Fax: (513) 494-1542

PUERTO RICO
Centro Medico
San Juan City Hospital
Pediatrics Department
PMB # 128 G.P.O., Box 70344
San Juan, PR 00936
Puerto Rico
(787) 764-3083 & (787) 274-0904
Fax: (787) 751-5143

TEXAS
Childrens Medical Center of Dallas
Department of Ambulatory Pediatrics
1935 Motor Street
Dallas, TX 75235
(214) 648-3720
Fax: (214) 456-5702

VIRGINIA
Children's Hospital of the King's Daughters
Pediatric Infectious Disease Division
601 Children's Lane
Norfolk, VA 23507
(757) 668-7238
Fax: (757) 668-8275

Senetra Norfolk General Hospital
601 Children's Lane
Norfolk, VA 23507
(757) 668-7238
Fax: (757) 668-8275

WASHINGTON
University of Washington
Children's Hospital and Regional Medical Center
Department of Pediatrics
4800 Sand Point Way, N. W., CH-32
Seattle, WA 98105
(206) 528-5140
Fax: (206) 527-3890

BAHAMAS
Princess Margaret Hospital
Shirley Street, P. O. Box 3730/N1784
Nassau, Bahamas
Bahamas
(242) 322-2839
Fax: (242) 356-2893

BRAZIL
Servico de Doencas Infecciosas – HUFF
Av. Brigadeiro Trompowski
S/N IIha do Fundao
Rio de Janeiro, CEP 21941-590
Brazil
55-21-562-61-48/49
Fax: 55-21-2562-6191

Hospital dos Servidores do Estado – RJ
Servico de Doencas Infecciosas e Parasitarias
Rua Sacadura Cabral
178 Anexo IV S° Andar
Saude, Rio de Janeiro, CEP 20221-161
Brazil
55-21-535-0493 (ALSO FAX)

Universidade Federal de Minas Gerais
Escola de Medicina
Av. Alfredo Balena 90-4 Andar
Belo Horizonte, Minas Gerais, CEP 30130-100
Brazil
55-31-3248-9822
Fax: 55-31-3273-0422

Universidade de Sao Paulo
Hospital das Clinicas da Faculdade da Medicina de Ribe
Av. Bandeirantes 3900
Ribeirao Preto, Sao Paulo, CEP 14049-900
Brazil
55-16-6330-136
Fax: 55-16-6022-700

Instituto de Infectologia Emilio Ribas
Av. Dr. Arnaldo 165-2 Andar-Sala 218
Sao Paulo, Sao Paulo, CEP 01246-900
Brazil
55-11-3085-0295
Fax: 55-11-3061-2521

Selected HIV-related internet resources

Leslie K. Serchuck, M.D.

Pediatric, Adolescent and Maternal AIDS Branch, NICHD/NIH, Rockville, MD

General AIDS information

AIDSinfo

http://www.aidsinfo.nih.gov
US Government sponsored portal with links to treatment guidelines and clinical trials (see below).

HIV InSite

http://hivinsite.ucsf.edu
A project of the University of California, San Francisco AIDS Program at San Francisco General Hospital and the UCSF Center for AIDS Prevention Studies. This is a comprehensive Web site for HIV and AIDS. This site also contains the AIDS Knowledge Base: an electronic textbook on AIDS and HIV that is frequently updated, with summaries of recent research on HIV and AIDS.

Johns Hopkins University AIDS Service

http://www.hopkins-aids.edu/
A wide-ranging collection of resources from Johns Hopkins University. Includes treatment updates, guidelines, plus full-text of the AIDS handbook, *Medical Management of HIV Infection*, as well as a bimonthly newsletter, *The Hopkins HIV Report*.

Division of AIDS, National Institute of Allergy and Infectious Diseases, National Institutes of Health

http://www.niaid.nih.gov/daids/
Links to treatment and prevention information, publications and meetings; vaccine, prevention, and treatment networks, and the Comprehensive International Program of Research on AIDS (CIPRA). Funding opportunities for both United States and International investigators, including those in poor countries with large HIV burdens.

United States Centers for Disease Control and Prevention

http://www.cdc.gov/
The CDCs website and its HIV homepage http://www.cdc.gov/hiv/dhap.htm, the definitive US source for epidemiologic information, downloadable publications and slide sets.

United States Food and Drug Administration

http://www.fda.gov/
Information about drug regulation and development.

AEGIS: AIDS Education and Global Information System

http://www.aegis.com/
This website features newsletters, HIV news from newspapers and wire services, and search capability for all documents. Contains an extensive publication library and many links.

AIDS Clinical Research Information Center

http://www.critpath.org/aric/
Contains an AIDS basic science information library and information and resources for People with AIDS (PWAs).

HIV Medicine Association

http://hivma.org
An organization of medical professionals caring for HIV-infected patients and a part of the Infectious Diseases Society of America. Site has links to IDSA practice guidelines and other resources.

International Association of Physicians in AIDS Care

http://www.iapac.org
This site is devoted to education of physicians and other healthcare providers. It advocates for the faster development and approval of treatments, vaccines, and technologies for the prevention and treatment of HIV/AIDS and provides good clinical information.

Project Inform

http://www.projinf.org/
A national, non-profit, community-based organization which provides information on diagnosis and treatment of HIV disease to HIV-infected individuals, their caregivers, and their healthcare and service providers. Project Inform provides excellent Fact Sheets and a frequently published journal *PI Perspective* which provides information from the most recent clinical trials and discussion regarding state of the art treatment and research issues. The site is in Spanish and English.

Medscape

http://www.medscape.com/hiv-aidshome
A commercial website with up-to-date information on HIV/AIDS as well as numerous other specialties. Contains international homepages as well.

Gay Men's Health Crisis

http://gmhc.org
Focus mainly on gay men, which may be helpful for gay adolescents, but also includes useful information on a variety of treatment-related topics. Educational information on HIV infection and AIDS pathogenesis for non-medical personnel.

All the Virology on the WWW

http://www.tulane.edu/~dmsander/garryfavweb.html
Site for virology resources on the web, with links to virology and microbiology courses, dictionaries, and specific virus sites (including emerging viruses and HIV/AIDS among numerous others).

Treatment centered sites

AIDSinfo

http://www.aidsinfo.nih.gov
Provides information about federally approved Treatment Guidelines for Use of Antiretroviral Agents in Adults and Adolescents with a separate document for Pediatric Patients infected with HIV. ATIS is staffed by bilingual (English and Spanish) health information specialists who answer questions on HIV treatment options.

AIDS Treatment Data Network

http://www.atdn.org/
National, not-for-profit, community-based organization. Extensive, comprehensive and up-to-date informational databases about AIDS treatments, research studies, services, and accessing care. Available in English and Spanish.

HIV-druginteractions.org

http://www.HIVdruginteractions.org
A service of the University of Liverpool, Department of Pharmacology and Therapeutics, features interactive drug interaction queries for antiretrovirals.

The Body

http://www.thebody.com/
A multimedia AIDS and HIV information resource. Its focus is on providing information for prevention and treatment of HIV infection but it includes some information on biology and immunology of HIV. The site features answers by experts to questions about AIDS and HIV.

Critical Path AIDS Project

http://www.critpath.org/
Critical Path AIDS Project was founded by persons with AIDS (PWAs) to provide treatment, resource, and prevention information in wide-ranging levels of detail – for researchers, service providers, treatment activists, and other PWAs. AIDS prevention, treatment, and referral information is available. Important site for patients and activists. Many links.

(Note: The manufacturers of antiretrovirals, HIV diagnostics, and agents for AIDS-related opportunistic infections maintain web sites with information pertaining to their products. These are often country-specific, but can generally be easily found using the popular search engines.)

Clinical trials

AIDSinfo

http://www.aidsinfo.nih.gov/
US Government-sponsored site containing current information on federally and privately sponsored clinical Pediatric ACTG and Adult ACTG trials open to accrual. Includes both treatment and prevention trials. Also contains links to treatment guidelines. Available in Spanish.

ClinicalTrials.gov

http://clinicaltrials.gov/
The U.S. National Institutes of Health, through its National Library of Medicine, has developed ClinicalTrials.gov to provide patients, family members and members of the public current information about clinical research studies for many diseases. The site currently contains thousands of clinical studies sponsored by the National Institutes of Health, other Federal agencies, and the pharmaceutical industry worldwide. Studies listed in the database are conducted primarily in the United States and Canada, but include locations in about 70 countries.

AIDS/HIV Treatment Directory (AMFAR)

http://www.amfar.org
The American Foundation for AIDS research. Contains information about conferences, grants, and a link to the AmFAR treatment directory, including information about treatment strategies and clinical trials.

The National Cancer Institute HIV and AIDS Malignancy Branch

http://aidstrials.nci.nih.gov
Links to the clinical trials in the HIV and AIDS Malignancy Branch, National Cancer Institute, for both adults and children.

National Institutes of Health Vaccine Research Center

http://www.niaid.nih.gov/vrc/

Basic and clinical research toward the development of vaccine for AIDS and other diseases. Enrolling patients in prophylactic and therapeutic vaccine clinical trials.

CENTER WATCH- Clinical Trials Listing Service

http://www.centerwatch.com/
A commercial web site offering a variety of information related to clinical trials in many disease areas. The site is designed to be a resource both for patients interested in participating in clinical trials and for research professionals.

International AIDS resources

UNAIDS-The Joint United Nations Programme on HIV/AIDS

http://www.unaids.org
Links to publications, surveillance, and response, WHO Initiative on HIV/AIDS and Sexually Transmitted Infections. Also contains news, upcoming events, and publications for the international community. Includes up-to-date country-specific HIV/AIDS statistics. Information is provided in English, Spanish, and French.

International AIDS Society

http://www.ias.se/
The International AIDS Society, a leading international professional society devoted to HIV/AIDS.

Global Fund to Fight AIDS, Tuberculosis and Malaria

http://www.theglobalfund.org/
International organization that collects and disburses funds to fight these serious infectious diseases in poor countries.

Pan American Health Organization (PAHO)

http://www.paho.org/Project.asp?SEL=TP&LNG=ENG&CD=AIDSS
PAHO is a UN agency. This site provides AIDS information by region from throughout Latin America and the Caribbean.

International AIDS Vaccine Initiative

http://www.iavi.ogr
Provides funding globally directed toward the development of an AIDS vaccine.

Gates Foundation

http://gatesfoundation.org
An important source of funding for HIV-related research globally.

Canadian HIV Trials Network

http://www.hivnet.ubc.ca/ctn.html
Links to Canadian clinical trials.

Onasida

http://www.ssa.gob.mx/conasida
This is the Mexican government health ministry HIV/AIDS server. This site is in Spanish.

The Body-International International HIV/AIDS Service Organizations and Resources

http://www.thebody.com/hotlines/internat.html
Includes international health organizations and resources and sites by region. Includes sites from Africa, Latin America, Asia, Russia, Europe, and Canada.

International Council of AIDS Services Organizations (ICASO)

http://www.icaso.org/
ICASO is a global network of non-governmental and community-based organizations. It has Regional Secretariats in Africa, Asia/Pacific, Europe, Latin America and the Caribbean, and North America.

Asian AIDS resources

http://www.utopia-asia.com/aids.htm
HIV/AIDS in the Asia/Pacific Region. Includes China, Thailand, Vietnam, and many others.

AIDSmap

http://www.aidsmap.com/
British HIV site, also with information on AIDS topics for continental Europe, Africa, and Asia.

Avert

http://www.avert.org/
A UK AIDS charity.

Pediatric AIDS resources

AIDS Alliance for Children, Youth and Families

http://www.aidspolicycenter.org/
The Alliance is a leading advocate for children, youth, and families affected by HIV/AIDS. Its mission includes policy analysis, advocacy, education, and training.

Children With AIDS Project

http://www.aidskids.org/
Good site for families and older children. Link to "Convomania," a place for seriously ill and disabled children on the Internet to connect with other children.

The Elizabeth Glaser Pediatric AIDS Foundation

http://www.pedaids.org/
This foundation is a non-profit organization that is an important funding source for pediatric AIDS research globally.

National Pediatric and Family HIV Resource Center

http://www.pedhivaids.org/
Non-profit organization serving professionals. Offers consultation, training, and teaching.

Research-oriented sites

National Library of Medicine: AIDS Publications

http://sis.nlm.nih.gov/HIV/HIVMain.html
Direct links to AIDLINE, AIDSDRUGS, and AIDSTRIALS databases at the National Library of Medicine with fact sheets

National Library of Medicine- PUBMED

http://www.ncbi.nlm.nih.gov and
http://gateway.nlm.nih.gov/. The National Center for Biotechnology Information. Provides free access to the MEDLINE medical literature database through PubMed and Entrez, and access to online versions of selected biomedical texts, online nucleic acid and protein sequence analysis tools, and online compilations of genetic information. Extensive links to voluminous collections of biomedical data. Links available to MedlinePlus, health information for consumers.

HIV Nucleic Acid Sequence and Immunological Databases

http://hiv-web.lanl.gov/
The HIV databases contain data on HIV genetic sequences, immunological epitopes, drug resistance-associated mutations.

NCI Drug Resistance Program

http://home.ncifcrf.gov/hivdrp/
The National Cancer Institute Drug Resistance Program, researching the mechanisms and implications of HIV drug resistance.

Harvard AIDS Institute

http://www.hsph.harvard.edu/hai/
The Institute has targeted four primary research areas related to HIV/AIDS: Basic Science (including molecular biology, virology and vaccines); Clinical Science (including pathogenesis and treatments); Epidemiology/Public Health and Prevention; Social Science and Policy.

Death and bereavement

Association for Death Education and Counseling

http://www.adec.org/
ADEC is an international, multidisciplinary organization dedicated to improving the quality of education, counseling and care-giving pertaining to dying, death, grief, and loss.

Growth House

http://www.growthhouse.org
This site provides public education and resources about hospice and home care, palliative care, pain management, death with dignity, bereavement, and related end-of-life topics. Includes international resources. Grief Sites are devoted to grief and bereavement, and include special pages for bereaved families, natal and infant loss, and helping children with grief and serious illness.

Hospice Foundation of America

http://www.hospicefoundation.org
HFA promotes hospice care and works to educate professionals and the families they serve in issues relating to care-giving, terminal illness, loss, and bereavement.

National Association for Home Care

http://www.nahc.org
This is the virtual headquarters of the National Association for Home Care (NAHC). Since its inception in 1982, NAHC has remained committed to serving the home care and hospice industry, which provides services to the sick, the disabled, and the terminally ill in the comfort of their homes.

Selected legal resources for HIV-infected children[1]

Carolyn McAllaster

ALABAMA

AIDS Task Force of Alabama, Inc.
Post Office Box 55703
Birmingham, AL 35255
(205) 324-9822
Legal referrals provided.

ALASKA

Alaskan AIDS Assistance Association
1057 West Fireweed Lane, #102
Anchorage, AK 99503
(907) 263-2050
Legal referrals provided; form documents with notary on site.

ARIZONA

AIDS Project Arizona
1427 N. 3rd Street, Suite 125
Phoenix, AZ 85004
(602) 253-2437
Legal referrals provided; estate planning and documents with notice.

HIV/AIDS Law Project (HALP)
Maricopa County Bar Association
Volunteer Lawyers Program
305 S. 2nd Avenue
Phoenix, AZ 85003
(602) 258-3434, ext. 282;
1-800-852-9075, ext 282
Direct legal services provided; legal referrals provided.

ARKANSAS

Arkansas AIDS Foundation
518 East 9th Street
Little Rock, AR 72202
(501) 376-6299
Legal referrals provided.

CALIFORNIA

North Coast AIDS Project
529 I Street
Eureka, CA 95501
(707) 268-2132
Legal referrals provided.

Central Valley AIDS Team
416 West McKinley
Fresno, CA 93728
(559) 264-2437
Legal referrals provided.

The Barristers AIDS Legal Services Project
1313 North Vine
Los Angeles, CA 90028
(323) 993-1640
Legal referrals provided.

HIV/AIDS Legal Services
    Alliance Inc. (HALSA)
3550 Wilshire Blvd., Suite 750
Los Angeles, CA 90010
(213) 201-1640
Legal referrals provided; direct legal services provided.

The Los Angeles Free Clinic Legal Dept.
8405 Beverly Boulevard
Los Angeles, CA 90048
(323) 655-2697
Direct legal services provided.

Los Angeles Gay and Lesbian Center
Legal Services Department
1625 North Schruder Boulevard
Los Angeles, CA 90028
(323) 993-7670
Direct legal services provided.

Desert AIDS Project Legal Services
1695 N. Sunrise Way, Bldg. 1
Palm Springs, CA 92262
(760) 323-2118
Legal referrals provided; direct legal services provided.

AIDS Service Center
1030 South Arroyo Parkway
Pasadena, CA 91105
(818) 441-8495; (626) 441-8495
Legal referrals provided.

AIDS Legal Referral Panel of the
San Francisco Bay Area
205 13th St.
San Francisco, CA 94104
(415) 291-5454
Legal referrals provided; direct legal services
  provided.

Legal Services for Prisoners with Children
  Women Prisoners with HIV/AIDS
  Project 100 McAllister Street
San Francisco, CA 94102
(415) 255-7036.

San Francisco AIDS Foundation
Financial Benefits Advocacy Program
Sixth St.
San Francisco, CA 94103
(415) 487-8000
Legal referrals provided; direct legal services
  provided; require clients to be 18 years old.

AIDS Legal Services
111 West St. John Street, Suite 315
San Jose, CA 95113
(408) 293-3135
Direct legal services provided; legal referrals provided.

Community Services AIDS Program
1601 East Hazelton Avenue
Stockton, CA 95201-2009
(209) 468-2235
Case management services.

Valley HIV/AIDS Center
6850 Van Nuys Boulevard, #110
Van Nuys, CA 91405
(818) 908-3840
Legal referrals provided.

AIDS Care Legal Clinic
73 North Palm Street
Ventura, CA 93001
(805) 643-0446
Legal referrals provided.

COLORADO
Boulder County AIDS Project Pro Bono
Attorney Team
2118 14th Street
Boulder, CO 80302
(303) 444-6121
Direct legal services provided.

Southern Colorado AIDS Project
1301 S. 8th Street, Suite 200
Colorado Springs, CO 80906
(719) 578-9092
Legal referrals provided.

Colorado AIDS Project Legal Program
701 East Colfax Avenue, Suite 212
Denver, CO 80203
(303) 837-1501
Legal referrals provided.

The Legal Center for People with Disabilities and
  Older People
HIV/AIDS Legal Program
455 Sherman Street, Suite 130
Denver, CO 80203
(303) 722-0300
Direct legal services provided; legal referrals provided.

CONNECTICUT
AIDS Legal Network for Connecticut
80 Jefferson St.
Hartford, CT 06105
(860) 541-5000
Legal referrals provided; direct legal services provided.

DISTRICT OF COLUMBIA

District of Columbia School of Law
HIV/AIDS Legal Clinic
4200 Connecticut Avenue, NW
Washington, DC 20008
(202) 274-7312
Direct legal services provided.

Whitman-Walker Clinic
Legal Services Department
1701 14th Street
Washington, DC 20009
(202) 939-7627
Direct legal services provided.

FLORIDA

Comprehensive AIDS Project
2222 West Atlantic Avenue
Delary Beach, FL 33445
(561) 274-6400
Legal referrals provided; direct legal services provided.

Jacksonville Area Legal Aid, Inc.
Ryan White Legal Project
126 W. Adams Street
Jacksonville, FL 32202
(904) 356-8371
Direct legal services provided.

AIDS Help, Inc.
Post Office Box 4374
Key West, FL 33041
(305) 296-6196
Legal referrals provided.

Legal Services of Greater Miami, Inc.
AIDS Legal Advocacy Project
3000 Biscayne Boulevard, Suite 500
Miami, FL 33137
(305) 576-0080
Direct legal services provided.

Big Bend Comprehensive AIDS Resources,
Education & Support, Inc.
Post Office Box 14365
Tallahassee, FL 32317
Legal referrals provided.

Legal Aid Society of Palm Beach County
HIV/AIDS Legal Project
423 Fern Street, Suite 200
West Palm Beach, FL 33401

(561) 655-8944, Ext. 286
Direct legal services provided.

GEORGIA

Atlanta Legal Aid Society
AIDS Legal Project
151 Springs Street, NW
Atlanta, GA 30303
(404) 614-3969
Legal referrals provided; direct legal services provided.

AIDS Law Project of Middle Georgia
111 Third Street, Suite 230
Macon, GA 31202
(478) 751-6261
Legal referrals provided; direct legal services provided.

HAWAII

Hawaii State Bar Association
Lawyer Referral & Information Service
1132 Bishop St., Suite 906
Honolulu, HI 96813
(808) 537-9140
Legal referrals provided.

ILLINOIS

AIDS Legal Council of Chicago
188 W. Randolph St., Suite 2400
Chicago, IL 60601
(312) 427-8990
Direct legal services provided; legal referrals provided.

Lambda Legal Defense & Education
Fund, Inc.
Midwest Regional Office
11 East Adams, Suite 1008
Chicago, IL 60603
(312) 663-4413
Legal contacts provided; direct legal services provided for
    precedent setting cases, often appellate level cases.

Legal Assistance Foundation, Inc. of
    Metropolitan Chicago
HIV/AIDS Project
111 W. Jackson. Suite 300
Chicago, IL 60604
(312) 347-8309
Legal referrals provided; direct legal services provided.

Cook County Legal Assistance Foundation, Inc.
AIDS Advocacy Project
828 Davis Street, Suite 201

Evanston, IL 60201-4489
(847) 475-3703
Legal referrals provided; direct legal services provided.

Springfield AIDS Resource Association
1315 North Fifth
Springfield, IL 62702
(217) 523-2191
Legal referrals provided.

INDIANA
AIDS Task Force, Inc.
2124 Fairfield Avenue
Fort Wayne, IN 46802
(219) 744-1144
Legal referrals provided.

Indiana HIV Advocacy Program
3951 North Meridian Street, Suite 200
Indianapolis, IN 46208
(317) 920-3190
Legal referrals provided; direct legal services provided.

Legal Services Organization of Indiana, Inc.
HIV/AIDS Legal Project
151 North Delaware, 18th Floor
Indianapolis, IN 46204
(317) 631-9410
Direct legal services provided.

AIDS Ministries/AIDS Assist
Post Office Box 11582
South Bend, IN 46634
(219) 234-2780
Legal referrals provided; direct legal services provided.

IOWA
University of Iowa College of Law
AIDS Representation Project
Iowa City, IA 52242-1113
(319) 335-9023
Legal referrals provided; direct legal services provided.

KENTUCKY
Legal Aid Society
HIV/AIDS Legal Project
810 Barret Avenue, Room 301
Louisville, KY 40204
(502) 574-8199
Direct legal services provided; legal referrals provided.

AIDS Volunteers, Inc.
AIDS/HIV Legal Project
Post Office Box 431
Lexington, KY 40588
(859) 225-3000
Legal referrals provided.

LOUISIANA
Mailing address:
AIDS Law of Louisiana, Inc.
Post Office Box 30203
New Orleans, LA 70190

Physical address:
144 Elk Place, Suite 1530
New Orleans, LA 70112
(504) 568-1631; 1-800-375-5035
Legal referrals provided; direct legal services provided.

MAINE
The AIDS Project, Inc.
615 Congress Street
Post Office Box 5305
Portland, ME 04101
(207) 774-6877
Legal referrals provided.

MARYLAND
Health Education Resource Organization
(HERO)
1734 Maryland Avenue
Baltimore, MD 21201
(410) 685-1180
Direct legal services provided.

University of Maryland Law School
AIDS Legal Clinic
500 West Baltimore Street
Baltimore, MD 21201-1786
(410) 706-8316
Legal referrals provided; direct legal services provided.

MASSACHUSETTS
AIDS Action Committee
131 Clarendon Street
Boston, MA 02116
(617) 450-1250
Legal referrals provided.

Gay & Lesbian Advocates & Defenders
AIDS Law Project
294 Washington Street, Suite 704
Boston, MA 02108
(617) 426-1350
Legal referrals provided; direct legal services provided.

North Shore AIDS Project
67 Middle Street
Gloucester, MA 01930
(978) 283-0101
Legal referrals provided.

AIDS Law Clinic
122 Boylston Street
Jamaica Plain, MA 02130
(617) 522-3003
Legal referrals provided; direct legal services
provided.

MICHIGAN
Wayne County Neighborhood
Legal Services
AIDS Law Center
51 W. Hancock St., #345
Detroit, MI 48201
(313) 832-8730
Direct legal services provided.

Michigan Protection and Advocacy Service, Inc.
HIV/AIDS Advocacy Program (HAAP)
106 West Allegan, Suite 300
Lansing, MI 48933
(517) 487-1755
Legal referrals provided; direct legal services provided.

MINNESOTA
Minnesota AIDS Project Legal Program
1400 Park Avenue South
Minneapolis, MN 55404
(612) 341-2060
Legal referrals provided; direct legal services
provided.

MISSOURI
Legal Aid of Western Missouri AIDS Legal Assistance
1005 Grand, Suite 600
Kansas City, MO 64106
(816) 474-6750
Direct legal services provided.

Legal Services of Eastern Missouri, Inc.
AIDS Project
4232 Forest Park Avenue
St. Louis, MO 63108
(314) 534-4200, ext. 1224
Direct legal services provided; legal referrals provided.

St. Louis University School of Law
Health Law Clinic
3700 Lindell Boulevard
St. Louis, MO 63108
(314) 977-2778
Direct legal services provided.

MONTANA
Butte AIDS Support Services
25 West Front Street
Butte, MT 59701
(406) 723-6507

NEVADA
Aid for AIDS Nevada
PO Box 478
Las Vegas, NV 89102
(702) 329-2437
Legal referrals provided.

Nevada AIDS Foundation
451 Roberts
Reno, NV 89504
(775) 329-2437
Legal referrals provided.

NEW HAMPSHIRE
Merrimack Valley AIDS Project, Inc.
Post Office Box 882
Concord, NH 03302
(603) 226-0607

Greater Manchester AIDS Project
Legal referrals provided
Post Office Box 59
Manchester, NH 03105
(603) 623-0710
Legal referrals provided.

NEW JERSEY
Hyacinth AIDS Foundation
78 New Street, 2nd Floor
New Brunswick, NJ 08901
(732) 246-0204
Legal referrals provided; direct legal services provided.

NEW MEXICO
AIDS Law Panel
Post Office Box 22251
Santa Fe, NM 84502
(505) 982-2021
Legal referrals provided; direct legal services provided.

NEW YORK
Bronx AIDS Services
Legal Advocacy Program
2633 Webster Ave.
Bronx, NY 10458
(718) 295-5690
Legal referrals provided; direct legal services
 provided.

Brooklyn Legal Services Corp. B HIV Project
105 Court Street
Brooklyn, NY 11201
(718) 237-5546
Direct legal services provided.

Nassau/Suffolk Law Services
Committee, Inc.
David Project
1757 Veteran=s Highway, Suite 50
Islandia, NY 11722
(516) 232-2400
Direct legal services provided; legal referrals
 provided.

Queens Legal Services Corporation
HIV Advocacy Project
8900 Sutphin Boulevard
Jamaica, NY 11435
(718) 657-8611
Legal referrals provided; direct legal services
 provided.

AIDS Service Center of Lower Manhattan
80 Fifth Avenue, 3rd Floor
New York, NY 10011
(212) 645-0875
Legal referrals provided; direct legal services provided.

The Family Center
66 Reade Street
New York, NY 10007
(212) 766-4522
Direct legal services provided; legal referrals provided.

Gay Men's Health Crisis
Legal Services Department
119 West 24th Street
New York, NY 10011
(212) 367-1040
Legal referrals provided; direct legal services
 provided.

HIV Law Project
161 William Street, 17th Floor
New York, NY 10038
(212) 674-7590
Direct legal services provided.

Lambda Legal Defense & Education Fund, Inc.
120 Wall Street. Suite 1500
New York, NY 10005
(212) 809-8585
Legal referrals provided; impact litigation.

Public Interest Law Office of Rochester
80 St. Paul Street, Suite 701
Rochester, NY 14604
(716) 454-4060
Direct legal services provided; legal referrals provided.

Volunteer Legal Services Project of Monroe County
80 St. Paul Street, Suite 640
Rochester, NY 14604
(716) 232-3051
Legal referrals provided; direct legal services
 provided.

Project Hospitality
Legal Advocacy Program
100 Park Avenue
Staten Island, NY 10302
(718) 448-1544, ext. 118
Direct legal services provided; legal referrals provided.

AIDS Law Project
472 South Salina Street, Suite 300
Syracuse, NY 13202
(315) 475-3127
Direct legal services provided; legal referrals provided.

Westchester/Putnam Legal Services
4 Cromwell Place
White Plains, NY 10601
(914) 949-1305
Direct legal services provided.

NORTH CAROLINA
AIDS Legal Assistance Project
Duke School of Law
Box 90360
Durham, NC 27708
(919) 613-7169
Direct legal services provided.

OHIO
Columbus AIDS Task Force
751 Northwest Blvd.
Columbus, OH 43212
(614) 299-2437
Legal referrals provided.

Toledo Bar Association
AIDS Assistance Committee
311 North Superior
Toledo, OH 43604
(419) 693-4423
Legal referrals provided; direct legal services provided.

OKLAHOMA
Legal Services of Oklahoma, Inc.
HIV/AIDS Legal Resources Project
2901 N. Classen Boulevard, Suite 110
Oklahoma City, OK 73106
(405) 524-4611
Direct legal services provided; legal referrals provided.

OREGON
Multnomah County Legal Aid Service
700 SW Taylor Street, Suite 300
Portland, OR 97205
(503) 224-4086
Direct legal services provided.

PENNSYLVANIA
AIDS Law Project of Pennsylvania
1211 Chestnut Street, Suite 600
Philadelphia, PA 19107
(215) 587-9377
Direct legal services provided.

Pittsburgh AIDS Taskforce
905 West Street, 4th Floor
Pittsburgh, PA 15221
Columbus, OH 43212-3856
(412) 242-2500
Legal referrals provided; direct legal services provided.

RHODE ISLAND
AIDS Project of Rhode Island
232 West Exchange Street
Providence, RI 02903
(401) 831-5522
Legal referrals provided.

SOUTH CAROLINA
Lowcountry AIDS Services
Legal Clinic
501 Manley Avenue
Charleston, SC 29405
(843) 747-2273
Direct legal services provided.

TEXAS
Dallas Legal Hospice
370 West Seventh St
Dallas, TX 75208
(214) 941-2600
Direct legal services provided.

AIDS Services of Austin
Post Office Box 4874
Austin, TX 78765
(512) 458-2437
Legal referrals provided; direct legal services provided.

La Fe CARE Center
1505 Mescalero
El Paso, TX 79925
(915) 772-3366
Direct legal services provided.

AIDS Outreach Center Legal Network
801 West Cannon
Fort Worth, TX 76104
(817) 355-1994
Direct legal services provided.

Houston Volunteer Lawyers Program, Inc.
AIDS Project
806 Main Street, 16th Floor
Houston, TX 77002
(713) 228-0735
Legal referrals provided; direct legal services provided.

UTAH
Utah AIDS Foundation
1408 South 1100 East
Salt Lake City, UT 84105
(801) 497-2323
Legal referrals provided.

VERMONT
AIDS Project of Southern Vermont
Post Office Box 1486
Brattleboro, VT 05302
(802) 254-8263
Legal referrals provided.

VIRGINIA
Whitman-Walker Clinic
Legal Services Department
5232 Lee Highway
Arlington, VA 22207
(703) 237-4900
Legal referrals provided; direct legal services provided.

AIDS/HIV Services Group
Post Office Box 2322
Charlottesville, VA 22902
(804) 979-7714
Legal referrals provided.

WASHINGTON
Volunteer Attorneys for Persons with AIDS (VAPWA)
AIDS Legal Access
900 Fourth Avenue, Suite 600
Seattle, WA 98164
(206) 340-2584
Legal referrals provided; direct legal services on an emergency basis.

WEST VIRGINIA
Charleston AIDS Network
Post Office Box 1024
Charleston, WV 25324
(304) 345-4673; 1-888-455-4673
Legal referrals provided.

WISCONSIN
AIDS Resource Center of Wisconsin
1212 57th Street
Kenosha, WI 53141
(414) 225-1578; 1-800-878-6267
Legal referrals provided; direct legal services provided.

Madison AIDS Support Network
Legal Services Program
600 Williamson Street
Madison, WI 53703
(608) 252-6540
Legal referrals provided; direct legal services provided.

AIDS Resource Center of Wisconsin
Legal Services Program
820 N. Plankinton Avenue
Milwaukee, WI 53203
(414) 273-1991; 1-800-359-9272
Direct legal services provided.

AIDS Law, Education, Research and Training ("ALERT")
Legal Aid Society of Milwaukee, Inc.
229 E. Wisconsin Ave., Suite 200
Milwaukee, WI 53202
(414) 765-0600
Direct legal services provided.

ENDNOTE

1. A primary resource for this compilation was the *Directory of Legal Resources for People with AIDS & HIV*, 2nd edn. ABA, AIDS Coordination Project (1997).

Index